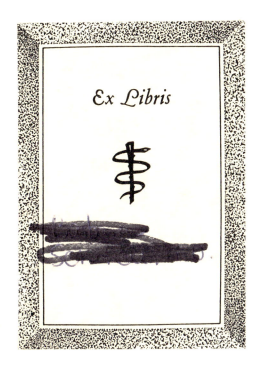

Ex Libris

AMERICAN HANDBOOK OF PSYCHIATRY

Volume Three

AMERICAN HANDBOOK OF PSYCHIATRY

SECOND EDITION

Silvano Arieti · Editor-in-Chief

VOLUME THREE

Adult

Clinical Psychiatry

SILVANO ARIETI and EUGENE B. BRODY · *Editors*

BASIC BOOKS, INC., PUBLISHERS · NEW YORK

Second Edition
© 1974 by Basic Books, Inc.
Library of Congress Catalog Card Number: 72-89185
SBN: 465-00149-1
Manufactured in the United States of America
74 75 76 77 78   10 9 8 7 6 5 4 3 2 1

CONTRIBUTORS

D. Wilfred Abse, M.D.
Professor of Psychiatry, University of Virginia, Charlottesville; Faculty member, Washington Psychoanalytic Institute, Washington, D.C.

Silvano Arieti, M.D.
Clinical Professor of Psychiatry, New York Medical College, New York; Training Analyst and Supervisor, William Alanson White Institute of Psychiatry, Psychoanalysis and Psychology, New York.

Eduard Ascher, M.D.
Associate Professor of Psychiatry, The Johns Hopkins University School of Medicine, Baltimore; Associate Clinical Professor of Psychiatry, University of Maryland School of Medicine, Baltimore.

Robert C. Bak, M.D.
Faculty member, New York Psychoanalytic Institute, New York; Attending Psychiatrist, Psychiatric Division, Montefiore Hospital and Medical Center, Bronx, New York.

George U. Balis, M.D.
Associate Professor of Psychiatry, University of Maryland School of Medicine, Baltimore; Director of Undergraduate Psychiatric Education, University of Maryland School of Medicine, Baltimore.

Aaron T. Beck, M.D.
Professor of Psychiatry, University of Pennsylvania, Philadelphia.

Jules R. Bemporad, M.D.
Director of Pediatric Psychiatry, Babies Hospital, Columbia-Presbyterian Medical Center, New York; Faculty member, Psychoanalytic Division, New York Medical College, New York.

David Berenson, M.D.
Research Psychiatrist, St. Elizabeth's Hospital,

Washington, D.C.; Assistant Professor of Psychiatry, Howard University, Washington, D.C.

Irving Bieber, M.D.
Clinical Professor of Psychiatry, New York Medical College, New York.

Eugene B. Brody, M.D.
Professor and Chairman, Department of Psychiatry, University of Maryland School of Medicine, Baltimore.

Norman A. Cameron, M.D.
Retired. Formerly, Professor of Psychiatry, Yale University School of Medicine, New Haven, Connecticut; Formerly Associate Psychiatrist, Yale Psychiatric Institute, New Haven, Connecticut.

James P. Cattell, M.D.
Associate Clinical Professor of Psychiatry, College of Physicians and Surgeons, Columbia University, New York; Director, District Court Clinic, Pittsfield, Massachusetts.

Jane Schmahl Cattell, R.N., M.A.
Psychotherapist and family therapist in private practice; Assistant Director, District Court Clinic, Pittsfield, Massachusetts.

Morris E. Chafetz, M.D.
Director, National Institute on Alcohol Abuse and Alcoholism, Department of Health, Education and Welfare, Rockville, Maryland.

Richard D. Chessick, M.D.
Professor of Clinical Psychiatry, Northwestern University Medical School, Evanston, Illinois; Senior Attending Psychiatrist, Evanston Hospital, Evanston, Illinois.

Gerard Chrzanowski, M.D.
Associate Professor of Clinical Psychiatry, New York Medical College; Training and Supervisory Analyst, William Alanson White Institute of

Psychiatry, Psychoanalysis and Psychology, New York.

David Davis, M.B., D.P.M., M.C.R. Psych.
Professor and Associate Chairman, Department of Psychiatry, University of Missouri School of Medicine, Columbia, Missouri.

Paul Friedman, M.D.
Deceased. Formerly, Preceptor in Psychiatry, Mount Sinai Hospital, New York; Formerly, Associate Clinical Professor of Psychiatry, Mount Sinai School of Medicine of the City University of New York.

Charles E. Frohman, Ph.D.
Director of Biochemistry, LaFayette Clinic, Detroit; Professor of Biochemistry, Wayne State University, Detroit.

Alvin I. Goldfarb, M.D.
Associate Attending Psychiatrist in charge of Geriatric Services, Mount Sinai Hospital, New York; Associate Clinical Professor of Psychiatry, Mount Sinai School of Medicine of the City University of New York.

Jacob Goldstein, DSSC
Psychologist, Mental Health Clinic, Family Court of the State of New York, New York.

Jacques S. Gottlieb, M.D.
Professor of Psychiatry, Wayne State University, Detroit; Director of the LaFayette Clinic, Detroit.

Marc Hertzman, M.D.
Executive Assistant to the Director, National Institute on Alcohol Abuse and Alcoholism, Department of Health, Education and Welfare, Rockville, Maryland; Associate Professor of Psychiatry, George Washington University, Washington, D.C.

Lawrence S. Kubie, M.D., D.Sc.
Deceased. Formerly, Senior Associate on Research and Training, The Sheppard and Enock Pratt Hospital, Towson, Maryland; Formerly, Clinical Professor of Psychiatry, University of Maryland School of Medicine, Baltimore.

H. E. Lehman, M.D.
Professor and Chairman, Department of Psychiatry, McGill University, Montreal; Director of Medical Education and Research, Douglas Hospital, Montreal.

J. Mendels, M.D.
Professor of Psychiatry and Chief, Depression Research Unit, University of Pennsylvania and Veterans Administration Hospital, Philadelphia.

Johannes M. Meth, M.D.
Member of American Institute of Psychoanalysis, New York; Associate at the Karen Horney Clinic, New York.

John Money, Ph.D.
Professor of Medical Psychology and Associate Professor of Pediatrics, The Johns Hopkins University School of Medicine, Baltimore; Psychologist, The Johns Hopkins Hospital, Baltimore.

Russell R. Monroe, M.D.
Professor of Psychiatry, Institute of Psychiatry and Human Behavior, University of Maryland School of Medicine, Baltimore.

John C. Nemiah, M.D.
Psychiatrist-in-Chief, Beth Israel Hospital, Boston; Professor of Psychiatry, Harvard Medical School, Boston.

Marie Nyswander, M.D.
Guest Investigator, The Rockefeller University, New York; Consultant, Beth Israel Hospital, New York.

Henry Pinsker, M.D.
Associate Professor of Psychiatry, Mount Sinai School of Medicine of the City University of New York, New York; Associate Director of Psychiatry, Department of Psychiatry, Beth Israel Medical Center, New York.

Sandor Rado, M.D., D.Pol. Sc.
Deceased. Formerly, President and Professor of Psychiatry, The New York School of Psychiatry; Formerly Clinical Professor of Psychiatry and Director, Columbia University Psychoanalytic Clinic, New York.

Jonas R. Rappeport, M.D.
Chief Medical Officer, Supreme Bench of Baltimore; Associate Clinical Professor of Psychiatry, University of Maryland School of Medicine, Baltimore.

David Rosenthal, Ph.D.
Chief of the Laboratory of Psychology, National Institute of Mental Health, Bethesda, Maryland.

Saul H. Rosenthal, M.D.

Clinical Associate Professor of Psychiatry, University of Texas Medical School, San Antonio.

W. Donald Ross, M.D., B.Sc. (Med.) FRCP, FAPA

Professor of Psychiatry and Associate Professor of Industrial Medicine, University of Cincinnati; Director, Psychiatric Consultation Service, Cincinnati General Hospital.

Leon Salzman, M.D.

Acting Director, Bronx State Hospital, Bronx, New York; Clinical Professor of Psychiatry, Albert Einstein College of Medicine, New York.

Charles W. Socarides, M.D.

Associate Clinical Professor, Albert Einstein College of Medicine, New York; Associate Attending Psychiatrist, Bronx Municipal Hospital Center, Bronx, New York.

Walter A. Stewart, M.D.

Faculty member, New York Psychoanalytic Institute, New York.

James L. Titchener, M.D.

Professor of Psychiatry, University of Cincinnati College of Medicine; Attending Physician, Cincinnati General Hospital.

James M.A. Weiss, M.D., M.P.H., F.R.C. Psych.

Professor and Chairman, Department of Psychiatry, and Professor of Community Health and Medical Practice, University of Missouri School of Medicine, Columbia, Missouri; Psychiatrist-in-Chief, University of Missouri Medical Center, Columbia, Missouri.

CONTENTS

Volume Three

PART SEVEN: *Unclassified Behavior and Syndromes and Those Intermediate between Neurosis and Psychosis*

PART ONE

General Concepts about Neuroses and Related Disorders

CHAPTER 1

THE NATURE OF THE
NEUROTIC PROCESS

Lawrence S. Kubie

THE NEUROTIC PROCESS has several major ingredients: (a) an affective potential which often is imposed early in life;[22] (b) patterns of obligatory repetition;[3] (c) various kinds of distortion of symbolic functions; and (d) which result in a loss or impairment of the freedom to change. This process never moves in a straight line. It reaches moments of critical obstruction out of which a wide variety of secondary symptoms precipitate. These take many forms: grave personality disturbances, antisocial behavior, self-destructive behavior, an array of symbolic distortions[14] with verbal or paralinguistic manifestations; distortions of body image and of body functions, such as longer and shorter periods of misuse of water, food, alcohol, drugs, sleep; exercise compulsions; overdriven rivalries; almost psychotic degrees of excessive and compulsive benevolence versus compulsive greed; compulsive overactivity or retardation, apathy and indifference, claustrophobia and agoraphobia. A moment's thought will make it clear that any

one of these symptoms has secondary consequences, both immediate and delayed, which give rise to new tertiary orders of symptoms which in turn produce new distortions of thought, feeling, purpose, and behavior, as a result of which a whole life may become distorted. This is why a life can become so much sicker than were the initial deviations. This is why every neurotic symptom, however simple it may seem, is a step in a long reverberating chain towards graver illness.

This is true even of intrinsically harmless symptoms. I think of an elderly lawyer, long since deceased, who had a compulsion to button, unbutton, and rebutton his vest, which nearly cost him his life while crossing a street. Moreover, this is why it is true that a socially valuable and creative work-drive can remain creative and productive only until the tax collector catches up with us to tumble us, for example, into an involutional depression. This is why inherently destructive symptomatic behavior, like the misuse of alcohol, extorts even graver penalties. Clearly, the feedback of destructive penalties varies widely, but they are always present.

There is still another ingredient in the neurotic process which is dependent upon the relationship of the symbolic process to the underlying perceptual and cognitive processes. Unhappily and unfortunately, this can begin the moment the toddler is able to use any form of symbolic representation of what reaches him from the outer world and also of what is going on in that continuous flow of imageless mentation, which we call the "preconscious stream." I speak of this as tragic, because those who have studied most closely the early desiccation of the creative potential in early childhood find that it is related closely to the way in which the free preconscious stream of analogic processing of experience becomes imprisoned between two wardens: on the one hand, is the conscious symbolic representation of weighted samples of the preconscious stream; and on the other hand, the distortions of the relationship of the symbol to what it was supposed to represent, which occurs whenever the link between the symbol and its referent is distorted or disrupted to give rise to what we call "unconscious processing." There is abundant evidence that the earlier the precocious child becomes able to use symbolic processes (and especially language, whether verbal or paralinguistic), the earlier does his vulnerability to neurotic distortions begin, and the more destructive their consequences for his subsequent development. It almost makes me wish that one could set up an effective ban on symbolic precocity in the interest of mental health.

One of its most destructive consequences, of course, is the imposition of patterns of obligatory repetition, which together with symbolic distortions and disruptions constitute the essence of the neurotic process from its inception in infancy, with the resultant limitation or even destruction of the freedom to change, to grow, to learn from experience, from trial and error, from success or failure, from hunger or satiation.

What I am presenting here is neither the method nor the results of research, but certain underlying principles which seem to me to furnish basic guides for research. Of these concepts perhaps the most important concern the unsolved problems that center around the nature of psychological change in individuals and deriving from that the consideration of the relationship of individual change to social and cultural change.

Here, I must introduce a working hypothesis about psychological health and illness.[21] My basic position is that psychological health is in essence synonymous with and in this sense also dependent upon the freedom to change, and furthermore, that in the long run the only freedom that counts is the freedom to go on changing in a continuous and evolving process. Otherwise, change is merely momentary and illusory. If this is a valid criterion of health, then to understand illness we have to ask ourselves, on what does this freedom for an ongoing and continuing process of change depend? And, in turn, what determines any limitation or impairment of this freedom to change as a first step in psychological illness.[2] From the study of children and the tragic early desiccation of their initial creative potential, we know that the impairment of the freedom to change can start early in life, actually as we learn to imprison the preconscious stream in symbolic language. In fact, this is one of the basic reasons why the neurotic process starts in infancy. Furthermore, it is one of the reasons why we lose this freedom to change repeatedly throughout life, and regain it repeatedly, and lose it again, over and over again, as long as we live. We know, furthermore, that this complex process which starts so early in life occurs not merely under externally destructive circumstances but even under the happiest and healthiest and most loving circumstances. Consequently, the struggle to prevent this impairment of the freedom to change, or to regain it when we have lost it, or when it has become impaired, is at the very core of man's spiritual and cultural Odyssey. When we put our quest in these terms we can begin to think about it usefully. Yet, most of these questions remain unanswered today, because they have never before been asked in this way. But it is essential to ask these questions insistently, especially those that we cannot answer. The quest for the answers to the unanswerable is our greatest moral and cultural imperative.

How is this freedom to change impaired? Here, we have to stop to describe for a moment what the essence of our psychological process consists of. It consists of a continuous processing of experiencing. The input from life, whether it reaches us via the distance receptors (the exteroceptive organs), or by the proprioceptors which bring us cues and signals from muscles and bones and joints and tendons and ligaments, or from enteroceptive organs which bring us news from the inside and supply the raw material of experience, furnishes a continuous supply of data which must be processed, with or without conscious participation and without words or visual or other representatives. This is the imageless thought of the old Würzburg School. It is a continuous process which goes on throughout life, whether we are awake or asleep, in mental health or in sickness. Samples of it must be taken; and then these samples must be represented. This, too, is a continuous process of symbolic sampling and whenever there is any disturbance in the process by which we select representatives from this continuous internal stream, or whenever there is any impairment or distortion of the symbolic processes by which we represent these samples, the freedom of the stream itself becomes distorted and impaired. Unhappily, this can begin in very early life, which is why a progressive imprisonment and distortion of the preconscious stream can start so early as the stream becomes trapped between the restrictions imposed by conscious symbolic representation on the one hand, and by the impact of unconscious distortions on the other. It is this which imposes on us that obligatory repetition which is the essential ingredient of the neurotic process.

Here, again, we face the destructive effects of certain of the entrenched and respectable techniques of drill and grill, on which unhappily our educational mores depend so largely; and this in spite of the fact that drill and grill

contribute to this loss of freedom by merging with the automatic repetition which is inherent in the neurotic process. Indeed, it is in this way that the educational process itself tends so often to entrench and reinforce the neurotic process. This is not a happy situation, yet educators have never devoted adequate thought to it. Nor have they designed experiments in efforts to break up this unholy alliance between the early steps in education and the early manifestations of the neurotic process. This is a strange oversight when we consider the fact that this challenge has been confronting us for generations in the educational problems of even the most highly endowed children.

My purpose here will not be to allocate to genetic, biochemical, or psychosocial variables, nor even to variables in intrapsychic conflicts, any specific separate or interdependent roles in the genesis and development of the neurotic process, but rather to make clear its extraordinarily subtle complexity.

All illnesses, whether somatic, psychological, or a mixture of both, are evolving processes, in which a chain reaction is established of secondary consequences which derive from the *primary symptoms*, plus the new symptom-clusters which the secondary consequences generate in turn;[18,23] followed by additional distortions which feed back tertiary symptoms into this stream of cumulative and progressive distortions of life. This is one of the many complications which make it difficult to trace the development of a process of neurotic illness to its precise origins and equally difficult to isolate the essential core and nature of the primary illness, or to select points in this continuous cybernetic chain at which invariable biochemical, genetic, or psychosocial correlations can be determined. A further result is the seemingly paradoxical fact that the secondary and tertiary consequences of an illness, whether somatic or psychological, can be so destructive to the pattern and quality of a life that the life which evolves can be much "sicker" than were the initial deviations with which it began. This is true not only in psychopathology but in somatic illness as well. A man who is still paralyzed in all four limbs because of an attack of poliomyelitis which may have occurred many years before no longer suffers from active infection by the polio virus, but he still leads a sick life because of his paralyzed limbs. A comparable anomaly can occur in psychopathological processes, although the interrelationships are subtler and even more complicated.

In psychopathological illnesses a seething turmoil of conscious, preconscious, and unconscious conflicts occurs, out of which several kinds of distortions precipitate. These distortions, which are usually called "symptoms," do three things simultaneously: They express the underlying conflicts in symbols, they hide the underlying unconscious conflicts, and they express veiled compromises among them. All of this takes the familiar forms of organized symptoms, i.e., the usual array of obsessions, compulsions, phobias, hysterical conversions, concurrent affective and somatic disturbances, etc., plus many, varied but recurrent, distortions in patterns of behavior. These include antisocial behavior, obligatory expressions of perverse libidinal impulses, disturbances in relationships to other people, dislocations between affects and their original precipitants, etc. Each of these in turn has its own distorting consequences. Uniquely human and important are the disturbances which arise in the relationships of the symbolic representatives of bits of the perceptual input to the samples of the preconscious stream which the symbolic process is supposed both to sample and represent: in short, disturbances in symbolic processing itself.[2,10] These symptomatic behavioral disturbances may take the form of acting out the unconscious conflicts, either impulsively or deliberately, or the form of direct expression of instinctual needs in perverse forms, or of disturbances in the affective coloring of all such experiences, or of disturbances in the relationships of symbols to their referents, i.e., to what they are supposed to represent. All of the ingredients of the neurotic process have two essential qualities in common: Each involves some degree of dissociation[32] among their many ingredients, and each component in the neurotic process is subject to automatic and obligatory repetition.[3]

Clearly the neurotic process is an extremely complex phenomenon. Most descriptions of these, whether in classical or in psychoanalytic psychiatry, have been flagrantly oversimplified.

The tendency to simplify is inescapable and even necessary in all scientific investigation and theory; yet it causes confusion. This is true not only in the "soft" sciences, but in the "hard" sciences as well. It is impossible to conduct any experiment without limiting the number and range of variables, in order to isolate other variables sufficiently to make it possible to test their influence one at a time. The theoretician has to do the same thing. Yet, in doing this both the theoretician and the investigator impose on complex natural phenomena an artificial simplicity. Actually, this is one of the essential functions of the scientist, whether in his armchair or in the laboratory. As long as we realize that we are doing this and that we *have* to do this, and as long as we never pretend to ourselves that the theoretical or laboratory facsimile is identical with its prototype in nature we will not be led too seriously astray, particularly in the study of clinical phenomena. Of course, as human beings we are fallible and often cling to the illusion that the simplified model and its prototype in nature are interchangeable. This leads to trouble; but I want to underscore the fact that these considerations are equally true for the experimentalist and for the formulator of hypotheses and theories. At best, these are metaphors, figures of speech, allegories if you will, efforts to find a verbal graph or diagram to serve as a working facsimile of the natural phenomena. I repeat that this is something that we have to do, but again that in doing so even the greatest scientific thinkers are in danger of becoming trapped in their own oversimplifications. It happened repeatedly to Freud himself, as it has to Linus Pauling.

This is not a criticism, an apology, or a defense. Whether these simplifications occur in the laboratory or in the armchair, they are necessary steps in the progress of science.

They help us to visualize the problems which we are trying to describe and ultimately to explain. Dangers threaten only if we pretend to ourselves or to others that they do not exist.

A Bit of Personal History

This brings me back to my original purpose, which is to try to spell out the enormous complexity and the wide range of the variables that enter into all processes of psychological development, both normal and neurotic. My own realization of this came slowly, over a period of about thirty years.

Naturally, to trace in detail the historical development of my own ideas would be of interest to me, but it would hardly be of general interest to others. Nevertheless, because I want to indicate how much more complex the problem is than the customary psychoanalytic formulations of it have allowed us to realize, I will have to make a brief résumé of the steps in my own thinking.

These began with the concept of "circus movements" in the brain.[1] The description of this was a happy accident which made me the midwife at the delivery of the concept of cybernetics. The real obstetricians were three, far greater, scientists, Jonas Friedenwald, Warren McCulloch, and Norbert Wiener, followed by many others. That reverberating circuits constitute essential steps in all psychological development, *both normal and pathological*, is no longer doubted. Yet, they raise many questions that are still unanswered. We know that under the influence of certain drugs and especially certain mixtures of drugs (such as barbiturates, alcohol, and others) some people become automata and develop a stereotyped and unvarying repetitiveness. We know that with the same medications and under apparently similar circumstances the psychological processes of others scatter and never become trapped in obligatory repetition. What we do not know is how this difference comes to exist. We do not know whether some brains are so organized anatomically as

to be more vulnerable to automatic repetition than others, and some less so, or whether this is due to differences in their chemistry, or in both. We know only that the difference exists and that a study of its nature is of critical importance for the clarification of any so-called constitutional factors in the development of neurotic illness. Adequate studies of these differences are so difficult that actually they have not yet been made.

The relevance of the concept of reverberating circuits to the phenomena of affective processes was not formulated until nearly twenty years later, in 1952, at one of the Macy Foundation Conferences on Cybernetics, in a paper called "The Place of Emotions in the Feedback Concept."[13] Other psychophysiological ingredients to which I find early experimental and clinical references in my own work had to do with the conditioned reflex in connection with analytical technique and also with analytical theory.[2] Here, again, we face many unanswered problems concerning the role of potential variables which determine the ease of conditioning and its persistence.[4,6,31,32]

The next ingredient that challenged me was the role of the general process of symbolization.[2,10] For the first time, I discussed the importance of any distortion or interruption of the link between the symbol of an intrapsychic event and that which the symbol was supposed to represent. In all normal psychological processes it is essential that the link between the symbol and its referent not be disturbed. This is especially true, because in the development of all symbolic processes, the symbolic representation of internal and external experiences, the symbolic representation of the near and the far, of the present, the past, and future, of changes that occur within the body and those which have their origins outside of the body, all provide multiple linkages, by means of which every symbol serves as a bridge between the past, present, and future, between the near and the far, and between the internal and external worlds, the "I" and the "non-I" worlds.[14,15,16] It should be clear that any disturbance in these representations will provide a basis for different kinds of dissociation that can lean to both neurotic and psychotic disorganizations of human mentation.[17,18,19]

This work was followed by and interspersed with a long series of studies involving the use of hypnotic processes for the artificial induction of dissociations that could lead to neurotic disturbances,[7,11] to the induction of a brief acute psychotic storm under hypnosis,[27] to the phenomena of automatisms in general,[28] and to dissociation of personality units into latent or manifest dual personalities, the larval existence of which has been previously sometimes suspected or recognized, and sometimes not.[29]

In 1945, in reporting on experimental work with the hypnotic process, Sydney Margolin and I pointed out that dissociations of various kinds play a role in all psychopathological phenomena.[32] If this is even approximately true, it forces us to challenge the idea that a dissociative process is in any sense unique for any given neurotic or psychotic process. Thus, the very term "schizophrenia" is a misleading misnomer.[25,26]

After the use of hypnotic processes for the experimental induction of various forms of dissociation leading to neurotic disturbances and regression[32] came the use of hypnotic processes, sometimes combined with drugs, in a more general study of the phenomena of regression, dissociation, and repression in the evolution of the neurotic process. This led to a further study of the interplay of hypnotic phenomena in both psychonoxious and psychotherapeutic processes. These studies were originally begun in close association with Richard M. Brickner, then with Milton H. Erickson, one of the most gifted students of hypnotic phenomena in this country, followed by a long series of experimental studies with Margolin.[5,6,20,24,29,30,32]

Shortly after World War II (and in part under the influence of the opportunities provided by the war for the study of both acute and chronic disorganizations and fragmentations of psychological functions), came the study of what I then called the "universal

masked neurotic potential and the problem of adaptation,"[8] followed in 1951 by a paper which separated these phenomena into a universal, masked, neurotic potential, the neurotic process, and the neurotic state.[12]

In some respects, I would formulate matters differently if I were writing those papers today. Nevertheless, they marked a turning point in my conceptions of the nature of the problem which confronts us.

(A Criterion of Psychological Illness or Health

Nothing in psychiatry and psychoanalysis has been characterized with less precision than the basic nature of the difference between health and psychopathology. I hope that through their cumulative effects my repeated efforts to clarify the problem may at least provide us with a few useful leads, as these successive formulations have shifted to a greater emphasis now on one, now on another aspect of the neurotic ingredient in human life. These shifting emphases are complementary and not inherently contradictory. Inevitably, my thinking did not follow a straight path, but wandered back and forth among these several components. I will try here to bring them into harmony as the basis for a consistent hypothesis based on clinical data.

An early formulation highlighted something which I will develop more fully here, namely, that the sine qua non of all psychopathology is *obligatory repetition*. Whenever any constellation of physiological and/or psychological processes which together produce any moment of thought, feeling, and/or action, predetermines at the same time its obligatory and automatic repetition, that moment of psychological behavior is pathological, and the underlying processes are ipso facto neurotogenic or more generally psychopathogenic.[19,21] To this early characterization an additional consideration must be added, namely, that whenever any thought, feeling, action, drive, instinct-serving impulse or purpose, or conglomerate mixture is itself subjected to obligatory repetition this fact alone will also have basic and inescapable (although variable) consequences for the evolving neurotic process itself. The primary symptoms might be called a first order of variables which have their own effects upon the patient's life. As they produce fresh consequences, these constitute a second order of variables, the nature of which will depend upon what specific ideas, actions, feelings, drives, etc., are subjected to obligatory repetition. For example, height phobias, claustrophobias, agoraphobias, dirt phobias, may have remarkably similar origins, and yet may have diametrically opposing yet equally disastrous consequences. This nuclear component in the neurotic process presents us with a new focus for both psychological and organic investigations, as I have pointed out in detail on several previous occasions.[19,20]

But, are all repetitions pathological? Obviously not. Indeed much repetition is essential for survival of the individual and/or race. If we did not repeat breathing, eating, drinking, and many other things, we could not survive. It is not abnormal to repeat anything as long as we retain the ability to change and to stop. It is only when repetition becomes so obligatory that not even total satiation makes it possible to stop that difficulties arise.

The questions that arise at once are, How does obligatory repetition become established? Are there many ways or only one? What determines its focus and its duration? Can psychological processes alone produce patterns of obligatory repetition? Or organic variables alone? Or both operating synergistically? And what is the role of intrapsychic conflict, whether conscious or unconscious, in the production of obligatory repetition?

Here we must note that obligatory repetition can also be induced by electrical stimulation of the median surface of the hemispheres of the brain,[16] or of the deeper layers of the temporal lobes,[9] or by alcohol, or by combinations of alcohol and barbiturates, or by cerebral concussions, or by encephalitis lethargica. What role then do conscious and unconscious conflicts play? The answers to all such questions demand precise and sustained clinical and experimental investigation.[19] Furthermore, how early in infancy do these obligatory repetitions become recognizable? And how do they vary?

❨ Symbolic Distortions

Quite naturally, the next focus was on the vulnerability of the symbolic process itself to different types of disturbance. The ability to draw statistically adequate and representative samples from the continuous preconscious stream of inner experience, and then to represent these samples by symbolic condensations, is certainly essential for the development of all psychological processes that are uniquely human, whether sick or well. This capacity is essential for our highest creative abilities. Yet, because of their high vulnerability to various kinds of distortion, the same symbolizing processes play an equally essential role in all human psychological illnesses. The two are linked in a direct fashion. Originally, I pointed out that if anything occurs to disturb the relationship of a symbol to that which it is supposed to represent, the symbolizing process becomes instead a misrepresenting, masking, misleading, and distorting tool. In place of accurate symbolic representation we have misrepresentation and then dissociation. If there is either a distortion or an interruption in that relationship, the symbolic process loses its ability to represent and ruminate and communicate about samples from the inner stream of preconscious mentation, along with its ability to test its relationship to reality. Thus, any distortions of the relationship of the symbol to what it set out to represent lead to increasingly complex further distortions in human psychology. And, where there is an interruption in the relationship of a symbol to its referent (i.e., to that which it was originally intended to represent), a discontinuity is introduced into psychological processing, which in general psychiatric language has been called "dissociation." In psychoanalysis, it has also been called "substitution," "displacement," "reversal," "repression," etc. All of these terms are metaphors. They do not indicate *how* it happens, but only *that* it happens, and that those important forms of symbolic distortion result which play such an essential role in the discontinuities that characterize all neuroses and psychoses. Yet, all such dissociations of linkages to time, space, objects, and persons produce secondary and tertiary dissociations in all other linkages of symbols to their referents.

Again, further questions confront us. How does the relationship of a symbol to what it is supposed to represent (i.e., to its roots or referents) become distorted or obliterated? Certainly, as I have said, there are distortions in time and place relationships. But are there others? Can distortions occur through the influence of organic as well as psychological processes? What is the role of conscious and/or preconscious conflict in such disruptions? Note that these are precisely the questions that have already been raised about the mechanisms by which obligatory repetition can be introduced into human behavior.

Subsequently, a third question occupied my thinking, namely, how do distortions occur in the affective components of experience?[13,22]

Out of these considerations came the hypothesis that everyone higher than the lower grades of defectives has a "neurotic potential," out of which an enormously variable yet inescapable neurotic process evolves, which, in turn, can lead either to the development of all manner of neurotic personality disturbances, to the precipitation of a neurotic state,[19] or, under special circumstances, to the occurrence of psychotic disorganization.[23]

It became my thesis that there are several primary ingredients in the neurotic process, and that under certain circumstances the obligatory repetition is the initiating disturbance, whereas in other instances the distortion of symbolic processes may be the first step in neurotic development. In still others, the first step is the imposition of a central emotional position[22] (or central affective potential), which leads thereafter to a central affective state to which that individual always tends to return, and which, in turn, can be set off by

one or more triggers. These central affective positions can vary from terror, rage, depression, or euphoria, to various mixtures of these.

❲ The Role of the Cybernetic Chain in the Continuation of the Neurotic Process and in the Distortion of Life

An understanding of how trouble starts is important for theoretical, practical, nosological, experimental, preventive, and therapeutic purposes. Yet, this alone is not enough. From the moment that the repetition of anything has become obligatory, the inflexible and insatiable repetition itself has consequences that vary with the nature of the repeated symptom, the situation, and the responses of those around it. These consequences, in turn, give rise to fresh deviations, which instigate new symptoms and new distortions of life. The examples that come to mind are literally endless. A child may develop a trivial repetitive pattern of behavior, such as getting out of bed and coming out to join the family, an insatiable need to be with the grown-ups, a need for their presence. This pattern may be linked to fear of the dark or of a sibling, of his own nocturnal impulses, whether conscious or unconscious, or of a fairy tale, but it can also arise in many other and subtler conflicts. The child may or may not be afraid. It may be a wholly natural impulse, as for instance to see what is going on, to feel close to others. But, whatever the reasons, once the pattern becomes one of obligatory repetition, an insatiable and repetitive necessity which he has to repeat endlessly, irrespective of rewards, punishment, teasing, joking, appeals to common sense or reason, loving, cuddling, or other substituted satisfactions such as a song or story, we know that a mechanism has taken over to produce the automatic repetition of what may have started as an intrinsically natural bit of behavior, thus converting it into a neurotic symptom. This launches a chain reaction, the nature of which depends upon many factors extrinsic to the initiating source.

In the past, when many adults lived under one roof in many families, the adults competed with one another in demonstrating their special talents for dealing with such disturbances. Today, on the other hand, there is usually only one senior person in any household to take care of such matters. It may be an anger-breeding burden to one person, but where it can be spread out among several, it can usually be handled with more patience. This is one of the profound differences between the old umbrella-shaped home and the conical family of today.

Further consequences depend not merely upon how many people there are to take turns in meeting the challenges of neurotically repeated demands, but also on the variable inner moods and feelings of those adults, specifically, the feelings about children in general which these demands evoke. These can range from rage, terrifying punishment, and humiliation, to bribery and excessive rewards in the form of overcuddling and overindulgence. In these ways, the feedback from the environment to the symptom plays a role in shaping the further feedback from the primary symptom to the evolution of further symptoms. The child, as well as the child's family, pay variable prices for even so banal and nearly universal a neurotic moment in childhood as this, and the prices will vary widely, in ways which mold the development of the process. Thus, there is a wide variety in the chain of neurotogenic experiences which can evolve out of even one single symptom, and wide differences in the consequences for an entire life which results from these differences. All of this is obvious; but the intricate complexity of the network of consequences which can evolve from the simplest neurotic symptom is something that even modern psychoanalytic psychiatry has tended to overlook.

Clearly, no neurotic symptom exists in a vacuum. It is set in a matrix, not only of people, but also of inanimate objects, which interact with the neurotic symptom and thereby play a role in the further evolution of the neurotic process. Therefore, the neurotic process depends not only on the nature of the initiating moment, nor on the focus of the initial obligatory repetition, nor on the point at which the symbolic process becomes strained, distorted, or disrupted, nor on the nature of the central affective potential which is imposed on the developing personality. It depends on all of these, but also on the nature of the complex network of their consequences, and on the feedback from these consequences which often establishes new conflicts (conscious, preconscious, and unconscious), which produce new neurotic symptoms secondary to the first, which, in turn, generate new secondary and tertiary consequences secondary to the new symptoms, to a third and fourth order of events.

In other words, the neurotic process is a continuously changing and evolving process, a reverberating or cybernetic chain reaction. All of this must be kept in mind when we ask what the effects of our therapeutic efforts are, whether they are somatic, pharmacological, psychotherapeutic in general, or psychoanalytic in particular, and with or without the introduction of organic adjuvants. Whatever techniques we use, we must ask what the influence of each of these ingredients is, not only on the originating or primary conflicts, but also on the affective components, their symbolic representations, and then on the chains of events which lead to all of the later consequences. Frequently, these later consequences can be interrupted with great benefit to the patient, yet without modifying the primary initiating ingredients in the neurotic process. Although symptomatic relief can be of great human value, from a scientific point of view it should never be confused with an attack on the heart of the matter.

⦗ The Universal Neurotic Potential and Process—The Less Frequent Neurotic State

Finally, I would like to say that before I understood any of this clearly, and particularly before I understood the role of the preconscious processing of human experience, which constitutes the essential continuum in human psychology, I wrote of a neurotic potential, a neurotic process, and a neurotic state.[19] At that time, this formulation was in a sense premature, and contained elements which I would modify today. Nevertheless, in its essence it has validity.

There is a neurotic potential in every human being who is capable of affective processsing, of generating obligatory repetitions, and of symbolic representation of these experiences. In my original formulation I laid primary emphasis on the symbolic distortion alone, because this is the characteristic which is unique to the human neurosis, whereas affective distortions can be induced experimentally in animals in many different ways, without necessarily involving the other two ingredients that are essential to the human neurosis. Such disturbances which can be produced in lower animals by special conditioning maneuvers have been called "an experimental neurosis"; but the late Howard Liddell said to me that this is not truly an experimental neurosis at all, but the "experimental production in lower animals of the affective concomitants of the human neurosis." Liddell said further that he regretted that he had fallen into the then popular fashion of speaking and writing of the "experimental neurosis" in sheep and other animals, because later he became convinced that there were better and less confusing terms to be used instead, to refer to the use of the techniques of conditioning by which emotional disturbances could be induced in laboratory animals.

On the other hand, the experimental superimposition of a fixed affective position is possible in the lower animals, in forms which are equally characteristic of human psychopathology. Whether or not we can induce in animals the other two ingredients of human neurosis is a challenge to which the animal experimentalists must soon turn their attention with greater specificity than they have done in the past.

However, there is surely in man a universal neurotic potential, out of which evolves inevitably, but with endless and infinite variety, a neurotic process that need never manifest itself in formal symptomatology. Thus, the obligatory repetitions, the fixed affective positions, and the symbolic distortions, may express themselves not through a symptom (like a counting compulsion, or a dirt phobia, or a conversion symptom), but rather in skillfully disguised and rationalized overemphases of some special pattern of life, such as in overdrives or underdrives, in rushing or dawdling. One need only think of the all-too-familiar compulsive work drive which may be highly productive, creative, and valuable from the point of view of society, and for which a man may receive honors and many rewards, until the day comes when the tax collector catches up with him and he goes into an involutional depression. This is the sad fate of success which was described long before the modern era of study of dynamic psychiatry and psychopathology.

The neurotic process may express itself in the choice of the kind of dwelling in which one lives, or in the choice of whether one lives in the city or in the country. One ingenious woman had a thousand extraordinarily good rationalizations for always taking her family on vacations to interesting and remote cities, where they could study different cultures, different art forms, different architectures, different languages, and observe the different ways in which people live. She was doing something very valuable for them, but she was also hiding her own paralyzing phobia, which was focused on everything that had to do with rural settings of life. A witty rationalization went with this, and she developed a magnificent theory as to why cities are beautiful and the country ugly and lacking in all essential aesthetic qualities. This did not change the fact that the pattern of her living was determined by a wholly unrecognized terror which afflicted her whenever she was in the country, hidden and protected by a brilliant, masking, counterphobic compulsion. Anyone with clinical experience could match this example with many others. These are the symptomatic manifestations of a skillfully disguised neurotic process, manifestations which may appear only as subtle distortions of the personality and of ways of living.

Sometimes, however, these personality distortions are not so simple. The compulsive do-gooder or the compulsive do-badder are gross examples. The juvenile delinquent is another; or the senile delinquent, for that matter. All forms of so-called sociopathy, all amoral or asocial personality disturbances are gross examples of the same principle.

It is of special interest and value to note that these skillfully masked neurotic manifestations that invade the personality and its ways of life can often be far more destructive to others than are any more formal symptoms. It is usually true that the frankly symptomatic mother does less damage to her children than does the mother who has neurotogenic personality exaggerations, but no frank symptoms. The former is less likely to impose her symptoms on others, than is the mother with a constellation of neurotic behavior which is rewarded (as is any working compulsion). It is extraordinarily difficult to render this alien to the patient's inner prideful feelings of adequacy, and it is extremely difficult therefore to persuade him to focus on it for therapeutic purposes. He wants instead to protect it, just as the patient in a euphoria claims to have the right to be elated (or for that matter to be angry). "I have a right to be angry, I mean hungry," said one woman.

Finally, there is the full-blown neurotic state, which is self-diagnosing. It is the easiest thing to recognize in all of medicine, because the patient comes in and tells you about it. "I am afraid of heights," or "I am afraid of depths," or "I am afraid of bugs," or "I am afraid of dirt," or "I cannot stop counting," etc. Although agoraphobia can be crippling to a patient's life, it is primarily the patient himself who is crippled. Only secondarily are the comfort and safety of the patient's family impaired. This is less important than are the other manifestations to which I have referred; yet, a knowledge of this whole area begins with a knowledge of the neurotic state. Unhappily, all too often this is where it ends, although this ought to be where such knowledge starts. The symptom cluster is only a cluster of consequences and should never be used as the basis for a nosological system. Again, it is for this reason that a given life is

so often far "sicker" than is the illness of the person who lives it.

❲ The Relation of the Neurotic Process to Psychotic Disorganization

Psychotic disorganization may be a direct outgrowth of an ongoing neurotic "chain reaction" which has led the patient into a trap, consisting of irreconcilable, conflicting, and unattainable drives, on which conflicting and irreconcilable symptoms are superimposed. Such a chain reaction has its roots in some of the primitive behavioral stereotypes (also called fixations) of infancy and/or early childhood.

The origins of stereotyped behavior are in an uncertain interplay among genetic, cultural, and familial factors, plus idiosyncratic experiential events, and also hypothetical somatic variables. Once established, such obligatory repetitions of any pattern of behavior produce distortions of life which, in turn, produce new, secondary symptoms, which have their own deforming consequences, which give rise to tertiary symptoms, and so on. The process is mediated by a continuous stream of preconscious processing of inner experiences under the concurrent influence of unconscious conflicts and preconscious sampling and control. As a result of the persisting dichotomy between symbolic units and their originating conflicts, these become inaccessible to conscious introspection or to correction by experience.

When all elements are conscious, their combined effect is to produce perplexity and sometimes inconsistent behavior, but not neurosis. As the years go on, however, one of the opposing pair usually attains dominant and manifest importance, the other becoming latent. At this point, the conflict between them becomes neurotogenic. Its conscious manifestations will take either the form of diffuse symptomatic behavior or symbolic symptom formations. In some instances, especially when the resultant symptoms also become conflicting and irreconcilable, there are psychotic sequelae.

Early conflicts focus on primary instinctual processes, such as ingestion and excretion, food phobias and compulsive gorging, compulsive sleeping and wakefulness. Becoming more complex as time goes on, such conflicts come to invade the processes of adult decision-making and thus may influence a person's choice of education, marital status, career, friends, etc. Perhaps the most frequent and highly charged dilemma encountered among psychotics is between gender identities, i.e., whether to become or remain a man or woman.

A woman patient's childhood had been marked by total rejection by her parents, who openly preferred her brother. As a result, she struggled throughout her life among conflicting unconscious drives to possess her brother, to kill him, to supplant him in her father's love by becoming a big blond boy like her brother; yet, she never totally abandoned all feminine goals or identifications. She struggled over whether to grow older or younger, whether to be boy or girl, or both. With each birthday, this struggle became sharper, and she became more depressed.

She was still able to function when she unconsciously sought a solution to her unresolved conflict through a surrogate relationship, namely, through marriage to a man who had been her brother's best friend. In addition, her new husband's father was a close friend of her own father; and prior to the marriage, he had always shown the patient far more affection than had her own father. But immediately after the marriage, the new father-figure turned away from her. With this repetition of her childhood pain and loss, she became bewildered and unhappy. Her husband's complete recovery from a dangerous illness came soon afterwards, and turned out to be a psychological catastrophe for her, by reactivating her buried death-wishes toward her brother and her need to replace him.

Thereupon, from having been freely active, she became anxiety-ridden and severely agoraphobic, so that she could hardly bring herself to move more than a few blocks from her home. With the passing years, and further deterioration of the marriage, she superimposed on this terror an equally violent claustrophobia. At this point, she was trapped between two terrors, so that she sometimes stood on the threshold of her home for hours, equally terrified to go in or to go out, to be among people or to be alone, to move or to remain motionless. Here, then, was a juxtaposition of irreconcilable drives and irreconcilable symptomatic defenses. This brought on the imminent threat of full-blown psychotic disorganization, which, fortunately, led her into intensive treatment just in time to save her.

One of the pitfalls in our theories about psychotic cases is the tendency to assume that the mechanisms which are at work during the psychosis *after* it has been established, had also initiated the psychosis, an error which can be seriously misleading. The phenomena of regression furnish frequent examples of this. Although regression is one of the more consistent components of psychotic disorganization, there is no clear evidence that it ever initiates the psychosis. What it does, is to set in motion and activate a new series of fantasies and a chain of new secondary and tertiary consequences.

Furthermore, regression can mean many things. It can mean an abandonment of adult life itself, with the unconscious implication that "If I go back to the beginning, I can start over and grow up different." It can be and often is linked to difficulties about gender identity and to the desire to change sides, to be the other sex, or both, or neither, which the psychotic patient so frequently expresses in many, varied, and transparent forms. It is not surprising, then, that one of the forms which the regressive movement can take is a suicide effort, which is not in reality an effort to die but rather to be reborn.

A distinction must also be kept in mind between mechanisms which touch off the process of disorganization, and those which are set in motion during that process, i.e., after it is under way, but which sustain and complicate it because of their own highly complex secondary consequences. To make this differentiation possible, it is important for us to begin systematically to collect examples of psychotogenic impasses which precipitate the gradual or acute decompensation of the neurotic process into psychotic episodes.

It will also be necessary to gather data on the nature of the noxious momentum, whether this consists of critical episodes or of gradual changes which cause latent double-binds to erupt into manifest forms. Sometimes, the inescapable concomitants of maturing will do it, e.g., the threat of emerging from home, school, hospital, or job; the threat of promotion, or advancement, or of loss. The conflict can be unmasked by the death of a close relative after a serious illness, or by his recovery, by pregnancies, and the end of pregnancies.

All of this will have to be correlated with the influence of drugs on the threshold for reverberating processes in the CNS, and on the organization and disorganization of symbolic processes, both in the waking state and during sleep. In some patients, the drugs with which we are experimenting today seem to terminate the psychosis and re-establish the pre-psychotic neurosis. Yet, in other patients the same drugs have an opposite effect. Sometimes, after a patient seems to have been pulled out of his psychosis by drugs, the lowering of the dosage may re-establish the psychosis. This is well-known, but another closely related fact has received insufficient attention; i.e., that during the transition back into psychosis or while it is taking place, the patient can sometimes report the transition step by step in the changes from normal waking thought processes to the type that occur in all of us during sleep. With reduction in medication, patients have described this sensation in many different words: "I can see it coming on"; "I am beginning to think differently"; "I am awake but I am thinking as though I were asleep."

From the point of view of psychopharmacology, this is an observation of an important paradoxical fact. It is as though a drug which is ultimately sleep-producing could also enable certain patients to think as a waking person thinks; whereas the withdrawal of the drug—which should awaken him still further

—causes his *thinking* processes during the waking state to become disorganized into sleep-like preconscious patterns. A study of many verbatim samples of these transitions in both directions is an area for basic research which should illuminate these observations.

(Bibliography

1. KUBIE, L. S. "A Theoretical Application to Some Neurological Problems of the Properties of Excitation Waves Which Move in Closed Circuits," *Brain*, 53 (1930), 166–178.

2. ———. "Body Symbolization and the Development of Language," *Psychoanalytic Quarterly*, 3 (1934), 430–444.

3. ———. "The Repetitive Core of Neurosis," *Psychoanalytic Quarterly*, 10 (1941), 23–43.

4. ———. Review of *Lectures on Conditioned Reflexes* Vol. 2: *Conditioned Reflexes and Psychiatry* by I. P. Pavlov. *Psychoanalytic Quarterly*, 11 (1942), 565–570.

5. ———. "The Use of Induced Hypnagogic Reveries in the Recovery of Repressed Amnesic Data," *Bulletin of the Menninger Clinic*, 7 (1943), 172–182.

6. ———. "The Value of Induced Dissociated States in the Therapeutic Process," *Proceedings of the Royal Society of Medicine*, 38 (1945), 681–683.

7. ———. Review of *War Neuroses in North Africa* by R. R. Grinker and J. J. Spiegel. *Psychosomatic Medicine*, 8 (1946), 67–69.

8. ———. "The Neurotic Potential and Human Adaptation," in J. Romano, ed., *Adaptation*, pp. 77–96. Ithaca: Cornell University Press, 1949.

9. ———. Discussion of Dr. Penfield's address on Memory Mechanisms, at 76th Annual Meeting of the American Neurological Association, Atlantic City, June 1951.

10. ———. Symbolic Distortion in Neurosis and Psychosis, Some Psychophysiological Considerations, *Transactions of the American Neurological Association*, 76th Annual Meeting, Atlantic City, June 1951, pp. 42–44.

11. ———. Communications Between Sane and Insane, Hypnosis, *Transactions of the*

Eighth Conference on Cybernetics, March 1951, pp. 92–133.

12. ———. "The Neurotic Potential, the Neurotic Process and the Neurotic State," *U.S. Armed Forces Medical Journal*, 2 (1951), 1–12.

13. ———. The Place of Emotions in the Feedback Concept, *Transactions of the Ninth Conference on Cybernetics*, March 1952, pp. 48–72.

14. ———. "The Distortion of the Symbolic Process in Neurosis and Psychosis," *Journal of the American Psychoanalytic Association*, 1 (1953), 59–86.

15. ———. "The Central Representation of the Symbolic Process in Psychosomatic Disorders," *Psychosomatic Medicine*, 15 (1953), 107; also in E. D. Wittkower and R. A. Cleghorn, eds., *Recent Developments in Psychosomatic Medicine*, pp. 126–133. London: I. Pitman & Sons, 1954.

16. ———. "Some Implications for Psychoanalysis of Modern Concepts of the Organization of the Brain," *Psychoanalytic Quarterly*, 22 (1953), 21–68.

17. ———. "The Concept of Normality and Neurosis," in M. Heiman, ed., *Psychoanalysis and Social Work*, pp. 3–14. New York: International Universities Press, 1953.

18. ———. "The Fundamental Nature of the Distinction Between Normality and Neurosis," *Psychoanalytic Quarterly*, 23 (1954), 167–204.

19. ———. "The Neurotic Process as the Focus of Physiological and Psychoanalytic Research," *Journal of Mental Science*, 104 (1958), 518–536.

20. ———. "Hypnotism: A Focus for Psychophysiological and Psychoanalytic Investigations," *Archives of General Psychiatry*, 4 (1961), 40–54.

21. ———. "Neurosis and Normality," in A. Deutsch, ed., *The Encyclopedia of Mental Health*, Vol. IV. New York: Franklin Watts, Inc., 1963.

22. ———. "The Central Affective Potential and Its Trigger Mechanisms," in H. S. Gaskill, ed., *Counterpoint, Libidinal Object and Subject, A Tribute to Rene A. Spitz on his 75th Birthday*, pp. 106–120. New York:

International Universities Press, 1963.

23. ———. "The Relation of Psychotic Disorganization to the Neurotic Process," *Journal of the American PSA Association*, 15 (1967), 626–640.

24. ———. Preface to J. Haley, ed., *Advanced Techniques of Hypnosis and Therapy: Selected Papers of M. H. Erickson*. New York: Grune & Stratton, 1968.

25. ———. "Multiple Fallacies in the Concept of Schizophrenia," in P. Doucet and C. Laurin, eds., *Problems of Psychosis, Part II*. The Hague: Excerpta Medica, 1971.

26. ———. "The Unfortunate Concept of Schizophrenia," in A. R. Kaplan, ed., *Genetic Factors in "Schizophrenia."* Springfield, Ill.: Charles C Thomas, 1972.

27. KUBIE, L. S., and R. M. BRICKNER. "A Miniature Psychotic Storm Produced by a Superego Conflict Over Simple Posthypnotic Suggestion," *Psychoanalytic Quarterly*, 5 (1936), 467–487.

28. KUBIE, L. S., and M. H. ERICKSON. "The Use of Automatic Drawing in the Interpretation and Relief of a State of Acute Obsessional Depression," *Psychoanalytic Quarterly*, 7 (1938), 443–466.

29. ———. "The Permanent Relief of an Obsessional Phobia by Means of Communications with an Unsuspected Dual Personality," *Psychoanalytic Quarterly*, 8 (1939), 471–509.

30. KUBIE, L. S., and S. G. MARGOLIN. "A Physiological Method for the Induction of States of Partial Sleep, and Securing Free Association and Early Memories in Such States," *Transactions of the American Neurological Association* (1942), 136–139.

31. ———. "An Apparatus for the Use of Breath Sounds as a Hypnagogic Stimulus," *The American Journal of Psychiatry*, 100 (1944), 610.

32. ———. "The Process of Hypnotism and the Nature of the Hypnotic State," *The American Journal of Psychiatry*, 100 (1944), 611–622.

33. ———. "The Therapeutic Role of Drugs in the Process of Repression, Dissociation and Synthesis," *Psychosomatic Medicine*, 7 (1945), 147–151.

CHAPTER 2

SYMPTOMATIC BEHAVIOR: EGO-DEFENSIVE, ADAPTIVE, AND SOCIOCULTURAL ASPECTS

Eugene B. Brody

⟦ Symptom, Defense, Culture, and Adaptation

A FEELING, THOUGHT, OR ACT designated "symptomatic" is considered reflective of something else. Just as fever, tachycardia, or tremor, it indicates an underlying process. This view assumes the existence of hidden (from both subject and observer) determinants and functions (probable consequences) of the visible behavior or reported subjective state. The psychoanalytically oriented (or psychodynamic) description of these determinants and functions is framed in terms of a conflict of unconscious or preconscious (more readily accessible to awareness) psy-chological forces. These forces may be two opposing but incompatible tendencies, e.g., a wish to be independent and autonomous versus a wish to be dependent (as upon a parent); or a wish to be passive, submissive, and compliant versus a wish to be active, dominant, and aggressive. Or they may be a socially unacceptable wish or drive (usually aggressive or sexual) versus an inhibiting force (often summarized in structural terms as the superego) on the other. The final behavioral pathway, i.e., the symptom, or index behavior itself, is shaped by the particular tendencies involved, the anxiety generated by conflict between them, and the ego-defense mechanisms which it activates. These last function to keep anxiety at a manageable level and unacceptable vectors of conflict from erupting undisguised into consciousness or being translated into action. This behavioral formulation or psychodynamic description is based on a group of interlocking concepts developed by Sigmund Freud. Major milestones in understanding the symptomatic (hidden) significance of privately experienced or publicly observable events were publication of *The Interpretation of Dreams* in 1900,[33] *The Psychopathology of Everyday Life*[34] in 1901, and *Jokes and Their Relation to the Unconscious*[35] in 1905. These works provide a basic chart for discovering the messages hidden in dreams, fantasies, affective states, ideas, and acts, including the most ordinary communications. The messages are obscured by condensation, derivative formation, and a series of typical distortions, regularities which suggest that they are systematically produced. The hypothetical distortion-producing processes were assumed to defend the subject from being confronted or overwhelmed by his own threatening, unacceptable wishes, impulses, or memories, *ergo* "defense mechanisms." Defense mechanisms are concepts constructed on the basis of detailed psychobiographies, with particular emphasis on inappropriate responses to external crises, or on psychological pain, or inappropriate behavior without apparent reason. The summary of psychoanalytic thinking forming the general basis of psychodynamics is Freud's work, *Inhibitions, Symptoms, and Anxiety*,[37] published in 1926. Anna Freud's summary of defense mechanisms, published in 1936,[32] also contains little which needs to be significantly modified. Psychological defense is conceived as one function of the ego: a coherent grouping or system of interrelated functions or activities, such as paying attention, making decisions, controlling motor action, or integrating whole complexes of thoughts, attitudes, and feelings, as well as managing anxiety and warding off impulses. Dysfunction in one aspect of the system is reflected in changes—sometimes of a compensatory nature—in the rest of the system.[5] The defensive functions of the ego

operate in concert with its integrative, executive, and other functions, conceived as part of this system of interrelated processes. Ego-functioning is also determined by a person's basic endowments, his equipment for receiving, processing, and integrating information from within and without, and for sending out new information. Perception, decision-making, defense, and conflict resolution depend to some degree on the intelligence, talent, knowledge, and special skills which the person has at his disposal.

Every element of a psychodynamic formulation of symptomatic behavior reflects immediate or remote cultural influences. Particular wishes or needs acquire significance, and ways of dealing with them and their associated tensions are based on a society's accepted rules for living. Nuclear families stimulate more intense attachments to and rivalries with the same sex and opposite sex parent than do extended families, or where many surrogate parents are involved in childrearing. Independence-dependence conflicts reflect the roles of adolescents in particular cultures. Childrearing practices are among the most faithful reflectors of traditional values, espoused by adults who ignore them in the actual conduct of their own lives. One example of an articulating hypothesis linking early developmental experience to adult (possibly symptomatic) behavior is that of Weisman[77] as summarized and interpreted by Caudill:[19] "Adult behavior is 'colored' by a recognizably different— according to the culture—set of derivatives coming from the particular, for the culture, solutions to pre-genital phases of development." Caudill and colleagues,[20,22] comparing Japanese and American mother-infant interaction, suggest strongly that differences in the motor and verbal behavior of Japanese and American infants during the first several months of life are learned (a function of culture), rather than genetic or maturational in origin. Caudill and Weinstein[22] noted:

If these distinctive patterns of behavior are well on the way to being learned by three-to-four months of age, and if they continue over the life span of the person, then there are very likely to be important areas of difference in emotional response in people in one culture when compared with those in another. Such differences are not easily subject to conscious control and, largely out of awareness, they accent and color human behavior.

The infants are considered by Caudill as having "learned some of the rudiments of their culture" by this age, "well before the development of the ability to use language in the ordinary sense." He views this as the acquisition of some aspects of the "implicit culture," as Linton[54] termed it, the ways of thinking and behaving which occur without conscious attention and are generally shared by people in the particular culture.

The core of the superego—the organized, internalized, unconscious standard-setting and inhibiting mechanisms—is what has been learned (during preverbal as well as later development) from culture-bearing parents. Socially transmitted values and symbols are crucial aspects of culture. The early acquisition of self-censoring and behavior-inhibiting tendencies (part of the process of socialization) was described by Wexler as incorporating the parent "garbed in the mythology of childhood."[78] Devereux[29] referred to the "relative degree of importance which a culture 'assigns' to various defense mechanisms," and utilized the concept of an "ethnic unconscious" composed ". . . of material which each generation teaches the next one to repress, in accordance with the basic demand patterns of the prevailing culture. . . . each society or culture permits certain impulses, fantasies and the like to become and remain conscious while requiring others to be repressed."

Wittkower and Fried[79] concluded that different clinical syndromes prominent in differing cultures may be related to differences in (a) the amount of aggression, guilt, and anxiety generated in regularly encountered life situations, and (b) the accepted techniques used in dealing with aggression, guilt, and anxiety. Thus, the relative acceptability of drives or wishes (the anxiety, guilt, shame, or disgust attached to them), as well as the repertory of defenses used to ward them off or manage the tension which they trigger, is

culturally influenced. These factors are recognized in the large literature on basic personality types or modal personalities. The modal personality concept implies that people exposed to certain regularities in childrearing and constraints and reinforcements on their adult behavior share certain response tendencies. As C. P. Snow, quoted by Leighton and Murphy,[50] has observed: "Without thinking about it, they respond alike. That is what culture means." Shared behavioral readinesses should logically be accompanied by shared vulnerability or resistance to particular types of symptomatic behavior. There is some support for this presumption, and an individual's habitual affective and cognitive styles developed within his familial or national cultural setting shape the form of his symptomatic behavior. Such patterns of shared behavior may, for example, increase the likelihood that any culture-bearer's overt disturbance will have a paranoid or an affective cast, or that his anxiety will be reflected in inner discomfort rather than outward action. However, the epidemiological evidence, especially in terms of the incidence of established syndromes, is as yet inconclusive.

Following the Freudian formulae, a symptom is a compromise formation. Symptomatic behavior represents an unsatisfactory compromise between unconscious wishes, the demands of the superego, and of reality (including aspects of culture and society). A series of defense mechanisms, with repression as the cornerstone, is activated by signal anxiety generated by the unconscious conflict. The final behavioral outcome, most prominently shaped by the leading defense mechanisms, reflects other factors as well. Significant among these are poorly dealt with anxiety or other tension emerging to the surface, and the disguised representation or gratification of the warded-off impulse. The symptom may have symbolic significance which allows it to function in this way; it may also be a symbolic communicative attempt, reflect unresolved identifications with important caretakers or love-objects, or involve culture-specific expressive or instrumental symbols. Psychological symptoms constitute a code to messages stated otherwise in cultural or individual historical terms.

Symptoms result in both primary and secondary gain. The former is the immediate intrapsychic consequence of the defensive process: anxiety and impulse control, as well as some disguised gratification of the warded-off wish. Because the latter gain is environmental, it provides another channel through which culture shapes symptoms. It includes the added control over important people which the person obtains by becoming sick. Reinforcing environmental rewards range from enslaving a dominant spouse—reversing roles—to temporary freedom from work demands.

The consequences of organic illness may be incorporated into a defense system, enhancing both primary and secondary gain. If the illness has resulted in cerebral deficit with impaired memory or reality evaluation, the deficit may function as an aid to the processes of repression and denial with environmental consequences. During the peak of prefrontal lobotomy usage in the United States, in the late 1940s, a middle-aged man received the operation for a severe, chronic, obsessive tension state. He had lived alone with his elderly mother who suffered from painful arthritis. Although the examining psychiatrist inferred the presence of significant unconscious hostility toward the mother, the patient's overt behavior had been docile, conforming, and unnecessarily polite, revealing underlying anger only through an excessive concern with her health and the possibility of her sudden death. This was sufficiently obtrusive to make her uncomfortable at times. Following surgery and significant relief from symptoms, his docile conforming behavior was replaced by a tendency to be boisterous and use crude language. He sometimes shouted at his mother (which he had never done before) when he experienced her as frustrating, and now acknowledged feelings of anger toward her to the psychiatrist. His overt concern for her health and comfort, however, remained and he could not acknowledge an aggressive intent in one new pattern of behavior which occurred repeatedly. That is, he would forget to stoke the coal furnace before going to work in the morning;

this meant that his mother, in her eighties, had painfully to crawl down the basement stairs and bit by bit fire the furnace herself. The patient would say only that since the surgery his memory had been so impaired that he was unable to remember to care for the furnace. (Psychological tests revealed no significant impairment six months after surgery, although it had been present for several weeks earlier.)

An emergency room experience also illustrates some of the elements of primary and secondary gain. A young woman was admitted with a quadriplegia that began when her husband left town. Eventually, it became clear that she was struggling with her unconscious and unacceptable love for her brother-in-law. The quadriplegia represented a symptomatic compromise between her love and the self-censoring (guilt-producing) mechanisms which kept it from emerging into consciousness. Her paralysis made it impossible for her on the one hand to go to her brother-in-law when her husband left town; on the other hand, it required him to come to her and made it impossible for her to ward him off if he were to decide to make love to her. Her symptom symbolized her wish to submit while allowing her to abdicate any responsibility for physical contact with him, should he initiate it. Aside from the primary gain (anxiety and guilt reduction, impulse control, need gratification), it obtained for her the secondary gain of limiting her husband's resented traveling for a time, unconsciously stimulating his anxiety about her, and increasing her real-life dominance over him.

Massive conversion reactions, such as the above, are most frequently reported in relatively unsophisticated populations. Hollingshead and Redlich[43] suggested that, in general, upper-class (I and II) psychiatric patients tend to be obsessive or depressed, middle-class (III) anxious, lower-middle or upper-lower (IV) hypochondriacal or somatically expressive, and the lowest classes (V) aggressive ("acting out" their conflicts) or resigned. These socioeconomic class-linked behaviors reflect the relative priorities of defense mechanisms determined by different developmental experiences, including the educational, as well as by the innate capacities, knowledge, and skills acquired by the person during development. Beyond the early cultural impact on ego development and communicative capacity, people in different social strata have variable access to sources of power and help. Social imperatives confine the effective cry for help of the lower-prestige person to one which is loud, dramatic, and sometimes threatening.

Ego-defensive processes following the Freudian formulae function mainly to achieve an intrapsychic steady state. Sullivan's[74] concept of security operations includes maneuvers aimed at interpersonal as well as intrapsychic factors. Hartman[42] emphasized individual-societal relations, defining psychological adaptation as the process of establishing and maintaining a reciprocal relationship with the environment. This implies a more active, creative attempt at dealing with the environment and its crises: active information-seeking, circumventing, and modifying, rather than adjusting to social conditions. Adaptive-coping behavior is sometimes mistaken for the symptomatic reflection of mechanisms defending against the emergence into consciousness or action of unacceptable unconscious wishes. A youngster growing up in a metropolitan ghetto, for example, may present himself to an examining doctor as wary, suspicious, and litigious. This behavior is the culmination of a long struggle to survive in a threatening environment in which readiness to attack is the best defense. It also reflects the hostile anxiety of a helpless person surrounded by strangers. The unaware physician may inadvertently describe the patient as paranoid, implying the presence of unconscious homosexual or aggressive wishes dealt with by disavowal and attribution to someone else (projection).

Some circumstances may require rigid self-monitoring to avoid the expression of hostile impulses. Over a period of time, having become habitual, adaptively necessary suppression may be confused with symptomatic defensive inhibition. This last involves the constant employment of repression and reaction-formation (resulting in a public display of inappropriate cheerfulness or docility), as a means of warding off the explosive eruption of unconscious hostile impulses. Behavior reflecting chronic reaction formation is often maladaptive in the long run, since it does not give others the responsive feedback which they need to maintain their own interpersonal orientation and security. This is an example of the way in which ego-defensive processes result in overt behavior which, evoking reactions from others, soon leads the patient to progressively disturbing and burdensome relationships. On the other hand, seriously symptomatic acts may occur over a lifetime without such social consequences, and they may exist without obvious impairment of creative performance. For example, the novelist Graham Greene[41] described his own patterns of risk-taking behavior aimed at relieving boredom and giving him the feeling of being alive. He feigned the symptoms of an abscess, deceiving a dentist into extracting a healthy tooth under ether: ". . . unconsciousness was like a holiday from the world. I had lost a tooth but the boredom was for the time being dispersed." Over several months he played solitary Russian roulette: "The discovery that it was possible to enjoy again the visible world by risking its total loss was one I was bound to make sooner or later. . . . I remember an extraordinary sense of jubilation. . . . My heart knocked in its cage, and life contained an infinite number of possibilities."

Adaptive behavior becomes symptomatic when it persists outside the context in which it was functional. The suspiciousness necessary for survival in an inner city alley is inappropriate in the hospital examining room. The tendency to blame misfortune on external occult forces, normative among the folk Catholics of rural Brazil, may interfere with survival in industrial São Paulo.[14] United States paratroopers in World War II were rewarded for killing Germans. Those who persisted in attacking German civilians after the war ended were labeled as aggressive psychopaths.[3] The behavior was no different, but it was no longer socially functional.

Behavior which is genuinely adaptive or coping may also have symptomatic significance or be incorporated into symptomatic fantasies. This can most readily be seen in the psychotherapeutic situation. A young professional man, for example, had realized for some time that he was entrapped in an unsatisfactory partnership arrangement. Although his self-esteem suffered because of the attitudes of his senior associate, he remained because of the financial security it offered. Finally, he severed the relationship, although not precluding the possibility of more favorable renegotiated terms. This was an overdue adaptive and coping act. In the course of the following therapeutic hours, however, its symptomatic significance became apparent through his repeated reference to the idea that he had "cut off" his income. At one level, it was an unconscious act of retaliation against his wife who had told him that she was stronger-willed than he and could control him. Now he had symbolically converted himself into a castrate, and she would not have the money she needed from him. He required her in concrete as well as symbolic terms to become the strongest. In the transference, his needs for the therapist were clear. He fantasied telling the therapist that he could not pay the bill, with the therapist agreeing in return to carry him without a fee as long as necessary. The unconscious need was for the therapist to express his love and his appreciation for him as a unique individual, not "just another patient," and someone of particular worth—in marked contrast to his father who always complained that he, the patient, didn't accomplish what father wanted. The patient had also noted that father "never listened" when he tried to tell him something.

The borderline between adaptation and ego-defense is most difficult to ascertain when the demands for survival are so severe and prolonged as to produce major psychological distortions. This has been reported in combat situation, concentration camps, and shipwreck survivors.

An example is a woman of superior intelligence who spent two of her late childhood years in a Nazi concentration camp and a third recovering from tuberculosis contracted there. Her parents died in the camp and she recalls vividly the attention to minutiae necessary for her own survival. Narrowing of atten-

tion facilitated highly focused alertness; it also aided in repressing and denying information of catastrophic significance. This was part of what was called "getting yourself organized." The persisting need to be organized, to remain attentive to potentially life-threatening circumstances, to find food and warmth, were accompanied by a massive repression of hostility against the camp commanders, their underlings, and a more attractive female friend who had been able to prostitute herself for favors in an earlier camp. Despite her musical talent and opportunities to play, despite her high intelligence and opportunities for executive or scholarly work, she has remained a bookkeeper engaged in routine tasks. Her personality is obsessive-compulsive, meticulous in detail, intolerant of ambiguity, anxious in the face of any uncertainty, mistrustful of the motives of others seeking her friendship, and wary of her own tremendous needs and capacity for unreal expectations and disappointment, should she allow a relationship to develop. Her obsessive-compulsive tendencies, social distancing behavior, and hypersensitivity to the possibly hidden motives of others, are symptomatic reflections of defensive processes which have their roots in her earlier adaptational struggle.

Ego-defensive behavior stemming from inner conflict may also be adaptive. Thus, the repression of unconscious sexual wishes could facilitate a stable reciprocal relationship with authoritative parents in a Victorian society. More commonly, obsessive-compulsive behavior which has not reached the point of producing paralysis is rewarded in those whose intelligence and talent, propelled in part by neurotic drives, lead them to complete arduous courses of study such as medicine or law, or, striving for unattainable perfection, to make scientific discoveries or achieve certain types of business success. Even more commonly, however, the behavior consequent to ego-defensive operations is maladaptive. A paranoid system based on projection may keep the person's anxiety at a manageable level, but as he acts upon it, he may alienate his boss, estrange his wife, and shatter his personal relations. The delusions and hallucinations as well as the physical immobility of the catatonic patient may help reduce his anxiety and ward off potentially explosive instinctual impulses. Without nursing care, however, they are followed by physical illness and death.

A frequently used example of an ego-defensive mechanism employed with ultimately adaptive consequences is "regression in the service of the ego." Ernst Kris,[47] following Freud's[36] hypothesis that artists are characterized by a "flexibility of regression," formulated this concept as an expression of his idea that the creative process requires access to fantasies, feelings, thoughts, memories, images, and other mental phenomena which are usually not in awareness, i.e., which are preconscious or unconscious. Both Freud and Kris regarded the capacity to occasionally relinquish one's tight hold on reality as indicative of mature, creative persons. Kris proposed that the artist can deliberately regress while remaining receptive to the preconscious primary-process flow of psychological events. In this way, he can arrive at new insights, novel orderings of relationships, or previously unsuspected groupings. This contrasts with the psychotic whose inability to experience humor in response to cartoons reveals his anxiety about relinquishing his fragmented reality hold because of the risk of being unable to recapture it or of being totally overwhelmed by fantasy.[17]

(Social and Cultural Appraisal of Symptomatic Behavior

Human behavior—thinking, feeling, acting— is constantly evaluated by the actor himself and his audience. But the ongoing evaluative process is usually outside the focus of awareness. The standards by which people categorize their experience are built into them through socialization and enculturation while they mature; sorting, matching, and classifying information, evaluating its congruence or fit with these standards, occur rapidly and automatically. The process is shared by most members of a community (because of regu-

larities in developmental and adult experience) and operates silently. It is part of an institutionalized behavior pattern. Institutionalized behavior, in Talcott Parsons' words, provides "a mode of 'integration' of the actions of the component individuals" of society.[63] Automatic consensus about the social significance of behavior is also implied by Clyde Kluckhohn's definition of culture as a society's blueprint for living: the socially transmitted behavior patterns utilized by everyone in relation to all of the important aspects of life from birth to death.[46] The standards or values at its base, statements of what is considered worthwhile by the society, determine its normative guidelines for living, whether contained in institutionalized patterns of behavior or embodied in a system of external restraints, such as a legal code. Parsons regards moral or obligatory standards in particular as ". . . the core of the stabilizing mechanisms of the systems of social interaction."[63] These, along with common knowledge, common psychological states, and common attitudes, constitute what Ralph Linton called the "covert or implicit aspects of culture."[54,55] Related is the definition of culture offered by Kroeber and Parsons: "the transmitted and created content and patterns of values, ideas and other symbolic-meaningful systems as factors in the shaping of human behavior, and the artifacts produced through behavior."[48] Jaeger and Selznick's definition of culture is more sharply focused as "everything that is produced by and capable of sustaining shared symbolic experience."[45] In short, all human behavior occurs in a cultural symbolic-meaningful matrix, of which values are an essential part. Within this context, a person may categorize his own behavior as symptomatic if he experiences it as alien or a foreign body in himself— it is not congruent with his own internalized norms, values, and expectations of himself. Having labeled himself he may then seek professional assistance to rid himself of his subjectively experienced discomfort or ego-alien behavior, even though it may not be apparent to others. (L. S. Kubie once noted that the true heroes of this civilization are the people who continue to work and carry out their social responsibilities despite intense feelings of anxiety, depression, obsessive ideas, compulsive acts, phobias, or other neurotic symptoms.)

Individual values are closely related to group values in this respect. For example, cultural factors, such as an emphasis on tolerance or stoicism, may determine subjective experience as well as the timing of help-seeking. Italian housewives with a tendency to focus on the immediacy of pain showed lower thresholds for electric shock according to Sternbach and Tursky than Jewish women with a future orientation or "Yankees" with a "matter of fact" orientation.[73] These latter groups exhibited more rapid adaptation of the diphasic palmar skin potential response to shock. Mechanic emphasized the role of fear, stigma, social distance, and feelings of humiliation in help-seeking, as well as the influence upon illness-linked behavior (particularly one's need to minimize it) of the extent to which a particular community holds its members accountable for fulfilling responsibilities, regardless of health status.[57] This last is closely related to Parsons' earlier conception of the sick-role as a socially acceptable though sometimes temporary solution to psychosocial impasses.[61] Parsons regarded exemption from the performance of certain normal social obligations, as well as from a certain type of responsibility for one's own state, as one of the features making it evident that "illness is not merely a 'condition' but also a social role." Different cultures and different social strata reinforce or counteract the sick-role in varying degrees. Self- as well as other-appraisal of behavior as symptomatic will depend to some degree upon the guilt- and shame-free availability, the usefulness or necessity, of the sick role as a conflict-resolving or otherwise rewarding position.[8] Beyond this, Zola has pointed out that signs ordinarily understood as indicating problems in one population may be ignored in others because of their congruence with dominant or major value-orientations.[80] An example of the "fit" of signs with major social values is the acceptance (by subject as well as observer) of hallucinatory experience in some less industrialized societies, in contrast to the anxiety and symptomatic labeling accompanying such experience in societies with greater emphasis on rationality and control. The variable appraisal of intense emotional display as symptomatic is illustrated by Anne Parsons' contrast between the prominence of dramatic expression as a preferred way of dealing with inner and outer conflict in Italian as compared with United States culture.[60] The importance of culture-specific values is illustrated by the same investigator's account of an excited young woman of South Italian descent who was not regarded by her family as mentally ill until she violated two crucial norms, respect for the dead and family solidarity.[59] Other illustrations include the location of bodily symptoms in accordance with dominant values inhibiting or permitting particular types of symbolic expression, and illness behavior and appraisal in relation to guilt and sin ideologies, with such associated needs as those for expiation, exhibition of one's worthlessness, and suffering, or ascetic self-abnegation.

Self-referral to mental health units, folk-healers, or their equivalents, may not always be a consequence of ego-alien behavior. People also refer themselves for psychological help because of the secondary anxiety attendant upon ego-syntonic behavior. This usually refers to acts defined socially but not experienced personally as deviant, i.e., evaluated as such by observers (the audience) rather than the subject (the actor). These acts may include compulsive stealing, various sexual activities, repeated self-narcotization, impulsive risk-taking, or self-defeating occupational or interpersonal patterns. The individual engaging in ego-syntonic behavior does not experience it as painful, alien, or symptomatic. In time, however, he may become anxious about its consequences: legal apprehension (as in the case of stealing), social condemnation (as in the case of a homosexual minister seducing adolescent male parishioners), the deterioration of physical health (as in chronic alcoholism), accidents (as in repeated speeding), unwanted pregnancy (as in impulsive intercourse without contraception), or economic failure (as in repeated job loss due to symptomatic errors or antagonizing superiors).

Such secondary anxiety can lead the person to appraise his own behavior as symptomatic, but his attention is usually focused on its symptomatic nature only between acts, especially in the somewhat depressed period which occasionally follows an episode.

Both ego-alien and ego-syntonic behavior may be subjectively appraised as sick or symptomatic in terms of the others, the referents, with whom the person compares himself.[58] The major *comparative* reference group is usually the particular subcommunity in which a person lives. Its institutional, organizational, and behavioral patterns are familiar, and a person has innumerable opportunities throughout the day and over years to evaluate, assess, and appraise himself, using intimately known others and patterns as standards. He receives constant affirmations of his stable identity from the responses of others to whose values and expectations he conforms. Objectively minimal changes in this stable context can produce major interpersonal consequences which may force the individual into drastic reappraisals of himself. Beyond the comparative reference group, the person's behavior may be determined by that of a more distant community which he values highly, but to which he does not belong. This wealthier, better-educated, or somehow more advantaged community functions for him as an *emulative* reference group. Historically, the white middle-class community has had emulative significance for the American black; since he could not aspire to become a member of the group, some of whose goals and values he had acquired, this had an impact not only on his self- and other-appraisal (for example, hating and deprecating himself and others like him), but on his actual behavior, for example, unconscious emulative attempts based on fragmented and inaccurate information often resulting in caricatures eliciting humorous contempt from whites.[24] Traditional goals of the dominant white North American, such as pecuniary, occupational, and educational achievement, are now being adopted and achieved, however, to an increasing degree by the black community.[25] More significantly, with the increasing value of the black identity,

fostered by socioeconomic and political militancy, whites *per se* have become less significant as an emulative reference group.[10]

Still others who come to clinics or private mental health practitioners, or are extruded from society at large into mental hospitals, do not evaluate their own behavior in this manner. They evoke discomfort in others who perceive them as socially or culturally alien. Socially identified as deviant, bizarre, or dangerous to themselves or others, they are ordered to go to the psychiatric facility; they may be forced to do so despite their vigorous resistance. In these instances the diagnosis of symptomatic behavior is made by the community. The line between self- and other-diagnosis is not totally clear, however, because the public expressions to which community agencies of social control respond can sometimes be understood as "cries for help." The communicative significance of the symptomatic act may be deeply repressed or accessible to the subject's awareness with little therapeutic effort. The cry for help is often not understood as such because community diagnoses and dispositions are capricious, reflecting prevalent beliefs and values. This is partly because the symptomatic or sick behavior series is logically continuous with other behaviors accepted as healthy (or customary), or defined in judgmental, religious, or other terms. Society's techniques for dealing with deviance, involving variable degrees of collaboration by the labeled deviant, include shunning, ridicule, nurturing, behavior change in place (as via outpatient treatment), extrusion from the system for punishment and deterrence (jail), or extrusion for behavior change (mental hospital). These are institutionalized ways of behaving which represent unthinking conformity to cultural norms defining proper, legitimate, or expected modes of action or social relationship.[11] The choice of social action depends in part upon the existence of "resources" or "facilities," such as mental hospitals, doctors, cult centers, and social agencies. These undertake many of the social control functions once carried out by families.[6] Their presence as well as norms and attitudes reflect the developmental state of the behavioral setting.[14]

Gibbs regards the likelihood of a person's being isolated for committing a deviant act as directly proportional to the degree to which he is a "social and cultural alien," i.e., one who differs in status and cultural traits from other members of the society, and particularly from the agents of social control and the power-holding dominant culture-bearers. In the United States, such persons have included those who are non-white, non-native, and in agricultural labor and other lower-class occupations. The validity of this proposition may rest upon the cumulative weight of a range of isolation stations. Thus, in Maryland a poor black man has been more likely to be sent to jail than a middle-class white exhibiting the same behavior who would more probably be sent to a hospital or a psychiatrist's office.[16] In New Haven, the police and the courts were more often the gateway to the mental hospitals for lower-class than for middle-class whites who were more apt to be referred to private physicians.[43] On the other hand, psychiatric diagnoses and hospitalizations (though not brief jail sentences for "disturbing the peace") were long delayed for Baltimore black men because of police tendencies to perceive their sick behavior as rule infractions requiring punitive action, family tendencies to see it (especially of a paranoid nature) as justified in terms of the social situation, and tolerance by police of even bizarre behavior by known persons so long as it was confined within the ethnic community ("inner city"). This last reflected their view of lowest socio-economic status blacks as primitive or child-like, as well as a relative lack of concern with the impact of their behavior on those around them.[16] Similarly, in Rio de Janeiro, the subordinate status of women, blacks, and youths, reflecting the paternalistic attitudes and values of husbands, fathers, and whites, often delayed psychiatric hospitalization until deviant patterns had become severe or habitual.[14] The families of the Rio de Janeiro patients, socialized largely in preindustrial semirural settings, often still living on the margin of the technological society, were more central decision-makers initiating the hospitalization process than often appears to be true for poor

people in United States inner cities.[26] This, along with the use of religious-spiritist centers rather than police stations as important relay points en route to mental hospitals, may account for the apparently high agreement between self and family or community appraisal, and the decision to seek professional assistance. The religious-spiritist centers are helping rather than disciplinary agencies and require the collaboration of the help seekers. As supportive and behavior-modifying systems they may indefinitely delay the isolation of deviants in hospitals or jails. Behavior regarded as deviant in the society at large may be freely emitted in the center, which also offers a variety of self-esteem-building gratifications making such behavior less necessary elsewhere.

Within the lower-class community, impaired capacity to contribute to family support often determines the appraisal of behavior as symptomatic or intolerable. In Rio de Janeiro, refusal or inability to work precipitated mental hospitalization more frequently among the recently migrant than the settled, the non-literate than the literate, and the uneducated than those with more schooling.[14] The common denominator is inability to care for a nonproductive family member, which may be associated with resentment at this further burden. The real threat, for which psychiatric hospitalization is the suggested cure, is to economic survival. This was also reported for Baltimore blacks.[16] Rogler and Hollingshead in Puerto Rico and Lewis and Zeichner in the continental United States, however, have reported diminished expectations of the patient, leading at times to role substitution by family members, which could indefinitely delay hospital admission.[64,53]

(Status, Role, and Symptomatic Behavior

A person's ways of thinking, feeling, and acting reflect his perceptions of and relationships with others who have particular meaning, i.e., are "significant" for him. George Herbert

Mead first stressed the importance of what he called the "generalized other," i.e., the interactive group to which an individual feels he belongs and which is basic to his sense of personal identity. One perceives himself and significant others to an important degree in terms of the statuses which he and they occupy. Status refers to one's position in society and most people have several. These are achieved, the result of what one does with his life, and ascribed or given, existing by reason of the accident of birth. Social class status is ascribed if a person remains in the stratum into which he was born, but can be considered as achieved if he has been upwardly or downwardly mobile in the class structure. Ascribed statuses, important in all societies, are age and sex. Self-perceptions and expectations of others are always determined by whether one is male or female, child or adult, young or old. Other ascribed positions are color, native or immigrant, and religious or ethnic statuses, insofar as a person remains identified with the position of his parents. With time, practice, and intelligence, a person can abandon many of the socially visible behavioral concomitants (e.g., manner of speech, gestures, clothing, food preferences) of some statuses, such as ethnic or religious. In early life, religion usually remains ascribed, bounded by parental sanctions; later, people can change their religion just as they can change their names and deny their ethnic origins. Such changes evoke modifications in the ways in which others perceive them, and in their own self-percepts. Nonetheless, internal conflict regarding parental identifications and other relatively unmodifiable residuals of early life may remain at the root of symptomatic behavior, ranging from dreams and slips of the tongue, to periods of depression or localized phobias.

Achieved statuses are marital, occupational, educational, and some temporary states, such as that of a hospital or office patient. Education, occupation, and available economic resources help in the process of self-change and are important aids to personal coping and adaptation, especially in industrialized societies. In these latter, especially those in the process of rapid change, occupational status (e.g., as a physician or psychiatrist) often supersedes the ethnic and religious statuses so important in more traditional societies. The achievement of socially valued statuses reflects successful coping. It brings concrete rewards and may be accompanied by a sense of fulfillment. Despite rewards, however, it may be accompanied by discomfort, e.g., depression or anxiety. Socially reinforced behavior may be regarded in such instances as having symptomatic aspects. The label "overachiever" is sometimes applied to those, for example, whose incessant work reflects an unconscious need to prove their self-worth, to affirm their masculinity, to compete with a father perceived only through the eyes of childhood, or to attain some goal which can never be reached because it is unconscious and can be identified. As a rule, though, this appraisal is not made by the community which sees and responds only to the person's status, and contributes to the rewards reinforcing his work. The appraisal may be loosely made by psychiatrists viewing the person's work career in narrowly defensive terms. They may ignore certain regularities in such careers, i.e., the pleasure in creative work, and the often encountered upswing in production in late middle life when the person becomes conscious of the limited time left him to accomplish certain projects. It is easier to appraise achieving behavior as symptomatic when it is accompanied by apparent costs, such as exhaustion in a person who compulsively overloads himself with too many tasks, or who does not have the capacity to accomplish the goals which he habitually sets for himself. In these instances, the psychiatrist is concerned with the person's hidden agenda: What are the unconscious goals he is trying to achieve in this way? Symptomatic achieving, while it may have defensive, anxiety-reducing, or impulse-controlling value despite its corollary discomfort, often has adaptive costs as well. These may be assessed in terms of disrupted relationships and broken families. These considerations are noted here, because achieved status often obscures underlying psychological pain.

The concept of social role in relation to social status exemplifies the interrelations between society, culture, and behavior. The role is the expected behavior pattern attached to the status, and a person has several roles attached to his several statuses. Thus, the variability of his behavior during a day, at work, with his family, with friends, or strangers, can be understood in part as social role behavior.[8] Behavior not congruent with a person's social role or status is apt to be perceived as deviant by others. A middle-aged, married male physician who behaves like an adolescent, unmarried chorus boy may be labeled at first as foolish or immature, and later as psychiatrically ill. In traditional societies, and more in the country than in the city, women are expected to behave as subordinates. Aggressive, independent behavior in females is viewed by others as markedly deviant, and may well reflect the onset of a psychiatric disturbance. Even the patient role is culturally conditioned. In a series of private hospitals in Japan, Caudill, for example, observed that the emotionally disturbed person who enters a mental hospital slips smoothly into a passive, dependent role, modelled by the structure of kinship relations, as between older and younger brother.[19] The doctor who, in terms of his own cultural norms, accepts and fosters this behavior would attribute special symptomatic significance to the egalitarian behavior of the middle-class United States analysand, should it occur in his own patient. One consequence of these role expectations has been that the Japanese patient's symptomatic behavior has been more apt to include irritation, depression, anxiety, and hypochondria, than open rage or anger. The disguised "cry for help," the open presenting complaint, and the nature of expressive behavior considered as sick, are influenced by the status and role of doctor and patient, and the way in which the doctor-patient relationship fits into the general social matrix of relationships.[8]

When a person occupies statuses with incompatible social roles, the ensuing conflict may contribute to symptomatic behavior.[7,12] Such problems are encountered on temporary bases in organizations. An example from the medical-psychiatric world is the man who acts simultaneously as departmental administrator and psychotherapist for a staff member. Efforts to reconcile the conflicting therapeutic needs of his patient or counselee with the administrative requirements of the organization may lead him to countertransference distortions in his role as therapist, or to inappropriate (symptomatic) organizational assignments for the patient-staff member in his role as administrator.

In the broader society, the likelihood of role conflict is increased by the number of subgroups it contains and its rate of social change.[12] The United States is a pluralistic, transitional society, in contrast to more isolated, primitive, or even to certain industrialized ones as Scandinavia, which is composed more of people of similar race, religion, and cultural heritage. The inhabitants of the various social worlds of the United States (based on national origin, race, and religion), especially growing children, are faced with the problem of reconciling the behavioral standards and goals acquired in families with those encountered in schools and elsewhere.[7,10] As Shibutani noted: ". . . when participating in societies in which the component group norms are not mutually consistent, it becomes progressively more difficult for any man to integrate his various self-images into a single unit."[68] This problem is most obviously present in marginal persons, those in transition between states. A marginal person, according to Kurt Lewin, is one who with a foot in each of two societies, does not feel completely at home in or belonging to either. Lewin was concerned with the children of immigrant European Jews coming to the United States at the beginning of the twentieth century.[52] They were caught between the culture and language of the parental home and those of the broader United States society. More recently, the concept has been applied to members of the Untouchable caste in India, who are experiencing the problems of upward mobility as the strictures of untouchability are loosened.[44] Similarly, marginality has become a significant problem for American blacks only since the restraints of caste based on racial visibility have been relaxed.[24,25] With this social change there appeared an increasing number of persons who were on the advancing "edge" or "margin" of their own sociocultural group as it was in contact with representatives of the surrounding power-holding white society. The marginal black person, as others in social transition, must be constantly vigilant for signs of avoidance, rejection, or hostility in his new (in this instance white) associates. Partial acceptance, with a chronic underlying threat of rejection, creates an ambiguous social situation, contributing to feelings of insecurity and an unstable sense of identity.[25] Some specific symptomatic behaviors encountered in marginal persons have been: disgust for food characteristic of childhood, acute sensitivity to anything reminding them of their origins, and anger at less sophisticated members of the culture of origin, whose actions elicit the distaste or humorous contempt of the (white) social power-holders.

The marginal person is in double jeopardy because he is also in danger of alienation from his social world of origin which, like the new social world, sees him as deviant, nonconforming, not fully belonging, and may make him the target of resentment generated elsewhere. Thus, the word "oreo," a chocolate cookie with a white inner layer has been applied by blacks to their upwardly mobile fellows who relate to whites and behave according to middle-class values. Similarly, American Indians serving as representatives of their people to the white establishment have been called "apples"—red outside and white inside.

❨ Symptomatic Participation in the Hospital Milieu

Mental hospitals have provided convenient settings for the study of patient behavior in relation to social and cultural factors. The statements and mood, actions and emotions of a hospitalized patient are not solely a function of his past personal history, his prior programming. They reflect, as well, the immediate social situation of which he is a part. Until the importance of the hospital context was recognized, behavior reflecting the patient's adapta-

tion to this milieu was labeled as symptomatic, stereotyped, or repetitive, and not related to environmental demands. Interest in the hospital milieu accelerated with the employment of social scientists in psychiatric units, especially after World War II. Hospitals have been conceptualized by many investigators as social systems in which patients, as well as professional helpers, administrators, and others, are mutually influencing actors. Among the early students of the vicissitudes of symptomatic behavior in hospital wards viewed in this manner were Rowland,[65,66] Devereux,[27,28,29] and Caudill and associates;[21] later Caudill[18] reviewed most of the significant literature before 1957. From the anthropological position, the hospital constitutes a subculture with its own values, belief-systems, myths, and norms, elements of which are transmitted from one generation of patients and staff to another. Stanton and Schwartz emphasized a particular dimension, the relationship of patient behavior, ordinarily interpreted in purely psychopathological terms (without reference to ongoing social phenomena), to covert conflict between staff members upon whom they were dependent.[72] Thus, a previously unexplained period of excitement in a chronically schizophrenic patient can be seen as an aspect of a total social field disturbance, the key element of which is an unconfronted disagreement between ward personnel.

While Stanton and Schwartz's major book on the subject did not appear until 1954, it was preceded by a series of papers beginning in the late 1940s.[67,69,70,71,72] These focused on the communicative and participative significance, in relation to the ward social process, of behavior such as incontinence, previously viewed by the staff in stereotyped pathological terms. A more recent study suggested that the patient's excitement following disagreement among staff members was due in part to the withdrawal from him of emotional support by a key staff member (now involved in conflict with a colleague) who was becoming a bridge for him to broader interpersonal involvement and reality contact.[4] Cumming and Cumming offer a general ego-psychological framework for the practice of environmental therapy.[23]

Their volume contains many examples of patient behavior which can be viewed as symptomatic in the sense of reflecting unresolved intrapsychic conflicts, but can be more profitably understood in relation to the hospital society and culture. As they note, ". . . the acting out of the patient role in complement to the roles of the others in the environment is the road to ego restitution" (p. 137).

Ullman reviewed United States mental hospital statistics for the early nineteenth century showing discharge or recovery rates of 80 and 90 per cent.[75] The "moral treatment" then in vogue was based on an expected and reinforced healthy role provided by the models of the superintendent, his family, and staff, who lived in close proximity to the patients. This treatment and its associated recovery rates declined after the 1850s with the building of large centralized hospitals and the increased inflow of immigrants, with whom the psychiatrist had difficulty communicating. The ensuing years witnessed a change in the expectations of physicians and their withdrawal as role models for institutionalized patients. This was due not only to the tremendous increases in the number of patients per doctor, but also to the rise of the medical model of illness. As Ullman noted, the patient was relegated to a passive role, awaiting the discovery of cure. Bockoven wrote: "The very idea of dead and decomposing brain cells carried with it the connotation of the patient's growing insensibility and unawareness of surroundings."[2] All of these factors summarized by Ullman contributed to the growth of what von Mering and King called the "Legend of Chronicity."[76]

The point of all of these studies for the present thesis is that the attitudes and behavior of staff reinforce particular aspects of patient behavior. In the era of moral treatment, patients were in effect taught to behave like integrated, healthy non-patients. Since then, particularly with the development of the aide culture, the predominance of the medical model, and the development of large custodial hospitals, they have been taught to behave as though they were sick and belonged in a hospital, i.e., as patients: conforming, submissive, suspicious, covertly circumventing. Occasion-

ally, "crazy" ways of acting, with their thinking and feeling corollaries which might be legitimately called symptomatic, are reinforced and functional in the hospital context. Sometimes, these symptomatic patterns help the patient achieve a new identity to replace that stripped from him by the homogenizing process of the hospital. A familiar example is the elderly woman with hypomanic tendencies who, quite aware of her role as a "clown," skillfully evokes the laughter and friendly interest, however patronizing, of the staff whom she meets at conferences. The staff, locked into this reciprocal perceptual and manipulative pattern, is amazed (and perhaps a little angry) to discover that an outside interviewer with a different set can evoke serious, coherent, and justifiably depressed responses from the patient who, it turns out, is highly sensitive to her hopeless role as a chronic inmate deserted by her relatives. Gentle probing clearly reveals the presence of unconscious and unacceptable rage against these relatives. In this instance, euphoric, overactive, or grotesquely comic behavior can be viewed in several conceptual frameworks: It reflects the defensive processes of denial and repression which keep her anxiety, guilt, and anger at manageable levels and help her self-esteem, while it simultaneously symbolizes her own self-hatred (turning rage against herself) as a contemptible court-jester; it is adaptive, stabilizing her relationship with the staff, achieving an acceptable social role within the anonymous patient mass; it is coping, allowing her to circumvent many administrative barriers and staff indifference, and to obtain certain concrete privileges as well as the facsimiles of love and regard, which also aid her fragile self-esteem.

These phenomena have been studied by Goffman[40] (with particular reference to the growth of the aide culture), Dunham and Weinberg,[31] and others. Goffman[39] has included the mental hospital in his category of "total institutions," i.e., jails, military units, and monasteries, in which the normally divided areas of living, such as working, playing, sleeping, and eating, are carried out together in one place under the guidance of an overall master plan. Under such circumstances, attempts at individual self-expression are viewed by those in control as deviant and non-normative and are treated as rule infractions. In this way, patients are encouraged to melt into the anonymous mass; those who have depended on social distancing mechanisms throughout life, especially those from the lower socioeconomic classes already in awe of authority and reluctant to stand out from the group, easily sink out of sight. They engage in a type of withdrawal which, regarded as regressive or symptomatic by examining psychiatrists, represents in fact a type of adaptation to a particular environment. Specific variations are imposed by the differing value orientations of staff upon whom patients are dependent, and who function for them in the role of parent-surrogates. Considerable differences in attitudes of aides, nurses, and resident psychiatrists in a small university psychiatric unit, for example, were documented toward sexual, aggressive, and other types of sensitively noted patient behavior.[1] Social attractiveness and consequent interpersonal choice among psychiatric patients and staff have also been demonstrated as a factor determining social isolation or acceptance, feelings of belonging or rejection, and even the determination of treatment goals by staff, and selection of patients for particular therapeutic attention.[30] These factors, reflecting complex relationships between biographical characteristics and values, have powerful effects on patient behavior, which may be considered simultaneously from symptomatic, adaptive, coping, or other frames of references.

(Society and Culture-Wide Forces and Symptomatic Behavior

Cross-cultural or Transcultural Approaches. Symptomatic behavior has been studied transculturally in the sense used by Wittkower to designate behavior which transcends a particular culture; it has also been studied in terms of behavioral comparisons between or across cultures.[79] Leighton and Murphy have summarized ideas as to how culture and cultural situations might exert causal or determining influences on psychiatric disorders.[50] Aside from the production of specifically vulnerable basic personality types, culture has been, according to their review, conceived as determining the pattern of certain specific disorders, e.g., *latah* in Malaya; producing disorders, latent for a time, through childrearing practices; selectively influencing patterns of disorder through particular sanctions which engender shame or guilt; confronting people with stressful roles; perpetuating disorder by rewarding it with prestigeful roles, e.g., as the shaman; changing at a rate too rapid for personal accommodation; inculcating beliefs and values that produce damaging emotional states, e.g., fears and unrealistic aspirations; affecting the distribution of disorders through breeding patterns; influencing the amount and distribution of disorder through patterns of poor hygiene and nutrition. A number of these factors are less tied to specific cultures than to socioeconomic status-related variables which may have similar significance in a variety of cultural settings. Some have been touched upon in previous sections of this chapter, others will be considered in varying degree. In every instance, the "disorder" may be viewed as a patterned syndrome of symptomatic acts.

Migration. * Migration provides a set of concrete operations for the study of adaptation and defense in relation to social change. A shift in residence involves not only new places, but new faces and new norms. As the person moves from one socioculture to another, behavioral modes useful in the old setting may prove maladaptive in the new. Acute sensitivity which permits empathic understanding in one group may be perceived as discomfort-provoking vigilance or paranoia in another. The culturally supported tendency to deal with the unknown or with the consequences of one's own inadequacy by attributing malevolent control to external forces, reinforced by magical belief systems in rural

* The material in this section has been adapted from E. B. Brody, Ref. 13, Bibliography.

areas, may interfere with the evaluation of one's actual capacities necessary for survival in the city. Under these circumstances, the person may so rationalize his adaptive failure in the new setting that he is not motivated to make the necessary coping effort. One index of such failure is incompatibility between the migrant's self-image on the one hand, and the status, of which he is unaware, given him by the new social system on the other.

Behavior in the new environment is a function of the push factors that contribute to the migrant's decision to leave the culture of origin, the pull factors that lure him to the new, the transitional experiences en route, the receptor networks or resistances encountered upon entry into the host system, the talents and personal and economic assets he brings with him, congruences between the old culture and the new, and internal motives for moving. Some of these last are the distillate of ungratified wishes and needs, undischarged tensions, and unresolved conflicts. Others are more easily related to a person's place in his individual social change career. Potential migrants are differentiated from their fellows with the first stirrings of dissatisfaction with the status quo. Once in the new environment, personal change may continue indefinitely, with the greatest acceleration not reached for several years. It is often difficult, given the resistance and discomfort of family and friends, to differentiate behavior accompanying rapid personal growth and the achievement of a new identity (usually accompanied by a change in social statuses) from symptomatic behavior. Similar growth phenomena may be encountered during the course of psychotherapy. The personal growth of later life accompanying the move to a new setting, with its new occupations and new friends, can be as turbulent as the growth occurring in adolescence, and can create as much discomfort in spouse and children as it once did in parents.

Some migrants are risk-takers, people willing to go a step beyond the ordinary or expected; the appraisal of risk-taking as self-defeating symptomatic behavior or as exploratory growing behavior may not be possible without detailed longitudinal data. Some are geographical escapers, people who deal with personal or environmental disaster by physical flight; these often carry their problems with them wherever they go. In this category are those for whom the move may be understood as symptomatic of pre-existing psychiatric illness.

Detailed reviews of the particular factors influencing a migrant's capacity to interact with the opportunity structure of his environment, and of the particular stress points he will encounter, are available elsewhere.

Minority Status, Low Socioeconomic Status, and Powerlessness. Minority status may be most meaningfully defined on the basis of access to or distance from sources of societal power. Thus, "a set of people who, capable of being distinguished on the basis of some physical or cultural characteristic, are treated collectively as inferior,"[56] may be socially visible on the basis of skin color, physiognomy, or ethnically or socioeconomically linked appearance. The specific vulnerabilities of minority groups to behavioral disorganization, as well as the symptomatic nature of prejudiced behavior, have been reviewed in this Handbook and elsewhere.[7,10,12,15,26] Exclusion from full participation in the majority culture,[9] lack of economic potency,[26] and awareness of blocked opportunities for upward mobility, all contribute to low self-esteem, retaliative anger against power holders, mistrust of those who do not belong to one's immediate social or family group, and a sense of alienation and powerlessness. A sense of powerlessness in the face of catastrophic natural as well as brutal or unpredictable human forces has been reported by Klein among Andean Indian serfs in Peru.[8] The most deprived of a Rio de Janeiro psychiatric patient sample revealed themselves through Rorschach and TAT responses as feeling completely at the mercy of forces beyond their control.[14] In both Peruvian nonpatients and Brazilian patients, symptomatic behavior patterns associated with lowest socioeconomic status and feelings of powerlessness were regressively defensive, withdrawn, self-insulating, inflexible. Non-hospitalized midtown Manhattan respondents of the lowest socioeconomic status studied by Langner and Michael[49] were described by them as "probable psychotics," rigid, suspicious, and passive-dependent, with some related depressive features. In contrast to "probable neurotics" of higher socioeconomic status, they had suffered more devastating early life stress, experiences favoring dependence upon externalized versus internal controls, self-esteem and ego-strength-weakening experiences, and failures in training for identity, communication, relating sexually, obtaining or postponing gratification, and planning for the future. These elements have their counterparts in the socioculturally disintegrated as compared with more integrated communities described by Leighton et al.[51] in the Stirling County study.

It is difficult to separate subculturally determined childrearing experiences from the social advantages and symbolic capacities associated with education and literacy as compared with partial or total lack of education and inability to read. The more capable and motivated literate Rio de Janeiro patients[14] showed a higher prevalence of psychophysiological symptoms, such as tachycardia or gastrointestinal dysfunction (in contrast to somatic pain, body or organ anxiety), diffuse anxiety, and fear of loss of control than the non-literates. While the resemblance was less clear than it is between the most deprived groups, they were more comparable in symptom formation to upper-class than lower-class New Haven patients[43] and midtown[49] Manhattan nonpatient respondents. Although the Rio patients showing these symptoms were not as socioeconomically privileged as the middle- and upper-class United States samples, in comparison to other groups in the Rio sample they were responsible, informed participants in the socioculture, with actively self-critical standards, the capacity to inhibit direct expression of feelings through action, fear of status loss, and higher value placed on rational, conscious control of behavior. Diffuse anxiety and fear of loss of control were most prevalent among the whites, educated, better housed, and non-manually employed, as well as the more literate Rio patients. In contrast,

acute anxiety attacks, as well as somatic complaints, and paranoid and other psychosis-related behavior were most prevalent among the least privileged, subject to the most pervasive social, economic, and physical survival threats. These were the patients most often described by projective testing as searching futilely for succor in an overwhelmingly stressful and coercive world. Those with acute anxiety attacks also exhibited situational fears about their jobs and families more frequently, often realistically. These observations fit the suggestion that behavioral consistency in the face of fluctuating environmental conditions is a function of an internalized set of evaluative standards. Conversely, behavioral dependence upon current environmental cues seems greatest in the absence of well-established internalized values and standards.[11]

(Concluding Remarks

This chapter is one aspect of an introduction to the study of psychiatrically significant behavior. It does not consider the process or entity aspects of neurosis to be compared, for example, with psychosis or character disorder. The focus is, rather, on behavior—feeling, thinking, acting, publicly observed and subjectively reported—how it is experienced by the subject, evaluated by others, and whether it makes sense in terms of the environment in which it occurs. Behavior is viewed in its symptomatic sense, i.e., as it reflects a hidden or underlying problem, or psychological event or process, is "symptomatic of" something else. In medical language, that "something else" may be described in disease terms as a bacterially engendered inflammation (reflected in symptomatic fever or pain), a neurosis, or an incipient schizophrenia. In the present chapter, the "something else" is a human problem and the person's attempts to solve it. Attempts at problem-solving reflected in behavior identified or experienced as uncomfortable or deviant and hence symptomatic are usually not successful. Or, if they are successful in one sphere of life, they may lead to disaster in others. Therefore, a systematic description in human problem language requires the use of a group of related concepts. These are ways of systematizing—permitting abstraction and generalization about—what is happening inside an individual in relation to what is going on outside. Inside and outside events are commonly referred to as "intrapsychic" and "interpersonal." Intrapsychic activity is conveniently described in psychodynamic conflictual terms, including ego-functioning, and particularly the operation of defense mechanisms. Interpersonal activity is conveniently described in adaptive and coping terms. The significance of the vectors of intrapsychic conflict, the use of defense mechanisms, characteristic cognitive, affective, and communicative styles, and the ability and opportunity to adapt and cope, are all influenced and shaped throughout life by society and culture. Society and culture are viewed longitudinally in relation to developing behavior patterns and potentials, and cross-sectionally in terms of behavior in a particular context, as a form of participating in an ongoing social process. The purpose of this chapter is to sensitize the student of psychiatry to these various ways of looking at behavior as he studies patterns identified as specific psychiatric disorders.

(Bibliography

1. BAND, R., and E. B. BRODY. "Human Elements of the Therapeutic Community: A Study of the Conflicting Values and Attitudes of People Upon Whom Patients Must Be Dependent," *Archives of General Psychiatry*, 6 (1962), 307–314.

2. BOCKOVEN, J. S. *Moral Treatment in American Psychiatry*. New York: Springer, 1963.

3. BRODY, E. B. "Psychiatric Problems of the German Occupation," *The American Journal of Psychiatry*, 286 (1948), 105.

4. ———. "Note on the Concept of 'Split Social Field' as a Determinant of Schizophrenic Excitement," *Journal of Nervous and Mental Disease*, 128 (1959), 182.

5. ———. "Character Disorder, Borderline State and Psychosis: Some Conceptual Problems," *Psychiatry*, 23 (1960), 75.

6. ———. "The Public Mental Hospital as a Symptom of Social Conflict," *Maryland State Medical Journal*, 9 (1960), 330–334.

7. ———. "Social Conflict and Schizophrenic Behavior in Young Adult Negro Males," *Psychiatry*, 24 (1961), 4.

8. ———. "Conceptual and Methodological Problems in Research in Society, Culture and Mental Illness," *Journal of Nervous and Mental Disease*, 139 (1964), 62–74.

9. ———."Cultural Exclusion, Character and Illness," *The American Journal of Psychiatry*, 122 (1966), 852–858.

10. ———. "Minority Group Status and Behavioral Disorganization," in E. B. Brody, ed., *Minority Group Adolescents in the United States*. Baltimore: Williams & Wilkins, 1968.

11. ———. "Culture, Symbol and Value in the Social Etiology of Behavioral Deviance," in J. Zubin, ed., *Social Psychiatry*. New York: Grune & Stratton, 1968.

12. ———. "Sociocultural Influences on Vulnerability to Schizophrenic Behavior," in J. Romano, ed., *Origins of Schizophrenia*. Excerpta Medica International Congress Series No. 151 (1970), 228–230.

13. ———. "Migration and Adaptation: The Nature of the Problem," in E. B. Brody, ed., *Behavior in New Environments: Adaptation of Migrant Populations*. Beverly Hills: Sage Publications, 1970.

14. ———. *Social Forces and Mental Illness in Rio de Janeiro*. New York: International Universities Press, 1973.

15. ———. Psychosocial Aspects of Prejudice. *American Handbook of Psychiatry*, 1st ed., Vol. 3. New York: Basic Books, 1966, pp. 629–642.

16. BRODY, E. B., R. L. DERBYSHIRE, and C. SCHLEIFER. "How the Young Adult Baltimore Negro Male Becomes a Mental Hospital Statistic," in R. R. Monroe, G. D. Klee, and E. B. Brody, eds., *Psychiatric Epidemiology and Mental Health Planning*. American Psychiatric Association Research Report No. 22, 1967.

17. BRODY, E. B., and F. C. REDLICH. "The Response of Schizophrenic Patients to Comic Cartoons Before and After Prefrontal Lobotomy," *Folia Psychiatrica Neurologica et Neurochirurgica Nederlandica*, 56 (1953), 623.

18. CAUDILL, W. *The Psychiatric Hospital as a Small Society.* Cambridge, Mass.: Harvard University Press, 1958.

19. ———. "Observations on the Cultural Context of Japanese Psychiatry," in Opler, M. K., ed., *Culture and Mental Health.* New York: Macmillan, 1959.

20. ———. "Tiny Dramas: Vocal Communication Between Mother and Infant in Japanese and American Families," in W. Lebra, ed., *Transcultural Research in Mental Health.* Honolulu: University Press of Hawaii, 1972.

21. CAUDILL, W., F. C. REDLICH, H. R. GILMORE, and E. B. BRODY. "Social Structure and Interaction Processes on a Psychiatric Ward," *American Journal of Orthopsychiatry,* 22 (1952), 314.

22. CAUDILL, W., and H. WEINSTEIN. "Maternal Care and Infant Behavior in Japan and America," *Psychiatry,* 32 (1969), 12–43.

23. CUMMING, J., and E. CUMMING. *Ego and Milieu.* New York: Atherton Press, 1962.

24. DERBYSHIRE, R. L., and E. B. BRODY. "Marginality, Identity and Behavior in the American Negro: A Functional Analysis," *International Journal of Social Psychiatry,* 10 (1964), 7–13.

25. ———. "Personal Identity and Ethnocentrism in American Negro College Students," *Mental Hygiene,* 48 (1964), 65–69.

26. DERBYSHIRE, R. L., E. B. BRODY, and C. SCHLEIFER. "Family Structure of Young Adult Negro Male Mental Patients," *Journal of Nervous and Mental Disease,* 136 (1963), 245–251.

27. DEVEREUX, G. "The Social Structure of a Schizophrenic Ward and Its Therapeutic Fitness," *Journal of Clinical Psychopathology,* 6 (1944), 231–265.

28. ———. "The Social Structure of the Hospital as a Factor in Total Therapy," *American Journal of Orthopsychiatry,* 19 (1949), 492.

29. ———. "Normal and Abnormal: The Key Problem of Psychiatric Anthropology," in *Some Uses of Anthropology: Theoretical and Applied.* Washington, D.C.: Anthropological Society of Washington, 1956.

30. DOHERTY, E. G. "Social Attraction and Choice Among Psychiatric Patients and Staff: A Review," *Journal of Health and Social Behavior,* 12 (1971), 279–290.

31. DUNHAM, H. W., and S. K. WEINBERG. *The Culture of the State Mental Hospital.* Detroit: Wayne State University Press, 1960.

32. FREUD, A. *The Ego and Mechanisms of Defense* (1936). New York: International Universities Press, 1946.

33. FREUD, S. *The Interpretation of Dreams* (1900). Standard Edition, Vol. 4. London: Hogarth Press, 1953.

34. ———. *The Psychopathology of Everyday Life* (1901). Standard Edition, Vol. 6. London: Hogarth Press, 1960.

35. ———. *Jokes and Their Relation to the Unconscious* (1905). Standard Edition, Vol. 8. London: Hogarth Press, 1960.

36. ———. *Introductory Lectures on Psychoanalysis* (1917). London: Allen and Unwin, 1929.

37. ———. *Inhibitions, Symptoms, and Anxiety.* Standard Edition, Vol. 20. London: Hogarth Press, 1959.

38. GIBBS, J. "Rates of Mental Hospitalization," *American Sociological Review,* 6 (1941), 217–222.

39. GOFFMAN, E. *The Characteristics of Total Institutions.* Symposium on preventive and social psychiatry, Walter Reed Army Medical Center. Washington, D.C.: U.S. Government Printing Office, 1957.

40. ———. *Asylums.* New York: Doubleday, 1961.

41. GREENE, G. *A Sort of Life.* New York: Simon and Schuster, 1971.

42. HARTMAN, H. *Ego Psychology and the Problems of Adaptation.* English translation by D. Rapaport. New York: International Universities Press, 1958.

43. HOLLINGSHEAD, A. B., and F. C. REDLICH. *Social Class and Mental Illness.* New York: Wiley, 1958.

44. ISAACS, H. R. *India's Ex-Untouchables.* New York: John Day, 1965.

45. JAEGER, C., and P. SELZNICK. "A Normative Theory of Culture," *American Sociological Review,* 29 (1965), 653.

46. KLUCKHOHN, C. *Mirror for Man.* New York: McGraw-Hill, 1944.

47. KRIS, E. *Psychoanalytic Explorations in Art.* New York: International Universities Press, 1952.

48. KROEBER, A. L., and T. PARSONS. "The Concept of Culture and of Social System," *American Sociological Review,* 23 (1958), 582.

49. LANGNER, T., and S. MICHAEL. *Life Stress and Mental Health*. Glencoe: Free Press, 1963.

50. LEIGHTON, A. H., and J. M. MURPHY. "Cross-Cultural Psychiatry," in J. M. Murphy and A. H. Leighton, eds., *Approaches to Cross-Cultural Psychiatry*. Ithaca: Cornell University Press, 1965.

51. LEIGHTON, D. C., J. S. HARDIN, D. B. MACKLIN, A. M. MACMILLAN, and A. H. LEIGHTON. *The Character of Danger. Psychiatric Symptoms in Selected Communities*. New York: Basic Books, 1963.

52. LEWIN, K. *Resolving Social Conflicts*. New York: Harper's, 1948.

53. LEWIS, V. S., and A. ZEICHNER. "Impact of Admission to a Mental Hospital on the Patient's Family," *Mental Hygiene*, 44 (1960), 503–510.

54. LINTON, R. *The Cultural Background of Personality*. New York: Appleton-Century, 1945.

55. ———. *Culture and Mental Disorder*. Springfield: Charles C Thomas, 1956.

56. MARK, R. W. *Class and Power*. New York: American Book Company, 1963.

57. MECHANIC, D. "Response Factors in Illness: The Study of Illness Behavior," *Social Psychiatry*, 1 (1966), 11–20.

58. MERTON, R. "Continuities in the Theory of Reference Groups and Social Structure," in *Social Theory and Social Structure*, Glencoe: Free Press, 1957.

59. PARSONS, A. Staff Conference at Institute of Psychiatry and Human Behavior, University of Maryland School of Medicine, 1963.

60. ———. Referred to by I. K. Zola; see Ref. #80 below.

61. PARSONS, T. "Illness and the Role of the Physician: A Sociological Perspective," *American Journal of Orthopsychiatry*, 21 (1951), 452–460.

62. PARSONS, T., and R. F. BALES. *Family Socialization and Interaction Process*. Glencoe: Free Press, 1955.

63. PARSONS, T., and E. A. SHILS. *Toward a General Theory of Action*. Cambridge, Mass.: Harvard University Press, 1961.

64. ROGLER, L., and A. B. HOLLINGSHEAD. *Trapped. Families and Schizophrenia*. New York: John Wiley and Sons, 1965.

65. ROWLAND, H. "Interaction Processes in a State Mental Hospital," *Psychiatry*, 1 (1938), 323–337.

66. ———. "Friendship Patterns in a State Mental Hospital," *Psychiatry*, 2 (1939), 363–373.

67. SCHWARTZ, M. S., and A. F. STANTON. "A Social Psychological Study of Incontinence," *Psychiatry*, 13 (1950), 399–416.

68. SHIBUTANI, T. *Society and Personality*. Englewood Cliffs: Prentice Hall, 1961.

69. STANTON, A. F. "Medical Opinion and the Social Context in the Mental Hospital," *Psychiatry*, 12 (1949), 243–249.

70. ———. "Observations in Dissociation as Social Participation," *Psychiatry*, 12 (1949), 339–354.

71. STANTON, A. F., and M. S. SCHWARTZ. "The Management of a Type of Institutional Participation in Mental Illness," *Psychiatry*, 12 (1949), 13–26.

72. ———. *The Mental Hospital*. New York: Basic Books, 1954.

73. STERNBACH, R. A., and B. TURSKY. "Ethnic Differences Among Housewives in Psychophysical and Skin Potential Responses to Electric Shock," *Psychophysiology*, 1 (1965), 241–245.

74. SULLIVAN, H. S. *Conceptions of Modern Psychiatry*. Washington, D.C.: William Alanson White Psychiatric Foundation, 1947.

75. ULLMAN, L. P. *Institution and Outcome*. New York: Pergamon Press, 1962.

76. VON MERING, O., and S. H. KING. *Remotivating the Mental Patient*. New York: Russell Sage Foundation, 1957.

77. WEISMAN, A. "Reality Sense and Reality Testing," *Behavioral Science*, 3 (1958), 228–261.

78. WEXLER, M. "The Structural Problem in Schizophrenia: The Role of the Internal Object," in E. B. Brody and F. C. Redlich, eds., *Psychotherapy with Schizophrenics*. New York: International Universities Press, 1952.

79. WITTKOWER, E., and J. FRIED. "Problems of Transcultural Psychiatry," *International Journal of Psychiatry*, 3 (1958), 245–252.

80. ZOLA, I. K. "Culture and Symptoms—An Analysis of Patients' Presenting Complaints," *American Sociological Review*, 31 (1966), 615–630.

PART TWO

Specific Neurotic and Character-Disordered Behavior and Syndromes

CHAPTER 3

ACUTE OR CHRONIC STRESS AS DETERMINANTS OF BEHAVIOR, CHARACTER, AND NEUROSIS

James L. Titchener and W. Donald Ross

Historical Introduction

PSYCHOLOGICAL reactions to stress have been studied with increasing sophistication during the twentieth century, although old-fashioned ideas, prejudice, and blind spots from wishes to ignore the effects of trauma and stress remain to plague clinical practice in this area.

The earliest explanations, in the 1800s, of conditions which we now recognize as neuroses following trauma were ones which postulated "molecular disarrangement" or vascular changes in the spinal cord. For example, John Eric Erichsen described symptoms "following (train) accidents which may assume the form of a traumatic hysteria, neurasthenia, hypochondriasis, or melancholia."[37] He called this syndrome "railway spine," attributing it to organic causes and the idea persisted in the literature as "Erichsen's disease." Brodie, in 1837, was probably the first physician to recognize that for some hysterical symptoms, "fear, suggestion, and unconscious simulation are primary factors."[37] In the 1880s, Oppenheim was the leading exponent of the organic etiology of "traumatic neurosis" while Charcot, pointing to the resemblance of the symptoms to the changes seen during hypnosis, hypothesized a psychogenesis of this condition. The idea of organic damage to the nervous system persisted, nevertheless, during

World War I in the term "shell shock," suggesting that the cumulative effects of noise and shock waves had caused damage in the central nervous system.

From re-examination of these conditions after World War I, the psychodynamic pathogenesis of the "war neuroses" gained increasing acceptance.[49] Psychoanalysts began to illuminate the psychological processes underlying these conditions largely from questions raised about the meaning of one of their features, the repetitive post-traumatic dreams. They noted how these nightmares replayed the traumatic episode up to the point of impact and ended in terror and awakening. These observations could be understood as attempts at mastering the trauma.[18,20,34]

Studies on "traumatic neuroses" in peace time[16,17] were greatly augmented during World War II and described in detail in publications during and after the war.[3,26,34,35,47,71] A more humanitarian attitude developed from recognition that these conditions needed treatment instead of a disciplinary approach and methods of treatment were conceived such as abreaction, using drugs, and dramatic presentation of the traumatic event to the victim.

Many reports have been published of symptoms and personality changes following industrial accidents, as summarized previously by one of the authors of this chapter,[50,51] and in a most comprehensive book by Lester Keiser,[37] indicating the reality and validity of psychic reactions to industrial accidents.

Reactions to disaster have been the object of many investigations in the last twenty years,[13,42,64,65,69] delineating the types and phases of these, with implications for preparedness even in the event of nuclear disaster.[14,43,52]

The term "gross stress reaction," as proposed in the 1952 official psychiatric nomenclature,[8] seemed a very appropriate diagnostic label for the conditions ensuing upon injury, psychic trauma, or disaster,[67] because it connoted the unusual circumstances in their development. It is to be regretted that for reasons of symmetry and classificatory neatness this term has been changed to the pallid "adjustment reaction of adult life" of the 1968 revision.[9]

Some of the effects of the most severe stresses imposed upon humans by other humans have been described for three groups of victims: adults held in Nazi concentration camps and their children;[5,12,25,29,39,52,58,66] survivors of atomic bombing in Japan;[14,43] and prisoners of war subjected to coercive indoctrination.[5,28,41,54,68]

Moral, ethical, and group pressures, as well as the usual physical punishment, threats to life, killing of relatives, overcrowding, starvation, and disease, were described as instruments of psychic trauma. "Survival guilt" is particularly prominent under the circumstances when relatives and other close associates have not survived. Also, there have been discoveries on how the will to survive could greatly increase ego strength when it became a moral value. Solzhenitsyn's *One Day in the Life of Ivan Denisovich* serves to inform us as an in-depth study of this crucial phenomenon.[60] Terrence Des Pres[11] presents a theory on the extreme situation in our times along the lines of the discoveries from studies of concentration camps, Solzhenitsyn's writings, and Robert Jay Lifton[41] on Hiroshima survivors.

Des Pres contrasts the tragic hero who, in Ernest Hemingway's phrase, is "destroyed but not defeated" with the survivor whose "task is harder, since for him destruction and defeat, like soul and body, cannot be separated." The "will to continue as a human being" constitutes victory for the survivor in the extreme situation. We see varieties of the tragic hero and the survivor in clinical work with victims of psychic trauma.

The reports on prisoners of recent wars have shown how powerful the effects of isolation and sleep deprivation could be, and how guilt over noncooperation with the indoctrinators could be used as a psychic trauma benefiting the interrogators if the prisoner was separated from his comrades. Meanwhile, a strong but self-righteous nation blamed its own younger generation for these "turncoats," perhaps setting up the rebellion and generation gap to come a decade or so later.

The most comprehensive coverage of psychoanalytic understanding of psychological stress is in a volume on *Psychic Trauma*, edited by Sidney Furst and including contributions by Anna Freud, Phyllis Greenacre, Marianne Kris, Peter Neubauer, Leo Rangell, Joseph Sandler, Albert Solnit, and Robert Waelder.[22]

Recommendations from industrial mental health studies have pointed out the responsibility of management for full awareness of the psychic effects of jobs,[31,33,46] including "executive stress,"[10,40,46] in order to design organizational measures for the avoidance of pathogenic stress or to provide early treatment of its symptoms. In fact, some court decisions have awarded compensation to employees with psychiatric disorders alleged to have been the consequence of stress on the job.[4,46] The Social Security Administration also awards compensations for these disorders, but there is great need for better scientific understanding to clarify the difficult questions of who should have compensation, and whether it is in the true, long-range interests of the victim to receive it.

The special stresses of space flight and the successful adaptation to these have been described from the study of astronauts through training and orbital flights.[53]

The war in Vietnam has also been contributing further experience with reactions to multiple stresses.[2,59]

There has been much clinical and experimental investigation of the biochemical accompaniments of stressful experiences.[45,69] The amount of "distress" and biochemical disturbance, such as the production rate of hydrocortisone, appear to relate to the degree of failure of ego defenses.[36] This research evokes speculation on the existence of chain reactions arising from stress-stimulating endocrine systems which in turn affect behavior. Could it be that some of the post-traumatic syndromes are the result of behavior patterned by endocrine systems altered by psychic stress? In laboratory experiments with rats, the psychic stress of overcrowded cages causes permanent changes in the rat's personality and is associated with clearly detectable alterations in the endocrine system.[1,6,7,44]

The conceptions and descriptions in the remaining sections will be based on clinical experience of both authors in industrial psychiatry and with surgical patients, from the reports of experience and ideas of many others, and from a recent study by one of the authors of patients admitted to a surgical service following injuries and burns.[62]

(A General Theory of Psychic Stress

Psychic trauma consists of these stages: first, an event or events, often threatening but sometimes just intense or demanding, and usually external; second, an intrapsychic process from the event; third, an emotional discharge from the process; and finally, the psychic consequences of the event, of the process, and of the discharge.[48] We cannot always identify traumatic events from their intrinsic nature as one man's trauma may be another's exciting and interesting episode, or the presumed stresses may be successfully warded off. Intrapsychic process means that the trauma is absorbed and a chain of reactions is set off within the mind, eventuating in varying intensities and qualities of emotional discharge. The consequences of trauma consist of temporary or permanent structural changes, such as psychological symptoms and changes in behavioral patterns. There is a reshaping of the resonating memories of the event. Changes occur in the course of intrapsychic process and in the intensities and qualities of the emotional discharge.

Trauma may start from the apparently trivial (a child's reaction to his mother's leaving the room) or from personally catastrophic happenings. In this chapter, we shall assume we are dealing with traumatic events *well beyond* "the average expectable environment,"[27] that is, with events that would put most women and men to the test, rather than with the subtle cumulative episodes in human relations which create predispositions in childhood to psychoneuroses in adulthood.

At its core, the basic theory of trauma and stress as an aspect of human experience is not complicated. The fundamental issue of psychic trauma is quite simple, and once we have grasped it we can then deal with the subtleties and ambiguities which always abound in reasonable concepts of human behavior.

The basic theory of trauma devolves upon the idea that the mind is equipped with a *stimulus barrier*, protecting it against sudden or excessive outside excitation which could upset the equilibrium or disturb the integration of essential functions. Psychic trauma occurs when the level of outside excitation or stimuli exceeds the capacity of the stimulus barrier to resist its intrusion, with the result of a breakthrough, disturbing integration, upsetting equilibrium, and leading to degrees of disorganization and imbalance of mental function.[23]

To investigate the nature of the stimulus barrier further, let us imagine, as Freud imagined, an organic vesicle suspended in atmosphere and receiving on its surface the random bombardment of stimuli from without. This continuing process soon causes a cornification or toughening of the outer layers of the vesicle. By the continuing passage of stimuli, the outer layers are changed (Freud said "baked through"), and the vesicle becomes resistant to stimuli.[21] Its inner processes are no longer so subject to the impinging changes of its environment. In this way, the human individual, at first subject to all excitations, which are partially controlled by a protective shield provided by parents and the nursing environment, gradually acquires his own stimulus barrier. The barrier or shield varies in resilience and toughness from the intensity and quality of excitations which have been allowed to impinge and change the perceptual layers of the mind. For most persons, the barrier functions effectively to protect the ego integration and personality organization in situations which are moderately stressful, that is, when the level of external excitation is above average but tolerable. These are situations of noisy confusion, burdensome threat,

or demand. If there are no special sensitivities, the protection offered by the stimulus barrier enables the individual to remain relatively cool and constructively responsive, without overwhelming the integration and organization of the mental systems. We have seen this behavior time and again in the experienced personnel of hospital emergency rooms.

From this point of view, psychic trauma may be understood as a purely *quantitative* mental phenomenon. Psychic trauma has occurred when the level of excitation from physical or emotional threat, from fear, from confusion and informational overload, is so great that the stimulus barrier is overcome. There follows an intrusion of these stimuli beyond the capacity of mental systems to maintain organization and integration of functions, thus a breakdown in mental receiving power and an inability to continue *orderly* processing of further stimuli. If we add the dimension of time to the concept of an intrusion of too much excitation causing disorder of the mind, we may observe that after an abatement of excessive excitation the disrupted stimulus barrier will be restored, reorganization will occur, disorder will end, and orderly processing by mental systems may resume. In many situations, the response to trauma can be described exactly this way, having only temporary effects, and the episode is recalled as an interesting life experience, leaving no more than a little shudder or a thrill at the base of the spine when it is remembered. In such cases, it may usually be recalled at will.

One of us can remember as an adolescent being a passenger in a car late at night in the country. The car veered gradually from the road and seemed to be methodically sheering a succession of fence posts. Then it turned to the other side, entering a soft and muddy pasture where it began to roll over slowly and deliberately, it seemed, three times. To this passenger it was the horizon turning. "Remarkable," he thought, "I'm dead when the horizon stops." The rolling ended and two of the three passengers faced one another on all fours on the roof of the overturned car. Speaking softly, they found no injuries, but the third person, the driver, was not there. The search for him was panicky with shouting, but brief. He was injured but not seriously. Shortly thereafter, help came and the psychic trauma was mostly over. For a few days to a week, there were very minor signs of leftover fear, but for the most part, whatever symptoms or residuals there were from this experience came from the pleasures of dramatizing and the attention it aroused. Note the indications of stimulus barrier from the perception that the destruction of fence posts seemed "methodical," that the rolling of the car seemed slow and deliberate, and in the philosophical attitude toward death, as though one were in a seminar on the subject during the second or two that the car bounced around in the pasture. The breakthrough occurred briefly during the disordered search for the driver. The overstimulation abated and the reorganization began when he was found and it continued for a few days afterward.

Continuing to speak from our approach to a central concept of psychic trauma, the quantitative point of view, we need to look for explanations of cases in which the painful effects of the traumatic experience are persistent. We are naturally attracted to an idea that first drew Freud and other early psychological theorists, not only as an explanation for the chronic effects of extraordinary stresses, but as an explanation for all kinds of neurosis. We may call it the *painful memory theory*.[32] This idea is that the psyche after trauma is eager to turn its back on the experience. It postulates that the persistent effects of a stress which no longer is exerting outside pressure come from trying hard not to encounter the memory, and also from painfully meeting it in dreams, in chance associations, and in samples or versions of it in occasions of real life. This theory is not quite right; it is too simple, though some aspects of it are correct, as we shall see from later views of the subtleties of behavior in the aftermath of stress. Our most immediate argument opposing this theory is that the capacity for memory of the whole traumatic scene and all its details actually correlates highly with full recovery, indicating that painful memories do not cause neurosis, and that the mind in these instances has been able to draw the unpleasantness from the experience. An impairment of memory for trauma seems more likely an indicator that a pathogenic response has occurred, rather than that the memory

disorder is a cause of continuing disturbance or excessive defensiveness.

Freud had to abandon the painful memory idea, though there are some professionals who still hold to it. Many traumatized patients are implicitly convinced of it; particularly those who are having difficulties they only partially recognize. "I only want (or need) to forget it; I don't want to talk about it," they say with some anger, if pressed to remember.

In place of the painful memory idea, we return to the concept of disorganization of psychic functions and loss of integration from a forcing of the stimulus barrier and flooding of the psychic apparatus with excitation.[19] As the flood abates and the mind is relieved of its overload, gaining order and strength to begin processing again, we may conceive that the reorganization could be imperfect. Just as the receding flood of a river which had overflowed its banks leaves damage upon the landed structures, or as the populace has not the resources to bring about repairs of dikes against further flooding, so the interior of the mind can be more or less permanently impaired in its functioning by the overload, and be without the inner resources to reconstruct a well-working stimulus barrier, and reorganize its functions as effectively as they worked before. The individual is then unable to strengthen defenses against much lesser stimuli than the trauma which caused the damage in the first place.

In other words, the persistent pathogenic effects of stress or trauma following excessive excitation through the stimulus barrier occur because reorganization of ego functions and reintegration have not achieved the efficiency and strength the ego had before the trauma. The damage has been too great or the reparative factors have not functioned well enough.

The processes of imperfect reorganization after trauma are relatively specific. They may often be observed during recovery from a serious injury. In the early aftermath of trauma or stress, reorganization appears to be most defective in reconstituting the stimulus barrier and in regulation of affect discharge, leaving the mind still hypersensitive to even minor stimuli, i.e., excitations that would not have disturbed personality equilibrium prior to trauma. In a second phase of pathogenic reconstitution, the reorganization may become imperfect in two ways: (1) An excessive need to avoid re-experiencing the trauma in any form, with modifications of defensive functions of the ego to deal with fears of re-experiencing these excitations, or (2) attempts to achieve impossibly absolute control and regulation over emotional discharge for the avoidance of possibly traumatic situations.

From this way of understanding acute, subacute, and chronic effects of stress, we see the psychic apparatus remaining too sensitive to stimulations from within (aggressive and sexual impulses requiring affect discharge and releasing anxiety signal), and from without (stimulations interpreted as possible recurrences of traumatic overload, or evoking the possibility of arousal and releasing anxiety signal). Or, the psychic apparatus may become increasingly rigid and organized around the requirement to protect against the possibility of an overwhelming stimulus. The result of these changes is an extremely restless, irritable, and anxious person, one complaining of a number of physical symptoms associated with autonomic discharge, or one with an extremely guarded and constricted personality.

While this purely quantitative point of view, the idea of "too much" as an understanding of the immediate impact and long-term effects of stress and trauma remains theoretically essential, there is much it does not explain in the clinical picture and in the process of reconstitution. This mode of theorizing helps little in clinical prediction regarding the recovery phase and in deciding which individuals will continue to have difficulty and which will not. It is helpful in thinking about prevention and treatment of the subacute and chronic effects of a traumatic experience, because it indicates that the overwhelmed individual needs a gradually dosed discharge of the anxiety aroused by trauma and dammed up by defenses. While the concept of excessive excitation is central to understanding trauma and stress, the subtleties and variations among individuals and the real clinical process of

reconstitution after impact require other points of view as well.

We need to add the following three approaches to our general psychological theory: (1) The *meaning* of the traumatic experience to the person at conscious and unconscious levels. (This is a psychodynamic point of view on trauma and stress.) (2) The nature of *relationships* of the traumatized individual with his environment, including its human and nonhuman aspects. (An adaptive point of view.) (3) The effects of *past experience* on the response to impact and the process of reconstitution. (A psychogenetic point of view.)

1. The primary problem with regard to the meaning to the individual of most forms of stress or trauma is the lack of meaning when it happens. When we wake up from a dream in which bad things are happening, we naturally experience relief when we have shaken off the clutches of the dream's vividness. The next thought in most cases is a reproach to the self for having been in the throes of the dream's imagery. How could one be so weak and stupid to have been taken in? "That really couldn't happen to me, why did I allow even my sleeping self to be so frightened and miserable?" said a man after relating such a dream. The reasons for such unpleasant dreams are not the province of this discussion, but the strong feeling that such things cannot happen to "me" is an indication of the feeling and attitude of *invulnerability* most people have before the trauma hits. But the invulnerability has gone then; it has happened, and the inner statement, "It couldn't happen to me," is altered to "Why me?" This question after the loss of the illusion of invulnerability, an illusion which many regain soon after recovery, is unanswerable in terms of external reality. Most forms of trauma occur in settings with which the victim is intensely familiar, on the job, on the way to work, and in the home, i.e., in settings where he feels comfortable, protected, and least expecting that the stress will occur. This external meaninglessness of it all is a special challenge to the feeling of invulnerability.

In support of the notion that the conviction

of invulnerability exists at all in the average human being, we have findings from our research studies which will not be detailed here. An investigator for the Federal Aviation Administration has noted how physician pilots are overrepresented in fatal small plane accidents and said, "These doctors must think nothing can happen to them!"

The external meaninglessness of trauma to the human mind which wants everything to have some meaning, the universal, if temporary, loss of the illusive invulnerability, and the question which first occurs to the awakening and relaxing mind, "Why me?" present problems for resolution to the individual, which add immensely to the levels of excitation brought on by the trauma itself. Each of these factors contributes to the feeling of helplessness, which will partly fade when the fear becomes less real, but which must be assimilated and worked through before reintegration can begin.

Beyond these problems, we come upon still others which are common, if not universal, in the process of initial or early response to trauma. Although the experience has no "real," that is, external, meaning to most, there are internal emotional meanings unconsciously evoked and attached to the stressful events. Like nature abhorring a vacuum, the human mind hates randomness and lack of meaning, so people suffering stress create a meaning for what has happened, often without regard to external reality. Thus the significance of the stress is formed from unconscious needs and thoughts. These assigned meanings, arising from the depths of personality, interact with pre-existing neurotic conflicts and strongly influence the subsequent processes of reconstitution.

For example, the situation of helplessness, as an aftermath of acute trauma and as an element of chronic stress, having both physical and emotional sides, is interpreted variously by trauma victims. The diminution of physical strength and control of the self because of immobilization, during the emergency and reparative treatment of physical injury, dovetails with serious concerns over deterioration

of social, vocational, and family roles. A basically trusting person, or one flexibly confident of his capacities in his current roles, may understand the helplessness as temporary and simply take help where and when needed. Another, with conflicts over basic trust, may interpret the situation as a deprivation beyond toleration, with an increase of anger or depression. Still another, with a fundamental difficulty in the area of self-doubt, may interpret the helplessness as a personal failure and become unaccepting of his dependency, or become increasingly depressed and anxious, rather than gradually relieved of these feelings with the lessening of stress.

The question everybody asks after or during an individual catastrophe, "Why me?" may be answered within, primitively, magically, and unconsciously, by a part of the self, an agency of the mind, functioning as critic and judge of the self, the superego: "Because you are guilty and deserve your fate." The attitude of deserving the trauma, unconscious but nevertheless powerfully influential in feeling and behavior, is parallel to the logic of primitive animistic belief and even some modern religions. Guilt comes to the surface in this way after trauma. It is also expressed in terms of excessive feelings of responsibility for an accident, in the form of not wanting to be aware of the causes of the stress because of possibly final and valid reasons to feel guilty.

The good fortune of surviving a stress which others do not almost always evokes guilt feelings overtly and unconsciously, too. The question of deserving to be saved is part of it, but the more severe forms of "survival guilt" derive from the natural prior wish that grenades or a prison guard's brutality, whatever it is, will fall on someone other than the self, even though the others may be close comrades. Magical thinking is an essential element of this kind of neurotic recovery from trauma, because one must believe that these personal and "selfish" wishes spare the self at the expense of others.

The external meaninglessness of most traumatic events causes individuals prone to self-condemnation to make the trauma part of a basic unconscious fantasy about themselves. In these persons the meaning of the trauma is that it is a "command."[61] This command to feel, think, and behave differently appears to be external, but is actually internal and due to the awakening of repressed memories of actual punishment or repressed fears of punishment. Here, the internal self-accusing forces of hypertrophied and harsh superegos have been projected upon this new external reality, the traumatic event, so that it is seen in the terms of unconscious fantasy as an indicator of personal badness, and the happening has been interpreted as a demand to rid the self of imagined evil. It means to such an individual that he must exorcise something, some feeling like sexual desire, from himself and from his future way of life. This kind of conceptualizing sounds primitive and magical, but it should be understood as an interpretation of deeply unconscious fantasies which give the trauma the meaning of a command. This kind of thinking comes to light in half-humorous statements like, "What did I do to deserve this?" but in a more brooding and serious way in patients who suffer obscurely from the idea that the powerful forces of fate have been directed at them for cause.

By the "physiodynamics" of a traumatic episode we mean the sequence and causal chain of events leading to impact, that is the *way* it happened. These physiodynamics tend to have psychodynamic significance, shaping conscious and unconscious feelings about the events which may persist for years or a lifetime. Also, the "intent" of the person responsible for the trauma, be it the self or another, the activity or passivity of the victim in the traumatic event, and the emotional disposition of the victim, have psychodynamic significance, with effects upon pre-existing emotional conflicts and a reshaping of defensive structure within the individual in years to follow. These factors require a case vignette for elucidation.

Mrs. D., a stable, intelligent, vigorous, forty-five-year old woman, was driving with her son on a wet winter evening. She came to an intersection, stopped, and waited for the green light. She accelerated when she saw it, and halfway through the intersection she noted a sudden brilliance on the streets and the approach of something from the right side of her car. The last she knew was her son saying, "What the. . . ." She suffered concussion, laceration, and bruises. Her son was comatose and remained so for thirteen months when he died. Several years later, following some further stresses, which were part of a chain reaction of family misfortune started by the original crisis, the woman sought help for recurrent feelings of depression and a number of bodily symptoms associated with autonomic dysfunction.

There were three trends with psychodynamic significance in her case, which also exemplify the conflict-causing factors in many cases of major stress. First of all, the wet and wintry streets were not brought into the vignette for dramatic effect. They were aspects of the scene later used by the woman as part of an obsessional blaming of herself and a wretched wishing that she had done differently, i.e., not driven on a wet night in winter. Then, every other circumstance of the night was used to charge her with crimes of omission or commission, for example, that she should not have gone to the meeting, that she should not have been with her son, and so forth. These ways of responding to and processing the history of the event and the night it happened, over the years, represent the problem of working over repetitively the complex and changing version of her own responsibility for what happened. In her case, there was no actual personal responsibility for what happened, yet her wishful need to undo the incident many years later was at the expense of assuming responsibility for the accident. (Distortions in the reverse direction, relieving the self of responsibility for the happening, have been observed. However, in those cases where individuals shrink from awareness of their own part in a traumatic happening there is even more severe deterioration in ego strength and capacities for social adjustment.) The evolving ways in which Mrs. D. felt about her choice of actions on the fateful night involve her spiritually and personally as a cause of the accident. This complex of thought and feeling is both wishful and includes suffering; wishful, because it means she could and can control events, and it perpetuates suffering, because she labors to undo each twist and turn of her decision-making that night, haunted continually by it and by the question of her responsibility.

Secondly, the last words, "What the . . ." of Mrs. D.'s son form the memory of a nearly unbearable loss. Such an experience of loss is a thread of meaning in almost all forms of psychic trauma. Some form of loss, even if it is but a part, a trait, or characteristic, of the self, is an element of all significantly stressful experiences. Something is lost or taken away as a result of trauma. There may be chances for compensatory recovery or regaining, but loss occurs in the form of a change in the body or the self, if not in the death of a son. Phantom phenomena with sensory input from severed limbs, or hallucinations of lost persons in otherwise non-psychotic persons, are examples of the psychodynamic effects of traumatic losses, with the matching powerful need to restore the loss by psychological means. Mrs. D. experienced a sometimes visible hallucination and sometimes just a "thereness" of her son; and she was not psychotic.[57]

Finally, we see in this case a vivid example of the significance of the psychological situation of passivity as an element of traumatic experience. In this woman, there was an awareness for a few seconds of the advance of the destructive force, but her normal mobilizing mechanisms could have no effect upon what happened. The psychophysiologic processes of emergency mobilization occurred, we can be sure, but they could not protect her against the trauma. Such is the essence of passivity in human experience, to know what is happening, to have an awareness of sequence, to be able to organize the emergency physiologic responses of fight or flight, but to have them mean nothing with respect to final consequences. From this point of view, the autonomic discharge in the form of neurasthenic symptoms long after the trauma could constitute continuing efforts to mobilize against the danger, because they were never shut off, never reaching their end point.

2. *Adaptive point of view.* The nature of the relationship of the individual to his environment and other persons may not be as central to the immediately pathogenic factors of trauma as the quantitative facets, or as the meaning of the happening to the victim, but it is as important as the other two with respect to the stages of reorganization, reintegration, and reconstitution.

As socializing animals with faculties for language, humans discover their personal significance as units in dyadic and group relations. In these systems, they experience feelings, attitudes, and thought, and in these fields of interaction, they realize personal values, strengths, and weaknesses. The individual's sense of his own environment and his patterns of human relations are the resources which the person has for responding to stress and for recovering from the impact of acute trauma.

The two extremes in the sensing of environments are hostile and friendly. The soldier faces a hostile and threatening environment in combat. His responding capacity is enhanced or eroded by the ratio of companionship to isolation with his fellow soldiers, and by the support or loneliness afforded by group morale and the will to survive together. A patient-victim after a serious injury may interpret the surgical facility as friendly or hostile. This interpretation of friendly or hostile environment derives in large part from the action and expression of all those responsible for his treatment.

Reorganization after the impact of trauma or during chronic stress is very much along the lines of the form and strength of relations with all those persons significant to the victim. Meaningful communication with other humans restores structure and redefines the self. The connection between fragmented parts of the self is restored in the renewal of social relations, and functions of adaptation are revitalized by the warmth, assurance, and orienting power of personal interchange. Resuming meaningful relations during or after stress is a giant resource for reorganization. The relationship to reality is most effectively restored through these connections with others. The realistic sense of the self is most strongly supported in the context of human interaction. Stress is often an isolating experience. Sometimes, it even means stimulus deprivation after the contrasting massive stimulation of the trauma, if immobilization in a hospital bed is required after a frightening accident. Breaking through this isolation affords orientation and a sense of continuity, as well as a means of gradual reduction of overstimulation, thus decreasing the fragmentation and loss of integration.

3. *Psychogenetic point of view.* An understanding of the past contributes to a theory of stress in three ways: (a) It allows an estimate of the psychic strengths and weaknesses that the ego has to meet the stress; (b) It uncovers the recollections of infancy in the helpless condition occasioned by stress; and (c) It acts as a screen for the re-enactment and re-explanation of prior conflict.

a. The early formative experiences in human development determine the strength a person has to fend off, or somehow process, and possibly discharge, the increased levels of excitation and demand upon ego function. The resilience and toughness of the stimulus barrier, versus its possible fragility or brittleness, are determined by these factors as well as by constitutional ones. The kind of stress to which a person is sensitive is similarly determined; for example, some soldiers may resist the horrors of threatened injury to themselves, but crack when they hear or see death or injuries to others.

Some of this sensitivity could be attributed to psychodynamic factors which were implanted in early times but remained relatively inactive before the stress. When a person carries with him a series of unresolved conflicts, one or more of which is awakened and revitalized by aspects of the stressful situation, there is an increased level of excitation to be managed by the traumatized ego. Also the nature of the stimulus barrier, its resilience and points of weakness, is derived from early family experiences and from the protection the family could afford the child as he developed his own stimulus barrier.

b. Actual and emotional helplessness is in some form and degree a part of the individual experience of a stressful situation. Since we have said that the central component of stress is the concept of excitation exceeding the ca-

pacity of the organism to integrate its functions, the response of helplessness follows naturally. The state of helplessness resulting from being seriously injured and immobilized, for example, repeats a condition of the past, the times of infancy, and some aspects of early childhood. This return physically and psychologically to a condition of a much earlier time can be an extremely significant factor in the stress and reorganization after impact, mostly determined by the individual's capacity to accept the physical and emotional situation of helplessness without being shattered absolutely by it, and without expecting that the recovery from it would be too great a task. The capacity to have a basic trust[15] (in the surgical treatment team, for example), acquired from early development in the mother-child interaction, provides strength for relieving the helplessness during and after the impact phase of a traumatic situation.

c. The use of the traumatic experience as a screen for emotional conflicts and defenses of the pre-stress personality is mostly significant for concepts of reconstitution and treatment, but is mentioned here since it brings the past, developmental, factors and the traumatic events together. Briefly, we usually see, in patients whose histories include evidence of significant neurotic problems prior to the traumatic event, that the recent experience takes over the previous neurosis. The trauma becomes a screen upon which the patient projects all previous problems.[24] It becomes a new explanation to the self, and a new way of defending against recognition of unconscious impulse and conflictual elements of the old neurotic difficulty. Thus, the adaptation to the new problem, reorganization after trauma, is shaped by the previous neurosis, and the two combine in intricate ways. Sometimes, the traumatic experience and the physical and emotional effects of it become a new way of life, a new way of living out neurotic patterns of adjustment. The unconscious use of the memory of trauma and its aftermath as a screen for the whole structure and pattern of a previous neurosis becomes a way of interpreting current experiences. ("I feel and behave this way because of what happened to me, not because of inherent problems.") This concept of the traumatic event as a screen for past conflict and defensive partial solutions explains why there are variations of reaction to trauma among individuals, which are based upon their way of dealing with previous neurotic difficulty. This idea also emphasizes that there are pathogenic factors leading to chronic disability, not based on mere secondary gain factors (from compensation or insurance payments), in a patient who relates all his symptoms to an injury and forgets pre-existing symptoms.

❲ Varieties of Stress

If stress is fundamentally a matter of overload, does it matter what kind of stress has been imposed? From the standpoint of theory it should not matter, since we are speaking only of a breaking point and it should not make any difference what does the breaking or how. The individual differences in reaction are explainable in theory by psychodynamic and psychogenetic factors.

Yet, the kinds of trauma, the varieties of stress, do make a difference psychologically. The social and physical settings, the expectations of the individual, and the rhythm and pace of living, are all different when, for example, we are comparing an auto accident with a mortar attack in a field of battle.

Accidents occur almost always in familiar settings, sometimes where they are least expected, at home, in automobiles, and at work.[55] The psychic trauma comes from actual physical injury or the intense threat of injury, and the possibility of loss of life immediately or for a while after the accident. Industrial accidents may differ slightly from others in that there may be certain occupational hazards to which the employee has learned to adapt and probably has some feeling of mastery over his fear of them. The accident occurs in these cases because of some lapse in the routines designed to insure safety on the part of the employee, often arising from excessive feelings of mastery over fears, or on the part of someone else.[30]

The stressful conditions of *combat* are the nearly constant fear of death and mutilation, amplified by loss of sleep, physical exhaustion, separation from family and personal hardship, and feelings about killing of other humans.[3,26,35,47,71] The great variety of neurotic symptoms or transient psychotic symptoms in the area of battle are responsive to the bloodshed and may require the individual's being removed from combat.

Rotation of duty from the front and back, giving a man something to anticipate with a degree of pleasure and some hope, may prevent some of these conditions.[3] Prompt return to duty in a noncombat assignment has been claimed by some military physicians to be helpful in relieving the pressure of the intense wish to employ symptoms as a means of getting away from the highly unpleasant situation, but this policy may have actually relieved the pressure of the medical officers from the line officers.

The conditions of military life, differing from those to which the individual was accustomed in civilian life, constitute the stresses for *noncombat military neuroses*.[3] Some military clinicians have noted that the proneness to neuroses in the support troops, the rear echelon noncombat soldiers, occurs because they are near the sounds of war, but do not have the aggressive outlet of the soldier in battle areas.

Disasters impose stress on groups, communities, cities, and counties, but the nature of the stress differs in the phases of reaction to it: (1) threat of impending disaster (a typhoon is moving in from the sea), (2) impact (the typhoon hits), (3) recoil (the typhoon has passed and people are recovering themselves, each other, and possessions), (4) post-traumatic period (people have returned to homes and begin reconstruction).[13,64,65,68]

The remoteness of a typhoon way out at sea may often encourage the unconscious defense of denial to misperceive the danger, but if denial is used as the threat becomes imminent the individual is less prepared to cope with the stress of impact than if he makes use of anticipatory rehearsal of steps to be taken in the emergency.

During impact, a minority of individuals (12–25%) remain cool and collected with full appreciation of the situation and able to carry through procedures for the safety of themselves and others. The majority (about 75%) manifest some degree of the "disaster syndrome," being stunned, bewildered, docile, and unresponsive. The rapidity of action and the seeming disorder of events restrict their field of attention and interfere with awareness of personal feelings, although they demonstrate physiological concomitants of fear. Another group (about 10–25%) shows inappropriate responses, such as paralysis from fear, or blind flight, or other varieties of excessive activity, flitting ineffectively from one task to another with great distractibility. According to these findings, "When in danger or in doubt/Run in circles; scream and shout," is the motto for some of us.

During recoil, when the survivors are getting to safety, there is more awareness and expression of emotions, such as anxiety, fear, and anger. Victims of disaster are described as contrasting to victims of accidents in this phase in respect to their appreciation for any help that is being given, rather than resenting others who were not singled out by the injury. In the period of recoil, there is a great need to be with others, and to give expression to feelings about the catastrophe.

Recognition of the meaning of disaster, of loss of loved ones, of home, possessions, of financial security, is the stress of the post-traumatic period. It is a drastically altered environment that the individual is facing, and he may continue to have symptoms of the disaster syndrome, or depression and other neurotic or psychotic sequelae.

Physical illness is a definite and common psychic stress leading, especially in psychologically defensive stages, to a much enhanced and regressive investment in the self, concomitant with less or a different investment in relations with others. This narcissistic regression will necessarily have a pervasive effect on personality adjustment. The fatal illness of a close relative is also a particularly potent stress agent.[70]

Some specific stressful features of *surgery*

may be illustrated by the immobilization and sensory deprivation following eye surgery, which must be countered by compensatory stimulation in the nursing care and by visitors.[63]

There have been many studies now of survivors after Nazi persecution in concentration camps, which have established the very persistent nature of the symptoms following upon the stresses of the most massive cruelty in the modern world.[5,39] The "Concentration Camp Syndrome" consists of a great deal of anxiety complicated by various defenses against anxiety, an obsessive ruminative state, psychosomatic manifestations, and depression and guilt. "Survival guilt" on the part of those who have remained alive when so many others have died seems to be an important factor in the perpetuation of symptoms and in negative therapeutic reactions to efforts in treatment.[5,12,25,29,39,58]

Survivors of the Hiroshima and Nagasaki bombings have presented symptoms and character changes not unlike those of the concentration camp victims.[14,43,52]

Several studies of returned *prisoners of war* of the Chinese Communists[5,28,41,54,68] have shown how powerful the effects could be of isolation and sleep deprivation, and alternating punishment and reward. They have also indicated how guilt over noncooperation with the indoctrinators could be used as a stress benefiting the interrogator if the prisoner was cut off from his fellows.

Examples of stresses in *work and school adjustments* include the presence of role conflict,[33] and the existence of discrepancies between expectations for the individual and his capacities to realize these expectations.[31] Various neurotic or psychosomatic symptoms may follow upon these stresses.

Experimentally induced stresses, such as *sensory isolation*, have been shown to induce acute hallucinations to be experienced by previously healthy subjects. It appears that information input underload constitutes a stress differing from the information input overload of other varieties of trauma. However, the findings of these experiments continue to support our psychoeconomic theory of trauma and the stimulus barrier concept, because it has been shown that the stressful aspect of sensory reduction is still formed from excessive excitation! This time, though, the hyperstimulation comes from within. When the equilibrium of outer interests and inner ones is thrown off by the considerable reduction of external stimuli, the mind becomes flooded with the demand of inner impulses and the affects and images which they excite, hence the hallucinations and peculiar feelings building up and disturbing internal order.

There have been cases of unpredictable behavior precipitated by sudden traumatic information, such as the news of the "shocking" assassinations in the United States in recent years, but these instances appear worth adding to the list only to illustrate the broad range of varieties of stress and the manifold reactions to them.

(Clinical Process of Acute or Chronic Stress

In an earlier section, we considered psychic trauma from a general theoretical point of view. Now, we must study it as a factor in psychopathology and see how and in what ways it is psychopathogenic.

Pre-Stress

Curiously, some trauma and some chronic stress appear to be the consequence as much as the cause of psychopathology. Certain individuals are the victims of stressful incidents far more often than others, and from study of such cases in comparison with controls, we are forced to the probable conclusion that their course of seeming misfortune and repeated "accidents" is not due to personal bad luck, but to internal psychological factors responsible for accident behavior. These persons use pathological action, impulsive, aggressive, belligerent and risk-taking behavior for the resolution of emotional conflict, or for adjusting problems with other people. These behaviors, which seem reasonable and eminently justifiable to them, are usually discovered to have

primitive roots in unconscious fantasy, when the whole pattern and the victim's communication about himself can be studied. Impulsive, aggressive, and risk-taking behavior, such as reckless, drunken driving, is not always or necessarily self-destructive in unconscious aim.[56] It may be intended as creative, though infantile, in the manner in which this basic motivation is carried through. The reckless driver may be creating for himself an image of power, virility and invulnerability, in the behavior leading to his trauma. In very brief summary form, this is a description of the repeating type of pre-stress personality.

Some pathological actions leading to trauma or chronic stress are not episodic, or repetitive, but occur only once in a person's life, and develop from situations of intense personal conflict or crisis in a family system, or from losses or changes in intense relationships. We rated histories of 65 subjects in our study of physical trauma victims, finding 68% of them to have experienced significant crisis or conflict just prior to the traumatic event. Some of the behavior came from explosions of feeling which were fended off by the victim, as some other behavior was caused by the powerful distraction of crises in which he was involved. At times, there was deep sadness about a current life situation, or the need to act strongly or wildly to relieve accumulating tension. These actions involved heavy risk to the victim's life and limb. (A mother jumped from a moving car during a bitter argument with her daughter.)

Some accident behavior is overtly or covertly suicidal. Three patients in our physical trauma series had been aware of suicidal intent, but concealed their intent from the emergency surgeons. As far as we have been able to observe, suicidal intent leading to trauma or chronic stress does not lessen the psychological effects of impact, although one might imagine that it would cushion the blow if the victim intended to do himself harm. Suicidal acts do not lessen problems of recovery, either. Instead, it is usually the case that the crisis or conflict precipitating the suicide attempt has not been reduced by the act, though it may appear to be temporarily so.

Impact

The possibly pathogenic aspects of impact have been indicated already from the viewpoints of excessive excitation, the internal psychodynamic problems, and the physiodynamics and varieties of stress that women and men may encounter.

Disorganization

This kind of pathogenesis occurs from every form of stress or trauma in everyone. If the capacities of the ego apparatus of the mind are exceeded, if the integration is broken down, some disorganization of ego function has occurred, if only briefly. The disorganization from trauma appears for a few seconds, a few hours, or days, or even months in the case of severe trauma or chronic stress. Even without brain impairment (which is sometimes a complicating accompaniment of trauma with shock or head injury), the disorganization shows in some disorientation and blunting of awareness, or disturbance in perception, in memory disturbance, in defects of judgment, in changes of the mode of relating, and in the regulation of affect discharge.

The disorientation and changes in perceptiveness are not of the kind seen when there is brain damage. They are more like a veil drawn over the capacity to understand a situation and to perceive clearly what is happening. There are likely to be distortions in thinking as a result of the disorganizing impact of trauma. For example, we may observe in stressful group situations, during natural disasters, and so forth, the ease with which rumors are fabricated, become exaggerated, and circulate. In medical and surgical stress situations, the explanations by physicians and others of the purpose and significance of diagnostic procedures and treatment become quickly and highly distorted. Memory disturbance from the mentally disorganizing effect of trauma is also not like that from brain impairment. It is selective, spotty, or amnesic, for brief or sometimes longer periods around the phase of impact and its immediate aftermath, suggesting an interference with certain functions of the mind, rather than changes in anatomical structure.

Beyond the moderate disorientation and memory disturbance, there is a loss of integration of thinking and a fragmentation which lowers comprehension and clarity of expression of thoughts. Some degree of forms of the disorganization occurs in everyone experiencing a psychic trauma worthy of the name. The longer term psychopathogenic effect of the acute disorganizing process is that it sensitizes the individual to adverse happenings in the phase of reconstitution, and becomes a part of the traumatic event which the victim would most want to avoid.

Psychic Regression

Except for the thorough falling apart of a major psychosis there is nothing so sure to induce regression in behavior, feeling, and mental function as a severe trauma or continuing stress.

Regression, a mainly intrapsychic process, is usually misunderstood in more than one sense. The process itself is not easily defined, and when in reality a patient is regressing, those around him will most likely not understand what is going on. But it is an extremely significant reaction with far-reaching and deep pathogenic effects, if not reversed.

Psychological development, as we have come to understand it, occurs along lines of unfolding potential with increasing refinement and sophistication. No one of the stages along a line of development is abandoned, rather it becomes a component and the basis for an advance in development. It is possible to move backwards along a particular line or along several and even all lines at once—resorting to earlier ways of adjusting, problem-solving, communication, feeling, relating, and behaving. This moving back along lines of development is regression and it happens usually or always as a response to stress. It is essentially intrapsychic but there are reflections in interaction with the environment and personal relations. The reactions of those in the environment to the relative helplessness and infantilizing of the subject will in turn influence the depth and reversibility of the regressive process.

Regression is at first a means of resilience with which the individual mind can resist the overwhelming stimuli. Later, if it becomes a fixed pattern and does not permit a resumption of more mature and age appropriate responses, these effects prevent psychological healing and become a basis for continuing symptoms and maladaptation after stress.

Two cases illustrate the contrasting courses of regression, with and without reversal of the process of reacting, with earlier modes of adaptation in recovery from stress.

A forty-two-year-old woman was about to enter her first marriage when she was hospitalized for emergency surgery for pancreatitis and gall bladder disease. About five weeks later, soon after leaving the hospital and while completing marriage plans again, she was a passenger in an auto out of control at high speed, striking a pole, which gave her a fractured hip and minor facial injuries. Her fiancé was more than discouraged. She became deeply morose, non-communicative, stared at the ceiling, and refused most of her food for about four weeks. As far as could be determined she interpreted her surgical condition as being as hopeless as her romantic life. However, physical rehabilitation was effective and it turned her sinking thoughts and feelings around to the point that her interests, her communicativeness, and her mode of relating all became much less withdrawn and sullen, and more appropriate to her age and sex role.

The process of regression was extremely functional and manifest in an eighteen-year-old high school girl suffering a jaw fracture in an accident in which her boyfriend was killed. About a year before the accident she had lost her father from a coronary attack. In the early interviews, when she did not know of the boyfriend's death and when she was dealing mostly with the concerns about herself and the isolation of the treatment unit, she formed an intense attachment with the interviewer in which she longed for physical as well as verbal contact. At times, she clutched the interviewer's tie while they talked. This outright need for a replacement for the dead father was the principal feature of the regressive process, providing some temporary strength and comfort in the early days of hospitalization. Demands on nurses for extra care and mutually accusatory arguments with them were less fortunate and less helpful aspects

of her regression. Some extraordinary interference from the family, including a bereaved mother and a bewildered sister, became a factor which prevented a reversal of the regressive process as the physical stress became less pressing. Recognition of the boyfriend's death was denied the girl for three weeks after she regained consciousness. She must have "known" he was dead, as his whereabouts were not known to her, but she was not allowed to recognize the fact and to feel it, since the decision had been made that she was not "ready" for the information. Some other forms of hushing things up had to do with complicated fears of legal reprisal. The stifling and overprotectiveness of the family in handling several of the circumstances evolving from the traumatic event prevented re-maturation after the regressive process, which seemed at first to be adding to the resilience of the patient's response. Later, her adjustment was built on non-recognition and no memory for the occurrence and significance of the trauma. As in the case of the dead boyfriend, who seemed never to have existed for her, the patient had absolutely no memory at all for the interviewer who had meant so much to her for a six-week period in her life.

In our discussion of a general theory of trauma we outlined its components, indicating what trauma or stress is. Now, in the clinical process of the response to trauma we have seen what trauma does, how the forces of disorganization, disintegration, and disorder may become weaknesses in the psychic apparatus. The other pathogenic force, regression, as illustrated in the two cases above, is at first a form of resilience in the individual response. However, it can also leave an ego weakness, becoming a maladaptation in the form of psychic or physical symptoms or character change if the regressive tendency does not reverse with recovery.

Reconstitution

Our final task is to consider reconstitution. This is all-important, because the way the mind is put back together will determine how it will function thereafter. The intensity and quality of the traumatic experience are of much less human importance than how the pieces fit in a functional unit when the trauma and the responses to it have passed. Since this phase of stress as a determinant of behavior is very much a matter of a person in interaction with the environment, it is the phase of the over-all traumatic process upon which we can have the most influence.

We, as professional staff, can be witnesses and participants in reconstitution from some forms of trauma, although not in all. When a person is recovering from trauma in a hospital, we can observe reconstitution. In the case of natural disaster, such as a mine disaster,[42] a team of investigators can go to interview and make observations.

Many other forms of trauma are seen after the fact of impact and reconstitution, when pathological consequences have already set in. That is why some faulty concepts of the consequence of trauma have been perpetuated in the literature. Head injury patients, discharged in a few days without plan for follow-up because brain damage had not occurred, may show up months or years later with headaches, tinnitus, and dizziness. Patients with back and other injuries in which the initial physical problems were well treated and the patients discharged but returned with symptoms later, are also victims of psychic trauma in which the reconstitution process was not observed and seen only when its outcome consisted of chronic symptoms or character change.

A twenty-nine-year-old construction worker fell three stories, striking scaffolding on his way down. He was admitted for a shoulder injury and concussion. He was discharged in a few days with the diagnosis of shoulder contusion and concussion, recovered. A year later he was found to have physical and psychological symptoms of a chronic traumatic neurosis.

The fact that the trauma problem has usually been studied after the reconstitutive work had been completed, has led to certain fallacious emphases in psychiatric knowledge and attitudes, for example, on the importance of "secondary gain" concepts and "compensation neurosis," to account for complex behavior patterns following stress. These ideas suggest a willful seeking or an unconscious drive to obtain compensation. While it may be true that a significant number of persons de-

mand financial support long after a trauma has occurred and when purely physical aspects of their injuries have been cured, it is short-circuited reasoning to assume that the symptoms are solely motivated by or dependent on the wish to be compensated. The term "compensation neurosis" appears to be claiming such mercenary etiology.

This way of thinking about reconstitution is based upon an incomplete understanding of "secondary gain" as a psychodynamic mechanism, and upon the tendency of some terminology used to replace true understanding and to perpetuate superficiality.

The term "secondary gain" is best understood as an unconscious resistance arising during treatment to the meaning of certain elements of a symptom. It is the resistance to the understanding of the self, saying, "Better I should suffer than face what I feel, and I shall even find a way to profit from my suffering!" The theoretical significance of this form of resistance, "secondary gain," is that the symptom is preferable to the individual than recognizing the meaning of it. It may transpire, in recovery from trauma, that the symptoms which obtain monetary gain are preferable to recognition of the very uncomfortable impulses and feelings which have been under poor control after the ego-weakening effect of trauma. Further, it may be true that the compensation won from industrial or governmental commissions by the severity of symptoms becomes an additional reinforcement to resistance against recognition of aspects of the self. However, there are also other resistances in a pathogenic reconstitution from trauma. The demand for compensation by the trauma victim may be the least neurotic part of his total behavior and the most realistic, because it is saying that the psychological effects of trauma can be as disabling as the physical. We psychiatrists often make the mistake of labeling the pursuit of monetary gain a "compensation neurosis" and thereby forget or ignore the problem underneath having to do with a self-image reduced by the traumatic experience. We may overlook the depression and rage suffered as a result of that reduction of self-esteem and we may ignore our own anger that a man should get money because he has depreciated himself. It is circuitous reasoning, then, to say that the drive for compensation is a cause of the neurotic complications rather than a consequence of them. We can easily recognize that the struggle with physicians and governmental boards over the award of compensation builds the resistances in the patient and, in fact, becomes a part of him, a new way of life, and even a world-view, not because his symptoms are designed to justify, but because he finds no other way of helping himself.

There are several other factors beyond the oversimplified one of secondary gain which have shaping effects on reconstitution after the disorganizing and regressive aftermath of impact. These factors toward a pathogenic or healthy remaking of the personality include the following: The form of object relations and the richness and effectiveness of communication in reconstitution; the modes of emotional expression and regulation; the "defensive style" emerging in the reconstitutive phase; the consciousness of the self emerging in the remaking. There is also the use of the traumatic experience as a screen in the same way that an early memory, a screen memory, is used to account within the self for an emotional disposition and conflict which actually preceded the trauma.

The most direct expression of the problem of object relations in reconstitution is when the person under stress and feeling helpless wonders whether he will be of use to people again, whether he will be attractive, acceptable, and wanted again. That idea, from the disorganizing and regressive pathogenic forces in recovery from trauma, reinforced by other physical or psychological changes in the person, may continue into the reconstitutive phase in the form of self-doubt in relations with others, and therefore less willingness to participate. A parallel force in the direction of less gratifying relations with others comes from the lack of capacity to turn outward, to invest energies in relations outside of the self, because of feeling a need to reserve these energies for protection and vigilance against recurrence of the trauma. It is common, for example, that sexual interests after a traumatic experience will be diminished. It appears in these cases that somehow the individual feels unable to afford such object-directed feelings and is conserving all his resources for tending to and defending the self. The same kind of constriction and degree of withdrawal of libido apply to other areas of interest: vacation, hobbies, social activities, and so on.

When we can observe reconstitution in cases of physical injury from a terrifying accident, the restoration of object relations from the stages of disorganization and regression appears to be predictive of the strength of the process and the degree to which the individual will become effective in adaptation. The deepest sorts of pathogenesis after trauma arising in the phases of reconstitution are associated with feelings of self-doubt and with doubt or lack of trust of others. The impact of the stress or trauma appears to excite most intensely these twin doubts: of the self in relation to others and of others in relation to the self. The restoration of both kinds of confidence seems deeply intertwined with the new organization of the mind. We cannot say whether reorganization depends on strength in gaining and keeping object relations, or the reverse, or whether there is a more complicated interaction of the two.

Through the family, and in the psychological milieu of a medical or surgical ward, the quality and significance of human relations for the reorganizing psyche of the traumatized individual are eminently influenceable. The case of the young woman who was not told of the loss of her friend and was kept in a kind of isolation with the best of intentions, and the case of the older woman whose last and best hopes for a wedding seemed dashed, are examples of the potential for modification of pathogenic currents in the process of reconstitution. When the members of the treatment team are sensitive to these aspects of healing, and when they are educated to intervene intelligently, it is possible to lessen self-doubt and mistrust of others in the re-establishment of mature human relations.

The principal affects left over from trauma and possibly causing pathological reconstitution are anxiety, depression, and anger. Anxiety is easy enough to understand. The experience has most likely been fearful. The overloaded mental organization may not have thoroughly processed the fear, and it remains as an anxiety which forces the person to act as though the traumatic situation were still active or would recur at any moment. Our previous discussion has also implied the persistence of anxiety from old problems and conflicts reawakened in the experience. Gradually, during reconstitution, anxiety will find differentiated modes of expression. It attaches itself to and reinforces doubts, mistrust, anger, or irritability, and other manifestations of the reorganized personality, making the clinician's job of finding the anxiety and disclosing its sources more difficult.

Depression may arise from the sense of loss after trauma. There may have been real losses in the traumatic event, of other persons or parts of the victim's body. This feeling also may come from guilt after trauma with a turning of anger on the self. Its most obscure form, and in the findings of our studies of physical trauma the most pervasive, comes from the notion of loss of invulnerability, the feeling of powerlessness, the disappointment, and sense of personal weakness, from the impact of the stress. This kind of depression is like a developmental problem in which there is sadness about losing a part of the self in going on to a new phase of maturity. For many victims, this sadness is brief, but others never quite regain their confidence from the loss of invulnerability. The unrealistic sense of weakness becomes a hidden and obscured part of their personalities in reconstitution.

The problem with anger is its channeling and means of expression. Most trauma victims have it in considerable quantities. Often, it seems that anger matches the violence of the unfortunate experience, as though the victim had been transfused with it. The danger of the victim's anger is that it seems to him to interfere with the object relations which he needs. He is afraid that the anger will bring about retaliation from those from whom he needs help. Thus, the problem with anger threatens the recurrence or at least the reawakening of

the traumatic situation. The disposition of quantities of aggression in trauma victims can be followed in their violent dreams. The problems from this aggression can be responded to therapeutically by understanding of these fears.

Kernberg has shown the emphasis in borderline patients on what he calls "first-order defenses."[38] Denial, projection, and reaction formation are first-order defenses, in contrast to isolation, rationalization, or affectualization, which are more "sophisticated" defenses. First-order defenses, especially denial, appear often and strongly in trauma patients whose defensive style is leading toward a pathological reconstitution. The young woman whose boyfriend died had her defense of denial massively joined and reinforced by the family, and this defense became a highly structured and sizeable component in the reorganization of her personality. Projection, mainly about feelings of responsibility for events, is a strong reshaping force with pathogenic consequence. Finally, reaction formation to feelings of hostility from what has happened causes a more rigid and brittle sort of person from the traumatic process. The settling-in of these defensive styles employing first-order defenses makes therapeutic resolution difficult.

Outcomes

The long-term result of these psychodynamic processes is a reintegration of the personality, either along the lines of the previous integration or with a chronic neurotic adjustment. Occasionally, there is improvement in personal integration from resolution of pre-traumatic problems as a result of realizing new ways of living and new insights from the traumatic or stressful experience. A chronic psychosis seems to be rare.

In most cases, the process of reintegration includes a working through of the traumatic episode in a verbal form, using the individual's memory of the events. This is a reconstruction in which the happenings and feelings are put in place. The struggle with anger or helplessness may be remembered in realistic ways, resolving guilt or shame over the feelings and seeing them in a new light. One of our patients was an electrician of considerable experience who worked over and over on the question as to why he had been so inexpert and foolish as to have allowed a piece of conduit in his hands to come in contact with a live wire. He could never answer the question but he had to confront himself with it to avoid this mistake from happening again.

The chronic neurotic adjustment is accompanied by persisting symptoms which developed as a defense against the traumatic anxiety. Commonly, these consist of a conversion type of hysterical neurosis, or a depressive neurosis, or a mixture of both. Less commonly, the persisting symptoms are of other types of neurosis, such as anxiety neurosis, or of psychophysiologic illnesses. Alcohol addiction sometimes develops as an attempt at self-treatment of anxiety or depression. Hyperthyroidism has been noted to ensue after an acute emotional trauma, and peptic ulcer occasionally begins during the reintegration after acute or chronic stress. Chronic reactive aggression or paranoid hostility are occasionally seen as the continuing outcome.

Chronic persistence of neurotic symptoms may be related to secondary gains being obtained by the individual in a regressed state with a constricted ego. The secondary gain may be dependent or retaliatory, according to the unconscious motives in seeking and obtaining compensation payments, a pension or other insurance, or some change in responsibility. When the trauma occurred at work, a phobia for the working situation may be contributing to dependency on the unearned income of workmen's compensation. The retaliation motive in the seeking of compensation is particularly present when the employee felt exploited by his employers, in addition to being overwhelmed and rendered helpless by the trauma of the accident.

Sometimes, the action on litigation or insurance has been initiated by another member of the family or by a professional adviser (for example, a doctor or a lawyer). The complexities of secondary gain can be illustrated by cases in which the dependency or retaliation is directed toward the family member or professional adviser, who then helps to perpetuate the neurosis by pursuing compensation or other legal redress, or encouraging the traumatic victim to do so. For example, the wife of an injured breadwinner may have gone to work while her husband was incapacitated, contributing to a shift in the family equilibrium. This shift may further a regression in which he becomes like a child or a substitute mother in the home, dependent on his wife, or retaliating for her assumption of his role. The wife may then push for compensation or insurance to reduce her own load.

If there has been painful physical injury with the acute emotional trauma, the pains may persist as sensory conversion symptoms, imposing what appears to be a physical disability, defending against the return to work, and against satisfactory rehabilitation and reintegration. If there is major physical disability after recovery from the acute effects of the injury, there may be a similar limitation to the reintegration of the personality. The individual is denied the opportunity of overcoming the phobia for the working situation and mastering his traumatic anxiety more completely. The crippled individual, more dependent on others than he was before the trauma, has a more difficult task to readjust and is more likely to present chronic depression or irritability.

In brief, there is a range of end results in behavior, character, and neurosis. The similarities and differences in these end results are understandable from our general theory of psychic stress and from the varieties of stress which occur. The end results are determined by factors in the various stages of the clinical process, through pre-stress, impact, disorganization, regression, and finally reconstitution.

⟨ Bibliography

1. BARNETT, S. A. "Physiological Effects of 'Social Stress' in Wild Rats: The Adrenal Cortex," *Journal of Psychosomatic Research*, 3 (1958), 1–10.

2. BOURNE, P. G. *Men, Stress and Vietnam.*

Boston: Little, Brown and Co., 1970.

3. BRILL, N. Q. "Personality Disorders IV: Gross Stress Reaction II: Traumatic War Neurosis," in A. M. Freedman and H. I. Kaplan, eds., *Comprehensive Textbook of Psychiatry*, pp. 1031–1035. Baltimore: Williams and Wilkens Co., 1967.

4. BRILL, N. Q., and J. F. GLASS. "Workmen's Compensation for Psychiatric Disorders," *Journal of the American Medical Association*, 193 (1965), 345–348.

5. CHODOFF, P. "Effects of Extreme Coercive and Oppressive Forces: Brainwashing and Concentration Camps," in S. Arieti, ed., *American Handbook of Psychiatry*, Vol. 3. New York: Basic Books, 1966.

6. CHRISTIAN, J. J. "Effect of Population Size on the Adrenal Glands and Reproductive Organs of Male Mice in Population of Fixed Size," *American Journal of Physiology*, 182 (1955), 292–298.

7. CHRISTIAN, J. J., and D. E. DAVIS. "The Relationship Between Adrenal Weight and Population Status of Urban Norway Rats," *Journal of Mammalogy*, 37 (1956), 475–485.

8. COMMITTEE ON NOMENCLATURE AND STATISTICS. *Diagnostic and Statistical Manual: Mental Disorders*. Washington, D.C.: American Psychiatric Association, Mental Hospital Service, 1952.

9. ———. *DSM II: Diagnostic and Statistical Manual of Mental Disorders* (Second Edition). Washington, D.C.: American Psychiatric Association, 1968.

10. DANIELS, R. A. "Executive Stress." Selected papers No. 38. Chicago: Graduate School of Business, University of Chicago, 1971.

11. DES PRES, T. "The Survivor," *Encounter*, 37 (1971), 3–19.

12. DE WIND, E. "Psychotherapy After Traumatization Caused by Persecution." Presented at Chicago Psychoanalytic Society, 1970.

13. DRAYER, C. S., D. C. CAMERON, A. J. GLASS, and W. D. WOODWARD. *Disaster Fatigue*. Washington, D.C.: American Psychiatric Association, 1956.

14. DRAYER, C. S., W. D. WOODWARD, and A. J. GLASS. *Psychological First Aid in Community Disasters*. Washington, D.C.: American Psychiatric Association, 1954.

15. ERIKSON, E. "Identity and the Life Cycle," in *Psychological Issues*, Vol. 1, No. 1. New York: International Universities Press, 1959.

16. FENICHEL, O. *The Psychoanalytic Theory of Neurosis*, Chapter 7. New York: Norton, 1945.

17. ———. *The Psychoanalytic Theory of Neurosis*, Chapter 21. New York: Norton, 1945.

18. FERENCZI, S., K. ABRAHAM, E. SIMMEL, and E. JONES. *Psychoanalysis and the War Neurosis*. New York: International Psychoanalytic Press, 1921.

19. FREUD, S. "Letters to Wilhelm Fliess," in M. A. Bonaparte, A. Freud, and E. Kris, eds., *The Origins of Psychoanalysis*. New York: Basic Books, 1954.

20. ———. "Introduction to Psychoanalysis and the War Neurosis" (1919), including an appendix (1920), in *Standard Edition*, Vol. 17. London: Hogarth Press, 1955.

21. ———. "Beyond the Pleasure Principle" (1920), in *Standard Edition*, Vol. 18. London: Hogarth Press, 1955.

22. FURST, S. S., ed., *Psychic Trauma*. New York: Basic Books, 1967.

23. GEDIMAN, H. "The Concept of Stimulus Barrier: Its Review and Reformulation as an Adaptive Ego Function," *International Journal of Psycho-Analysis*, 52 (1971), 243–250.

24. GLOVER, E. "The 'Screening' Function of Traumatic Memories," *International Journal of Psycho-Analysis*, 10 (1929), 90–93.

25. GRAUER, H. "Psychodynamics of the Survivor Syndrome," *Canadian Psychiatric Association Journal*, 14 (1969), 617–622.

26. GRINKER, R. R., and J. P. SPIEGEL. *Men Under Stress*. New York: Blakiston (McGraw-Hill), 1945.

27. HARTMANN, H. *Ego Psychology and the Problem of Adaptation*. New York: International Universities Press, 1958.

28. HINKLE, L. E., JR., and H. G. WOLFF. "Communist Interrogation and Indoctrination of 'Enemies of the State,'" *Archives of Neurology and Psychiatry*, 76 (1956), 115–174.

29. HOPPE, K. D. "Chronic Reactive Aggression in Survivors of Severe Persecution," *Comprehensive Psychiatry*, 12 (1971), 230–237.

30. ISKRANT, A. P., and P. V. JOLIET. *Accidents and Homicide*. Cambridge, Mass: Harvard University Press, 1968.

31. JACQUES, E. *Work, Creativity and Social Justice*, Chapter 9. New York: International Universities Press, 1970.

32. JONES, E. *The Life and Work of Sigmund Freud*, Vol. 1. New York: Basic Books, 1953.

33. KAHN, R. L. "Stress from 9 to 5," *Reflections*, 4 (1969), 39–47.

34. KARDINER, A. *War, Stress and Neurotic Illness*. New York: Hoeber, 1947.

35. ———. "Traumatic Neuroses of War," in S. Arieti, ed., *American Handbook of Psychiatry*, Vol. 1. New York: Basic Books, 1959.

36. KATZ, J. L., H. WEINER, T. F. GALLAGHER, and L. HELLMAN. "Stress, Distress, and Ego Defenses: Psychoendocrine Response to Impending Breast Tumor Biopsy," *Archives of General Psychiatry*, 23 (1970), 131–142.

37. KEISER, L. *The Traumatic Neurosis*. Philadelphia: Lippincott, 1968.

38. KERNBERG, O. "The Treatment of Patients with Borderline Personality Organization," *International Journal of Psycho-Analysis*, 49 (1968), 600–610.

39. KRISTAL, H., ed., *Massive Psychic Trauma*. New York: International Universities Press, 1968.

40. LEVINSON, H. *Executive Stress*. New York: Harper and Row, 1970.

41. LIFTON, R. J. "'Thought Reform' of Western Civilians in Chinese Communist Prisons," *Psychiatry*, 19 (1956), 173–195.

42. LUCAS, R. A. *Men in Crisis: A Study of a Mine Disaster*. New York: Basic Books, 1969.

43. MARTIN, M. "Psychologic Aspects of Nuclear Disaster," *Canadian Medical Association Journal*, 87 (1962), 1384–1386.

44. MASON, J. W. "Psychological Influence on the Pituitary-Adrenal Cortical System," *Recent Progress in Hormone Research*, 15 (1959), 345–353.

45. ———. "A Review of Psychoendocrine Research on the Pituitary-Adrenal Cortical System," *Psychosomatic Medicine*, 30 (1968), 576–607.

46. MCLEAN, A. A., ed. *To Work Is Human: Mental Health and the Business Community*. New York: Macmillan, 1967.

47. MENNINGER, W. C. *Psychiatry in a Troubled World*. New York: Macmillan, 1948.

48. RANGELL, L. "The Metapsychology of Psychic Trauma," in S. S. Furst, ed., *Psychic Trauma*. New York: Basic Books, 1967.

49. ROSS, T. A. *Lectures on War Neuroses*. London: Arnold, 1942.

50. ROSS, W. D. "Neuroses Following Trauma and Their Relation to Compensation," in S. Arieti, ed., *American Handbook of Psychiatry*, Vol. 3. New York: Basic Books, 1966.

51. ———. "Differentiating Compensation Factors from Traumatic Factors," in J. J. Leedy, ed., *Compensation in Psychiatric Disability and Rehabilitation*. Springfield, Ill.: Charles C Thomas, 1971.

52. ———. "The Emotional Effects of an Atomic Incident," *Cincinnati Journal of Medicine*, 33 (1952), 38–41.

53. RUFF, G. E. "Space Psychiatry," in S. Arieti, ed., *American Handbook of Psychiatry*, Vol. 3. New York: Basic Books, 1966.

54. SCHEIN, E. H. "Patterns of Reactions to Severe Chronic Stress in American Army Prisoners of War of the Chinese" in *Symposium No. 4: Methods of Forceful Indoctrination: Observations and Interviews*, pp. 253–269. New York: Group for the Advancement of Psychiatry, 1957.

55. SCHULZINGER, M. A. *The Accident Syndrome*. Springfield, Ill.: Charles C Thomas, 1956.

56. SELZER, M., and C. E. PAYNE. "Automobile Accidents, Suicide and Unconscious Motivation," *The American Journal of Psychiatry*, 119 (1962), 237–240.

57. SHAFER, R. *Aspects of Internalization*. New York: International Universities Press, 1968.

58. SIGAL, J. J., and V. RAKOFF. "Concentration Camp Survival: A Pilot Study of Effects on the Second Generation," *Canadian Psychiatric Association Journal*, 16 (1971), 393–397.

59. SOLOMON, G. F., V. P. ZARCONE, JR., R. YOERG, N. R. SCOTT, and R. G. MAURER. "Three Psychiatric Casualties from Vietnam." *Archives of General Psychiatry*, 25 (1971), 522–524.

60. SOLZHENITSYN, A. *One Day in the Life of Ivan Denisovich*. New York: Bantam Books, 1963.

61. SPERLING, O. E. "The Interpretation of the Trauma as a Command," *Psychoanalytic Quarterly*, 19 (1950), 352–370.

62. TITCHENER, J. L. "Management and Study of Psychological Response to Trauma," *Journal of Trauma*, 10 (1970), 974–980.

63. ———. "Psychological Aspects of Surgery," in A. M. Freedman and H. I. Kaplan, eds., *Comprehensive Textbook of Psychiatry*,

pp. 1130–1138. Baltimore: Williams and Wilkins, 1967.

64. TYHURST, J. S. "Individual Reactions to Community Disaster," *The American Journal of Psychiatry*, 107 (1951), 764–769.

65. WALLACE, A. F. C. "Tornado in Worcester: An Exploratory Study of Individual and Community Behavior in an Extreme Situation." Washington, D.C.: Committee on Disaster Studies, *Disaster Study No. 3*, National Academy of Sciences. National Research Council, Publication No. 392, 1956.

66. WARNES, H. "The Traumatic Syndrome," *Canadian Psychiatric Association Journal*, 17 (1972), 391–396.

67. WEISS, R. J., and H. E. PAYSON. "Personality Disorders IV: Gross Stress Reaction I," in A. M. Freedman and H. I. Kaplan, eds., *Comprehensive Textbook of Psychiatry*,

pp. 1027–1031. Baltimore: Williams and Wilkins Co., 1967.

68. WEST, L. J. "United States Air Force Prisoners of the Chinese Communists," in *Symposium No. 4: Methods of Forceful Indoctrination: Observations and Interviews*, pp. 270–284. New York: Group for the Advancement of Psychiatry, 1957.

69. WOLFENSTEIN, M. *Disaster: A Psychological Essay.* Glencoe, Ill.: Free Press, 1957.

70. WOLFF, C. T., M. A. HOFER, J. W. MASON, et al. "Relationship between Psychological Defenses and Mean Urinary 17-Hydroxycorticosteroid Excretion Rates: I A Predictive Study of Parents of Fatally Ill Children." *Psychosomatic Medicine*, 26 (1964), 576–591.

71. ZETZEL, E. R. *The Capacity for Emotional Growth*, Chapter 2. New York: International Universities Press, 1970.

CHAPTER 4

DEPRESSIVE NEUROSIS

Aaron T. Beck

❲ The Clinical Picture

DEPRESSION, one of the major health problems of today, is the most common psychiatric disorder treated in office practice and outpatient clinics. The study of depression is important, not only because of the human misery it causes, but because its by-product, suicide, is a leading cause of death in certain age groups.

Until the past century, depression was described under the label of "melancholia." In the second century A.D., Plutarch vividly described the melancholic as a man who "dares not employ any means of averting or of remedying the evil, lest he be found fighting against the gods." He drives away his friends and physician and "rolls naked in the dirt confessing about this and that sin."[227] Pinel, at the beginning of the nineteenth century, described the symptoms of depression as "taciturnity, a thoughtful pensive air, gloomy suspicions, and a love of solitude."[164]

These accounts are remarkably similar to modern textbook descriptions of depression. The symptoms used to diagnose depression today are found in the ancient descriptions of disturbed mood, self-blame, self-debasing behavior, wish to die, physical symptoms, and delusions of having committed unforgiveable sin.

There are few psychiatric disorders whose clinical descriptions are so constant throughout history. Because the disturbed feelings are usually a striking manifestation of depression, psychiatrists have generally tended to regard this condition as a "primary mood disorder." This designation is misleading, since there are many components of depression other than emotional deviation, and in some cases depressed patients do not report feeling sad or apathetic.

An individual who describes his mood as "depressed" may be referring to normal sadness. On the surface, pathological depression may appear to be an intense, exaggerated form of sadness accompanied by anorexia, insomnia, fatigue, and other symptoms. While depression is regarded by some authorities as a discrete disease entity based on biological disorder,[96] others believe that depression and sadness are two extremes on a continuum of mood reactions.[133]

The key factor in diagnosing depression is *change* in the psychobiological systems—changes involving emotion, motivation, cognition, physiology, and behavior.

A sample of 966 psychiatric patients was

studied by the Beck Depression Inventory and semi-structured interviews by experienced psychiatrists to determine the differentiating characteristics of depressed patients. The signs and symptoms listed below occurred from two to ten times more frequently among depressed than nondepressed patients.[10]

Emotional: Sadness or apathy; crying spells; self-dislike; loss of gratification; loss of feelings of affection; loss of sense of humor.

Cognitive: Negative self-concept; negative expectations; exaggerated view of problems; attribution of blame to self.

Motivational: Increased dependency; loss of motivation; avoidance; indecisiveness; suicidal wishes.

Physical and Vegetative: Loss of appetite; sleep disturbance; fatigability; loss of sexual interest.

Emotional changes

The emotional changes which accompany depression must be viewed in the context of the individual's premorbid behavior and mood level, as well as what might be considered the "norm" in the patient's age, sex, and social group. For example, crying spells in a patient who rarely cried before becoming depressed might point to a greater level of depression than it would in a patient who habitually cried even before the depression.

Beck found[10] that 88 percent of severely depressed psychiatric patients versus 23 percent of nondepressed psychiatric patients reported some degree of unhappiness or sadness. Though the dejected mood is sometimes couched in somatic terms, such as a lump in the throat or an empty feeling in the stomach, terms such as "miserable," "blue," or "downhearted" are generally used. Of course, individuals who are in no way clinically depressed may use these adjectives; the dejected mood may range from feelings of mild, transitory sadness to a profound feeling of hopelessness and worry. The *dysphoric* emotions may also stem from a patient's feelings about himself; that is, he may feel useless or disappointed in himself.

Loss of gratification, at first involving only a

few activities and later encompassing almost everything the patient does, is a distressing feature of depression. Social activities and biological drives are not spared. Saul[186] noted that demands from activities involving responsibility and productivity (for example, college assignments) may upset the "give-get balance." Initially, the imbalance may be corrected by recreational activities. In more advanced depressions, however, even passive, regressive activities fail to provide gratification.

Loss of gratification is usually accompanied by reduction of emotional attachments to other people or activities. A decline in the degree of affection for family members may worry a patient and cause him to seek professional help. Some patients have described this feeling as a "wall" between themselves and others. In some cases, love is replaced by apathy or resentment. In an analysis of suicide notes, Bjerg[20] reported that 81 percent of the writers had unfulfilled wishes (other than suicidal).

Depressed women in particular are likely to experience increased periods of crying. Some patients with recurrent depressions mark the onset of depression by a sudden impulse to weep. However, the severely depressed individual may find that he cannot cry even though he wants to.

Many depressed patients report that they have lost their sense of humor. Rather than having lost the ability to perceive the "punchline" of a joke, the depressed patient seems instead to have lost the ability to respond emotionally to humor; in short, he does not feel like laughing. Nussbaum and Michaux[144] found that their clinical ratings of improvement of depression correlated well with improvements in the affective response to riddles and jokes.

Cognitive Changes

Although thought disorders are traditionally associated with schizophrenia and paranoia, recent work has uncovered systematic distortions of reality in depression. These findings may cast doubt on the classification of depression as a primary mood disorder and may also provide clues for the treatment of the disease.[9]

The cognitive manifestations of depression include the patient's distorted views of himself, his world, and his future. I have called this group of thoughts the "cognitive triad."[11] Low self-evaluation, distortions of body image, negative expectations, self-blame, and indecisiveness are characteristic cognitive changes.

Depressed individuals view themselves as deficient in qualities that they consider important: popularity, intelligence, physical attractiveness, ability, or financial resources. This sense of personal inadequacy is reflected by complaints of deprivation of love or material possessions.[23] The depressed individual finds evidence of his own worthlessness in every experience and feels compelled to blame himself for his faults.

Pessimism and a gloomy outlook on life have been found to correlate highly with suicidal tendencies.[162,78,10] Depressed patients believe that their present state of deprivation is irreversible,[185] and 75 percent of them believe they will never recover.[33] A negative view of the self and the future was found to be highly correlated with depression and dissipated when the depression improved.[209] Engel[53] described the "helplessness-hopelessness" axis in depression—the patient cannot help himself and is unlikely to be helped by outside forces. Wohlford[224] found that depressed patients see the future as highly constricted.

The depressive blames adverse experiences on some deficiency within himself, and then he criticizes himself for having the alleged defect. In the severe state, he may view himself as a criminal or social leper and is prone to blame himself for events that are in no way connected with him. He makes statements such as, "I'm responsible for the violence and suffering in the world."

Vacillation, difficulty in making decisions, and changing decisions are also prominent in the depressive. Several factors contribute to the indecisiveness: (1) the patient anticipates making an incorrect decision, and (2) he would rather evade the situation than go through the mental operations required to make conclusions.

Another cognitive aberration is the patient's distorted image of his physical appearance. This characteristic is found more frequently in depressed women. The patient regards herself as ugly and repulsive, and she may even expect people to turn away from her in disgust.

Motivational Changes

The typical motivations of the depressed patient are "regressive" in nature. He seeks activities that are the least demanding for him (either in terms of the amount of energy required or the degree of responsibility involved). His wishes to escape may carry him to the point of suicidal wishes, and his desire to shun responsibility may lead him to abandon his family, friends, and vocation.

Another common manifestation of depression is the desire to withdraw from the routine things in life. The depressed person regards his tasks as boring and meaningless and wishes to seek refuge from them; thus, the housewife yearns to leave her daily chores, the clerk longs to get away from his paperwork, the student dreams of faraway places. To the severely depressed individual even the most elementary tasks, such as eating or taking medication, seem to be overwhelming. Although he is aware of what he should do, he does not experience any internal stimulus to do it. In short, a "paralysis of the will" sets in.

Increased dependency has also been noted in some depressed patients, and accentuation of dependency has been assigned a major etiological role in some theories of depression.[1,170] Dependency, in our sense of the word, refers to the desire for help rather than the process of relying on someone else. Receiving guidance appears to carry special emotional significance and is often gratifying to the depressive.

Physical and Vegetative Changes

Behavioral manifestations in themselves can often lead to a diagnosis of depression.[104]

Most persons who are depressed have sad facial expressions (though some may hide their feelings behind a cheerful mask in "smiling depression"), and women, in particular, tend to weep often. Another characteristic of the depressive is a stooped posture. In retarded depression, movements are slow and calculated, verbal output decreases, and the level of spontaneous actions diminishes. The severe state may even be characterized by stupor or semistupor. The agitated patient, on the other hand, is incessantly active and restless. While retardation appears to be a reflection of passivity, agitation seems to be a fight against actual and anticipated torture and pain.

Loss of appetite, which may result in substantial weight loss, loss of sexual responses, and sleep disturbance with early morning wakening, are also included in the physical and vegetative symptoms of depression. Loss of motivation and escapism seem to be associated with increased fatigue, which correlates highly with lack of gratification and pessimism.

The vegetative symptoms of depression are considered by some writers to be signs of "vital depression" and are viewed as evidence that a biological disorder is the basis of depression.[30,96] However, this theory may be erroneous, since the physical symptoms do not correlate well with each other or with the clinical ratings of the depth of depression. Furthermore, the somatic symptoms may be a manifestation rather than a cause of the disorder.

(Classification of Affective Forces

In the nomenclature of the American Psychiatric Association's *Diagnostic and Statistical Manual* (DSM-II),[6] involutional melancholia and manic-depressive illness are categorized as "major affective disorders." These two forms of depression are distinguished from the depressive neuroses and psychotic depressive reactions in that they do not seem to be precipitated by life stresses.

The diagnostic label "involutional melancholia" has practically disappeared from recent clinical reports and research, and DSM-II recommends that the diagnosis be given only if other types of affective illness do not apply. The other "major affective disorder" included in DSM-II is manic-depressive illness, which is subdivided into manic, depressed, and circular types. Extreme mood swings, recurrence, and remission characterize the illness. While the manic type consists exclusively of manic episodes with accelerated motor activity and speech, extreme elation, and irritability, the depressed type is marked by mental and motor inhibition. A patient with the circular type of manic-depressive illness may alternate between these two extremes and has experienced at least one manic and one depressive episode.

Perris[161] suggested that bipolar and unipolar depressive psychoses are two separate disorders. Manic and depressive phases characterize the bipolar cases, while the unipolar are marked by depressive episodes only. According to Perris, the two groups differed in terms of age, personality traits, course of illness, response to ECT, flicker threshold, and color-form preference.

Some writers have distinguished types of depression by the way patients react to external events. Gillespie[65] studied several groups of depressed individuals and labelled those who responded favorably to environmental influences as "reactive." The cases which showed no response to encouragement or favorable stimuli were labelled "autonomous." Another division is that of agitated vs. retarded depression. In this case, the disorder is classified according to the predominant activity level.

The unitary school does not believe in a sharp division between neurotic and psychotic depressions, or between reactive and endogenous depressions. These writers[111,191] maintain that the distinctions between the two groups are quantitative rather than qualitative in nature.

In the literature, there has been a tendency for psychotic depression to be associated with endogenous depression, while neurotic depression is associated with exogenous (reactive) depression. These distinctions have etiological connotations: endogenous refers to cases caused by some biological disorder, and exogenous refers to those caused by external stress. The former includes involutional melancholia and manic-depressive psychosis, and the latter consists of psychogenic, neurotic, or reactive depressions.

Factor Analyses of Depressive Phenomena

Many investigators believe that the isolation of "types" or subgroups of depression is necessary before the essential nature of affective disorders can be revealed. Some recent research has been directed to the question of whether the symptomatology of depression is unitary in nature, or whether it represents an intricate pattern of related but mutually exclusive syndromes.

The development of techniques for measuring depression has led to attempts to classify depressive phenomena by factor analysis. After quantitative scores on individual test items are intercorrelated and a correlation matrix is prepared, factors are rotated until they are isolated. In some cases, each isolated factor is tested for orthogonality (independence) and ranked according to the magnitude of factor loadings with respect to a particular test instrument. The so-called major factors are given unitary labels which are purported to imply clinical significance.

Several factor analyses of rating scales and depressive symptom inventories have been reported. Hamilton[77,76] factor-analyzed his depression scale and extracted six orthogonal factors, the first four of which he called "retarded depression," "agitated depression," "anxiety reaction," and "psychopathic depression."

Grinker et al.[74] studied the intercorrelations of checklists labeled "current behavior" and "feelings and concerns." The data yielded five factors from the feelings and concerns list and ten factors from the current behavior list. When all fifteen factors were combined, four patterns emerged which characterized depres-

sion as "retarded empty," "anxious," "hypochondriacal," or "angry."

The following orthogonal factors were reported by Overall:[147] (1) depression in mood; (2) guilt; (3) psychomotor retardation; (4) anxiety; (5) subjective experience of impairment in functioning; (6) extreme preoccupation with physical health; and (7) physical reaction to stress.

Another study of depressed patients yielded five orthogonal factors. Friedman et al.[61] described these factors as (1) "classical mood or affective depression with guilt, loss of esteem, doubting, and psychological internalizing;" (2) "retarded, withdrawn, apathetic depression;" (3) "a primarily biological reaction characterized by a loss of appetite, sleep disturbance, constipation, work inhibition and loss of satisfaction;" and (4) "oral demanding depression," which was defined as a "querulous hypochondriacal type."

Two factors were extracted in another factor analysis of a depressive symptoms checklist.[93] Besides a general factor of depression, the authors obtained a bipolar factor that distinguished between endogenous depression and exogenous (neurotic) depression. Carney et al.[31] later extracted a third factor called "paranoid psychotic." The bipolar factor was found to correlate highly with a "general factor of endogenous depression" reported by Rosenthal and Klerman.[180]

In a factor analysis of the Beck Depression Inventory,[40,212] four patterns were reported: (1) "guilty depression;" (2) "retardation;" (3) "somatic disturbance;" and (4) "tearful depression."

Other studies[173,174] used the Ward Behavior Rating Scale, the Inventory of Somatic Complaints, and a mood scale which was compiled by the researchers from several sources. Significant correlation clusters, such as "friendliness" and "carefree" were extracted, but seemed to be unrelated to depression. These clusters may indicate that a more well-defined list of factors is isolated with instruments which sample a wider range of behavioral traits.

Paykel[157] classified depressed individuals according to a special cluster analysis procedure. The findings indicated a hierarchy of groups. The first level consisted of two groups, one older and more severely depressed, and one younger and more mildly depressed. Subsequent division of these categories produced four approximate groups. One was characterized by severe illness and corresponded to psychotic depressives as described in the literature. A second group consisted of moderately depressed patients with high neuroticism scores and anxiety. The third group of depressives had a considerable element of hostility, and the last group, comprised of young patients, were mildly depressed with backgrounds of personality disorder.

The factor analytic studies described thus far have dealt with questionnaires, rating scales, and symptom inventories. Weckowicz et al.[213] have attempted to relate the factors obtained from intercorrelation of clinical evaluations, symptoms, and complaints, to measures of psychomotor and physical functions. Patients were administered the Beck Depression Inventory, objective psychomotor tests, the Shagass sedation threshold test, amount of salivation tests, and autonomic nervous system activity tests. Twenty first-order factors and six second-order factors were derived. Of the seven canonical correlations found, the first was a pattern of bodily complaints and somatization, and the second was a pattern of guilt, anxiety, and depressed mood. Two other patterns were indicated, the first consisting of psychomotor retardation with symptoms of atypical depression; the second characterized by psychomotor retardation with disturbance in the autonomic nervous system and typical depression. Two other canonical correlations emerged which suggested depression in an involutional setting with anxiety prominent in one pattern and guilt in the other.

❰ Course and Prognosis

The onset of depression is generally well defined. In most cases, the symptoms progressively increase in severity until they "bottom out" and then steadily improve until the episode is over. While the intervals between attacks are generally free of depressive symptoms, there is a trend toward recurrence.

Rates of complete recovery from affective disorders range from 80 to 95 percent.[120,176] Younger patients have the highest recovery rate—in one study,[120] 92 percent of patients less than thirty years of age recovered, while the rate was 75 percent in the thirty to forty age group.

Studies relevant to the duration of depressive episodes vary, partly because of differences in methodology and diagnostic criteria. Lundquist[120] found a median duration of 6.3 months in patients younger than thirty, and 8.7 months for those older than thirty. He reported no significant difference between men and women in regard to duration. Rennie's[176] results were similar: the first episode lasted an average of 6.5 months. The average duration of hospitalization, according to Rennie, was 2.5 months. Paskind[150,151,152] studied non-hospitalized depressives and found the median duration to be three months.

In regard to duration of multiple episodes of depression, earlier studies suggested that there is a tendency toward prolongation of episodes with each successive attack.[95] More recent studies by Paskind[152] and Lundquist[120] however, found no significant increase in duration with recurrences.

Variations relevant to frequency of recurrence among depressives are also reported in the literature. Rennie[176] found that 79 percent of hospitalized depressives subsequently had a relapse. Stenstedt [203]and Lundquist,[120] however, reported respectively, 47 percent and 49 percent incidence of recurrence. Rennie's more stringent diagnostic criteria probably account for his higher percentage of recurrences. In his series, more than half of the depressives had three or more relapses.

Recurrences of depressive episodes may occur after years of apparent good health; Kraepelin[95] reported a recurrence 40 years after recovery from an initial episode of depression. Rennie found that the highest percentage of relapses occurred ten to twenty years following the initial depression. Kraepelin found that with each successive relapse, the symptom-free intervals tended to become shorter. This trend was also observed by Paskind.[151,152]

Suicide

Depressive episodes may end in suicide; however, the actual risk of suicide among depressed patients is difficult to establish because of problems in determining cause of death. Rennie[176] and Lundquist[120] reported that approximately five percent of patients diagnosed as depressive later committed suicide. A more recent study[160] however, found that 14 percent of patients diagnosed as psychotic depressive died from suicide.

Pokorny[168] studied the suicide rate among former psychiatric patients in a Texas veterans' hospital. He found the suicide rate for depressed patients to be twenty-five times the expected rate and substantially higher than the rate among patients with other psychiatric disorders. Temoche et al.[205] found that the suicide rate for depressives was about three times higher than that of schizophrenics and alcoholics, and thirty-six times higher than that of the general population. The risk of suicide is greatest during weekend leaves from the hospital and shortly after discharge from the hospital. Temoche et al. reported that half of the suicides they studied occurred within eleven months after discharge.

The best indication of a suicidal risk appears to be the communication of suicidal intent.[178] Thus, the idea that the person who talks about suicide will never carry out his wishes is a fiction. In addition, an unsuccessful suicidal attempt greatly increases the chances of a successful attempt some time in the future.[135]

(Measurement of Depression

Rating scales and self-report measures can be extremely useful tools in the research and treatment of depression, especially when one considers the inherent difficulties in obtaining consistent diagnoses. One such scale, designed to measure the psychological, physiological, and behavioral manifestations of depression, was developed by Beck et al.[17] and factor-analyzed repeatedly.[43,46,163,40,212] Three studies[132,183,124] reported relatively high correlations between the Depression Inventory and clinicians' ratings of depression. The Depression Inventory discriminated among groups of patients with varying degrees of depression. The scale also reflects changes in the severity of depression following an interval of time.[17]

Similar scales have been reported by Hamilton,[76] Wechsler et al.,[215] and Zung.[228] Hamilton's scale has been used for assessing depression in medical inpatients,[189] and for measuring psychiatric inpatients' reactions to antidepressant medications.[103] Another scale by Humphrey[86] is a combination of some of Zung's items and some of his own, which were designed to assess functional disturbances resulting from depression, such as performance at work.

Some instruments which were developed to measure general pathology include items on depression. Examples are the Malamud-Sands Psychiatric Rating Scales,[122] the Minnesota Multiphasic Personality Inventory,[79] the Lorr Multi-Dimensional Scale,[117] and the Wittenborn Scales.[223] These general scales are usually considered inadequate for purposes of research or therapy in the specific area of depression. The MMPI, for example, is based on the old psychiatric nomenclature, and factor analytic studies reveal that its Depression Scale contains only one heterogeneous factor which is consistent with the clinical concept of depression.

Other instruments, such as the Lubin Scale[118] and the Clyde Mood Scale,[35] are examples of adjective checklists designed to measure depression alone or in combination with other mood states. One advantage of the Lubin Scale is the incorporation of a number of parallel versions.[119]

(Psychoanalytic Theories of Depression

The early psychoanalytic view of depression was primarily a description of the interaction between drives and affects, such as feelings of loss, guilt, and orality. In his writings of 1911[1] and 1916,[2] Abraham postulated that the depressive's capacity for affection is undermined by feelings of hatred and hostility brought about by unsatisfied sexual desires. Unable to love, the depressive's hostility is turned inward by means of reverse projection, i.e., "I am hated because of my defects." He tends to be irritable, seeks revenge, and feels intense guilt. In his later works, Abraham supported Freud's ideas regarding pregenital sexuality, and suggested that the refusal to eat could be explained by the unconscious wish to eat up the love object. To document his thesis, Abraham described several patients who continued to associate sexual gratification with the act of eating.

Freud's paper of 1917,[59] "Mourning and Melancholia," analyzes depression in analogy to normal grief. While both reactions may be the result of a lost love object, in melancholia the loss occurs within the ego. The depressive's hostility toward the lost love object is manifested in his self-accusations. The ego is identified with the abandoned object and feelings of aggression towards the object cause the melancholic to feel deep guilt. A marked decrease in self-esteem, which distinguishes depression from normal mourning, develops in an attempt to punish the incorporated object. The widely accepted role of "anger-in" in the development of depression is largely an outgrowth of Freud's concept of hostility turned inward.

Abraham[3] expands on some of Freud's formulations and draws upon his concept of the psychosexual stages of development. According to Abraham, the depressive's development is fixed at the oral stage, due to an inherited predisposition to oral eroticism and childhood disappointments in love. In his comparison of manic-depressive psychosis and obsessional neurosis, Abraham noted that the obsessional tries to retain his loved object while the melancholic expels the object which has disappointed him. The depressive may then try to repossess the lost object orally and sadistically punishes it within him.

Depression is described by Rado[170] as "a great despairing cry for love." He wrote that the depressive is an individual with a precarious self-concept and a narcissistic need for approval. When the love object is lost, the depressive's first reaction is that of rebellious anger; when the rebellion fails, he tries to recapture his self-esteem through the punishment of the ego by the superego. Because of his aggressive nature, the depressed individual believes that he is to blame for his loss; simultaneously, however, he blames the "bad part" of the love object in his ego. The internal conflict between the good and bad parts of the introjected object result in guilt and self-reproach.

Melanie Klein[94] theorized that predisposition to depression is rooted in the mother-child relationship in the first year of life, rather than in a series of traumatic experiences. The weak ego of the deprived infant is susceptible to sadness, helplessness, and frustration ("the depressive position"), and there is a failure to build up a strong self-concept independent of the mother's affection. Klein also depicted the dependent infant's unconscious fantasies of sadism.

While Rado described depression as a "cry for love," Fenichel[56] characterizes depressives as "love addicts," whose self-esteem is generated by external supplies. Depression is the attempt to coerce the orally incorporated object to return the supplies upon which self-esteem depends, and also to grant protection, forgiveness, security, and love. Like other psychoanalytic writers, Fenichel views depression in adults as a repetition of the "primal depression" in early childhood experience.

Recent psychoanalytic thinkers de-emphasize the drive theory and concentrate on the ego states. Bibring,[18] for example, emphasized the loss of self-esteem within the ego, and viewed helplessness to achieve goals as the primary characteristic of depression. According to Bibring, the disorder is the "emotional correlate of a partial or complete collapse of the self-esteem of the ego, since it feels unable to live up to its aspirations while they are strongly maintained." The three major areas of aspiration are the wish to be loved and valued, the desire to be strong and secure, and the wish to be loving and good. Depression results when these goals are not realized, and the conflict occurs within the ego rather than between the superego and the ego.

Edith Jacobson's ideas[88,89] are an outgrowth of Bibring's ego-centered views, with loss of self-esteem as the central feature of depression. She states that self-esteem represents the degree of discrepancy between "ego ideal" and "self-representation." In an attempt to delineate the nature of ego regression in depression, Jacobson theorized that early disappointment and its concomitant self-reproach occur in the early life of a depressive. The prepsychotic personality is extremely defensive and cannot tolerate disappointment. The depressive responds to hurt with denial; when this and other mechanisms fail, the self withdraws from reality and becomes helpless and childlike.

In his historical picture of psychoanalytic theories of depression, Gaylin[64] traced the emphasis on decreased self-esteem back to Freud's formulation of the lost love object. According to Gaylin, the loss of self-esteem is a loss of self-confidence which occurs with deprivation or disappointment.

Similarly, Engel[53] described the "giving-up–given-up complex," including these characteristics: (1) helplessness or hopelessness—the affects of giving up; (2) depreciated self-image; (3) lack of gratification from roles or relationships; (4) lack of continuity between past, present, and future; and (5) reactivation of memories of previous periods of giving up.

Relevant criticisms have been directed at some of the psychoanalytic theories described above. Mendelson,[131] for example, has pointed to their tendency to incorporate all psychological behavior into a single vast formula, thus overly simplifying a complicated problem. The formula is often derived from insufficient data, and the emphasis on very early childhood events is a shortcoming. Not enough attention is paid to events in later life, and empirical validation is scanty. Also, rather than using data to arrive at a theory, analysts have been prone to interpret data to support the a priori theory. One hypothesis in psychodynamics, however, has been subject to systematic study; namely, the relation of "object loss" to depression.

Parental Deprivation and Depression

Many authors have commented on the relationship between early parental separation and the subsequent development of depression. This area of research has been characterized by discrepancies among various studies; for example, the inclusion of endogenous or manic-depressive groups may color the findings. In addition, control data are often absent or inadequate since rates of childhood bereavement in the general population may vary widely.

Brown[26] found a significant relationship between parental deprivation (particularly paternal) in childhood and adult depression. Forty-one percent of the depressed adults he studied had lost a parent before the age of fifteen, while the incidence of orphanhood in England's general population was 12 percent. In a control group of 267 medical patients, the incidence of early orphanhood was 19.6 percent. However, the use of medical patients as controls in this and other studies has been questioned, since depressive symptoms are quite common in medical inpatients.[189]

In a group of 297 depressed patients studied to determine the relationship of orphanhood to depression, 27 percent of severely depressed patients were found to have lost a parent before age sixteen, while the nondepressed group had an incidence of 12 percent.[14]

Birk[19] compared 331 depressed outpatients with 296 medical patients and found a significantly greater number of orphans among the depressives. Dennehy[46] reported that depressed females had an excess of paternal loss while depressed males had an excess of maternal loss. Since Dennehy, Birk, and Brown used the 1921 British Census as their source of control data, the comparability of their controls to depressed patients has been questioned by Munro.[137]

Parent-child separation does not appear to be a significant factor in endogenous depression: Gay and Tonge[63] report that parental loss is more frequent in psychogenic than in endogenous depression. No comparison was made with normal controls. Hill and Price[81] compared depressives with other psychiatric patients; they report no excess of maternal loss, but a significant excess in paternal loss.

Munro[136] suggested that parental deprivation could be related to the *severity* of the depression. This finding was also reported by Wilson, Alltop, and Buffaloe.[219]

These positive findings seem impressive, but there have been studies which failed to establish any significant relationship between separation and depression. Pitts et al.[165] found no significant association between psychiatric illness and childhood bereavement; however, problems arise in the interpretation of this study, due to the aforementioned problems of using medical inpatients as control. It would be necessary, in these cases, to control for the presence of depression in non-psychiatric groups.

A systematic comparison of psychiatric diagnoses and parental loss was made by Gregory[72] using MMPI high points and clinical diagnoses. No significant correlation between any diagnostic group and parental loss was established. Negative findings have also been reported by Brill and Liston.[25]

In a study of 152 depressed patients matched with controls, Abraham and Whitlock[4] found no significant difference in childhood loss of one or both parents. The authors claim that it was not the physical loss of the parent, but rather the poor interaction between child and parent or between both parents that may have caused the depression.

Further research is necessary before the etiological relationship of parental loss in childhood to adult depression can be definitely established.

Life Stress and Depression

Much of the literature on depression has attempted to assess the relationship between life events and depression. While Freud[59] attributed depression to the loss of a loved object, Bibring emphasized the loss of self esteem in his theory of depression.[18] More recently, other investigators[180,128] have attempted to define as endogenous those depressions that occur without an actual loss.

Since we have little satisfactory data regarding the incidence of stressful life events in the general population, carefully controlled studies in this area have been scarce. The following three groups of authors have used medical inpatients as control groups: Forrest et al.,[58] Hudgens et al.,[84] and Morrison et al.[134]

Forrest et al. compared 158 depressives with 58 controls. In the three years prior to hospitalization, depressed patients had an excess of stress factors. Hudgens and associates compared 40 hospitalized depressives with 40 hospitalized medical controls and found stressful events to be infrequent in the six months preceding onset of illness. Since patients were excluded if their symptoms disappeared in a few days with the removal of stress, a selective definition of depression was used. A later study by the same group of authors[134] also found few differences between the depressed group and the control group. However, these findings may be questioned, due to the fact that life events are frequently associated with other physical illnesses,[171,172] and depression occurs among medical inpatients.[189]

While the three studies mentioned above used medical controls, Paykel et al.[158] used controls from the general population. On the average, the depressed group reported almost three times as many life stresses in the six months preceding onset of illness as did the controls. Paykel's findings suggest that certain kinds of events on the Holmes and Rahe Social Readjustment Rating Scale,[83] such as increase in arguments with spouse, marital separation, new job, etc., are more likely than others to occur prior to a depressive episode. Exits from the social field preceded clinical depression significantly more frequently than did entrances. Desirable events (marriage, promotion, engagement) were more common in the control group than in the depressives. The familiar psychoanalytic theme of a lost love object, then, is supported by these findings.

❲ Cognitive Theories of Depression

Depression may be viewed in terms of the activation of three major cognitive patterns that lead the individual to see himself, his surroundings, and his future in an idiosyncratic manner. The content of these patterns revolves around the themes of loss and deprivation.

The first component of the "cognitive triad" is the negative view of self: deprived, defective, or defeated. The depressed individual regards himself as lacking in gratification, inadequate, or worthless. He believes that he is undesirable and rejects himself because of his alleged defects. The second component is the negative view of experiences. The patient interprets all of his interactions with his environment as representative of deprivation and defeat. Finally, the negative view of the future permeates his ideation. As he looks ahead, the patient sees an indefinite continuation of his present difficulties and a life of unremitting deprivation, frustration, and hardship.

The other phenomena of depression may be considered as consequences of the activation of the negative cognitive patterns. The affective group of depressive symptoms (feeling sad, hopeless, lonely, bored) can be analyzed in terms of these negative concepts. If a patient simply *thinks* he is being rejected, he will react with the same negative affect that occurs with actual rejection. Similarly, if the individual believes he is a social outcast, he will feel lonely.

The motivational changes in depression (paralysis of the will, suicidal wishes, increased dependency, and escapist and avoidance wishes) are also related to cognition. "Paralysis of the will" may be considered as a result of the patient's pessimism and hopelessness; since he expects a negative outcome, he is reluctant to commit himself to a goal or undertaking. Conversely, when he is persuaded that he can succeed at a particular task, he may be stimulated to pursue it.

Avoidance and escapist wishes are also outcomes of the negative expectations. Suicidal wishes are an extreme expression of the desire to escape from what appear to be insoluble problems or an unbearable situation. Since he sees himself as a worthless burden, the depressed patient believes that everyone, including himself, will be better off when he is dead.

Increased dependency may also be attributed to negative concepts. The patient sees himself as inept and undesirable; he tends to overestimate the difficulty of normal tasks in life, and expects things to turn out badly. Under these circumstances, many patients yearn for help from other persons whom they consider to be strong.

Some of the physical correlates of depression may be related to cognitive patterns. Profound motor inhibition appears to be associated with the negative view of the self. When a patient can be encouraged to initiate an activity, however, the retardation and the subjective sense of fatigue are reduced.

How does an individual form the concepts that predispose him to depression? Early in life, a child develops many attitudes about himself and his surroundings. Some of these concepts are realistic and facilitate healthy adjustment, while others deviate from reality and make the individual vulnerable to possible psychological disorders.

Since the formation of the three types of concepts central to depression (those regarding the self, the world, and the future) is similar, we can use the example of self-concepts as a model for the other two.

An individual's self-concepts are clusters of favorable and unfavorable attitudes derived from his personal experiences, from his identification with significant others, and from the attitudes of others towards him. Once a particular concept is formed, it may influence subsequent judgments. Each negative judgment, for instance, tends to reinforce the negative attitude toward the self. Thus a cycle is set up. If this negative concept persists, it becomes an enduring structure in the individual's cognitive organization.

The vulnerability of the depression-prone individual is a result of these enduring negative concepts. Although the schemas may be latent at a given time, they are activated by particular kinds of circumstances and consequently may lead to a full-blown depression. Situations reminiscent of the experience responsible for embedding a negative attitude may trigger a depression. For instance, disruption of a marital situation may light up the idea of an irreversible loss that followed death of a parent in childhood.

Situations that lower a person's self-esteem (such as failing an examination or being fired from a job) are frequent precipitators of depression. Another type of precipitating event involves thwarting of important goals or confrontation with an "insoluble" problem. Depression may also be triggered by a physical abnormality or disease that activates the notion that the patient can never have a happy life.

While any of these circumstances might be painful to the average person, they would not cause a depression, unless the person is particularly sensitive to the situation because of his specific predepressive constellation. While a normal individual may experience such a trauma and be able to maintain interest in other aspects of life, the depression-prone person experiences such a constriction of his cognitive field that he is hit by negative ideas about everything in life. It should be noted that depression is often the result of a series of stressful situations rather than one particular situation.

Depressions, as they occur in the preceding description, are due to *specific stress* situations. However, an individual may develop a depression when exposed to a *nonspecific stress* situation of overwhelming proportion, or a series of traumatic events. Depending on the content of the predisposing factors, stress situations may lead to depression or to other pathological reactions, such as paranoid reaction, psychosomatic disorders, etc., or no psychological disorder at all.

To clarify further the relationship between cognition and affect, it is necessary to explore how depressive thinking becomes dominant, and why the patient seems to cling to his pain-

ful attitudes, despite the evidence of positive factors in his life.

In conceptualizing any life situation composed of many stimuli, an individual extracts certain aspects and combines them into a specific pattern. Different people reach dissimilar conclusions, but a particular individual tends to be consistent in his responses to similar types of events.

A cognitive *structure* is a more or less permanent component of the cognitive organization, while a cognitive *process* is transient. The term "schema" has been generally used in the literature on cognition. A schema is used for screening out, differentiating, and coding the stimuli that confront the individual. Through the matrix of schemas, he orients himself in relation to space and time, and categorizes and evaluates his experiences. When a person is faced by a particular stimulus, a schema related to the stimulus is activated. The data are molded into cognitions, which are defined as any mental activity with verbal content. A schema may be applied to a small pattern involved in a concrete conceptualization, such as tying a shoelace, or to large patterns, such as self-concepts or prejudice.

Although a schema may be inactive at a given time, it is activated when energized. A specific schema can be energized or de-energized by rapid changes in the environmental inputs. The content of a schema is usually a generalization relating to the individual's goals, values, and attitudes. From an analysis of the individual's style of structuring different experiences, from his free associations, his daydreams and dreams, and his responses to psychological tests, we may infer the content of a schema.

A depressed patient's ideation is marked by typically depressive themes. As the depression deepens, his thought content is increasingly saturated with these ideas, even though there may be no logical connection between the actual situation and the interpretation. This cognitive impairment is due to idiosyncratic schemas which assume a dominant role in the thought processes of a depressed individual.

The systematic errors which lead to distortion of reality in depressed patients include arbitrary interpretation, selective abstraction, exaggeration, incorrect labeling, and over-generalization. The orderly matching of stimulus and schema is upset by the intrusion of the overactive idiosyncratic schemas which displace the more appropriate schemas. As the idiosyncratic schemas become more active, they are evoked by stimuli less congruent with them; the reality situation is distorted to fit the schema. The patient loses control over his thinking processes and is unable to energize other more appropriate schemas.

In the milder stages of depressive illness, the patient may be able to view his negative thoughts with objectivity, but in the more severe stages, he finds it difficult to even consider the idea that his interpretations might be erroneous. This loss of objectivity may be explained by the fact that the stronger idiosyncratic schemas tend to interfere with the cognitive structures involved in reality-testing and reasoning.

The activated schemas have a direct relationship to the affective response to a situation. If the content is relevant to being deserted, thwarted, undesirable, or negligent in one's duties, the schemas will produce, respectively, feelings of loneliness, frustration, humiliation, or guilt.

The formulation of a feedback model can provide a more complete explanation of depressive phenomena. This system operates as follows: An unpleasant life situation triggers schemas related to loss, negative expectancies, and self-blame. These schemas produce a stimulation of the affective structures connected to them once they are activated. The activation of the affective structures, in turn, further energizes the schemas to which they are connected. In phenomenological terms, the depressive's negative ideation leads to sadness; he labels the sadness as a sign that his life is painful and hopeless. These negative interpretations of the affect further reinforce his negative attitudes. Hence, a vicious cycle is produced.

A cognitive formulation presented by Lichtenberg in 1957[112] hypothesized that depression is the result of felt hopelessness to achieve one's goals when the individual blames himself for the failure. In this case, hope was defined as "the perceived probability of success with respect to goal attainment." Lichtenberg believed that neurotic, agitated, and retarded depressions were each related to a specific type of goal—an expectancy associated with the particular situation, an expectancy associated with a style of behavior, or an expectancy associated with a generalized goal. In each type of depression, the hopelessness is placed in the context of phenomena such as interpersonal relations, perceptions of secondary gains and losses, time perspective, and perception of personal responsibility.

Cognitive Studies of Depression

Beck and Valin[15] reported that ideas of self-punishment were extremely frequent in the delusions and hallucinations of psychotic depressives. A pilot study by Beck and Hurvich[13] and a more comprehensive study by Beck and Ward[16] revealed higher incidences of "masochistic dreams" in depressed patients than in nondepressed patients. These dreams were identified as those which included themes of thwarting, rejection, punishment, disappointment, injury, personal unattractiveness, etc.

Rather than ascribe these "masochistic dreams" to the Freudian notion of the patient's need to suffer, the conclusion of these studies was that the depressive actually pictured himself as a "loser." He regarded himself as deprived of an important source of gratification and as defective in certain important attributes. It was also found[10] that early memories, various self-ratings, and responses to pictorial stimuli were pervaded by the concept of loss. A Focused Fantasy Test[8] presented sets of drawings in which one twin has a pleasant experience and the other is a "loser." Depressed patients identified more frequently with the "loser" twin than did a nondepressed group of patients.

Another study of self-concept in depression was conducted by Laxer,[99] who showed that depressed patients were characterized by low self-esteem and self-blame. Laxer[100] compared depressives with other psychiatric patients; depressives showed a lower self-concept on being admitted to a hospital, but their self-concept improved more at discharge. Plutchik et al.[167] asked manic-depressive patients to describe their ideal self, their least-liked self and their normal self on a forced choice test of emotions. They found that the emotion profile for the depressed state correlated highly with the least-liked self.

One hypothesis derived from the work of Lichtenberg and Beck is that a successful experience will improve certain depressive symptoms such as low mood, pessimism, and low self-esteem. Loeb et al.,[116] for example, devised a study which involved the manipulation of success and failure with a verbal task. After a success experience, the depressed group showed a greater increase in level of aspiration, level of mood, and expectations of success, as compared with nondepressed subjects. In addition, the depressed group's scores on these indices decreased after failure. In a later study,[115] it was reported that the depressed patients' performance on a subsequent task improved more after success than did the performance of nondepressed subjects.

When a depressed patient believes that he will fail in every undertaking, apathy sets in; thus, cognitive distortions may explain the motivational as well as emotional manifestations of depression. If the depressive sees himself as inept and unable to meet his responsibilities, he may engage in escapism or become overly dependent on others. Loeb et al.[116] found that depressed patients who were led to believe that their performance on a given task was inferior to others were less motivated to volunteer for the experiment again. The lack of motivation may also be related to psychomotor retardation.

The existence of a thinking disorder in depression has been supported by systematic studies. Two such studies[184,68] demonstrated an impairment of abstract conceptualization, while Neuringer[141] pointed out rigid thinking in depressives. The tendency of depressed individuals to think in bipolar opposites (dichotomous thinking) was also reported by Neuringer.[140,142,143]

The concept that the depressed patient has a negative view of the future and low self-esteem was supported by a systematic study.[209] These negative concepts disappeared when the patient recovered from his depression. Melges and Bowlby[126] reported time constriction in depression, and more recently, Melges et al.[125] have reported a high correlation between self-esteem and optimism.

(Behavioral Theories of Depression

Behaviorally oriented writers have only recently presented their concepts of depression. Ferster[57] asserted that the loss of a "significant other" causes a sudden reduction in the output of behavior and a decreased rate of positive reinforcement. He also observed the tendency of depressives to restrict the number of persons with whom they interact; this tendency makes the depressed individual especially vulnerable to the loss of a loved person or object.

Lazarus[102] proposed that depressions which could not be explained by learning theory principles are probably organic in nature. He viewed depression as a "function of inadequate or insufficient reinforcers." Thus, therapy should help the depressive to take advantage of all available reinforcers or provide a change in the reinforcement schedule. This recommendation is similar to an approach outlined by Burgess;[28] the therapy is based on the S-R model and has as its goal the extinction of depressive behavior.

According to Patterson and Rosenberry,[153] an individual is predisposed to depression if he lacks social skills. Since he has fewer available sources of reinforcement, loss of a source is a greater deprivation for him than for the socially skilled person. In addition, the individual lacking in social skills finds it more difficult to replace a lost reinforcer.

Personal characteristics, such as a lack of social skills, or environmental factors may cause the low rate of positive reinforcement, according to a recent study.[110] Testing the hypothesis that depressed individuals are lacking in social skills, the authors reported that depressed individuals interact with fewer people than do nondepressed individuals; depressives also emit shorter messages which are often timed inappropriately. A therapeutic approach was designed by these researchers to positively reinforce constructive behaviors and social skills, while negatively reinforcing depressive behaviors.

Ullmann and Krasner[208] view depression as occurring when previously reinforced behavior no longer results in reinforcement. For example, when a person ages, his role status changes and his rate of positive reinforcement is reduced. The claim that depressive behavior itself stimulates positive reinforcement in the form of kindness and sympathy is contradictory to the position[110] that depressive behavior alienates other people.

The behavior theorists have been criticized for their neglect of the subjective components of depression, such as sadness, hopelessness, and suicidal wishes. In addition, much of the data used to substantiate various behavioral concepts has been contradictory. In general, behavior theory has been applied only to limited aspects of the phenomena of depression.

❨ Sociological and Demographic Aspects of Depression

Sex

Most studies have shown that depression is approximately twice as frequent in females than in males.[191] Recent studies have revealed that the peak years for women with reactive depression are earlier than those for men and occur prior to menopause.[92] In terms of endogenous depression, Watts[211] found the peak age for women to be concurrent with the menopause, while in men it appears much later.

In a study with medical inpatients, it was found[190] that only slightly more females are depressed and that definite sex-related profiles of depression emerge. Findings indicated that females tend to somatize, while males refer more often to feelings of personal despair.

One interesting feature of studies which attempt to relate depression and sex is that depression is more common in women, but that suicide is more frequent in men. High morbidity with low mortality in women, and low morbidity with high mortality in men has been observed in other health fields.[49]

Age

Traditionally, depression has been considered an illness of the middle-aged and elderly. It is thought to be rare in infancy and childhood, first appearing clinically in adolescence, reaching its greatest proportions in middle years, and declining to some extent in the later years.[198] In recent years, however, greater attention is being paid to depression in young adults because of a rising suicide rate in persons of this age.[47]

Although depression is thought to occur more frequently in older persons, Redlich and Freedman[175] wrote that depression may be found in all age groups and is not uncommon in young adults. Other studies have found the peak age for reactive depression to be between twenty-six and forty.[92]

The factor of age is important because it may influence the diagnosis of psychotic affective disorders and, thus, the reported age distributions of these conditions.[198] Schizophrenia, for example, is often thought of as a disease afflicting younger persons, while depression is considered an ailment of the middle-aged and elderly.

Race

Stainbrook[202] noted that as far back as 1895 melancholia was relatively uncommon in blacks. In the 1963 fiscal year, reports from all mental hospitals, psychiatric clinics, and psychiatric services of general hospitals in Maryland showed the rates for all mental disorders *except* the affective disorders to be higher among blacks than among white groups.[139]

There have been discrepancies in studies which compare rates of depression in whites and blacks. One[55] found no great racial differences in depressed individuals of different races except for the low percentage of blacks with the depressed type of manic-depressive psychosis. Another[206] studied 220 depressed patients in New Haven and found no significant difference in the incidence of depression among blacks and whites, nor in the symptomatology.

Prange[169] compared the incidence of depression among blacks and whites in the northern and southern United States, and found that southern Negroes have the lowest rates of all the groups. He believes that the incidence of depression in southern blacks will rise as urbanization and the disruption of local cultural patterns occur. McGough et al.[121] studied the changing patterns of mental illness among blacks in the South and predicted a rise in reported frequency of depression as treatment facilities become more accessible to blacks.

Social Class

Class studies of frequency of depression are relatively recent. Hollingshead and Redlich[82] found that the psychotic depressions were two and a half times more frequent in the lower classes than in the upper, while neurotic depressions were twice as common in the upper. The Midtown Manhattan Study of symptom prevalence in the general population[98] reported a consistent inverse correlation between social class and depressive illness.

Marital Status

It is commonly thought that psychiatric disorders occur more frequently among the unmarried. However, most studies show that depression, unlike the other psychiatric illnesses, is more common in married individuals.[191] In a study of neurotic depressive women in psychiatric hospitals, Briggs[24] found that more were married than the general population. Schwab et al.[189] found that depression was almost twice as frequent in the married as compared with the unmarried.

Ethnic Group

It is important to be cautious in interpreting the vast amount of literature on mental illness in peoples of various cultures. Observations in these studies are often impressionistic and misleading because of discrepancies in form and content of mental conditions and also societal attitudes towards psychiatric disorders.[198]

A study of the Hutterites[51] is of particular interest because of the isolation of these colonies and the small degree of intermarriage. The Hutterites are an Anabaptist group with marked religious restrictions who live in the Dakotas and central Canada. The study found that manic-depressive illness was four times as frequent as schizophrenia in these communities. However, this high frequency may be due to inbreeding, which increases the chances of any genetic factors emerging. In addition, prevalence rates decreased significantly when cases active at the time of survey were separated from recovered cases.

Murphy et al.[138] conducted a questionnaire survey of psychiatrists around the world. He concluded that the frequency of depression does not appear to be related to religion, culture, social class, etc., but rather to the cohesiveness of the community. It must be noted, however, that the methodological shortcomings of this study make it extremely difficult to accept these findings.

Another ethnic study[34] refers to the "air of mild depression that pervades Japanese life" and the high number of suicides in that country, most of which occur between the ages of fifteen and twenty-four.

Depressive disorder was thought to be virtually nonexistent on the African continent until the 1950s. In a review of the literature on the incidence of depression in various parts of Africa, Collomb[37] found incidence rates which varied from 1.1 percent to 15 percent; the discrepancies are due to methodological differences in the studies.

A study of the Yoruba of western Nigeria[106] found many of the symptoms of depression, even though the illness itself was unknown there. In Ghana, comparatively high rates of hospitalized manic-depressives, depressives, non-hospitalized depressives, and attempted suicides have been observed.[214] Depression is also reported to be common in Ethiopia.[207]

Biological Approaches to Depression

Kraines[97] has presented an elaborate theory which stresses the role of biological disorder in the development of depression. He infers that the frequency of depressive attacks in later life, and the occurrence of post-partum and premenstrual depressions are due to hormonal changes. In addition, a physiological basis is suggested because depression may occur in personalities that appear to be well-adjusted. The symptoms, onset, and course of the illness are basically identical in most patients, despite radical differences in culture, status, etc.

Other evidence that seems to confirm the possibility of biological disorder in depression consists in: (1) the beneficial results of physical therapies (ECT and drugs); (2) seasonal peaks of onset in the spring or fall; (3) the precipitation of depression in certain individuals by the administration of large doses of phenothiazines.

The role of the hypothalamus is central to Kraines's theory. Depression occurs when the cerebral cortex stimulates the hypothalamus, which in turn excites the somato-visceral system. The feedback from this system is further integrated in the thalamus and limbic system and stimulates the reticular system. The impulses terminate in the cerebral cortex. Kraines believes that mood is derived from this "emotional circuit" and that pathology of the hypothalamus is responsible for manic-depressive illness. Psychopathological symptoms are secondary in this theory, and are considered to be a defense induced by the physiopathology of the diencephalon.

Kraines's theory, however, is based on fragmentary and questionable evidence. Genetic studies have not clearly delineated the role of heredity in depression; no consistent hormonal abnormalities, except for steroid excretion, have been found; and much of his evidence may also be interpreted to support a psychogenic explanation of depression.

Despite the tremendous amount of research that has attempted to delineate the relationship between depression and biological disorder, there is little solid knowledge of the specific biological correlates of depression. Initial positive results have not been replicated in many cases, and methodological shortcomings often cast doubt on the original findings.

Some studies have been concerned with depression and autonomic function. Funkenstein[62] demonstrated a relationship between depression and blood pressure reactivity by measuring the response in blood pressure to an injection of Mecholyl. However, more precise measures, proper controls, and blind ratings are necessary before these findings can be unequivocally accepted.

Other studies have been conducted to determine whether there is any evidence of a decrease in salivary secretion among depressed individuals.[204,159,29,42,148] While most of these findings were positive, longitudinal studies[70] show a discrepancy; once again, better controls are needed to fully interpret the results.

In the area of neurophysiology, one group of studies has attempted to determine the sedation threshold of depressed patients.[194, 5,145,60] This work has yielded contradictory data, and no solid evidence has supported the hypothesis that there is a significant difference between the sedation thresholds of neurotic and psychotic depressives.

Electromyograph (EMG) studies[216,217,67] measured the muscle action of depressed patients and found that mute and retarded patients show increased muscular activity. In contrast, Rimon et al.[177] found an inverse correlation between muscle tension and severity of depression. Larger samples and control for age are necessary before definite conclusions may be reached.

Studies of the sleep EEG's of depressed patients show that they tend to have excessive periods of light or restless sleep, a shorter period of total sleep, and are more sensitive to noise when asleep.[48,146,229,73,130,129] These studies are hampered by the use of normal controls instead of nondepressed psychiatric patients and the small number of patients used in each study.

Contradictory results have been obtained in studies of the reactivity of the central nervous system in depression. EEG arousal response studies[156,195,220,218] found an increased threshold for external stimulation during depression and a reduction in the threshold on recovery. Many of these findings have methodological inadequacies, and their findings have been contradicted by one study.[50]

There is some evidence that genetics may predispose an individual to depression. By examining the rates of depression among pairs of identical twins, Kallmann[90] found that 22 of 23 twins of patients with manic-depressive illness were also diagnosed as manic-depressive. However, the usefulness of this study is decreased by methodological problems. Slater[200] found a 57 percent concordance rate for fraternal twins, but his sample was even smaller than Kallmann's. Shields[196] compared identical twins reared together with those reared separately. He found that concordance rates for the separated and nonseparated twins were the same for cyclothymic features, anxiety traits, emotional lability, and rigidity, though none of his results were significant statistically.

Another technique used to determine the influence of heredity in affective disorder is to assess the incidence of the illness in children of psychotic parents. Elsasser[52] found that 33 of 47 children of such parents were normal. However, since his cases were drawn from a wide variety of sources, the diagnoses are inconsistent and consequently unreliable.

Family studies have also been used to determine the role of genetics in depression. Stenstedt[203] found a 15 percent incidence of manic-depressive illness in the parents, siblings, and children of 288 manic-depressive patients. The estimated morbidity risk for the general population was 1 percent. Winokur[221] found that alcoholism and affective disorder were significantly more frequent in the first-generation relatives of patients with affective disorder than in a group of controls. Comparing patients whose families had a history of affective illness, Winokur found that almost all of the manic patients belonged to the former

group. He also found that daughters of depressed mothers were more likely than sons to be depressed. No such finding occurred in the sons or daughters of depressed fathers.

Biochemical Studies

The study of the biochemistry of depression has been difficult because the tissue of interest —the brain of the depressed individual— cannot be chemically examined. Instead, concentrations of compounds active in brain metabolism must be indirectly estimated by measuring their concentrations in body fluids, usually urine or blood. Many tissues other than the brain contribute to the total concentration of the compounds of interest in body fluids, and thus urine or blood levels do not necessarily offer an accurate index of the amounts of these compounds in the central nervous system.

In general, when a biochemical basis is sought for a particular disorder, it is expected that there will be a single, unique biochemical explanation. In work on the biochemistry of depression, this assumption has tacitly not been made. Studies in the field have not sought (nor found) a "depressed range" for some biochemical parameter in which all individuals diagnosed as depressed will score, and in which normal control groups will not score. Rather, these studies have looked for overlapping depressed–normal ranges in which there is nonetheless a statistically significant difference between the two groups for the particular parameter. Such statistically significant differences in overlapping ranges clearly do not offer an immediate possibility for a unique biochemical explanation of depression. However, searching for statistical biochemical differences seems both valid and necessary at this time, given the possible heterogeneity of disorders and diagnostic categories in depression, and the statistical (rather than consistent) effectiveness of antidepressant drugs.

The most extensive work done in recent years on the biochemistry of depression has attempted to test the "catecholamine hypothesis." This hypothesis proposes that in depression there is a depletion of catecholamines (particularly norepinephrine) functioning at adrenergic receptor sites in the brain. In mania, functional brain catecholamine levels are hypothesized to be elevated. The catecholamine hypothesis was originally suggested on the basis of studies of the biochemical effects of antidepressant drugs (MAO inhibitors, tricyclics) in animals. A very considerable amount of data has now been collected on catecholamine levels in humans.

Urinary excretion studies have resulted in a variety of findings. Early studies showed that urinary norepinephrine and epinephrine were lowered in depression.[187] However, Curtis et al.[41] found increased norepinephrine levels in depressed patients (though mainly those with agitated or anxious depressions). Similarly, Bunney et al.[27] found elevated urinary norepinephrine in psychotic but not neurotic depression. Normetanephrine and 3-methoxy-4-hydroxy-phenylglycol (MHPG), two metabolic products of norepinephrine, were shown to be low in the urine of depressed patients and to increase as the depression improved.[188,71]

Plasma concentrations of catecholamines were measured by a sensitive new technique in a recent study.[225] It presented convincing data that plasma levels of catecholamines correlated well with anxiety ratings for the patient, but the correlation with depression ratings was not significant. Epinephrine has not been found in the brain of humans, and norepinephrine does not cross the blood-brain barrier in either direction.[66] Thus, the measurement of epinephrine and norepinephrine in the blood or urine probably has little relevance to the catecholamine hypothesis, which states that catecholamines are depleted in the central nervous system. The levels of normetanephrine or MHPG in urine may or may not reflect central nervous system noradrenaline turnover,[187] so these levels (which are decreased in depression) are also of unproved relevance.

Concentrations of noradrenaline have been determined in the *cerebrospinal fluid* by Dencker et al.[44] Their study did not present a statistical treatment of the data, but did show a mean noradrenaline level in depressed patients three times higher than the mean in a control group. (The control group of four subjects was unfortunately small).

Post-mortem examination of the brains of individuals committing suicide has been done by two different groups.[149,22] Both groups found noradrenaline levels in the suicides comparable to those in the same brain areas of control groups that had died of a variety of physical illnesses. Bourne et al.[22] discuss limited reasons to believe that amine levels have not changed drastically from the moment of death to the time of assay (an average of six months), but neither study presents convincing arguments that body storage, brain removal, freezing, long-term storage, and thawing of brain samples do not significantly alter noradrenaline concentrations.

Precursor administration to depressed patients has been attempted in the thorough study by Goodwin et al.[69] The immediate precursor of brain catecholamines is L-DOPA, an amino acid which can cross the blood-brain barrier. L-DOPA has been successfully used in the treatment of Parkinson's disease, in which dopamine levels are known to be lowered. In the experiments of Goodwin et al. only 4 of 16 depressed patients showed clinical improvement on high doses of L-DOPA, and one of these may have undergone spontaneous remission. The authors suggest that the improvement may have been the result of L-DOPA causing psychomotor activation. They also point out that on the basis of animal studies, even the high dosage of L-DOPA they gave the patients might be expected to change centrally functioning noradrenaline levels only slightly. Dopamine levels would be raised to a greater extent, but in some part the dopamine increase might be localized in capillary walls. Thus, there are also expected weaknesses in this method (precursor load) of examining the catecholamine hypothesis.

In summary, the catecholamine hypothesis is difficult to definitively test. Measurements have been made of catecholamines (and their metabolic products) in blood, urine, cerebrospinal fluid, and stored brain slices. However, the relationship of these measurements to the actual concentration of catecholamines functioning as neurotransmitter in the brain has not been established.

The catecholamine hypothesis has given rise directly to two other important lines of research. The first concerns urinary concentrations of the nucleotide cyclic 3', 5'-adenosine monophosphate (cAMP) in depressed patients. Catecholamines are known in many tissues to activate the enzyme adenyl cyclase which catalyzes the production of cAMP. A recent study has shown that cAMP levels in urine are statistically low in severely depressed patients and high in manic patients. Furthermore, the values return toward normal upon clinical improvement.[155] The same group of authors has also reported that urinary cAMP dramatically rose in seven patients on the day of a switch from depression to mania.[154] They suggest that rapid cAMP elevation may be a "trigger" for a sustained metabolic process responsible for mania. Although these authors claim that physical activity does not significantly affect urinary cAMP concentrations, this point is controversial. Furthermore, it is unknown to what extent urinary cAMP levels reflect central nervous system cAMP levels. Another group has reported normal cAMP concentration in the cerebrospinal fluid from depressed and manic patients.[179]

Some investigators, considering that imipramine and MAO inhibitors increase other amine levels, have broadened the catecholamine hypothesis to a more general hypothesis, relating depleted transmitter amines of several kinds to depressed mood. In particular, many of the studies examining catecholamine levels have also measured indoleamine concentrations.

In the urine, 5-hydroxyindoleacetic acid (5-HIAA) levels are decreased in agitated depressions, and increased in retarded depressions and in manic conditions. However, much urinary 5-HIAA is known to come from the gastrointestinal tract and diet would be an important factor in these studies.[187]

In cerebrospinal fluid, Dencker et al.[45] and Ashcroft et al.[7] reported a lowered level of 5-

HIAA in a depressed group compared to a normal group. However, Ashcroft et al. were very careful in interpreting this difference, noting that a five-fold concentration gradient of 5-HIAA in the CSF made sampling difficult, and effects of physical activity could not be ruled out.

The post-mortem examination of brains of suicides was done for indoleamines as well as noradrenaline. Pare et al.[149] found that 5-HIAA levels were the same in the brains of the suicides compared to the controls, while there was a slight 5-hydroxytryptamine (5-HT) decrease. They state that the 5-HT decrease is possibly accountable for by suicide-control age differences. Bourne et al.[22] found the opposite; lowered 5-HIAA levels and the same 5-HT levels in the suicide group compared to controls.

It is difficult to reach any strong conclusion on indoleamine metabolism in depression at this time, because of the contradictory findings and the same complexities of interpretation associated with the catecholamine data.

Recent contributions on the role of corticosteroids in depression have been reviewed by Sachar,[182] Coppen[38] and Shopsin and Gershon.[197] The main steroids studied have been limited to 11-hydroxycorticosteroids and 17-hydroxycorticosteroids; plasma and urine determinations of their levels in depression and mania have been made. There is controversy surrounding two central points: Are there abnormally high levels of corticosteroids in depression, and does cortisol synthesis in depression respond normally to hypothalamic-pituitary-adrenal feedback as measured by "dexamethasone suppression"? (The steroid analogue dexamethasone when ingested by normal subjects lowers their level of plasma cortisol measured nine hours later.) Shopsin and Gershon take the position that though many studies have found elevated plasma or urinary corticosteroids in a depressed population compared to normal, this elevation is not large and can probably be attributed to general stress and anxiety suffered by the patients. Stress will also cause short-term elevations in normal subjects. Sachar and Coppen echo the view that elevated corticosteroid levels found in most studies of depression are a nonspecific aspect of the condition related to stress. Shopsin and Gershon found normal dexamethasone suppression of plasma cortisol in depressed patients and are unable to explain why Carrol et al.[32] had found that half the patients in their depressed sample did not show normal dexamethasone suppression.

⟮ Bibliography

1. ABRAHAM, K. "Notes on Psychoanalytic Investigation and Treatment of Manic-Depressive Insanity and Allied Conditions," in *Selected Papers on Psychoanalysis*, pp. 137–156. New York: Basic Books, 1960.

2. ——. "The First Pregenital Stage of the Libido," in *Selected Papers on Psychoanalysis*, pp. 248–279. New York: Basic Books, 1960.

3. ——. "A Short Study of the Development of the Libido," in *Selected Papers on Psychoanalysis*, pp. 418–501. New York: Basic Books, 1960.

4. ABRAHAM, M. J., and F. A. WHITLOCK. "Childhood Experience and Depression," *British Journal of Psychiatry*, 115 (1969), 883–888.

5. ACKNER, B., and G. PAMPIGLIONE. "An Evaluation of the Sedation Threshold Test," *Journal of Psychosomatic Research*, 3 (1959), 271–281.

6. AMERICAN PSYCHIATRIC ASSOCIATION. *Diagnostic and Statistical Manual: Mental Disorders*. Washington, D.C.: 1952.

7. ASHCROFT, G. W., T. B. B. CRAWFORD, D. ECCLESTON, D. F. SHARMAN, D. J. MacDOUGALL, J. B. STANTON, and J. K. BINNIS. "5-hydroxyindole Compounds in Cerebrospinal Fluid of Patients with Psychiatric or Neurological Diseases," *Lancet*, 2 (1966), 1049–1052.

8. BECK, A. T. "A Systematic Investigation of Depression," *Comprehensive Psychiatry*, 2 (1961), 162–170.

9. ——. "Thinking and Depression: 1. Idiosyncratic Content and Cognitive Distortions," *Archives of General Psychiatry*, 9 (1963), 324–333.

10. ——. *Depression: Clinical, Experimental, and Theoretical Aspects*. New York: Paul B. Hoeber, Inc., 1967.

11. ——. "The Core Problem in Depression: The Cognitive Triad," *Science and Psychoanalysis*, 17 (1970), 47–55.

12. ——. "Cognition, Affect, and Psychopathology," *Archives of General Psychiatry*, 24 (1971), 495–500.

13. BECK, A. T., and M. S. HURVICH. "Psychological Correlates of Depression. 1. Frequency of 'Masochistic' Dream Content in a Private Practice Sample," *Psychosomatic Medicine*, 21 (1959), 50–55.

14. BECK, A. T., B. B. SETHI, and R. W. TUTHILL. "Childhood Bereavement and Adult Depression," *Archives of General Psychiatry*, 9 (1963), 295–302.

15. BECK, A. T., and S. VALIN. "Psychotic Depressive Reaction in Soldiers Who Accidentally Killed Their Buddies," *The American Journal of Psychiatry*, 110 (1953), 347–353.

16. BECK, A. T., and C. H. WARD. "Dreams of Depressed Patients: Characteristic Themes in Manifest Content," *Archives of General Psychiatry*, 5 (1961), 462–467.

17. BECK, A. T., C. H. WARD, M. MENDELSON, J. MOCK, and J. ERBAUGH. "An Inventory for Measuring Depression," *Archives of General Psychiatry*, 4 (1961), 561–571.

18. BIBRING, E. "The Mechanism of Depression," in P. Greenacre, ed., *Affective Disorders*, pp. 13–48. New York: International Universities Press, 1953.

19. BIRK, A. "The Bereaved Child," *Mental Health*, 25 (1966), 9–11.

20. BJERG, K. "The Suicidal Life Space," in E. S. Shneidman, ed., *Essays in Self-Destruction*, pp. 475–494. New York: Science House, 1967.

21. BÖÖK, J. A. "A Genetic and Neuropsychiatric Investigation of a North Swedish Population with Special Regard to Schizophrenia and Mental Deficiency," *Acta Geneticae Medicae*, 4 (1953), 1–100.

22. BOURNE, H. R., W. E. BUNNEY, JR., R. W. COLBURN, J. M. DAVIS, J. N. DAVIS, D. M. SHAW, and A. J. COPPEN. "Noradrenaline, 5-hydroxyindoleacetic Acid in Hindbrains of Suicidal Patients," *Lancet*, 2 (1968), 805–808.

23. BREED, W. "Suicide and Loss in Social Interaction," in E. S. Shneidman, ed., *Essays in Self-Destruction*, pp. 188–203. New York: Science House, 1967.

24. BRIGGS, P. F. "Working Outside the Home and the Occurrence of Depression in

Middle-aged Women," *Mental Hygiene*, 49 (1965), 438–442.

25. BRILL, N. Q., and E. H. LISTON, JR. "Parental Loss in Adults with Emotional Disorders," *Archives of General Psychiatry*, 14 (1966), 307–314.

26. BROWN, F. "Depression and Childhood Bereavement," *Journal of Mental Science*, 107 (1961), 754–777.

27. BUNNY, W. E., JR., J. M. DAVIS, H. WEIL-MALHERBE, and E. R. B. SMITH. "Biochemical Changes in Psychotic Depression: High Norepinephrine Levels in Psychotic vs. Neurotic Depression," *Archives of General Psychiatry*, 16 (1967), 448–460.

28. BURGESS, E. P. "The Modification of Depressive Behaviors," in R. Rubin and C. Franks, eds., *Advances in Behavior Therapy, 1968*, pp. 193–199. New York: Academic Press, 1969.

29. BUSFIELD, B. L., and H. WECHSLER. "Studies of Salivation in Depression: A Comparison of Salivation Rates in Depressed, Schizoaffective Depressed, Nondepressed Hospitalized Patients, and in Normal Controls," *Archives of General Psychiatry*, 4 (1961), 10.

30. CAMPBELL, J. D. *Manic-Depressive Disease*. Philadelphia: Lippincott, 1953.

31. CARNEY, M. W. P., M. ROTH, and R. F. GARSIDE. "The Diagnosis of Depressive Symptoms and the Prediction of ECT Response," *British Journal of Psychiatry*, 111 (1965), 659–674.

32. CARROLL, B. J., F. I. R. MARTIN, and B. DAVIES. "Resistance to Suppression by Dexamethasone of Plasma 11-OHCS Levels in Severe Depressive Illness." *British Medical Journal*, 3 (1968), 285–287.

33. CASSIDY, W. L., N. B. FLANAGAN, and M. SPELLMAN. "Clinical Observations in Manic-Depressive Disease: A Quantitative Study of 100 Manic-Depressive Patients and 50 Medically Sick Controls," *Journal of the American Medical Association*, 164 (1957), 1535–1546.

34. CAUDILL, W., and L. T. DOI. "Psychiatry and Culture in Japan," in I. Goldston, ed., *Man's Image in Medicine and Anthropology*. New York: International Universities Press, 1963.

35. CLYDE, D. J. *Clyde Mood Scale Manual*. Coral Gables, Fla.: University of Miami, Biometrics Laboratory, 1963.

36. COHEN, B. M., and R. E. FAIRBANK. "Statistical Contributions from Mental Hygiene Study of Eastern Health District of Baltimore," *The American Journal of Psychiatry*, 94 (1938), 1377–1395.

37. COLLOMB, H. "Methodological Problems in Cross-Cultural Research," *International Journal of Psychiatry*, 3 (1967), 17–19.

38. COPPEN, A. "Pituitary-Adrenal Activity During Psychosis and Depression," *Progress in Brain Research*, 32 (1970), 336–342.

39. COSTELLO, C. G., and A. L. COMREY. "Scales for Measuring Depression and Anxiety," *Journal of Psychology*, 66 (1967), 303–313.

40. CROPLEY, A. J., and T. E. WECKOWICZ. "The Dimensionality of Clinical Depression," *Australian Journal of Psychology*, 18 (1966), 18–25.

41. CURTIS, G. C., R. A. CLEGHORN, and T. L. SOURKES. "The Relationship Between Affect and the Excretion of Adrenaline, Noradrenaline, and 17-Hydroxycorticosteroids," *Journal of Psychosomatic Research*, 4 (1960), 176–184.

42. DAVIES, B. M., and J. B. GURLAND. "Salivary Secretion in Depressive Illness," *Journal of Psychosomatic Research*, 5 (1961), 269–271.

43. DELAY, J., P. PICHOT, T. LEMPERIERE, and R. MIROUZE. "La Nosologie des États Depressifs. Rapport entre l'Étiologie et la Semiologie. 2. Résultats du Questionnaire de Beck," *L'Encéphale*, 52 (1963), 497–505.

44. DENCKER, S. J., J. HAGGENDAL, and U. MALM. "Noradrenaline Content of Cerebrospinal Fluid in Mental Diseases," *Lancet*, 2 (1966), 754.

45. DONCKER, S. J., U. MALM, B. E. ROSS, and B. WERDINIUS. "Acid Monoamine Metabolites of Cerebrospinal Fluid in Mental Depression and Mania," *Journal of Neurochemistry*, 13 (1966), 1545–1548.

46. DENNEHY, C. M. "Childhood Bereavement and Psychiatric Illness," *British Journal of Psychiatry*, 112 (1966), 1049–1069.

47. *Depression and Suicide in Adolescents and Young Adults*. Proceedings of a Conference at Bonnie Oaks Lodge, Fairlee, Vt., June 6–8, 1966. A Technical Assistance Project sponsored by three northern New England states and the NIMH.

48. DIAZ-GUERRERO, R., J. S. GOTTLIEB, and

J. R. KNOTT, "The Sleep of Patients with Manic-Depressive Psychosis, Depressive Type: An Electroencephalographic Study," *Psychosomatic Medicine*, 8 (1946), 399–404.

49. DORN, H. F. "Some Problems for Research in Mortality and Morbidity," *Public Health Reports*, 71 (1956), 1–5.

50. DRIVER, M. V., and M. D. EILENBERG. "Photoconvulsive Threshold in Depressive Illness and the Effect of ECT," *Journal of Mental Science*, 106 (1960), 611–617.

51. EATON, J. W., and R. J. WEIL. *Culture and Mental Disorders: A Comparative Study of the Hutterites and Other Populations.* Glencoe, Ill.: Free Press, 1955.

52. ELSASSER, G. "Ovarial Function and Body Constitution in Female Inmates of Mental Hospitals; Special Reference to Schizophrenia," *Archives of Psychiatry*, 188 (1952), 218.

53. ENGEL, G. "A Life Setting Conducive to Illness: The Giving-Up—Given-Up Complex," *Bulletin of the Menninger Clinic*, 32 (1968), 355–365.

54. ESSEN-MOLLER, E. "Individual Traits and Morbidity in a Swedish Rural Population," *Acta Psychiatrica Scandinavica*, Suppl. 100 (1956), 1–160.

55. FARIS, R. E. L., and H. W. DUNHAM. *Mental Disorders in Urban Areas: An Ecological Study of Schizophrenia and Other Psychoses.* Chicago: University of Chicago Press, 1939.

56. FENICHEL, O. *The Psychoanalytic Theory of Neurosis.* New York: Norton, 1945.

57. FERSTER, C. B. "Classification of Behavioral Pathology," in L. Krasner and L. P. Ullmann, eds., *Research in Behavioral Modification*, pp. 6–26. New York: Holt, 1965.

58. FORREST, A. D., R. H. FRASER, and R. G. PRIEST. "Environmental Factors in Depressive Illness," *British Journal of Psychiatry*, 111 (1965), 243–253.

59. FREUD, S. "Mourning and Melancholia" (1917), in *Collected Papers*, Vol. 4. pp. 152–172. London: Hogarth Press, 1950.

60. FRIEDMAN, A. S. Personal Communication, 1966.

61. FRIEDMAN, A. S., B. COWIT, H. W. COHEN, and S. GRANICK. "Syndromes and Themes of Psychotic Depression," *Archives of General Psychiatry*, 9 (1963), 504–509.

62. FUNKENSTEIN, D. H. "Discussion of Chapters 10–11: Psychophysiologic Studies of Depression: Some Experimental Work," in P. H. Hoch and J. Zubin, eds., *Depression.* New York: Grune and Stratton, 1954.

63. GAY, M. J., and W. L. TONGE. "The Late Effects of Loss of Parents in Childhood," *British Journal of Psychiatry*, 113 (1967), 753–760.

64. GAYLIN, W. *The Meaning of Despair: Psychoanalytic Contributions to the Understanding of Depression.* New York: Science House, 1968.

65. GILLESPIE, R. D. "Clinical Differentiation of Types of Depression," *Guy Hospital Report*, 79 (1929), 306–344.

66. GLOWINSKI, J., I. J. KOPIN, and J. AXELROD. "Metabolism of H^3-Norepinephrine in the Rat Brain," *Journal of Neurochemistry*, 12 (1965), 25–30.

67. GOLDSTEIN, I. G. "The Relationship of Muscle Tension and Autonomic Activity to Psychiatric Disorders," *Psychosomatic Medicine*, 27 (1965), 39–52.

68. GOLDSTEIN, R. H., and L. F. SALTZMAN. "Cognitive Functioning in Acute and Remitted Psychiatric Patients," *Psychological Reports*, 21 (1967), 24–26.

69. GOODWIN, F. K., D. L. MURPHY, H. K. H. BRODIE, and W. E. BUNNY, JR. "L-Dopa, Catecholamine, and Behavior: A Clinical and Biochemical Study in Depressed Patients," *Biological Psychiatry*, 2 (1970), 341–366.

70. GOTTLIEB, G., and G. PAULSON. "Salivation in Depressed Patients," *Archives of General Psychiatry*, 5 (1961), 468–471.

71. GREENSPAN, K., J. J. SCHILDKRAUT, E. K. GORDON, L. BAER, M. S. ARONOFF, and J. DURELL. "Catecholamine Metabolism in Affective Disorders. III. MHPG and Other Catecholamine Metabolites in Patients Treated with Lithium Carbonate," *Journal of Psychiatric Research*, 7 (1970), 171–183.

72. GREGORY, I. "Retrospective Data Concerning Childhood Loss by a Parent: II. Category of Parental Loss by Decade of Birth, Diagnosis, and MMPI," *Archives of General Psychiatry*, 15 (1966), 362–367.

73. GRESHAM, S. C., H. W. AGNEW, and R. L. WILLIAMS. "The Sleep of Depressed Patients: An EEG and Eye Movement Study," *Archives of General Psychiatry*, 13 (1965), 503–507.

74. GRINKER, R. R., J. MILLER, M. SABSHIN, R. NUNN, and J. C. NUNNALLY. *The Phe-*

nomena of Depressions. New York: Harper and Row, 1961

75. HAGNELL, O. *A Prospective Study of the Incidence of Mental Disorder.* Lund: Svenska Bokforlaget Norstedts, 1966.

76. HAMILTON, M. "A Rating Scale for Depression," *Journal of Neurology, Neurosurgery & Psychiatry,* 23 (1960), 56–62.

77. HAMILTON, M., and J. M. WHITE. "Clinical Syndrome in Depressive States," *Journal of Mental Science,* 105 (1959), 985–997.

78. HARDER, J. "The Psychopathology of Infanticide," *Acta Psychiatrica Scandinavica,* 43 (1967), 196–245.

79. HATHAWAY, S., and C. McKINLEY. *Minnesota Multiphasic Personality Inventory.* New York: Psychology Corp., 1951.

80. HELGASON, T. "The Frequency of Depressive States in Iceland as Compared with the Other Scandinavian Countries," *Acta Psychiatrica Scandinavica,* Suppl. 162 (1962), 81–90.

81. HILL, O. W., and J. S. PRICE. "Childhood Bereavement and Adult Depression," *British Journal of Psychiatry,* 113 (1967), 743–752.

82. HOLLINGSHEAD, A. B., and F. C. REDLICH. *Social Class and Mental Illness: A Community Study.* New York: John Wiley and Sons, 1958.

83. HOLMES, T. H., and R. H. RAHE. "The Social Readjustment Rating Scale," *Journal of Psychosomatic Research,* 11 (1967), 213–218.

84. HUDGENS, R. W., J. R. MORRISON, and R. BARCHHA. "Life Events and Onset of Primary Affective Disorders," *Archives of General Psychiatry,* 16 (1967), 134–145.

85. HUGHES, C., M. TREMBLAY, R. RAPAPORT, and A. H. LEIGHTON. *People of Cove and Woodlot. The Stirling County Study,* Vol. 2. New York: Basic Books, 1960.

86. HUMPHREY, M. "Functional Impairment in Psychiatric Patients," *British Journal of Psychiatry,* 113 (1967), 1141–1151.

87. IVANYS, W., S. DZDKOVA, and J. VANA. "Prevalence of Psychoses Recorded Among Psychiatric Patients in a Part of the Urban Population," *Ceskoslovenká Psychiatrie,* 60 (1964), 152–163.

88. JACOBSON, E. "Contributions to the Metapsychology of Cyclothymic Depression," in P. Greenacre, ed., *Affective Disorders,* pp. 49–83. New York: International Universities Press, 1953.

89. ———. "Transference Problems in the Psychoanalytic Treatment of Severely Depressive Patients," *Journal of the American Psychoanalytic Association,* 2 (1954), 595–606.

90. KALLMANN, F. "Genetic Aspects of Psychoses," in *Biology of Mental Health and Disease,* pp. 283–302. New York: Hoeber, 1952.

91. KENDELL, R. E. *The Classification of Depressive Illnesses.* London: Oxford University Press, 1968.

92. KIELHOZ, P. "Diagnosis and Therapy of the Depressive State," *Acta Psychosomatica Documenta Geigy,* No. 1, American Series, 1959.

93. KILOH, L. G., and R. F. GARSIDE. "The Independence of Neurotic Depression and Endogenous Depression," *British Journal of Psychiatry,* 109 (1963), 451–463.

94. KLEIN, M. "A Contribution to the Psychogenesis of Manic-Depressive States (1934)," in *Contributions to Psychoanalysis, 1921–1945,* pp. 282–310. London: Hogarth Press, 1948.

95. KRAEPELIN, E. "Manic-Depressive Insanity and Paranoia," R. M. Barclay, trans., *Textbook of Psychiatry.* Edinburgh: Livingstone, 1913.

96. KRAINES, S. H. *Mental Depressions and Their Treatment.* New York: Macmillan, 1957.

97. ———. "Manic-Depressive Syndrome: a Diencephalic Disease." Presented at Annual Meeting of American Psychiatric Association, New York, May 6, 1965.

98. LANGNER, T. S., and S. T. MICHAEL. *Life Stress and Mental Health: The Midtown Manhattan Study.* New York: Free Press, 1963.

99. LAXER, R. M. "Self-Concept Changes of Depressive Patients in General Hospital Treatment," *Journal of Consulting Psychology,* 28 (1964a), 214–219.

100. ———. "Relation of Real Self-Rating to Mood and Blame and Their Interaction in Depression," *Journal of Consulting Psychology,* 28 (1964b), 538–546.

101. LAZARE, A. "The Difference Between Sadness and Depression," *Medical Insight* (February 1970), pp. 23–31.

102. LAZARUS, A. "Learning Theory and the Treatment of Depression," *Behavior Research and Therapy,* 6 (1968), 83–89.

103. LE GASSICKE, J., W. BOYD, and F. MCPHERSON. "A Controlled Out-Patient Evaluation with Fencamfamin," *British Journal of Psychiatry*, 110 (1964), 267–269.

104. LEHMANN, H. E. "Psychiatric Concepts of Depression: Nomenclature and Classification," *Canadian Psychiatric Association Journal*, Suppl. 4 (1959), S1–S12.

105. LEIGHTON, A. H. *My Name is Legion. The Stirling County Study of Psychiatric Disorder and Sociocultural Environment*, Vol. 1. New York: Basic Books, 1959.

106. LEIGHTON, A. H., T. A. LAMBO, C. C. HUGHES, D. C. LEIGHTON, J. M. MURPHY, and D. B. MACKLIN, *Psychiatric Disorder Among the Yoruba*. Ithaca, N.Y.: Cornell University Press, 1963.

107. LEIGHTON, A. H., J. S. HARDING, D. B. MACKLIN, A. M. MACMILLAN, and A. H. LEIGHTON, *The Character of Danger: Psychiatric Symptoms in Selected Communities. The Stirling County Study of Psychiatric Disorder and Sociocultural Environment*, Vol. 3. New York: Basic Books, 1963.

108. LEMKAU, P. V., C. TIETZE, and M. COOPER, "Mental Hygiene Problems in an Urban District. 1. Description of the Study," *Mental Hygiene*, 25 (1941), 624–646.

109. ———. "Mental Hygiene Problems in an Urban District. II. The Psychotics and the Neurotics," *Mental Hygiene*, 26 (1942), 100–119.

110. LEWINSOHN, P., M. SHAFFER, and J. LIBET. "A Behavioral Approach to Depression." Presented at the meetings of the American Psychological Association, University of Oregon, 1969.

111. LEWIS, A. "Melancholia: A Clinical Survey of Depressive States," *Journal of Mental Science*, 80 (1934), 277–378.

112. LICHTENBERG, P. "A Definition and Analysis of Depression," *Archives of Neurology and Psychiatry*, 77 (1957), 516–527.

113. LILIENFELD, A. M. "Epidemiological Methods and Inferences in Studies of Noninfectious Diseases," *Public Health Reports*, 72 (1957), 51–60.

114. LIN, T. "A Study of the Incidence of Mental Disorders in Chinese and Other Cultures," *Psychiatry*, 16 (1953), 313–336.

115. LOEB, A., A. T. BECK, and J. C. DIGGORY. "Differential Effects of Success and Failure on Depressed and Non-depressed Patients," *Journal of Nervous and Mental Disease*, 152 (1971), 106–114.

116. LOEB, A., S. FESHBACH, A. T. BECK, and A. WOLF. "Some Effects of Reward Upon the Social Perception and Motivation of Psychiatric Patients Varying in Depression," *Journal of Abnormal and Social Psychology*, 68 (1964), 609–616.

117. LORR, M., R. L. JENKINS, and J. O. HOPSOPPLE. "Multidimensional Scale for Rating Psychiatric Patients, Hospital Form," *U.S. Veterans Administration Bulletin*, TB 10–507, Veterans Administration, Washington, D.C.

118. LUBIN, B. "Adjective Checklist for Measurement of Depression," *Archives of General Psychiatry*, 12 (1965), 57–62.

119. LUBIN, B., V. A. DUPRES, and A. W. LUBIN. "Comparability and Sensitivity of Set 2 (Lists E, F, and G) of the Depression Adjective Checklists," *Psychological Reports*, 20 (1967), 756–758.

120. LUNDQUIST, G. "Prognosis and Course in Manic-Depressive Psychoses," *Acta Psychiatrica et Neurologica*, Suppl. 35.

121. McGOUGH, W. E., E. WILLIAMS, and J. BLACKLEY. "Changing Patterns of Psychiatric Illness Among Negroes of the Southern United States," Sixth World Congress of Psychiatry, Madrid, Spain, 1966. Abstracts, International Congress Series No. 117. Amsterdam: Excerpta Medica.

122. MALAMUD, W., and S. L. A. SANDS, "A Revision of the Psychiatric Rating Scale," *The American Journal of Psychiatry*, 104 (1947), 231–237.

123. MAOZ, M. D., S. LEVY, N. BRAND, and H. S. HALEVI. "An Epidemiological Survey of Mental Disorders in a Community of Newcomers to Israel," *Journal of the College of General Practitioners*, 11 (1966), 267–284.

124. MAY, A. E., A. URQUHART, and J. TARRAN. "Self-Evaluation of Depression in Various Diagnostic and Therapeutic Groups," *Archives of General Psychiatry*, 21 (1969), 191–194.

125. MELGES, F. T., R. E. ANDERSON, H. C. KRAEMER, J. R. TINKLENBERG, and A. E. WEISZ. "The Personal Future and Self-Esteem," *Archives of General Psychiatry*, 25 (1971), 494–497.

126. MELGES, F. T., and J. BOWLBY. "Types of Hopelessness in Psychological Process,"

Archives of General Psychiatry, 20 (1969), 690–699.

127. MENDELS, J. *Concepts of Depression.* New York: John Wiley and Sons, 1970.

128. MENDELS, J., and C. COCHRANE. "The Nosology of Depression: The Endogenous Reactive Concept," *The American Journal of Psychiatry*, 124 (1968), Suppl., 1–11.

129. MENDELS, J., and D. R. HAWKINS. "Sleep Studies in Depression," *Proceedings of the Symposium on Recent Advances in the Psycho-biology of Affective Disorders.* Bethesda, Md.: National Institute of Mental Health, 1970.

130. MENDELS, J., D. R. HAWKINS, and J. SCOTT. "The Psychophysiology of Sleep in Depression." Presented at annual meeting of the Association for the Psychophysiological Study of Sleep, Gainesville, Fla., March, 1966.

131. MENDELSON, M. *Psychoanalytic Concepts of Depression.* Springfield, Ill.: Charles C Thomas, 1960.

132. METCALFE, M., and E. GOLDMAN. "Validation of an Inventory for Measuring Depression," *British Journal of Psychiatry*, 111 (1965), 240–242.

133. MEYER, A. "The Problems of Mental Reaction Types (1908)," in *The Collected Papers of Adolf Meyer*, pp. 591–603. Baltimore, Md.: Johns Hopkins Press, 1951.

134. MORRISON, J. R., R. W. HUDGENS, and R. BARCHHA. "Life Events and Psychiatric Illness," *British Journal of Psychiatry*, 114 (1968), 423–432.

135. MOTTO, J. A. "Suicide Attempts: A Longitudinal View," *Archives of General Psychiatry*, 13 (1965), 516–520.

136. MUNRO, A. "Parental Deprivation in Depressive Patients," *British Journal of Psychiatry*, 112 (1966), 443–457.

137. ———. "Parent-Child Separation: Is It Really a Cause of Psychiatric Illness in Adult Life?" *Archives of General Psychiatry*, 20 (1969), 598–604.

138. MURPHY, H. G. M., E. D. WITTKOWER, and N. CHANCE. "Cross-Cultural Inquiry Into the Symptomatology of Depression: A Preliminary Report," *International Journal of Psychiatry*, 3 (1967), 6–22.

139. NATIONAL INSTITUTE OF MENTAL HEALTH, Biometry Branch, Public Health Service, U.S. Department of Health, Education, and Welfare. Unpublished data.

140. NEURINGER, C. "Dichotomous Evaluations in Suicidal Individuals," *Journal of Consulting Psychology*, 25 (1961), 445–449.

141. ———. "Rigid Thinking in Suicidal Individuals," *Journal of Consulting Psychology*, 28 (1964), 54–58.

142. ———. "The Cognitive Organization of Meaning in Suicidal Individuals," *Journal of General Psychology*, 76 (1967), 91–100.

143. ———. "Divergencies Between Attitudes Towards Life and Death Among Suicidal, Psychosomatic, and Normal Hospitalized Patients," *Journal of Consulting Clinical Psychology*, 32 (1968), 59–63.

144. NUSSBAUM, K., and W. W. MICHAUX. "Response to Humor in Depression: A Prediction and Evaluation of Patient Change?" *Psychiatric Quarterly*, 37 (1963), 527–539.

145. NYMGAARD, K. "Studies on the Sedation Threshold: A. Reproducibility and Effect of Drugs, B. Sedation Threshold in Neurotic and Psychotic Depression," *Archives of General Psychiatry*, 1 (1959), 530–536.

146. OSWALD, I., R. J. BERGER, R. A. JARAMILLO, K. M. G. KEDDIE, P. C. OLLEY, and G. B. PLUNKETT. "Melancholia and Barbiturates: A Controlled EEG, Body and Eye Movement Study of Sleep," *British Journal of Psychiatry*, 109 (1963), 66–78.

147. OVERALL, J. E. "Dimensions of Manifest Depression," *Psychiatric Research*, 1 (1962), 239–245.

148. PALMAI, G., and B. BLACKWELL. "The Diurnal Pattern of Salivary Flow in Normal and Depressed Patients," *British Journal of Psychiatry*, 111 (1965), 334–338.

149. PARE, C. M. B., D. P. H. YEUNG, K. PRICE, and R. S. STACEY. "5-Hydroxytryptamine, Noradrenaline, and Dopamine in Brain Stem, Hypothalamus, and Caudate Nucleus of Controls and of Patients Committing Suicide by Coal Gas Poisoning," *Lancet*, 2 (1969), 133–135.

150. PASKIND, H. A. "Brief Attacks of Manic-Depressive Depression," *Archives of Neurology and Psychiatry*, 22 (1929), 123–134.

151. ———. "Manic-Depressive Psychosis as Seen in Private Practice: Sex and Age Incidence of First Attacks," *Archives of*

Neurology Psychiatry, 23 (1930a), 152–158.

152. ———. "Manic-Depressive Psychosis in Private Practice: Length of Attack and Length of Interval," *Archives of Neurology and Psychiatry*, 23 (1930b), 789–794.

153. PATTERSON, G., and C. ROSENBERRY. "A Social Learning Formulation of Depression." Unpublished Study.

154. PAUL, M. I., H. CRAMER, and W. E. BUNNEY, JR. "Urinary Adenosine 3′, 5′-Monophosphate in the Switch Process from Depression to Mania," *Science*, 171 (1971), 300–303.

155. PAUL, M. I., J. CRAMER, and F. K. GOODWIN. "Urinary Cyclic AMP Excretion in Depression and Mania," *Archives of General Psychiatry*, 24 (1971), 327–333.

156. PAULSON, G. W., and G. GOTTLIEB. "A Longitudinal Study of the Electroencephalographic Arousal Response in Depressed Patients," *Journal of Nervous and Mental Disease*, 133 (1961), 524–528.

157. PAYKEL, E. S. "Classification of Depressed Patients: A Cluster Analysis Derived Grouping," *British Journal of Psychiatry*, 118 (1971), 275–288.

158. PAYKEL, E. S., J. K. MYERS, M. N. DIENELT, G. L. KLERMAN, J. J. LINDENTHAL, and M. P. PEPPER. "Life Events and Depression: A Controlled Study," *Archives of General Psychiatry*, 21 (1969), 753–760.

159. PECK, R. E. "The SHP Test: An Aid in the Detection and Measurement of Depression," *Archives of General Psychiatry*, 1 (1959), 35–40.

160. PEDERSON, A., D. BARRY, and H. M. BABIGIAN. "Epidemiological Considerations of Psychotic Depression," *Archives of General Psychiatry*, in press.

161. PERRIS, C. "A Study of Bipolar (Manic-Depressive) and Unipolar Recurrent Depressive Episodes," *Acta Psychiatrica Scandinavica*, 42 (Suppl.) (1966), 1–88.

162. PICHOT, P., and T. LEMPERIERE. "Analyse Factorielle d'un Questionnaire d'Autoevaluation des Symptomes Depressifs," *Revue de Psychologie Appliquée*, 14 (1964), 15–29.

163. PICHOT, P., J. PIRET, and D. J. CLYDE. "Analyse de la Symptomatologie Depressive Subjective," *Revue de Psychologie Appliquée*, 16 (1966), 103–115.

164. PINEL, P. (1801). *A Treatise on Insanity*, trans. by D. D. David. New York: Hofner, 1962.

165. PITTS, F. N., J. MEYER, M. BROOKS, and G. WINOKUR. "Adult Psychiatric Illness Assessed for Childhood Parental Loss and Psychiatric Illness in Family Members," *The American Journal of Psychiatry*, 121 (Suppl.) (1965), i–x.

166. PLUNKETT, R. J., and J. E. GORDON. *Epidemiology and Mental Illness*. New York: Basic Books, 1960.

167. PLUTCHIK, R., S. R. PLATMAN, and R. R. FIEVE. "Self-Concepts Associated with Mania and Depression," *Psychological Reports*, 27 (1970), 399–405.

168. POKORNY, A. D. "Suicide Rates in Various Psychiatric Disorders," *Journal of Nervous and Mental Disease*, 139 (1964), 499–506.

169. PRANGE, W. A. "Cultural Aspects of the Relatively Low Incidence of Depression in Southern Negroes," *International Journal of Social Psychiatry*, 8 (1962), 104.

170. RADO, S. "The Problem of Melancholia," *International Journal of Psycho-Analysis*, 9 (1928), 420–438.

171. RAHE, R. H., and R. S. ARTHUR. "Life Change Patterns Surrounding Illness Experience," *Journal of Psychosomatic Research*, 11 (1968), 341–345.

172. RAHE, R. H., J. D. McKEAN, and R. J. ARTHUR. "A Longitudinal Study of Life Change and Illness Patterns," *Journal of Psychosomatic Research*, 10 (1967), 355–366.

173. RASKIN, A., J. SCHULTERBRANDT, N. REATIG, and J. McKEON. "Replication of Factors of Psychopathology in Interview, Ward Behavior, and Self-Report Ratings of Hospitalized Depressives," *Journal of Nervous Mental Disease*, 148 (1967), 87–97.

174. RASKIN, A., J. SCHULTERBRANDT, N. REATIG, and C. RICE. "Factors of Psychopathology in Interview, Ward Behavior, and Self-Report Ratings of Hospitalized Depressives," *Journal of Consulting Psychology*, 31 (1967), 270–278.

175. REDLICH, F. C., and D. X. FREEDMAN. *The Theory and Practice of Psychiatry*. New York: Basic Books, 1966.

176. RENNIE, T. "Prognosis in Manic-Depressive Psychoses," *The American Journal of Psychiatry*, 98 (1942), 801–814.

177. Rimon, R., A. Stenback, and E. Huhmar. "Electromyographic Findings in Depressive Patients," *Journal of Psychosomatic Research*, 10 (1966), 159–170.

178. Robins, E., S. Gassner, J. Kayes, R. H. Wilkinson, and G. E. Murphy. "The Communication of Suicidal Intent: A Study of 134 Consecutive Cases of Successful (Completed) Suicide," *The American Journal of Psychiatry*, 115 (1959), 724–733.

179. Robison, G. A., A. J. Coppen, P. C. Whybrow, and A. J. Prange. "Cyclic AMP in Affective Disorders," *Lancet*, 1 (1970), 1028.

180. Rosenthal, S., and G. L. Klerman. "Endogenous Features in Depressed Women," *Canadian Psychiatric Association Journal*, 11 (Special Suppl.) (1966), 11–16.

181. Roth, W. F., and F. H. Luton. "Mental Health Program in Tennessee," *The American Journal of Psychiatry*, 99 (1943), 662–675.

182. Sachar, E. J. "Psychological Factors Relating to Activation and Inhibition of the Adrenocortical Stress Response in Man: A Review," *Progress in Brain Research*, 32 (1970), 316–324.

183. Salkind, M. R. "Beck Depression Inventory in General Practice," *Journal of the Royal College of General Practitioners*, 18 (1967), 267.

184. Salzman, L., R. Goldstein, H. Baloigian, and R. Atkins. "Conceptual Thinking in Psychiatric Patients," *Archives of General Psychiatry*, 14 (1966), 55–59.

185. Sarwer-Foner, G. J. "A Psychoanalytic Note on a Specific Delusion of Time in Psychotic Depression," *Canadian Psychiatric Association Journal*, 2 (Special Suppl.) (1966), S221–S228.

186. Saul, L. J. *Emotional Maturity*. Philadelphia: Lippincott, 1947.

187. Schildkraut, J. J. *Neuropharmacology and the Affective Disorders*. Boston: Little, Brown, and Co., 1970.

188. Schildkraut, J. J., R. Green, E. K. Gordon, and J. Durell. "Normetanephrine Excretion and Affective State in Depressed Patients Treated with Imipramine," *The American Journal of Psychiatry*, 123 (1966), 690–700.

189. Schwab, J. J., M. R. Bialow, J. M. Brown, and C. E. Holzer. "Diagnosing Depression in Medical Inpatients," *Annals of Internal Medicine*, 67 (1967), 695–707.

190. Schwab, J. J., J. M. Brown, and C. E. Holzer. "Depression in Medical Inpatients: Sex and Age Differences," *Mental Hygiene*, 52 (1968), 627–630.

191. Schwab, J. J., J. M. Brown, C. E. Holzer, and M. Sokolof. "Current Concepts of Depression: The Sociocultural," *International Journal of Social Psychiatry*, XIV (1968), 226–234.

192. Schwab, J. J., R. S. Clemmons, B. Bialow, V. Duggan, and B. Davis. "A Study of the Somatic Symptomatology of Depression in Medical Inpatients," *Psychosomatics* 6 (1965), 273–277.

193. Sethi, B. B. "Relationship of Separation to Depression," *Archives of General Psychiatry*, 10 (1964), 486–496.

194. Shagass, C., J. Naiman, and J. Mihalik. "An Objective Test Which Differentiates Between Neurotic and Psychotic Depression," *Archives of Neurology and Psychiatry*, 75 (1956), 461–471.

195. Shagass, C., and M. Schwartz. "Cerebral Cortical Reactivity in Psychotic Depressions," *Archives of General Psychiatry*, 6 (1962), 235–242.

196. Shields, J. *Monozygotic Twins Brought Up Apart and Brought Up Together*. London: Oxford University Press, 1962.

197. Shopsin, B., and S. Gershon. "Plasma Cortisol Response to Dexamethasone Suppression in Depressed and Control Patients," *Archives of General Psychiatry*, 24 (1971), 320–326.

198. Silverman, C. *The Epidemiology of Depression*. Baltimore, Md.: Johns Hopkins Press, 1968.

199. Sjögren, T. "Genetic-Statistical and Psychiatric Investigations of a West Swedish Population," *Acta Psychiatrica et Neurologica*, Suppl. 52 (1948).

200. Slatter, E. "Psychiatric and Neurotic Illnesses in Twins," Medical Research Council Special Report Series, No. 278. London: Her Majesty's Stationery Office, 1953.

201. Sørenson, A., and E. Strömgren. "Frequency of Depressive States Within Geographically Delimited Population Groups. 2. Prevalence (The Samsø Investigation)," *Acta Psychiatrica Scandinavica*, 37 (Suppl. 162) (1961), 62–68.

202. Stainbrook, E. "A Cross-Cultural Evalua-

tion of Depressive Reactions," in P. H. Hoch and J. Zubin, eds., *Depression*. New York: Grune and Stratton, 1954.

203. STENSTEDT, A. "A Study in Manic-Depressive Psychosis: Clinical, Social, and Genetic Investigations," *Acta Psychiatrica Scandinavica*, Suppl. 79 (1952).

204. STRONGIN, E. I., and L. E. HINSIE. "Parotid Gland Secretions in Manic-Depressive Patients," *The American Journal of Psychiatry*, 94 (1938), 1459.

205. TEMOCHE, A., T. F. PUGH, and B. MAC-MAHON. "Suicide Rates Among Current and Former Mental Institution Patients," *Journal of Nervous and Mental Disease*, 136 (1964), 124–130.

206. TONKS, C. M., E. S. PAYKEL, and G. L. KLERMAN. "Clinical Depression among Negroes," *The American Journal of Psychiatry*, 127 (1970), 329.

207. TORREY, E. F., ed. *An Introduction to Health and Health Education in Ethiopia*. Addis Ababa: Berhanena Selam Printing Press, 1966.

208. ULLMANN, L. P., and L. KRASNER. *A Psychological Approach to Abnormal Behavior*. Englewood Cliffs, N.J.: Prentice-Hall, 1969.

209. VATZ, K. A., H. R. WINIG, and A. T. BECK. "Pessimism and a Sense of Future Time Constriction as Cognitive Distortions in Depression." Mimeographed.

210. WALDRON, J., and T. J. N. BATES. "The Management of Depression in Hospital," *British Journal of Psychiatry*, 111 (1965), 511–516.

211. WATTS, C. A. *Discussion Two in Depression*. (Ed. by E. Beresford Davies.) Cambridge: Cambridge University Press, 1964, pp. 55–69.

212. WECKOWICZ, T. E., W. MUIR, and A. J. CROPLEY. "A Factor Analysis of the Beck Inventory of Depression," *Journal of Consulting Psychology*, 31 (1967), 23–28.

213. WECKOWICZ, T. E., K. A. YONGE, A. J. CROPLEY, and W. MUIR. "Objective Therapy Predictors in Depression: A Multivariate Approach," *Monograph Suppl. No. 31*, Clinical Psychology Publishing Co., Inc., 1971.

214. WEINBERG, S. K. "Cultural Aspects of Manic-Depression in West Africa," *Journal of Health and Human Behavior*, 6 (1965), 247–253.

215. WECHSLER, H., G. H. GROSSER, and B. L. BUSFIELD, JR. "The Depression Rating Scale," *Archives of General Psychiatry*, 9 (1963), 334–343.

216. WHATMORE, G. B., and R. M. ELLIS, JR. "Some Neurophysiologic Aspects of Depressed States: An Electromyographic Study," *Archives of General Psychiatry*, 1 (1959), 70–80.

217. ———. "Further Neurophysiologic Aspects of Depressed States: An Electromyographic Study," *Archives of General Psychiatry*, 6 (1962), 243–253.

218. WHYBROW, P. C., and J. MENDELS. "Toward a Biology of Depression: Some Suggestions from Neurophysiology," *The American Journal of Psychiatry*, 125 (1967), 1491–1500.

219. WILSON, I. C., L. B. ALLTOP, and W. J. BUFFALOE. "Parental Bereavement in Childhood: MMPI Profiles in a Depressed Population," *British Journal of Psychiatry*, 113 (1967), 761–764.

220. WILSON, W. P., and N. J. WILSON. "Observations on the Duration of Photically Elicited Arousal Responses in Depressive Illness," *Journal of Nervous Mental Disease*, 133 (1961), 438–440.

221. WINOKUR, G. "Genetic Principles in the Clarification of Clinical Issues in Affective Disorders," in A. J. Mandell and M. P. Mandell, eds., *Psychochemical Research in Man*. New York: Academic Press, 1969.

222. WINOKUR, G. and F. PITTS, "Affective Disorder: 1. Is Reactive Depression an Entity?" *Journal of Nervous and Mental Disease*, 138 (1964), 541–547.

223. WITTENBORN, J. R. *Wittenborn Psychiatric Rating Scales*. New York: Psychological Corp., 1955.

224. WOHLFORD, P. "Extension of Personal Time, Affective States, and Expectation of Personal Death," *Journal of Personal and Social Psychology*, 3 (1966), 559–566.

225. WYATT, R. J., B. PORTNOY, D. J. KUPFER, F. SNYDER, and K. ENGELMAN. "Resting Plasma Catecholamine Concentrations in Patients with Depression and Anxiety," *Archives of General Psychiatry*, 24 (1971), 65–70.

226. YOO, P. S. "Mental Disorders in Korean Rural Communities," in *Proceedings of the Third World Congress of Psychiatry*, pp. 1305–1309. Montreal, Canada, 1961.

227. ZILBOORG, G. *A History of Medical Psychology*, p. 67. New York: Norton, 1941.

228. ZUNG, W. W. K. "A Self-Rating Depression Scale," *Archives of General Psychiatry*, 12 (1965), 63–70.

229. ZUNG, W. W. K., W. P. WILSON, and W. E. DODSON. "Effect of Depressive Disorders on Sleep EEG Responses," *Archives of General Psychiatry*, 10 (1964), 439–445.

CHAPTER 5

ANXIETY: SIGNAL, SYMPTOM, AND SYNDROME

John C. Nemiah

I N *The Anatomy of Melancholy*, that vast, quixotic, and entrancing early seventeenth-century lumber room of psychiatric lore, Robert Burton speaks of fear as "cousin-german to sorrow . . . or rather a sister, *fidus Achates*, and continual companion, an assistant and a principal agent in procuring of this mischief; a cause and symptom as the other."

Many lamentable effects, [he continues] this fear causeth in men, as to be red, pale, tremble, sweat; it makes sudden cold and heat to come over all the body, palpitation of the heart, syncope, etc. It amazeth many men that are to speak or show themselves in public assemblies, or before some great personages . . . It confounds voice and memory. . . . Many men are so amazed and astonished with fear, they know not where they are, what they say, what they do, and that which is worst, it tortures them many days before with continual affrights and suspicions. It hinders most honourable attempts, and makes their hearts ache, sad and heavy. They that live in fear are never free, resolute, secure, never merry, but in continual pain: that as Vives truly said, *Nulla est miseria major quam metas*, no greater misery, no rack, nor torture like unto it; ever suspicious, anxious, solicitous, they are childishly drooping without reason . . . It causeth oftentimes madness, and almost all manner of diseases. Fear makes our imagination conceive what it list, invites the devil to come to us . . . and tyranizeth over our phantasy more than all other affections, especially in the dark.

Burton has included in his crowded sentences most of the phenomena associated with anxiety, an eloquent witness to the fact that human nature changes little, if at all, over the centuries. Burton wrote about what he read and what he saw, and was content to remain an empirical reporter of the varieties of human emotional suffering. Since his time, anxiety has been reified, deified, and vilified. Impossible to define with any precision,[29] it has been viewed as the mere awareness of a physiological state,[21] as a central force in mental functioning,[12,13] as the ontological core of man's being,[33] and it has been denied any existence at all.[40] In the midst of what has been pridefully proclaimed "The Age of Anxiety," the anxiety neurosis, to which Freud gave birth in 1895, has recently been quietly laid to rest as "excess baggage," a "colorful metaphor" in the "romantic mystique" of psychoanalysis.[42] It is, therefore, with some diffidence, not to say anxiety, that one approaches a systematic exposition of such an elusive subject.

❴ Clinical Aspects of Anxiety

The psychiatric clinician, forced by his patients' complaints to pay attention to their subjective woes, has long been aware that anxiety is a major source of human discomfort. If he has been less critically precise in his conceptualizing than his more scientifically minded colleagues, he has at least tried accurately to record and describe what his patients have told him and what he has observed, and it is to the clinician we must go for a broad operational definition. In what follows we shall briefly review the historical evolution of clinical knowledge about the emotion of anxiety as a prelude to a consideration of its general characteristics and of its more specific relation to the anxiety neurosis.

Historical

Hysteria and hypochondriasis (the latter long considered to be the male counterpart of hysteria) had for centuries been recognized as clinical entities, but it was not until the nineteenth century that clinical investigators began to focus on the more discrete, nonpsychotic symptom complexes of neurasthenia, the phobias, obsessions, and compulsions. Janet was perhaps the first to try to systematize these in a comprehensive scheme of classification. In his view, there were two major categories: *hysteria*, which included all of the classical mental and sensorimotor dissociative phenomena, and *psychasthenia*, a congeries of all the other neurotic manifestations parcelled out by modern diagnosticians among the various psychoneuroses.

Among Janet's multitude of case histories (which are often unusually full, detailed, and vivid) there are reports of several patients suffering from anxiety, but in his experience this was rarely found in pure culture. On the contrary, it was generally part of a larger complex of symptoms, including obsessions, compulsions, tics, phobias, and a wide spectrum of hysterical phenomena. Of the one hundred and fifty-odd patients whom Janet described in *Les Névroses et Idées Fixes*,[23] only one manifested anxiety alone, a woman of thirty-nine, who developed a heightened emotional responsiveness to minor stimuli following the serious illnesses of her husband and son.

If you saw her during a period of calmness [writes Janet] you would not detect any pathological symptom, all of her organs functioning normally: there is no apparent nervous difficulty or anesthesia—in the special senses, the skin, the muscles, and, as far as one can determine, there is no disturbance in visceral sensation. She feels well, although greatly fatigued, has no headache, and no change in memory or her thought processes. But for this state of well-being to continue, it is necessary, as she says herself, "that nothing happens"—that is to say, every occurrence, no matter what, causes an upset. When someone goes in or out, when someone speaks to her, or does not speak to her, when her children cough or sniffle, when a carriage passes, etc., she very shortly experiences phenomena that are always identical: she senses a tightness in her throat along with a desire to cry, and feels suffocated and labored breathing as in an attack of asthma. Her stomach and lower abdomen become distended, she trembles, has palpitations, and breaks into a cold sweat, etc. Simultaneously her thoughts become vague and seem to escape her. She is afraid of something without knowing what it is. The attack generally lasts for a short time, a half hour or so; she cries copiously, which eases her, and finally becomes fairly calm until the next emotional outburst (which is triggered off by anything at all) occurs within an hour or two.

It was Freud who first suggested that anxiety belonged to a diagnostic entity *sui generis*, which he termed *anxiety neurosis*, "because all of its components can be grouped round the chief symptom of anxiety."[11] Particularly to be distinguished from neurasthenia, of which it had been considered to be a part by earlier clinicians, its symptoms comprised general irritability, anxious expectation, and gastrointestinal symptoms (particularly diarrhea) as its more chronic manifestations, on which were superimposed acute attacks accompanied by a variety of somatic symptoms.

An anxiety attack of this sort [wrote Freud] may consist of the feeling of anxiety, alone, without any associated idea, or accompanied by the interpretation that is nearest to hand, such as ideas of the extinction of life, or of a stroke, or of a threat of madness; . . . or, finally, the feeling of anxiety may have linked to it a disturbance of one or more of the bodily functions—such as respiration, heart action, vasomotor innervation or glandular activity. From this combination the patient picks out in particular now one, now another, factor. He complains of "spasms of the heart," "difficulty in breathing," "outbreaks of sweating," "ravenous hunger," and such like; and, in his description, the feeling of anxiety often recedes into the background or is referred to quite unrecognizably as "being unwell," "feeling uncomfortable," and so on.

Although his concept of the central role of anxiety in psychic functioning was accepted by psychoanalysts, and anxiety itself was generally recognized as a neurotic symptom by clinical psychiatrists, Freud's proposal of anxiety neurosis as a distinct diagnostic entity was slow to catch on, and it was not until the 1930s, especially in American texts, that the term "anxiety neurosis" began to be used with any regularity. Medical experience with military personnel during World War II was a major factor in subsequently sensitizing clinicians at large to the prevalence and importance of anxiety in human illness, and since that time "anxiety neurosis" (or "anxiety reaction") has been a standard diagnostic category in both the *Diagnostic and Statistical Manual of Mental Disorders* of the American Psychiatric Association[2] and the *International Classification of Diseases* promulgated by the World Health Organization.[50]

One further fact of historical interest must be mentioned. In 1871, J. M. DaCosta[9] published an article in the *American Journal of the Medical Sciences* in which he described a "functional disorder of the heart" to which he gave the name "irritable heart." On the basis of his clinical experience with soldiers in the Union Army during the Civil War, he described a syndrome characterized by precordial pains, palpitations, and giddiness, occurring either when the patient was at rest, or following slight exertion. He attributed the condition to a "disordered innervation" of the heart, resulting from periods of "excitement" in the patient and leading to cardiac "overaction." "Irritable heart," or "DaCosta's Syndrome," as it was also termed, was subsequently described during the Franco-Prussian and Spanish-American Wars, and in World War I a new label, "Disordered Action of the Heart" ("D.A.H.") was attached by internists to the same symptom complex.[30] Although they were unable to assign a specific etiology to the disorder, they were evidently unaware of Freud's earlier comment that "the feeling of anxiety may have linked to it a disturbance of one or more of the bodily functions," and they classified the syndrome as a "functional" cardiac illness without recognizing it as being psychogenic or related to anxiety.

Epidemiological Considerations

These excursions into the past have an important bearing on the epidemiology of the anxiety neurosis. Although transient anxiety as a symptom is widespread, it is (as with the neuroses generally) virtually impossible to determine the true incidence of the specific disorder itself in the population at large, partly because it is rarely severe enough to require psychiatric hospitalization, partly because patients suffering from the symptoms are often treated by private medical physicians or psychiatrists from whom statistics are unavailable, and partly because the syndrome is still not infrequently misdiagnosed as a cardiac disorder. At the same time serious doubt must be cast on the notion that anxiety is more characteristic of contemporary society than that of previous generations. It has been said, for example, that anxiety constituted a major portion of the psychiatric casualties in World

War II in contrast to those of World War I, which were primarily hysterical in nature. Consider, however, the fact that during World War I there were 60,000 cases of "Disordered Action of the Heart" in the British Army alone. Diagnosed by internists unaware that they were dealing with anxiety, these patients were viewed as suffering from a cardiac disorder, and the fact that their problem was neurotic anxiety went unnoticed and unrecorded. It was not that anxiety was absent, but that it was unrecognized.

General Characteristics of Anxiety

From the glimpses we have had of it thus far, it is clear that anxiety has many faces. Its several major features must be made explicit here:

1. Anxiety may be viewed either as a *symptom* or as a specific neurotic *syndrome*. As a symptom, it is found to a greater or lesser degree throughout the entire spectrum of psychiatric disorders. Thus, it is a central feature of the phobic neurosis, is a common accompaniment of the obsessive-compulsive neurosis, is frequently seen in patients with depression, especially of the agitated variety, and often is associated with the early stages of schizophrenia. In the syndrome of anxiety neurosis, it constitutes the central and predominant symptom, and is characteristically "free-floating" in nature—that is, the patient experiences anxiety without any evident reason for it or without its being referred to any object or situation.

2. Anxiety may be either acute, occurring in discrete attacks, or chronic, or a mixture of both, the attacks arising out of a background of longer-lasting, less intense symptoms.

3. The manifestations of anxiety are both somatic and experiential. The somatic phenomena are mainly the result of autonomic nervous system discharges and the release of epinephrine and norepinephrine producing observable changes appropriate to the organ systems affected, such as tachycardia, increased blood pressure, flushing, sweating, diarrhea, or urinary frequency. In addition, deepened, sighing respirations and increased

muscular tension, often with trembling and motor restlessness, may be seen. From an experiential point of view, many of the symptoms of anxiety consist of the patient's conscious awareness of the somatic processes just described. Palpitations, a sharp precordial pain, and a sensation of suffocation and "air hunger" are common complaints, especially in acute attacks, and the patient often feels impelled to open a window or go outdoors in order to get adequate air. In addition, there are certain phenomena that appear to be more than merely a consciousness of body functioning. Patients often complain of dizziness and lightheadedness, mental confusion, an inability to concentrate, memory impairment, and disorganization of logical thought; perhaps most characteristic of anxiety is a sense of inner, nameless dread that in its extreme form reaches panic.

Before moving on to an exploration of the clinical details of the anxiety neurosis, we must first turn our attention to certain aspects of the symptom that have a bearing on the difficulties attached to studying the phenomena that constitute it. There is little problem among investigators in agreeing on the existence and the nature of the somatic manifestations, for these are not only open to public inspection, but are in a rough way measurable, quantifiable, and reproducible. When it comes to the subjective experience of anxiety, the situation is quite different; here the terms "anxiousness," "dread," or "panic," have as their referent a state of conscious awareness that is qualitative in nature, and their meaning cannot be truly conveyed to another person unless he, too, has experienced the inner state to which they refer. To the uninitiated, to define anxiety as a feeling of anxious apprehension, of dread, or of panic, is a nearly meaningless tautology, and he is liable to dismiss as an airy nothing that which to the patient who has suffered it is one of the most intense, real, and painful experiences he has ever lived through. Some observers are probably constitutionally incapable of ever knowing with any immediacy what the patient is trying to tell them. Most of us, even though we may not have exactly shared his experience, are able intuitively to get at least some faint inkling of what he means as he tries desperately to say the ineffable. It is for that reason that we shall rely heavily in what follows on the autobiographical statements of patients who have known anxiety at first hand.

The Syndrome (Anxiety Neurosis)

The anxiety neurosis, in which the symptom of anxiety is featured in the leading part, occurs in an acute and chronic form.

ACUTE ANXIETY

As the term implies, acute anxiety is usually sudden in onset and occurs in attacks. These may last for only a few moments and disappear without major sequelae, or they may continue with waxing and waning intensity for many minutes or hours at a time. In some, the attack is an isolated episode that occurs rarely if ever again; in others a series of attacks may occur in cycles lasting for days or weeks. Generally, the patient is unable to specify any precipitant of his symptoms, though in some a clue is provided from their associations, if one allows them to talk freely about the experience. In this connection, mention should be made here of one special form of anxiety that is encountered with some regularity and frequency, the so-called homosexual panic. Occurring usually in late adolescent or young adult males, often at a time when they are first exposed to the intensive contact with other men, such as exists in army barracks, male dormitories, or camps, homosexual panic is characterized by particularly severe anxiety associated with the idea that one may be homosexual or that other people think so. Those afflicted with this condition may verge on being delusional, are at times strongly impelled to suicidal acts, and are frequently driven by the emotional pain of their symptoms to seek medical help, especially in general hospital emergency wards.

The quality of an acute anxiety attack is well described in the following account by a patient of his experience during such an episode.

I was about half an hour into giving a lecture when it suddenly came over me. I had been perfectly well up until that time. There was nothing unusual about the situation, the lecture was the fourth or fifth in a series I was giving to a class I knew, and I had not been worried or concerned about anything before I began. All at once, without any warning, I felt something start up in me. It was as if a sudden, slight impulsion had simultaneously hit my upper chest and head. I was momentarily thrown off balance and felt I was swaying to the left (although I am sure my body did not really move), and I experienced a mild fullness in my throat. I kept on talking, following the text of my lecture, but automatically, without really being aware of what I was saying, since my attention was now focused on what was happening within me. Almost immediately my heart began to race, I broke into a sweat, especially across my forehead, around my eyes and upper lip, and felt flushed in the face and a fullness in the front of my head that seemed almost to be an inner confusion. Central to this was a feeling of what I would almost call panic, which seemed to fill my whole awareness. Despite the fact that this was intensely vivid and real, I find it almost impossible to describe it in words. It was a kind of dire apprehension of I know not what, and I felt almost overwhelmingly moved to run, to get away, to escape, lest I collapse then and there. I was now aware that my legs were shaking (fortunately hidden from the audience by the lectern), and I took several deep breaths in the pauses between the phrases of what I was saying, swallowing hard as if to force back down what was rising up inside me. There was, curiously, a small part of me that was outside of all of this, observing it and telling myself that it was really nothing, was quite unnecessary, and that I should hang on, get control of myself, and calm down. This I was able to do by what seemed an exertion of my will power, and the panic and my body's reaction rather rapidly ebbed to a point where I realized I could carry on with what I was doing. The whole business took no longer than fifteen to twenty seconds, and I am sure that no one there knew anything was happening to me. I finished the lecture, which went on for another twenty minutes or so. Once or twice I thought the symptoms were coming back, but managed to abort them by the same will power that had overcome the attack itself. I remained inwardly somewhat tense and continued to have the flushed feeling in my face and a mild fullness in my head till the end of the class. Thereafter, I felt only as if I were being rather mechanical in my speaking, going through the motions without being wholeheartedly involved in what I was saying, and remaining emotionally somewhat distant from and out of contact with the audience. Afterwards, I felt perfectly all right, but was aware for the rest of the day of tension and fatigue.

CHRONIC ANXIETY

For every person who experiences an acute anxiety attack like that just described, there are dozens, probably hundreds who suffer from the symptoms of chronic anxiety, which, if less dramatic in their manifestation, can be equally unpleasant and debilitating. Indeed, almost all people undergo transient anxiety at one time or another in their lives, and it can hardly be called pathological unless it reaches a degree of chronicity or intensity that interferes with the individual's life and functioning. Referred to usually as "tension" or "nervousness," the manifestations are a lower-keyed version of what has been detailed above, as is evident in the responses of a class of normal students who, when asked to state what they felt like when they were "nervous," described the following phenomena: "shortage of breath," "tightness in the chest," "difficulty breathing," "stomach uneasy," "rumbling stomach," "fluttering stomach like butterflies," "stomach shaking," "had to keep swallowing," "diarrhea," "loss of appetite," "nausea," "retching, gagging," "sweating," "palpitations," "heart pounding," "dizziness," "lightheadedness," "trembling," "shakiness of voice," "tongue-tied," "stuttering," "tightening of the neck muscles with resulting headache," "jumpy all over," "fidgetiness," "body feels speeded up and full of energy," "had to do something with my hands all the time," "legs wanting to move," "twisting hair," "tired," "inability to concentrate," "feel like exploding."

The individual suffering from chronic anxiety does not, of course, complain of all of these phenomena. Each manifests his own combination of symptoms grouped in patterns (the ordering of which is not entirely understood) that focus in some on the cardiovascular system, in others on the neuromuscular apparatus or gastro-intestinal tract, in yet others on the more subjective aspects of mental functioning. The appearance of chronic anxiety may be insidious in onset or may start with an acute anxiety attack; it can last for weeks and months on end, and comes and goes without obvious reference to external events; and it may be punctuated in its course by outbursts of the more acute variety of symptoms.

William James has left for us a vivid account of chronic anxiety (admixed with depression), the beginning of which was heralded by the sudden outbreak of an acute anxiety attack. Attributed in *The Varieties of Religious Experience*[22] (where it was first recounted) to an anonymous Frenchman, it was later revealed in his edited letters to be autobiographic.[20]

Whilst in this state of philosophic pessimism and general depression of spirits about my prospects, I went one evening into a dressing-room in the twilight to procure some article that was there; when suddenly there fell upon me without any warning, just as if it came out of the darkness, a horrible fear of my own existence. Simultaneously there arose in my own mind the image of an epileptic patient whom I had seen in the asylum, a black-haired youth with greenish skin, entirely idiotic, who used to sit all day on one of the benches, or rather shelves against the wall, with his knees drawn up against his chin, and the coarse gray undershirt, which was his only garment, drawn over them inclosing his entire figure. He sat there like a sort of sculptured Egyptian cat or Peruvian mummy, moving nothing but his black eyes and looking absolutely nonhuman. This image and my fear entered into a species of combination with each other. *That shape am I,*[*] I felt, potentially. Nothing that I possess can defend me against that fate, if the hour for it should strike for me as it struck for him. There was such a horror of him, and such a perception of my own merely momentary discrepancy from him, that it was as if something hitherto solid within my breast gave way entirely, and I became a quivering mass of fear. After this the universe was changed for me altogether. I awoke morning after morning with a horrible dread in the pit of my stomach, and with a sense of the insecurity of life that I never knew before, and that I have never felt since. It was like a revelation; and although

---

[*] Italics in original.

the immediate feelings passed away, the experience has made me sympathetic with the morbid feelings of others ever since. It gradually faded, but for months, I was unable to go out into the dark alone.

In general I dreaded to be left alone. I remember wondering how other people could live, how I myself had ever lived, so unconscious of that pit of insecurity beneath the surface of life. My mother in particular, a very cheerful person, seemed to me a perfect paradox in her unconsciousness of danger, which you may well believe I was very careful not to disturb by revelations of my own state of mind. I have always thought that this experience of melancholia of mine had a religious bearing.

I mean that the fear was so invasive and powerful that if I had not clung to scripture-texts like "The eternal God is my refuge," etc., "Come unto me, all ye that labor and are heavy-laden," etc., "I am the resurrection and the life," etc., I think I should have grown really insane.

HYPERVENTILATION SYNDROME[10]

An occasional complication of anxiety is seen in those patients who experience respiratory distress as a part of their syndrome. The resulting rapid, deep breathing that accompanies an acute attack of anxiety leads to a respiratory alkalosis secondary to the blowing off of excessive carbon dioxide. Most commonly this produces a modest sensation of tingling in the fingers, but in more extreme situations tingling in the toes and around the mouth, and even mild tetanic flexion contractions of the distal extremities may occur. In addition, the patient feels a tightness and fullness in the head and a sense of lightheadedness that compounds the already existing panicky anticipation of disaster—fainting, a heart attack, or dropping dead. Those patients with chronic anxiety who exhibit frequent, intermittent deep sighing may live on the threshold of a respiratory alkalosis that renders them particularly liable to develop the overt symptoms of hyperventilation with only a few more deep breaths during an attack of acute anxiety. Having the patient hyperventilate during the physical examination will demonstrate his sensitivity in this regard by reproducing the symptoms that characterize the hyperventilation syndrome—a finding that

will indicate to both doctor and patient a significant factor in the production of symptoms, often to the considerable reassurance of the latter.

The Anxious Character

When we speak of the hysterical or the obsessional character, we are referring to a grouping of behavioral traits that can be designated with some precision, persist over a period of time, have a certain degree of internal consistency, and are commonly associated with symptoms sharing the same diagnostic category. Thus, we view the person with a hysterical character as being emotional, seductive, imaginative, etc.; the person with an obsessional character as being rational, precise, obstinate, ambivalent, etc.; and obsessional and hysterical symptoms, when they are present, as occurring with a fair degree of correlation in conjunction with the appropriate character traits.

The term "anxious character" is used less frequently and with a lesser degree of exactitude, and generally refers to a person with moderate chronic anxiety—that is, to an individual exhibiting symptoms rather than specific character traits. The manifestations of the "anxious character" are not related solely to the anxiety neurosis but may accompany a variety of neurotic syndromes (the phobic or obsessive-compulsive neurosis, for example), hypochondriasis, or certain kinds of depression. It characterizes the individual who approaches everything with apprehension, the chronic worrier, or those with social insecurity or doubts about their own capacities to perform successfully. The term, then, has little denotative specificity and is less useful clinically than the more commonly employed designations of character types.

❨ The Nature of Anxiety

Anxiety and Fear

An issue that is frequently raised by investigators and clinicians alike concerns the relation between fear and anxiety. Are they the same or different? The question, as one might expect, elicits answers that take dramatically opposite sides.

Anxiety is distinguished from fear by many observers on the basis of the nature of the stimulus that elicits the emotional reaction. Fear, it is said, is the response to a real external threat to life, limb, or security. Anxiety, on the other hand, is a similar reaction to an internal stimulus (an impulse or drive with its associated emotions and fantasies), or to an external event that is not in reality threatening but merely appears so to the individual's neurotically distorted perceptions. This distinction is well exemplified in the fragment of a dialogue captured for us by George Borrow:[5]

"What ails you, my child?" said a mother to her son, as he lay on a couch under the influence of the dreadful one; "What ails you? You seem afraid!"

BOY. "And so I am; a dreadful fear is upon me."

MOTHER. "But of what? There is no one can harm you; of what are your apprehensive?"

BOY. "Of nothing that I can express. I know not what I am afraid of, but afraid I am."

MOTHER. "Perhaps you see sights and visions. I knew a lady once who was continually thinking that she saw an armed man threaten her, but it was only an imagination, a phantom of the brain."

BOY. "No armed man threatens me; and 'tis not a thing like that would cause me any fear. Did an armed man threaten me I would get up and fight him; weak as I am, I would wish for nothing better, for then, perhaps, I should lose this fear; mine is a dread of I know not what, and there the horror lies."

MOTHER. "Your forehead is cool, and your speech collected. Do you know where you are?"

BOY. "I know where I am, and I see things just as they are; you are beside me, and upon the table there is a book which was written by a Florentine; all this I see, and that there is no ground for being afraid. I am, moreover, quite cool, and feel no pain—but, but—"

Some within the camp of the separatists would go even further than those who distinguish fear from anxiety by the nature of the precipitant, and seizing on the vocabulary of

patients who, like Borrow's boy, use words such as "horror" and "dread," maintain that anxiety as an experience is qualitatively different from fear—that it has an eery power, an ineffable aura of evil, an almost supernatural intensity that sets it apart from the more mundane but understandable emotion of the fear of danger in the real world.

Other observers have tended to overlook the distinction we have just been considering and to emphasize the similarities between fear and anxiety. Both, it is pointed out, share the same kind of autonomic response, the same apprehensive expectation of what is to come, the same gradations in intensity from low level concern to compelling panic and horrified dread. They see no reason for basing a differentiation on the nature of the stimulus.

There is merit and reason on both sides of the argument—which, as arguments go, is not a very acrimonious one, and which, like so many disagreements, results from incomplete data and oversimplified generalizations. The nature of emotion in general is complex and poorly understood, and our knowledge of anxiety shares in the confusion of information that comes from studies of the physiological, psychological, and social aspects of emotional processes. A review of some of the highlights of these studies should help us to put the disagreements concerning fear and anxiety in perspective. For the sake of simplification, the term "anxiety" will be used throughout what follows, except where "fear" is clearly more appropriate.

Physiological Aspects of Anxiety

Much of the interest in the physiology of anxiety, as has just been suggested, must be placed in the larger contest of the study of the nature of emotions in general, a study to which the specific investigation of anxiety and fear has made major contributions. Fear was only one of the emotions on which William James[21] focused his attention when (concurrently with the independent work of Lange in Germany), he formulated what has come to be known as the James-Lange theory.

James's own exposition of his ideas is notable for its simplicity and clarity:

> Our natural way of thinking about these coarser emotions, is that the mental perception of some fact excites the mental affection called the emotion, and that this latter state of mind gives rise to the bodily expression. My theory, on the contrary, is that *the bodily changes follow directly the perception of the exciting fact, and that our feeling of the same changes as they occur is the emotion.*° Common-sense says, we lose our fortune, are sorry and weep; we meet a bear, are frightened and run; we are insulted by a rival, are angry and strike. The hypothesis here to be defended says that this order of sequence is incorrect, that the one mental state is not immediately induced by the other, that the bodily manifestations must first be interposed between, and that the more rational statement is that we feel sorry because we cry, angry because we strike, afraid because we tremble, and not that we cry, strike, or tremble, because we are sorry, angry, or fearful, as the case may be. Without the bodily states following on perception, the latter would be purely cognitive in form, pale, colorless, destitute of emotional warmth. We might then see the bear, and judge it best to run, receive the insult and deem it right to strike, but we should not actually *feel*° afraid or angry.

James's paradoxical relegation of emotion to a mere state of awareness of somatic processes led to considerable controversy and investigation. A significant challenge to his views came several decades later in the work of Marañon.[31] Observing the responses of experimental subjects to the injection of adrenalin (which produced the fundamental functional bodily changes associated with fear), Marañon discovered that a majority of his subjects experienced only the physical symptoms produced by adrenalin *without emotion*, or, if they did have emotion, described it in a "cold," removed manner and spoke of themselves only as feeling "as if" they were afraid.

Not long after the publication of Marañon's work, Cannon[7] enunciated what has become a classic criticism of the James-Lange theory. In opposition to its propositions, he cited the following facts derived both from Marañon's findings and his own already extensive investigations into the emotions:

1. The total separation of the viscera from the central nervous system does not alter emotional behavior.
2. The same visceral changes occur in very different emotional states and in nonemotional states.
3. The viscera are relatively insensitive structures.
4. Visceral changes are too slow to be a source of emotional feelings.
5. The artificial induction of the visceral changes typical of strong emotions does not produce those emotions.

Instead of James's focus on the periphery as the locus of emotions, Cannon postulated the thalamus as the primary site of origin. In his theory, stimulation of the dorsal thalamus resulted in the feeling of emotions and, via the activation of hypothalamic structures, in their peripheral expression in specific patterns of visceral responses to autonomic discharge. In subsequent developments of the theory, which took into account the more recent neurophysiological findings concerning the cortical control of viscera, Papez[37] and McLean[34] each extended Cannon's notion of the central mediation of emotions to include the limbic system as being the "visceral brain" and the seat of emotions.

More recent findings have provided evidence that the Papez-McLean theory, although obviously having an important bearing on the phenomena of emotions, is too restricted to explain all of the facts. The work of those concerned with the reticular-activating system has tended to emphasize the quantitative over the qualitative aspects of emotional arousal. Pribram[39] has suggested that memory (related as well as the emotions to limbic system function) is an important component of emotional phenomena. Furthermore, contemporary research on the catecholamines and other endocrines indicates a complexity not hitherto suspected. The sympathetic nerve endings, for example, secrete norepinephrine whereas both epinephrine and norepinephrine are released from the adrenal medulla. Each

---

° Italics in original.

of these is not only controlled by different areas of the hypothalamus, but has a specific and selective effect on the target organs responsive to them.[25] Ax,[3] relating epinephrine to fear, and epinephrine-norepinephrine to anger, comments that the "finest nuances of psychological events may be found to have a corresponding differentiation at the physiological level." The way is paved by such findings for the reintroduction of the concept that the nature of the peripheral visceral response plays a part in the determination of the quality of experienced emotions.[47]

In a recent study, furthermore, it has been suggested that an excessive amount of blood lactate (the levels of which are raised by epinephrine) can contribute to the production of anxiety through the lowering of the level of ionized calcium. Patients with the symptoms of anxiety, it has been demonstrated,[38] manifest an excessive production of lactate after exercise, they are unduly sensitive to a standard infusion of sodium lactate, and their symptoms of anxiety can be prevented by adequate parenteral doses of calcium ion. The significance of these findings, however, and their specificity for clinical anxiety have been called into question,[17] and it is clear that the etiology of the symptoms involves more than a single metabolic abnormality. Indeed, not only are a variety of physiological as well as emotional factors implicated in the production of anxiety and other emotional states, but cognition and influences from the social milieu play a role as well, as has been shown in the work of Schachter and Singer to which we must now briefly turn.

Social and Cognitive Determinants of Emotion

Using mice that had been injected with either epinephrine or a placebo, Singer[45] demonstrated a difference in the response to environmental stimuli. "In an unstressful situation (the non-fear condition)," he reported, "differential drug injection has no effect upon behavior, but in a fear producing situation, the greater the drug-induced sympathetic arousal, the greater the amount of fright displayed."

To test further the implications of this experiment that physiological arousal alone does not necessarily produce an emotional state, Schachter and Singer[44] turned to a study of man. In an elaborately controlled experiment they gave a number of subjects a subcutaneous injection of ½ cc. of a 1:1000 solution of epinephrine. Part of the subjects were told what to expect in the way of visceral symptoms; the others were not. All of the subjects were then exposed first to a "stooge" who behaved in an elated, hyperactive fashion, then to a second who pretended to be angry. As compared with the informed subjects, a significantly larger number of those in the uninformed group became euphoric or angry as they were exposed to the one or the other "stooge," the informed group tending merely to be aware of the visceral effects of the injection without being emotionally aroused. Similarly, when the figures were adjusted for artifactual responses, a group of subjects given a placebo injection of normal saline were significantly less emotionally responsive than those given adrenalin and kept uninformed.

On the basis of these and related experiments, Schachter has suggested that the capacity to experience emotion requires visceral arousal, but that given such arousal, the experience of the presence and the quality of the emotion would depend on cognitive factors determined in part by the social environment. In Schachter's words:[43]

1. Given a state of physiological arousal for which an individual has no immediate explanation, he will "label" this state and describe his feelings in terms of the cognitions available to him. To the extent that cognitive factors are potent determiners of emotional states, one might anticipate that precisely the same state of physiological arousal could be labeled "joy" or "fury" or any of the great number of emotional labels, depending on the cognitive aspects of the situation.

2. Given a state of physiological arousal for which an individual has a completely appropriate explanation (e.g., "I feel this way because I have just received an injection of adrenalin"), no evaluative needs will arise and the individual is

unlikely to label his feelings in terms of the alternative cognitions available.

Finally, consider a condition in which emotion-inducing cognitions are present but there is no state of physiological arousal. For example, an individual might be completely aware that he is in great danger but for some reason (drug or surgical) might remain in a state of physiological quiescence. Does he experience the emotion of "fear"? This formulation of emotion as a joint function of a state of physiological arousal and an appropriate cognition, would, of course, suggest that he does not, which leads to my final proposition.

3. Given the same cognitive circumstances, the individual will react emotionally or describe his feelings as emotions only to the extent that he experiences a state of physiological arousal.

In the light of these observations it should be clear that there is no certain way of defining the physiological correlates of emotions in general, or anxiety in particular, and that, indeed, if Schachter is correct, it is cognitive and social factors that are the primary determinants of the emotional coloring to be given the visceral processes. Even more futile, in our present state of knowledge, is the hope of differentiating between anxiety and fear on any objective or measurable basis. If they cannot be separated out by subjective, experiential criteria, there is no sure method for distinguishing between them. For the clinician or the psychologist, however, this is perhaps not so catastrophic as it might at first glance appear. Both terms refer to introspective phenomena that have much in common and can be differentiated empirically from emotions that lie along other dimensions, such as joy, anger, and sorrow. Given the presence of anxiety or fear in his patients, the clinician can use that as a starting point for investigating those psychological and environmental determinants to which Schachter has called attention. This, of course, has always been the practice of the pragmatic psychiatrist, who has been more concerned with elucidating the personal and social sources of his patient's emotions than with exploring their physiological underpinnings. It is time, then, to turn to an examination of the psychological aspects of anxiety, with the understanding that the term

will be used henceforth in full recognition of the difficulties inherent in defining it exactly.

Psychological Aspects of Anxiety

Although the phenomena of anxiety had been recognized for centuries, anxiety itself was not singled out as a specific object of study until well into the nineteenth century. Internists and military surgeons, as we have seen, focused on its somatic manifestations (especially those involving the cardiovascular system), but their naïve ignorance of the central position of emotions in the production of the disorder they called "DaCosta's Syndrome" or "Disordered Action of the Heart" (and more recently "Neurocirculatory Asthenia"[8]) relegates them to a byway of psychiatric history. With the introduction by Beard[4] in 1880 of the term "neurasthenia," attention was drawn to a loose grouping of symptoms, among which those of anxiety were frequently found. Beard's explanations of the disorder centered on the pathognomonic complaints of weakness and fatigue, and it was not until Janet's introduction of the concept of *psychasthenia* that any attempt was made to discuss the etiology of anxiety.

For Janet, neurotic illness was, as we have seen, divided into the two major categories of *hysteria* and *psychasthenia*, a rich, neurotic stew of phobias, obsessions, compulsions, anxiety, fatigue, depression, etc. In Janet's theoretical scheme,[24] the concept of a loosening of mental structure was the keystone to his explanation of emotional illness. Every individual, he postulated, is hereditarily endowed with a quantum of nervous energy that binds together all the mental elements under the dominance and control of the conscious ego. In those with hereditary degeneracy of the nervous system, either spontaneously or as the result of an excessive expenditure of the nervous energy from the demands of life, the quantity of energy is lowered to a point where the synthesis of mental elements begins to dissolve and specific mental functions escape from the ego's control. An early sign of this is *dissociation*, in which clusters of memories and mental associations fall away from consciousness, resulting in the amnesias, anesthesias, and motor disturbances that characterize hysteria. A yet further dissolution of the synthesis permits more primitive forms of mental functioning to emerge in the form of phobias and obsessive-compulsive phenomena, and, as the anarchy spreads, in the symptoms of anxiety, which represent the autonomous discharging of the "vegetative" nervous system.

Freud kept the prevalent quantitative notion of nervous energy, but his concept of the structure and functioning of the mental apparatus, which was dynamic and functional where Janet's had been static and mechanical, introduced a radical change into the theoretical explanation of symptom formation. It had been recognized by numerous investigators toward the end of the nineteenth century that following their dissociation, mental elements, though unconscious and inaccessible to voluntary recall, could nonetheless indirectly influence conscious awareness and bodily functioning in the form of symptoms like obsessions, compulsions, and the large variety of hysterical phenomena. The problem was to explain the etiology of the process of dissociation itself. Janet, as we have seen, invoked a passive falling away of the mental elements as the mental synthesis was weakened following a lowering of the nervous energy. Freud[14] postulated a different mechanism: Mental elements, he proposed, that were unacceptable to the ego (because they were shameful or frightening, for example) were *actively* pushed and held out of conscious awareness by a mental counterforce, subsequently termed *repression*, that rendered them unavailable to conscious awareness.

As Freud was developing these new conceptions that heralded the onset of dynamic psychiatry, he was also introducing innovative suggestions for the reclassification of neurotic disorders.[11] In particular, dissatisfied with Janet's catch-all diagnosis of psychasthenia, Freud, as we have mentioned earlier, advanced the idea that the anxiety neurosis was a psychiatric entity in its own right, characterized by the central affect of anxiety. Furthermore, as his clinical observations indicated,

the anxiety occurred whenever there was a blocking of the release of sexual energy through orgasm, whether this was the result of continence or coitus interruptus. Putting these two sequential facts together, he proposed that anxiety represented a transformation of the undischarged sexual libido.

In a subsequent development of his theory, the blocking of libidinal discharge was seen as occurring not so much from the external circumstances just alluded to, but rather through the operation of the repression of unacceptable libidinal drives. Freud called the resulting syndrome of anxiety an *aktuel neurose*— the German *aktuel* not having the English connotation of "actual" or "real," but meaning "current," "present," "here-and-now." Implicit in the adjective *aktuel* was the idea that the processes leading to the symptoms involved forces that arose only out of factors to be found in the patient's existing, contemporaneous situation—the blocking, that is, of currently existing libidinal drives pressing then and there for discharge. This was viewed as being in contradistinction to the psychoneuroses, in which the psychological phenomena of repressed memories and emotions from *past* situations played a central role in determining the symptoms. Furthermore, the psychoneuroses were viewed as resulting from complex, higher-order mental phenomena like memories and fantasies, whereas the *actual neurosis* was seen as involving biological and somatic processes nearer to the physiological end of the mind-body spectrum.

Freud's views of the nature and etiology of anxiety remained unchanged for nearly three decades after their first formulation. It was not until the third decade of this century, and only after he had developed the foundations of an ego psychology, that Freud revised his concept of anxiety.[12] Reviewing the case of Little Hans, the phobic little boy whose story he had first told in 1909, Freud came to recognize that anxiety played a special role in the functioning of the psychic structure. Anxiety was now viewed as the ego's response to an unconscious id impulse which, if experienced or expressed, would expose the individual to a real or fantasied danger. Anxiety in this setting was seen as anticipating a future event and acted as a signal of an impending danger, leading to the setting in motion of ego defense mechanisms to control and keep unconscious the impulse that threatens to emerge into expression and discharge. Anxiety in this scheme was seen as the cause rather than the result of repression, and from that point on was given a central place in the psychic structure where, as an *ego affect*, it constituted both a symptom in itself and a force that set in motion other psychological processes underlying neurotic symptom formation.

Although Freud himself never completely gave up his earlier, more physiological, conception of anxiety, those who have since developed the theory have focused on its psychological aspects. As a signal of psychic dysequilibrium, the presence of anxiety leads to the asking of two questions: (1) What internal drive is the anxious individual afraid of? and (2) What are the consequences he fears if the drive were to be discharged? The answer to the first question is less complicated than that to the second. The drives most commonly implicated in psychic conflict and symptom formation are either sexual or aggressive in nature, whereas the consequences feared fall into four major categories which have been labeled according to the nature of those consequences:

1. *Superego anxiety*, as the term implies, is the ego's anticipation of the experience of guilt if the individual transgresses the ethical standards of behavior he has adopted for himself. By extension, if he has actually behaved as his forbidden impulse has directed, the individual then lives in anxious expectation of being found out, even when in reality other people may not be at all concerned about or critical of what he has done. ("The wicked flee when no man pursueth.")

2. *Castration anxiety* is a shorthand term used to refer to the anxious expectation of harmful retaliatory punishment. At the core of this anxiety are often to be found fantasies expressly representing an irrational fear of actual, physical castration, which by extension may be manifested in a derivative way in fears of injury to other bodily parts, or of a more general diminution of one's power, skills, and capabilities. A businessman, for example, had recurrent fears and doubts about his capacity to perform adequately in his work. Gradually, in the course of therapy he became aware of his fears of impotence, and finally, in one therapeutic session, to the accompaniment of intense anxiety, he recalled a long-repressed fantasy that some unknown person was driving a large spike through his penis.

3. *Separation anxiety*, as the name suggests, represents the dread of being ostracized or abandoned as a consequence of one's transgressions.

4. *Id anxiety* refers to an anxious foreboding, often amounting to panic, that one will not only lose control of one's impulses, but that the very integrity of one's ego and one's identity will be overwhelmed and destroyed by the strength of the drive's pressure for discharge and satisfaction. Anxiety of this sort is frequently seen in the early stages of an acute psychotic episode and in that event can be veridical.

It should be emphasized that in the adult these various anxieties are often entirely unrealistic and do not represent a response to threats that exist in their actual human or physical environment. On the contrary, they derive from *fantasied* expectations that have their source in long-past childhood phases of development. In childhood itself, although numerous anxieties stem from inner, autogenous fantasies, many represent a response to real external dangers. There is, for example, often actual punishment inflicted by parents and others, who spank or isolate the naughty child and thereby potentiate his internal tendencies to fear abandonment or castration. Fear of these threats from the external environment subsequently becomes internalized, and is incorporated along with the autogenous fantasies into the child's developing psychic structure, these together then being carried with him, largely unconscious in nature, into adulthood, where they form the basis of the anxiety that motivates his defenses and contributes to neurotic symptom formation.

The concept of anxiety was further developed by a number of Freud's colleagues and followers. For Rank,[41] the central issue was the fear of separation, a threat that dogged the individual throughout his years as he lived out the process of individuation. In his view, it was first and perhaps most intensely experienced in the process of being born. The vagaries of the "birth trauma," a universal human event, set the stage and pattern for all subsequent episodes of anxiety and became the hallmark of Rank's conception of that affect. Adler,[1] for whom anxiety was never a central element in his theory, saw it as being closely linked to the feelings of inferiority, weakness, and helplessness, that were for him the prime motivating factors in human behavior. Horney,[18] Fromm,[15] and Sullivan[48] have all focused on separation as the basic factor in anxiety and have laid more explicit stress than previous theorists on the importance of the individual's human and social environment. The child's conflict between dependence and independence on his mother, and the hostility that is an inevitable part of his struggle, are seen by Horney as playing the major role in the production of anxiety. For Fromm, the issues are similarly colored by the dependence-independence dialectic, but the contest is carried out against the larger backdrop of society as a whole, as man now strives for autonomy in freedom from cultural dictates, now, anxious and lost, retreats back into the crowd. Sullivan narrows the interpersonal stage down to the mother-child relationship and sees anxiety as arising in the earliest phases of that relationship as the infant almost intuitively senses his mother's disapproval in regard to elements of his behavior, and recognizes it as a threat to his security.

Although volumes have been written in support of the different views just summarized, the position of the various proponents, despite the acrimony of the debates that have ensued, are not basically unreconcilable. A little reflection suggests that the attention of each of the investigators whose concepts have been briefly reviewed is focused on one aspect of anxiety, all aspects of which are included in the broader, more inclusive scheme of the more strictly Freudian theory. Adler, for instance, seems to be dealing with what, in other terms, would fall into the category of "castration anxiety," while the other authors are more concerned with the general issue of "separation anxiety." And, while there are genuine differences among them in their theoretical positions, they appear to be in substantial agreement as to the clinical nature of anxiety, and its role in symptom production and psychological conflict.

Anxiety and Learning Theory

At first sight, it may appear paradoxical to include a consideration of learning theory in a discussion of anxiety, since learning theorists (especially those with a strong behavioral bent) are inclined to view subjective emotions as chimeras, to deny any scientific relevance to whatever processes go on within the skull, and to base their theoretical statements only on observable behavior. In actual fact, numerous learning theorists weave statements about emotions into their expositions, and fear has been elevated into a central place in the theory explaining operant conditioning. Mowrer was one of the first to move in this direction. In connection with the conditioning processes related to painful stimuli, Mowrer[36] wrote as follows:

When a buzzer sounds in the presence of a laboratory animal and the animal then receives a brief but moderately painful electric shock, we can be sure that the reaction of *fear*,° originally aroused by the shock, will, after a few pairings of buzzer and shock, start occurring to the buzzer alone. Only when the subject, not motivated by the secondary (acquired, conditioned) drive of fear, starts *behaving*° (as opposed to merely feeling) he is likely to hit upon some response which will "turn off" the danger signal and enable the subject to avert the shock. This, however, is no longer conditioning, or stimulus substitution, but habit formation. Here it seems that the subject first learns to *be afraid*° and then what to *do*° about the fear.

Fear, in other words, becomes bound to a signal other than the painful stimulus through the process of stimulus substitution, a central concept in the classical Pavlovian theory of

° Italics in original.

stimulus-response conditioning. But more has taken place—the now conditioned fear, anticipatory of the painful stimulus to come, becomes an acquired drive to purposeful action designed to avoid that stimulus.

With the development of this "two-factor" or "two-stage" concept, which included the stimulus substitution of Pavlovian conditioning and the phenomenon of the "shaping" of behavior through learned responses, the way was opened to the rational application of learning theory to the explanation and treatment of a variety of clinical psychiatric problems. It became possible to alter undesirable behavior through operant-conditioning shaping techniques, employing "rewards" and "punishments," and to combat anxiety (here considered synonymous with fear) by deconditioning procedures based on Pavlovian theory, especially when the anxiety was manifested in the form of a phobia. Learning theory and behavior therapy, already a significant addition to the knowledge and therapeutic armamentarium of the clinician, need further development, both in regard to their treatment techniques and their integration with the existing solid body of psychodynamic fact and theory.

The Existential View of Anxiety

Finally, a word must be said about a more philosophical approach to anxiety which, tracing its roots to Kierkegaard[26,27] in the nineteenth century, has provided an intellectual meeting ground for a variety of modern artists, philosophers, and psychiatrists. For the existentialist thinker and clinician, anxiety is not merely a sign of psychopathology. On the contrary, it is viewed as being a central element in normal human existence, closely bound up with man's psychological, moral, and spiritual growth away from the dependent state of childhood into the self-directed autonomy of truly responsible adulthood. Entailing as it does the frequent and frightening loss of security as the individual gives up one comfortable and familiar situation after another, the development of maturity necessarily produces repeated periods of anxiety,

which is not only a response to the uncertainty about what lies ahead, but also a positive and valuable stimulus to the individual's continued growth and to his solution to basic and universal human conundrums. The ultimate existential anxiety has to do with man's awareness of the fragility of his identity, the transience of his being, and the immensity of the nothingness that lies just beneath the surface of his existence. In the hierarchy of anxieties, this is the most profound and most real, and it is seen as being irreducible to other forms of anxiety or to other elements of human mental functioning. In the words of May,[32] one of the foremost English-speaking exponents of the existentialist view:

Authentic existence is the modality in which a man assumes the responsibility of his own existence. In order to pass from unauthentic to authentic existence, a man has to suffer the ordeal of despair and "existential anxiety," i.e., the anxiety of a man facing the limits of his existence with its fullest implications: death, nothingness. This is what Kierkegaard calls the "sickness unto death."

❲ Differential Diagnosis

Presented with a patient complaining of anxiety, the clinician is faced with two primary diagnostic problems: (1) to determine whether the complaints are the result of physical disease producing anxiety-like symptoms, and (2) having ascertained that the symptoms are in fact anxiety, to decide whether the patient is suffering from anxiety neurosis or another psychiatric syndrome of which the presenting anxiety is merely a part.

Psychiatric Syndromes

It should be evident from what has been said thus far that anxiety is to be found throughout the whole range of psychiatric disorders. If it occurs alone in either its acute or chronic form, the diagnosis of anxiety neurosis is made; if in conjunction with other symptoms, the latter usually predominate in defining the diagnostic category to which the illness is to be assigned. Thus, the patient in whom phobias are paramount is viewed as suffering from a phobic neurosis, even though anxiety may be a prominent feature of his disorder. Similarly, the diagnosis of schizophrenia, which in its acute form may be heralded by the outbreak of severe anxiety attacks, is established by the characteristic disorganization of thought and affect that soon follows. Of practical clinical importance is the fact that anxiety may form an integral part of depressive states. In two carefully studied series of patients with primary depressive illness,[28,35] acute anxiety attacks, at times reaching the intensity of panic, occurred in over 10 percent. In patients suffering from mid-life agitated depressions, anxiety forms an integral part of the syndrome, and individuals with neurotic reactive depressions often manifest considerable anxiety, the depressive affect being referable to the situational loss that has precipitated the illness, the anxiety to the uncertainties about the future created by the loss.

Physical Illness

ACUTE MYOCARDIAL INFARCTION

The symptoms and signs of chest pain, breathlessness, tachycardia, palpitations, and sweating, that characterize many anxiety attacks, may at times be confused with an acute myocardial infarction, especially by the physician who is unaware of the nature of anxiety and whose attention is too exclusively focused on somatic processes. Patients who have been dramatically rushed to a general hospital emergency ward in the midst of an acute attack of anxiety have sometimes been hurriedly admitted to the coronary intensive care unit where, on the accumulated evidence of negative diagnostic laboratory examinations, it is gradually recognized that the problem is one of a psychological disorder. If the physician does not include the symptoms of anxiety in his diagnostic considerations, and if he fails in his history-taking to look for recent life events that may be anxiety-provoking in nature, he may subject some of his patients to unnecessary hospitalization, diagnostic studies, and expense.

HYPERTHYROIDISM

Chronic anxiety is often a central complaint in the clinical evolution of hyperthyroidism, and the physician should consider this condition in searching for the cause of his patient's symptoms. At the same time, it should be recognized that many patients with thyroid disease remain anxious even after all the physiological parameters of thyroid function have been restored to normal. The exact relation between emotional stress and hyperthyroidism is still unclear, but there is sufficient evidence that emotional factors are involved to warrant an evaluation of each such patient's psychological and social situation.

PHEOCHROMOCYTOMA

In this rare tumor of the adrenal medulla, epinephrine and norepinephrine may be episodically poured into the circulating bloodstream in sufficient quantities to produce an acute diffuse visceral response that has all the peripheral autonomous signs and symptoms of an anxiety attack. These do not necessarily carry with them the subjective experience of anxious dread, but in patients with the proper cognitive set (as described by Marañon[31] and Schachter[43]) it is conceivable that the presence of the peripherally induced visceral sensations might arouse the central feeling of anxiety. On a statistical basis, it is unlikely that any given patient complaining of anxiety will be harboring a pheochromocytoma, but if there are reasonable grounds for suspecting it clinically, the further appropriate physical and radiologic examinations should be made.

OTHER CONDITIONS

The anxious patient's complaint of "dizziness" or "faintness" may lead the clinician to think of Menière's Syndrome or hypoglycemia. These conditions should be easily ruled out by glucose metabolism studies in the case of the latter disorder, and by careful history and physical examination in the former. In patients with anxiety, the dizziness is not a true vertigo, but is rather a sense of swaying or lightheadedness, and is unassociated with nystagmus or deafness, or the other signs of middle ear disease that are characteristically a part of Menière's Syndrome.

Treatment

Medication

The use of medication is aimed at controlling the symptoms. Theoretically, drugs might be employed that acted either centrally or peripherally, but the proposed use of propanalol,[16] an adrenergic reaction-blocking agent acting on the peripheral autonomic nervous system, has not been given an adequate clinical trial, and current pharmacotherapy is generally limited to the centrally acting tranquilizers. Those commonly in use are meprobamate, chlordiazepoxide hydrochloride (Librium), and diazepam (Valium), the stronger phenothiazines being reserved for the agitation and anxiety found in schizophrenia and certain toxic or drug-withdrawal states. Barbiturates are useful for patients who include insomnia among their symptoms, but with the advent of the newer tranquilizers are now much less frequently prescribed for the control of anxiety. In view of their soporific effects and the danger of addiction, especially in dependent patients, this represents an advance in the chemotherapy of anxiety.

Psychological Measures

SUPPORTIVE THERAPY

Many patients find that their anxiety responds merely to the establishment of a supportive relationship with their doctor, a vital element in the treatment of all illness, whether physical or psychological in nature. The physician may, when indicated, potentiate the beneficial effect of the doctor-patient relationship by certain more active psychological measures, such as encouraging the patient to talk about his anxieties, giving reassurance, information and advice, or manipulating the environment when it is possible to change external anxiety-provoking situations. It should also be recognized that psychological support is an important element in the effectiveness of anti-anxiety medications, and these should generally not be used without providing the appropriate adjunctive supportive measures.

SUGGESTION AND RELAXATION

A variety of techniques and exercises have been proposed which can be learned by anxious patients to help them reduce anxiety by consciously induced physical and mental relaxation.[19] In all of these, suggestion probably plays an important role, the patient responding both to his anticipation of the results to be obtained and to his ideas of what the physician expects of him. In those with a capacity for hypnotic trance,[46] the effectiveness of suggestion and relaxation can often be greatly increased through the techniques of self-hypnosis, which can readily be taught many patients, thus giving them an important measure of self-control over their symptoms.

DECONDITIONING

Based on the concepts of learning theory, a technique has been devised for the treatment of phobias that is aimed at undoing the learned, conditioned linkage between anxiety and an environmental stimulus that is not in itself essentially anxiety-provoking in character. The patient is instructed to construct a hierarchy of phobic objects and situations in ascending order of their potential to produce anxiety. He is then required sequentially to imagine each step in the hierarchy from the least to the most disturbing, while at the same time the anxiety associated with each step is reduced to tolerable and controllable levels through the use of tranquilizers, relaxation exercises, or hypnosis—a technique referred to as *reciprocal inhibition*.[49] Considerable success has been reported in thus rendering once phobic objects incapable of arousing anxiety, and the growing interest in these currently experimental therapeutic techniques should ultimately provide sufficient information to enable one more accurately to determine both the indications for their use and their long-term effectiveness.

INSIGHT PSYCHOTHERAPY

The decision to treat anxiety with psychoanalysis or one of its derivative shorter forms of insight psychotherapy cannot be based on the presence of the symptom alone. On the contrary, the effectiveness of such methods of treatment is determined by a variety of factors that include the individual's capacity to tolerate painful emotions, his psychological-mindedness, his ability to express his feelings and to make lasting human relationships, a reasonable stability in his patterns of work, his control of his impulses, and his general level of intelligence. Unlike the forms of treatment that have just been reviewed, insight psychotherapy is aimed at altering the underlying internal psychological mechanisms that produce anxiety, rather than at the removal or control of the symptom alone. It should be emphasized that the development of insight requires the patient to examine the anxiety-provoking elements in his psychic structure. This inevitably arouses anxiety, which, as indicated, he must be able to tolerate, and which acts for both patient and therapist as an indicator of the locus and nature of the pathologic psychological conflicts. In this setting, anxiety can no longer be viewed as merely a symptom to be suppressed or dispelled, but rather as a pathway to psychological growth and maturation. It is perhaps here that the psychotherapist comes closest, if in a limited way, to those existential philosophers who see in anxiety a positive force for individual human good.

⟪ Bibliography

1. ADLER, A. *Problems of Neurosis*. New York: Cosmopolitan Book Corp., 1930.
2. AMERICAN PSYCHIATRIC ASSOCIATION. *Diagnostic and Statistical Manual of Mental Disorders* (DSM-II). Washington, D.C.: American Psychiatric Association, 1968.
3. AX, A. F. "The Physiological Differentiation Between Fear and Anger in Humans," *Psychosomatic Medicine*, 15 (1953), 433.
4. BEARD, G. *A Practical Treatise on Nervous Exhaustion (Neurasthenia)*. New York: William Wood, 1880.
5. BORROW, G. *Lavengro*. London: Oxford University Press, 1947.
6. BURTON, R. *The Anatomy of Melancholy*. 3 Vols. London: Dent, 1964.
7. CANNON, W. B. "The James-Lange Theory of Emotions: A Critical Examination and an Alternative Theory," *American Journal of Psychology*, 39 (1927), 106.
8. CRAIG, H. R., and P. D. WHITE. "Etiology and Symptoms of Neurocirculatory Asthenia," *Archives of Internal Medicine*, 53 (1934), 633.
9. DaCOSTA, J. M. "On Irritable Heart; a Clinical Study of a Form of Functional Cardiac Disorder and Its Consequences," *American Journal of Medical Science*, 61 (1871), 17.
10. ENGEL, G. L., E. B. FERRIS, and M. LOGAN. "Hyperventilation: Analysis of Clinical Symptomatology," *Annals of Internal Medicine*, 27 (1947), 683.
11. FREUD, S. "On the Grounds for Detaching a Particular Syndrome from Neurasthenia under the Description 'Anxiety Neurosis,'" in Standard Edition, Vol. 3. London: Hogarth Press, 1962.
12. ———. *Inhibition, Symptom and Anxiety*, in Standard Edition, Vol. 20. London: Hogarth Press, 1959.
13. ———. *New Introductory Lectures on Psycho-Analysis*, in Standard Edition, Vol. 21. *Complete Psychological Works of Sigmund Freud*. London: Hogarth Press, 1964.
14. FREUD, S. and J. BREUER. *Studies on Hysteria*, in Standard Edition, Vol. 2. London: Hogarth Press, 1955.
15. FROMM, E. *Escape from Freedom*. New York: Discus Books, 1969.
16. GRANVILLE-GROSSMAN, K. L., and P. TURNER. "The Effect of Propanalol on Anxiety," *Lancet*, 1 (1966), 788.
17. GROSZ, H. J., and B. B. FARMER. "Blood Lactate in the Development of Anxiety Symptoms," *Archives of General Psychiatry*, 21 (1969), 611.
18. HORNEY, K. *New Ways in Psychoanalysis*. New York: W. W. Norton & Co., 1939.
19. JACOBSON, E. *Progressive Relaxation*. Chicago: University of Chicago Press, 1938.
20. JAMES, H. *The Letters of William James*. 2 Vols. Boston: The Atlantic Monthly Press, 1920.
21. JAMES, W. *The Principles of Psychology*.

2 Vols. New York: Henry Holt & Co., 1890.

22. ———. *The Varieties of Religious Experience.* New York: Random House, 1902.

23. JANET, P., and F. RAYMOND. *Les Névroses et Idées Fixes.* 2 Vols. Paris: Félix Alcan, 1898.

24. JANET, P. *Les Obsessions et la Psychasthénie.* 2 Vols. Paris: Félix Alcan, 1903.

25. KETY, S. "Psychoendocrine Systems and Emotion: Biological Aspects," in D. C. Glass, ed., *Neurophysiology and Emotion.* New York: Rockefeller University Press and Russell Sage Foundation, 1967.

26. KIERKEGAARD, S. *Fear and Trembling.* Trans. by Walter Lowrie. Garden City, N.Y.: Doubleday & Co., 1955.

27. ———. *The Concept of Dread.* Trans. by Walter Lowrie. Princeton: Princeton University Press, 1957.

28. LEWIS, A. "Melancholia: a Clinical Survey of Depressive States," *Journal of Mental Science,* 80 (1934), 277.

29. ———. "The Ambiguous Word 'Anxiety,'" *International Journal of Psychiatry,* 9 (1970–71), 62.

30. LEWIS, T. *The Soldier's Heart and the Effort Syndrome.* New York: Paul B. Hoeber, 1919.

31. MARAÑON, G. "Contribution a l'étude de l'action émotive de l'adrénaline," *Revue française d'endocrinologie,* 2 (1924), 301.

32. MAY, R. *The Meaning of Anxiety.* New York: The Ronald Press, 1950.

33. MAY, R., E. ANGEL, and H. F. ELLENBERGER, eds. *Existence.* New York: Basic Books, 1958.

34. McLEAN, P. D. "Psychosomatic Disease and the 'Visceral Brain': Recent Developments Bearing on the Papez Theory of Emotion," *Psychosomatic Medicine,* 11 (1949), 338.

35. MITCHELL-HEGGS, N. "Aspects of the Natural History and Clinical Presentation of Depression," *Proceedings of the Royal Society of Medicine,* 64 (1971), 1171.

36. MOWRER, O. H. *Learning Theory and Behavior.* New York: John Wiley and Sons, 1960.

37. PAPEZ, J. W. "A Proposed Mechanism of Emotion," *Archives of Neurology and Psychiatry,* 38 (1937), 725.

38. PITTS, F. N., JR., and J. N. McCLURE, JR. "Lactate Metabolism in Anxiety Neurosis," *New England Journal of Medicine,* 277 (1967), 1329.

39. PRIBRAM, K. H. "Emotion: Steps Toward a Neuropsychological Theory," in D. C. Glass, ed., *Neurophysiology and Emotion.* New York: Rockefeller University Press and Russell Sage Foundation, 1967.

40. RABKIN, R. "An Embarrassing Situation," *International Journal of Psychiatry,* 9 (1970–71), 98.

41. RANK, O. *The Trauma of Birth.* New York: Harcourt, Brace & Co., 1929.

42. SARBIN, T. R. "Anxiety: Reification of a Metaphor," *Archives of General Psychiatry,* 10 (1964), 630.

43. SCHACHTER, S. "The Interaction of Cognitive and Physiological Determinants of Emotional State," in P. H. Leiderman, and D. Shapiro, eds., *Psychobiological Approaches to Social Behavior.* Stanford: Stanford University Press, 1964.

44. SCHACHTER, S., and J. E. SINGER. "Cognitive, Social and Physiological Determinants of Emotional State," *Psychological Review,* 69 (1962), 379.

45. SINGER, J. E. "Sympathetic Activation, Drugs and Fear," *Journal of Comparative and Physiologic Psychology,* 56 (1963), 612.

46. SPIEGEL, H. "A Single Treatment Method to Stop Smoking," *Journal of Clinical Experimental Hypnosis,* 18 (1970), 235.

47. STEIN, M. "Some Psychophysiological Considerations of the Relationship between the Autonomic Nervous System and Behavior," in D. C. Glass, ed., *Neurophysiology and Emotion.* New York: Rockefeller University Press and Russell Sage Foundation, 1967.

48. SULLIVAN, H. S. *The Interpersonal Theory of Psychiatry.* New York: W. W. Norton and Co., 1953.

49. WOLPE, J. *Psychotherapy by Reciprocal Inhibition.* Stanford: Stanford University Press, 1958.

50. WORLD HEALTH ORGANIZATION. *International Classification of Diseases.* Washington, D.C.: U.S. Department of Health, Education and Welfare, 1968.

CHAPTER 6

PHOBIC REACTIONS

Paul Friedman and Jacob Goldstein

THE TERM "PHOBIA" is derived from the Greek word *phobos*, meaning flight, dread, panic, or fear. When a fear becomes attached to objects or situations which objectively are not a source of danger—or, more precisely, are known by the individual not to be a source of danger—we designate it as a phobia. The patient, as a rule, realizes the irrationality of his behavior but feels compelled to avoid those specific situations which expose him to overpowering anxiety.

The concomitant physiological symptoms usually present in anxiety states and in reactions of fear and panic—tachycardia, rapid breathing, tremor, sweating, etc.—may likewise accompany acute phobic reactions.

⟨ Historical Remarks

The earliest known case history of a phobic patient is recorded in one of the books attributed to Hippocrates.[62]

One of the first attempts to deal systematically with the origin of phobic reactions was made by John Locke in the chapter entitled "Of the Association of Ideas," included for the first time in the fourth edition of *An Essay Concerning Human Understanding*.[91]

"Antipathies" and fears, Locke reasoned, often arise from associations of ideas, and, if such "antipathies" were acquired in childhood, their causes may later be forgotten:

The ideas of goblins and sprites have really no more to do with darkness than light, yet let but a foolish maid inculcate these often on the mind of a child, and raise them there together, possibly he shall never be able to separate them again so long as he lives, but darkness shall ever afterwards bring with it those frightful ideas, and they shall be so joined, that he can no more bear the one without the other.

Locke recognized that it is not within the power of reason to relieve the "antipathies" thus acquired, but added that they could sometimes be cured by time. (Incidentally, he was quite explicit in stating that besides the acquired "antipathies" there are also some which depend on constitution.)

Within the field of psychiatry proper phobic phenomena began to receive increasing attention during the second half of the nineteenth century. One of the historically important papers was published by Westphal[128] who introduced the term "agoraphobia" to describe fear of wide streets, squares, or open spaces, and presented data on three agoraphobic patients.* Westphal described the agoraphobic reaction as determined by a fear that is "psychologically unmotivated"; that is, by an idea of danger which appears irrational and strange to the individual, but which dominates his behavior as he approaches the feared area. He also argued against some earlier theories which ascribed such fears to attacks of dizziness or to epilepsy.

The phenomenological similarity between phobias and obsessions led the descriptive psychiatry of the late nineteenth and early twentieth century, as represented in the writings of Oppenheim,[100] of Kraepelin,[79] and (to a lesser extent) of Pitres and Régis,[102] to lump them together, a tendency already implicit in Westphal's discussion of agoraphobia. The phobias, as well as obsessions and "impulsions," were regarded as being, to a large extent, constitutionally determined, although Pitres and Régis placed considerable stress on the importance of the precipitating incident and on the emotional aspects of both the phobic and the obsessive reactions. In the early editions of Kraepelin's *Lehrbuch* these conditions were classified under the neurasthenias; later they were reclassified under "compulsive insanity," which in turn was designated as a psychopathic state. Although he considered these states as a form of degeneration of the nervous system, Kraepelin admitted that such "degenerative" symptoms could occur in persons of superior intelligence whose intellectual capacity appeared otherwise unimpaired. Kraepelin, as well as Oppenheim, regarded the prognosis of phobias as unfavorable, although both mentioned that recoveries occasionally took place. The therapeutic measures recommended by Oppenheim included

exercises aiming to accustom the patient to the phobic situation; in the case of agoraphobia, he suggested that the physician accompany the patient in walking across the feared open places. However, he also advised various somatic measures, such as washing the head in cold water and removal of nasal polypi.

A study of fears utilizing the questionnaire method was published in 1897 by G. Stanley Hall.[58] His statistical analysis, based essentially on a classification of the feared objects, led Hall to advance the view that some fears represent vestigial traces of ancestral experiences, perhaps antedating limbs and visual space perception. According to him, the best evidence for the phylogenetic antiquity of the predisposition for fear rests on "the proportional strength of different fear elements and tendencies. Their relative intensity fits past conditions better than it does present ones."

Pierre Janet[68,69] submitted the phobic reactions to a more thorough psychological study, relating them closely to hysterical paralyses, since both have—according to him—the function of preventing the individual from carrying out some task he does not want to perform. In this conception, the fear aspect is a secondary phenomenon rather than a cause of the phobia. Janet was the first to present a massive amount of observational data on the phobic and obsessional symptoms.†

However, it was Freud who introduced the truly dynamic conception of phobia. As early as 1895, in his paper "Obsessions and Phobias: Their Psychical Mechanisms and Their Aetiology",[47] he sharply differentiated these two conditions from one another, designating phobias as part of anxiety neurosis. But the fundamental psychoanalytic formulation concerning the mechanisms underlying the phobias is contained in his clinical study "Analysis of a Phobia in a Five-Year-Old Boy,"[45] which remains a classic exposition of the subject. It will serve here as a basis for a detailed discussion of these mechanisms.

---

* The term "claustrophobia" was introduced in the same year (1877) by Raggi.[106]

† Limitations of space prevent a more detailed exposition of Janet's hypotheses, which originated in Charcot's theory of the hypnoid states of hysterical patients.

❪ Experimental Studies of Acquired Fears

Experimental study of the acquisition and elimination of fear reactions in infants was one of the foci of interest of the behavioristic school, as represented in the work of J. B. Watson and his followers[122,123,124] and M. C. Jones[72,73,] 1924 a & b). Thus, Watson and Rayner—using a technique based on the conditioning procedures developed by Pavlov—found that a fear reaction to a white rat (which was initially a neutral object) could be established rather easily in an eleven-month-old infant by repeatedly producing behind the infant's head a loud sound which was presumably frightening to the infant whenever the animal was shown; and that the fear reaction thus established was then also manifested in relation to other similar objects, such as a rabbit. Although Watson's antimentalistic and elementaristic brand of psychology has long since been rejected, there has recently been a resurgence of interest in this early work on fears, largely under the influence of behavior therapists, who regard these authors as important forerunners of the behavior therapy approach.

A more sophisticated approach, involving an attempt to translate psychoanalytic concepts into learning-theory terms, is found in the work of Dollard and Miller,[25] who interpret phobias as learned avoidance reactions. (For a critique of Dollard and Miller's approach see Rapaport.)[107]

In the years which have elapsed since the publication of Dollard and Miller's volume, many experimental studies have dealt with traumatic avoidance reactions (avoidance reactions established through the administration of an electric shock or some other noxious stimulus to the animal subject), as well as with conditions under which such reactions can be eliminated (or "extinguished," to use conditioned-response terminology). Some investigators regard these studies as providing a close experimental analogue of the phobias. It should, however, be noted that there are still wide differences of opinion between those in-

vestigators who favor behavioristic interpretations of experimental findings on avoidance learning and those who favor cognitive explanations. For relevant literature summaries see Baum[10] and Wilson and Davison.[130]*

While the experiments on traumatic avoidance learning appear to be of relevance for the understanding of some of the simpler phobic reactions, their relationship to the more deep-rooted phobias in which symbolic displacement plays a prominent role appears more remote.

❪ Differential Considerations

At this point, it is necessary to introduce some distinctions whereby the phobias can be more carefully differentiated from other types of fear reactions.†

Today we distinguish sharply between anxiety neurosis and anxiety hysteria (phobia).

* Quite apart from these differences in interpretation, the available evidence suggests that some fears which typically manifest themselves at particular developmental stages cannot easily be reduced to the traumatic avoidance model. One is the fear of visual patterns which simulate the danger of falling. The available findings[121] indicate that this fear is typically present in an intense form in sighted human infants by the age of six months. Some of the evidence[21] suggests that this fear reaction is not yet present in the two-month-old infant who—as far as can be determined from behavioral and physiological indications—typically reacts to a similar optical pattern with curiosity rather than fear. Since some animal species display a fear reaction to comparable optical patterns within a day after birth (without the benefit of experience of the kind envisaged by the conditioned avoidance model), a plausible case can be made for the assumption that maturation plays a role in the development of this fear reaction in the human infant. However, there is reason to believe that improved cognitive grasp of the properties of perceived space also plays a role in the emergence of this fear. It should, incidentally, be noted that the six-month-old infant's fear of the danger represented by the visual pattern is quite realistic, though in the experimental situation the infant is protected against the actual dangers of falling by a transparent surface.

It may be conjectured that this early fear of the dangers of downward extension is one of the factors which may contribute to the subsequent development of height phobias in some persons.

† Problems of differential diagnosis of phobias by means of the Rorschach test are discussed by Schafer, by Klopfer and Spiegelman,[78] and by Deri.[23]

The clinical forms of anxiety neurosis may range all the way from acute kakon-crisis* characterized by sudden onset and by violent excitation to milder states of generalized anxiety. The anxiety neurotic suffers from a general fear of dying rather than from fear of a specific object. His anxieties are of a floating form, whereas the phobic's fears center on a specific object or group of related objects, and subside when the object is removed. This is why phobic patients carefully avoid the anxiety-arousing object or situation.

Phobic reactions should also be distinguished from paranoid apprehensiveness in which suspicion of evil intentions of others is a prominent feature. Of course, phobic reactions such as agoraphobia or claustrophobia can sometimes be overdetermined by paranoid tendencies.

Still another fear reaction which should be distinguished from phobia is an exaggerated fear of disease which is more likely to be of a narcissistic-hypochondriacal rather than of a genuinely phobic nature. In a true phobia the fear can be reduced by avoiding the phobic object; but there is no such possibility of avoidance of his own body by the patient who fears cancer or a heart attack. (However, while one's own body, as such, cannot be avoided, an avoidance reaction may be manifested in a less direct fashion, e.g., through avoidance of a medical examination on the part of persons who fear that they may be found to have a malignant disease or may be in need of surgery.) The possibility of avoidance is only slightly better for the person with a pathological fear of germs. In cases with a strongly obsessive component, the fear of germs may take the form of elaborate precautions against infection. In the more narcissitic or hypochondriacal cases, the fear of germs is more likely to take the form of a preoccupation with the notion that an invasion of the body by the germs has already taken place. (Of course, precautionary measures against infection are not pathological unless they take an exaggerated form.)

The difference between true phobias and

hypochondriacal disturbances is not to be understood merely in terms of a different choice of the phobic object; rather, the difference in the choice of the phobic object is a function of more basic differences in the level of regression.

Phobic fears must be differentiated from fears based upon realistic danger as well as from fears involving primarily an intellectual belief in the dangerous character of certain objects or situations. For example, a person is not necessarily manifesting a phobic reaction if he hesitates to travel by air because of his knowledge that plane accidents do sometimes happen. It is true that this rational consideration, which is based on statistical facts, may occasionally be overdetermined by a genuine phobia of flying. But then, the phobic component is precisely that part of the avoidance reaction which is independent of the intellectual estimate of danger and whose intensity is disproportionate to such intellectual judgment. An excellent description of these relationships can be found in *The Love and Fear of Flying* by Bond.[13] Of course, culturally accepted beliefs about the dangerousness of certain objects or situations sometimes differ sharply from objective reality, but fear of such culturally defined dangerous objects does not necessarily constitute a phobia in the sense of individual pathology. (For relevant anthropological data see Hallowell.)[59,60]

The fact that phobic reactions can take place in the absence of a conscious belief in the dangerousness of the object is highlighted by the findings—e.g., those summarized by Bandura[6]—which indicate that phobic reactions may be evoked by pictorial representations of the phobic object.

A distinction must also be drawn between the true phobias and the so-called panophobic reactions. The latter are usually pseudophobias, in which the fear is not attached to a particular object, although the patients seem to be afraid of many objects and situations. Indeed, such individuals fear anything and everything, especially any change.

The phobias proper may be broadly grouped, according to their content, into those relating to objects and those relating to situa-

* Von Monakow[97] derived the appellation of this acute anxiety state from the Greek *kakon* = evil.

tions. Among the former, we may cite the animal phobias; among the latter, stage fright, the fear of blushing in public (erythrophobia), of going out into the street, etc. Sometimes, as in the case of erythrophobia, the fear is phenomenologically focused not so much on the objective situation as such as on anticipated embarrassment resulting from one's own uncontrolled reaction. The phobias can also be classified in terms of the degree of displacement which they represent or in terms of developmental fixation or regression involved in the phobic symbolism. Thus, as Sperling's[114] findings indicate, a spider phobia often reflects a pregenital fixation with anal-sadistic features and with an ambivalent relationship to the mother; and it also represents a substantial degree of displacement, since the typical spider phobia is not a result of an actual injury by a spider.

Another important distinction among the phobic reactions, which has proved the most practical of all classifications, was formulated by Freud[47] when he divided them into:

(1) Common phobias, an exaggerated fear of all those things which everyone detests or fears to some extent, such as night, solitude, death, illness, dangers in general, snakes, etc.; and (2) specific phobias, the fear of special circumstances that inspire no fear in the normal man; for example, agoraphobia and the other phobias of locomotion.

The common—or, as Freud later designated them—*universal* phobias are thus fears which are common to most human beings but which, in the case of the phobic patient, have become intensified and have assumed neurotic proportions. Any normal person might, for instance, experience fear at the sight of a snake or when caught unprotected in a thunderstorm.

There is a wide range of variation with respect to the objects of phobic fears. Some of the more frequently encountered phobias involve fear of animals, of open and closed spaces (agoraphobia or claustrophobia), or of heights (acrophobia). But a phobia may involve virtually any object. Hence Hall's[58] notion of classifying phobias according to the feared object or situation and endowing each with a Greek name (gynophobia, peccatipho-

bia, botophobia, photophobia, etc.) is no longer considered useful, as one would have to add an infinite number of such names to the list.

While cultural factors appear to have some influence on the choice of some specific phobic objects, the incidence of other phobic fears seems to be much less subject to culturally determined fluctuations. The latter are essentially the phobias that correspond to the more universal experiences of space, darkness, water, etc., which in large measure extend to early infancy.*

(Pathogenesis

The processes involved in the formation of phobic symptoms are especially well illustrated in Freud's "Analysis of a Phobia in a Five-Year-Old Boy",[45] commonly known as the case of "Little Hans." Usually, the origin of a neurosis can be traced only through a reconstruction of remote events, but in this instance the phobia came under study almost as soon as its manifestations appeared, and the boy's father, who conducted the treatment under Freud's guidance, was in a much better position than are most therapists to supple-

---

* In a volume published in 1956, Laughlin[82] noted that syphilophobia, common in the 1920s, had since become extremely rare and was by 1956 being encountered only in association with schizophrenia; and that, in contrast, the frequency of phobic fears of cancer had apparently risen. These changes, he pointed out, seem to have paralleled changes in the relative danger from the two diseases, and also have reflected the greater publicity "recently" (as of 1956) given to cancer. On the other hand, he notes that the popularity of some phobic objects—water, heights, closed spaces, open saces—had apparently remained unchanged during the same period.

In the interval since the publication of Laughlin's remarks, VD rates had again risen, and in response to the rising VD rates anti-VD educational efforts have become intensified. During the same period, beginning approximately with the publication of the Surgeon General's 1957 statement on the subject, wide publicity has been given to the relationship between smoking and cancer. Whether these factors have had an effect on the incidence of syphilophobia and cancerophobia is a question that cannot be answered at this time. It can, however, be stated that water, heights, closed spaces, and open spaces still remain among the frequent phobic objects.

ment the patient's statements with his own knowledge of certain relevant events.

Freud's classic case study deals with a child who refused to go out into the street for fear that a horse might bite him. At the root of the phobia, as the analysis revealed, was a conflict between the boy's instinctual strivings and his ego demands. His oedipal conflict and strong hostility toward the father gave rise to intense fears of punishment, that is, to castration fears, which became transformed into the phobic fear of being bitten by a horse, as well as into a fear that a horse pulling a heavily loaded vehicle will fall down. The horse was substituted for the father, an internal danger was changed into an external one, and the fear was displaced onto the substitute. It is easier to avoid an external danger than to cope with an inner danger that cannot be avoided.

These processes are characteristic of the phobic structure in general.[*]

(Repression and Displacement

In phobia, the original object of the fear is typically replaced by some other object, and the original source of the fear reaction becomes repressed. In the case of "Little Hans," death wishes against the father and fear of punishment for such wishes were repressed, because consciously they were unacceptable to this boy who also had strong positive feelings toward the father. However, his death wishes and fear of punishment (as well as still other components of the psychological constellation) re-emerged in the form of a phobia consisting of fears that a horse would fall down and that a horse would bite him. The choice of a horse as the phobic object appears to have been overdetermined by various factors, including the precipitating incident in which Hans saw a horse fall.

[*] Dixon *et al.*[24a] (1957) maintain that it is "both incorrect and misleading" to consider phobias as isolated symptoms, and that "any apparent specificity of the complaint may in fact be due to unconscious displacement." While the statistical analysis presented by these authors is highly interesting and instructive, exception must be taken to their conclusion that the phobia is not a distinct entity. The fears dealt with in their study seem to be symptoms of various clinical conditions.

The child was unaware of the symbolic meaning of his fear. Thus, the displacement provided a double advantage: He could go on loving his father, while the fear was concentrated on a more easily avoided object.

As already indicated, his choice of the horse as the phobic object was by no means accidental. Before the outbreak of the phobia Hans had shown a lively interest in horses. He had observed that they (and other large animals) had large "widdlers" (penises). This item of information led him to conclude that his father likewise had a large "widdler," and, as yet unfamiliar with the facts of sexual differentiation, he reached a similar conclusion about his mother. Such observations, moreover, served to reassure the little boy that his own "widdler" would grow larger as he grew older. But it is noteworthy that after the phobic symptoms had emerged, the work of repression extended also to his recollection of his observations of the "widdlers" of large animals, that is, of observations that undoubtedly had played a role in the choice of the horse as the substitute object in his phobic symptom.

In fact, the repression not only caused this substitution to be made but also encompassed the original affects. As Freud points out, the child's *hostile feelings* toward the father were replaced by a *fear* of the horse, so that the aggression was displaced (projected) to the outside.[†] Nor were his sexual feelings toward the mother manifestly present in the phobic symptom, although the castration fear, symbolized by the fear of the horse, was in part derived from a fear of punishment for these feelings.

The degree of displacement in phobia may vary. Fenichel[39] mentions several categories, such as "sex phobia," eating phobias, fighting phobias, which primarily involve fear of temptation and where relatively little displacement occurs. In other types, the degree of displacement is much greater, so that the symbolic meaning of the phobia is more effectively concealed and can be discovered only through

[†] Actually the fear that a horse might fall reflects the hostile feelings more closely than does the fear of being bitten by a horse. However, here also the hostility is masked through projection.

prolonged analytic work. Thus, the agoraphobic symptom may have a variety of remote meanings, including the idea of an open street as an opportunity of sexual adventure; the idea of leaving home; the idea that on an open street one may be seen and caught; the idea that some other person (usually a parent or sibling) may die while one is away from home; or the idea of being born. In a less symbolic sense, agoraphobia may also represent a reaction to "equilibrium eroticism," that is, to a sexualized pleasure in the sensations of equilibrium while walking.[1]

Displacement is likewise a prominent feature of claustrophobia, a symptom often traceable to fantasies of intrauterine existence. According to Ferenczi,[41,42] there is a close association between claustrophobia and the idea of being inside the mother; the fear of being buried alive is often a transformation of the wish to return to the womb. He also cites a case where claustrophobia and fear of being left alone in any enclosed space acted as a defense against masturbatory temptation. Observing that skin and chest sensations are particularly prominent in claustrophobic anxiety, Lewin[86] attributes this fact to the fantasy of being inside the mother and to ideas concerning the tactile sensations and breathing of the fetus. This fantasy is also described by him as one of partial identification through oral incorporation.

These are but a few examples where displacement is prominent. It is actually a characteristic feature of most phobias. The assumption that the choice of the phobic object is determined by displacement is consistent with the view that fears of early infancy affect the subsequent choice of the phobic object.

Concomitantly with displacement, projection plays an important role in the phobic symptom formation. "Little Hans," as already indicated, harbored aggressive impulses against his father. These impulses he projected onto the object of his hostility, the father, thence displacing them onto the horse by which he feared would bite him.

One might say that the general human tendency to create the outer world in the image of the inner world is one of the prominent features of the phobic's defense against anxiety.* However, although in phobia the ego structure is more severely impaired than in conversion hysteria, the projection in phobia is far less extensive than it is in psychosis. Unlike the paranoiac, the phobic remains capable of reality testing, and is usually aware that his anxiety is subjective rather than based on objective danger (Nunberg[98a]).

❨ Identification and Regression

The role of identification in phobia has been described by many authors. Deutsch[24] showed that the phobic fear of going out alone in the street is closely bound up with ambivalence, which frequently can be traced back to the oedipal situation. In some instances of animal phobia (for example, the hen phobia described by Deutsch), analysis revealed the existence of an earlier identification with the animal, which subsequently became the phobic object.[24]

In the case of "Little Hans," the realization that large animals have large "widdlers" became fused with his own wish for a large "widdler." This occurred by way of identification, thus paving the way for the replacement of the father by the horse in the phobic symptom.

The process of identification may also take a more primitive form. Thus, the idea of being devoured by animals, a common phobic fear in childhood, is based upon a regression to the oral stage of development. The classical illustration is the fear of being eaten by the wolf, described in Freud's paper, "From the History of an Infantile Neurosis."[46] (The popular children's story of the "Little Red Riding Hood" probably derives part of its appeal from the reassurance it offers to the young child against this fear.) Moreover, the theme of oral incorporation also characterizes many

* According to Fenichel,[39] even "the physical state of sexual or aggressive excitement" may be projected and experienced in sensations of equilibrium and space. (Whether this kind of projection can still be characterized as anxiety hysteria seems doubtful.)

phobias of adults. For instance, a male patient related his phobic fear of bridges to a fantasy of crossing into a dangerous country where he might be devoured by prehistoric animals. Since phobic reactions are indicative of regressive processes in the same measure as they place the person in a situation of infantile dependency, this regression is especially marked in phobic syndromes which restrict the patient's locomotion and make him continuously dependent upon a companion.[3,24,39]* But to some extent it is inherent in all phobias; they all impose some restriction of action not caused by objective reality. Viewed from this standpoint alone, regression would seem to be minimal where the phobic object is quite remote and easily avoidable, as in a phobia of some rare exotic animal. This general consideration, however, is not the only criterion for the existence of regression in phobic reactions.

Evidence of regressive features is frequently found in the symbolism utilized by the phobia. For example, in the case of "Little Hans," the repressed impulses themselves—sexual wishes toward the mother, death wishes toward the father—were predominantly of an oedipal kind, in keeping with the child's developmental stage. But his fear of being bitten by a horse contained, along with the castration symbolism, a strong oral-sadistic component characteristic of an earlier age.

❲ Symbolism in Phobias

To understand the meaning of a phobic symptom we must delve into the complex and multifaceted structure of its symbolic content. Only thus can we uncover the real source of the patient's fear.

---

* It may be relevant, in this connection, to note Abraham's[2] comment that the fear of walking in the street usually occurs in persons who are also afraid of being left alone indoors. The common feature of the two situations is seen in the fact that "the unconscious of such patients does not permit them to be away from those on whom their libido is fixated," and that "any attempt by the sufferer to defy the prohibitions set up by his unconscious is visited by an anxiety state." Thus, in the cases covered by Abraham's generalization, the term "agoraphobia" describes only one aspect of the manifest phobic picture.

Coming back to the case of "Little Hans," we find that his fear was a result of a combination of many elements. He was not simply afraid of horses as such or of the street as such. He was afraid that a specific kind of horse would bite him and that a horse would fall down in the street. But his phobia also included heavily loaded furniture vans and other vehicles that might cause the horse to fall; and at one point he was afraid, moreover, that a horse would come into the room and bite him.

Freud convincingly argued that this diffuseness of the boy's phobia was "derived from the circumstance that the anxiety had originally no reference at all to horses but was transposed onto them secondarily and had now become fixed upon those elements of the horse-complex which showed themselves well adapted for certain transferences." The idea of the falling horse represented a death wish against his father, while the idea of being bitten by a horse having some specified characteristics represented a punishment for this wish. On another level, which emerged only later, the heavy furniture vans represented pregnancy and the falling horse represented his mother having a baby.†

---

† Freud's interpretation of "Little Hans's" phobia in terms of symbolic displacement of oedipal strivings has been challenged by Wolpe and Rachman[133] and by Bandura[6] who interpret Hans's fear of horses, as well as phobias in general, in terms of conditioning. The general position of the Wolpe and Rachman paper is also applied by Rachman and Costello[105] to several other psychoanalytic studies of childhood phobias (specifically, to the studies by Bornstein[15,16] and by Schnurmann[111b]).

This is not the place for a detailed critique of Bandura's, Wolpe and Rachman's, and Rachman and Costello's formulations. A brief comment is, however, in order. Noting that "Little Hans" was afraid of one horse pulling a heavy vehicle but not of two horses pulling such a vehicle, Bandura attributes this difference to the greater similarity of the former to the external conditions present in the traumatic situation, i.e., the occasion on which "Little Hans" saw a horse fall. While Bandura assumes that on the occasion in question the vehicle was driven by one horse, a reference to Freud's paper indicates that the vehicle was reportedly being driven by *two* horses on that occasion. Thus, at least with reference to this one variable (number of horses pulling a heavy vehicle), the data show exactly the opposite of what one would expect if the degree of similarity to the traumatic situation were the only relevant factors.

These ideas found their clear formulation in Freud's *Introductory Lectures,* where he compared the content of the phobia to the manifest content of the dream, characterizing it as a "façade." Lewin, using this view as a point of departure for his illuminating study of "Phobic Symptoms and Dream Interpretation",[87] showed that the overdetermination of the phobic symptom is the work of the primary process, as is also true of the dream fabric. He treats the façade of the phobia the way the psychoanalyst is used to treat the manifest content of the dream. Indeed, as the case of "Little Hans" exemplifies, true phobias frequently consist of a condensation of various symbols which seem to be interrelated in a meaningful way. Moreover, as one of the authors has shown elsewhere,[51] and as Jones[71] had previously observed in his paper on symbolism, in the phobia (as in the dream) there is a certain affinity between the person and the symbols he chooses to express his unconscious imagery.

The following example is an illustration of phobic symbolism. An unmarried woman of twenty-six sought psychoanalytic treatment because of a fear of walking down a flight of stairs, an affliction from which she had suffered since adolescence. The clinical picture could be described as follows. When approaching the first step on her way downstairs, she became frightened and her legs stiffened, as though paralyzed. She could not move her feet. Clinging to the bannister, she would move her left leg with great effort, by lifting it first to the left, then to the right, before she could finally put her foot down on the step. Exactly the same procedure was then performed by the right foot, etc. Throughout her descent the patient's eyes were centered on her movements, as though she were a child learning to walk.

Her phobia had first appeared at about sixteen, in high school, when a teacher had warned the class to be careful in walking downstairs, as the stairs were rickety and had caused some minor accidents. Since then, the phobia had persisted continuously for more than ten years.

The patient had an only brother three years her junior, who apparently was favored by the mother. When he was very small, the patient had hated him, teased him, and often threatened to leave him in the woods at night. She also used to frighten him by telling him that he was not the real child of her parents but a foundling, and she felt gratified when the little boy would run crying and complaining about it to the mother. She remembered having been scolded and punished by her mother, whom she had feared and disliked since early childhood.

Nevertheless, she felt pity for the mother who, she believed, was being cruelly attacked by the father. When she was about eight or nine, she used to overhear conversations between her parents, and would not fall asleep until all noise had stopped completely. Many times she became frightened, felt anxious, wanted to scream, and wished her father would die.

At about six, she once walked into the bathroom and surprised the piano tuner while he was urinating. The man then showed her his erect penis, and she told him that she had seen the same thing before on her father. It is significant that in the early stages of her analysis, the patient found it difficult to remember having seen her father nude or having observed him in the bathroom; nor could she remember having indulged in masturbation before the age of ten or eleven, when she started to masturbate regularly. However, she remembered an incident which apparently took place when she was about nine. She had been playing with some other girls and boys in an empty carriage that stood abandoned in the backyard of their house. A boy slightly older than she tried to put his hand under her skirt. She became frightened, wanted to jump down from the carriage, but for some reason felt unable to do so. However, in her state of fright, she somehow did leave her companions and went to complain to her mother.

When she was eighteen she worked as a secretary for a much older man who once attacked her from behind while she was standing near the files. She became frightened and left the office.

From that time on, there were several unsuccessful love affairs. One, with a young intern in medicine, lasted about two years. She hoped to marry him, but when he suggested a separation she accepted it without any protest or ill feeling; she understood, she said, that he could not afford to marry a poor girl because he needed money to establish himself in practice. She then had an affair with a much older man who likewise left her with some rationalization, which she again accepted. A third affair followed, with precisely the same pattern and the same outcome. In all these relationships she was completely frigid. As she put it, most of the time she would comply with the man's insistent desire to have intercourse, and then consent to go on with the affair only because she was very much afraid of being blackmailed.

The patient's early jealousy of her brother persisted during adolescence; it became further increased when he was allowed to go to engineering school, whereas she had to renounce her own aspiration to study medicine. When he enlisted in the Air Force at the outbreak of World War II, she wanted to join the WACs or some other women's military auxiliary, but she was forced to give up this project because of a sudden increase of phobic symptoms.

The conflict about her femininity and her identification with the brother was brought out in many revealing dreams during the analysis. Very often she dreamed of being pursued by men who threatened to kill her; she would flee from the man in fright, then gloat as he ran into a mortal danger, but she would finally rescue him from this plight.

At a certain phase of the transference situation, the patient had a dream in which she stood on a small, round platform at the top of a long, narrow, endless flight of stairs. The entire structure was suspended in mid-air in a vast, arena-like space. As she stood on top, she became frightened, nervous, heard a voice telling her to go down the stairs. She felt unable to move and, looking down, thought that nobody could walk down these stairs. But the voice was telling her to go down, to move. Finally, she figured out that by sitting down she would gain more security: "If I were

closer to the stairs, I would feel surer of myself." She then imagined that there were railings, and very cautiously somehow she began to descend. She kept her eyes closed until she had moved down some distance. Opening them, she saw that the stairs were beginning to close up at the bottom and were growing nearer and nearer to her. Then she heard another voice, telling her to turn around and go back. She felt paralyzed and unable to release her hold on the rails. With great effort she managed to take her right hand off the rail and to grasp the other rail with both hands, attempting to turn around. She did not remember going up, but thought that somehow she had done so, for she remembered then lying on the platform at the top of the stairs and sobbing. At the same moment, the stairs seemed to twist like a snake, but they were stationary the rest of the time.

This dream, in which the patient's phobic experience was minutely enacted, became fully understandable only through the analysis of another anxiety dream soon thereafter. This time no stairs appeared in her dream; the dilemma consisted in having to cross a bridge, but of being threatened with death if she did so. Her associations to this dream led to hitherto inaccessible childhood memories, including the recall of two decisive experiences at the age of five or six.

In the first memory, the patient remembered that she had slept in the same bed with her parents. Half awake, she had witnessed intercourse between them. She remembered exactly how her mother had pushed her father away, saying to him: "Turn your back, it's enough." The father then had turned toward herself, put his arms around her, and touched her with his wet penis. She had been frightened, as if paralyzed, wanting to jump out of bed, to scream and holler at her parents, but being unable to do so.* This was all she could remember about this incident. But she immediately related the words spoken by her mother, "Turn your back," to the dream in which an invisible voice told her to "Turn around and go

* This dream and its interpretation were previously reported by Friedman in a paper on bridge symbolism.[51]

back." She was as paralyzed in the dream as she had been when lying in bed with her parents. It became clear that the movement of the stairs and the trembling of the platform represented the shaking of the bed during the parents' intercourse.

The second memory concerned an incestuous game with her brother, which had taken place on several occasions near a window overlooking a bridge. While engaged in this forbidden sexual activity the little girl had guiltily looked through the window, watching lest someone should come.

Thus, the analysis of these two dreams showed that the bridge and the stairs were really interchangeable. Both were symbols crystalizing the conflict at the base of the phobia: desire and punishment for incestuous sexual pleasure.

This brief fragment from the patient's history and analysis has served to demonstrate the sadistic and self-punitive trends underlying the structure of her phobia. From a tender age she had harbored hostile and aggressive impulses, and the analysis revealed intense murderous wishes toward the brother, whom she had used in her incestuous play. Her guilt feelings and self-punishment were at the basis of her masochistic behavior.

The symbolism of the stairs, so often discussed by Freud, is especially transparent in the staircase dream supplied by Rank (and included only in Freud's last (1930) edition of The Interpretation of Dreams). It is interesting to note that the connotation of this symbol here is not static but kinetic, a concept described in Friedman's aforementioned paper.[51] There, too, the bridge symbolism represents a dynamic process of crossing.*

Stairways and bridges seem to be closely connected and often used interchangeably. Both represent links (one vertical, one horizontal) between one place or condition and another. (For further relevant comments, see Friedman,[52] Friedman and Goldstein.)[53]

There are other sets of symbols presenting

similar affinities; for example, all vehicles or all animals are respectively interchangeable. By the same token, an original monophobia may progressively spread to other objects belonging to the same associative or symbolic constellation.

Having noted before that virtually any object can become the object of a phobia, we may now add that any symbol can be used to express a variety of meanings. Taking the phobia of the elevator as an example, it may stand for a fear of the *claustrum*; it may stand for a fear of height; or it may, like any phobia involving means of locomotion, stand for a fear of sexualized sensations of equilibrium and space.[39]

The foregoing considerations are of importance because they shed light on the obscurities behind the façade of the phobic symptom.†

While the psychoanalytic theory places considerable emphasis on symbolic substitution in phobic symptoms' formation, some authors, notably Rado‡ and Lief,[88] stress the role of the "sensory context" in the acquisition of phobias. Indeed, phobic reactions may become attached to the "sensory context" of a traumatic experience, but upon closer scrutiny the latter may prove to be a precipitating rather than a causative factor. However, as previously suggested, there may well be some phobic reactions in which symbolic substitution plays a less prominent role and which correspond more closely to the model of avoidance learning.

(Phobias in Children and Adults

Phobias "are *par excellence* the neuroses of childhood" (Freud[45]). Indeed, there is scarcely a human being who has not, at some time early in life, experienced fear of a phobic nature.

The case history of "Little Hans" is illumi-

---

* Gerhart Hauptmann, in his book *Griselda*, makes use of the symbolism of stairs, giving it also a sexual meaning. This was cited by Reik in *The Secret Self*.[108]

† For a theoretical formulation stressing other symbolic meanings of fear of heights, see Bergler.[11]

‡ Rado, S. "Emergency Behavior, with an introduction to the dynamics of conscience," in P. Hoch and J. Zubin *Anxiety* New York: Grune & Stratton, 1950. Pp. 150–175.

nating also because it demonstrates a typical causative factor which often gives rise to infantile phobias—the little boy's castration fear. In girls we may find a corresponding factor in fantasies of previous injury to the genitals. Bornstein[16] reports a case of this kind, where the child's belief that her genitals had been injured produced a phobia as early as the third year of life.

Castration anxiety and its feminine counterpart, however, are by no means the only major source of childhood phobias. Symbolic threat of sexual attack plays an important pathogenic role in girls[118] and in boys with passive homosexual tendencies. Moreover, phobic reactions in both sexes frequently originate in separation anxiety. Thus, Abraham[2] reported a case of childhood agoraphobia that could easily be traced to the child's desire to be with the mother, and observation which is corroborated by interpretations of agoraphobia by Weiss,[125] Deutsch,[24] and other psychoanalytic authors.

Separation anxiety seems to be responsible for a variety of phobic reactions which in recent years have received a great deal of attention under the general heading of "school phobia." As suggested by Johnson et al.,[70] and corroborated by more recent studies, school phobia is a syndrome occurring under very definite circumstances which include: (1) "A history of a poorly resolved dependency relationship between a child and its mother"; (2) an acute anxiety in the child, "produced either by organic disease or some external situation . . . and manifested in hysterical or compulsive symptoms"; and (3) a recent frustration or threat suffered by the mother, increasing her need to exploit the child's dependency relationship, with the result that separation from her when going to school becomes a traumatic experience.* However, separation anxiety is certainly not the only causal factor in school phobia.†

Because of the young child's identification with the important persons of his environment, we often find a predisposition to phobia in children of phobic parents. Hence the child psychiatrist may find it necessary to recommend treatment for his patient's parents in order to remove such pathogenic influences.

A childhood phobia may be a transitory disturbance or may continue into adult life. However, not all phobias start in childhood. In treating adult patients we are often confronted with the question whether the development of a phobic symptom actually represents a new disturbance or a reactivation of an earlier neurosis, a point that may be important in the choice of therapeutic procedures.

In a retrospective study of adult phobic patients, Marks and Gelder‡ found that in the case of specific animal phobias the mean age of onset of the symptom was placed at 4.4 years, while the mean age of onset of specific situational phobias, social anxieties, and more idiosyncratic phobic structure, is reported in Freud's case history of the "Wolf Man."[46] This patient, while in school, developed a fear of a teacher who was quite critical of him and whose name happened to be Wolf. As the patient had had a wolf phobia (or, more precisely, a fear of a picture of a wolf drawn in a particular position) in early childhood, the teacher's name apparently reactivated some of those early fears. Even much later in life the patient reacted with panic when he consulted a dentist named Wolf.[92]

School phobia, which represents a genuine anxiety reaction to the school situation, should be carefully distinguished from other personality factors which make for poor school attendance. The available evidence suggests that in the large majority of cases school truancy is due to a combination of interdependent factors, including in varying degrees a low level of interest in school learning, a low level of achievement motivation, a lack of basic skills needed for meaningful participation in school work, and to oppositional attitudes toward the authority figures represented by the school. Sometimes, the pattern may be complicated by drug use (and by participation in a drug subculture which draws much of the individual's attention away from normal school activities) or by glue sniffing (in the case of younger children). In contrast, the school phobic child tends to be above average in intelligence and average or higher in achievement.[61,85,111] There are, however, some cases of school phobic adolescents whose achievement level is extremely low, though their intelligence may be average or higher.

* Katan[75] has suggested that a mild form of agoraphobia may be considered a normal phenomenon in the development of the adolescent girl.

† An interesting manifestation which at one level might be regarded as a school phobia, but which in reality was merely a reactivation of an earlier and

‡ Marks, I. M. and M. G. Gelder. "Different Ages of Onset in Varieties of Phobias," Amer. J. of Psychiatry, 123 (1966), 218–221.

agoraphobia was placed much higher (22.7, 18.9, and 23.9, respectively). Because of the retrospective nature of the data these figures cannot, of course, be taken as representing anything more than a rough estimate of the age of onset. Moreover, the possibility cannot be excluded that those phobias which Marks and Gelder found to have a typically later onset may have been preceded by earlier related phobic manifestations that were either subsequently repressed, or not consciously connected with the later phobia. However, even after an allowance is made for this possibility, Marks and Gelder's findings corroborate clinical experience which indicates that animal phobias originate in childhood. It is of interest in this connection to note that the majority of the patients with animal phobias in Marks and Gelder's sample placed the onset of the phobia within the age range which corresponds roughly to the oedipal period. Some of the available evidence suggests that fears of large animals are especially prevalent in early childhood, and that, if anything, such fears tend to decline by the time the child has reached the age of four or five.* In the light of this evidence consideration should be given to the possibility that Marks and Gelder's subjects may have (on the average) developed their animal fears at an earlier age than their recollection indicates, but that the onset of the phobia tended to be retrospectively placed within the oedipal period because at that time the fear may have acquired a new significance. (It should, of course, be noted that since the large majority of childhood animal phobias disappear spontaneously in the process of development, the cases studied by Marks and Gelder, in which animal phobias persisted for a number of years, are probably of more than average severity.)

Just as in the case of animal phobias, phobic fear of dental treatment in adults apparently also usually goes back to childhood. In a study of dental patients with dental phobias,

* It should be noted that the time interval dealt with retrospectively in this study extends to the period before television came into use, and there is a possibility that the visual experiences provided by that medium may have altered to some extent the developmental pattern of fears in young children.

Lautch[83] found that in each of the thirty-four cases in his phobic sample there was a history of at least one traumatic dental experience in childhood. However, except in a few cases in which there was an earlier history of neurotic manifestations, two traumatic visits to a dentist were apparently needed for the development of the phobia. In the few cases with prior neurotic manifestations a single visit to a dentist was sufficient to establish the dental phobia. However, ten of Lautch's thirty-four control subjects (dental patients who did not have a dental phobia) also claimed a history of traumatic dental treatment in childhood.

Lautch's findings are particularly instructive in that they highlight in a statistical fashion the relationship between specific painful events and other factors in the development of dental phobia. On the one hand, it would appear—within the limits of Lautch's sample—that a traumatic dental experience in childhood is a regular (though perhaps not actually necessary) condition for the occurrence of a dental phobia that persists into adulthood. On the other hand, Lautch's findings indicate just as clearly that such a traumatic experience is not sufficient for the development of the phobia. Since Lautch also found that dental phobics tended to have a lower pain threshold than did the control subjects, it is possible that this lower pain threshold contributed to their greater susceptibility to the development of the phobia as a response to the painful treatment experience. However, there is also the possibility (supported by some other aspects of Lautch's findings) that neurotic predispositions (possibly involving displacements from other areas) may have contributed to the formation of the phobic symptom. Finally, Lautch's findings suggest that repeated dental trauma may have a greater effect than a single such trauma in the development of the phobia.

It may further be observed that dental phobias differ from animal phobias in that relatively few of the children who develop animal phobias have had the experience of having been hurt by animals (though some of them, like "Little Hans," may have had the experience of being frightened by some event involving the subsequently feared animal). Moreover, a child who is hurt by an animal does not necessarily develop a phobia of that animal. Thus, Sperling[114] reports a case of a two-year-old girl who was bitten by a dog and did not develop either a dog phobia or even a fear of the particular dog, but did develop (for other reasons) a spider phobia. Apparently the dog bite did not have in this case the kind of symbolic meaning that would lead to the development of a dog phobia.*

Counterphobia

In some cases, a phobic fear is masked by an attempt to actively seek out the phobic situation. In its more moderate forms, a wish to face the phobic situation may represent in part a healthy desire to put the phobia to a test in the hope of mastering the fear. In its more extreme forms, however, the tendency to seek out the phobic situation represents an active attempt at denial of the fear, and it is also often tied up with self-destructive impulses, e.g., in the case of an individual with a masked height phobia who becomes a diver or a pilot. The term "counterphobia" has been used (e.g., by Fenichel[37] and by Szasz[119]) to refer to the condition which is characterized by such masking of phobic fears. It should be noted that the counterphobic is not satisfied with merely facing situations which the non-phobic individual does not fear, but rather seeks out situations involving real danger (which, however, fall along the same dimension as the underlying phobic fear).

Therapy

Psychoanalytic Approach

Except for the need for more active intervention at an appropriate stage of treatment, psychoanalytic therapy of phobias is guided

* For a historically interesting study of fears in young children see Fackenthal.[35]

by the same general principles as is psychoanalytic therapy of other psychoneuroses. However, there is always some fluctuation and haziness in the manifest content of a phobia, and considerable probing may be needed before this manifest content can be accurately described.

In some cases of early childhood phobias it may be necessary for the therapist to include certain educational measures, such as explanation of the anatomical differences between the sexes, reassurance to the little girl that her sexual organ is intact, to the young boy that he is in no real danger of being castrated. In dealing with such infantile anxieties, the educational and the analytical part of the work cannot be rigidly separated. The cases reported by Bornstein[15,16] and by Sterba[118] illustrate the need for some initial analytic work to determine precisely what the child fears or to establish a pattern of communication best designed to convey the needed reassurance.

Sometimes, symptoms can be eliminated by supportive measures alone. In some childhood phobias, for instance, such measures may consist essentially in accustoming the child gradually to the feared situation. Thus, it has been found that in some cases a child's fear of school can be gradually overcome if he is brought to the school every day but not forced to attend classes or to participate in any prescribed activities.[77] Under these conditions "going to school," as such, becomes less threatening, and this decrease in the child's fear may then be extended to the specific object or situation on which the phobia really centers.† However, in cases with a more deep-rooted disturbance such a simple procedure may not be sufficient. Moreover, one should be on guard against the error of assuming that compliance in school attendance is a sufficient indication that the phobia has been cured. As

† It may be interesting to cite here the following passage from Locke: "Many children, imputing the pain they have endured at school to their books they were corrected for, so join these ideas together, that a book becomes their aversion, and they are never reconciled to the study and use of them all their lives after; and thus reading becomes a torment to them which otherwise possibly they might have made the great pleasure of their lives."[91]

Sperling[113] has noted, the school-phobic child who attends school may develop substitute symptoms which sometimes take the form of psychosomatic complaints.

Particularly in the case of children who had previously attended school without such difficulty, the emergence of a school phobia can often be assumed to represent something other than a mere reaction to an unfamiliar school environment, although the latter feature may, of course, be involved in the child who has just been transferred from a familiar to an unfamiliar school setting. Moreover, the likelihood of a more severe disturbance which cannot be adequately treated through superficial measures becomes greater if there is evidence that the onset of the phobia has followed closely some traumatic event, such as actual or threatened object loss, or if there are some features in the family constellation which would tend to favor the development of a school phobia.* Psychological tests may also be helpful in distinguishing between the more superficial phobic disturbances which require a more basic type of treatment.

In children, as well as in adult patients, genuine phobias marked by a high degree of symbolic displacement require systematic psychoanalytic treatment. This method atttempts to uncover the symbolic meanings of the symptom and to interpret changes in these meanings in terms of the changing transference situation.

Although the use of other techniques is sometimes imperative in order to provide early relief (e.g., from disabling phobias, as in the case of individuals whose fear of travel interferes with their ability to hold a job or even to undergo treatment), such symptomatic treatment does not necessarily obviate the need for a subsequent psychoanalytic exploration of factors which may have contributed to the phobia. This point is illustrated by a case reported by Kubie[80] in which the emergence of a height phobia was precipitated by a homicidal fantasy which was directed against

* For evidence relating school phobia to a depressive family constellation see Eisenberg;[28] for evidence relating school phobia in older children and adolescents to object loss see Tietz.[120]

the patient's wife. In this case the alleviation of the phobia (which was apparently accomplished by a nonpsychoanalytic procedure) did not do away with the need for dealing with the patient's hostility towards his wife. Without going into the details of the case it may be noted that the phobia first emerged while the patient was on a balcony of a chalet in the Alps, shortly after some events had taken place which had rendered obsolete his original motivation for his marriage, and that just prior to the experiencing of the phobic fear he had a fantasy of hurling his wife from the balcony. Thus, the hostile feelings towards his wife which were reflected in the phobia in a disguised form were important not only from the standpoint of the genesis of the phobia but also in terms of the patient's current marital relationship. It would appear that problems of this kind—involving as they do complex and partly unconscious interpersonal attitudes—fall outside the scope of techniques which aim merely at elimination of the symptom as such.

In his paper, "Turnings in the Ways of Psychoanalytic Therapy," Freud[48] stressed the necessity of exposing the phobic patient to the dreaded situation or object, and he warned that "one can hardly ever master a phobia if one waits till the patient lets the analysis influence him to give it up. He will never in that case bring for the analysis the material indispensable for a convincing solution of the phobia."

Therefore, it is often necessary for the analyst to intervene more actively and to insist that the patient brave the phobic situation. In this way, the full strength of the underlying conflict can be evoked in the associative material. Evidently, the analyst will await a propitious phase when the patient's positive transference may help to reduce the phobic fear. This more active intervention in the analysis of phobias constitutes an exception to the standard psychoanalytic procedure.

To give an example: An agoraphobic patient was referred to one of the authors (Friedman), after having been treated by several other therapists over a period of several years. She had always been accompanied to their offices by her husband, and for a short time this arrangement was permitted to continue. But as soon as the transference situation appeared propitious the patient was requested to come alone. She complied readily, but had to telephone the analyst before each session to assure herself that he was expecting her. After a few months, she was even able to go unaccompanied to her place of work, although she still had to call the analyst very frequently to feel secure.* Her evident dependency needs and defensive devices, as well as the strong hostility underlying her dependency, could then be analyzed in the light of the transference situation. It thus transpired that the phone calls served to reassure the patient that her death wishes against the analyst as a transference object had not materialized. Her transference manifestations revealed the characteristic ambivalence toward identification figures which had been described by Deutsch,[24] Katan,[75] and other authors as among the basic factors in agoraphobia. It may be added that this patient's feelings of dependence displayed, in rather transparent form, a "linkage fantasy,"[101] whereby an identity between herself and the analyst (as symbolic parent figure) was asserted by magical means.

An adequate psychoanalytic approach to the interpretation and treatment of phobias must take cognizance of the fact that phobias are often multiply determined, and that an understanding of the origins of the phobic symptom often needs to be supplemented by a grasp (on the part of both the therapist and the patient) of the role which the phobia plays in the patient's current functioning. Thus, a phobia may become intensified under conditions where realistic factors contribute to the general level of anxiety. It should also be noted that a phobia, such as a fear of heights, may play a self-preservative role in the case of a patient who has a self-destructive impulse to jump, and that when this is the case an in-

crease in the strength of the phobia may reflect an increase in the strength of the suicidal impulse. In cases of this kind, the patient should not be encouraged to face the phobic situation until the therapist is reasonably convinced that the suicidal impulses are under control.

In some cases, secondary gains from a relationship of dependence on others—e.g., in the case of phobias which restrict the individual's locomotion—may contribute to the persistence of phobias whose origin is due to other factors. It is of interest to note in this connection that, according to the findings of a number of studies (for a summary see Andrews[5]), dependence is a frequent characteristic of phobic patients. As the case on page 124 cited illustrates, the phobic need for dependence on others may also have a strongly hostile underlying quality.

Another type of contemporaneous influence consists in fluctuations in the patient's general level of anxiety. An existing phobia may become reactivated under conditions of stress. Fluctuations in the strength of a phobia during psychoanalytic treatment cannot always be taken at face value as indications of changes in the severity of the disturbance. Thus, as Glover[55] has noted, an apparent increase in the strength of a phobic symptom, after a date for termination of treatment has been set, may represent a transference reaction reflecting a wish for continuation of the therapy. As Glover points out, it may be necessary in cases of this sort to extend several times the tentatively set termination date until the patient is able to accept the termination without this type of reaction.

The length of time and amount of therapeutic effort needed for psychoanalytic or psychoanalytically oriented treatment of a phobia varies considerably. In some cases[50, 113] the patient's acquisition of insight into the meaning of the phobia leads to the disappearance or substantial alleviation of the symptom, although further treatment may be needed to deal with the residual neurosis. In other cases a good deal of working through may be needed before the insight brings about a substantial alleviation of the phobic symptom. In still other cases, the phobias are extremely

* In a somewhat similar vein, Deutsch[24] mentions an agoraphobic patient who, in a state of positive transference, was able to go unaccompanied to the analyst's office, and whose fear of walking alone was considerably attenuated with respect to the analyst's neighborhood.

resistant to treatment. Among the patients whose phobias are so resistant to treatment there are some who have good intellectual insight into the origins of their fears.* In general, it would appear that the ease of treatment of a phobia is inversely related to its duration (and particularly to its continuity since childhood), as well as to the patient's over-all degree of disturbance. At least in the case of young children, prompt psychoanalytically oriented intervention after the phobia has first made its appearance in response to emotional stress can sometimes result, as Sperling's[113] findings illustrate, in a prompt disappearance of the symptom. On the other hand, a phobic symptom may be extremely difficult to treat if it is part of a long-standing obsessive or schizophrenic pattern.

Since phobic patients realize the irrationality of their fears, direct suggestive therapy is not effective. Sometimes, it may even strengthen the patient's guilt feelings, or intensify his hostility to the therapist or resistance to the treatment. And when such attempts at rational persuasion seem successful, this is usually due to rapport rather than to logical reasoning.

(For further material relevant to the psychoanalytic theory and treatment of phobias see[3, 27,36,38,40,44,89.])

Behavior Therapy

In contrast to psychoanalytic and other dynamic approaches that view neurotic symptoms as a function of inner conflict, the behavior therapy approach—at least in its more orthodox forms[132,131,103,33,34,32]—views neurosis as essentially nothing more than a set of maladaptive habits. Although there are important differences among these orthodox exponents of behavior therapy both with regard to the learning theories they espouse and the specific therapeutic procedures they favor, they all share a view of the therapeutic process as involving either unlearning of maladaptive habits, or as learning of new habits that would render the maladaptive habits ineffective. Most of them also reject the notion of displacement, and regard insight on the part of the patient as irrelevant to the success of the treatment. Although they grant that psychoanalytic treatment can sometimes result in symptom alleviation, they maintain that this is due to the operation of principles of learning which are accidentally built into the procedure (e.g., to "extinction" of fear responses, which presumably takes place when thoughts which previously gave rise to anxiety are verbalized without punishment), rather than to anything specific to the psychoanalytic approach.† The behavior therapy approach to phobias has by now become the subject of a voluminous and rapidly growing literature. (For an extensive bibliography see Eysenck and Beech.[33])

One of the techniques of behavior therapy widely used in the treatment of phobias is the technique of *progressive or systematic desensitization* developed by Wolpe[131,132] and derived in part from his earlier experiments with cats. This technique is based on the assumption that fear of the phobic object can be reduced by confronting the subject with a succession of objects representing increasing degrees of phobic threat under conditions of deep muscle relaxation, which presumably inhibits anxiety. (The notion that deep muscle relaxation inhibits anxiety is derived by Wolpe

---

* Since phobic symptoms are usually multiply determined, and since, in principle, the therapist can never be certain that all the determinants of a phobia have been explored in a given case, the question as to whether the patients have acquired insight into the origin and meaning of the phobia can only be understood in a relative sense. Moreover, in some of the cases described by J. H. Friedman[50] and by Sperling,[114] where a relatively brief period of therapy was needed to interpret the symptom to the patient, one may assume that no attempt was made to explore the meaning of the symptom in an exhaustive fashion. Thus, it would appear that a necessarily selective interpretation given in the course of brief treatment can in some cases be effective in dealing with a phobic symptom. Of course, it is likely that positive transference may also have contributed in these cases to the success in the treatment of the phobia.

† The foregoing characterization of behavior therapy approaches does not apply fully to *implosive therapy*, which is classified by its originator[116] as a form of behavior therapy, but which does entail the notion that the original source of phobic avoidance may be repressed.

in part from Sherrington's[112] concept of reciprocal inhibition which, however, originally referred to pairs of antagonistic muscles, rather than to emotional states.)

In the usual desensitization procedure the graded intensities of phobic threat are presented indirectly by asking the subject to imagine relevant situations or objects (stairways, bridges, etc.), or (sometimes) by showing the subject pictures of such situations or objects. Sometimes, however (e.g., in the case of subjects who have difficulty in complying with the instructions to visualize), real objects are used—a procedure known as desensitization *in vivo*. The (real or vicarious) graded series of objects—or a "hierarchy," as it is called—presumably corresponding to different intensities of the subject's fears is usually established on the basis of interviews with the subject and/or of the subject's questionnaire response obtained prior to the initiation of the desensitization procedure. Before the initiation of the desensitization series, the subject is also taught the technique of deep muscle relaxation.[67] Sometimes, hypnosis or a drug is used to help the patient reach the relaxed state, but neither is essential to the procedure. Some findings, e.g.,[103] suggest that muscular relaxation is also not essential for desensitization, but that desensitization is favored by a psychological state of calmness.

Inasmuch as the procedure rests on the assumption that the experiencing of the previously feared situation under conditions of no anxiety (or, more precisely, minimal anxiety) is the crucial factor in the elimination of the phobic fear, the subject is instructed to interrupt the presentation whenever the anxiety becomes too disturbing. When this happens, the therapist shifts to a less disturbing item. This procedure is kept up (often in a series of sessions) until the patient can face with relative freedom from anxiety the most disturbing item in the hierarchy.

Sometimes, more than one hierarchy is used either to deal with several symptoms (each of which is treated separately) or to deal with several "dimensions" of fear involved in a given symptom, as determined in the interview. Thus, if a patient is afraid of steep stairways in narrowly enclosed areas the fear of steepness may be dealt with through one hierarchy and the claustrophobic aspect through another hierarchy.

As a rule, at least when the procedure is carried out for research purposes, an attempt is made to minimize the role of therapist-patient interaction. In some cases,[81] this has involved the use of tape-recorded instructions in lieu of a live therapist during the desensitization sessions.

In recent years, a vast literature on desensitization has accumulated and various modifications of the procedure have been introduced, in addition to the variations already noted. Thus, in lieu of muscular relaxation, Lazarus and Abramovitz[84] have used a procedure which involves instructing the subject to imagine pleasant objects in alternation with the items in the anxiety-arousing series, on the assumption that pleasant moods will reduce the anxiety level aroused by the feared object. The desensitization procedure has also been adapted to group therapy. Behavior therapy techniques based on principles other than desensitization have also been employed. (For discussions of other techniques of behavior therapy, some of very recent origin, see Rachman,[108] Marks,[93] Wells,[127] Gurman,[57] Orwin,[99] Edlund,[26] Lang,[81] Migler and Wolfe.[49])

Exponents of behavior therapy, such as Eysenck, have emphasized the link between behavior therapy and learning theory in claiming for the former the status of an approach solidly based on science.* However, as critics of behavior therapy (e.g., Breger & McGaugh[18,19]) have pointed out, there is no one generally accepted theory of learning. Moreover, the assumptions of learning theory typically utilized by behavior therapists often represent oversimplified or outdated models, and their use of analogies based on animal

* In the recent formulation by Eysenck and Beech,[33] the claims with respect to the status of learning theories are considerably toned down. Instead, the emphasis is placed on the tentative nature of many scientific hypotheses, which serve as useful working models but soon become obsolete after they have served their purpose in giving direction to experiments.

experimentation is often questionable in its applicability to human neurosis.*

Critics (e.g., Locke[90]) have also pointed out that the procedures of behavior therapy are much less behavioristic in fact than they are in principle. (In this connection see also Wilkins,[129] Wilson and Davison,[130] and Grossberg,[56] Andrews.[5]) For instance, the behavior therapist relies on the patient's introspective accounts to determine the nature of the phobia and to establish the fear hierarchy, and except when *in vivo* procedures are used, he also relies on imagery, rather than on manipulation of external physical variables, to provide the hierarchy of "stimuli." Moreover, except in special instances, he uses the patient's reports rather than direct physical observation or physiological measurement to evaluate the degree of relief from anxiety. It has also been noted, e.g., by Weitzman,[126] that such verbal reports are used by Wolpe primarily to provide data about the subject's psychological state, rather than as an indirect way of obtaining information about physiological manifestations of anxiety. Moreover, case reports by behavior therapists indicate that they occasionally resort to persuasion and to educational measures which, strictly speaking, fall outside the scope of behavior therapy as usually defined. This line of criticism does not necessarily imply that the procedures as such are objectionable. It does imply, however, that whatever effectiveness these procedures might have may be due to factors other than those envisaged in the theoretical formulations of behavior therapists.

The available evidence suggests, moreover, that the psychological processes involved in imagining the object suggested by the therapist are in reality much more complex than the behavior therapist assumes. In theory, the patient is supposed to turn on the image when he is instructed to do so by the therapist, and to hold it until he is instructed to turn it off; but Weitzman's findings suggest that the patient's imagery under these conditions tends to undergo continuous changes, somewhat in the nature of free association. It thus appears possible that, at least in some cases, progressive desensitization produces significant psychological effects for reasons that are not necessarily related to the rationale of the procedure.

The effectiveness of a therapeutic procedure is, of course, not always dependent on the validity of its theoretical underpinnings. In the case of behavior therapy, a considerable degree of success in short-term treatment of phobias has been claimed in various research reports, although some of these reports, e.g., Evans and Liggett,[30] indicate that certain kinds of phobias, such as agoraphobia, have been more resistant to this form of treatment. One of the claims frequently made in this connection is that in the large majority of cases symptom removal has not resulted in the substitution of some other symptom.†

* Quite apart from the general problem of generalizing from animal to human subjects, there are some more specific problems which apply to the generalization from animal experiments to behavior therapy techniques. In Wolpe's animal experiments on desensitization, food was used to counteract anxiety in the presence of the objects on the phobic hierarchy. It is an open question to what extent the procedures used to induce relaxation in humans are comparable to the feeding of the experimental animals. It may, however, be of historical interest to note that in an early study which utilized what today would be called desensitization in dealing with fears of young children[72] food was in fact used in a manner somewhat analogous to that of Wolpe's animal studies. Of course, the fact that the human subject in a typical desensitization experiment is a voluntary participant who has some advance information about the procedure makes for conditions that are very different from those of the animal studies.

† It has often been maintained, both by psychoanalysts and by behavior therapists, that psychoanalytic theory would lead to the expectation of symptom substitution in cases where a pathological manifestation is removed through treatment which is directed at the symptom rather than at underlying causes. Thus, behavior therapists have often cited the low incidence of symptom substitution in their studies as evidence against psychoanalytic theory, while psychoanalytic critics have often expressed skepticism concerning behavior therapy on the ground that apparently successful treatment directed against specific symptoms is bound to lead to the emergence of other symptoms. However, Weitzman[126] has recently presented several arguments in support of the view that psychoanalytic theory is in fact quite consistent with the notion that symptom removal may bring about more general therapeutic benefits (e.g., that improved mastery of the environment resulting from an alleviation of a phobia may result in increased ego strength). It has also been argued[95] that the objections originally raised by Freud against treatment

Although in some of the studies[74,94] behavior therapists have made a special effort to minimize the effects of patient-therapist interaction, the possibility cannot be excluded that transference, as well as patient expectations of successful cures, may have played a role in some of the favorable outcomes. It should be noted in this connection that an impersonal attitude on the part of the therapist does not necessarily prevent the patient from creating fantasies in which the therapist is endowed with a special significance.

Moreover, in evaluating the reports of successful treatment of phobias by behavior therapists it is important to bear in mind that the selective factors that make up the patient population with which they deal are often quite different from those operative in the selection of patients for psychoanalytic or other dynamically oriented forms of therapy. In a number of studies the behavior therapy patients were students whose phobic symptoms were discovered by means of questionnaires administered to college classes, and many of whom would probably not have sought treatment for these symptoms if they had not been offered such treatment as research subjects; moreover, in some of the studies, the phobias dealt with (e.g., snake phobias) were such as to have little, if any, maladaptive significance in the subjects' environment. In contrast, the phobic patients studied by psychoanalysts and other dynamic therapists are generally individuals who have actively sought treatment (or, as in the case of young children, have been brought to treatment) because of disturbing presenting symptoms. Consequently, it is to be expected that the latter group would tend to have a larger propor-

tion of individuals with more severe disturbances that may require more complex treatment. It may also be conjectured that those college students who accept the offer of treatment tend to have favorable expectations of the outcome of treatment, and that this itself contributes to a positive result.

In the light of some of these considerations it would appear that whatever success is achieved in the treatment of phobias through the use of progressive desensitization can be reinterpreted in cognitive terms, and also in terms that allow for the operation of unconscious processes. (Thus, it may be supposed that the reassurance gained through the experiencing of the phobic object in a protected setting is operative both on conscious and on unconscious levels.) As regards the role of free associations, Weitzman's findings clearly indicate that the processes of desensitization cannot be adequately understood without taking such associations into account, but considerably more research will need to be done in order to determine (a) to what extent such associations contribute to the therapeutic process; (b) whether there is anything specific to the desensitization procedures which contributes to the value of free associations in this context; and, (c) assuming that the answer to the preceding question is in the affirmative, whether anything can be done to develop new techniques that would make optimal use of such findings.

Implosive Therapy

In contrast to desensitization, which involves gradual habituation to the anxiety-arousing situation under conditions where the subject is presumably protected against the impact of the anxiety, the implosive or "flooding" technique[115,116,63,64,65,74,104] involves the use of massive exposure (though usually in imagination rather than *in vivo*) to the phobic object (or to the presumably repressed fear objects which the phobic object is assumed to represent).

Implosive therapy is usually classified as a form of behavior therapy because its rationale is derived from a learning-theory model.

---

aimed at the symptoms rather than at underlying causes were focused primarily on a specific kind of treatment in which symptom removal was brought about through the therapist's authority, and that the same considerations need not necessarily hold when symptom removal or alleviation is brought about through some other means.

In this connection, it may be suggested that insofar as a therapeutic method brings about personality changes other than symptom alleviation or removal, it cannot be considered "merely" symptomatic, even if it ostensibly deals only with the symptoms. For other relevant comments, see Yates,[135,136] Bookbinder,[14] and Camoon.[20]

However, unlike the more typical behavior therapy approaches, the implosive therapy approach also makes use of some psychoanalytic concepts, including the distinction between the manifest and the repressed objects of anxiety. In line with the foregoing, the implosive approach also rejects the behavior therapists' claim that a neurosis consists merely of the symptoms.

The learning theory model underlying implosive therapy is that of extinction of traumatic avoidance reactions. As used in conditioned-response literature, the term "extinction" refers to a decrease or disappearance of a previously conditioned reaction as a consequence of presentations of the conditioned stimulus without the unconditioned stimulus. In the case of avoidance reactions, the unconditioned stimulus is a noxious stimulus, such as electric shock. With minor modifications, the foregoing definition of extinction would also apply to the "instrumental" learning situation in which the noxious stimulus is contingent on the completion of some act by the subject. According to experimental findings with animals, learned avoidance reactions are extremely difficult to extinguish under conditions where the animal is free to avoid or escape the situation in which the noxious stimulus was originally administered; but (with some exceptions which are not as yet well understood[98,110]) extinction tends to proceed much more easily if the opportunity for avoidance is blocked and the animal is, so to speak, forced to subject its fear to "reality testing."[10]

While the principle of extinction of anxiety responses appears simple when stated in an abstract fashion, its application to concrete clinical situations presents some complications. In the first place, there is, as in the case of desensitization, the question as to whether the image evoked in response to the therapist's instructions is functionally equivalent to an external phobic object. (On the analogy of Weitzman's[126] findings with respect to desensitization, it seems plausible to conjecture that the instructions given in implosive therapy similarly tend to give rise to a chain of associations in which the visual image does not necessarily remain stable.) It may also be noted that, according to some findings, e.g., Barrett,[9] implosive instructions occasionally give rise to "run-away" imagery which continues beyond the therapy sessions. Moreover, even if one disregards the foregoing problem, it may be difficult in practice to draw a sharp line of demarcation between anxiety-arousing experiences which might theoretically be expected to lead to the "reality testing" of existing fears, and those which might lead to the development of new fears. In this connection Bandura[6] has drawn a distinction between imaginal evocation of the phobic object as such, and imaginal evocation of disastrous consequences of an (imaginal) evocation of the phobic object or situation. (This distinction may be exemplified, in the case of a stairway phobia, by the difference between the subject's being told to imagine that he is walking down a steep stairway, and his being told to imagine that he is falling from the stairway or that the stairway is collapsing.) Bandura suggests that the latter type of imaginal evocation may have the effect of extending rather than reducing the fear, particularly if the noxious consequences had not previously been envisioned by the subject, and he notes that the procedures used in such evocation resemble closely the procedures used in aversion therapy.* Of course, the therapist who instructs the patient to imagine the phobic object might find it difficult in some cases to prevent the emergence of imagery representing noxious consequences of the phobic situation.†

* In this connection, a further distinction can be made, however, between imagined noxious consequences which were truly unfamiliar to the patient, and those which had been repressed or suppressed but are significantly related to the origins of the phobic fear. Evocation of material of the latter type could possibly be helpful under some conditions, provided that the patient's ego strength is sufficient to withstand the emergence of such potentially threatening content.

† The rationale of implosive therapy must be carefully distinguished from that of Freud's previously mentioned recommendation that the phobic patient be confronted *in vivo* with the phobic situation. Freud saw such a confrontation primarily as a means of utilizing the anxiety thus elicited, as a means of evoking associations which would help in understanding the origins and meaning of the phobia. The implosive therapist utilizes the massive evocation of the phobic imagery as a means of reducing the anxiety. Moreover, while

Similarly, it has been conjectured by some investigators that instructions to imagine the phobic situation along with the fear reaction and its somatic accompaniments may be quite different in its effects from instructions which specify the phobic situation but not the fear and its somatic accompaniments (see page 130). Actual studies which have utilized instructions intended to arouse highly noxious imagery, including imagery involving somatic accompaniments of fear, have yielded conflicting results.

Staub[117] has attempted to reconcile these conflicting results by citing evidence which suggests that flooding procedures tend to be more effective with longer intervals of continuous exposure to imaginal stimuli. He conjectures that longer exposure exerts this effect through reduction of the intensity of the physiological accompaniments of the fear reaction during the exposure interval, and through providing the human subject with an opportunity to realize that the adverse consequences are not forthcoming. While Staub's argument deserves serious consideration, there is reason to believe that it involves an oversimplified view of the processes involved in implosion. Thus, as already noted, it is by no means clear that the duration of the imagined stimuli can be controlled through instructions with any degree of precision. Moreover, Staub's formulation takes no account of individual differences in reactions to implosive instructions. However, other interpretations of the conflicting results are also possible. It is perhaps of relevance to note that the main negative results thus far were obtained in a study[104] which dealt with the spider phobia, while some of the positive results came from studies using other phobias, such as the snake phobia.[134] Perhaps the deeper level of regression in the spider phobia is the factor that accounts for the negative results.

By way of summary, it can be stated that

the implosive technique offers some interesting possibilities for further research, but that as of now the factors that make for success or failure in implosive treatment of phobic symptoms have not been sufficiently elucidated. In addition to the factors already mentioned, the role of the patient's attitude towards the therapist and towards the imaginal task, as well as of subtle factors in patient-therapist interaction, needs to be systematically explored.

Modeling and Related Techniques

This procedure consists in having the phobic subject observe another person (the "model") perform the phobic act (e.g., playing with a dog, in the case of a dog phobia) in a fearless manner and without aversive consequences. One of the major assumptions underlying this procedure is that such viewing results in a "vicarious" extinction of the fear.[16]

As already implied, some of the key concepts used by proponents of modeling, e.g., the concept of extinction, are derived from conditioned response terminology. However, since the postulated fear reduction in the observing subject is presumably mediated by a change in attitude towards the feared object, rather than by direct extinction of the avoidance responses, the modeling procedure can be more adequately classified as representing a cognitive rather than a behavioristic approach. (Of course, as already noted, the behavior therapy approaches are also not consistently behavioristic). It should, however, be noted that some of the major proponents of modeling[6] share the behavior therapists' opposition to the concept of symbolic displacement as applied to neurotic symptoms.

As in the case of desensitization, the modeling procedure often involves a progression from the less feared to the more feared act. A less gradual exposure to the phobic stimulus would presumably result in an increase rather than a decrease of anxiety.

Insofar as modeling involves providing the subject with visible evidence that the feared object is not in fact dangerous, it may appear to represent a form of persuasion, which,

---

Freud advocated the exposure to the phobic situation only under conditions where the degree of phobic fear had already been reduced through therapeutic work, in implosive therapy the imaginal presentation of the feared object is initiated as soon as possible after the preliminary interviews.

however, is implicit rather than explicit. Such a view, if it should turn out to be correct, would run counter to clinical experience which indicates that persuasion is largely ineffective in the treatment of phobias. However, the evidence suggests that something other than persuasion, in the usual sense, is at least in part involved in the treatment of phobias through modeling. One reason for this supposition is that most adult subjects are already convinced of the irrationality of their phobias by the time they come for treatment. It thus appears plausible that the visual factor involved in the experience of seeing the phobic act performed by another person without adverse consequences has an effect over and above its rational function of providing evidence that the feared act is not dangerous. Perhaps something in the nature of empathy or identification is involved here.

The available evidence[7,6,8] suggests that modeling can be quite effective as a means of alleviation of some phobic fears, such as fears of dogs in children, and that its effectiveness can be enhanced when it is used in conjunction with other techniques, such as desensitization or physical guidance of the subject in the performance of the feared act.

A procedure known as contact desensitization and utilizing a combination of modeling, desensitization, and physical aid in the performance of the phobic act, has been developed by Ritter,[109] who has used it with some degree of success in the alleviation of acrophobia in a nonpatient sample. Ritter's findings indicate that physical contact with the experimenter while facing the phobic situation was a significant factor in the success of the procedure. In this connection, it seems plausible to assume that the physical contact may have had for some of the subjects psychological significance beyond that of physical protection against the danger of falling.

Ritter's study is of considerable interest because it is one of the very few systematic studies indicating that a space phobia can be alleviated by a procedure that does not involve exploration of the origins or individual meaning of the fear. However, Ritter herself explicitly avoids the claim that her procedure has succeeded in eliminating the phobia.*

Existential Therapy

In sharp contrast to learning-theory approaches, which view human personality in strictly deterministic terms, existential psychiatry places a great deal of emphasis on man as a free and responsible agent. In spite of this wide difference in theoretical starting points, the best known technique for the treatment of phobias to have come out of the existential school—Frankl's method of *paradoxical intention*[43,54]—bears a considerable resemblance to implosion, and more specifically to the type of implosive therapy that involves imagining disturbing consequences of the phobic situation. However, while implosive therapy typically makes use of imaginal presentation of the feared object, the method of paradoxical intention is usually applied *in vivo*.†

The technique of paradoxical intention consists essentially in having the patient make a voluntary effort to magnify his fear reactions, such as sweating or acceleration of the heart rate, in the phobic situation. Frankl makes the assumption that the attempt to augment physiological reactions will fail, but that in making the attempt the patient will attain a greater distance from his phobic symptom, and that he will derive a therapeutic benefit from his ability to laugh at himself in this situation. (Frankl credits G. W. Allport[4] with the notion that the patient's ability to laugh at himself represents the first step toward the cure of neurosis). In part, Frankl's rationale is also based on the (correct) assumption that phobic anxiety is increased by the effort to resist it. One of the examples of this approach is pro-

* The previously mentioned procedure of getting a school-phobic child gradually accustomed to the school setting may be considered as involving features of desensitization, modeling, and guided participation. Of course, when the child is exposed to the natural school setting, the operation of these factors cannot be controlled to the same extent as under experimental conditions.

† While Frankl's approach is known as "logotherapy," it is usually classified as representing the varieties of existential therapy.

vided by a patient of Gerz, who feared a heart attack, and whose fear was relieved after he was told by the therapist to try to accelerate his heart rate so as to produce a heart attack.*

Frankl recognizes that the method of paradoxical intention is not applicable to all phobias, but he insists (and here there is a definite parallel to behavior therapy approaches) that the success of the method is not dependent on the personality of the therapist or on a correct understanding of the history of the phobia. He reports, however, that recall of the traumatic events sometimes occurs *after* the technique of paradoxical intention has brought relief.

It would appear that Frankl's method is primarily applicable in those cases where the phobia is not so severe as to prevent the patient altogether from facing the phobic situations, and apparently also in some cases, e.g., fear of a heart attack, in which the phobic object is internal and thus cannot be avoided. On the other hand, it may be conjectured that there are some phobias in which the application of the method would be quite dangerous. For instance, encouraging an acrophobic patient to amplify his fears while he is walking down a steep stairway might well lead to a loss of control, which in turn might result in falling. Such a procedure would be especially contraindicated in cases where there is reason to believe that the acrophobia is overdetermined by unconscious or preconscious suicidal tendencies. As a general rule, paradoxical intention should not be applied in those cases where there is reason to believe that loss of control resulting from the amplified fear reaction would represent a realistic danger to the subject.

Although other existential therapists have also dealt with phobias, there is no one theory of phobias, or of treatment of phobias, that could be said to characterize the existential

* It is one of Frankl's and Gerz's contentions that instructions to accelerate the heartbeat, etc., do not represent a danger because these automatic functions are not subject to voluntary control. In view of recent findings which indicate that autonomic functions are to some extent subject to voluntary control,[96,81] it may be best to reserve judgment on this point.

school as a whole. One theme which is encountered in the writings of several existentialists and phenomenological psychiatrists involves the notion that a phobia, such as a claustrophobia or an agoraphobia, reflects the individual's way of perceiving visual space, and, in a more general way, of seeing his relationship to the world. While some of these authors[12] interpret this relationship in terms that are at least broadly consistent with psychoanalytic notions of symbolic representation, others, especially Boss,[17] reject the notion of symbolic displacement, and maintain that there is no real distinction between the symbol and that which is symbolized. On a more concretely empirical level, Colm,[22] who makes extensive use of psychoanalytic concepts, has presented some interesting insights, e.g., concerning the role of parental insecurity in the genesis of phobias in children, and has also outlined some of the implications of these insights for the therapy of children's phobias.

Hypnotherapy

The use of hypnosis in the treatment of phobias includes a variety of techniques, which may be thought of as ranging on a continuum from those aiming more or less exclusively at symptom relief (with little or no reference to the genesis of the symptom) to dynamically oriented approaches, which include measures directed at symptom relief, but which place this aim in a broader context. At one end of this continuum are techniques that utilize the therapist's authority to reassure the patient against the phobic fear or to command the patient to perform the feared act. At the other end of the continuum are the approaches[29,49] that involve intensive exploration of the genesis of the symptoms and seek to facilitate the development of insight. The development of techniques of hypnotic age regression has contributed significantly to the range of techniques available for intensive hypnotherapy. In contrast to the techniques that rely primarily on authoritative suggestions, these more intensive techniques may require a much more prolonged effort, at least in some cases, although the time involved would still be considerably below that required for psychoanalytic treatment.

In addition to hypnotic therapies proper hypnosis is also used as an adjunct to other techniques in the treatment of phobias, e.g., as a means of uncovering repressed material for subsequent use in the waking state, or as a means of inducing a state of relaxation.

Hypnotic treatment that relies primarily on authoritative suggestion or on positive transference can sometimes produce prompt and spectacular results. But as long as the underlying conflict remains untouched, the patient is prone to develop a new phobic symptom.* However, according to clinical reports thus far available, the more dynamically oriented forms of hypnotherapy tend to result in more durable improvement, including symptom relief.

A detailed description of a dynamically oriented hypnotherapy of a case with phobic symptomatology has been published by Freytag,[49] whose volume includes an introductory comment by Erickson. A detailed discussion of Freytag's procedure would fall outside of the scope of this presentation. However, since one of the features of her procedure involves the use of desensitization, it will be instructive to compare her use of desensitization with systematic desensitization as used by Wolpe, discussed earlier.

The significant common feature of the two procedures is that they both involve gradual exposure to phobic stimuli of increasing intensity under conditions of reduced anxiety, with provision for interruption of the series whenever there is an increase in the anxiety level. One of the major differences between the procedures is that in Wolpe's technique desensitization is the major focus of the therapy, while in Freytag's approach desensitization is a technical device which is used when an ap-

propriate situation presents itself, but which has meaning only within a larger context that includes hypnotic regression, etc. A second difference consists in the fact that instead of using a prearranged hierarchy Freytag applies the desensitization procedure to material which emerges in the hypnotic trance, and which is presumably significant in relation to the genesis of the phobia.† A third difference is that in Freytag's procedure the desensitization is applied to hallucinated material rather than, as in Wolpe's procedure, to images, which, one gathers, are clearly distinguishable in their phenomenal qualities from perception of reality. (As previously noted, Wolpe occasionally uses desensitization *in vivo*. The *in vivo* technique does not, however, always permit the same degree of control by the therapist as does the hypnotic procedure. For instance, it would not be feasible to have a patient with a bridge phobia walk through a series of bridges of various lengths.) As Erickson points out in the introduction to Freytag's book, hypnotically induced hallucinations are less subject to artifacts due to the subject's attitudes than are waking images produced as a result of instructions[9]. To use Erickson's example, a subject who is told to imagine that he is cold while the weather is hot in reality might experience the request as artificial or absurd, but this problem would not arise for the subject in a deep trance, who would feel the cold temperature as if it were really there. A fourth point of difference pertains to the role of post-hypnotic amnesia; one gathers from Wolpe's case reports that he makes no effort to induce amnesia for the treatment. On the other hand, post-hypnotic amnesia plays a major role in Freytag's procedure. In this connection, Freytag expresses the view that the amnesia makes it possible for the patient to avoid a good deal of unpleasant experience which would otherwise be associated with psychotherapy.

The results reported by Freytag and by Erickson[29] are quite impressive. However, since very few studies dealing with intensive psychoanalytically oriented hypnotherapy of

---

* As it has been previously noted, there are good theoretical reasons for assuming that under some conditions the removal of a symptom without exploration of its etiology would not necessarily lead to symptom substitution. However, such substitution is particularly likely to develop when the symptom removal is based on authoritative suggestion or on positive transference.

† These differences are not explicitly discussed by Freytag, but they emerge quite clearly from a comparison of Wolpe's and Freytag's procedures.

phobias are thus far available, the range of applicability of the method still remains to be determined. (One may note here that Freytag's patient had had some psychoanalytic treatment before entering hypnotherapy. Although this treatment apparently had not brought about a major alleviation of the symptoms, it may very well have contributed to the subsequent progress of the hypnotherapy.) The fact that a deep trance is required for this approach would, of course, preclude its application to patients who are unable or unwilling to attain such a trance. Moreover, further research is needed to explore the possibility of undesirable side effects, such as the development of excessive dependence on the therapist, in this form of treatment. Also, the advantages and disadvantages of posthypnotic amnesia as a feature of intensive hypnotherapy of phobias represent a problem which is in need of further investigation. One may wonder whether the insight attained in the trance can become optimally utilized if it is dissociated from the conscious personality. In the case described by Freytag the treatment took place entirely while the patient was in the trance state, except, of course, for the initial explanation of the procedure and for the procedure involved in getting the patient into and out of the trance at each session. However, this is not necessarily always the case in psychoanalytically oriented hypnotherapy. Sometimes, for instance, recordings of material obtained in a trance and then subjected to post-hypnotic amnesia are played back to the patient while he is in the waking state.

(For a recent study utilizing hypnosis in the reduction of phobias see Horowitz.[66])

◖ Closing Comments

A wide range of techniques is now available for the relief of phobic symptoms. However, even though symptom relief obtained through short-range measures may lead to more general therapeutic benefits, such as an increase in ego strength, it does not obviate the need for more intensive dynamically oriented therapy in many of the cases where a deeper long-standing disturbance is involved. On the other hand, as Kubie's[80] previously cited case illustrates, the use of short-range measures to relieve a severely disturbing or disabling phobic symptom is not inconsistent with subsequent psychodynamic exploration of the meaning of that symptom.

At the moment, the practical knowledge of techniques that can be used to alleviate phobic symptoms outstrips the theoretical understanding of how the various techniques work. To be sure, there is no dearth of theories which attempt to explain how these techniques work, but, even apart from the specific criticisms that have been advanced against some of these theories, the very diversity of the techniques that apparently work in some cases leads one to suspect that the reasons for whatever effectiveness some of them might have may be quite different from those postulated by some of the theories. Thus, we know that phobic symptoms have been successfully treated both by techniques that attempt to minimize anxiety in the presence of stimuli resembling the phobic object and by techniques that involve massive exposure to anxiety-arousing stimuli. And, to complicate matters still further, we also know from at least one study[31] that administering an electric shock while the subject imagines the feared object can also lead to the mitigation of a phobic symptom. While it would be tempting to ascribe the apparently successful use of these various methods to the "placebo" effect involving interaction with the therapist, and perhaps also to the expectation of success, such a conclusion is rendered unlikely by the findings of various studies which utilized "pseudotherapy" control groups. These control group data indicate, on the whole, that little or no improvement occurs when the interaction with the therapist involves no attempt at treatment. (Of course, the nature of the problem precludes the use of a double-blind design in which neither the therapist nor the subject would be able to differentiate between the experimental and the control procedure.)

The phobic patient, more than any other

neurotic, can become a faithful ally of his therapist in the struggle against his ego-alien and tormenting symptom. His need for dependency and protection, and his will to recover, offer excellent chances for successful treatment, if it is undertaken in the early stages of the illness. But only the therapist's skill and understanding of the dynamics will enable the patient to overcome his resistance and to give up his neurotic defenses.

The ambivalent struggle of an agoraphobic patient, as she anticipated her first unaccompanied visit to her therapist's office, was expressed in the following verses:

Which Epitaph Shall Be Mine?
She couldn't try
For fear she'd die;
She never tried
And so she died.

or

She couldn't try
For fear she'd die;
But once she tried
Her fears—they died.

❨ Bibliography

1. Abraham, K. "A Constitutional Basis of Locomotor Anxiety," in *Selected Papers on Psychoanalysis*, pp. 235–243. New York: Basic Books, 1953. (Originally published in 1913)

2. ———. "On the Psychogenesis of Agoraphobia in Childhood," in *Clinical Papers and Essays in Psychoanalysis*, pp. 42–43. New York: Basic Books, 1955. (Originally published in 1913)

3. Alexander, F. "Psychoanalysis Revised," *Psychoanalytic Quarterly*, 9 (1940), 1–36.

4. Allport, G. W. *The Individual and His Religion*. New York: Macmillan, 1956.

5. Andrews, J. D. W. "Psychotherapy of Phobias," *Psychological Bulletin*, 66 (1966), 455–480.

6. Bandura, A. *Principles of Behavior Modification*. New York: Holt, 1969.

7. ———, J. E. Grusee, and F. L. Menlove. "Vicarious Extinction of Avoidance Behavior," *Journal of Personality and Social Psychology*, 5 (1967), 16–23.

8. ———, and F. L. Menlove. "Factors Determining Vicarious Extinction of Avoidance Behavior Through Symbolic Modeling," *Journal of Personality and Social Psychology*, 8 (1968), 99–108.

9. Barrett, C. L. "Runaway Imagery in Systematic Desensitization Therapy and Implosive Therapy," *Psychotherapy*, 7 (1970), 233–235.

10. Baum, M. "Extinction of Avoidance Responding Through Response Prevention (Flooding)," *Psychological Bulletin*, 74 (1970), 276–284.

11. Bergler, E. "Fear of Heights," *Psychoanalytic Review*, 44 (1957), 447–451.

12. Binswanger, L. "The Existential Analysis School of Thought," translated by E. Angel. In R. May, E. Angel, and H. F. Ellenberger, eds., *Existence: A New Dimension in Psychiatry and Psychology*. New York: Basic Books, 1958.

13. Bond, D. D. *The Love and Fear of Flying*. New York: International Universities Press, 1952.

14. Bookbinder, L. J. "Simple Conditioning vs. the Dynamic Approach to Symptom Substitution: A Reply to Yates," *Psychological Reports*, 10 (1962), 71–77.

15. Bornstein, B. "The Analysis of a Phobic Child," in *The Psychoanalytic Study of the Child*, Vol. 3/4, pp. 181–226. New York: International Universities Press, 1949.

16. ———. "Phobia in a Two-and-a-Half-Year-Old Child," *Psychoanalytic Quarterly*, 4 (1935), 93–119.

17. Boss, M. *Psychoanalysis and Daseinsanalysis*. New York: Basic Books, 1963. (Originally published in 1957)

18. Breger, J. L., and J. L. McGaugh. "Critique and Reformulation of Learning Theory Approaches to Psychotherapy and Neurosis," *Psychological Bulletin*, 63 (1965), 338–358.

19. ———. "Learning Theory and Behavior Therapy: A Reply to Rachman and Eysenck," *Psychological Bulletin*, 65 (1966), 170–173.

20. Camoon, D. "Symptom-substitution and the Behavior Therapies: a Reappraisal," *Psychological Bulletin*, 69 (1968), 149–156.

21. Campos, J. J., A. Langer, and A. Krowitz. "Cardiac Responses on the Visual Cliff in

Prelocomotor Human Infants," *Science*, 170 (1970), 196–197.

22. COLM, H. *The Existential Approach to Psychotherapy with Adults and Children.* New York: Grune and Stratton, 1966.

23. DERI, S. *Introduction to the Szond: Test.* New York: Grune and Stratton, 1949.

24. DEUTSCH, H. *Psychoanalysis of the Neuroses.* London: Hogarth Press, 1951.

24a. DIXON, J. J., C. DE MONCHAUX, and J. SANDLER. "Patterns of Anxiety: the Phobias." *British Journal of Medical Psychology*, 30 (1957), 34–39.

25. DOLLARD, J., and N. E. MILLER. *Personality and Psychotherapy.* New York: McGraw-Hill, 1950.

26. EDLUND, C. V. "A Reinforcement Approach to the Elimination of a Child's School Phobia," *Mental Hygiene*, 55 (1971), 433–436.

27. EIDELBERG, L. "On the Genesis of Agoraphobia and the Writer's Cramp," in *Studies in Psychoanalysis*, New York: International Universities Press, 1948.

28. EISENBERG, L. "School Phobia: Diagnosis, Genesis and Clinical Management," *Pediatric Clinics of North America*, 5 (1958), 645–666.

29. ERICKSON, M. H. "Pseudo-orientation in Time as a Hypnotherapeutic Procedure," *Journal of Clinical and Experimental Hypnosis*, 2 (1954), 261–283.

30. EVANS, P., and J. LIGGETT. "Loss and Bereavement as Factors in Agoraphobia: Implications for Therapy," *British Journal of Medical Psychology*, 44 (1971), 149–154.

31. EVANS, W. O. "The Effectiveness of Visual Imagery When Accompanied by Electric Shock in Reducing Phobic Behavior." Unpublished doctoral dissertation, Fuller Theological Seminary, 1968.

32. EYSENCK, H. J. "Learning Theory and Behavior Therapy," *Journal of Mental Science*, 105 (1959), 61–75.

33. ———, and H. R. BEECH. "Counterconditioning and Related Methods," in A. E. Bergin and S. L. Garfield, eds., *Handbook of Psychotherapy and Behavior Change: An Empirical Analysis.* New York: Wiley, 1971.

34. EYSENCK, H. J., and S. J. RACHMAN. *The Causes and Cures of Neurosis.* San Diego: Knapp, 1965.

35. FACKENTHAL, K. "The Emotional Life of Children," in (Wellesley College Psychological Studies), *Pedagogical Seminary*, 3 (1895), 319–330.

36. FELDMAN, S. S. "On the Fear of Being Buried Alive," *Psychiatric Quarterly*, 16 (1942), 641–645.

37. FENICHEL, O. "The Counterphobic Attitude," *International Journal of Psychoanalysis*, 20 (1939), 263–274.

38. ———. "The Dread of Being Eaten," *International Journal of Psycho-Analysis*, 10 (1929), 448–450.

39. ———. *The Psychoanalytic Theory of Neurosis.* New York: Norton, 1945.

40. ———. "Remarks on the Common Phobias," *Psychoanalytic Quarterly*, 13 (1944) 313–326.

41. FERENCZI, S. *Contributions to Psychoanalysis.* Boston: Badger, 1916.

42. ———. *Further Contributions to the Theory and Technique of Psycho-Analysis.* New York: Basic Books, 1952.

43. FRANKL, V. E. "Paradoxical Intention—A Logotherapeutic Technique," *American Journal of Psychotherapy*, 14 (1960), 520–535.

44. FREUD, S. *A General Introduction to Psychoanalysis* (1917), Garden City: Doubleday, 1943.

45. ———. "Analysis of a Phobia in a Five-Year-Old Boy (1909)," in *Collected Papers*, Vol. 3, pp. 149–289. New York: Basic Books, 1959.

46. ———. "From the History of an Infantile Neurosis (1918)," in *Collected Papers*, Vol. 3, pp. 473–605. New York: Basic Books, 1959.

47. ———. "Obsessions and Phobias: Their Psychic Mechanisms and their Aetiology (1895)," in *Collected Papers*, Vol. 1, pp. 128–137. New York: Basic Books, 1959.

48. ———. "Turnings in the Ways of Psychoanalytic Therapy (1919)," in *Collected Papers*, Vol. 2, pp. 392–402. New York: Basic Books, 1959.

49. FREYTAG, F. F. *The Hypnoanalysis of an Anxiety Hysteria.* Foreword by M. H. Erickson. New York: Julian Press, 1959.

50. FRIEDMAN, J. H. "Short-Term Psychotherapy of Fear of Travel," *American Journal of Psychotherapy*, 4 (1950), 258–278.

51. FRIEDMAN, P. "The Bridge: A Study in Symbolism," *Psychoanalytic Quarterly*, 21 (1952), 49–80.

52. ———. "On the Universality of Symbols," in J. Neusner, ed., *Religions in Antiquity: Essays in Memory of Edwin Ramsdell Goodenough*. Leiden: E. J. Brill, 1968, 609–618.

53. ———, and J. Goldstein. "Some Comments on the Psychology of C. G. Jung," *Psychoanalytic Quarterly*, 33 (1964), 194–225.

54. Gerz, H. O. "The Treatment of the Phobic and the Obsessive-Compulsive Patient Using Paradoxical Intention," in V. E. Frankl, ed., *Psychotherapy and Existentialism: Selected Papers on Logotherapy*. New York: Washington Square Press, 1967. 199–201.

55. Glover, E. *The Technique of Psychoanalysis*. New York: International Universities Press, 1955.

56. Grossberg, J. M. "Behavior Therapy: A Review," *Psychological Bulletin*, 62 (1964), 73–88.

57. Gurman, A. S. "A Note on the Use of 'Expanded' Emotive Imagery in Desensitization," *Psychotherapy*, 7 (1970), 226–227.

58. Hall, G. S. "A Study of Fears," *American Journal of Psychology*, 8 (1897), 147–249.

59. Hallowell, A. I. "Fear and Anxiety as Cultural Variables in a Primitive Society," *Journal of Social Psychology*, 9 (1938), 25–47.

60. ———. "Psychic Stress and Culture Patterns," *American Journal of Psychiatry*, 92 (1936), 1291–1310.

61. Hersov, L. A. "Persistent Non-Attendance in School," *Journal of Child Psychology and Psychiatry*, 1 (1960), 130–136.

62. Hippocrates. *On Epidemics*, V., Section LXXXII, translated by S. Farr. London: Cadel, 1780.

63. Hogan, R. A. "The Implosive Technique," *Behaviour Research and Therapy*, 6 (1968), 423–431.

64. ———. "Implosively Oriented Behavior Modification: Therapy Considerations," *Behaviour Research and Therapy*, 7 (1969), 177–183.

65. ———, and J. H. Kirchner. "Preliminary Report of the Extinction of Learned Fears via Short-Term Implosive Therapy," *Journal of Abnormal Psychology*, 72 (1967), 106–109.

66. Horowitz, S. L. "Strategies Within Hypnosis for Reducing Phobic Behavior," *Journal of Abnormal Psychology*, 75 (1970), 104–112.

67. Jacobson, E. *Progressive Relaxation*. Chicago: University of Chicago Press, 1938.

68. Janet, P. *Les Neuroses*. Paris: Bibliothèque de Philosophie, 1909.

69. ———. *Les Obsessions et la Psychasthenie*. Paris: Alcan, 1919.

70. Johnson, A. M., E. Falstein, S. A. Szurek, and M. Svendsen. "School Phobia," *American Journal of Orthopsychiatry*, 11 (1941), 702–711.

71. Jones, E. "The Theory of Symbolism," in *Papers on Psycho-Analysis*. 5th ed. London: Bailmière, Tindall & Cox, 1948.

72. Jones, M. C. "A Laboratory Study of Fear: The Case of Peter," in H. J. Eysenck, ed., *Behavior Therapy and the Neuroses*, pp. 45–51. Oxford: Pergamon, 1960. (Originally published in 1924)

73. ———. "The Elimination of Children's Fears," in H. J. Eysenck, ed., *Behavior Therapy and the Neuroses*, pp. 38–44. Oxford: Pergamon, 1960. (Originally published in 1924)

74. Kahn, M., and B. Baker. "Desensitization With Minimal Therapist Contact," *Journal of Abnormal Psychology*, 73 (1968), 198–200.

75. Katan, A. "The Role of 'Displacement' in Agoraphobia," *International Journal of Psycho-Analysis*, 32 (1951), 41–50.

76. Kirchner, J. H., and R. A. Hogan. "The Therapist Variable in the Implosion of Phobias," *Psychotherapy*, 3 (1966), 102–104.

77. Klein, E. "The Reluctance to Go to School," in *The Psychoanalytic Study of the Child*, Vol. 1, pp. 263–279. New York: International Universities Press, 1945.

78. Klopfer, B. G., and M. R. Spiegelman. "Differential Diagnosis," in B. Klopfer et al., eds., *Developments in Rorschach Technique*, Vol. 2. New York: World Book, 1956, 282–317.

79. Kraepelin, E. *Lehrbuch der Psychiatrie*. Leipzig: Barth, 1903.

80. Kubie, L. S. "Case Presentation: A Patient with a Height Phobia," in R. Porter, ed., *The Role of Learning in Psychotherapy: a CIBA Foundation Symposium*, pp. 320–321. Boston: Little, Brown & Co., 1968.

81. Lang, P. J. "Stimulus Control, Response Control, and the Desensitization of Fear," in D. J. Levis, ed., *Learning Approaches to*

Therapeutic Behavior Change, pp. 148–173. Chicago: Aldine, 1970.

82. LAUGHLIN, H. P. *The Neuroses in Clinical Practice*. Philadelphia: Saunders, 1956.

83. LAUTCH, H. "Dental Phobia," *British Journal of Psychiatry*, 19 (1971), 151–158.

84. LAZARUS, A. A., and A. ABRAMOVITZ. "The Use of 'Emotive Imagery' in the Treatment of Children's Phobias," *Journal of Mental Science*, 108 (1962), 191–195.

85. LEVENTHAL, T., and M. SILLS. "Self-Image in School Phobias," *American Journal of Orthopsychiatry*, 34 (1964), 685–695.

86. LEWIN, B. D. "Claustrophobia," *Psychoanalytic Quarterly*, 4 (1935), 227–233.

87. ———. "Phobic Symptoms and Dream Interpretation," *Psychoanalytic Quarterly*, 21 (1952), 295–322.

88. LIEF, H. A. "Sensory Association in the Selection of Phobic Objects," *Psychiatry*, 18 (1955), 331–338.

89. LITTLE, R. B. "Spider Phobias," *Psychoanalytic Quarterly*, 36 (1967), 51–60.

90. LOCKE, E. A. "Is 'Behavior Therapy' Behavioristic? An Analysis of Wolpe's Psychotherapeutic Methods," *Psychological Bulletin*, 76 (1971), 318–327.

91. LOCKE, J. "An Essay Concerning Human Understanding," in J. A. St. John, ed., *The Philosophical Works of John Locke*. London: G. Bell, 1913.

92. MACK-BRUNSWICK, R. "A Supplement to Freud's 'History of an Infantile Neurosis,'" in R. Fliess, ed., *The Psychoanalytic Reader*, Vol. 1, pp. 86–126. New York: International Universities Press, 1948.

93. MARKS, I. M. *Fears and Phobias*. London: Heinemann Medical, 1969.

94. MIGLER, B., and J. WOLPE. "Automated Self-Desensitization: A Case Report," *Behaviour Research and Therapy*, 5 (1967), 133–135.

95. MILLER, N. E. "Chairman's Closing Remarks," In R. Porter, ed., *The Role of Learning in Psychotherapy: a CIBA Foundation Symposium*, pp. 320–321. Boston: Little Brown & Co., 1968.

96. ———. "Learning of Visceral and Glandular Responses," *Science*, 163 (1969), 434–445.

97. VON MONAKOW, C., and R. MOURGUE. *Introduction biologique à l'étude de la neurologie et la psychopathologie*. Paris: Alcan, 1928.

98. NAPALKOV, A. V. "Information Process of the Brain," in N. Weiner, and J. C. Schade, eds., *Progress in Brain Research: Nerve, Brain and Memory Models*. Amsterdam: Elsevier, 1963.

98a. NUNBERG, H. *Principles of Psychoanalysis: Their Application to the Psychoneuroses*. New York: International Universities Press, 1955.

99. ORWIN, A. "Respiratory Relief: A New and Rapid Method for the Treatment of Phobic States," *British Journal of Psychiatry*, 119 (1971), 635–637.

100. OPPENHEIM, H. *Textbook of Nervous Diseases for Physicians and Students*. New York: Stechert, 1911.

101. OSTOW, M. "Linkage Fantasies and Representations," *International Journal of Psycho-Analysis*, 36 (1955), 387–392.

102. PITRES, A., and E. RÉGIS. *Les Obsessions et les Impulsions*. Paris: O. Doin, 1902.

103. RACHMAN, S. *Phobias: Their Nature and Control*. Springfield, Ill.: Thomas, 1968.

104. ———. "Studies in Desensitization. II. Flooding," *Behavior Research and Therapy*, 4 (1966), 1–6.

105. RACHMAN, S., and C. J. COSTELLO. "The Etiology and Treatment of Children's Phobias: A Review," *The American Journal of Psychiatry*, 118 (1961), 97–105.

106. RAGGI, A. "Tre casi di clitrofobia" *Rivista Clinica*, 7 (2nd series) (1877), 257–261.

107. RAPAPORT, D. Review of J. Dollard and N. E. Miller, *Personality and Psychotherapy: An Analysis in Terms of Learning, Thinking and Culture*. *American Journal of Orthopsychiatry*, 23 (1953), 204–208.

108. REIK, T. *The Secret Self: Psychoanalytic Experiences in Life and Literature*. New York: Farrar, Straus & Young, 1952.

109. RITTER, B. "Treatment of Acrophobia with Contact Desensitization," *Behaviour Research and Therapy*, 7 (1969), 41–45.

110. ROHRBAUGH, M., and D. C. RICEIO. "Paradoxical Enhancement of Learned Fear," *Journal of Abnormal Psychology*, 75 (1970), 210–216.

111. SARASON, S. B., K. S. DAVIDSON, F. F. LIGHTHALL, R. R. WAITE, and B. K. RUEBUSH. *Anxiety in Elementary School Children: A Review of Research*. New York: Wiley, 1960.

111a. SCHAFER, R. *Psychoanalytic Interpretation in Rorschach Testing*. New York: International Universities Press, 1954.

111b. SCHNURMANN, A. "Observation of a Phobia," *Psychoanalytic Study of the Child*, Vol. 3–4 (1949), 253–270.

112. SHERRINGTON, C. S. *The Integrative Action of the Nervous System*. New Haven: Yale University Press, 1906.

113. SPERLING, M. "School Phobias: Classification, Dynamics and Treatment," in *Psychoanalytic Study of the Child*, Vol. 22, pp. 375–401, 1967.

114. ———. "Spider Phobias and Spider Fantasies: A Clinical Contribution to the Study of Symbol and Symptom Choice," *Journal of the American Psychoanalytic Association*, 19 (1971), 472–498.

115. STAMPFL, T. G., and D. J. LEVIS. "Essentials of Implosive Therapy: A Learning Theory Based Psychodynamic Behavioral Therapy," *Journal of Abnormal and Social Psychology*, 72 (1967), 496–503.

116. ———. "Implosive Therapy: A Behavioral Therapy," *Behaviour Research and Therapy*, 6 (1968), 31–36.

117. STAUB, E. "Duration of Stimulus Exposure as a Determinant of the Efficacy of Flooding Procedures in the Elimination of Fear." *Behaviour Research and Therapy*, 6 (1968), 131–132.

118. STERBA, E. "Excerpts from the Analysis of a Dog Phobia," *Psychoanalytic Quarterly*, 4 (1935), 135–160.

119. SZASZ, T. S. "The Role of Counterphobic Mechanisms in Addiction," *Journal of the American Psychoanalytic Association*, 6 (1958), 309–325.

120. TIETZ, W. "School Phobia and the Fear of Death," *Mental Hygiene*, 54 (1970), 565–568.

121. WALK, R. D., and E. J. GIBSON. "A Comparative and Analytical Study of Visual Depth Perception," *Psychological Monographs*, 75 (1961), 1–44.

122. WATSON, J. B. *Behaviorism*. New York: Norton, 1924.

123. ———, and J. B. MORGAN. "Emotional Reactions and Psychological Experimentation," *American Journal of Psychology*, 28 (1917), 163–174.

124. ———, and R. RAYNER. "Conditioned Emotional Reactions," *Journal of Experimental Psychology*, 3 (1920), 1–14.

125. WEISS, E. "Agoraphobia and Its Relation to Sexual Attacks and to Traumas," *International Journal of Psycho-Analysis*, 16 (1935), 59–83.

126. WEITZMAN, B. "Behavior Therapy and Psychotherapy," *Psychological Review*, 74 (1967), 300–317.

127. WELLS, W. P. "Relaxation-rehearsal: A Variant of Systematic Desensitization," *Psychotherapy*, 7 (1970), 224–225.

128. WESTPHAL, C. "*Die Agoraphobie: Eine Neuropathische Erscheinung*," *Archiv für Psychiatric und Nervenkronkheit*, 3 (1871), 138–161.

129. WILKINS, W. "Desensitization: Social and Cognitive Factors Underlying the Effectiveness of Wolpe's Procedure," *Psychological Bulletin*, 76 (1971), 311–317.

130. WILSON, G. T. and G. C. DAVISON. "Processes of Fear Reduction in Systematic Desensitization," *Psychological Bulletin*, 76 (1971), 1–14.

131. WOLPE, J. *The Practice of Behavior Therapy*. New York: Pergamon Press, 1969.

132. ———. *Psychotherapy By Reciprocal Inhibition*. Stanford: Stanford University Press, 1958.

133. ———, and S. RACHMAN. "Psychoanalytic 'Evidence': A Critique Based on Freud's Case of Little Hans," *Journal of Nervous and Mental Diseases*, 131 (1960), 135–148.

134. WOLPIN, M., and J. RAINES. "Visual Imagery, Expected Roles and Extinction as Possible Factors in Reducing Fear and Avoidance Behavior," *Behaviour Research and Therapy*, 4 (1966), 25–27.

135. YATES, A. J. "A Comment on Bookbinder's Critique of 'Symptoms and Symptom Substitution,'" *Psychological Reports*, 11 (1962), 102.

136. ———. "Symptoms and Symptom Substitution," *Psychological Review*, 65 (1958), 371–374.

CHAPTER 7

NEURASTHENIA AND HYPOCHONDRIASIS

Gerard Chrzanowski

NEURASTHENIA AND HYPOCHONDRIASIS are descriptive concepts, dating back to an era when mental disorders were obscure, inexplicable phenomena whose origin was almost exclusively linked to non-psychological aspects. In the intervening years, the discrepancy has widened between the original terminology and our current understanding of neurasthenic and hypochondriacal manifestations. Today, the nosological boundaries of neurasthenia and hypochondriasis have become vague to the point of being more of a burden than a diagnostic help.

Optimally, psychiatric terms serve as sophisticated, professional working tools designed to aid in the task of providing information about the nature and the expected outcome of a particular mental disorder. They represent a coded language pertaining to difficulties in living with the capacity of evoking appropriate thoughts in skilled psychiatrists as to how best to deal with the prevailing situation ther-apeutically, as well as to offer an educated guess about the prognosis. In addition, the terms are essential for interprofessional communication, as well as for epidemiological considerations. It is mandatory to establish a working consensus about the proper usage of terms, lest one diagnostician's neurasthenia become another diagnostician's schizophrenia.

One can appreciate the significance of nosological concepts in realizing the powerful impact on psychiatric theory and practice when Eugen Bleuler[3] rejected the fatalistic term *dementia praecox* in favor of the diagnostic category schizophrenia. In spite of Bleuler's fundamentally organic point of view, the change of term opened the door to a broad exploration of schizophrenic disorders as a basically human condition, rather than an a priori organic defect. It paved the way for consideration of interpersonal, sociocultural, chemical, hereditary, and other components within the totality of human transactions.

(Neurasthenia

When we come to the nosological classification of neurasthenia, we are confronted with a confusing picture. There is not even complete agreement in regard to the definition of the clinical syndrome. It is usually characterized by a wide variety of symptoms. Ordinarily, there are chronic feelings of weakness and fatigue, various aches and pains, as well as strange physical sensations. Insomnia and irritability may occur in conjunction with a feeling of more or less chronic distress in an organ or organic system of the body. Whereas some patients experience vague, general discomfort, others center their attention upon a particular organ. Any part of the body may be affected. However, there is a high percentage of gastrointestinal symptomatology. The clinician who is compelled to arrive at a psychiatric diagnosis does not have an easy task when confronted by a multitude of symptomatic manifestations.

When Freud dealt with the syndrome of neurasthenia, he considered the following symptoms to be characteristic: headache, spinal irritation, and dyspepsia with flatulence and constipation. In regard to hypochondriasis he said, "It is the form favored by true Neurasthenics when they fall victim to anxiety neurosis as they often do."

In "An Attempt at Analysis of the Neurotic Constitution," Adolf Meyer[28] stated that the term "neurasthenia" should be reserved for the cases combining the symptoms of great exhaustibility and irritability, depending largely on the mental attitude of lack of repose and of ready recoverability, frequent head pressures, palpitations and uneasiness of the heart, gastric disorders, phosphaturia and oxaluria, and in men especially, abnormality of sexual responsiveness. He went on to state:

Frequently, associated with other traits of nervousness, we meet with hypochondriasis, usually built on a feeling of ill-health which leads to self-observation and explanations. These are apt to become the center of thought and interest, are elaborated, or the person merely is troubled with vain fears over trifles, consults quack literature, etc. On the whole, the impressions are apt to become dominating.

Neurasthenia means literally nervous debility or weakness. The notion of weakness of the nerves harks back to the nineteenth-century concepts of mental disorder.

Historically speaking, it is significant that earlier considerations in regard to the etiology of mental disorders did not distinguish between somatic aspects and metaphysical conceptualizations. This mode of thinking gave way to rationalistic and mechanistic models of mental disorders. Thus, in his *Elementa Medicina*, published in England in the eighteenth century, John Brown described the nervous system in terms of eighteenth-century mechanistic concepts, and postulated that "irritability" of the nervous system could cause mental illness. Following this theory, neurasthenia came into existence as a diagnostic syndrome that referred to a weakness or exhaustion of the nervous system. As such, neurasthenia was regarded as the forerunner of all the more severe nervous disorders, e.g., hysteria, epilepsy, locomotor ataxia, general paralysis, etc.

The term "neurasthenia," to denote nervous exhaustion, was subsequently introduced into American psychiatry by George Miller Beard in 1869. Beard maintained that the nerves might "run down" as a result of overexertion or overwork. Thus, according to Beard's theory, the nerve cells operated in much the same way as a battery: When their supply of stored nutriment was depleted, they lost their natural "charge." As an outgrowth of this concept, S. Weir Mitchell developed his rest treatment which prescribed complete rest to cure "anemia of the brain."

The influence of George Miller Beard's hypothetical model is evident in Freud's early formulations concerning the etiology of neurosis. Freud believed that Beard's concept of neurasthenia was too inclusive, and proposed instead the broader classification of "actual neuroses," which would encompass three separate syndromes, namely, neurasthenia, anxiety neurosis, and hypochondriasis. (Hypochondriasis resulted when an anxiety neurosis was superimposed on neurasthenia.) At the same time, however, like Beard, he attributed these phenomena to physicochemical forces, rather than psychological factors. Thus, in Freud's first theory of anxiety, he distinguished between the etiological factors which produced anxiety in specific clinical entities: The psychoneuroses were psychogenic in origin whereas actual neuroses had a physical basis. More specifically, in the actual neuroses, abnormal sexual practices prevented the adequate somatic discharge of chemical substances, or "toxins." Concomitantly, there was an interference with the adequate discharge of the psychic component of sexual tension, which gave rise, in turn, to anxiety. In contrast, in the psychoneuroses, the abnormal sexual functioning which produced anxiety was due to psychic factors, specifically, to repression.

Subsequently, Freud recognized the psychological nature of anxiety and neurosis. Throughout his life, however, he continued to believe that psychical and physical processes were closely interrelated and that physical processes preceded psychological manifestations. Accordingly, Freud's later theory of anxiety did not rule out the possibility that there was a direct somatic relationship between sexual conflicts and anxiety in certain neurotic conditions or, more accurately, that these conditions resulted from the toxic effect of dammed up sexual energy.

He also maintained that there was a potential link between actual and psychoneurosis, that the symptoms of an actual neurosis might precipitate psychoneurotic symptoms in many instances. And, in this connection, he postulated a possible relationship between neurasthenia and conversion hysteria on the one side, and between hypochondriasis and paranoia on the other. For example, initially, the pain which accompanies a neurophysiological symptom, such as a headache, is "real"; that is, it is somatic in origin and due to sexual "toxins." This actual physiological disturbance may then become a future source of focal irritation which might serve as the basis for psychoneurotic symptom formation. Freud further postulated that hypochondriasis represents a withdrawal of interest or libido from

objects in the outside world; instead, the libido formerly connected with the ideas of objects now intensified all ideas concerning body organs. In paranoia, too, an organ becomes the representative of an external object, as a result of narcissistic regression. Thus, Freud hypothesized that hypochondria is the somatic basis of paranoia, just as the anxiety neurosis, that is, a continual readiness to "explode," is the somatic basis of hysteria.

Freud's theoretical foundation for the relationship between the conditions mentioned above is to be found in his concept of narcissism. He distinguished between ego libido and object libido. The former is a withdrawal of interest from object relations and runs counter to the capacity of gaining genuine satisfaction. Freud[17] stated in "On Narcissism:"

The relation of hypochondria to paraphrenia is similar to that of the other actual neuroses to hysteria and the obsessional neurosis: which is as much as to say that it is dependent on the ego-libido . . . and that hypochondriacal anxiety, emanating from the ego-libido, is the counterpart of neurotic anxiety.

Since Bleuler's day, there has been an increasing awareness of the clinical observation that neurasthenia and hypochondriasis may serve as a mask for severe mental illness. Both symptoms occur frequently as precursors of depressions, schizophrenic states, obsessions, and hysteria. In other situations, hypochondriasis and neurasthenia serve as a displacement for a wide variety of difficulties of living, as well as indicating the existence of miscarriages in human relations.

In regard to hypochondriasis, Bleuler[3] stated categorically that "we do not know a disease hypochondriasis." He found the occurrence of hypochondriacal phenomena in schizophrenia, depressive states, in neurasthenia, in early organic psychosis, and in all forms of psychopathy.

A glance at our present psychiatric textbooks does not add much to the picture. Henderson and Gillespie[21] contribute little to our knowledge of neurasthenic and hypochondriacal conditions. They allude to heredity, constitution, autointoxication, and prolonged emotional disturbances as major etiological factors. Noyes[30] is dissatisfied with the term "neurasthenia" which he attributes to deep-lying personal maladjustment. Hypochondriasis is, in his opinion, an organ neurosis. Masserman[27] speaks of neurasthenia as an exhaustive-regressive state, which he believes to be due to unrecognized, cumulative, internal tensions. Harry Stack Sullivan[35] states that, as a student of personality, he finds no virtue in the conception of neurasthenia. From a psychiatric viewpoint, chronic fatigue and preoccupation with fancied disorders which cannot be explained on an organic basis form merely a panoply, obscuring the nature of various interpersonal events. Although Sullivan rejected the concept of neurasthenia, he referred to certain interpersonal phenomena related to this syndrome. In particular, he described somnolent detachment, apathy, and lethargy in this connection.

The appearance of psychogenetic fatigue assumes special significance in regard to the concept of hostile integration. This phenomenon is akin to a sadomasochistic transaction in which both partners relate to each other's insecurities, rather than to their respective strengths. The integration centers on the mutual capacity to evoke anxieties in the other person and markedly lowers their respective feelings of self-esteem. In a hostile integration, neither party can give encouragement, comfort, or support. A hostile integration is a mutual dependency on undermining each other. The result is frequently a manifestation of security operations, ranging from "not feeling well" to "feeling excessively tired," "fatigued," and what have you, as a mask for the malevolent interpersonal atmosphere.

In addition, we have a host of protective devices which are designed to attenuate tension and lower the threshold of painful awareness. Here we encounter the phenomena of apathy, lethargy, and somnolent detachment. Each of the above mentioned manifestations occurs in the face of inescapable and protracted severe anxiety. The result is a decrease in vulnerability to profound interpersonal stress and strain. In apathy and lethargy, the person is out of touch with his most elemen-

tary needs after a state of severe frustration. In other words, fatigue is a complex phenomenon with many different faces. It may reflect a variety of interpersonal malintegrations in which both partners tend to undermine each other's basic security.

From a historical viewpoint, it seems appropriate to include Janet[23] in a discussion of neurasthenia and hypochondriasis. He introduced the term "psychasthenia" in denoting practically all neurotic manifestations which he did not group as those of hysteria. Janet described neurasthenia as a prolonged state of fatigue, without somatic basis. He postulated the notion that neurasthenia was due to a psychic depression in which there is a general depletion of mental energy and a lowering of mental tension.

❲ Hypochondriasis

In its general usage, hypochondriasis or hypochondria denotes the subjective preoccupation with suffering a serious physical illness which cannot be verified objectively on a physiological or organic basis. Hypochondriasis refers also to a chronic tendency of being morbidly concerned about one's health and of dramatically exaggerating trifling symptoms, as if they were a dreaded disease. The name "hypochondriasis" stems from a topographic, anatomical point of view. It was once thought that the soft part of the abdomen below the ribs and above the navel was the seat of the disorder.

In regard to hypochondriasis, Freud was greatly dissatisfied with the osbcurity of the concept. He complained to Ferenczi about it in a letter dated March 18, 1912. Freud formulated hypochondriasis as a withdrawal of interest and libido from the objects in the outer world. The relatedness of certain hypochondriacal symptoms to schizophrenia was recognized early. Freud thought that hypochondriasis has the same relation to paranoia as anxiety neurosis has to hysteria.

The concepts of neurasthenia and hypochondriasis have remained relatively unchanged in analytic literature. Fenichel[11] gave a lucid description of these syndromes but stuck closely to the economic concept of libido theory. He affirmed that many an actual neurosis required only adequate sexual outlets. It is interesting that he recognized alterations in the muscular attitudes of people with neurasthenia. He appreciated the inability of such people to concentrate, because they are unconsciously preoccupied with defensive activities. He pointed to the impoverished life activities leading to restriction of the personality, etc. There were many other important insights offered by him, including the appearance of apathy against aggressiveness. However, he still considered an improved sexual technique to be an adequate treatment in some of these patients. The fact that a change in sexual pattern indicates a reorientation in the total personality was not mentioned.

As far as hypochondriasis is concerned, Fenichel saw it primarily as a transitional state between reactions of a hysterical character and those of a delusional, clearly psychotic one.

Regardless of how misleading the terms may be, the fact remains that neurasthenic and hypochondriacal manifestations are almost ubiquitous in all types of psychiatric practice. Furthermore, the phenomena associated with these concepts are widely represented in our culture, without being given much psychopathological significance. Feeling excessively tired, as well as being deeply concerned about one's health, are relatively conjunctive aspects of our social pattern.

Many people feel righteous about being entitled to a reactive state of weariness as a result of labor and exertion. For instance, it is considered quite respectable for a professional person to feel worn out at the end of the day; for the housewife and mother to be exhausted from her many chores; for the businessman, after a day of pressure at the office, to be very tired. On the other hand, we can frequently observe how certain interpersonal aspects can aggravate the fatigue markedly, whereas others can make the person forget how tired he is. I am not talking here about occasional states of overwork, etc. What matters is the recur-

rent nature of the syndrome—a state of affairs where feeling exhausted forms a more or less consistent pattern. As far as the reaction of the environment is concerned, it ordinarily does not seem to be practical or in good taste to quarrel with people's justification for being tired, regardless of the circumstances. Furthermore, it is to be understood that special allowances are to be made for the person who is afflicted by debility and potential ill health. The victims of neurasthenic and hypochondriacal symptoms can always claim that they wish it were otherwise, but they just can't help feeling the way they do. Obviously, the more absorbed a person is with his mysterious predicament, the less available is he for personal relatedness to others. The "I don't feel myself" preoccupation impoverishes the nature of all other communication and insulates the person from more direct contact with the environment.

Despite this obvious dilemma, the nature of the insulation is such that it still permits a tenuous relatedness to others at a time when more meaningful contact might not be possible. As long as at least one marginally structured channel of communication is preserved, this may suffice to prevent a disintegration of the personality.

Another significant aspect is demonstrated by the fact that almost every practicing psychiatrist has seen patients who seemingly feel tremendous relief when a "real" organic villain is found. The patient who gets X-ray evidence of duodenal ulceration, kidney stones, herniated disk, etc., may be almost pleased. The point is that he has something which he considers to be beyond his personal control. It exonerates him from a peculiar kind of blame by himself or others. Such people often are hounded with the illusion of imaginary ailments. They frequently believe that they can turn symptoms on or off at will, if there is no specific organicity involved. Everything is done to conceal from themselves and others long-standing, unhappy life experiences involving the total personality. The compulsion to negate personal misfortunes is so great that some of these patients readily submit to a surgeon's knife, painful treatments, prolonged use of medication, etc., in situations that therapeutically do not demand drastic steps.

Here is a situation illustrative of the point made. I saw a sensitive and troubled woman patient in her late thirties who had suffered a transient psychotic episode. Part of this profound upheaval was triggered off by her belated awareness that her husband had much in common with an older sibling of hers whom she despised. On the surface, it all started with an attack of acute abdominal distress. She was admitted to a general hospital and kept for ten days' observation. There was some idea of a gall bladder disorder. The findings, however, were inconclusive, and she was told that she was severely run down. From the time she returned home, things went from bad to worse. Finally, she accused her husband of having poisoned her food, and of similar uncharitable acts. The situation deteriorated to the point where he felt compelled to institutionalize her. Her hospitalization was relatively short. During her illness, it was brought home to her that she owed deep gratitude to her husband's kindness and thoughtfulness. It turned out later that she had never faltered in her conviction that the mental hospital had been a punitive act on his part. At a later point, when my patient had made major strides toward recovery, her husband began to ail. He had always been known as a hypochondriacal person who suffered from headaches, backaches, gastric ulcers, and neuralgias. Sudddenly, he developed an excruciating back pain, which his wife suspected to be psychogenic in nature. Despite her urging, he refused to consult a psychiatrist. After several weeks of acute misery, he had an orthopedic surgeon operate on him for a dislocated *nucleus pulposus*. The result of the surgical intervention was miraculous. Now the dragon's tooth which had been bothering him for years had been extracted. His relief was so great that he did not even complain about having to maintain prolonged sexual abstinence. My patient was not unduly affected by this restriction. It soon came out that there had been no sexual relations for more than two years prior to the operation. When my patient became fleetingly interested in sex again, her husband's physical symptoms reappeared temporarily.

As the history unfolded in therapy, several aspects in the situation became clearer. In the past, my patient had experienced several spells of depression and ill health, which usually coincided with her husband's feeling on top of the world. There were times when my patient had been highly successful, and her devoted husband almost invariably came down with a physical illness. Furthermore, it became clear that my patient's feelings of well-being were usually enhanced by feeling needed. This seesaw pattern had been familiar to the patient within the setting of her own family. In their later years, both of her parents had taken turns in feeling down in the dumps. At such times, the low-ebb marital partner was taken to a shock therapist by the solicitous spouse. As a matter of fact, there had been a similar interplay between the patient and her oldest brother. She always came to his help when he was physically ill or in a jam. Once he was well again, she felt all worn out. He would, however, always make her feel she had not done enough for him. On the whole, he led a glamorous life and had always been his parents' favorite. Anyhow, certain aspects of the hostile integration between the siblings had found their way into the marriage. We can see, then, a highly intricate and morbid interplay in a family setting, where alternating hypochondriasis and neurasthenia occur. By the time the husband seemingly blew a spinal fuse, a serious crisis had occurred which threatened to break up the old, familiar pattern. The surgical removal of the man's emotionally exaggerated pain served as a *deus ex machina*. An obvious villain for much obscure difficulty in living had been found. Everybody could point to the tangible intervention and the resulting success. One might add sadly that the patient's psychosis had almost been suffered in vain. Nobody talked, however, of mutual suspicions, resentment, power struggles, and humiliations. A cause had been found that could be reactivated if necessary, but which was placed outside of psychological boundaries.

So far, the terms "neurasthenia" and "hypochondriasis" have been used separately. It is not always easy to draw a line of demarcation between these two conditions. However, when we follow the respective roles these two concepts have played in the evolution of psychiatric theory and practice, the situation is somewhat different.

As pointed out previously, the notion of fatigue and overwork as a cause for mental disorders was prevalent at one time. With the advent of psychoanalysis, the etiological focus shifted to the area of sexual behavior. In regard to neurasthenia, Freud wrote that "it arises whenever a less adequate relief takes the place of the adequate one, thus, when masturbation or spontaneous emission replaces normal sexual intercourse." Freud thought that every neurosis has a sexual etiology. However, he postulated a major difference between the actual neuroses and the psychoneuroses. The former group of disorders has its origin in the here-and-now, while the psychoneurotic conditions relate back to traumatic experiences in infancy. Finally, Freud also contended that the actual neuroses (i.e., neurasthenia, hypochondriasis, and anxiety neurosis) frequently functioned as a focus for neurotic symptom formation.

Bleuler, too, rejected Beard's hypothesis that exhaustion of the nervous system caused neurasthenia. On the contrary, he believed that work was beneficial, and he noted that individuals who work hard seldom fall victim to neurasthenia. Bleuler also noted that neurasthenia was frequently a precursor of schizophrenia.

(Current Etiological Concepts

Brenner[4] summed up the situation as follows: ". . . the category of the actual neuroses has ceased to be a significant part of psychoanalytic nosology." The same author, in collaboration with Arlow,[1] expressed renewed interest in hypochondriasis, which is the third of the actual neuroses. According to Brenner and Arlow, ". . . hypochondriacal impulses are not properly explainable as the result of libidinal regressions and displacement . . . they are

more satisfactorily explained in terms of the conceptual framework of the structural theory, with its emphasis on anxiety, conflict and defense." Otherwise, current psychoanalytic literature has largely ignored the actual neuroses, in spite of the great interest in ego psychology with its emphasis on reality factors. For the most part, references to neurasthenia and hypochondriasis in the current literature do not extend beyond the description of these conditions. Concomitantly, when they are included, discussions of etiology are usually limited to a brief allusion to heredity, constitution, autointoxication, and prolonged emotional disturbances as major etiological factors. There has also been a growing dissatisfaction with outmoded terminology in recent years. Noyes,[30] for one, has taken issue with the concept that neurasthenia represents an exhaustion of the nervous system. Rather, he believes that, invariably, neurasthenia is due to personal maladjustment. On another level, Masserman[27] has described neurasthenia as an exhaustive-regressive state, due to unconscious, cumulative, internal tensions.

Harry Stack Sullivan's concern with the etiology of neurasthenia and hypochondriasis reflected his interest in the reformulation of psychiatric syndromes in interpersonal terms. To begin with, he contended that the diagnosis should pertain to an ongoing process which would be considered indicative of the way in which personal situations have become integrated in more or less durable patterns. The integration has its roots in significant interpersonal constellations of the past, as well as of the present. Furthermore, personal encounters in the immediate future are an integral part of the situation, for past and present events tend to determine future experiences. Viewed from this perspective, Sullivan could find no virtue in the diagnosis of neurasthenia as a one-dimensional, somatic concept which made no reference to maladjustments in patterns of living. He postulated, instead, that certain factors, such as deficiency states, malnutrition, and chronic intoxication, might produce neurasthenic symptoms that were purely physiological in origin. On the other hand, psychiatric or interpersonal phenomena might produce symptoms, such as fatigue, apathy, and somnolent detachment, which resembled neurasthenia to some degree. Apathy and somnolent detachment were conceived of as protective operations against a lowering of self-esteem. More specifically, by taking refuge in sudden, overwhelming sleepiness, the individual withdraws from a tension-producing situation and is no longer vulnerable to feelings of inadequacy, worthlessness, or hostility. In apathy, all the individual's responses become less intense as a reaction to severe frustration.

Sullivan viewed hypochondriasis as a particular kind of security operation. The self-esteem of the hypochondriac has been organized in such a fashion that bodily phenomena are given a great deal of highly pessimistic attention. For the hypochondriac, an intense, morbid preoccupation with his body serves as a distraction from a stressful interpersonal situation. And, concurrently, the recognition of anxiety is minimized or avoided. The hypochondriacal person has difficulty in achieving any genuine satisfaction, because he is constantly haunted by the shadow of impending doom. Hypochondriasis is further characterized by an implicit symbolism which is body-centered and reflects a regression of cognition. It is this regression of the cognitive operations that links the hypochondriacal thought processes to certain schizophrenic thought processes. Sullivan formulated his ideas on the subject as follows:

It is as if the hypochondriacal patient had abandoned the field of interpersonal relations as a source of security, excepting in one particular. He has to communicate data as to his symptoms; the illness, so to speak, becomes the presenting aspect of his personality.

It was also Sullivan's opinion that, in all likelihood, paranoid, algolagnic, hypochondriacal, depressive, and obsessional states were different manifestations of the same maladjustive processes. He observed that in many patients there was a blending of these conditions and an alternation between one state and another.

Another etiological basis for neurasthenic and hypochondriacal preoccupations may be the existence of unexpressed anger, which leads to concealed resentment. This concept has been stressed in particular by Rado,[32] who believes that hypochondriasis serves to obscure the feelings of repressed rage and hurt pride.

Finally, symbolic feelings of rejection and worthlessness may be communicated in characteristic patterns of nonverbal and verbal communication. For example, Weinstein[39] pointed out that the statement "I am tired" results from a complex interpersonal transaction that expresses a particular relationship to the environment. Similarly, a hypochondriacal preoccupation may be understood as a symbolic expression of feeling disliked, not approved of, and isolated from other people.

It has proved helpful to study human personalities on the basis of mutual activities in a field. By stressing the operational aspects, our interest has turned toward how people affect each other and what impact the social and cultural setting has upon them. This has largely taken the place of being predominantly preoccupied with intrinsic factors. There has been less need to think in terms of strict causality alone. Today, it does not suffice to diagnose an organic disorder or rule out overt somatic involvement. Even in the predominantly organic disorder there are involved some sociocultural as well as some interpersonal components. The individual and his environment are an interdependent system at all times. Any effort to isolate one or the other produces major artifacts. Every disorder tells something about the persona in terms of specific life experiences. It points to potential vulnerabilities or sensitivities in the total life history. The area which is of interest to the psychiatrist is always of a strictly personal nature. It has to do with personalistic, experiential data which can become communicable in increasingly more meaningful terms.

When we encounter neurasthenic and hypochondriacal manifestations in our patients, we have to think largely in terms of symbol processes. They tell something about what the patient thinks of himself and of his personal world in his communal existence. There has been increasing interest in denial of illness and bodily feelings in general. The nature of people's self-image ("I and my body," visual, tactile, auditory modes of perception) is a wide-open field for study. As a conceptual scheme, the notion of a nexus (as used by Whitehead), a central relay station where all sorts of things get together, is a fascinating concept.

The clinical study of neurasthenia and hypochondriasis brings another consideration to mind. It is as if the person were attempting to cling to some reality when the world seems in danger of slipping away. There seems to be a focusing on that which is closest as a means of warding off interpersonal tension or losing oneself. Much of the bodily preoccupation has the appearance of a miscarried effort at finding oneself. The more intrapersonal fear is experienced, the less attention will be paid to interpersonal difficulties. Some of the symptoms found in neurasthenia and hypochondriasis can best be understood in terms of the patient's role in his family constellation, in addition to sociocultural and other factors. It is of interest that certain somatic preoccupations are widely fostered in our cultures. The interest in weight for reasons of health is highly acceptable. To climb on a bathroom scale twice a day is not an unusual occurrence in the American family. For women, the intense interest in the surface measurements and contours of legs, breasts, waist, etc., is encouraged; the way eyelashes are curled, hair-dos are fussed about—all these are deeply rooted in the culture. For this reason, it may be more difficult to detect severe personality disorders in women where there is a camouflage of socially acceptable preoccupations. Some people are aspirin, laxative, patent-medicine, or Christian Science addicts. It may be possible to get by on this basis without showing overt symptoms of hypochondriasis or neurasthenia.

There has been an increasing awareness of the interdependence of environmental factors and personal, adaptational aspects in the continuum of an individual's life space. We have a great number of variables to consider, and the conceptualization of static units closes the door to meaningful new insights.

We have long been aware that fashions are not confined to the outer wrappings of people, but that neurosis and psychosis, in all their diversity, have something of "a latest look" of their own. The modern way of life in our fast-changing culture will undoubtedly produce relatively novel aspects of human aberrations which are not yet in vogue. It is that much more remarkable how durable the phenomena called neurasthenia and hypochondriasis have remained.

⟪ Considerations of Social Psychiatry

We still have a great deal to learn about the intricate relationship between culture and symptomatology. However, several pilot studies by social psychologists and allied scientists have thrown light on possible connections between the Gestalt of psychopathological phenomena and cultural determinants. Epidemiological investigations have been used to focus attention on the occurrence of certain psychiatric manifestations in various cultural and social settings. Much interest has been shown in the part that the traditions of an ethnic group, sex, age, level of social achievement, etc., play in the particular shape and form of mental illness. There has also been increasing understanding of the degree to which the definition of mental disorder constitutes a social phenomenon.

Opler[31] has alluded to how certain ethnic groups tend more toward some symptoms than do others. For instance, he points to the difference in attitude toward illness of Italians and "Yankees." Then we have the New Haven study by Hollingshead and Redlich.[22] This study is limited to people under psychiatric treatment and, accordingly, is not a study of the community at large. It stresses the influence of social and cultural conditions on the development of sundry deviations in behavior. Particular interest is shown in the impact of different class levels of a given society on the type of disorder which can be observed. In the New Haven study the percentage of patients who tended toward somatizing their complaints was highest among the lowest two classes in the group studied. These two groups consisted mainly of the people whose educational and economic level was at the bottom of the scale. Although the tendency toward somatization is not synonymous with the existence of neurasthenia and hypochondriasis, it seems to be a factor worthy of consideration.

In private psychoanalytic office practice, where patients from middle- and upper-middle-class groups are prevalent, I have encountered a fairly large number of hypochondriacal patients. However, the great majority of these patients suffered from recurrent episodes of preoccupation with their health. There were some patients in whom the symptoms of concern over ill health were more or less constant. These people invariably showed severe pathology and were very slow as far as speed of recovery is concerned. Despite grave distortions in the personality, these patients usually did not create an impenetrable wall by means of their somatic complaints. Similar observations were made in supervising the work of some of my colleagues.

The situation was quite different in consultation work in a community clinic located in a low-income borough of Greater New York. There the incidence of somatic preoccupation as a primary complaint was much higher. In several instances, it seemed most difficult to get beyond the level of neurasthenic and hypochondriacal preoccupation. Many of these patients had been referred by general practitioners who prescribed psychiatric treatment. Not infrequently, the patient insisted on side-stepping any interpersonal complications and expected to be magically liberated from physical distress.

Anna Freud[14] found that hypochondriasis occurred only rarely in children, unless they were motherless and had been institutionalized. On the other hand, precursors of neurasthenia and hypochondriasis, in the form of "growing pains," fatigue, and sleep disturbances, are fairly common in children.

❮ Management and Therapy

Earlier reference was made to the frequent occurrence of neurasthenia and hypochondriasis in psychiatric and medical practice, as well as in the culture in general. In some communities, patients wih this symptomatology constitute a large number of referrals to the psychiatrists. Others go around and change physicians frequently, or they become more or less permanent fixtures in a doctor's practice. Some of these patients show up in a psychiatrist's office with the challenge, "I have tried everything else, this is my last resort!" The urgent question arises as to what to do with these patients. Should they all be analyzed or tranquilized? Would it be in their best interest to receive mild reassurance by the medical practitioner, or would they do better with expert psychiatric help? Is it helpful to distract them, help them change their environment if possible, stimulate other interests, etc.?

I need not state specifically here that it is not possible to devise one formula for all cases. The management or method of therapy depends on a multitude of factors.

Generally speaking, I have not found tranquilizers given in moderate amounts to be very helpful. Most patients today have tried one kind or another by the time they come to the psychiatrist's attention. It seems that relief is usually not adequate or lasting. There is undeniable merit, however, in having the psychiatrist attempt chemotherapy that does not make the patient unduly drowsy. (Great care must be taken not to offer the medication as a miracle pill.) I am opposed to all forms of shock treatments in these conditions. In hospital, clinic, and private work, I have seen no indication of even minor improvement in hypochondriasis and neurasthenia as a result of various shock methods. On the other hand, I have encountered distinct difficulties in psychiatric and psychoanalytic treatment with patients who had undergone this procedure. Every neurasthenic and hypochondriacal patient requires individual consideration. In a somewhat schematic evaluation, we might distinguish between the following possibilities: Neurasthenia and hypochondriasis may occur in connection with structural visceral changes. Regardless of whether the organic or the psychic malfunction comes first, by the time there is a demonstrable preorganic or organic situation, we do not have a primary psychiatric problem at hand.

Occasionally there can be considerable relief, or even cure, as a result of straight medical treatment. In a great many people, however, there is a concomitant disturbance of the personality. This may require attention in its own right.

We may find neurasthenic and hypochondriacal phenomena in conjunction with character disorders, neurotic difficulties, etc. Here we have a different situation. Not all patients have the motivation to change; not all patients have the opportunity to rearrange their lives. There are people who would have to undergo tremendous changes of the personality. Their pattern of relating to others would have to be grossly modified if they were to become less neurasthenic and less hypochondriacal. The decision as to whether the patient is amenable to treatment should be left to highly experienced psychiatrists. Doubtful cases should be worked up carefully, including projective psychological tests, whenever possible. There is grave responsibility involved in arriving at a thoughtful and adequate conclusion.

Some patients can be found to be preschizophrenic; others to be full-blown schizophrenics, some with delusional ideation. The latter group frequently is markedly paranoid, and some offer a poor prognosis. Among the preschizophrenic or schizophrenic patients (without a fixed delusional system), treatment by a highly skilled analyst in office practice may be successful. Occasionally, a patient has to be hospitalized if all communication is broken off as a result of suicidal tendencies, preternatural preoccupations with somatic symptoms etc.

We may also encounter people with neurasthenic and hypochondriacal complaints who develop the characteristic symptoms after experiencing an acute existential predicament, that is, a state of affairs where professional, marital, or other difficulties have been prominent. Once the crisis is over, these people are apt to suffer from neurasthenic and hypochondriacal symptoms. In other words, it can be observed that pressing reality problems are capable of obscuring the existence of neurasthenia and hypochondriasis. At the end of an emergency situation, we may find a flare-up of difficulties, which had been at times sub-clinical until then.

Some people are prone to have a chain reaction of highly unfortunate life experience. Once the external pressures subside and life seems to offer more satisfaction and happiness, that is the time when long-standing personal insecurities come to the fore. As long as there is a powerful distraction by more or less constant, external misfortunes, there is less opportunity for coming in contact with unfortunate aspects of the person's self-image. The low self-esteem inculcated early in childhood was always there, but the patient did not suspect his grave personal vulnerabilities and hypersensitivities until actual living conditions became much more promising.

We have to appreciate that there can be actual, current conflicts largely beyond the individual's control. People cannot be expected to undergo excessive stress and strain without showing some after-effects. It should be kept in mind, however, that many situational factors have to be understood in terms of people's character patterns. The vicissitudes of life which call for change of environment, if possible, for less strenous activity, more rest, and other managerial rearrangements, etc., are not in the realm of psychiatric practice. More often, history tends to repeat itself, and personal difficulties have to be analyzed, so that there will not be just a shift of symptoms.

I should like to add here that some people in our culture are bored, find their living conditions dull, and entertain themselves with interesting physical symptoms. To some of these patients the psychiatrist has little or nothing to offer. They often go on and on, without improving or deteriorating much.

It should also be emphasized that the distinction between so-called real and so-called imaginary illness is unfortunate. All symptoms are real, whether or not our methods are adequate in explaining them. We seldom find hypochondriasis and neurasthenia among people who are just plain fakers. Whatever a person feels is based on some perception and some experience. We do not have the right to suggest figments of the mind, precisely because our over-all understanding of the nature of the complaint may be lacking. The assumption that a complaint without demonstrable organic basis is a senseless complaint needs to be dispelled.

In considering therapeutic intervention, we need to keep in mind that neurasthenic and hypochondriacal manifestations are usually a mask for basic personality problems. It is doubtful that the formation of either syndrome is connected with any standard set of circumstances responsible for the syndrome's existence. There seem to be variable traumatic events which manifest themselves in more or less circumscribed patterns. As is common with syndromes and symptoms in medicine and in psychiatry, they cannot ordinarily be cured as such. In psychiatry, the elucidation of particular, personal life experiences is a highly skillful and time-consuming procedure. When Mr. Jones complains of always feeling tired, and Mrs. Smith of never enjoying good health, we must assume that common-sense approaches have been tried in most instances. Patients should not be expected to waste good money and time just to be told the obvious. It is not advantageous to be told that the trouble is in the head and not in the body. We have to realize that patients frequently cannot hear us when they are highly defensive about the nature of their actual difficulty. Standard clichés of our common language are often sterile channels, precluding mutually meaningful understanding. The patient who says "fatigue" and the psychiatrist who hears "neurotic syndrome" obviously are not talking in the same tongue. Any attempt to exchange the word "fatigue" for "neurosis," or vice versa, will do nothing to improve communication. As long as there is no common meeting ground, it does not even matter whether the patient nods his head in approval, or shakes it in disbelief.

In discussing therapy, I object strongly to any kind of do-it-yourself manual in psychiatry. At the same time, I recognize the necessity for formulating technical procedure. It seems to me that illustrations are best offered in terms of a particular approach without creating a model for direct imitation.

Suppose Mrs. Smith consults you with the following story: She has been to many medical doctors for pain around her heart, headaches, backaches, and thyroid trouble; she had been treated for gastric ulcers, but she has always feared it might be cancer. Nobody so far had been able to help her. A chiropractor offers her occasional relief, but it is never for very long. Her family physician has prescribed tranquilizers and barbiturates, but they do absolutely nothing for her. Another physician had recommended a different medication, which helped only in the very beginning. Finally, she had come to see a psychiatrist. She repeats her complaints to him, but the quality of her voice is such that she sounds as if she did not actually expect to be believed. After taking in her recital, with an occasional query here and there, the psychiatrist deliberately changes the focus of the interview. He comments something to the effect, "I hear that you have not been well for some time. Suppose you tell me how it all started." If there is a more or less definable starting point, he may go on to inquire what life was like at that time. Was fate smiling, or were there hardships or misfortunes? If all goes well, interest may be stimulated in relating experiences of stress and strain of a familial, social, economic, or other nature. The emphasis is not on a single traumatizing event, but on repeated experiences of unhappiness, friction, disappointment, etc. Then, a brief glance is attempted into the past, with such nonthreatening questions as, "How happy a childhood did you have?" If you get a rigidly defensive answer, then, "I suppose there were at least some fleeting moments of unhappiness, as we find in the life of all children?" Should all answers point to a Hollywood Class C movie with a happy ending, it would be appropriate to say so.

Anyhow, the attempt is made from all directions to get the patient interested in talking about herself in areas which present potential difficulties in living. You may find that you have gently and skillfully helped point to the way in which the patient may eventually find help. Almost invariably, however, such a patient will counter with some sundry version of, "That is all very well and very interesting, but how about my various ailments?" Then it seems appropriate to explain that psychiatrists do not know how to cure tangible or intangible physical disorders as such. They do know, however, something about frustrations, tensions, and anxieties. It is often possible to get a new slant on what gets in a person's way. There can be no promise of the disappearance of the physical symptoms, but it has been found that in some instances discomfort has been greatly reduced when certain difficulties in living were better understood. Under no circumstances can we afford to have the patient sit back while the psychiatrist is expected to do his stuff and melt the patient's complaints away. If there is to be any measure of success, the principle of collaboration has to be stressed from the very beginning.

It is most important that we do not offer things to patients which we cannot deliver. The reassurance is much more profound when it is made clear that direct verbal communication may lead to a better understanding of one's life situation, but that one cannot assume that bodily complaints will fall by the wayside as soon as insight is gained. The psychiatric facts are often otherwise, and it is our duty to inform our patients honestly and knowledgeably.

I wish to emphasize the fact that successful intervention related to neurasthenic and hypochondriacal manifestations does not necessarily mean a cessation of symptoms. Some people may have acquired a style of life which includes a measure of neurasthenic or hypochondriacal preoccupation. What matters is the capacity not to be unduly distracted by the familiar manifestations, which now assume a peripheral significance, without interfering with constructive aspects of person-to-person relatedness. It is understood, that the ability to sense one's own, as well as one's partner's, feelings of inadequacy provides a more effective protection against an ongoing hostile integration.

Bibliography

1. ARLOW, J. A., and C. BRENNER. *Psychoanalytic Concepts and the Structural Theory.* New York: International Universities Press, 1964.
2. BLAU, A. "In Support of Freud's Syndrome of 'Actual' Anxiety Neurosis," in S. Lorand, ed., *Yearbook of Psychoanalysis*, Vol. 9. New York: International Universities Press, 1954.
3. BLEULER, E. *Lehrbuch der Psychiatrie.* Berlin: Springer, 1937.
4. BRENNER, C. *An Elementary Textbook of Psychoanalysis.* New York: International Universities Press, 1955.
5. CHRZANOWSKI, G. "The impact of interpersonal conceptions on psychoanalytic technique," in *International Yearbook for Psychoanalysis*, Vol. 1. Goettingen: Hoffgard, 1964.
6. ———. "Neurasthenia and Hypochondriasis," in A. Freedman and H. Kaplan, eds. *Comprehensive Textbook of Psychiatry.* Baltimore: Williams & Wilkins Co., 1967.
7. ———. "An Obsolete Diagnosis," in J. Aronson, ed. *International Journal of Psychiatry*, Vol. 9. New York: Science House, 1970–1971.
8. ———. *Presentation of the Basic Practical Features in the Application of the Psychoanalytic Method.* New York: Grune & Stratton, 1960.
9. DUNBAR, F. *Mind and Body: Psychosomatic Medicine.* New York: Random House, 1955.
10. FEDERN, P. *Ego Psychology and the Psychoses.* New York: Basic Books, 1952.
11. FENICHEL, O. *The Psychoanalytic Theory of Neurosis.* New York: Norton, 1945.
12. FERENCZI, S. (Tr. by J. I. Suttie), "Actual and Psycho-Neuroses in the Light of Freud's Investigations and Psycho-Analysis" (1908), in *Further Contributions to the Theory and Technique of Psycho-Analysis* (Comp. by J. Rickman). New York: Basic Books, 1952.
13. ———. (Tr. by E. Jones), *Sex in Psycho-*

analysis. New York: Basic Books, 1950.

14. FREUD, A. "The role of bodily illness in the mental life of children," Psychoanalytic Study of the Child, 7 (1952), 69.

15. FREUD, S. *A General Introduction to Psycho-Analysis.* Garden City, New York: Liveright, 1938.

16. ———. (Tr. by J. Rickman), "The Justification for Detaching from Neurasthenia a Particular Syndrome: The Anxiety Neurosis" (1894), in *Collected Papers,* Vol. 1. New York: Basic Books, 1959.

17. ———. (Tr. by C. M. Baines), "On Narcissism: an Introduction" (1914), in *Collected Papers,* Vol. 4. New York: Basic Books, 1959.

18. ———. (Tr. by M. Meyer), "Obsessions and Phobias: Their Psychical Mechanisms and Their Aetiology" (1895), in *Collected Papers,* Vol. 1. New York: Basic Books, 1959.

19. ———. (Tr. by J. Rickman), "A Reply to Criticisms on the Anxiety-Neurosis" (1895), in *Collected Papers,* Vol. 1. New York: Basic Books, 1959.

20. GLOVER, E. *Psycho-Analysis.* London: Staples, 1939.

21. HENDERSON, SIR D., and R. D. GILLESPIE. *A Text-Book of Psychiatry.* Oxford, 1956.

22. HOLLINGSHEAD, A. B., and F. D. REDLICH. *Social Class and Mental Illness, A Community Study.* New York: Wiley, 1958.

23. JANET, P. M. F., *Psychological Healing.* New York: Macmillan, 1925.

24. JONES, E. *Essays in Applied PsychoAnalysis,* Vol. 1. London: Hogarth, 1951.

25. ———. *The Life and Work of Sigmund Freud,* Vols. 1 and 2. New York: Basic Books, 1955.

26. KLEIN, M. *Contributions to Psycho-Analysis.* London: Hogarth, 1948.

27. MASSERMAN, H. J. *The Practice of Dynamic Psychiatry.* Philadelphia: Saunders, 1955.

28. MEYER, A., in A. Lief, ed. *The Commonsense Psychiatry of Dr. Adolf Meyer.* New York: McGraw-Hill, 1948.

29. MULLAHY, P., ed. *A Study of Interpersonal Relations.* New York: Hermitage Press, 1949.

30. NOYES, A. P. *Modern Clinical Psychiatry.* Philadelphia: Saunders, 1953.

31. OPLER, M. K. *Culture, Psychiatry and Human Values.* Springfield, Ill.: Charles C Thomas, 1956.

32. RADO, S. *Psychoanalysis of Behavior.* New York: Grune & Stratton, 1956.

33. SELYE, H. *The Stress of Life.* New York: McGraw-Hill, 1956.

34. SULLIVAN, H. S. *Clinical Studies in Psychiatry.* New York: Norton, 1940.

35. ———. *Conceptions of Modern Psychiatry.* New York: Norton, 1940.

36. ———. *The Interpersonal Theory of Psychiatry.* New York: Norton, 1953.

37. SZASZ, T. S. "A Contribution to the Psychology of Bodily Feelings," Psychoanalytic Quarterly, 26 (1957), 1.

38. WEINSTEIN, E. A., and R. L. KAHN. *Denial of Illness.* Springfield, Ill.: Charles C Thomas, 1955.

39. WEINSTEIN, E. A. "Linguistic Aspects of Delusions," in *Progress in Psychotherapy,* J. Massermand, ed., Vol. 3, p. 132. New York: Grune & Stratton, 1958.

40. ZILBOORG, G., and H. W. GEORGE. *A History of Medical Psychology.* New York: Norton, 1941.

CHAPTER 8

HYSTERICAL CONVERSION AND DISSOCIATIVE SYNDROMES AND THE HYSTERICAL CHARACTER

D. Wilfred Abse

⟨ Terms and Symptoms

HYSTERIA is a term loosely appiled to a wide variety of sensory, motor, and psychic disturbances which may either appear in the absence of any known organic pathology, or accompany organic illness and grossly exaggerate its effects. The term is also used to describe certain forms of group excitement (mass hysteria). Hysterical phenomena, such as convulsions, pareses, and sensory disturbances, often appear among participants in frenetic religious, political, or erotic group activity. Although the term usually designates a type of psychoneurosis, many persons who exhibit hysterical phenomena either in a sustained and solitary fashion or more transiently within a group may also show evidence of psychotic disorder, including paranoid delusions—that is, false beliefs of persecution and of grandeur.

The term "hysteria" is derived from the Greek *hustérā*, which means "uterus", reflecting an ancient Greek notion concerning the sexual nature of the disorder. Related terms are "hysteriform" and "hysteroid," used often in an attempt at greater precision, the former to designate conditions which in some respects suggest the hysterical type of psychoneurosis but in others suggest psychotic disorder, the latter to indicate a general resemblance to hysteria. In clinical practice, hysterical symptoms may be found associated with other kinds of neurotic disturbances, or may occasionally occur together with florid manifestations of psychosis. Hysterical symptoms frequently appear in males, children, and elderly people; however, they are most commonly seen in women who are in the early adult period of life.

It is to be noted that the term "hysterical" is often used as a defamatory colloquialism and that this usage is to a varying extent carried over inappropriately into the medical sphere. Various forms of psychic excitement and various inhibitions are sometimes comprised under the folk description "hysteria," and often the folk description does overlap with the word as it is used as a psychiatric diagnostic term.

In *conversion hysteria* there are dramatic somatic symptoms into which the mental conflict of the individual is "converted," whereas in *dissociative reactions* there is an attempt to avoid mental conflict at the cost of disturbance of memory and the stream of consciousness. In conversion hysteria there may be gross paralytic, spasmodic, and convulsive motor disturbances, exaggeration, diminution, or perversion of sensation, or dumbness, deafness, or blindness. In dissociative reactions, amnesia, fugue, or somnambulism may first attract attention. Any of these symptoms may occur together, although there are characteristic ensembles, or a symptom may present separately or in alternation with others. Such flamboyant symptoms may subside temporarily in response to equally striking modalities of magical or magico-religious treatment. Historically, the "cure" of such symptoms has been exploited both consciously and unconsciously in the quest for power over others by the magician, the priest, the king, and the quack, or in order to exalt this nostrum or that god.

(Brief History

The ancient Greeks accounted for the instability and mobility of physical symptoms and otherwise unaccountable attacks of emotional disturbance in women by a theory that the womb somehow became transplanted to different positions. This theory of the wandering of the uterus referred to disease phenomena characterized by mobility and fugacity, especially when the course included the creation of scenes in which strong emotions were expressed. In accordance with this view, Hippocrates (460–375 B.C.) considered such states as peculiar to women. In Plato's *Timaeus*, it is stated more even-handedly:

In men the organ of generation—becoming rebellious and masterful, like an animal disobedient to reason, and maddened with the sting of lust—seeks to gain absolute sway; and the same is the case with the womb of women; the animal within them is desirous of procreating children, and when remaining unfruitful long beyond its proper time, gets discontented and angry and wandering in every direction through the body, closes up the passages of the breath, and by obstructing respiration, drives them to extremity, causing all varieties of disease.

Hippocrates also held a naturalistic view of those priestesses, allegedly afflicted with the "sacred disease," who chanted their oracles after convulsing. In many cases, the sacred disease was not epilepsy but hysteria; however, Hippocrates, like many a modern physician, found it difficult to distinguish convulsive hysteria from idiopathic epilepsy.

In the second century A.D., Galen noted that similar kinds of mental and physical distress occurred in men; in these cases, he assumed that the cause was retention of sperm.[100]

The physiological idiom in which these ancient theories are couched indicates an emerging understanding, clouded during the Middle Ages, but developed in modern times by Freud, that hysteria is derived from a disturbance of sexuality resulting from an impediment to adequate sexual expression.

During the Middle Ages, the naturalistic viewpoint of the ancient Greeks was overshadowed by the attribution of hysterical phenomena to demonic possession, sometimes associated with witchcraft. This belief in the demoniacal origin of hysteria was widely held in Europe, and with associated superstitions attained epidemic proportions, resulting in an outbreak of persecution that might be interesting to compare with the rapid and widespread diffusion of popular delusions by means of mass communication in our own time. In the medieval witch trials, the hysterical "stigmata" were relied upon as a method of ascertaining possession by the devil, or else of a pact with him. Later, at the close of the seventeenth century, the populace of Massachusetts (with notable exceptions) became convinced that the Devil had achieved a foothold in Puritan New England, and a witchhunt ensued. Available accounts indicate strongly that the alleged witches and those who were "bewitched" suffered from hysterical disorder. Some of the "witches" apparently practiced black image-magic. This witchcraft, centered in Salem, engendered the wider communication of hysterical disorder within the community of Massachusetts.[57]

With the resurgence of an age of reason, the more educated and influential rejected these medieval notions. Although the womb theory of Hippocrates could no longer be maintained in its crude form in the eighteenth and nineteenth centuries, many observers continued to find a connection between hysterical symptoms and the sexual emotions. According to Ellis,[30] Villermay asserted in 1816 that deprivation of the pleasures of love, griefs connected with this passion, and disorders of menstruation are the most frequent causes of hysterical symptoms.

The development of the sciences of anatomy and physiology in the nineteenth century created a tendency in medical circles to interpret all mental phenomena in terms of diseased structure of the brain. The main current of opinion agreed with Briquet,[15] who denied any connection between hysteria and sexuality. In short, after two thousand years of discussion, hysteria came to be regarded as an organic disease rather than as primarily a mental ailment, and the role of sexual disorder in its pathogenesis was minimized. However, this narrow conception of the disease was soon challenged by the work of Charcot.[19,20] The traumatic power of emotional disturbance in provoking the manifestations of the disease, and the elimination of the manifestations through suggestion under hypnosis, were clearly demonstrated by Charcot's work. Thus, the ground was laid for renewed investigation of the psyche of the patient suffering from hysteria.

Janet,[62] a pupil of Charcot, proceeded to investigate with great care the psychological aspects of hysteria. As a pertinent example of his case studies, here is an abridgment of the report he gives of his patient, Irene.

This girl nursed her mother assiduously during terminal illness, at which time she also toiled away at a sewing machine in order to earn a livelihood. The mother died, and Irene attempted to revive the corpse. The body slipped to the floor and she desperately attempted to drag it back into the bed. Shortly after these events, Irene commenced to have somnambulistic attacks. Janet writes of these attacks:

The young girl has the singular habit of acting again all the events that took place at her mother's death, without forgetting the least detail. Sometimes she only speaks, relating all that happened with great volubility, putting questions and answers in turn, or asking questions only, and seeming to listen to the answers; sometimes she only sees the sight, looking with frightened face and staring at the various scenes, and acting accordingly. At other times she combines hallucinations, words and acts and seems to play a singular drama. [Janet writes of his patient between such attacks:] We shall soon notice that even in these periods she is different from what she was before. Her relatives who had conveyed her to the hospital stated: "She has grown callous and insensible, she has soon forgotten her mother's death, and does not remember her attacks." That remark seems amazing; it is, however, true that this young girl is unable to tell us what brought about her illness, for the good reason that she has quite forgotten the dramatic events that took place three months ago.

Janet concluded from cases of this kind that one series of ideas had become isolated from consciousness generally, in a process of dissociation. Thus, in the case of Irene in the periods between attacks, she knew nothing of what had happened at the time of her mother's death. There was a gap between the idea of her mother's death (and associated ideas), and the system of ideas she evinced in the intervening periods.

Janet concluded that hysteria may be defined as "a malady of the personal synthesis." He emphasized the factors of retraction and of dissociation of consciousness evident in the disease. These he thought to be essentially due to a "preliminary ailing tendency." In postulating this inherited ailing tendency, he followed the view of his master, Charcot, who had insisted upon the hereditary predisposition of the nervous system of sufferers from conversion hysteria, both in its convulsive and nonconvulsive forms, and in the forms of the disease now designated as dissociative reactions. Janet, however, proceeded to connect this inherited predisposition with a failure of mental tension to hold together under conditions of stress (toxic, exhaustive, or psychological) partial systems of thought, which thus separated from the main body of consciousness.

In 1893, Breuer and Freud published an account of their experiences in a new method of investigation and treatment of hysterical phenomena. This preliminary communication, entitled "The Psychic Mechanism of Hysterical Phenomena," was followed by a series of case histories and theoretical explanations, constituting the *Studies on Hysteria*,[14] published in 1895. These studies presented evidence for their view that disturbance of sexuality, as a source of psychic traumas and as a motive of defense in the repression of ideas from consciousness, was of outstanding importance in the pathogenesis of hysteria.

Breuer and Freud found that individual hysterical symptoms subsided when, in hypnotherapy, they had succeeded in thoroughly awakening the memories of the causal process with its accompanying affects, and when the patient in a detailed way discussed circumstantially the emotionally exciting situations, giving verbal expression to the affects. It was necessary that the original emotionally exciting memories be reproduced as vividly as possible, so as to bring them back *in statu nascendi,* whereupon they could be thoroughly "talked out." Recollections without affects were of little therapeutic value. Thus, they found that "the hysteric suffers mostly from reminiscences." Often the critical experiences dated back to childhood, and were experiences that had established the soil out of which further emotional excitation in later years could produce more or less intensive morbid phenomena.

It is apparent that in their joint work on the problem of hysteria Breuer and Freud were opening up a path to the crepuscular field of psychoanalysis, a path shortly to be followed energetically by Freud alone. They found, in brief, that the pathogenic efficacy of the original nonabreacted ideas was abrogated when strangulated affects were vented through speech, and brought to "associative correction by drawing them into normal consciousness."

⟮ Clinical Manifestations

Hysteria is manifest in many different forms, some of which are readily confused with patterns of organic disease. In order to avoid confusing it with organic disease, it is necessary not only to comprehend its characteristics but also to be familiar with the manifestations of organic disease. The protean forms assumed by hysterical disease have given rise to a carnival of literary expansiveness, whereas the problems of diagnosis have been comparatively neglected. For this reason, only its more common and some of the more dramatic forms are dealt with briefly here; the important related topics of psychopathology and diagnosis will occupy our attention later. In any case, the possible symptoms are so numerous that it would be impossible to discuss them all without making the text encyclopedic. It often happens that the disease is not seen in pure culture; although predominantly hysterical, an illness may, as already noted, simultaneously present features of other neuroses, of psychosis, or of organic disease. This serves only to increase the need for accurate diagnosis. Typically, the clinical features are:

1. A group of physical symptoms without an ascertainable structural lesion.
2. Complacency in the presence of gross objective disability (*la belle indifférence* of Janet).
3. Episodic disturbances in the stream of consciousness when an ego-alien homogeneous constellation of ideas and emotions occupies the field of consciousness. This may exclude the normative stream of consciousness in the individual so affected.

It is characteristic of hysteria that, whatever the result of dissociation, be it a localized muscular paralysis or an alternate personality, the operative mental function is a homogeneous whole; affect and ideation are not utterly incongruous, and there is no primary thought disorder, as in schizophrenia. In hysteria, the splitting of the personality is molar—not, as in schizophrenia, molecular. Some cases evince a transition from hysterical disorder to schizophrenia; in transitional phases, it may be difficult to predict the movement, whether in a reaching back to reality accompanied, however, by a consolidation of hysterical symptoms, in a deepening withdrawal accompanied by molecular disintegration, or in integrative progression. The direction of change often depends largely upon management and psychotherapy.

The diagnostic problem of the differentiation of hysteria from organic disease on the one hand, and from schizophrenia on the other, will be apparent from consideration of these clinical features; it is a point of crucial concern to which we will return later. With this general orientation as a background, specific symptoms will now be discussed.

Amnesia and Multiple Personality

The simplest form of dissociation is shown in the absence of recall of a circumscribed series of events in the patient's life, events which later investigation reveals as having been associated with strong emotion. As Freud[44] noted, the temporary forgetting of names is the most frequent of all parapraxes. Examination of such common instances often reveals a need to repress associated thoughts which would otherwise result in anxiety or other dysphoric emotion. In a circumscribed amnesia, a similar but stronger motive operates to keep at bay the remembrance of a series of events. These events may have been either directly evocative of painful feelings, or, paradoxically, involved at the time with pleasurable ones which would now, however, evoke either a sense of guilt or a painful sense of loss in the patient because of adverse changes in his situation in life.

Thus, a young man who fainted shortly after performing vigorously in a football trial, could later remember little about several years prior to the beginning of the football season; when this gross gap in memory was filled again, he could remember nothing of the short segment of time during which he had tested his athletic prowess at this level of increased competition. As he gradually recalled his fanatical yearnings and hope during high school years for fame as a football player, and his energetic and pleasurably successful practice during that time, there was this curious reversal of amnesia: He became amnesic for the most recent three months of time, but remembered his entire life before that. These three months included the final strenuous time of testing of the prepared metal in the fire. It became apparent that during this time he had been beginning to fear that severe injury might result from his fanatical efforts, as indeed his father had warned him. At the same time, he had wanted to continue thinking of himself as unafraid, and it was this enmeshment in conflict and its associated painful feelings, including threatened loss of self-respect, that he was seeking to exclude from consciousness by means of repressive forgetting.

Amnesia is sometimes the sequel of a fugue, a restriction of the field of consciousness, which becomes dominated by a homogeneous series of ideas and emotions hitherto excluded from awareness. During fugue, a patient may leave his usual abode and way of life for a journey which has no immediate connection with his former activity. The patient typically complains later of a complete amnesia for this episode. Such cases occur not infrequently under the stress of military conditions. In one case, a soldier was found wandering at a sea-side resort by the military police and was unable to give a satisfactory account of himself. Psychiatric investigation revealed that one day he had suddenly left his unit and boarded a train, presumably for his home in another part of the country. However, he changed trains at a junction and made for the seaside resort. This resort had many pleasant associations for him. He had spent his honeymoon there, and he and his wife were in the habit of going there for their annual holiday. In the army, he had become preoccupied with the impulse to leave, to the exclusion of all other considerations. His activity in making for the resort could only be made meaningful to him as an attempt to recapture symbolically the palmiest of palmy days of peace, pleasure, and security. Before the psychiatric intervention, he could give no adequate account of himself to the police, for he could not recall how he had got into the situation with them.

This example demonstrates the usual findings in dissociative reactions limited to a hysterical level. The reaction is not aimless, as the wandering might at first appear, but symbolically purposive. Moreover, the present is exchanged for the past and is met partially as though it were indeed the past. The patient sought to return to a time and place in which gratification had been maximal, and to escape from his frustrating current military situation. Janet's somnambulic Irene, in contrast, combined hallucinations, words, and acts in a dramatic reliving of the traumatic and painful situation which precipitated her illness. Her case demonstrates also the exchange of the present for a remembered situation, in this instance, however, in an effort to master its pain.

When these somnambulic episodes are not spontaneous, they can be evoked in hypnotherapy to help the patient to abreact the strangulated affects, and to bring the memories to associative correction by drawing them into the normative stream of consciousness.

A more complex and extravagant clinical manifestation of severe dissociation than that exhibited in fugue and somnambulic states with amnesia is that of multiple alternating personality. Stevenson's *Dr. Jekyll and Mr. Hyde* is the literary fictional model of this type of severe dissociation. The rarely reported actual cases often achieve comparable fame. William James[61] has given an account of double personality which has become famous: The Reverend Answell Bourne disappeared from a town in Rhode Island. Two months later a man calling himself A. J. Brown woke up in a fright asking where he was. This was in Pennsylvania, where six weeks earlier he had rented a confectionery shop. A. J. Brown, the confectioner, then started to claim that his name was Bourne, that he was a clergyman, and that he knew nothing of the shop or Brown. Subsequently, he was identified as the Reverend Answell Bourne by his relatives. He remained unable to explain this episode in his life, which seemed to him uncanny.

Morton Prince,[83] who introduced into medical literature the concept of multiple alternating personality, investigated such a case in the person of Miss Beauchamp, who exhibited at various times three separate fragmentary personalities. A self-righteous, moralistic, and masochistic personality was usually dominant, but alternated with a strongly ambitious, aggressive, distinctive character, which created a perplexing cleavage in the life and personality of Miss Beauchamp. In working with this patient, Prince used hypnotherapy. Under hypnosis, a third personality fragment, calling herself "Sally," came to occupy the field of consciousness. Sally was aware of the saintly personality, though the saintly Miss Beauchamp was unaware of Sally, the impish child. Prince, over a period of six years' work, was able to achieve an integration in the character of Miss Beauchamp.

A more recent well-known example, that of

a housewife reminiscent of Prince's Miss Beauchamp, is provided by a study of Thigpen and Cleckley,[98] *The Three Faces of Eve.* Masserman[76] also reported a case of alternating personality. There are, in fact, about two hundred accounts of alternating and multiple personality in the literature of psychiatry and psychology. In some cases, there is evidence from persons other than the patient of the manifestation of two or more personalities that differed significantly before psychotherapy;[40] in other cases, the emergence of multiple personalities has occurred in the course of hypnotic or of other psychotherapeutic investigation.[74] Congdon et al.[25] have described a case studied and treated at the University of Virginia Hospital (also discussed further by D. W. Abse[1]):

This patient was a twenty-three-year-old housewife who had suffered convulsive attacks following proceedings for divorce. In the hospital, the patient recovered from the convulsive attacks and from depression, and was then discharged and treated as an outpatient. During subsequent psychotherapeutic interviews, the patient, Betty, revealed that as a lonely child she had created an imaginary playmate whom she called "Elizabeth." About two months after discharge from the hospital, during one interview, when she was again describing her imaginary playmate, she suddenly sat upright in her chair and then assumed a relaxed and friendly attitude quite unlike her usual self, and said: "I think it's about time I started to tell you about me." The astonished therapist said, "What do you mean?" and the patient replied, "About me, not about her." She then proceeded to describe herself (Elizabeth) and her career. From this time on until the eclipse of Elizabeth four months later, it was possible for several observers to study both Betty and Elizabeth under a number of different circumstances. Psychological tests of the two personalities supplemented the clinical observations.

Hypnoid States

The phenomena of amnesia and of multiple personality are often associated with distinctive alterations of consciousness, including fugue and somnambulism, and these alterations of consciousness often resemble or are identical with states of hypnotic trance. It is indeed remarkable that notions about and attitudes towards hysterical phenomena have been inextricably interwoven historically with views concerning the nature of hypnosis. In some periods, the art of hypnotizing was regarded as a special attribute of particular persons, a divinely granted and sanctioned power or gift. At other times, it was held to be an instrument of dark powers and a force of evil. Attitudes toward hysteria have similarly and sometimes synchronously oscillated. Sometimes, the relation has been reciprocal, for example, the good power of the priest-physician exorcizing the Devil held responsible for the hysteria.

In the early nineteenth century, Braid[13] eventually succeeded in getting recognition in orthodox medical circles for the facts of mesmerism. He became convinced that it was essentially a narrowing of the attention, a "monoideism," that ushered in the trance. He also began to understand something of the nature of the relation between hypnotist and patient, and of the peculiar effects of hypnosis on memory. After Braid's death in 1860, his discoveries were taken up in France. Soon there were two great schools of thought regarding hypnotism. The Paris School, under the leadership of Charcot,[21] took the view that hypnotism was a phenomenon characteristic of hysteria, and could be induced only in persons suffering from, or at least prone to, that disease. The Nancy School, led by Bernheim and Liebeault,[7] followed more closely the practice and theory of Braid, maintaining that hypnosis could be induced by suitable methods in almost anyone, and that it was a phenomenon dependent on the general psychological trait of suggestibility. They tried to keep the problems of hypnotism and hysteria apart, despite Moebius' dictum: "Everyone is a little hysterical."*

The fact is that in both hypnosis and in hysterical disease there are phases that show

---

* *Jedermann ist ein bisschen hysterisch,"* as quoted by Jones.[64]

alterations in consciousness. Braid, for example, stressed the restriction of consciousness as a prelude to trance. Both the Paris and Nancy schools emphasized the importance of suggestibility in both hypnosis and hysteria. Again, the effects on memory in hypnosis and in hysterical disease may be those of an extraordinarily restrictive or amplifying kind. Moreover, the stages of hypnosis described by Charcot[21]—lethargy, catalepsy, and somnambulism—can be seen quite independently of hypnosis as symptoms of hysterical disease. The view that Janet came to espouse, namely, that the hysteric personality is unstable in its integration, so that dissociative phenomena result, is also pertinent, since these phenomena can readily be shown in the trance state of persons who disclose no evidence of hysterical disease in their usual mode of life.

Breuer and Freud[14] in their preliminary communication pointed out repeatedly that in hysteria groups of ideas originate in hypnoid states, each state being characterized, as is hypnosis itself, by very emotionally intense notions dissociated from all else that the usual consciousness contains. Associations between these hypnoid states may take place, and their ideational content can in this way reach a high degree of psychic organization. Moreover, Breuer and Freud noted that the nature of hypnoid states and the extent to which they are cut off from other conscious processes varies as it does in hypnosis, ranging from complete recollection to total amnesia. They wrote:

We have stated the conditions which, as our experience shows, are responsible for the development of hysterical phenomena from psychical traumas. In so doing, we have already been obliged to speak of abnormal states of consciousness in which these pathogenic ideas arise, and to emphasize the fact that the recollection of the operative psychical trauma is not to be found in the patient's normal memory but in his memory when he is hypnotized. The longer we have been occupied with these phenomena the more we have become convinced that the splitting of consciousness which is so striking in the well-known classical cases under the form of *double conscience* is present to a rudimentary degree in every hysteria, and that a tendency to such a dissociation, and

with it the emergence of abnormal states of consciousness (which we shall bring together under the term "hypnoid") is the basic phenomenon of this neurosis.

They presumed that these hypnoid states developed out of reveries, so frequent in everyone, and for which feminine handwork offered so much opportunity. Breuer wrote in the same work:

I suspect that the duplication of psychical functioning, whether this is habitual or caused by emotional situations in life, acts as a substantial predisposition to a genuine pathological splitting of the mind. This duplication passes over into the latter state (splitting) if the content of the two coexisting sets of ideas is no longer of the same kind, if one of them contains ideas which are inadmissible to consciousness—which have been fended off, that is, or have arisen from hypnoid states. When this is so, it is impossible for the two temporarily divided streams to reunite, as is constantly happening in healthy people, and a region of unconscious psychical activity becomes permanently split off. This hysterical splitting of the mind stands in the same relation to the "double ego" of a healthy person as does the hypnoid state to a normal reverie. In this latter contrast what determines the pathological quality is amnesia, and in the former what determines it is the inadmissibility of the ideas to consciousness.

And Breuer observed of Anna O. that the girl seemed in perfect health but had the habit of letting fantastic ideas accompany her usual activities, and that an anxiety affect would sometimes enter into her daydreaming and create a hypnoid state for which she later had an amnesia. This repeated itself on many occasions, acquiring a richer ideational content, alternating with states of normal consciousness.

Later, Freud[50] wrote of their joint theory as follows:

I have gone beyond that theory, but I have not abandoned it; that is to say, I do not today consider the theory incorrect, but incomplete. All that I have abandoned is the emphasis laid upon the so-called "hypnoid state" which was supposed to be occasioned in the patient by the trauma, and to be the foundation for all the psychologically abnormal events which followed. If, when a piece of joint work is in question, it is legitimate to make a subsequent division of property, I should like to take this opportunity of stating that the hypothesis of "hypnoid states"—which many reviewers were inclined to take as the central portion of our work —sprang entirely from the initiative of Breuer. I regard the use of such a term as superfluous and misleading, because it interrupts the continuity of the problem as to the nature of the psychological process accompanying the formation of hysterical symptoms.

Freud was more concerned with those unconscious genetics and dynamics of hysterical symptom formation, which were more startling and alienating to scientific circles. He minimized the notion of "hypnoid states" in order to focus on the resistance with which his inferences were confronted. As will be detailed here, he elaborated and demonstrated the view that the body language of the conversion reaction could be translated back to word language in the process of psychotherapy, and he showed how the partial failure of repressive defense had led to conversion. At this time, he turned away from giving due consideration to obvious and marked fluctuations in the symbolizing, integrative, defensive, and conscious aspects of ego functioning. This was, of course, before he turned his attention more definitively to ego psychology.

Breuer[14] had previously remarked on Freud's interest in defense in the following noteworthy paragraph:

Freud's observations and analyses show that the splitting of the mind can also be caused by "defence," by the deliberate deflection of consciousness from distressing ideas: only, however, in some people, to whom we must therefore ascribe a mental idiosyncrasy. In normal people, such ideas are either successfully suppressed, in which case they vanish completely, or they are not, in which case they keep on emerging in consciousness. I cannot tell what the nature of this idiosyncrasy is. I only venture to suggest that the assistance of the hypnoid state is necessary if defence is to result not merely in single ideas being made into unconscious ones, but in a genuine splitting of the mind. Auto-hypnosis has, so to speak, created the space or region of unconscious psychical activity into which the ideas which are fended off are driven.

Here Breuer suggests that there is a place for understanding the hypnoid state as a way-station which appears during partial repression and before conversion reduces the psychic tension. Thus, the concept of the hypnoid state does not interrupt the continuity of the problem of identifying the psychological processes that accompany the formation of hysterical symptoms. Besides, the concept is based on an actual phenomenon of striking change in the quality of consciousness, one that is important to understand in order to follow more adequately the vagaries of the hysterical personality.

As introspection quickly reveals, there are different levels of intensity of consciousness and different qualitative states of consciousness. The dreaming consciousness, the hypnagogic, the hypnopompic, and others, including the postprandial, are certainly statistically normal phenomena. In hysterical disorder, there are sometimes decisively pathological alterations of consciousness, including depersonalization and a variety of hypnoid states.

The person afflicted with depersonalization complains that he is no longer the same, that he has somehow changed and is no longer himself. Sometimes, he may complain he is a mere puppet, that things just happen, and that he has no joy or sorrow, hatred or love. He might feel dead, without hunger, thirst, or other bodily needs. The world also appears changed and somehow strange to him. We might sum it up by saying that there is a rejection of ego experience in the autopsychic, allopsychic, and somatopsychic spheres. As Schilder[88] states, however:

All depersonalized patients observe themselves continuously and with great zeal; they compare their present dividedness-within-themselves with their previous oneness-with-themselves. Self-observation is compulsive in these patients. The tendency to self-observation continuously rejects the tendency to live, and we may say it represents the internal negation of experience.

A further paradox is that the depersonalized person continuously observes not only his autopsychic functions but also his own body, and he continuously reports hypochondriacal sensations. Here, too, according to Schilder, a rejection of bodily experience is involved.

In regard to the paradoxical phenomenology of depersonalization, it is as though there were the cry, "Wolf! Wolf!" before the wolf has yet descended upon the fold. Depersonalization is sometimes a syndrome ushering in schizophrenic disorganization or severe forms of ego loss or constriction. The patient begins to talk as if this disorganization or constriction had already occurred, but also expresses his intensified self-observation both in the auto-psychic and somatopsychic fields and in his heightened observation of what goes on around him. He samples, as it were, some degree of impoverishment of ego experience, and restitutionally observes himself and the world around him with heightened vigilance. Besides, in this way he makes an appeal for help, like the shepherd in the fable, who suspects that his sheep are threatened by the wolf. He is, of course, also trying to summon help to prevent dissociation and to enable him to maintain integration.

Wittels[105] has emphasized that the hysteric experiences difficulty attaining actuality as a grown-up human being; in consequence, she confuses fantasy and reality, that is to say, allows the law of the id to enter into the ego. In the depersonalization syndrome, on the contrary, we note the law of the superego entering the ego. The self-observation and internalized threat of negation are pervasive; the strangulation of affect and the unpleasantness of bodily sensations are clearly apparent.

When modalities of function more characteristic of the id enter more completely into the way the hysteric perceives herself and the world, when a more archaic and even more id-ridden ego functioning begins to emerge in the hysteric, a hypnoid state of consciousness, qualitatively quite different, reflects this state of affairs. Self-observation is deleted, ideation is often vague, affect-charged, and restricted. In this state, ideational and verbal performance becomes quite inadequate. The process of symbol-making departs in varying degrees from the denotational towards greater saturation with the mythic mode.

Goldstein[55] has made us familiar with the clinical significance of the abstract attitude and its relation to speech. From his work with brain-damaged patients, he came to distinguish two ways of using words in connection with objects: the real naming of objects, which is an expression of the categorical attitude towards the world in general, and pseudo-naming, which is simply a use of words held in memory. The incidence of pseudo-naming depends on the extent of the individual's verbal possessions. In it, words are used as properties of objects, just as other properties—color, size, hue—are used; they belong to concrete behavior. Often, in the mild, prolonged hypnoid states of some severe hysterical personalities, treatment has to be modified very considerably because much of the time the patient is incapable of adequately achieving the abstract attitude, as it is involved, for example, in psychoanalytic procedure. This is particularly important, as it relates to the analysis of the transference. Such persons often become completely and concretely involved in the transference, without having sufficient means to achieve any distance and sense of time that would enable them to realize that they are caught up in a reliving of the past.

We have sketched the antithetical nature of some qualities of consciousness in the depersonalization syndrome and in other hypnoid states. In the former, the phenomenological characteristics of vigilance and anhedonia were briefly outlined. In other hypnoid states, a confusion and haziness of varying degrees of severity are more often obvious.[26] In all human beings, there is from hour to hour considerable fluctuation in alertness and many other qualities of consciousness. The state of mind of a man busily engaged in his professional activities might contrast remarkably with his state of mind at a later hour during a cocktail party; the reality principle might loosen some of its hold even before the effects of alcohol could facilitate the increasing sway of the pleasure principle. In the hyponoic and sometimes (in some fugue states) anoetic qualities of the hypnoid state, the dominance of repetition compulsion becomes apparent. The state of mind is comparatively blind and issues in acting-out, dissociated from previous learning, in accordance with the reality and pleasure-pain principles.

Today, the possibilities for reverie, which Breuer and Freud saw as being present to a woman engaged in handiwork, and conducive to hypnoid states, appear during the well-nigh automatic driving of an automobile, which affords opportunities for musing and for fantasy expansion, first with increasing id dominance. This accompaniment to driving may sometimes lead to "highway hypnosis" and then to traffic accidents. Myerson[81] recently described a male hysteric who, while driving, sometimes paid less attention to the road than to his rebellious, pleasurable involvement with speed and with the admiring women and the disapproving policemen who focused on him in his fantasy. His preoccupation with the imaginative derivatives and symbols of sadistic phallic wishes of the oedipal situation led him to reckless driving and once to bodily injury, the latter indicating a primitive superego reaction.

Convulsive Hysteria

Charcot[19,20] categorized hysteria into two types, convulsive and nonconvulsive, indicating the high incidence of hysterical convulsions in the patients who came to his notice in Paris in the last decades of the nineteenth century. Briquet[15] earlier showed in his statistics that nearly three-quarters of his hysterical patients suffered convulsive attacks. From 1942 to 1945, the present writer found convulsive attacks to be a frequent manifestation of conversion hysteria in Indian soldiers, in contrast to their occasional incidence as a manifestation of hysteria in British soldiers during the same time in India. Janet[62] traced the connection between convulsive attacks and somnambulisms, showing that convulsive attacks were merely degraded forms of somnambulism where the outer expression of the somnambulic idea in physiognomy, attitude, and act was no longer clear. He showed also in his case studies that hysterical convulsive attacks have the same "moral causes" as somnambulisms, or other expressions of hysteria, and that these hysterical accidents, like others, "begin on the occasion of particularly

affecting events, genital perturbations, sorrows, fears, etc."

Although hysterical convulsive attacks may be relatively infrequent in the United States, as compared to their reported incidence in Paris a century ago, there is clinical evidence of an increment in their actual incidence, or at least of their detection, recently. For example, Bernstein[8] reports case examples of adolescent girls from the Massachusetts General Hospital, who presented to neurologists complaints suggesting epileptic disorder. These young women were struggling with sexual pressures and severe anxieties, and their symptoms served as an angry dramatization of their plight.

Convulsive hysteria may indeed closely simulate idiopathic or symptomatic epilepsy. Hysteria may sometimes be suspected on the following grounds: The patient is not completely unconscious during the attack; the attack occurs only in the presence of onlookers; the patient does not fall in a dangerous situation; the corneal, pupillary, and deep reflexes are present; the patient does not bite his tongue or micturate; he becomes red in the face rather than blue or white; attempts to open the eyes are resisted; pressure on the supraorbital notch causes withdrawal of the head. However, it must be stated that hysteria is manifest in so many forms, some of which so closely imitate organic disease of the nervous and other systems that without the distinctive marks of its etiology and psychopathology symptomatology alone can be misleading. Where epilepsy is associated with the development of abnormal rhythms in the cerebral cortex, the electroencephalograph can be helpful in making a differentiation.

It is often clear on investigation that the hysterical fit represents partly a rage reaction or temper tantrum due to frustration or fear of genital sexual wishes. Often, too, one can find evidence of erotic discharge in the form of the attack (*attitudes passionelles*, ecstatic poses, etc.). The case of a young woman of nineteen who suffered frequent "fits" provides an illustration: The fits occurred about 6:30 P.M. every evening when she was listening to the radio. The attacks had commenced following the dissolution of a love affair. The young man, it was ascertained, had formerly appeared at her house regularly at this time and had listened with her. The fit was preceded by painful sensations in the right side of her body. Here she had formerly experienced pleasurable sensation, for her boyfriend had sat closely at her side. In conversation, this patient at first expressed the view that she did not care at all about her friend's defection. This defense against her affective disturbance had proved adequate during the day when she was at work. Returning home in the evening, she was assailed by her memories of the young man, and the convulsive attack then provided the outlet she required for her outraged feelings.

Kretschmer[69] points out that in living beings the "tantrum violent-motor-reaction" is a typical reaction to situations that menace or impede the course of life. He sees its purpose as basically enabling the organism to make a rapid selection, from among the many at its disposal, of that motion which will meet the situation. Should one of the many irregular motions by chance separate the animal from the zone of danger, this single motion will be continued, with a speedy resumption of quietness. Being an instinctive reaction which expires quite schematically, it may either disappear or become directly harmful. In the course of evolution, the "violent-motor-reaction" as a biological defense reaction retires more and more into the background. More recent and more expedient formations replace the older reaction type. In adult human beings, selective voluntary action is the chief reaction type to new situations. In panic, shocking experiences momentarily paralyze the higher psychic functions, and a phylogenetically older adaptive mechanism, the "violent-motor-reaction," comes once more automatically into activity in their place. In an earthquake or other catastrophe, a crowd will display "headless" hyperkinesias—screaming, trembling, convulsions, twitchings, aimless running. If among the many motions initiated there is one which by chance takes the person away from the sphere of tumbling houses or the zone of danger, quiet ensues; the "violent-motor-reac-

tion" has attained its regulative aim. In children's response to painful stimuli, the "violent-motor-reaction"—pushing, screaming, sprawling, striking—is often evident, instead of the deliberative speech and deportment of adults.

Alongside these two groups of responses—panic and childish behavior—are the hysterical hyperkinesias—the twilightlike running away, the tremors, and the convulsive paroxysms. The hysterical convulsive attack, Kretschmer insists, represents an atavistic "violent-motor-reaction." He points out that in general such psychogenic reaction forms are hysterical where psychic aims in man avail themselves of reflex, instinctive, or otherwise biologically preformed mechanisms.

Paralysis, Involuntary Movements

Many varieties of hysterical paralysis occur. In some, the paralysis is more or less complete. Sometimes, it is associated with tremor of the affected limbs, or contractures; it often takes the form of astasia-abasia (inability to stand and to walk). In this condition, movements may be carried out when lying down or even when sitting down, although standing and walking cannot be performed. Such a symptom as astasia-abasia may thus provide clear evidence of a dissociation characteristic of hysteria. In other cases of conversion reaction, a number of signs that occur in organic paralysis are absent; among these may be mentioned those elicited by testing the tendon reflexes. Dyskinesias, such as tremor, may often accompany paralysis or paresis, and there may be an accompanying bizarreness of gait. Tics and muscular spasms may accompany a paresis, or may occur alone. Disturbance of speech is another common type of hysterical motor disturbance. Sometimes, this is limited to one language, whereas another language (usually the mother tongue) is spoken without difficulty. In such a case, a dissociation characteristic of hysteria is already evident on the basis of symptom observation. Usually, however, the certain diagnosis of hysteria requires closer investigation than is afforded by the mere observation of symptoms. On the one hand, most symptoms are readily confused with the manifestations of other diseases; on the other hand, hysteria frequently occurs in concert with other diseases and its contribution to the manifestations of disease has to be determined.

Kretschmer points out how widely spread in nature is the immobilization or "sham-death-reflex"—the occurrence in animals of motor rigidity in response to threatening danger. As previously stated, he groups convulsive hysteria around the biological radical of the primitive violent-motor-reaction. Immobilization, on the other hand, in one form or another, he groups around the biological radical of the phylogenetically important sham-death-reflex. Hysterical paralysis is often accompanied by an obvious restriction of the field of consciousness. Sometimes, this reaches the degree of stupor. These hypnoid-stuporose hysterical states, together with paralytic conversion reactions, Kretschmer thinks are anchored in the old, general, animalistic reflex mechanism of sham death. Thus, he believes that hysterical reactions group themselves around these two fundamental animal reactions to danger. He further believes that in human beings the danger may be external and/or may be bound up with the emotions and conflicts which accompany the sexual life. He states:

Wishes, struggles, and disappointments of an erotic nature form the large main group of experiences which produce hysteria in ordinary civil life, especially in women; the war neuroses, and a part of the accident neuroses, contribute the other very large half of hysterical reactions.

Such a dichotomy, however, is apt to be misleading, as actual experience of physical violence is also resymbolized following the mobilization of mnemic traces of anxious fantasies linked with the forbidden erotic wishes of early childhood.

In order to illustrate characteristic findings in a case of conversion paralysis, the following case summary shows how the diagnosis may be established on positive grounds from the point of view of symptom observation and etiology, as well as psychopathology:

The patient, a married man, aged fifty-nine, complained of paralysis of the left leg and weakness of the left arm. Examination disclosed the left upper and lower limbs to be slightly spastic. When the patient was encouraged to flex the left thigh at the hip joint, the antagonistic muscles went into increased spasm. The patient was next required to raise himself into the sitting position in bed, his arms being folded and his legs separated. Under these conditions the paralyzed left leg remained firmly on the bed. (The paralyzed leg rises higher than the other under these conditions in organic disease of upper motor neurone type—"Babinski's second sign.") The plantar reflex was flexor (Babinski's sign negative), and the tendon reflexes were present and equal on both sides.

In discussion it was ascertained that the patient's illness commenced during the bombing of London, at which time he had become acutely fearful. Moreover, the illness required giving up work just as he was approaching the time for retirement on full pension. The only other noteworthy item of information in this discussion was that his father had died in his eighties of cerebral thrombosis with left-sided paralysis. This patient was later given sodium amytal intravenously for the purpose of further psychological exploration. Under narcosis, he prayed for the forgiveness of his sins, giving an account of the use of contraception since the birth of his second son (twenty-five years of age). The doctors had at that time advised against further children on account of his wife's ill health, and he had since used contraceptive techniques, although this was against his religious convictions and those of his father. He also spoke of his struggles against masturbation prior to marriage, and wept bitterly. He felt he had committed grave errors and was not entitled to enjoy retirement, as his father had before him. During the bombing he had felt convinced that retribution was at hand. In further discussions without narcosis, the patient at first denied any sense of having done wrong, and defended his conduct during marriage on the grounds that he had to think of his wife's health, and that in any case she was quite satisfied with her two boys, etc. He appeared quite reasonable in his attitude toward his sexual problem, although he admitted he had always spoken in public against any form of contraception, and went on to talk of moral dangers.

Interview with his wife disclosed his great dependence on her in all respects, including an incapacity for decision without her. Moreover, she gave an account of her honeymoon thirty years before, which had been marred by her husband's worry lest he had cancer.

In this case, the signs were characteristic of hysteria. We may also note that there was a temporal connection between the onset of his paralysis and the dangerous situation of bombing. A conflict of a sexual nature evoked by this stress was uncovered, and the meaning of the symptoms became clearer. Moreover, his personality background showed evidence of overdependence and neurotic traits, the latter presenting chiefly in the form of hypochondriasis at the time of his marriage, which, incidentally, he had delayed for a considerable time. (The diagnostic importance of the chronological correlation of stress and conflict with the onset of symptoms in the setting of hysterical character background will be emphasized later.)

Further Notes on Involuntary Movements

As has been emphasized, observation of symptoms may not in itself be sufficient to diagnose hysteria; for this purpose further investigation along both psychologic and physical lines may be requisite. For example, in a child, the distinction between the diagnosis of a relapse of Sydenham's chorea and that of a hysterical mimesis is sometimes extremely difficult to make, and quite impossible on the basis of symptom observation alone. Not uncommonly, hysteria is responsible for evanescent hyperkinesis definitely choreiform in type in young children. In such children, an impression of choreiform movements may have been previously produced by an attack of rheumatic chorea, or the child may have observed such an attack, usually in hysterical cases in another member of the family. Sensitivity of the physician to the underlying psychodynamics of the neurosis is essential in arriving

at such difficult differentiations, and the psychopathology of conversion reactions is discussed below.

Nonchoreiform movements, that is, typical movements which might be performed normatively but which are performed excessively and inappropriately, may also, of course, be part of hysterical disorder. When such movements are circumscribed, single, or few in number, and have become stereotyped by repetition, the terms "tic" and "habit spasm" are often synonymously applied. In older children and adults, systematized tics are usually found in the setting of obsessive-compulsive neurosis or of severe obsessive character disorder. It seems that in such cases of persistent tics the original hysterical symptom has become assimilated within the deeper regression of compulsive disorder. Tics frequently involve the head and neck; spasm of some of the facial muscles or rotation of the head are often observed. The latter symptom may present in full flower as "spasmodic torticollis." Frequently, this is a symptom of conversion hysteria as revealed in intensive investigative psychotherapy.

A man, age forty-four, was suffering from severe spasmodic torticollis. The conditions had been present for a year and had gradually worsened. During this time, he had received thorough physical investigation, including radiographic and neurological examinations with negative findings. He presented a pathetic picture. The head and neck would twist to the right about eight times a minute, the neck appeared swollen, and his face wore an anxious pained expression. In conversation, he complained bitterly of the pain and the impossibility of his attending to his work as chief clerk in a large office. A careful history showed the following facts: His illness had begun at a time when he was greatly worried about his son, aged fourteen. The boy had been ill with acute appendicitis and had been removed to hospital. Following appendectomy, his life hung in the balance. The patient frequently telephoned to the hospital to ask about his son's condition, and he persisted in this when the boy was already out of danger and after repeated reassurances of the boy's recovery. It was indeed at this time that the neck movements commenced. He was working at his desk in the office when he found that his head moved to the right so that he could not keep his eyes on his work. It was further elicited that his marriage presented considerable difficulties. At first, in the early days of his marriage, he had enjoyed passionate happiness. Following the birth of this only child, his wife's attitude changed. She had, for example, informed him that they now had something serious to occupy their attention, and that the "nonsense" of their mode of life must now cease. She renounced sexual intercourse, and in consequence he had been sexually abstinent since.

From this short account it will be clear that the patient had been subject to protracted stress, and that the spasmodic torticollis had crystallized in response to further stress.

In such cases, obsessive-compulsive features are usually also prominent, and one is obliged to use in diagnosis the inelegant term "mixed neurosis," or some synonym. Similar considerations apply frequently to "occupational cramp." This is a progressively severe disability due to spasm of the muscles employed in finely co-ordinated movements essential to the fundamental skills of the particular occupation of the patient: "writer's cramp" is but one example. Occupational cramp often yields to psychotherapeutic intervention when the hysterical nature of the symptoms becomes apparent. Sometimes, such cramps also yield in response to favorable shifts in the patient's life situation when the increasingly incapacitating course is dramatically interrupted and reversed.

Sensory Disturbances

Somatic conversion symptoms often include subjective and objective sensory disturbances. Pain is the most common and persistent complaint, occurring anywhere in the head, body, or limbs, and described sometimes in quite horrific terms, though the patient may at the same time evince a complacent attitude. At other times, florid histrionic behavior accompanies the complaint of pain. Severe pain and

hyperesthesia of the scalp may be localized in the temporal or parietal regions and described as a sensation of a nail being driven into the head (clavus). Pain in the back is common, sometimes accompanied by rigidity of the muscles and curvature of the spine, as in bent back (camptocormia); this often follows minor trauma to the spine. Abdominal pains may simulate organic disease, leading to erroneous diagnoses and useless surgical interventions. The symptom of localized hysterical tenderness gave rise to the concept of hysterogenic zones, formerly utilized alternatively to stimulate or terminate a hysterical attack. These tender spots are sometimes found over the breasts, the inguinal regions (ovarian), the head, or the spine. Allochiria, the perception of sensation on the opposite side of the body corresponding to that stimulated, is sometimes elicited.

Diminution of sensation is common, sometimes amounting to more or less complete anesthesia. These anesthesias do not follow typical neural distributions but involve, for example, a limb or part of it (glove and stocking), or may be sharply limited by the midline to one half of the body.

The so-called stigmata sometimes accompany other symptoms of hysteria, and consist mainly of sensory disturbances. Localized reduction of cutaneous sensation, or pharyngeal anesthesia may be discovered. Hyperesthetic spots on the abdominal skin over the ovaries and absence of reflex closure of the eye when the cornea is touched, have often been described. Concentric contraction of the field of vision and the feeling of a lump in the throat (globus hystericus) are other anomalies. Traditionally, these anomalies were held to be characteristic of hysteria and, on this account, were designated stigmata. They came to form the positive grounds for the diagnosis of hysteria. Babinski,[5] however, weakened this base for diagnosis when he showed that they often arose as a result of iatrogenic suggestion (pithiatism). Sometimes, one or more of the stigmata do occur independently of the physician's examination, and accompany other symptoms of hysteria. Ferenczi[38] has shown that the body sites where they occur are peculiarly adapted for the symbolic representation of unconscious fantasies, and it is for this reason that they may occur, or readily arise, on suggestion.

Affective Disturbance

Patients suffering from conversion reaction are often quite complacent in the presence of gross objective disability, presenting a proverbially puzzling paradox which is encountered in the early phase of psychotherapy. Usually, if pain is prominent, much anxious concern is focused upon this, although a complacent attitude about the accompanying disability, or the possibilities of organic disease which the patient often suggests himself, may remain. *La belle indifférence* simulates, sometimes, the flattened affect of some forms and phases of schizophrenia. Janet[62] noted the disposition to "equivalences" in hysteria. When, for example, a somatic conversion symptom was deleted following suggestion, anxiety or depression or, in some cases, confusion appeared in its place, shattering the façade of striking indifference which had formerly accompanied the somatic symptom. Seitz[92] has more recently investigated the conditions of replacement of one symptom by another. Somatic symptoms may be replaced wholly or in part by the expression of anxiety or depression or, in some cases, by feelings of victimization. Symptom formation in hysteria represents the unconscious solution, or attempted solution, of emotional conflict. The symptoms serve more or less as a protection against the perception of anxiety and depression associated with this conflict. When the somatic conversion reaction is incompletely protective, anxiety and/or depression are then also apparent. It is to be noted, too, that anxiety which arises on recession of somatic conversion symptoms, or which accompanies such symptoms, is usually displaced from its source in the conflict and may be displayed in phobic reactions. Freud[47] termed such displaced anxiety, specifically connected with a special situation, anxiety hysteria.

As will be detailed later, the physical disorder in conversion hysteria is sought partly as a protection against dysphoric affects. However, it must be emphasized that the development of these affects is inextricably bound up with the excitement of instinctual strivings, or symbolic derivatives of them, which produce inner mental conflict. In any event, the somatic symptoms are seldom sufficiently persistently protective under all circumstances.

Anxiety may be exhibited as a vague fear of impending disaster or, more specifically, of death, heart failure, or insanity. In such cases, the somatic accompaniments of anxiety, such as dilated pupils, sweating, palpitations, and digital tremor, may be apparent in addition to the conversion symptoms. Other patients exhibit their martyrdom and resignation with a keen sense of the dramatic value of pathos, expressing feelings of sadness and self-pity. Indeed, some patients, in sharper contradistinction to the usual classical indifference, exhibit periodical affect storms. Many of these patients secondarily come to utilize an imperfect and reduced image of these uncontrolled and uncontrollable emotional floodings as a means of controlling others and of impressing them. This latter kind of emotionality was described by Seigman[91] as a hysterical character defense. Later, the term "affectualization," coined by Bibring et al.,[9] was explained as the overemphasis on and the excessive use of the emotional repercussions of unwelcome issues confronting the patient, in order to avoid a rational understanding of them. Valenstein[99] has pointed out that affectualization usually occurs in hysterics who not only have a strong propensity for fantasy life and acting out, but who also are prone to have powerful and relatively primitive affect responses. Volkan[101] recently discussed the significance, the usefulness, and the relationships of abreaction, affectualization, and emotional flooding, especially in treatment sessions with hysterical, borderline, and schizophrenic patients.

Severe and protracted attacks of copious weeping in response to an adverse situation sometimes belong to the category of spuriously exaggerated feelings of sadness, an appeal for help and sympathy, over which, however, the patient may entirely lose control. In one such case, that of continuous, copious weeping by an accountant newly inducted into the army, the momentum of the crying persisted beyond the time of induced favorable change in his situation, namely, his release from the army and return to his usual employment.

(The Nature of the Symptoms of Hysteria, and Freud's Discovery of Psychoanalysis

Psychoanalysis connotes the techniques devised and evolved by Sigmund Freud for investigating the human psyche, and the body of theory that has emerged from the data thus collected. Its beginnings can readily be traced to the working association of Breuer and Freud at the close of the nineteenth century, when together they worked out a method of treating hysterical phenomena. It was found that if instead of being hypnotized and receiving direct suggestions of cure the patient was simply encouraged to talk while under hypnosis, hysterical symptoms were often more effectively relieved. It was found, too, that this talking out under hypnosis was laden with emotional charge, whereas the same patient would be lacking in affective expression under waking conditions. More than this, it was discovered that important events connected with the emotional life of the patient which were otherwise forgotten, were recalled and expressed under hypnosis. This method of talking out of emotionally charged and otherwise forgotten events was called "mental catharsis," as it operated to eliminate from the psychic system sources of disturbance that would, without this, result in symptoms. The process of affording an outlet for emotion in talking was called "abreaction."

The fact that a patient suffering from hysteria was unable in the waking state to recall significant and emotionally charged events that would, with encouragement, appear under hypnosis, gave rise to the psychoanalytic concept of resistance which opposed such recall, and which was lessened by the hypnotic procedure. The fact that the patient came to develop an intense emotional relationship to

the physician was one component of the concept of transference. Freud found that this development in the patient-physician relationship was due to the transfer of emotion from earlier objects of the patients's feelings to the personality of the physician. Later, Freud used the technique of "free association" to replace hypnosis as a method of lessening, or attempting to lessen, resistance, and thus psychoanalysis emerged. Although, in general, the method of free association accomplishes less than hypnosis in the factual recall of early events and experiences even when the resistances are unveiled, emotional revival is, in the long run, facilitated. The emotional revival involved in transference became the prime means of success in Freud's later psychoanalytic work. The technique of psychoanalysis has encompassed ways and means of developing and utilizing transference, of effecting its dissolution by interpretation, and of unveiling resistances in the process of resolving emotional difficulties out of the range of the patient's awareness. This technique has emerged from the mental catharsis method of treating patients suffering from hysteria.

In the foregoing brief genetic account of the formulation of the concepts of resistance and transference apprehended from clinical work with patients suffering from hysteria, it will be noticed that these same findings have additional implications. Thus, the fact that certain events of the past were recalled under hypnosis, or as a result of analytical work, indicates that such events were somehow and somewhere recorded and stored within the psyche, though not immediately available to consciousness. Access to consciousness was at first barred by resistance. Such exclusion from consciousness as a result of the operation of an inner resistance is known as repression and is an important manifestation of resistance.

With Freud's theory of dreams,[43] psychoanalysis was enlarged from a psychotherapeutic method to a psychology of the depth of human nature. Freud showed that dreams were meaningful, that each one represented the disguised expression of an attempted wish fulfillment. He contrasted the manifest content, that is, the dream as related directly, with the latent dream thoughts reached by the techniques he devised to deal with resistance. In the young child, the manifest and latent content may be identical, the dream plainly representing the imaginary fulfillment of an ungratified wish. Usually, in adults, the wish is a repressed one, disguised in the manifest dream because of resistance. Freud showed that human life was dominated by conflict between conscious appraisal of reality plus ethical values (including the unconscious conscience), and the repressed unconscious. In sleep—a temporary withdrawal from the external world—the energy of repression-resistance is diminished, so that the unconscious forces obtain some degree of hallucinatory satisfaction. This is "safer" during sleep, since the avenues to motor expression are then blocked; in any case, some degree of repression-resistance persists, so that even in hallucination the latent thoughts are disguised. In this way, disturbance emanating from ungratified unconscious conative processes is drained off, and sleep is safeguarded. Of course, this function of the dream sometimes fails; the disguise is not sufficiently heavy, and the watcher awakes in anxiety. On the other hand, when the disguises have worn too thin, there can be the comforting thought, in sleep, "After all, this is only a dream." Thus, sleep is permitted to continue despite the threat of revelation.

The following is a clinical example to illustrate some of the foregoing points and their connection with the psychopathology of hysteria:

A middle-aged male patient was brought to psychiatric interview on account of total paralysis of his legs. Seated in a wheel chair, he explained calmly that two weeks previously he had awakened in the morning to find himself paralyzed. In view of the prevalence of an epidemic of poliomyelitis, he assumed that he had the disease and summoned his physician. He now understood that the diagnosis was in considerable doubt, and that, following intensive organic investigation, no definite organic basis was discoverable. The patient expressed this situation in his own way, and at the same time expressed his doubt concerning the opinion of the physicians. During the further course of interview, the patient explained that he had had considerable difficulty in getting to sleep since his wife had left him three months previously. He also expressed the view that he did not care very much about this, and spoke with bitterness about the faithlessness of women. The events of the day before the paralysis were recounted as having been routine, but a dream had occurred during the night. In this dream, the patient went away from his house and found himself struggling with two people in a strange neighborhood; shots were fired, he had a gun in his hands, and then he woke up in anxiety to find himself paralyzed.

During the course of treatment, this dream was further investigated and was found to represent his wish to pursue his wife and wreak revenge upon her and her lover. Consciously, he was very much against any such course of action. It was, indeed, found that his paralysis was a massive defense against any possibility of his moving to kill his wife and her lover, and the massive nature of the defense was partly a measure of the intensity of his vengeful wishes. The "strange" neighborhood turned out, in fact, to be the old familiar neighborhood of his childhood at a time when the patient thought himself to be an unwanted child, because his father had been released from the army and his mother had given over all her attention to the father.

This fragmentary account illustrates that a forceful repressed wish found hallucinatory satisfaction in his dream, and that, the disguise being too thin, he awakened in anxiety. His inability to get to sleep showed his need for inner vigilance to ward off these dangerous wishes, which were being repressed with increasing difficulty. Later, the repression partially failing, it needed to be supplemented in the waking state by the conversion reaction of paralysis. There was much self-punishment in this paralysis, too, as became apparent from the patient's associations in the process of psychotherapy. It is noticeable here that the dream is the first member of a series that includes among its members the hysterical symptom, the obsession, and the delusion. As Freud states,[43] it is differentiated from the others by its transitory nature and by the fact that it occurs under conditions that are part of normal life. In this pathological case, the connecting link with a hysterical conversion symptom is clear.

It is also clear in this case that the dream was related not only to current events in the life of the patient but also to childhood experience. The patient in his childhood had found his passionate wish for exclusive possession of his mother's love threatened by the return of his father from a lengthy absence in the army, and this threat turned out to be well grounded in reality. In later years, this experience led to his very reserved attitude toward women, and it was only in middle life that he had found his way to marriage with a much younger woman who later deserted him for a younger man. This had revived all the emotions constellated around his childhood oedipal-phase experiences, the murderous wishes being transferred from his "faithless" mother and his father to his wife and her lover. Sleep became difficult, because he was afraid to relax lest these ego-alien wishes should succeed in breaking through from repression. In the dream, the disguise was not sufficiently heavy to safeguard his sleep adequately, and he woke in anxiety. The succeeding hysterical symptom was a compromise formation compounded of the repressed wishes and the repressive forces, including those of unconscious conscience. In this case, some of the repressed wishes are more obvious in the dream, are the defense against them and the self-punishment in the symptom of conversion paralysis. It is also to be noted, in this particular case, that the symptoms of paralysis defend against the expression of hostile wishes which result from the frustration contingent upon the disruption of the patient's marital life. In many cases, the symptom has a more clearly evident sexual-symbolic reference. In this case, too, however, the paralysis symbolically represents castration—loss of the power to satisfy genital-sexual needs through their unconscious acquisition of a forbidden charac-ter by association with earlier incestuous wishes.

(Psychopathology of Hysteria

Following consideration of the dream of the patient with conversion paralysis, we are in a position to take more fully into account the previously described case of spasmodic torti-collis. In this case, on account of the neurotic attitude of his wife following the birth of their only child, the patient was confronted with sexual abstinence unless he ventured into extramarital digression or divorce. Analysis revealed that he submitted to sexual abstinence in these restrictive circumstances because of an awakening of a deep-seated sense of guilt in relation to genital sensual enjoyment, a sense of guilt founded upon a grossly inadequate resolution of the Oedipus complex. In brief, his wife, by becoming a mother and proclaiming a sexual taboo, combined to activate this unconscious complex and to re-establish inappropriately the old prohibition of sensuality, namely, the exclusion of genitality, which had been achieved with difficulty in his relationship with a possessive and controlling mother in childhood.

The normal wish for sexual intercourse with his wife was repressed only with the greatest difficulty, and the patient required another defense mechanism to support this repression. For years, since the adoption of sexual abstinence, he had suffered from difficulty in going to sleep. When lying in bed with his wife, he would concern himself in largely unproductive preoccupation with office problems. As he said, he had kept his mind very closely on his work. This was obviously a heroic effort to continue to exclude from consciousness, to crowd out, any ideational representation of genital sexual craving, an effort which indicates that the repression was only tenuously held in operation over the fourteen years that preceded the outbreak of his painful torticol-lis. The symptom was due to a partial break-down in his repressive resistances, brought about, as we have seen, by the illness of his son. Analysis further revealed that he had unconsciously come to resent the intruder who had upset his affectionate and sexually gratifying relationship with his wife, much as he had resented his father. Indeed, unconsciously, he had wished his own son out of the way. This wish, too, remained excluded from consciousness, and this exclusion was supported by another defense, namely reaction formation. He had always consciously felt and expressed excessive anxiety about the health and welfare of his son.

The severe illness of his son resulted in erosion of the repressive barriers, because the unconsciously charged sadistic wish to get rid of him came near to realization. In fact, he became very anxious, redoubled his efforts to care for his son, whom, it must be added, he also basically loved and identified with. He made a nuisance of himself with the hospital personnel, and continued to question the surgeon even when the son was out of danger.

Closer investigation came to reveal that the torticollis was a disguised expression of his repressed phallic sadistic impulses, and that the repressive resistances had been sufficiently overcome by the increased charge of these impulses, resulting from a complex reaction to his son's appendectomy, to permit this expression. The movements of his neck were of an autoerotic nature, that is to say, he had pleasurable sensations on account of them. The neck had come to represent the erected genital organ, was a symbol for it. Vasomotor disturbances resulted in swelling, and the rhythmic movements aped those in coitus, an upward displacement anatomically. The symptom represented more than this, for it also condensed elements derived from his sense of guilt and need for punishment. He also suffered considerable pain. In short, he was punishing himself also, and the fury of this punishment had the quality of his repressed hostility toward his son. He was turning his hostility against himself. Thus, the symptom was a compromise formation between the two vectors of his unconscious conflict. More than this, it had an attention-attracting function. It was a dramatic expression also of his wish for sympa-

thetic acceptance of his appalling psychological situation, a wish at first directed especially toward his wife. A complex state of affairs is indeed covered by a hysterical flight into illness, and uncovered during analytic types of psychotherapy. The symptoms of hysteria should be treated with respect, for they represent a deep disturbance in the psychic life of the suffering patient. It is remarkable with what contempt these symptoms may be treated by some physicians because they cannot find any anchorage for them in organic nosology.

When traced to its roots, hysteria in all its forms is predominantly related to the climax of infantile sexuality, the Oedipus situation, with the struggle to surmount incestuous genital-sexual and hostile strivings. Some conversion symptoms represent a materialization of unconscious fantasies concerned with forbidden genital-sexual wishes. Genitalization may consist in tissue changes, including hyperemia and swelling, representing erection, or of muscle spasms, representing the movements of coitus, or of sensations resembling genital sensations, although these are often complicated by the perception of pain. On the other hand, as in the cases described above, the symptoms may also represent the reactive hostility to frustration of genital-sexual wishes, and in such cases anal-sadistic fantasies may find expression. Sometimes, pregenital expression of predominantly genital wishes may also occur; bed-wetting, a frequent masturbation equivalent in children, is a common example of this. Often interpolated between the original oedipal experiences and fantasies, and the symptoms of the adult, are daydreams connected with masturbatory activities.

The symptoms consist of an autoplastic attempt to discharge the tension created by intrapsychic conflict, and express drive and defense simultaneously, short-circuiting conscious perception of conflict related basically to the Oedipus complex. This last statement covers the primary or paranosic gain. Secondary or epinosic gain is involved in the alloplastic ego endeavor to utilize the symptoms for manipulating other people and the current life situation. Often the attention-attracting function is conspicuous: By physical symbolic exhibition of conflict, the patient indirectly attracts sympathy for his plight. The flight into illness may provide escape from an intolerable job or family situation, or from military service. In other words, some gain might sometimes be related to a precipitating factor. In the latter event, a passive mastery might ensue, with later recession of the symptoms. Following injury, hysterical perpetuation or exaggeration of symptoms may have a conspicuous secondary gain factor motivated by the wish for compensation. In some cases, the secondary gain persists only as long as the symptoms persist, and in such a situation the disease may become chronic and present an additional important resistance in treatment.

(Further Considerations

Orality and Hysteria

As indicated earlier, in the study and treatment of hysterical phenomena Freud invented the method of psychoanalysis and its basic concepts. The concepts of fixation and regression also grew out of these early studies, and there arose a formulation that the personality of those liable to exhibit hysterical symptoms when frustrated was fixated at the phallic or early genital phase. In the onset of neurosis, regression to this point of fixation, with its infantile object relationships and its attendant castration anxiety, took place. The anxiety had motivated repression which, however, later failed to be effective, and symptom formation ensued.

Marmor[75] has emphasized that, in many cases of hysteria, fixations in the oedipal phase of development are themselves the outgrowth of pre-oedipal fixations, chiefly of an oral nature.

The kind of parent whose behavior keeps a child at an "oral" level is apt to be the kind of parent whose behavior favors the development of a strong Oedipus complex. The pre-oedipal history of most of the hysterias I have seen has revealed one of two things—either intense frustration of their oral-receptive needs as a consequence of early defection or rejection by one or both parent figures, or excessive gratification of these needs by one or both parent figures.

Fitzgerald[39] emphasized early "love deprivation" and consequent "love craving" as a basic character trait of the hysterical personality. Similarly, Halleck,[56] in discussing the personality traits of adult female hysterics, brings into special prominence, from his clinical experience, the view that the hysterical patient has usually suffered severe maternal deprivation. Accordingly, she never develops an adequate basic trustfulness, and is incapacitated in her search for intimacy. Seeking the satisfaction of basic oral needs from her father and later from other males, she has learned to use seductiveness and helplessness to control men. Halleck stresses the hysterical woman's search for the answers to life in the strength of an ideal man. However, she uses her femininity as a weapon to control the man she finds, destroying the possibility of finding the strength she seeks. Her troubles are aggravated when men disappoint or reject her. Complaining of physical symptoms, she may then visit a physician.

The concept of multiple points of fixation, and, in particular, in hysteria, of the importance of oral fixation, explains psychodynamically the clinical associations noted in many cases between hysteria and schizophrenia, hysteria and depressive disorder, and hysteria and addiction, especially alcoholism. There is often a narrow margin between hysterical introversion or dissociative reactions and schizophrenic autism, or between hysterical materialization and schizophrenic hallucination; under certain circumstances, as already noted, the transition from classical conversion hysteria to florid schizophrenic psychosis takes place. Where the oral fixation factor is of greater importance, the ego-integrative capacity is weaker, and psychotic regression occurs more easily.

It is to be noted, too, in the opinion of this writer, that the importance of secondary gain factors in the psychoeconomy of the patient is often underestimated because of inadequate realization of the quantitative loading of pregenital fixation. For attention-attracting and sympathy-gaining, the compensation-managing and the acquisition of dominance are related, in the complex stratification of psychic life, to the frustrated oral dependency and anal-manipulative needs for, respectively, narcissistic supplies and mastery.

Language and Hysteria

We have noted above that in conversion reactions the symptomatic changes in physical function unconsciously give distorted expression to the instinctual strivings that had previously been more fully repressed. At the same time, the symptoms indirectly represent the defensive force in conflict with the derivatives of instinctual impulses, and the retribution or punishment for forbidden wishes. Freud found that the symptoms are substitutes for ideational representation of these strivings and of the forces opposing them, and that, accordingly, the symptoms could be gradually translated into word language from their "body language," with accompanying affective expressions. Sometimes this translation is partly but a retranslation into the patient's own actual words, comprising a thought formation, during the incubation period of symptom formation. The following example illustrates:

Mrs. X, a thirty-five-year-old white, married, and physically very attractive woman was admitted to the medical wards of a large university hospital, referred by her family physician for repeated fainting attacks and complaints of severe pain in the neck. At the time this patient was first interviewed by a psychiatrist, she was in bed, constrained by an ingenious traction apparatus which pulled on her neck muscles. There was considerable spasm of these muscles, although exhaustive physical examinations had failed to reveal any basic organic pathology. The patient complained that despite the apparatus and the various medications, she still had a severe pain in the neck. She proceeded to say that before admission to the hospital, in addition to this neck pain which had progressively worsened, she had had alarming "blackouts." She was asked what she meant by a "blackout," and the patient, looking puzzled by the psychiatrist's apparent ignorance of the vernacular, explained about her faints. It was indicated that this was understood, but attention was directed to the phrase "blackout," and inquiry was made as to whether she herself had thought of using this expression. It seemed the patient was not at all sure as to the first application of this term to her faints, whether by her husband, herself, or one of the doctors. She was then asked whether when she was "out" in the faint, did she see black? Hesitating a moment, the patient stated thoughtfully, "No, in fact, I pass out and see red." In further conversation, she gave a restrained account of her widowed mother-in-law who was living in her home. The patient's husband was this woman's only offspring, and there ensued a talk about the close attachment of this woman to her only son, the patient's husband, and the possible difficulties this might have led to. The conversation became increasingly animated, and at one point the patient was told that despite her conciliatory and laudably understanding attitude towards her mother-in-law, in fact this lady had begun to give her a pain in the neck, and the first occasions when she had seen her mother-in-law breakfasting alone with her husband had made her see red.

As the emergency psychotherapy progressed in later interviews, more adequate affective expression of her rage against and jealousy of her mother-in-law became clearly evident, as well as expressions of guilt feelings. These strong feelings were the affect indicators of strong and conflicting conative trends, which had roots, it was later revealed in analytic psychotherapy, in her early family drama with a tyrannical mother who excluded her even from expectable communication with her father as she was growing up.

It became evident that her wish for her mother-in-law to live elsewhere, if she was to live at all, came into conflict with her sense of duty. Once there were beginnings of translation of her symptoms into affect-laden metaphoric language, she protested that she ought to be able to get along with her mother-in-law, whom she respected, though the presence of this lady disturbed her feelings of well-being. She soon acknowledged that she herself had thought what a pain in the neck the good woman was, and that sometimes she had made her see red. Thus, this translation of her symptoms into word language was but a re-translation back to the unspoken language of her own thoughts, thoughts that had later become forbidden. Later, this conflict was found to have many ramifications, including the fact that it was but a re-edition of an older unresolved conflict with her own mother.

As discussed elsewhere,[2] the acquisition of discursive language, with its power of generality and abstraction, is the result of a complicated series of developments. From primitive naming, that is, basic phonetic-symbolic representation, there is a semantic movement through metaphor and the fading of metaphor. We are not concerned here with these complicated developments; we are concerned with the sort of metaphoric symbolism that functions largely to convey feelings. Its adequacy depends on how well it performs this function. Often, in the preliminary retranslation of hysterical somatic symptoms to word language, it performs this function vividly and only less dramatically than the symptoms themselves. The essential messages in a conversion reaction are embodied cryptically in the somatic symptoms, which do not involve primarily any words at all, and only relatively infrequently the laryngeal apparatus. Word language is reduced and compressed in inaudible symbols of a more primitive character, in such a way that the subject is unaware of their essential meaning, and his reference group is very likely misled. We have, of course, the concepts of repression and of the unconscious (of the repressed unconscious), as well as of regression, to aid us in our quest for understanding. The disorder of expression and of communication, internal and external, is indeed a function of pathological disturbance in repression and regression, as we have learned from Freud. Besides the messages readily translatable to a verbal metaphoric symbolic level, other messages are couched in a more primitive (cryptophoric) symbolism, as when the neck indirectly represents another part of the body, the erect genital—as noted in the case of spasmodic torticollis.

The somatic symptoms of conversion hysteria condense a variety of levels of meaning and a variety of messages, the emphasis differing in various symptomatic expressions. The following example will illuminate this statement:

A middle-aged Negro woman whose life had become one of increasing hardship, economically, socially, and sexually, developed a clouded (hypnoid) mental state associated with peculiar movements of the arms and fingers. She was referred for neurological investigation for the possible determination of brain tumor or a presenile organic dementia. This investigation, which was quite thorough and included air-encephalography, yielded no positive pathological findings. The resident conducted a conversation with her while she was in amytal narcosis, at which time she discussed in a vague and disconnected way her father's encouragement of her education and her once-upon-a-time interest in the piano. At first sight of this lady, the psychiatrist said to the resident who had reported the ramblings of the patient in amytal narcosis, "But she is now playing the piano." In the ensuing short interview, the patient, with initial direction, went into considerable and vivid detail about her father's looking at her admiringly as she was playing the piano, and about how proud he was of her at this time during her school years—all described by the patient in the present tense.

In brief, in response to adverse life circumstances, this patient had retreated to a time of maximal happiness in her life, a time effectively symbolized by her piano playing with an encouraging, admiring, affectionate father at her side, with whom she confused the psychiatrist. Clinically, this case was a hysteriform borderline state, the conspicuous features being a hysterical pseudodementia, and apparently weird movements of the arms and fingers. These movements were in fact pantomimic in their essential nature. In discussing hysterical symptomatic attacks in 1909, Freud[46] wrote:

When one psychoanalyses a patient subject to hysterical attacks one soon gains the conviction that these attacks are nothing but phantasies projected and translated into motor activity and represented in pantomime.

It sometimes happens, too, that there is a revival in memory of actual events, rich in associated fantasy and feeling, a revival which in a truncated way is pantomimically expressed in body movements, as in the piano playing of the patient in the severe dissociative reaction just described.

In summary, clinical experience indicates six interrelated aspects of movement and of sensory phenomena in conversion reactions:

1. Sexual symbolic references.
2. Distorted affect expressions—e.g., of appeal, rage, resentment, weeping, joy, etc.
3. Condensation of identifications (see below).
4. Associated connotations relating to wish-fulfilling and punitive fantasies.
5. Denotative propositional pantomimic movements—often truncated, or with reversals in sequence, or other disguises.
6. Metaphoric embodiments.

Identification in Hysteria

It is a notorious fact that hysteria is a great imitator and may thus set an awkward trap for the unwary medical diagnostician. The sensations or movements constituting the conversion symptoms may relate to observations of others made by the patient. For example, Freud's patient Dora[45] developed a cough which was found to be traceable to her observations of Mrs. K's coughing attacks. She unconsciously wished to put herself in Mrs. K's position as the wife of Mr. K, but felt guilty about her rivalry. She selected Mrs. K's affliction as the point of identification, thus caricaturing her envy in the service of self-punishment. Oedipal wishes may, however, result also in an identification with the signifi-

cant person of the opposite sex. When the forbidden and desired object must be relinquished, a partial identification with the object may ensue. Multiple identifications often occur. Freud deciphered the movements of one patient as an attempt to take her clothes off with one hand, while trying to keep them on with the other. While identifying with a woman being sexually assaulted, she identified partly, too, with the male sexual aggressor. Bonnard,[11] similarly, has interpreted the peculiar gestures of some disturbed children as partial identifications with both an aggressor and a victim. These children had been exposed repeatedly to the severe quarreling, including physical combat, of their respective parents.

Multiple identifications may assume dimensions of partial personality systems in more severe dissociative reactions, as described previously.

Pathological identification with the physical infirmity of another person frequently occurs in group situations. Freud cited a hysterical epidemic in a girls' school as an example. One girl who received a love letter fainted, whereupon other girls soon fainted, too. In this instance, the purpose of the symptom identification was vested in the other girls' wishes for the same experience; they thus dramatized forbidden wishes, and accepted punishment as well. Indeed, in such group situations, anyone who offers some libido-economic advantage as a prototype, at a time of heightened inner conflict and tension, may be thus imitated. More recently, Moss and McEvedy[79] described an epidemic of over-breathing among schoolgirls in Britain. Approximately a third of a total of 550 girls were affected, and about a third of these required inpatient care. It became apparent that the epidemic was hysterical. A previous polio epidemic had rendered the schoolgirls emotionally vulnerable, and a three-hour parade, producing twenty faints on the day before the outbreak, had been the precipitating cause. McEvedy et al.[77] contrasted two other school epidemics, one of vomiting, the other of abdominal pain. One (hysterical) occurred in a school for girls; it was manifest almost exclusively in school hours, its maximum incidence showed a swing from older to younger classes, and it correlated with conduct disorders. The other epidemic did not show accord with any of the circumstances noted, and was found to be due to infection with *Shigella sonnei*.

The important role of identification in the sociology of the body image is discussed by Schilder,[90] who emphasized that the image of the body is not static but in constant flux, changing according to reactions to circumstances. There is a continuous process, underlying the evident changes of experience—a process of construction, dissolution, and reconstruction of the body image. Unconscious processes of identification, and of projection, are of considerable importance in bringing about such changes. In hysteria, the mechanism of identification expresses the close relation of the patient to different postural models of different persons. Innumerable condensations of object relations may be expressed in a hysterical change in one organ of the body. Schilder draws attention, too, to Freud's patient Dora. Her coughing attacks, it seems evident, also expressed genital wishes to be infected and to take the place of her mother, who had vaginal catarrh.

Fenichel[37] states that identification is the very first type of reaction to an object. All later object relationships may, under certain circumstances, regress to identification. The hysterical identification is characterized by the fact that it does not involve the full amount of cathexis available. Jacobson[59] and, earlier, Foulkes,[51] attempted to show the relation between less (hysterical) and more regressive forms of identification. In the opinion of this writer, it is often by study of the types of identifications the patient has made, and of the correlative fate of the object relationships involved, that it is possible to obtain a better notion of how far from psychosis a particular case of hysteriform disorder may be. Identifications may, however, elude understanding, especially in short-contact work with a patient, or when psychotherapy is of a "repressive-inspirational" type, utilizing, perhaps unwittingly, further primitive forms of identification in the suppression of symptoms.

Group Hysteria

The suggestibility of individuals is basically of varying degree; that is to say, there are marked individual differences. Moreover, in regard to a particular individual, his suggestibility varies considerably both with factors that are internal and physiologically based (e.g., fatigue, degrees of mental alertness related to circadian rhythms), and with external factors that notably include the behavior of people in his immediate environment. The strongest suggestibility is often a feature of the hysterical personality. So much has this feature impressed clinicians that in the early part of the century, one of the foremost accepted theories of hysteria, that formulated by Babinski,[5] defined it along this parameter alone. Hysteria was held to be basically a mental disposition to be affected by the suggestive force of imagination, and hysterical symptoms to be the result of suggestion. Moreover, pithiatism, that is, forced suggestion, was the method prescribed by Babinski for the removal of hysterical symptoms, the idea being to fight fire with fire. It happens, however, that some hysterics are under many circumstances especially resistant to suggestion. As will be detailed later, there are variations in the compendium of manifest traits that characterizes the hysterical personality.

High suggestibility is very largely the result of uncontrolled processes of unconscious identification and is associated with a fragile ego fundament; sometimes a hyperexic defense against vulnerability to suggestion includes an emotional detachment. Even in the latter eventuality, however, the impact of events in a group may rupture such a massive defense.

In the formation and maintenance of groups, primitive processes of unconscious identification may become very active and may escalate beyond the control of many people. Moebius' dictum that everyone is a little hysterical is frequently illustrated by behavior in groups. We can but briefly consider here simple crowds and highly organized groups, but there are, of course, many varieties of grouping of human beings. The character of both simple crowds and more permanent organized groups also varies considerably. Often, the individual in becoming one of a crowd loses in some degree his self-consciousness and he may even become depersonalized. Enveloped and overshadowed and carried away by forces he is powerless to control, he may fail to exercise self-criticism, self-restraint, and more refined ideals of behavior. It is often the case, too, in simple crowds that the order of reasoning employed is that of the lowest common denominator, and this facilitates suggestibility. A further ground of heightened suggestibility in a crowd is the prevalence of emotional excitement. The kinds of regression in the collective ego adumbrated above are, of course, contingent upon many factors, including the type of leadership. In the highly organized group, with its greater control of impulses and with a continuity of direction of activity, with a differentiation and specialization of the functions of its constituents, emotional excitement may yet be periodically evoked, with accompanying hysterical excrescences. The hysterical phenomena are then apt to occur in a setting of group paranoid formations, which serve to enhance group narcissism and to direct hostility outwards. We are, of course, here considering only the pathological aspects of group functioning, often associated with pathological, especially hysterical and paranoid, leadership, and frequently with the occurrence of hysterical phenomena.

Hypnoid alterations of consciousness occur transiently in group religious excitement. Although these dissociative reactions are for the most part temporary, sometimes they issue in a persistent conversion reaction or in psychotic disturbance. Thus, for example, following each periodic visit to Raleigh, North Carolina, of a world-famous revivalist, several casualties of the mass meeting are admitted to the Dorothea Dix Mental Hospital. Another North Carolina example, glossolalia, the "speaking in tongues," which occurs in a state of happy excitement, may persist beyond its due time with a particular religious group and its evangelical leader.[1] It requires note, too, that sometimes a conversion reaction abates fol-

lowing a hypnoid state induced through group religious excitement. Thousands of sick come to pray at the feet of Our Lady of Lourdes. Some, after participating in the procession of the Holy Sacrament, others after worshiping at the famous grotto, find their prayers answered.

In the ceremonial rites of religious groups as, for example, in the Voodoo cult in Haiti, the trance state is a sanctioned means of release and communication within the group. Only when the activities generated during the hypnoid state persist beyond, originate outside, or exceed the ritual, do they communicate anything abnormal, or sickness, to other members of the group. In particular, the phenomenon of possession usually occurs within the context of ritual exhibition, as the dances and roles become increasingly frenetic; often, the priest himself enacts the spirit-role, sometimes another member of the group does so. However, this socially sanctioned mode of behavior is occasionally made use of in an individual attempt to express and reduce mental conflict. Such cases have been reported in many parts of India where an individual so "possessed" may be designated as a patient and brought to a psychiatric clinic.[97] The phenomenon was encountered mostly in young women of low socioeconomic and educational class. Such symptoms of possession, of governance by a strange soul, occurred alone in hysterical instances, and the abnormal behavior was readily understandable as a response to a frustrational life situation. In other instances, the symptoms of possession formed only a minor part of the total clinical picture of schizophrenia or of mania. The authors of the Indian study separate "hysterical psychosis" from the major psychoses.

Hysterical possession symptoms are sometimes a feature of many culture-bound syndromes. Besides Voodoo, the Piblokot of Eskimos and Whitiko of Ojibwas may be cited; in the latter, a morbid craving for human flesh is accompanied by a conviction of transformation into a supernatural being.

Extremist political meetings and avant-garde encounter group therapy sessions also precipitate their quantum of hysterical acting and behaviors and of later conversion and dissociative reactions. We have already noted the occasional occurrence of an epidemic of hysteria in girls' schools.

Hysteria in Childhood

Abstracting data from the charts of all inpatients treated and discharged with a diagnosis of conversion reaction in the North Carolina Memorial Hospital at Chapel Hill between September 1952 and September 1958, Somers,[93] working with me, noted that there were 612 such recorded conversion reactions. The majority of these patients had been on the medical service and a high percentage of these had been diagnosed and treated with psychiatric consultation. The next group in size had been on the psychiatric service itself, with the pediatric, obstetric, and surgical services contributing smaller groups of patients with this diagnosis on their charts. The ages of these patients ranged from seven to seventy-two. There were 22 patients under sixteen years of age, that is 4 percent of the total number. Proctor,[84] during this same period, reviewed 191 unselected, consecutively diagnosed cases in the child psychiatric outpatient unit of the Department of Psychiatry, and 25 cases of frank conversion and/or dissociative reactions were recorded, an incidence of 13 percent. These findings of Somers and of Proctor indicate that the observations of some others,[32] that hysteriform conditions in childhood are uncommon, must be modified, at least in terms of the area in which the observations are made.

In the study of Proctor, only the frank conversion and dissociative reactions were counted and studied, inasmuch as these were phenomenologically consonant with the descriptions of hysteria of Charcot, Babinski, Janet, and Kretschmer; in that of Somers, the diagnostic criteria generally applied were those incorporated in the definition of conversion reaction in Strecker's *Fundamentals of Psychiatry,** this also being descriptively and

* E. A. Strecker, *Fundamentals of Psychiatry*, 6th edition, M. M. Pearson, ed. Philadelphia: Lippincott, 1963.

dynamically, so far as it goes, similar to those offered by the earlier investigators mentioned in connection with the Proctor study.

LaBarre[71] has pointed out that ethnographic and psychiatric records reveal that *Tobacco Road* is no artistic caricature but a faithful portrait of some regions of the South. He writes of the intricate interplay, including the discrepancies, between the rigidly compulsive cultural background of the Bible Belt and the individual's actual adaptation. The picayune fanaticism of some of the rural folk operates within the context of a fundamentalist rural religion which frowns on smoking, drinking, and sex, although these are all in fact heavily indulged in. In the mountains of North Carolina, as in other Appalachian areas, there is widespread belief in hex doctors and in faith healing. Side by side with widespread overt belief in magic and punitively repressive antisexual attitudes are the further factors of early stimulation of the child by discussion of original sin and by disapproval of the body, both of which at the same time hint at, and emphasize, the temptations and the desirability, of gross sensual pleasures. Such inconsistencies are often acted out. Thus, the familial style of life, including the sleeping arrangements associated with the poor housing, results in the frequent early observation by the children of sexual scenes between the adults. In addition to repeated exposures to the "primal scene," which is in any case associated with heightened difficulty in surmounting the oedipus complex and with later vulnerability to frustration, so that major hysterical attacks readily occur in adult life, sons sometimes sleep with their mothers and daughters with their fathers throughout a large part of childhood. This involves enormous stimulation with concomitant denial of verbal expression, so that regression to primitive modes of somatic discharge readily occurs in childhood itself.

Winnicott[102] showed the close relationship of convulsive phenomena in the first year of life to frustrated orality. He demonstrated with case material that infantile convulsions can at times be precipitated and perpetuated by an adverse mother-child relationship, especially when associated with clumsy and abrupt attempts at weaning. As early as 1882, Gillette[53] carefully documented a functional paralysis of an arm in an eighteen-month-old child, and there is a similar case report by Anna Freud[41] of a twenty-seven-month-old child. Proctor[84] comments that a primitive discharge mechanism in the somatic sphere in the earliest infantile period (under a year), although descriptively similar to convulsive hysteria, is not structurally and dynamically the same, since at this time there is less distinction between id and ego and between the mental and bodily ego. Moreover there is no word representation to be repressed as a prelude to somatic regression and disguised expression.

Somatic dissociation in the slightly older child, such as the cases reported by Gillette or Anna Freud, raises many questions regarding faulty ego development, especially relating to the adequate construction of the boundaries of the image of the body, the core of the mental ego, which may be disturbed in the continuous interaction between the child and the mother. Indeed, Schilder[89] emphasized that hysterical phenomena in all children show with marked clarity the continuous interaction of the attitudes of the particular child with his parents. However, it would seem that a hysterical psychoneurosis does not properly form before latency with the consolidation of the superego following the Oedipus conflicts.

Kaufman[66] gives an especially vivid account of conversion hysteria in the latency period in psychoanalytic treatment. At the age of eight and a half years, a patient, a girl, was referred for psychoanalysis because of hysterical blindness. The mother described the events preceding the referral: Catherine had been caught by two old ladies investigating a six-year-old boy to see if he was built the same way as her baby brother. In brief, the patient was caught peeping and made to feel guilty about forbidden activity shortly before the onset of blindness. During the course of her two years of analysis, she elaborated and worked upon the classical dynamic features of a conversion hysteria. She had an unresolved wish for the penis from her father expressed symbolically in terms of a gift from Santa

Claus. She portrayed herself as damaged and castrated. In her transference reaction, she wanted to take the analyst's finger from him, expressing her desire to be a boy. Later, she was able to elaborate a feminine identification and convey her wish for a baby. Additional material illustrated her blocked hostility against her mother and her fear of retaliation. The unconscious oedipal complex had been activated and then repressed following the trauma, and had become associated with being caught and punished for her sexual curiosity about the differences between boys and girls.

In summary, it is to be noted that primitive identification, dissociation, and discharge phenomena may occur in early childhood and resemble hysterical phenomena of later life. However, these phenomena occur in response to separation anxiety in the relatively undifferentiated psyche in a diadic context; in the differentiated psyche of later childhood, formed defenses of repression, displacement, and conversion (with cryptophoric bodily and metaphoric bodily symbolization in a regression from word symbolism) are deployed in response to castration anxiety in a triadic context. There are many cases in later childhood in which both oral and phallic-oedipal aspects of psychopathology are evident. In the repetitive promiscuous patterns of many adolescent girls, the sexual acting out is less an expression of a genital need than an oral acquisitive process associated with the wish to receive care and attention from a mothering figure.

Incidence and Prevalence of Hysteria

Hollingshead and Redlich,[58] in their study of the relationship of social class to the prevalence of mental disorder, found more psychotics and fewer neurotics in the lower classes of this country than in the upper classes. Srole and his co-workers[94] found a similar difference in the prevalence of neurosis and psychosis in the lower and upper socioeconomic classes. However, according to Hollingshead and Redlich, hysterical reactions, unlike the other neurotic disorders, show an inverse relationship with class position. Although cases occur in all socioeconomic classes of the population, they are more frequently found in the lower classes, predominantly in classes IV and V in their designations, which are based on areas of residence, occupations, and levels of educational achievement.

There has been considerable discussion concerning the incidence of classic hysteria in Western society. Chodoff[23] has maintained that an actual diminution in the incidence of conversion hysteria has occurred, because of changes in the cultural climate, including a wider dissemination of education and a less authoritarian social structure. However, Stephens and Kamp[96] show that the admission rates for hysteria at the Henry Phipps Psychiatric Clinic during the periods 1913–20 and 1945–60 are not appreciably different. It may be that though dramatic conversion reactions are less frequent than formerly in the upper classes, hysterical character disorder, with identity diffusion and borderline qualities, is more common than earlier in the twentieth century. Anyway, the bulk of the disorders of a hysterical nature is not seen by psychiatrists. This segment of the population, perhaps at least 10 percent of those seeking medical help, applies to other medical practitioners and is often referred to neurologists. Further, injuries sustained in road accidents which often, if to an undetermined extent, occur following transient hypnoid alterations of consciousness— alterations that interfere with accident-avoiding attention and intention—obviate the psychic need for conflict reduction in classical hysterical symptom formation. These patients are usually treated by the orthopedic surgeons, though some of them are later referred for psychiatric help.[1]

Whether there is an actually decreased incidence of hysteria in urban Western society thus remains debatable. Certainly, classical forms of hysteria are common in the more outlying rural areas of this country, and are quite highly visible in clinics in such areas as Puerto Rico. Bart[6] has shown that women who were admitted to the Neurology Service of the U.C.L.A. Neuropsychiatric Institute, and who emerged with psychiatric diagnoses, usually belonged to rural subcultures unlikely to have

ambient "psychiatric vocabularies of discomfort," and this was reflected in the way they presented themselves as physically ill. These women, with psychogenic physical complaints, were usually of lower social status, rural, and poorly educated, whereas members of another comparable group who on admission offered psychiatric reasons for their distress were usually of higher social status and of urban residence.

As already noted, hysterical symptoms appear in males, children, and elderly people, but they are most commonly seen in women who are in the early period of adult life— except, of course, under military conditions in wartime.

An elemental passionateness with an excessive love-craving forms part of one type of hysterical personality, as will be discussed, and hysterical neurosis is often encountered in women of this type. In regard to this liability to hysteria, certain problems in feminine development may be briefly adumbrated here. The girl, like the boy, passes through a phallic phase. Later, she attains a feminine position and this entails a change of libidinal object, from the mother to the father, and another erotogenic zone, the vagina. As Freud[49] elucidates, there is a difference between the sexes in the relation of the Oedipus complex and the castration complex. The boy's oedipal strivings develop out of the phase of phallic sexuality. The threat of castration results in a decisive repression of these strivings, and a severe superego in regard to the incest taboo is inwardly established as the legacy of the rivalrous relationship with the father. In contrast, in the case of the girl, the castration complex, including penis envy and increased hostility towards the mother, prepares the way from the preoedipal attachment to her mother to an intensified positive relationship with her father; in this "Oedipus" or, as is more accurate parabolically, Electra situation, she remains more indefinitely than does the boy. These complications which beset woman's development are responsible for greater liability to hysteria, which not infrequently remains on the plane of specifically sexual disability, including all degrees of frigidity.[82] On the other hand, under the stress of military conditions in wartime, especially in battle, the stage is set for the increased incidence of male hysteria.

❲ Hysterical Personality

Charcot[22] emphasized the role of heredoconstitutional factors in the pathogenesis of hysterical neurosis and might thus have proceeded to a detailed investigation of the inborn characteristics of the personality of those suffering hysterical symptoms. However, he directed his interest to the classification of symptoms and the differentiation of hysteria from organic neurological disease, so that apart from drawing attention to the unstable nervous system and the exaggerated suggestibility of those suffering hysterical symptoms he did not offer a more detailed analysis of the behavioral or anamnestic characteristics of his hysterical patients. At this time, the known etiological field consisted of constitutional factors and of environmental factors which were not especially related to early emotional transactions in childhood. The important role of the early personal environment was largely hidden from the view of clinicians before Freud's investigations. Freud was in fact also impressed with the importance of heredoconstitutional factors in the etiology of the neuroses, but in unraveling the meaning of symptoms in terms of the patient's experience, he penetrated the amnesia for events in early life, and recognized also the crucial formative importance in personality development of these early happenings. More attention thus came to be paid to the personality characteristics of patients suffering from symptom neuroses.

The first psychoanalytic contribution to characterology was Freud's paper in 1908* on the anal character. As it became apparent that the optimal goal of therapy went beyond the relief of symptoms to resolving the need for symptom formation, psychoanalytic characterology increasingly assumed clinical impor-

tance. Reich,[86] in his book on character analysis, attempted to depict the character structures in symptom neuroses, including hysteria. He described the behavior of the hysterical character as obviously sexualized, including coquetry in women and softness and effeminacy in men. Even locomotion, he considered, was sexualized so that movements are soft, graceful, and sensually provocative. As the sexual behavior came closer to attaining its apparent goal, apprehensiveness became evident. Reich also described unpredictability, strong suggestibility, sharp disappointment reactions, imaginativeness, lack of conviction, compliance readily giving way to depreciation and disparagement, compulsive need to be loved, overdependency on others for approval, powerful capacity for dramatization, and somatic compliance. He attempted to explain these features as being determined by fixation in the early genital phase of infantile development with incestuous attachment, but as we have noted, Marmor[75] and others have with more cogency related some of these features to pronounced orality in the hysterical personality.

Chodoff and Lyons[24] challenge the close relationship adduced by others between conversion phenomena and the hysterical personality. Of 17 patients with unequivocal conversion reactions, only 5 satisfied criteria (similar to those of Reich's description above) they laid down for the diagnosis of the hysterical personality. They therefore concur with Kretschmer[69] and Bowlby[12] in the opinion that conversion reactions do not occur solely, by any means, in patients who present the characteristics of the designated hysterical personality. They suggested that instead of conversion hysteria there may be substituted one of the three more precisely defined diagnoses: conversion reaction, hysterical personality, or hysterical personality with conversion reaction, whichever may be appropriate. In the 1968 edition of the Diagnostic and Statistical Manual of Mental Disorders (DSM-II), authorized by the Council of the American Psychiatric Association, "Hysterical Neurosis, Conversion-Type," "Hysterical Neurosis, Dissociative-Type," and "Hysterical Personality

* Freud, S. (1908) "Character and Anal Erotism," in Standard Edition, Vol. 9. London: Hogarth Press, 1959. Pp. 169–175.

(Histrionic Personality Disorder)," are separately listed—a maneuver which enables adequate classification without separating conversion reaction from its venerable association with hysteria at any time, but with the option of either separating conversion-type hysteria from the hysterical personality, or citing them together.

In regard to Chodoff and Lyons' divorce of conversion reactions from "hysterical personality," the following comments are appropriate. Freud[48] noted that instances of neurotic illness fall into a "complemental series," within which the two factors of type of personality and adverse experience (discussed as the fixations of the libido and frustration) are represented in such a manner that if there is more of the one, there is less of the other. As stated above, some of the features of the hysterical personality belong to derivatives of pregenital points of fixations, and where these are absent it might be expected that the etiological role of the actual conflict would be more emphatic. Secondly, while the predisposition to acquire hysterical illness is built up very largely from undue emotional attachment to one or both parents, with difficulty of later displacement of this attachment, the dependent and other correlative patterns of personality are often not so simple and obvious. To understand deviations from such a pattern it is necessary to study the total repertoire of unconscious defenses and to take into account that the evident achievements in external adjustments and independence may show the marks of overcompensation. Basically, such patients remain unconsciously dependently fixated on the infantile object (in fact or in fantasy), and are vigorously defending themselves against this fixation. An example from military psychiatric experience is briefly outlined below.

Following enlistment in the army, the patient, aged thirty, developed pains in the stomach. Later, he began to suffer trouble with his eyes, especially when riding his motorcycle. He could not keep them open and complained they kept "screwing up," which, indeed, they did. He was of a very aggressive character-type. Prior to enlistment, he often performed in fairgrounds on the "wall of

death," demonstrating his skill and daring on a motorcycle, and was proud to be earning much more money than his father. He had always been a daredevil, amateur motorcycling being his hobby from an early age. His usual employment was that of a butcher, and he was the mainstay of the home. He had never taken up a sustained relationship with any woman other than his mother, to whom he remained very attached. In discussions he made it clear that he was ready for anything in the army and could perform wonders on his motorcycle—were it not for the spasms of his eyes.

In this case, both the unconscious underlying overdependency and passive homosexual strivings were vigorously countermanded by character defenses. These gave an appearance of remarkable and heroic virility and independence, with others depending upon him, prior to his separation from his mother and the onset of symptoms, including conversion reaction.

Brody and Sata[17] suggest that a semantic solution may be achieved by using the term "histrionic personality" to describe that type of hysterical personality background identified by Reich and by Chodoff and Lyons. They give the following useful clinical description:

> The people described in this manner are vain, egocentric individuals displaying labile, and excitable, but shallow affectivity. Their dramatic, attention-seeking, and histrionic behavior may encompass lying and pseudologia phantastica. They are conscious of sex and appear provocative, but they may be frigid and are dependently demanding in interpersonal situations. They have a lifelong history of seriously disturbed relationships with others. The loss of a parent through divorce, desertion, or death is often reported.
>
> Histrionic personalities under stress may exhibit impaired reality testing, intensive fantasy production, and convictions about the motives of others bordering on delusion. In moments of repose, they are characteristically vague and imprecise about emotionally significant matters. They cannot express their inner feelings with accuracy and often utilize bodily action for communicative purposes.
>
> Although histrionic personalities may exhibit conversion reactions, the latter can occur in association with almost any type of character struc-

ture. Histrionic character features occur more frequently in Western society among women. They are, indeed, considered feminine by our societal standards, and male histrionic characters are frequently described in this way.

In a transcultural survey of 21 female patients, 7 from San Francisco, 7 from London, and 7 from Copenhagen, Blinder[10] found that they all exhibited the characteristics of hysterical personality adumbrated above. A picture emerged of a group of women, often the youngest children in their families, born of mothers who seem to have had scant time or talent for serving as models for identification and of fathers even less able to interact favorably with their growing daughters. These women exhibited a significant number of persistent childhood neurotic traits, and their medical histories revealed an uncommonly high incidence of abdominal surgical procedures. Particularly in the sexual sphere, they were strikingly underdeveloped or inhibited.

Blinder was impressed with their superficially cheerful childlike manner, their emotional lability, their dramatic use of overstatement, or of stoic understatement when this could be used for dramatic effect, the incongruence of their verbal communication with their actual behavior, their emphasis on feminine characteristics to the point of caricature, and their widespread use of denial.

It is clear that in the West there exists transculturally a histrionic female character (to be observed in fact also in the East) liable to hysterical neurosis. However, there are other character structures not so well or so frequently discussed in the literature, and the soldier described briefly above is an example. Such men do not exhibit "softness and effeminacy" as described by Reich. On the contrary, character traits of persistent insistence on being the strong man, of exaggerated exhibition of sadistic masculinity, are anamnestically revealed prior to hysterical symptom formation. It is indeed remarkable that Reich omitted a discussion of the consolidated reactive defense (including identification with the male aggressor) against unconscious feminine identification of these men who are liable to hysterical attacks and symptoms. Some of them, though by no means the majority, pursue women vigorously, are hyperactive, even athletic, sexually, thus feverishly countermanding castration anxiety and remaining busy a large part of their time constructing and reconstructing a "he-man" image for themselves, and to purvey to others.

Many women liable to hysterical attacks and symptoms are quite overtly inhibited sexually; on account of deep-seated guilt and anxiety related to incestuous fantasies which continue to saturate their sexual strivings unconsciously, they strenuously avoid sexual provocation and sexual contact, dress drably, and far from being aggressively exhibitionistic, are excessively modest and masochistic in their style of life. When symptom formation occurs, the sexual symbolic references are ample.

It will be recalled that the same Oedipus who eventually killed his father and married his mother began life by being exposed on a mountain, deprived of maternal care. While the final stages of the Oedipus drama are more representative of one broad category of hysterical character disorder and neurosis, one generally accessible to psychoanalysis of relatively limited duration, there is a second broad category for which the beginnings of the legend are more pertinently parabolic. This second broad category contains those with pronounced oral character traits, sometimes also undergirded by severe narcissistic ego disorder. These latter cases may often be better considered as hysteriform borderline personalities. In the course of treatment psychotic problems may become apparent. It has been noted by Reichard[87] that 2 of the 5 patients reported in the *Studies on Hysteria* showed schizophrenic features. Easser and Lesser[27] differentiate "hysteroid" from hysterical characters and especially remark on the painful masochistic elements in the fantasies of these more pregenitally oriented patients.

(Diagnosis

Glover[54] sums up the pathogenesis of symptom formation in hysteria by citing roughly in sequence the major factors usually involved. These are: (1) somatic compliance; (2) frustration; (3) introversion; (4) regression; (5) reactivation of Oedipus strivings; (6) failure of repression; (7) displacement, symbolization, and/or identification with the incestuous object; (8) breakthrough of innervations; (9) inhibition or exaggeration of somatic function, giving rise to crippling or painful symptoms; and (10) somatic dramatization of unconscious fantasy formations, including repetition of some elements actually associated with Oedipus-phase development.

Examples of somatic compliance are the localization of symptoms in accordance with fixation of body libido (erotogenic zones) and localization due to libido disturbance, the result of organic disease. Thus, conversion symptoms of an oral kind may readily occur in a patient of constitutionally strong oral libido with oral fixation. On the other hand, an organ affected by organic disorder is readily chosen to express symbolically a reactivated oedipal conflict. This last is an important warning to the clinician not to adopt an "either-or" frame of reference in the differential diagnosis of hysteria from organic disease.

Conflict induced by frustration results in the reactivation of an Oedipus complex which has been held in faulty repression and of which the negative (homosexual) aspects are strongly emphasized.

With these major points in mind, it can be stated that the positive grounds upon which a diagnosis of hysteria is established consist in the distinctive marks of its etiology and psychopathology which psychiatric investigation of the patient and his symptoms affords. The disorder is the result of mental conflict, and there are connections between the conflict and the symptoms. Hysteria is manifest in so many forms, some of which closely imitate organic disease of the nervous and other systems, that without the distinctive marks of its etiology and psychopathology symptoms may be misleading. It often happens that the symptoms themselves are no more characteristic of hysteria than of other diseases. In some cases, however, where there are characteristic symptoms such as astasia-abasia, anesthesia en manchon, clavus, globus hystericus, or the changing of one to another symptom, it is necessary to consider the extent to which hysteria is responsible for the illness of the patient. The stigmata only occasionally accompany other symptoms of hysteria. Rarely, pharyngeal anesthesia may be discovered, and cutaneous anesthesia is sometimes demonstrable, for example, in case of hysterical convulsive attacks.

The occurrence of mental conflict prior to the manifestations of the disease, or of its exacerbation, may be revealed by a painstaking history of the present illness. Such conflict is provoked by changes in the life situation of the patient. It is necessary to determine the temporal connections of periods of stress with the conflicts and symptoms. Following this chronological correlation, which is positive in cases of hysteria, the nature of the conflict and its possible symbolic relation to the symptoms needs to be more closely studied. In hysteria, the meaning of the symptoms thus becomes evident, for they express regressively (and often in a body language) both the repressing forces and the repressed Oedipus strivings in the field of conflict. Next, the personality characteristics of the patient need to be evaluated. Dependence aspects may disclose attitudes derived from the persisting, albeit unconscious, strong emotional attachments to the parents or their surrogates. The repressed Oedipus complex of early childhood may express itself in the record of events of later life which the patient is able to recall. Overdependence in the spheres of occupational, social, and sexual adjustment is often clear. In some cases, this is masked by a reactive insistence upon independence, which, however, betrays the character of overcompensation and shows the marks of unresolved aggression toward the parent (or parent figures).

It is also possible in diagnostic interviews to increase understanding of the patient and his illness by a consideration of the neurotic traits that he has evinced during the process of growth and development. These are prominent and, in cases of hysteria, often persist into adult life. In some instances, too, there is a history of previous frank neurosis which can be correlated with the life situation and the conflicts evoked at that time. No interview schema should be rigidly followed, but the data are all required. It may be necessary to have more than one distributive discussion, in which the patient is helped to talk freely in his own way and at his own pace, in order to elicit the information.

As repeatedly stated above, hysteria and organic disease may be contemporaneously present. Organic disease may follow hysteria, as for example when refusal of food proceeds to anorexia nervosa[63] and subsequent physiological derangement. In other cases, physical disease is primary, with disturbances of the body image and an induced regressive ego orientation—a state of affairs conducive to conflict in many people with symptoms comprising, perhaps, an overlay of hysteria.

It is sometimes difficult to differentiate hysteria from organic nervous disorder. In general, an organic lesion of lower-motor-neurone type is one of individual muscle elements, whereas hysterical paralysis is usually a paralysis en masse.[42] An upper-motor-neurone lesion, however, often results in a paralysis which superficially resembles that which occurs in conversion reaction, but there usually are important symptomatic differences. Thus, lower-face paresis, hemianopsia, and circumduction of the leg at the hip, are common in an upper-motor-neurone lesion. Pronounced changes in the tendon reflexes, sustained ankle clonus, and the sign of Babinski, usually point toward organic involvement of the nervous system. Hysteria has to be diagnosed, however, on its own characteristics and not merely by the exclusion of organic disease, which, at times, it may accompany. The following schema summarizes the requirements in history-taking for the diagnosis of hysteria.

Directive Scheme for History-Taking in Diagnostic Interview *

1. Present Illness:
   a. Consideration of chronological correlations of onset and exacerbation

* Reproduced by permission of the publishers, from D. W. Abse, *The Diagnosis of Hysteria.* Bristol: John Wright & Sons, Ltd., 1950.

of symptoms with changes in life situation (or traumatic experiences).
   b. Consideration of conflicts evoked by such changes in life situation. The connections of these conflicts with particular symptoms as far as can be consciously disclosed in discussions by the patient when his attention is directed thereto.
2. Personality Background:
   a. Dependence Aspects:
      i. Nature of current interpersonal relationships, especially family and affianced.
      ii. Current occupational, social, and sexual adjustment, including recreational and cultural interests.
      iii. Employment and school record and achievement.
   b. Neurotic Traits:
      Predominant type, time of appearance, disappearance, or persistence.
   c. Previous Nervous Breakdown: type, correlation with life situation at that time.
3. Family and Hereditary History, and the patient's view of it.

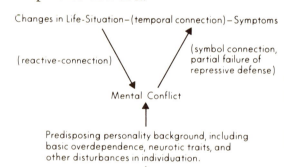

Figure 8-1.   Associative anamnesis in hysteria.

In certain forms and phases of schizophrenia, with delusions, hallucinations, disfigurements of speech, and the generalization of automatization, the disease is readily distinguished from hysteria. Incipient schizophrenia may occasion difficulty in differentiation, especially because the resemblances depend upon an initial similarity of psychological mechanism.[63] The difficulty is enhanced by the fact that, occasionally, hysteria ushers in a schizophrenic psychosis, that hysterical phenomena may cover, or occur with, schizophrenic disease, and by certain forms of hysteria, including dissociative reactions, such as fugue, Ganser's syndrome, pseudodementia, puerilism, and stupor. These last are sometimes part of a transient psychotic disturbance, but there is usually no regression to fixed schizophrenic disorganization. Hypochondriasis in schizophrenia is usually of a bizarre nature, which may be accompanied by a subjective experience of a change or duality of sex, perplexity, and a peculiar overideation. If any of these symptoms accompany somatic conversion symptoms, schizophrenia should be suspected.

Ganser's syndrome is not infrequently observed in people charged with crime, of which they may or may not be actually guilty. The patient is unable to answer simple questions with accuracy, although he is not altogether incoherent, as in hysterical pseudodementia, which, however, may ensue. He compulsively answers all questions approximately, including ones of no relevance to the circumstances of his arrest. Thus, if at 3 P.M. the patient is shown the examining doctor's watch, which is accurate, asked the time of day he may say 4 P.M. In such instances, there is a hypnoid alteration of consciousness which is clouded and suffused with anxiety. The patient may become panic-stricken and excited if questioned very much. Usually he is unfit to plead and requires sedation and supportive psychotherapy before he can focus his thoughts at all adequately. The example offered above in regard to an approximate answer as to the time of day demonstrates, as other such answers do, an overwhelming motivation against organizing events in time and space. This, of course, would be required of the patient in the course of investigation of the events at the time of the alleged offense. In regard to the latter, a particular patient may be caught up

in it in his fantasy or associated with it in actuality; the syndrome is a sequel of accusation.

Depressive or paranoid episodes may punctuate the course of a predominantly hysterical illness. In such cases the diagnosis may more properly be designated as "borderline state," and the treatment may require appropriate modification.[68]

Prognosis, Management, and Treatment

Conversion hysteria, especially when associated with some mild manifest anxiety, is often best treated in individual psychoanalysis. In retrospect, it would seem that analyzable hysterical patients successfully brought to termination of their treatment were usually characterized by adequate ego strength and flexibility, by drive organization predominantly fixated at the phallic-oedipal rather than at pregenital levels, with a good measure of basic self-esteem, and they were well motivated for both treatment and recovery. Psychoanalysis usually succeeds in such cases in not only the deletion of symptoms but in minimizing the need for symptom formation in response to frustrational life situations. Various conditions, however, may indicate the suggestive methods of psychotherapy for relief of symptoms, and others may contraindicate classical psychoanalysis. Immediate medical help may be mandatory as, for example, in acute conditions, such as anorexia with bodily emaciation, or when anxiety is intense and confusion prominent. In such cases of acute hysteria, tranquilizing medication by day and sedation at night may for a time be necessary. Consideration of these cases for psychoanalytic therapy must wait until symptoms have been relieved and the patient is calmer. Advanced age, exceptionally great secondary gain from the illness, or feeble-mindedness, are contraindications to analysis. In instances of conversion or dissociative reaction which follow a severely stressful precipitating situation, the simpler supportive methods of psychotherapy may suffice for recovery to the *status quo ante*. The question of psychoanalysis may in such cases be raised by the patient himself, and may be best left, for the most part, to his own consideration and decision to visit and discuss with a psychoanalyst his suitability for psychoanalysis.

In some cases complicated by the exhibition of psychotic mechanisms, psychoanalytically oriented psychotherapy with modification of the usual technique of psychoanalysis is beneficial.[68] This is frequently the case in the more severe dissociative reactions.

In selected instances of conversion hysteria, especially at phases of a readiness for recovery, following adequate investigation, hypnotherapy, with direct suggestion of symptom relief under hypnosis, may be usefully employed. Some therapists also utilize hypnosis in "uncovering" types of psychotherapy with remarkable success.[106,33,34]

Hysterical character disorder is often usefully treated in group analytic psychotherapy in a carefully composed therapy group.[52] For some patients, weekly individual sessions are also desirable to prevent antitherapeutic acting-out episodes.

It frequently happens in families of lower socioeconomic class, and sometimes in others, that if an individual is to change sufficiently, so that he is not easily liable to recurrence of hysterical symptoms, the context in which he lives must also change. The patient cannot be brought forth from the family soup, so the soup also has to be doctored. There is insufficient basic individuation and socialization and over much deep collective family dependency, so that only temporary improvement may result from individual or even from group psychotherapy—when the group is not composed of the family. Family therapy is thus an important modality of treatment in community mental health clinics.[3]

There are some cases of conversion reaction with an unfavorable prognosis, no matter what treatment is attempted.[107] The conversion reaction may be the only possible emotional solution for the patient, because the real life situation excludes healthier possibilities of gratification. Even in these cases, psychother-

apy on a weekly or more infrequent basis may be considerably ameliorative.[95] Other cases, formerly designated "chronic degenerative hysteria" and characterized by an intense and profoundly pervasive masochism, deteriorate into a massive form of emotional dependence, even parasitism, upon others. When the victim or victims separate or are separated, institutionalization may become necessary, sometimes because of a supervening psychotic disorder of depressive or paranoid type.

❨ Bibliography

1. ABSE, D. W. *Hysteria and Related Mental Disorders: An Approach to Psychological Medicine.* Baltimore: Williams & Wilkins, 1966.

2. ———. *Speech and Reason.* Charlottesville: University Press of Virginia, 1971.

3. ACKERMAN, N. W., ed. *Family Process.* New York: Basic Books, Inc., 1970.

4. ALLEN, D. W., and M. HOUSTON. "The Management of Hysteroid Acting-Out Patients in a Training Clinic," *Psychiatry,* 22 (1959), 41–49.

5. BABINSKI, J. F. F. "My Conception of Hysteria and Hypnotism (Pithiatism)," *Alienist and Neurologist,* 1 (1908), 1–29.

6. BART, P. B. "Social Structure and Vocabularies of Discomfort: What Happened to Female Hysteria?" *Journal of Health and Social Behavior,* 9 (1968), 188–193.

7. BERNHEIM, H. *Suggestive Therapeutics: A Treatise on the Nature and Uses of Hypnotism,* C. A. Herter, transl. Westport: Associated Booksellers, 1957.

8. BERNSTEIN, N. R. "Psychogenic Seizures in Adolescent Girls," *Behavioral Neuropsychiatry,* 1 (1969), 31–34.

9. BIBRING, G. L., et al. "A Study of the Psychological Processes in Pregnancy and of the Earliest Mother-Child Relationship," *The Psychoanalytic Study of the Child,* 16 (1961), 9–72.

10. BLINDER, M. G. "The Hysterical Personality," *Psychiatry,* 29 (1966), 227–235.

11. BONNARD, A. "Testificatory Gestures of Children." Presented at research meeting of Department of Psychiatry, University of North Carolina, April, 1957.

12. BOWLBY, J. *Personality and Mental Illness.* London: Kegan Paul, Trench, Trubner & Co., 1940.

13. BRAID, J. *Neurypnology, or the Rationale of Nervous Sleep, Considered in Relation with Animal Magnetism.* London: J. Churchill, 1843.

14. BREUER, J., and S. FREUD. *Studies on Hysteria* (*1893–1895*), J. Strachey, transl. New York: Basic Books, Inc., 1957.

15. BRIQUET, P. *Traité clinique et therapeutique de l'hystérie.* Paris: J. B. Ballière, 1859.

16. BRODY, E. B. "Borderline State, Character Disorder, and Psychotic Manifestations— Some Conceptual Formulations," *Psychiatry*, 23 (1960), 75–80.

17. BRODY, E. B., and L. S. SATA. "Personality Disorders. I: Trait and Pattern Disturbances," in *Comprehensive Textbook of Psychiatry*, Chapter 25, pp. 937–950. Baltimore: Williams & Wilkins, 1967.

18. BYCHOWSKI, G. "Psychoanalytic Reflections on the Psychiatry of the Poor," *International Journal of Psycho-Analysis*, 51 (1970), 503–509.

19. CHARCOT, J. M. *Leçons sur les maladies du système nerveaux faites à la Salpêtrière.* Paris: Delahaye, 1873.

20. ———. *Lectures on the Diseases of the Nervous System*, G. Sigerson, transl. London: New Sydenham Society, 1877.

21. CHARCOT, J. M., and G. GILLES DE LA TOURETTE. "Hypnotism in the Hysterical," in D. H. Tuke, ed., *A Dictionary of Psychological Medicine.* Philadelphia: Blakiston, 1892.

22. CHARCOT, J. M., and P. MARIE. "Hysteria," in D. H. Tuke, ed., *A Dictionary of Psychological Medicine.* Philadelphia: Blakiston, 1892.

23. CHODOFF, P. "A Re-examination of Some Aspects of Conversion Hysteria," *Psychiatry*, 17 (1954), 75–81.

24. CHODOFF, P., and H. LYONS. "Hysteria, the Hysterical Personality, and 'Hysterical' Conversion," *The American Journal of Psychiatry*, 114 (1958), 734.

25. CONGDON, M. H., J. HAIN, and I. STEVENSON. "A Case of Multiple Personality, Illustrating the Transition from Role-playing," *Journal of Nervous and Mental Diseases*, 132 (1961), 497.

26. DICKES, R. "The Defensive Function of an Altered State of Consciousness: A Hypnoid State," *Journal of the American Psychoanalytic Association*, 13 (1965), 356–403.

27. EASSER, B. R., and S. R. LESSER. "Hysterical Personality: A Re-Evaluation," *Psychoanalytic Quarterly*, 34 (1965), 390.

28. ———. "Transference Resistance in Hysterical Character Neurosis—Technical Considerations," in G. Goldman, and D. Shapiro, eds., *Developments in Psychoanalysis at Columbia University.* New York: Hofner Publishing Co., 1966.

29. EHRENWALD, J. "Neurosis in the Family," *Archives of General Psychiatry*, 3 (1960), 232–242.

30. ELLIS, H. *Studies in the Psychology of Sex*, Vol. 1, Part I, Chapter 2. New York: Random House, 1936.

31. ENGEL, G. L. "A Reconsideration of the Role of Conversion in Somatic Disease," *Comprehensive Psychiatry*, 9 (1968), 316–326.

32. ENGLISH, O. S., and G. H. J. PEARSON. *Common Neuroses of Children and Adults.* New York: W. W. Norton, 1937.

33. ERICKSON, M. H., S. HERSHMAN, and I. I. SECTER. *The Practical Application of Medical and Dental Hypnosis.* New York: Julian Press, Inc., 1961.

34. ERICKSON, M. H., and L. S. KUBIE. "The Successful Treatment of a Case of Acute Hysterical Depression by a Return Under Hypnosis to a Critical Phase of Childhood," *Psychoanalytic Quarterly*, 10 (1941), 583–609.

35. FAIRBAIRN, W. R. D. "Observations on the Nature of Hysterical States," *British Journal of Medical Psychology*, 27 (1954), 105–125.

36. FEDERN, P. "The Determination of Hysteria versus Obsessional Neurosis," *The Psychoanalytic Review*, 27 (1940), 265–276.

37. FENICHEL, O. *The Psychoanalytic Theory of Neurosis*, Chapter 12. New York: W. W. Norton, 1945.

38. FERENCZI, S. "Hysterical Manifestations," Chapter 6 in *Further Contributions to the Theory and Technique of Psychoanalysis.* New York: Basic Books, Inc., 1952.

39. FITZGERALD, O. W. S. "Love Deprivation and the Hysterical Personality," *Journal of Mental Science*, 94 (1948), 701.

40. FRANZ, S. I. *Persons One and Three: A Study in Multiple Personalities.* New York: McGraw-Hill, 1933.

41. FREUD, A. "An Hysterical Symptom in a

Child of Two Years and Three Months," *International Journal of Psycho-Analysis*, 7 (1926), 227.

42. FREUD, S. "Some Points in a Comparative Study of Organic and Hysterical Paralysis (1893)," in *Collected Papers*, 3rd Ed., Vol. 7. London: The International Psychoanalytical Press, 1946.

43. ———. "The Interpretation of Dreams (1900)," in Standard Edition, Vols. 4, 5. London: Hogarth Press, 1953.

44. ———. "The Psychopathology of Everyday Life (1901)," in Standard Edition, Vol. 6. London: Hogarth Press, 1960.

45. ———. "Fragment of an Analysis of a Case of Hysteria (1905)," in Standard Edition, Vol. 7. London: Hogarth Press, 1953.

46. ———. "Some General Remarks on Hysterical Attacks (1909)," in Standard Edition, Vol. 9. London: Hogarth Press, 1959.

47. ———. "Analysis of a Phobia in a Five-Year-Old Boy (1909)," in Standard Edition, Vol. 10. London: Hogarth Press, 1955.

48. ———. "Some Thoughts on Development and Regression—Aetiology (1916)." Lecture XXII of *Introductory Lectures on Psychoanalysis*, in Standard Edition, Vol. 16. London: Hogarth Press, 1963.

49. ———. "Femininity (1933)," Lecture XXXIII of *New Introductory Lectures on Psychoanalysis*, in Standard Edition, Vol. 22. London: Hogarth Press, 1964.

50. ———. "Fragment of an Analysis of a Case of Hysteria," in *Collected Papers*, 3rd Ed., Vol. 3, p. 35n. London: Hogarth Press, 1946.

51. FOULKES, S. H. "On Introjection," *International Journal of Psycho-Analysis*, 18 (1937), 269–293.

52. ———. *Therapeutic Group Analysis*. New York: International Universities Press, 1965.

53. GILLETTE, W. R. "Hysteria in Early Childhood," *New York Medical Journal*, 36 (1882), 66.

54. GLOVER, E. "Psycho-Neuroses," in *Psycho-Analysis*, 2nd Ed., Chapter 10, p. 145. London: Staples, 1949.

55. GOLDSTEIN, K. "On Naming and Pseudo-Naming," *Word* 2, 1 (1946), 1–7.

56. HALLECK, S. L. "Hysterical Personality Traits," *Archives of General Psychiatry*, 16 (1967), 750–757.

57. HANSEN, C. *Witchcraft at Salem*. New York: George Braziller, Inc., 1969.

58. HOLLINGSHEAD, A. B., and F. C. REDLICH. *Social Class and Mental Illness: A Community Study*. New York: John Wiley & Sons, Inc., 1958.

59. JACOBSON, E. "Contribution to the Metapsychology of Psychotic Identifications," *Journal of the American Psychoanalytic Association*, 2 (1954), 239–261.

60. JAFFE, D. S. "The Role of Ego Modification and the Task of Structural Change in the Analysis of a Case of Hysteria," *International Journal of Psycho-Analysis*, 52 (1972), 375–399.

61. JAMES, W. (1890) *Principles of Psychology*. New York: Dover Publications, 1950.

62. JANET, P. *The Major Symptoms of Hysteria: Fifteen Lectures Given in the Medical School of Harvard University*, 2nd Ed. New York: Macmillan, 1920.

63. JESSNER, L, and D. W. ABSE. "Regressive Forces in Anorexia Nervosa," *British Journal of Medical Psychology*, 33 (1960), 301–312.

64. JONES, E. "The Action of Suggestion in Psychotherapy," in *Papers on Psychoanalysis*. London: Balliere, Tindall & Cox, 1938.

65. JUNG, C. G. "Dementia Praecox and Hysteria (1906)," in *The Psychology of Dementia Praecox*, Chapter 4, A. A. Brill, transl. New York: Nervous and Mental Disease Publishing Co., 1936.

66. KAUFMAN, I. "Conversion Hysteria in Latency," *Journal of the American Academy of Child Psychiatry*, 1 (1962), 385–396.

67. KERNBERG, O. "Borderline Personality Organization," *Journal of the American Psychoanalytic Association*, 15 (1967), 641–685.

68. KNIGHT, R. P. "Management and Psychotherapy of the Borderline Schizophrenic Patient," *Psychoanalytic Psychiatry and Psychology*, Vol. 1. New York: International Universities Press, 1954.

69. KRETSCHMER, E. *Hysteria*. New York: Nervous and Mental Disease Publishing Co., 1926.

70. LABARRE, M., and W. LABARRE. " 'The Worm in the Honeysuckle:' A Case Study of a Child's Hysterical Blindness," *Social Casework*, 46 (1965).

71. LaBarre, W. *They Shall Take Up Serpents.* Minneapolis: Minnesota University Press, 1962.

72. Lazare, A. "The Hysterical Character in Psychoanalytic Theory," *Archives of General Psychiatry,* 25 (1971), 131–137.

73. Lazare, A., G. L. Klerman, and D. J. Armor. "Oral, Obsessive, and Hysterical Personality Patterns," *Archives of General Psychiatry,* 14 (1966), 624–630.

74. Leavitt, H. C. "Case of Hypnotically Produced Secondary and Tertiary Personalities," *Psychoanalytic Review,* 34 (1947), 274.

75. Marmor, J. "Orality in the Hysterical Personality," *Journal of the American Psychoanalytic Association,* 1 (1954), 656–671.

76. Masserman, J. H. *Principles of Dynamic Psychiatry,* pp. 33–35. Philadelphia: Saunders, 1946.

77. McEvedy, C. P., A. Griffith, and T. Hall. "Two School Epidemics," *British Medical Journal,* 2 (1966), 1300–1302.

78. Minuchin, S. "The Plight of the Poverty-Stricken Family in the United States," *Child Welfare,* 49 (1970), 124–130.

79. Moss, P. D., and C. P. McEvedy. "An Epidemic of Overbreathing Among Schoolgirls," *British Medical Journal,* 2 (1966), 1295–1300.

80. Mucha, T. F., and R. F. Reinhardt. "Conversion Reactions in Student Aviators," *The American Journal of Psychiatry,* 127 (1970), 493–497.

81. Myerson, P. G. "The Hysteric's Experience in Psychoanalysis," *International Journal of Psycho-Analysis,* 50 (1969), 373–384.

82. Nash, E. M., L. Jessner, and D. W. Abse. "Sexual Disorder and Marriage," in *Marriage Counseling in Medical Practice.* Chapel Hill: The University of North Carolina Press, 1964.

83. Prince, M. *The Dissociation of a Personality.* New York: Longmans, 1905.

84. Proctor, J. T. "Hysteria in Childhood," *American Journal of Orthopsychiatry,* 28 (1958), 394–407.

85. ———. "The Treatment of Hysteria in Childhood," in M. Hammer, and A. Kaplan, eds., *The Practice of Psychotherapy with Children.* Homewood: Dorsey Press, 1967.

86. Reich, W. *Character Analysis.* 3rd Ed., T. Wolfe, transl. New York: Orgone Institute Press, 1949.

87. Reichard, S. "A Re-Examination of 'Studies in Hysteria,'" *Psychoanalytic Quarterly,* 25 (1956), 155.

88. Schilder, P. *Medical Psychology,* p. 306, D. Rapaport, transl. New York: International Universities Press, Inc., 1953.

89. ———. "The Concept of Hysteria," *American Journal of Psychiatry,* 95 (1939), 1389–1413.

90. ———. *The Image and Appearance of the Human Body.* New York: International Universities Press, 1950.

91. Seigman, A. J. "Emotionality—A Hysterical Character Defense," *Psychoanalytic Quarterly,* 23 (1954), 339–354.

92. Seitz, P. F. D. "Experiments in the Substitution of Symptoms by Hypnosis," *Psychosomatic Medicine,* 15 (1953), 405–424.

93. Somers, J. E. "Conversion Reactions—600 Cases." Presented at American Psychiatric Association Divisional Meeting, Scientific Program, Miami Beach, Florida, 1958.

94. Srole, L. et al. *Mental Health in the Metropolis.* New York: McGraw-Hill, 1962.

95. Stein, M. I., ed. *Contemporary Psychotherapies.* New York: Free Press, 1961.

96. Stephens, J. H., and M. Kamp. "On Some Aspects of Hysteria: A Clinical Study," *Journal of Nervous and Mental Disease,* 134 (1962), 305.

97. Teja, J. S., B. S. Khanna, and T. D. Subrahmanyan. "'Possession States' in Indian Patients," *Indian Journal of Psychiatry,* 12 (1970), 71–87.

98. Thigpen, H., and H. M. Cleckley. *The Three Faces of Eve.* New York: McGraw-Hill, 1957.

99. Valenstein, A. F. "The Psycho-Analytic Situation," *International Journal of Psycho-Analysis,* 43 (1962), 315–323.

100. Veith, I. *Hysteria: The History of a Disease.* Chicago: The University of Chicago Press, 1965.

101. Volkan, V. D. *Emotional Flooding and Related Emotional States.* Presented at the Annual Meeting of the American Psychoanalytic Association, San Francisco, Cal., May 1970.

102. Winnicott, D. W. *Clinical Notes on Disorders of Childhood.* London: Wm. Heinemann, 1931.

103. Winokur, G., and C. Leonard. "Sexual Life

in Patients with Hysteria," *Diseases of the Nervous System*, 24 (1963), 337–343.

104. WISDOM, J. O. "A Methodological Approach to the Problem of Hysteria," *International Journal of Psycho-Analysis*, 42 (1961), 224–237.

105. WITTELS, F. "The Hysterical Character," *Medical Review of Reviews*, 36 (1930), 186–190.

106. WOLBERG, L. R. *Medical Hypnosis*. New York: Grune and Stratton, 1948.

107. ZIEGLER, D. K., and N. PAUL. "Natural History of Hysteria in Women," *Diseases of the Nervous System*, 15 (1954), 301–306.

CHAPTER 9

OBSESSIVE BEHAVIOR

A. So-called Obsessive-Compulsive Neurosis

Sandor Rado

THE FIRST PSYCHIATRIC OBSERVATIONS on obsessive behavior date from the 1860's,[9] but it was not until after the turn of the century that Freud opened the way to a deeper understanding of this disorder and its recognition as a well-defined clinical entity.* His classical description of the clinical picture, published in 1917,[4] follows:

The obsessional neurosis takes this form: the patient's mind is occupied with thoughts that do not really interest him, he feels impulses which seem alien to him, and he is impelled to perform actions which not only afford him no pleasure but from which he is powerless to desist. The thoughts (obsessions) may be meaningless in themselves or only of no interest to the patient; they are often

---

* Freud, like Kraepelin before him, called this entity *Zwangsneurose*; by way of different translations, *Zwang* became "obsession" in London and "compulsion" in New York. Subsequent authors, apparently unaware of this fact and eager to ascertain what is meant by "obsessive" and what by "compulsive," settled for the unhappy designation "obsessive-compulsive." The Standard Edition of Freud's work, abides by rendering *Zwangsneurose* as "obsessional neurosis"; hence my term "obsessive behavior."

absolutely silly; in every case they are the starting-point of a strained concentration of thought which exhausts the patient and to which he yields most unwillingly. Against his will he has to worry and speculate as if it were a matter of life or death to him. The impulses which he perceives within him may seem to be of an equally childish and meaningless character; mostly, however, they consist of something terrifying, such as temptations to commit serious crimes, so that the patient not only repudiates them as alien, but flees from them in horror, and guards himself by prohibitions, precautions, and restrictions against the possibility of carrying them out. As a matter of fact he never literally, not even once, carries these impulses into effect; flight and precautions invariably win. What he does really commit are very harmless, certainly trivial acts—what are termed the obsessive actions—which are mostly repetitions and ceremonial elaborations of ordinary every-day performances, making these common necessary actions—going to bed, washing, dressing, going for walks, etc.—into highly laborious tasks of almost insuperable difficulty. The morbid ideas, impulses and actions are not by any means combined in the same proportions in individual types and cases of the obsessional neurosis; on the contrary, the rule is that one or another of these manifestations dominates the picture and gives the disease its name; but what is common to all forms of it is unmistakable enough.

. . . he [the patient] can displace and he can exchange; instead of one silly idea he can adopt another of a slightly milder character, instead of one ceremonial rite he can perform another. He can displace his sense of compulsion, but he cannot dispel it. This capacity for displacing all the symptoms, involving radical alteration of their original forms, is a main characteristic of the disease; it is, moreover, striking that in this condition the *"opposite-values"* (polarities) pervading mental life appear to be exceptionally sharply differentiated. In addition to compulsions of both positive and negative character, doubt appears in the intellectual sphere, gradually spreading until it gnaws even at what is usually held to be certain. All these things combine to bring about an ever-increasing indecisiveness, loss of energy, and curtailment of freedom; and that although the obsessional neurotic is originally always a person of a very energetic disposition, often highly opinionated, and as a rule intellectually gifted above the average. He has usually attained to an agreeable high standard of ethical development, is over-conscientious, and more than usually correct.

❴ Clinical Picture

The designation "obsessive behavior" will be applied to patients who have obsessive attacks and obsessive traits. For convenience, I shall subdivide obsessive attacks into spells of doubting and brooding, bouts of ritual making, and fits of horrific temptation. In time, the form of attacks may shift from one to the other. They may be mild or severe, last half an hour, an hour, or longer; may be quiescent for a while or occur many times a day. Obsessive traits, however, once evolved, do not change significantly. I shall describe and illustrate first the three forms of attacks, and then the traits.

Spells of doubting and brooding may be described as a swinging back and forth between the same set of pros and the same set of cons without being able to reach a decision. They are thought activities that tend to defeat the purpose of thinking. Doubt may invade a belief, proposition, observation, or recollection, spreading from one to the other. The patient can trust neither his memory nor the testimony of his own eyes. Upon leaving home, he may feel forced to rush back to make sure that he turned off the light or locked a certain door, eventually repeating this "making sure" trip several times; or, upon sealing an envelope, he may have to open it over and over again to reassure himself that he has signed the enclosed check, etc.

In his bouts of ritual-making, the patient repetitively executes a sequence of motor acts. Most often these sequences are ceremonial and distortive elaborations of some routine of daily life, such as going to bed, getting up, taking a bath, dressing and undressing, settling down to work or finishing work. They may, however, also be composed of out-of-place or apparently nonsensical motor acts. Repetition of the sequence tends to be continued until the patient is exhausted.

The term "ritual-making" includes obsessive hand-washing, washing or cleansing of pieces of wearing apparel or other objects of daily use, as if they had been soiled or somehow contaminated; the obsession to count (for example, the number of parked cars), to touch (for example, every lamppost on the street). or, on the contrary, to avoid touching certain objects (for example, doorknobs), or to step on or avoid stepping on certain spots (for example, the pavement cracks) and the like; ceremonial and stereotyped elaborations of sexual performance, in particular, of its "before" and "after" phases; of the patient's table manners and eating habits; of his toilet habits; of the way he makes and keeps social engagements, parts with money, makes purchases or presents gifts, etc.

In his "fits of horrific temptation" the patient, suddenly beset by the urge or idea to kill someone (characteristically a close and beloved relative), shrinks back in horror from a temptation so alien to his entire being.

Turning to the obsessive traits, we observe that the patient is overconscientious in his own particular way. What he is mostly concerned about are the minutiae, the inconsequential details, the meticulous observance of minor rules and petty formalities. Specializing as he does in trifles, he is always in danger of missing the essentials. Similarly, his orderliness tends to be excessive and inappropriate, costing valuable time and effort; in his life, the clock is a menace. He may, for instance, keep papers on file that should be discarded, and save or record matters of little or no importance. Upon arriving at his office, he may spend hours putting his desk in "order," arranging utensils and papers; turning at last to his job, he is capable of making important decisions hurriedly, without qualms. A scientist, though never noticing that his shoelaces were untied, was so meticulous in his literary documentation that his colleagues dubbed him a footnote fetishist. A patient recorded all his railroad travels from grammar school to high school, listing all the station stops, even when repeating the same trip. Another had his secretary keep a pyramid of indexes to his private files—a regular index, an ever-growing series of cross indexes, and an index of the indexes. Regardless of how rushed he may have been, whenever he consulted the files himself, he had to take time out to see whether the item concerned was indexed to perfection. Another, the product of a Victorian upbringing, from adolescence on kept a meticulous record in secret signs about his orgasms and failures—long before Kinsey and without the latter's point of view. Another, so instructed by his equally obsessive mother who always worried that he might catch cold, kept his supply of socks in the drawer in carefully separated piles marked "heavy," "light heavy," "heavy light," and "light."

A rough sketch of the obsessive patient would depict him as highly opinionated and proud of his superior intelligence, avowed rationality, keen sense of reality, and "unswerving integrity." He may indeed be an honest man, but he may also turn out to be a sanctimonious hypocrite. He is the ultimate perfectionist. While very sensitive to his own hurt, he may, at the same time, be destructively critical, spiteful, vindictive, and given to bitter irony and to bearing grudges in trivial matters. Or, on the contrary, he may be overcautious, bent on avoiding any possibility of conflict. His "common sense" militates against what he views as fancies of the imagination: he is a "man of facts," not of fancies. He smiles condescendingly at people who are fascinated by mysticism, including "the unconscious" and dreams, but let him undergo some psychoanalytic treatment of the classical type, and he will switch to attributing oracular significance to slips of the tongue or the pen. As a "man of reason" he cannot admit even to himself that he is superstitious. His interest in fine arts is slight or pretended; his true admiration is reserved for mathematics, the exact sciences, technology, the new world of electronic computing machines. In contrast to the expressional (so-called hysterical) type, he rarely has artistic gifts and conspicuously lacks genuine charm and grace. His amatory interests are laden with ulterior motivations and pretense. His envy of a successful rival—in work, for example—may carry him to dangerous lengths: if the opportunity arises, he may subtly cut the man's throat—a token of his admiration and respect. This sort of thing is usually termed "ambivalence"—a term itself in need of clarification. Finally, the obsessive patient is almost never completely free from tension and irritability, though in general the degree of these characteristics fluctuates from slight to severe.*

⟨ Pathology

The Dynamics of Obsessive Behavior

We are now prepared to turn to the pathology of obsessive behavior. Overreactive disorders arise from the organism's inability to handle danger situations effectively by its available means of emergency control: In this event, instead of acting as signals, its emergency emotions themselves inflict, or threaten to inflict, damage upon the organism. Thus, in

---

* Part A is an abbreviation of the original chapter in the first edition of this handbook. Dr. Rado presented a summary of the adapational framework which has subsequently been published in detail: Rado, S. *Adaptational Psychodynamics Motivation & Control.* J. Jameson and H. Klein, eds. New York: Science, 1969.

the face of an external danger, far from increasing the organism's efficiency, they come to disorder its systemic operations, adding trouble within to the trouble without. We call this development "emergency dyscontrol." It begins in childhood with the parents' prohibitive measures, their punishments and threats of punishment. The disorder so created may continue or may flare up again in later life. It is then complicated by the consequences of the organism's own miscarried repair work which always includes unnecessary inhibitions and a reactivation of the long since outdated adaptive pattern of infantile dependence. Obsessive behavior is a subdivision of the class of overreactive disorders.

In Freud's view, all neuroses originate in childhood, from conflicts between the child and his parents. Dependent upon loving parental care, the child is, at the same time, subject to parental discipline. Though the conflict and its consequences become repressed, they may nonetheless disturb the patient's development and produce his neurosis.[4] These findings, now widely recognized, are embodied in adaptational psychodynamics. As regards the specific etiology of obsessive neurosis, Freud held that the patient's development was to some extent arrested and thrown back to an earlier stage. The patient's "genital level" was weakened by "fixation" at the previous level; his regression to that level, at which the child's life was dominated by "anal-erotic and sadomasochistic impulses," was considered the key to his obsessive neurosis.[3,4,5,6,8]

Freud's theory calls attention to the processes of bowel training. The child must be helped to bring evacuation under voluntary control. However, bowel control presupposes maturation of the requisite neuromuscular apparatus. If the mother is overambitious, demanding, and impatient, and if the child is marked by a particular combination of characteristics, then the stage is set for the battle of the chamber pot.

Irritated by the mother's interference with his bowel clock, the child responds to her entreaties with enraged defiance, to her punishments and threats of punishment with fearful obedience. The battle is a seesaw, and the mother, to fortify her position, makes the disobedient child feel guilty, undergo deserved punishment, and ask forgiveness. This indoctrination transforms the child's fear into guilty fear, and impresses upon him the reparative procedure of expiatory behavior. The mother-child conflict provokes in the child a struggle between his own guilty fear and his own defiant rage. It is a characteristic of the type of child under consideration that his guilty fear is always somewhat stronger; sooner or later, it represses his defiant rage. Henceforth, his relationship to the mother, and soon to the father, will be determined by this motivating system: *guilty fear over defiant rage* or, *obedience versus defiance*. The severity of the conflict, sustained by the inordinate and unrelenting strength of fear and rage, perpetuates this outcome. In our view, with the establishment of this motivating system, the child acquires a crucial factor toward a predisposition to obsessive behavior.

Freud's theory of obsessional neurosis features a "sadistic super-ego" and a "masochistic ego,"[3,5] a dramatization unquestionably inspired by observations similar to the ones from which our interpretation derived. Thus, our interpretation is a development of Freud's early insight. On the other hand, his emphasis on the destinies of evacuative pleasure, their significance in the causation of obsessive behavior, is refuted by clinical experience. He assumed that bowel obedience forces the child to relinquish evacuative pleasure by "sublimating" the desire for it or by stemming its tide by "reaction-formations." These developments were then reflected in the shaping of obsessive symptoms. Bowel defiance, he thought, increases the child's evacuative pleasure. The fact is, however, that children forced into bowel obedience enjoy the evacuative act just as heartily as other children, whereas bowel defiance is often enough strengthened by the intent to avoid an act rendered painful by an anal fissure or some other local disturbance. With her insistence on bowel regularity, the mother hurts not the child's evacuative pleasure but his pride in having his own way. Furthermore, one sees obsessive patients whose bowel training has been uneventful, but they are nonetheless marked by the same severe conflict between guilty fear and defiant rage; it originated in other behavior areas. The future obsessive patient's emphatic obedience and stubborn defiance, far from being limited to his bowel responses as a child, are spread over his entire behavior.*

The pathological development of conscience is directly traceable to the unusual strength of two presumably inherited traits, hopelessly at variance with each other. One is the child's craving for autonomous self-realization, a derivative of his primordial belief in his own omnipotence that drives him to reshape the world about him in his own image, which may also be described as a strong bent for alloplastic adaptation. The other trait is his rationalism, his realistic foresight that forces him to take no chances when it comes to preserving the parent's loving care. In adult life, this trait is manifested as a strong desire to be treated by one's social environment as an admiring parent treats a favorite child. Since, however, the parents insist on obedience, and later, society on adherence to its laws and mores, the organism so constituted will eventually do its utmost to conform.

That a child is born to stubborn and tenacious self-assertion may be surmised from the inordinate strength of his rage. This provokes the parents into severe retaliatory measures which, in turn, elicit his defiant rage and even stronger fears. He is thus forced to move with undue haste from ordinary fear of punishment contingent upon detection to fear of conscience, that is, fear of inescapable punishment, and then to guilty fear and the reparative pattern of expiatory self-punishment. Automatization at such an early stage makes these mechanisms overstrong as well as rigid. Healthy conscience fulfills its adaptive function smoothly; it has little need for guilty fear and the reparative work of repentance. But with early automatization, conscience grows into an organization dominated not by the healthy mechanisms of self-reward but by the

morbid mechanisms of expiatory self-punishment. The latter are morbid because they are automatized operations not of, but in, the patient; he does not initiate them, nor is he or his environment aware of their meaning; he is aware of only the damaging effects these nonreporting processes inflict upon him. A conscience so constituted will diminish rather than increase the organism's capacity for happiness. It is an example not of autoplastic adaptation but of autoplastic maladaptation.

A closer look at these developments is indicated. Endangered by its rage, and forced to control it, the organism does not rely on merely repressing it; through accumulation, repressed rage may, indeed, reach the point of explosive discharge. To forestall this possibility, as its next precautionary move, the organism turns the larger part of its repressed rage against itself, or, more precisely, against the rest of its repressed rage—the strategy of defeating the enemy with the help of its deserters. The retroflexion is achieved by assimilating repressed rage with the now-prevailing mood of repentance. This explains the clinical fact that the child's (and later the adult's) self-reproaches may far exceed in vehemence the reproaches his parents ever leveled against him, and that his self-punishments may be far more severe than were his parents' threats. The strength of these mechanisms of self-control is determined not by the actual attitude taken by the parents but by the strength of the child's own retroflexed rage.

Fear of conscience and its derivative, guilty fear, rest on the belief in inescapable punishment. This belief cannot stem from experience. The child knows he was punished only when caught. Nor can religious indoctrination be its ultimate source, for it flourishes in agnostic patients as well.

The chain of psychodynamic inferences leads us back to the infant. Elated by the success of his early muscular activities, the infant pictures himself as an omnipotent being. The hard facts force this grand illusion to recede slowly into the range of nonreporting processes. Sensing that his beloved omnipotence is about to evaporate, the child fancies that he has merely delegated it to his parents: they

---

* The manifestations of defiance were meticulously investigated by David Levy who speaks of them as "oppositional behavior."[10]

exercise *his* magic powers *for* him. He is then terrified to discover that the parents can turn *his* omnipotence *against* him; he has no way of telling what they can now do to him. The dread of inescapable punishment, appearing within his fear of conscience and within his guilty fear, is basically a dread of his own omnipotence, which he now feels the parents can cause to work in reverse. It is powerful enough to retroflex the bulk of his repressed rage. We must assume that stronger-than-average residues of primordial omnipotence are a factor in the predisposition to obsessive behavior.

In the healthy individual, the supreme pleasure of genital orgasm gives rise to a host of affectionate desires, which soften rage by their counterbalancing effect. In the obsessive patient, in whom the pleasure of genital orgasm is seen to be comparatively weak, these derivative motivations are enfeebled, without power to soften rage; the job must be done, and is being done, by conscience alone.

One must assume that a shortage of sexual love is genetically determined; in any case, we consider this deficiency a factor in the predisposition to obsessive behavior. It may well be that, genetically, it is linked with the innate strength of rage.

The early rigidity of conscience vitiates its adjustment to the conditions of adult existence. One must qualify the oft-repeated statement that the obsessive patient is over-conscientious: he is that chiefly, if not only, in the areas of infantile discipline. His silly excesses in cleanliness, orderliness, regularity, and punctuality show that his conscience still operates in the world of the nursery—ruled most often by an obsessive mother.

Some twenty-five years ago, listening to the jeremiad of a tortuous and self-tortured patient, the idea struck me that his obsessive attacks derived from the rage attacks of his childhood.[15] This discovery, abundantly corroborated by subsequent experience, sparked the entire investigation here presented.

In a temper tantrum the discharge of rage is explosive. In an obsessive attack we see the organism struggling with the imperative task of ridding itself of its morbid tensions. Here the discharge of rage, continuously interrupted by counterdischarges of guilty fear, is extremely slow and always incomplete.

The dynamic structure of such attacks is best seen in a simple bout of obsessive ritual-making. Here, driven by his tension, the patient performs a sequence of two motor acts and then goes on repeating this same sequence over again. For example, going to bed, he places his shoes on the floor first at right angle, then side by side; then again at right angle, then side by side again, etc. Analysis shows that both acts are symbolic. One expresses the intent of defiant rage to carry out a prohibited desire; the other, the opposite intent of guilty fear. Consequently, one act achieves a fragmentary discharge of morbid rage tension; the other, of morbid fear tension. Repetition of the sequence is continued until tension is somewhat reduced and the patient is exhausted. In its entirety, the process is a mechanism for the alternating discharge of opposite tensions. We call it an interference pattern of discharge;[16] its mode of organization explains why it is so slow and tortuous. If the patient tries to stop, his tension becomes so unbearable that he must yield to it and continue. In other forms of obsessive ritual-making, the two opposite tensions are discharged by repeating a single act or a stereotyped series of acts; though the motor picture is different, the pattern of discharge is built on the same principle.

The interference pattern of discharge also operates in the brooding spell. Here the discharge is mediated not by seesawing motor acts but by trains of thought traveling in opposite directions. However, doubt and brooding may eventually open the door to mechanisms which are familiar to us from the nonschizophrenic form of paranoid behavior. While, as a rule, their appearance in this context is transient and their form rather rudimentary, such a development is an unwelcome complication of the obsessive picture. In these mechanisms the patient discharges not naked tensions but, in prolonged separate phases, the full-blooded emergency emotions of guilty fear and guilty rage. Through the quasi-delusions of the hypochondriac mechanism, he releases excessive guilty fear at the organismic level; through the quasi-delusional self-preoccupations of the referential mechanism, he likewise releases excessive guilty fear, but this time at the social level; on the other hand, through the quasi-delusions of the persecutory mechanism, he vents, in presumed self-defense, his guilty rage.[15]

The problem of discharge in fits of horrific temptation will be considered later.

At this point the relation of full-blooded emotions to their denuded tensions must be clarified by completing our examination of the organism's repressive activities. The patient is just as unaware of his guilty fear as he is of his defiant rage. As stated before, excessive guilty fear prompts the organism to repress its slightly less excessive defiant rage. We must now add: Humiliated by its guilty fear, the organism soon represses its guilty fear as well. The outcome is a tripartite motivating system: restored pride over repressed guilty fear over more strongly repressed defiant rage. In contradistinction to the brute pride that the organism takes in its self-assertive rage, we call this restored pride domesticated or moral pride; now proud of its virtuous conduct, the organism does not choose to remember that it has been forced into morality by its guilty fear of inescapable punishment.

These repressions do not, however, sufficiently control the patient's excessive, if not altogether inappropriate, emergency emotions. Though the repressive mechanism succeeds in inhibiting their characteristic feeling tone and peripheral expression, as well as the thoughts engendered by them, nevertheless, the overflowing tensions of the patient's fears and rages penetrate his consciousness. Though his tension fluctuates in degree, he feels tense most of the time, complains about it, and recognizes it when it is brought to his attention. Excessive emergency emotions tax the power of the repressive mechanism. Healthy persons, too, experience naked tensions arising from an imperfectly repressed emotional turmoil, though far less frequently, but in the obsessive patient this failure is chronic and produces far more serious consequences.

Our next task is to trace the multifarious influences that contribute to the shaping of obsessive attacks and traits. The rage that filters through in an obsessive attack is the characteristic reaction to frustration. Some of the patient's present resentments repeat the ones he had experienced in childhood when his parents denied him fulfillment of his most highly valued desires. His rage was then, as it is now, his instrument for making them give in or go away. He wished they were dead. Of course, he took it for granted that when needed they would promptly return—and behave. The child's quick death wishes, reflecting his ignorance, are not really murderous; they are only coercive, as are so many other expressions of his rage.

At first the child uses rage to force satisfaction of a particular prohibited desire. Later, as a matter of policy, he wishes to keep the parents under permanent control; they should let him have his own way and still love him. While continuing to serve other ends, the desire to dominate becomes a goal in itself. Next, the child wishes to eliminate, or at least dominate, his siblings; they must not be allowed to compete with him for the position of the favorite child. This motive produces the clinical pictures of "sibling rivalry."[11] The obsessive patient is the child who has, despite innumerable defeats, retained these attitudes for life. His ritual-making and brooding perpetuate the struggle for dominance, drawing their original dramatic contents from the long-since-repressed conflict situations of his early years. This remarkable fact shows that its repressed rage glues the organism to humiliating experiences of its past. Its thirst for wiping out those humiliations takes precedence over its desire to repeat routine gratifications: Triumph is a stronger self-reward than routine pride.

The child's first orgastic experience, made often by chance, awakens his desire for genital self-stimulation. This applies to boys and girls alike. The mother (father) counters the child's practice with a campaign of deterrence, threatening, among other things, punitive removal of his (her) guilty hands and of the boy's penis (Freud's "threat of castration"). He (she) is now caught in the clash between two groups of forces of almost equal strength: *prohibited sexual desire plus defiant rage* versus *fear of conscience plus guilty fear*. This is a precarious situation; to touch or not to touch is now the question. He (she) may find a mode of orgastic arousal that does not depend for its success upon touching the genital organ. He outsmarts the parents by sticking to their words. Later, he will try to circumvent, in the same manner, prohibitions of whatever kind.

If however, guilty fear prevails and he represses his prohibited genital desire, he may switch his pleasure-seeking tendency and self-stimulatory practices to his anus, or resign and develop a tic, or go into ritual-making. It is almost unbelievable to what extent the obsessive ritual may draw its basic conflicts from the now-repressed tragedies of the past. This is particularly true of the struggle, begun in childhood and resumed at puberty, to achieve the genital abstinence demanded of him.

The child may advance his forced precautionary moves to an earlier target point. His parents' intimacies, which he witnessed by chance if not surreptitiously, aroused him. Were it not for his parents' example, he would not have to struggle with his temptation. His effort to keep the parents sexually apart may continue under the guise of an obsessive ritual.

In passing, it should be noted that motives of this kind may produce socially valuable results rather than disorder. A brilliant electrical engineer, in his middle twenties, had more than a dozen patents to his credit. His inventions ranged over a wide variety of technologically unrelated problems. Until his treatment, he never realized that, each time, his success hinged upon preventing the formation of an electric spark. He was an only child who, as an adolescent, had managed to break up his parents' marriage; his infantile obsession to prevent them from having another child eventually besieged his scientific imagination.

The organs the obsessive patient most often uses in his ritual-making are the four extremities. Their psychodynamic significance dates from the corresponding stages of neuromuscular maturation and derives from the se-

quence of illusions which the child develops about his newly won powers. Gorged with his success in co-ordination, he grandiosely overestimates the might of his hands and feet, in particular, of his trampling feet. This illusion persists in the patient's ritual-making, whose procedures, as we shall see, are performed not for their physical but for their hoped-for magical effect.

Earlier, the child believes that his mouth, in particular the biting teeth, is his most powerful weapon. He will have fear-ridden dreams —as will later the adult—in which he loses his teeth; this means that he loses the magic power of his coercive rage to secure domination for him and the magic power of his sexual organ to give him orgastic satisfaction. Attempts to control the dangerous power of teeth may eventuate in their compulsive grinding in sleep. The charm may spread to saliva (compulsive spitting) and to speech. Verbal attack knows no limits when words have magic power. This is seen in the obsessive patient's resort to magic words and in the ordinary citizen's use of cursing. As we shall later see, the magic of words is also a significant component in the dynamics of stammering.

To spit, void, or defecate upon someone are the expressions used in the vernacular to signify contempt. This language usage derives from the annihilating magical effect attributed by the child to his excretions and evacuative acts. But, in the contrary emotional context of yearning for help, the same excretions are relied upon to produce a healing effect. The puzzle of their antithetical meaning and significance is solved by the simple fact that they are utilized as tools by love and hate alike. In ritual-making, no nonreporting motive occurs more frequently than the fear of having been contaminated by someone's secretions or excretions, or the desire thus to contaminate someone else.

The fact that magic thought appears in the shaping of obsessive behavior was discovered at an early date by Freud and Ferenczi.[2,7] We have shown that magic's deepest root is the infant's belief in his own omnipotence, in his primordial self which we view as the nucleus of the action self. From this source derive the obsessive patient's superstitions which he is reluctant to admit even to himself.

Our theory of primordial self also explains the fact that magic is universal. In our culture, its most common manifestations are our wishful or fear-ridden dreams and daydreams, the creative arts, the performing arts, the born leader's charism, etc. In emotional thought—be it lovebound, ragebound, or fearbound—the power of the wish corrects reality. To a degree, all emotional thought is magic thought. In pathology, however, the purpose for which magic is used depends upon the nature of the disorder. The obsessive disorder specializes in coercive magic; the expressional (so-called hysteric), in the performance magic of illusory fulfillment. In the former, unknown to himself, the patient seeks to break his prohibitive parent, intent on turning him into a first-class slave; in the latter, likewise unknown to himself, he materializes his adolescent dreams of drama, romance, and glory.[15]

We shall now revert to the patient's fits of horrific temptation. Though hardly more than a signal of rage below, his temptation shakes the patient's proud morality. His reaction of horror amounts to a voluminous discharge of guilty fear; it may take him hours to regain his composure. His groping for safeguards tends to disrupt the pattern of his routine activities; he is distracted, makes mistakes, loses himself in aimless repetitions, and does not really know where to turn.

It would be a serious mistake to surmise that the patient bursts with repressed rage. On the contrary, closer examination shows that his outward-bound rage has been almost completely retroflexed, turned upon himself; all he can do with it now is to torture himself. To be able to vent it, instead, upon the environment would be his salvation. This inspiration of despair is, indeed, the secret message that his horrific temptation to kill conveys: "I wish I were a murderer."

Extreme retroflexion of rage may be precipitated by opposite errors in education. Too harsh discipline is bound to break the child; oversolicitousness is likely to disarm him: "My parents are so nice to me, I cannot allow myself to get angry at them even when I should." A patient who suffered from the horrific temptation to kill the grandchild she loved most had been overindulged all her life.

Horrific temptation may take the form of obsessive confession, a mechanism first described by Theodor Reik.[17] Learning about a crime from the newspapers, the patient may at once be convinced that it was committed by himself. Nonreporting guilty fears may accumulate from an endless series of nonreporting temptations. To relieve such insupportable guilty fears, to secure deserved punishment and eventual forgiveness, the patient may confess to a crime he never committed. Fëdor Dostoevski, our best pathologist of conscience so far, described memorable examples of this obsession. Police chronicles literally abound with such cases.

If the patient develops a severe depression, his morbid self-accusations not infrequently refer to a beloved person whose actual wrongdoings he blames on himself. Such self-inculpatory fits have, invariably, an ironic intent.[16]

Under the accidental influences of his changing life situation, the patient may shift his doubts and broodings from one favored subject matter to another, and move the seesaw of his symbolic transgressions and repentances further and further away from the original contents of his conflict. But the motivating system responsible for these activities remains the same, showing that the obsessive attack must be understood in terms not of its dramatics but of its function of discharge.

From the model of the patient's obsessive attacks, we can readily understand his obsessive traits, for, in one way or the other, most of these permanent marks derive from the same motivating system—perpetuation of the infantile conflict between the child's overstrong tendency to self-assertive domination versus his still stronger clinging to the security of being loved and cared for. The more environment-directed rage slips through, the stronger the self-assertive aspect of his traits; and, on the contrary, the keener his rational foresight and prudence, the more prevalent will be his traits of cautious avoidance.

The patient's craving for perfection is a direct expression of his primordial almightiness; to the warning that no one can be perfect in an imperfect world, he will respond with a polite smile.

Special mention must be made of the attitude the obsessive patient displays toward the competitive aspects of life. He may be prudent enough to limit his fierce competitive efforts to his major areas of aspiration. He often professes the doctrine of fair play which calls for competitive cooperation, victory through superior performance. At the same time, not always unwittingly, he may quietly employ all the tricks of sibling rivalry, seeking to discourage if not to disqualify his most dangerous competitors from staying in the race, then rush to offer assistance to his victims. When in a slightly elated state, he may be seen competing indiscriminately for almost anything.

In the obsessive patient, the manifold and widespread motivations ordinarily sustained by affection and sexual love are diminished in both strength and scope, presumably because his genital orgasm lacks the overwhelming force and pleasure it has in healthy people. We suspect strongly that this is an innate trait. It must not be confused with the patient's capacity for sexual performance, which may be unimpaired. Unwittingly, the patient is prone to make up for his romantic impoverishment by pedantic execution of the act. He is not exactly a lover, but he is a dependable ritual-maker. If an impairment of performance is present, however, its pathological mechanisms are the same as elsewhere.[13,14] The question of sexual pain dependence will be dealt with in another context.

A few words should be added about the obsessive patient's "ambivalence." Bleuler, who coined the term in his work on schizophrenia, distinguished between intellectual, emotional, and volitional ambivalence.[1] We trace these manifestations uniformly to the severity of the underlying obedience-defiance conflict. Bleuler stressed the fact that the schizophrenic patient, like the child, tolerates the coexistence of conflicting thoughts or feelings or impulses in his consciousness. The opposite is true of the obsessive patient. While the schizophrenic patient is, or appears to be, unaware of such conflicts in him, the obsessive patient is, more often than not, only too keenly aware of them. He ponders unendingly: Must he give in, or could he gain the upper hand without giving offense? Facing the same question, the ordinary citizen makes a decision and sticks to it. But to the obsessive patient this question is a dilemma that throws him into endless broodings and keeps him engaged in countless postmortems. Since the two tendencies concerned are almost equally overstrong, he will always believe that he made the wrong decision. He could have won, why didn't he try? If he wins, he is afraid he will have to pay for it. He cannot make up his mind: Does he love his wife or does he hate her? If he loves her, why does he resent almost everything she does? And if he hates her, why does he cling to her so firmly? He is aware that his indecision is both widespread and chronic.

The obsessive patient excels in repeating the component acts of performance. Repetition enters as an organizing principle into his ritual-making, brooding, and, to some extent, the entire routine of his daily life. Its origin is unmistakable. Repetition is pre-eminently the technique employed in the learning process. Whatever the child has to or wants to learn must be repeated and practiced. The point is that it is the parents who impose this maxim upon him. The defiantly obedient child, the future obsessive patient, carries it, in utmost seriousness, to absurdity: "All right, all right, if this is how you want me to do it, I shall go on and on until *you* get sick and tired of it." His senseless use of repetition is a travesty of the learning technique. Aside from this, repetition is forced upon him by the prompt interdictions of conscience. Interrupted by them as soon as he starts, he must make a fresh start over and over again. He never gets beyond the first step toward the nonreporting goal of his forced effort. Without loss of ironic intent, repetition thus becomes an integral feature of the interference pattern of discharge.

Stammering is a speech disorder closely related to obsessive behavior. They have two dynamic features in common—motivating system and interference pattern of discharge. The stammerer gives a drastic illustration of the afore-mentioned point: He, too, gets stuck at the start—in the first letter or syllable—and repeats it until he is able to complete the word. In stammering, the organism acts upon the early illusion that its most powerful weapon is the mouth; its rage is channeled into speech. Naturally, in the motivational context of rage, the magic of words is coercive or vindictive. To the nonreporting range, the letters or syllables in which the patient most often gets stuck signify the beginning of a verbal assault—obscenity, cursing, etc. Without knowing why, he gets scared. Guilty fear promptly stops his speech, as if to warn, "Watch your words." This mechanism explains why stammering disappears in situations which obviate the necessity of precautions. As is generally known, the stammerer's speech is undisturbed when he is alone, or recites the same lines together with an entire group, or when he sings, etc. Otherwise, humiliated by his defect, he tends to withdraw and reduce his speech to a minimum; this phobic avoidance is, of course, a secondary development. Or, if the patient is angered by his defect, he will stubbornly insist on speaking and finishing what he wants to say. In this effort, one of my patients pressed his teeth together, blushed, his cheek muscle vibrating restlessly and going into spasm. I should like to close these remarks on stammering with a personal reminiscence. When I was a young psychoanalyst, a dear friend and mentor of mine referred a severe stammerer to me for treatment, explaining the nature of this disorder as follows: "Stammering is a conflict between the urethral-erotic tendency to expulsion and the anal-erotic tendency to retention, displaced upward to the mouth. *Eine Verschiebung von unten nach oben*, that's what it is." In this explanation, my friend's romantic enthusiasm for the libido theory eclipsed his native brilliance; he was, in human quality as well as in scientific achievement, the towering figure among Freud's early disciples.

Like all chronic disorders, obsessive behavior imposes unfavorable modifications upon the organism's pattern of interaction with its social environment. It forces the patient to live on an ever-rising obsessive note of tension, lowering his adaptive efficiency, capacity for enjoyment, and active achievement in life.

The onset and further course of the disorder, as well as the measure of its severity, vary widely. In evaluating the degree, we have to consider three pathological factors: The first is the degree to which the self-punitive mechanisms of conscience have become automatized; the second is the degree of the patient's pleasure deficiency, which is indirectly responsible for his severity of conscience; the third, closely linked with the first, is the presence and degree of pain dependence.

Clinically, we can readily appraise degrees of automatization and residual flexibility, by watching, as we do in a laboratory experiment, the influence that stress, absence of stress, and other factors have upon an established response. But about the organization of these highly significant processes we are completely in the dark and will probably remain there until behavior physiology comes to our aid. Unfortunately, as far as mechanisms of conscience are concerned, little help can be expected from animal studies.

Pain dependence is a chronic disturbance imposed upon the organism chiefly by its own retroflexed rage, which, in turn, is an outcome of restrictive upbringing.[12,13,14] Its various forms may be observed in the pathological context of any disorder. In the obsessive patient, the form called moral pain dependence is most frequent. Its development may be summed up as follows: His omnipresent and unrelenting fear of conscience—fear of inescapable punishment—and his refusal to take chances with his security force the patient to shy further and further away from activities that could lead him into temptation. From its original area, the inhibition thus spreads to include the approaches to this area, thence to include approaches to these approaches, and so on in ever-widening circles of precautions.

A graphic and typical illustration of this process is supplied by a patient who, as an adolescent, was prohibited from visiting a house of ill repute. He avoided the house as ordered, then he felt compelled to avoid the street in which the house was located, and eventually he avoided the entire section of the city. By coincidence, he subsequently had to move to a town in which there was no house of ill repute; he departed with a sigh of relief. Unfortunately, in this town he discovered a former schoolmate who had since acquired an unsavory reputation; step by step, he developed the same series of precautions. Changing circumstances are powerless to terminate obsessive preoccupation; the same idea will force itself upon the patient in another form. In this patient, his house-of-ill-repute experience became the hidden content of an obsessive ritual.

Yet no man can stay alive without satisfying, one way or another, the organism's minimal hedonic requirements, and so the patient is forced to find solace and high moral gratification in the fact that he is a "fine man." He discovers more and more opportunities to "fulfill his duty," imposing upon himself burdens and sacrifices which often enough do no good either to him or to anyone else. He becomes a self-styled martyr—without a cause. In moral pain dependence, under the supremacy of retroflexed rage, conscience defeats its purpose.

However, the obsessive patient may also suffer from sexual pain dependence. As a source of pleasure, genital orgasm is unrivaled. If, as they usually do, the parents interfere, the organism puts up a hard fight to protect it. We have already seen that the child may circumvent the parental prohibition by indirect modes of stimulation. But there are other methods. Defeated as a child by the campaign of deterrence, the adolescent may find himself incapacitated for standard sexual performance. By chance, he then discovers that his submission to humiliation or other abuse has a disinhibitory effect upon his performance. Analysis reveals the reason: He has taken the inescapable punishment beforehand; now he is entitled to prove that he deserved it. He develops the practice of inviting abuse (short of serious injury) from the mate, thereby restoring his (her) capacity for performance. We call this practice the fear-ridden

or submissive version of sexual pain dependence.

Another patient may discover that coercive rage takes care of his trouble. Assuming the role of the authority, he (she) inflicts the dreaded punishment upon the mate, enjoying vicariously the mate's suffering. The triumph unfreezes and strengthens his (her) sexual potency even more. This practice is called the enraged or triumphant version of sexual pain dependence. The two versions of this disturbance are far less self-destructive than is moral pain dependence.

I shall now sum up the etiologically significant results of this analysis. Obsessive behavior is based on a predisposition which is acquired in childhood and includes five clearly discernible factors: (1) overstrong rage; (2) guilty fear made stronger by retroflexion of the larger part of repressed rage; (3) stronger-than-average residues of primordial omnipotence that make rage strong and its paradoxical retroflexion possible; (4) relative pleasure deficiency in the area of genital orgasm, with its consequent enfeeblement of genital love and affection—a deficiency that makes it imperative to control repressed rage by retroflexion; (5) intelligent foresight leading to realistic fears. Presumably, the acquired predisposition to obsessive behavior is based on a genetic predisposition in which the overstrength of rage may be linked with the pleasure deficiency of sexual orgasm.

Parental punishment initiates a pathological development of conscience—repression of defiant rage, first by fear of punishment contingent upon detection, and, later, by fear of conscience—of inescapable punishment and guilty fear. The child's fear that the parents can make his omnipotence work in reverse increases his fear of conscience and guilty fear to such a degree that they become capable of retroflexing, as an added safety measure, the larger part of his repressed rage. Retroflexed rage makes remorseful self-reproaches and expiatory self-punishments all the more severe.

Accumulation of excessive emergency emotions in the nonreporting range—guilty fear and the rest of outward-bound rage—forces the organism to create an outlet. His denuded tensions filter through the pain barrier of repression and produce the obsessive attacks with their interference pattern of discharge. Horrific temptations arise when the retroflexion of rage is carried to an extreme. They show that, in his despair, the tortured patient would perfer to be a murderer.

Looking once again at the motivating system, we find rage at the bottom, in the key position: restored pride over repressed guilty fear over more strongly repressed defiant rage. Beyond a shadow of a doubt, in the etiology of obsessive behavior, the ultimate psychodynamically ascertainable factor is rage.

In 1926 Freud[5] summed up his etiological theory of neurosis in the following beautifully phrased (in the German original) passage that ends on a disarming note:

These minor rectifications cannot in any way alter the main fact that a great many people remain infantile in their behaviour in regard to danger and do not overcome age-old determinants of fear [*Angst*]. To deny this would be to deny the existence of neurosis, for it is precisely such people whom we call neurotics. But how is this possible? Why are not all neuroses episodes in the development of the individual which come to a close when the next phase is reached? Whence comes the element of persistence in these reactions to danger? Why does the affect of *fear* [*Angst*] *alone* seem to enjoy the advantage over all other affects of evoking reactions which are distinguished from the rest in being abnormal and which, through their inexpedience, run counter to the movement of life? In other words, we have once more unexpectedly come upon the riddle which has so often confronted us: whence does neurosis come—what is its ultimate, its own peculiar meaning? After whole tens of years of psychoanalytic work we are as much in the dark about this problem as ever. [Italics supplied.]

In the above paragraph, Freud does not so much as mention rage, or even imply it, say, by some reference to his so-called "death instinct," that "instinct of destruction and self-destruction."

I have shown here that persistence and excessive strength of the child's fears are necessary consequences of the fact that the child—and later the adult—is forced to hold his rage

in check. My examination of the other psychoneuroses (the overreactive and mood-cyclic disorders of our classification) has led me to the same conclusion. Summing up a series of studies, I wrote in 1955:[12]

Caught in the clash between their own defiant rage (violence from within) and the retaliatory rage of their parents (violence from without), these patients [suffering from overreactive and mood-cyclic disorders] have emerged from childhood with an established pattern of adaptation that forces them unawares to damage themselves in order to avoid the dreaded danger of damaging others. Their suffering is increased if they develop pain-dependence.

The primary task of education is to domesticate the infant, to make him fit for social life by taming his rage. If this process miscarries, the child's inadequately controlled rage will cause behavior disorders. Trapped for decades in a labyrinth of misconstructed theories, it may well be that we are at last finding our way back to the obvious.

From the analysis of obsessive behavior, we derive a general insight. Since, in all overreactive and mood-cyclic disorders, the root disturbance is emergency dyscontrol, the principal dynamic function of these disorders is to discharge the insupportable tensions created by emergency dyscontrol. Or, to put it more precisely, these disorders are created by the biological necessity to discharge insupportable tensions; in each of them, formation of the characteristic clinical picture is then influenced by contributory causes.

The physiological pathology and the genetics of obsessive behavior have hardly reached even the preparatory stage of development. To offer clues to such investigations is a psychodynamic task of paramount importance.

Bibliography

1. BLEULER, E. *Dementia Praecox or the Group of Schizophrenias.* New York: International Universities Press, 1950.

2. FERENCZI, S. "Stages in the Development of the Sense of Reality," in *Sex in Psychoanalysis*. New York: Basic Books, 1950.

3. FREUD, S. *The Ego and the Id*. London: Hogarth Press, 1927.

4. ———. *A General Introduction to Psychoanalysis*. New York: Liveright, 1935.

5. ———. *Inhibitions, Symptoms and Anxiety*. London: Hogarth Press, 1936.

6. ———. "The Predisposition to Obsessional Neurosis," in *Collected Papers*, Vol. 2, p. 122, New York: Basic Books, 1959.

7. ———. *Totem and Tabu* in Standard Edition, Vol. 13, London: Hogarth Press, 1955.

8. JONES, E. "Hate and Anal Eroticism in the Obsessional Neurosis," in *Papers on Psychoanalysis*, Baltimore: Wood, 1923.

9. KRAEPELIN, E. *Psychiatrie*, Vol. 4, p. 1823, Leipzig: Barth, 1915.

10. LEVY, D. "Development and Psychodynamic Aspects of Oppositional Behavior," in S. Rado, and G. E. Daniels, eds., *Changing Concepts of Psychoanalytic Medicine*, New York: Grune and Stratton, 1956.

11. ———. *Studies in Sibling Rivalry*. New York: American Orthopsychiatric Association, 1937.

12. RADO, S. "Adaptational Psychodynamics: A Basic Science," in *Collected Papers*, New York: Grune and Stratton, 1956.

13. ———. "An Adaptational View of Sexual Behavior," in *Collected Papers*, New York: Grune and Stratton, 1956.

14. ———. "Evolutionary Basis of Sexual Adaptation," in *Collected Papers*, New York: Grune and Stratton, 1956.

15. ———. Lectures at the Columbia University Psychoanalytic Clinic 1945–1955, unpublished record.

16. ———. "Psychodynamics of Depression from the Etiologic Point of View," in *Collected Papers*, New York: Grune and Stratton, 1956.

17. REIK, T. *Geständniszwang und Strafbedürfnis*, Leipzig: International Psychoanalytische Verlag, 1925.

B. Integration of Psychoanalytic and Other Approaches

Russell R. Monroe

❲ Phenomenological (Existential) Model

I n Part A of this chapter, Rado lucidly reported the Freudian description of obsessive behavior, as well as the post-Freudian adaptational psychodynamic explanation for the development of obsessive traits and obsessive attacks. The other significant framework within which obsessive behavior has been described is that of the phenomenological or existential analysis as elaborated in the writings of Jaspers,[14] Straus,[28] and von Gebsattel.[8] The fundamental prerequisite of a phenomenological analysis of obsessive behavior is to clear one's mind of preconceptions of both clinical descriptive psychiatry as well as psychoanalytic theory. In this sense, then, phenomenological analysis is the radical empiricism of observing overt behavior without either concern for biographical data or reliance on a motivational analysis of behavior (psychodynamics), with its assumption of unconscious mental activity. The phenomenologists insist upon this because a biographical report is data only in the sense that it is the individual's memory of his past and not the situation as it actually occurred; hence it has little explanatory reliability in determining etiologic mechanisms.[28] Phenomenologists also believe that inferences regarding the un-

conscious more likely reflect the thoughts of the observer than the observed; thus, there is the danger of forcing data into the mold of old hypotheses, rather than developing new ones to fit the facts.[28]

The psychoanalyst answers that the phenomenologist's radical empiricism seeks for an illusory intellectual security in restricting extrapolations to the domain of the thoroughly tested, without taking the risk of hypothesis formation and future-testing.[15] Despite this avowed difference in observational attitudes, the conclusions arrived at by both the phenomenologists and psychoanalysts, such as Rado, are surprisingly similar. Perhaps this is so because both are rigorous observers of clinical behavior. Some "pure" phenomenologists, however, question whether morbid attitudes or psychopathology is a proper field of inquiry for their study, because phenomenology depends upon the "verdict of immediate experience," which suggests that the only legitimate areas for phenomenological analysis are such universals as consciousness, anxiety, volition, etc., and not the unique or deviant phenomenon represented by psychopathology, which precisely because of its uniqueness is not a universally immediate experience.[26]

Jaspers[14] treats this dilemma by analyzing the morbid experiences in comparison to the nonmorbid or universal experience. From his analysis, we can identify five essential characteristics of compulsive symptoms: (1) a nonsensical, meaningless, or absurd quality to the thoughts and actions of the obsessive, which is recognized by the obsessive himself; (2) despite this recognition of the meaningless quality of the symptoms, the thoughts and acts have a compelling force; (3) a belief that thoughts and actions can influence events in some magical, omnipotent way; (4) a need for certitude and order associated with a brooding doubt; (5) a preoccupation with terrifying, unacceptable impulses usually of an aggressive nature; that is, the patient fears he will harm someone else or be harmed himself. There is no essential difference, therefore, between the phenomenologist's description of the obsessive, and Freud's original description quoted by Rado.[6]

After description, however, the next steps are quite different in the phenomenologic and the classical psychoanalytic models. For instance, within the libido theory, the ultimate explanation of obsessive behavior is that the obsessive individual has regressed to the anal sadistic level of libidinal organization and therefore is not solving his oedipal conflict with phallic gratification, but utilizing punitive and expiatory symptoms because of his sadistic superego.[3] In a somewhat more elaborate statement, Anna Freud[4] says that obsessional neurosis in children closely resembles its adult counterpart; she then explains the development of the obsessional neurosis within the libido framework:

[There is] initial developmental progress to a comparatively high level of drive and ego development (i.e., for the child to the phallic-oedipal, for the adult to the genital level); an intolerable increase of anxiety or frustration on this position (for the child castration anxiety within the Oedipus complex); regression from age-adequate drive position to pregenital fixation points; emergence of infantile pregenital sexual aggressive impulses, wishes, and fantasies; anxiety and guilt with regard to these, mobilizing defense reactions on the part of the ego under the influence of the superego; defense activity leading to compromise formation; resulting character disorders or neurotic symptoms which are determined in their details by the level of the fixation points to which regression has taken place; by the content of rejected impulses and fantasies, and by the choice of the particular defense mechanisms which are being used.

These defense mechanisms in terms of the psychoanalytic ego psychology are displacement, reaction formation, isolation, and undoing, together with the excessive use of intellectualization, rationalization, and denial. Many feel that such "explanations" within the libido framework are not truly explanations, but tautologies, understandable only to those steeped in psychoanalytic language, and, in fact, not even of much use to the psychoanalyst. The complexities of such theoretical considerations are illustrated in two psychoanalytic symposia on the subject.[5,7]

Rado's motivational analysis proposes that obsessive behavior develops from conflicts between the child's defiant rage and fearful obedience in a struggle with parents who attempt to control the child's rages and fears in order to make him fit for a civilized society. If this training proves successful, it teaches self-control and co-operativeness; but if unsuccessful, the child responds with either defiant rebelliousness or fearful submission, reinforced by an omnipotent belief of inescapable punishment. This is to Rado the essence of obsessive behavior.

On the other hand, the phenomenologist investigates the obsessive's versus the normal's view of the world, and establishes how this view influences their "I-world" relationships. Thus, the phenomenologist looks at what makes the world nonsensical, meaningless, or absurd to the obsessive, what gives this view a compelling force, and how his belief that thoughts and actions have a magical omnipotence arises. In doing this, Straus[28] feels that most obsessives belong in one of two groups: those with what he calls "contamination obsessions," or those who fear they are "compulsive" killers. Those with "contamination obsessions," Straus says, have no feelings of abundance, harmony, softness, growth, vigor, beauty, or love, as found in the normal individual; the physiognomy of their I-world relationship is completely reversed from the living to the dying, from the blooming to the failing, from abundance to scarcity, from vigor to apathy, from appetite to disgust. The world becomes decay in a thousand shapes: disease, dirt, decomposition, germs, dust, mud, excrement, sweat, sperm, sputum. Straus identifies the central theme as a feeling of disgust and decay, and analyzes these feelings in terms of the normal's view of the world. He points out that what is disgusting to the obsessive may also be disgusting to the normal in certain contexts:

The sweat of the athlete who has just won the contest will not prevent his girlfriend from embracing him, the perspiration which covers the face of the sick has quite another effect; the difference is determined by the context to which the parts belong.

In the first instance, the context is strong, healthy life; in the latter instance, it is sickness and death. Thus, the sick or weak man is disgusted by a plate heaped high with delicious food, as may be the normal person whose appetite is satiated, but not the person who is hungry and healthy. Straus sees the "sympathetic relations" of the contamination obsessives as limited and feels that the contamination obsession is psychotic behavior with an inherent genetic deficit of sympathetic, abundant, warm, loving feelings. This is similar to Rado's conclusion from his motivational psychodynamic analysis, that there is a lack of pleasurable emotions in the obsessive's life. In summary, Straus says that the world in which the contamination obsessives live is such that their behavior is dominated by horror and dread, not because of fear of imminent death, but because of the presence of death in the sensory immediateness, which is warded off by the feelings of disgust.

Concerning the obsessive "killer," Straus believes their symptoms are characteristic of the neurotic obsessional. Briefly summarized, the perfectionism of the obsessive serves to overcome his paralysis of action; that is, "Perfectibility alone permits action, for only if something were perfect would it be immune against attack." Likewise, in his orderliness the

obsessive defends himself in a struggle against omnipresent attacks, just as he uses isolation to avoid struggle with the hostile world. The ritual represents a primitive magic by which the obsessive protects himself against this hostile world, where, helpless and alone, he hopes that the magic of repetitious acts, that is, the ritual, will protect him from aggression. Straus, then, offers an answer to the problem of distinguishing the neurotic obsessive from the schizophrenic patient with obsessional symptoms, a distinction important for both prognostic and therapeutic reasons. However, I know of no follow-up study which substantiates Straus's impression that the contamination obsessions are always or even usually schizophrenic, although clinical experience suggests such a possibility.

The deficiency in the phenomenological model is that although it may help us understand the world view of the obsessive, it does little to explain it, nor does it clearly identify a course of corrective action to either prevent or modify obsessive behavior. Psychoanalytic theory would predict that obsessive parents will likely rear obsessive children, and this certainly is supported by clinical observations. Nevertheless, the psychodynamic model is not a sufficient explanation, because children reared in the same predisposing environment with obsessive parents do not invariably develop obsessive neurosis or even obsessive traits. By and large, investigators in the field of psychopathology have committed themselves to either the psychoanalytic (psychodynamic) model or the phenomenological model. Both models, however, leave the student with a feeling that there is still much to be learned about obsessive behavior.

There is an obvious alternative to this dichotomy; that is, perhaps psychodynamic and phenomenologic methods are complimentary; an integration of the two might shed light on the development of obsessive behavior, which, in turn, might provide clues as to how such behavior can be prevented or modified.[18] An attempt at such an integrated analysis follows.

Rado states that one is predisposed to obsessive behavior if there is a stronger than average residue of primordial omnipotence (primary narcissism), and a deficiency in the usual pleasurable emotions that would otherwise counteract intense emergency feelings, such as fear and anger. In another context, Rado points out that the basic emergency emotions of fear and anger are inevitably associated; usually one is more obvious, but the other is present, even if covert. Others[16,17,18] modify this concept by adding that the truly significant factor in the development of the obsessive is that neither fear nor anger dominates the other, although both are excessive. Each affect, that is, fear and anger, is felt and overtly responded to simultaneously or in rapid succession. The result is a constant vacillation between polar opposites of fear-dominated obedient behavior and anger-dominated coercive behavior. MacKinnon and Michels[17] described this succinctly:

> The obsessive individual is involved in a conflict between obedience and defiance. It is as though he constantly asks himself, "Shall I be good or may I be naughty?" This leads to a continuing alternation between the emotions of fear and rage. Fear that he will be caught at his naughtiness and punished for it, rage at relinquishing his desires and submitting to authority. The fear stemming from defiance leads to obedience, while the rage derived from obedience leads back again to defiance.

This formulation is supported by the clinical observation that if anger comes to dominate the obsessive's behavior he develops paranoid, referential, persecutory behavior, while if fear dominates he is more likely to develop a depression with guilty protests of unworthiness as expiatory attempts to recapture love. A dramatic example of this fear-anger conflict is illustrated in the following treatment situation:

An obsessive patient in analysis had only two rules to follow. One was that he come regularly to his appointment five times a week, and the other that he report as candidly as possible all thoughts that came to his mind, no matter how irrelevant they seemed, or how difficult they were to reveal. As might be expected of the obsessive, for two years he was prompt for appointments and seldom missed

one for any reason. However, there were long silences during which the patient admitted to many thoughts which he deemed irrelevant or unimportant, hence would not report. Despite repeated interpretation of this resistance to therapy, he entered a phase in treatment where for eleven successive sessions he came promptly, left promptly, but during the hour did not say a word. His therapist, too, remained silent. At the twelfth session, the patient finally blurted out in frustration the absurdity of his behavior; that is, coming regularly, yet sitting a full hour in silence. He spontaneously recognized that attending regularly was his obsequious, obedient attitude, but refusing to communicate in these sessions represented his angry, rebellious behavior.[18]

It is easy to understand how the constant vacillation between fear-dominant and anger-dominant behavior leads to the bizarre inconsistencies in the life patterns of the obsessive. We can also realize his consequent need for certitude and order, associated with brooding doubt. However, motivational analysis does not explain the nonsensical meaninglessness of the obsessive behavior. Perhaps a phenomenological analysis will help in understanding at least the neurotic obsessional patient, that is, the patient Straus calls the obsessive "killer." Dynamically we can understand from where fear and anger arise, but we cannot understand the affects themselves, which requires a phenomenological analysis.

Much is written in the existential literature concerning fear and dread, but surprisingly little about rage and anger. Space only allows a cursory phenomenological analysis of these affects. Pertinent to our considerations is Heidegger's concept of *Angst*, translated in the existential literature as "dread," and distinguished from fear.[11] Heidegger used the word fear in the sense of being afraid about something or afraid of something; that is, the fearful man is "always bound by the thing he is afraid of and in his efforts to save himself from this something, he becomes uncertain in his relationship to other things. In fact he loses his bearing generally." On the other hand, dread is always a dreadful feeling about something vague, but not about a specific thing or a specific person. The feeling of dread has something uncanny about it, it crowds around us, leaves nothing for us to hold on to, and in fact is the ground of our very being and reveals the existential concept of "Nothing." This dread cannot be denied or avoided, except through neurotic behavior. This all-pervasive dread sometimes is described as "spellbound peace" or "blissful" peace. The continuity of these apparent polar opposites is hard to understand, but can be experienced in the "peak" experience (psychedelic or religious experience). To Heidegger, this dread was the very ground of our Being. Although it is an oversimplification, we can say that not accepting this dread distorts our Being. Could it be that this very lack of what Straus calls "sympathetic emotions," or what Rado says is a deficiency of pleasurable emotions, that is, the feelings of abundance, warmth, understanding, growth, etc., denies the association between dread and blissful peace, leaving this basic human emotional tone unacceptable to the obsessive? The dread then is shifted to fear; that is, afraid about something or afraid of something. Thus, the obsessive, as Heidegger says, becomes uncertain in his relationship to other things.

There is surprisingly little written about the competing emotions of rage, hate, anger, and resentment. Boss,[1] however, identifies anger and rage as affects, hate not an affect but rather a passion; both he calls emotions. To paraphrase, he says that we cannot decide and undertake to have a fit of anger. It assaults us, falls upon us, and effects us suddenly and tempestuously. Anger rouses us up, lifts us above ourselves in such a way that we are no longer in control of ourselves. We say of someone who is in a fit of anger, "He is not really himself." The passion of hate also cannot be produced by decision. Like an affect, it, too, seems to fall upon us suddenly. Nevertheless, the assault of the passion hate is essentially different from the fit of anger. It can break out suddenly in deed or utterance, but only because it has long been rising within us. It has, as we say, been nourished within us.

On the other hand, we do not say and never believe that anger, for example, is being nourished, while a passion such as hate is. A fit of anger, on the other hand, subsides again as fast as it comes over us—it blows over. Hatred does not blow over; after its outbreak, it grows and hardens, eats into, and devours our entire feelings. This collectiveness of our being, brought about by the passion of hate, does not close us off, does not blind us (like the affect anger), but makes us see more clearly, makes us deliberate. The angry man loses his senses, the hating man's senses are heightened. The great hatred of the paranoiac, for instance, makes him aware of the slightest traces of hostility in his fellow human beings. Anger is blind, while a passion such as hate heightens one's being and opens one up to the world. It is rare that the obsessive becomes enraged, just as it is rare that he panics, but he is constantly fearful and simultaneously persistently hateful or resentful. Perhaps it is not only the lack of pleasure that augments the intensity of fear and hate, but also the fact that the obsessive seldom allows himself to become enraged or panicky, which, in turn, would allow the affect to "blow over" and dissipate the passion, which otherwise is nurtured and persists. As Boss suggests, then, the passion hate concentrates and extends the obsessive's view of the world, even if it narrows his field of vision. The obsessive's cognitive and behavioral deviations defend him against the subjective awareness of this hate, but his concentrated view of the world gives malevolent meaning to even the most extraneous circumstances. As Heidegger says,[12] "It goes without saying that this collecting moves in a direction which depends upon the passions by which it is brought about." To repeat, then, the intensity of the passion hate becomes particularly obvious when the obsessive's defenses against the passion are thwarted, or release through anger or inhibited panic.

What are the further implications if the obsessive's view of the world is concentrated and directed by the basic passions of hate and fear, neither being attenuated nor counteracted by the passions of love, nor dissipated by a "fit of anger or panic"? What does this do to the illumination of the world as seen by the obsessive? If the world is illuminated solely by the passions of fear and hate, with no counteracting feelings of love, joy, abundance, growth, it is a world of malevolent forces filled with decay, contamination, persecution, and killing. Because of the vacillation between fear-dominated and hate-dominated passions, one moment the obsessive is the victim of these malevolent forces, and the next the instigator, one minute fearfully obedient, and the next angrily coercive, one moment killed, the next the killer.

Does an analysis of the effects of these passions clarify other obsessive symptoms, such as the nonsensical, meaningless, and absurd nature of the obsessive behavior? To examine this we have to understand what we mean by meaning or what makes something nonsensical. (Here, we give credit to Strasser[27] for his lucid discussion on the subject.) Meaning, even in the practical sense, is always the meaning of Being, and one makes this Being visible by discovering it through one's actions. While this is an intentional achievement, the intentions in themselves are not creative. Nevertheless, a discovered object owes its Being for me to my "dis-covering" acts. For example, the meaning of a glass of ice water in front of me becomes clear as I reach for it on a hot summer day and lift it to my parched lips. What would happen then if my intentions were contradictory? If, for example, I make contradictory judgments concerning Being, as revealed through intentions which were in turn contradictory. If my intentional acts are vacillating, with the vacillating basic passions of fear and hate, then everything would be nonsense, as a result of this defective intentional achievement. The discovered object is one minute this, the next that, with "this" and "that" usually at polar extremes; hence, the nonsensical nature of my behavior and the meaninglessness of the world about me. For example, in my fear-dominated intentional act, the glass is filled with tepid, cloudy, contaminated water, or in my rage-dominated act picking up the glass is to throw it in the face of my host who has humiliated me; there

would be no gratification, no clarity, no consistency in my intentional behavior, therefore, the world becomes meaningless and my actions inconsistent and nonsensical.

As we establish meaning through our intentional acts, the horizons of our knowledge extend and that which was previously beyond this horizon (i.e., not previously experienced as an object of our intentional acts) loses its meaninglessness. We know, however, that we cannot encompass the whole in its entirety; that is, there will always be a horizon or a limit to our consciousness (a world filled with potential intentional but not yet consummated acts). Even though we do not yet know the meaning of that which is beyond the horizon, we do not assume it is nonsense, but believe it could become meaningful through intentional acts, once they occurred. However, if our intentional acts are always contradictory, then this world beyond our horizon is likewise contradictory; that is, nonsense, mysterious, unpredictable, and threatening. To elaborate further, if we could ascend to the heights of a transcendent cognitive attitude, that which has become meaningful for us through our intentional acts might be compared by analogy to a mere nutshell floating on a fathomless and tumultuous sea. But this tumultuous sea, still meaningless to us, is not empty of meaning. It has a still hidden and unspoken meaning which Strasser refers to as "premeaning" or "fundamental meaning," in contradistinction to the "signified" meaning which has already revealed itself through our discovering acts. There is an element of dread in this vague premeaning, which seems to be a basic human condition. Those who cannot accept this dread, according to Tillich,[29] deny this mystery by substituting a false certitude, often in the form of neurotic, particularly obsessive, behavior. The obsessional individual refuses to accept the mystery of this ontological truth. Others see this mystery in terms of growth, abundance, and becoming, but the obsessive, in his vacillation between fear and hate, sees it only as malevolent and leading to death, destruction, decay, and disease. With this view of the world, it is not surprising that the obsessive has an intolerance for the indefinite, undetermined character of what is beyond the horizon and still beyond his intentional acts. He denies this mystery and, instead, fills his world with intentional acts that become increasingly mundane, repetitive, routine, and nonsensical. He hopes to control the mystery which he cannot face through the magic of rituals. Thus, in order to avoid the unknown, the complexities of the world are made certitudes by precise intellectualizations, rationalizations, and simplified causes and effects, while the mysteries of the premeaning beyond the horizon are made certitudes through the concretization of magic. The obsessive then fills up his world with trivial intentional acts; the frightening void of the unknown becomes a meaningless known of mundane activities. If this sounds too metaphysical, remember that the obsessive is preoccupied with metaphysics. Support for such metaphysical ruminations seems to lie in the surprising similarity of obsessives' rituals, regardless of culture and developmental background. This strongly suggests that the obsessive's behavior might be more than that which Rado proposes, namely, a displacement of the overly strict morality of the nursery which, in turn, leaves an overly strict infantile superego.

Finally, we must consider the obsessive's sense of omnipotence. This omnipotence pervades not only normal behavior but also many pathological states. Primary omnipotence (primary narcissism) is inferred from the behavior of the very young infant and reaches its peak of absurdity in the grandiose delusions of the paranoid. Omnipotence is adaptive when it provides a necessary security during periods of relative helplessness, with survival depending not on an individual's efforts, but on fortuitous circumstances beyond his control. The sailor, when washed overboard, swims aimlessly, convinced that death will pass him by and rescue is imminent. Returning to the analogy of the meaningful world as a mere nutshell on the fathomless sea, we can see how dread of the ontological mystery can also be relieved through a personal sense of omnipotence. Such a sense of omnipotence not only has healing value, but is essential in viewing the "totality-of-what-is." Only through this sense of omnipotence can we be aware of the

infinite, the perfect, pure actuality, as opposed to the frightening and unpredictable potentiality. Painful renunciation of this omnipotence, however, is part of human maturation, apparently made easier by the perception of love, abundance, and growth, all of which imply a benevolent fate. If the obsessive sees only destruction and disintegration, then maintaining one's personal omnipotence is the only defense for such a terrifying world, giving one power to coercively control the destructive fates through even more powerful personal magic. The fact that the obsessive's magic rituals are unceasing and only temporarily relieve anxiety indicates that unlike the grandiose paranoid individual, he has no real conviction of his personal omnipotence, only hopes for it, while fearing that if he does not possess it someone else does.

The vacillation between angry coerciveness and fearful submission leaves a pervading sense of inconsistency and confusion in the obsessive's view of the world. There is no stable ground phenomenon upon which he stands. The obsessive drives unceasingly to the point of exhaustion to find a secure foothold. Decisive action becomes more and more trivial, totally lacking in adaptive value, but quite cogently reflecting the need to find consistency in a world illuminated by the conflicting and threatening passions of fear and hate.

Thus, it seems that after identifying through a motivational analysis the conflicting passions of fear and hate, neither counteracted by pleasurable emotions, further explanation for the obsessive's behavior can be sought by a phenomenological analysis of the basic passions fear and hate. Then, what is poorly explained by psychodynamics, that is, the nonsensical quality of the obsessive's behavior, as well as his tireless struggle for meaning and his need for magical omnipotence, becomes clear.

❲ Differential Diagnosis

Obsessive Neuroses

The most widely accepted definition of obsessive neuroses is that of Lewis:[20] "Whenever a patient complains of some mental experience which is accompanied by a feeling of subjective compulsion so that he does not willingly entertain it, but on the contrary does his utmost to get rid of it, that is an obsession." The three essential elements, then, are a feeling of subjective compulsion, the resistance to it, and retention of insight. Some differentiate the obsessive neuroses from the compulsive neuroses, the latter defined as a stereotyped, usually innocuous behavior which the patient feels compelled to carry out. The urge to carry out the act is pressing, even imperative, and if the patient resists this urge he becomes tense and anxious. These obsessive-compulsive symptoms may occur in many different mental illnesses, neurotic and psychotic, functional and organic, but in the obsessive-compulsive neurosis they form the kernel of the illness and are the presenting symptoms. The subjective feeling of compulsion, the *sine qua non* of the obsessive-compulsive neurosis, may not be present in other disorders where obsessive-compulsive symptoms are nevertheless described. For instance, in the obsessive-compulsive personality, although the individual may subjectively feel the compulsion, he does not unwillingly entertain nor resist these ideas, in fact accepts them as part of his routine existence.

As described later, the unacceptable subjective aspects of obsessive-compulsive symptoms may become acceptable through a shift to the "delusion-like ideas" of the psychotic depression or to the delusion proper characteristically related to schizophrenia. Likewise, in organic brain syndromes and other neurologic defects, there may be both a denial of the basic illness itself, as well as the obsessional behavior patterns, which are egosyntonic to the individual.

Confusion in precisely applying the words "obsession" or "compulsion" occurs because any symptom, such as an intrusive, maladaptive thought, recurring affect, or repetitious habit, all characteristic of psychopathology in general, is sometimes labeled obsessive, merely because it is repetitious. For instance, a strongly developed habit, a tic, or stereotyped behavior, is erroneously labeled an ob-

session or compulsion. It must be remembered that all symptoms are intrusive and repetitive (the repetition compulsion of Freud). Even such firmly fixed habits as smoking, nail-biting, or thumb-sucking, have been labeled as obsessive, but if the word is to have meaning, some discrimination in its application must be made. There is no consensus among psychiatrists as to this precision, but from a review of standard usage it would seem that the following discrimination might be helpful: (1) Obsessive-compulsive neuroses should be limited to those situations where the individual has a feeling of subjective compulsion, does not willingly accept the idea or behavior, and in fact does his utmost to get rid of it. The individual feels forced to complete an act, even though he does not like to do it, and recognizes that it is meaningless, despite his compulsion. This should be distinguished from the perverse act where the individual feels forced to enjoy some behavior against his will. Thus, in the compulsive act the individual appears to perform the act in order to avoid anxiety, while in the perverse act he completes the act in the hope of obtaining pleasure. (2) If the individual does not resist the obsessive act or thought, that is, if his behavior is egosyntonic, the behavior can be an obsessive symptom or an obsessive trait only if it is otherwise similar in form to the behavior of the obsessive neurotic; that is, the repetitions occur frequently, usually many times a day; the acts or thoughts are complete; and they are usually mundane, routine activities which are bizarre because of their repetitiousness and inconsistency.

Obsessional symptoms should be distinguished from phobias, which are pure inhibitions of behavior; that is, the phobic minimizes anxiety by avoiding a real or symbolically frightening situation; the obsessive minimizes anxiety by the ritualistic magical act. Many individuals demonstrate both phobic and obsessive behavior, but others show clearly one or the other.

Some motor behavior is pathological not only because it is repetitious, but because it represents incomplete acts, for example, tics or mannerisms. Often, these are erroneously labeled obsessive or compulsive acts, but it would be better to follow the traditional differentiation, namely, that a partial act is a symbolic act if it is a partial or incomplete motor pattern associatively connected with some past experience of a *nonconflictual* nature, and it is a symptomatic act if it is a partial act associatively connected with past *conflictual* experiences. In both instances, the action represents only a fragment of an intention, and for this reason lacks adaptive value. But it is best not to label these partial acts as compulsions, just because of their repetitive nature.

Another aspect of compulsive behavior is a symbolic doing and undoing, wherein the underlying impulse that is avoided by this behavior is never carried to fruition. Thus, the obsessive-compulsive is seldom the "killer," although he often fears that he will be the "killer." The obsessive-compulsive act, then, should be differentiated from the irresistible impulse where the unacceptable impulse has been carried through to completion, even though there may have been a long period of defensive resistance to this action, utilizing obsessive-compulsive symptoms. Likewise, habits that are repetitive behaviors often accepted by the individual with little or no awareness of their repetitious nature, should not be designated as compulsions.

To reiterate, in considering the diagnosis of obsessional neurosis and its relationship to other disorders with obsessional symptoms, it is important to evaluate the patient's resistance to the obsessional ideas and rituals. As long as there is a recognition of the nonsensical quality of the symptoms and an attempt to resist the symptoms, it is a true obsessional neurosis. When the rituals become egosyntonic, a number of factors must be considered. There may be the denial of the symptom of the obsessional rituals without delusional elaboration, such as occurs in patients with underlying neurologic or central nervous system disorder, or in the individual with an obsessive personality. There may be a change from obsessions to delusion-like ideas, described by Jaspers as typically associated with affective disorders; these should be distinguished from the change in obsessions to the delusions characteristically related to schizophrenia.[14]

Obsessive Personality

The individual described as an "obsessive character" demonstrates behavioral patterns typical of the obsessive neurotic, but does not see his behavior as symptomatic. When others accept such behavior, it may have adaptive value, and when others reject it, it will be maladaptive in terms of the individual's interpersonal relations. These character traits are labeled in the psychoanalytic literature as "anal-erotic traits," denoting the point in the libidinal development of an individual where such behavior is predominant.

For instance, the boss of an obsessive character may describe his underling as a person who loves order, is thorough, accurate, fastidious, and organized. He may note that his employee has definite opinions, stands up for his rights, is self-confident, intelligent, and critical, has a keen sense of reality, is objective and unemotional. He will say that this person has unswerving integrity, abides by the rules, has a strong sense of duty, and is cautious. Furthermore, he will describe his employee as conservative, formal, and reserved, adding that he is thrifty and takes pleasure in his possessions, as well as shows perseverance, endurance, and a tremendous capacity for work. As can be seen, this is an ideal person for middle management, or the kind of person you would like to work on your car or television set, or perhaps perform surgery on you. This is an individual you would look for when hiring an accountant or quality control engineer.

At home, however, his wife describes this same person as pedantic, wasting time in meaningless indexing and note-taking. She may complain that her husband is defiant and stubborn, seeing only one way to do things, adding that he is a miser, hoards things unnecessarily, and treats people like possessions. Furthermore, she says he is self-centered, scornful of others, and convinced he can do things better than anybody else. She complains bitterly that he lacks warmth, charm, and grace, noting that he is a hair-splitter, indecisive, inflexible, unimaginative, and lacking in the normal capacity for pleasurable relaxation.

Those of us who do family therapy are struck by the frequency with which hysterical women marry men with obsessive characters. Before marriage, they see in these men fatherly attitudes of strength, reliability, conscientiousness, and control, which will reinforce their own lack of control and compensate for their own emotional instability. It is only after marriage that they realize the price paid for this external control. Then, they become resentful and dissatisfied with their marriage, hoping to manipulate their spouse with hysterical outbursts, which unfortunately elicit only more stubborn, defiant behavior. With the disintegration of their interpersonal relationship, the individual with obsessive personality traits may experience anxiety and depression due to threatened desertion, but still may not see his obsessive character traits as symptomatic. In such instances, the diagnosis should not be obsessive-compulsive neurosis, but rather an anxiety or depressive neurosis in an individual with an obsessive-compulsive personality. As already mentioned, both obsessive neurotics and obsessive personalities may be associated with phobic anxiety, but rarely are patients with obsessive character traits or obsessive neuroses associated with the hysterical personality or the hysterical neurosis.

Obsessions and Depression

There are frequent reports concerning the relationship between obsessive personality traits and the appearance of depressive neuroses and psychoses, as well as the frequent occurrence of obsessive symptoms during both psychotic and neurotic depressions. Obsessions may appear episodically or cyclically, much as manic-depressive psychosis does, as well as during intervals between manic-depressive cycles. In fact, Tokes[30] points out that many recurrent obsessional episodes

probably mask an underlying psychotic depression, inasmuch as these individuals show other symptoms characteristic of this disorder, such as diurnal variations, poor appetite, weight loss, and early morning wakening.

This relationship between obsessions and depression has been investigated extensively by Gittleson[9] in 359 patients with depressive psychosis. He points out that in the literature only 3.5 percent of schizophrenics are reported to have obsessive symptoms, while between 5.4 to 23 percent of psychotic depressions are associated in some way with obsessive symptoms or character traits. Gittleson found that 42 percent of his patients with depressive psychosis had obsessional personalities (although not necessarily obsessional symptoms) prior to the onset of their depressive episodes, and that 31.2 percent of the patients with depressive psychosis were obsessive during their depressive episodes. Of the individuals with a premorbid history of obsessional sysmptoms, 75 percent continued with these symptoms during the depressive episodes, while 25 percent of the psychotic depressive patients developed obsessive symptoms for the first time during their depression. In the psychotic depressives, shifts from obsessional thoughts to delusional ideas occurred in 5.3 percent; when this occurred, the individual was more likely to make a suicidal attempt. In fact, Gittleson felt that obsessive-compulsive symptoms during depression seemed to have some protective effect against suicide. However, the content of the obsession during depressive episodes was often of a suicidal or homicidal nature. Gittleson noted the greater incidence of depersonalization among patients with psychotic depression with premorbid obsessive symptoms, which suggests that many American psychiatrists might consider this group not as psychotic depressives but as schizophrenics.

Obsessions and Schizophrenia

Both Straus[28] and Rado (Part A) pointed out the frequency with which extreme obsessive symptoms are really a manifestation of an underlying schizophrenic process. Straus considered those obsessives preoccupied with contamination as probably representing a basic schizophrenic process wherein the individual has an underlying deficit in his pleasurable emotions. This is a concept similar to Rado's belief that anhedonia is common to both the obsessive-compulsive neurotic and the schizophrenic. Rado added that if there were a further deficit in body image, due to proprioceptive deficits, schizophrenic behavior was likely. The contradictory nature of some of the genetic studies to be described may be due to the failure to distinguish between the schizophrenic with obsessive-compulsive symptoms and the true obsessive-compulsive neurotic. Identifying the schizophrenic obsessive-compulsive is extremely important because it considerably modifies prognosis and treatment. For instance, dramatic improvements have been noted in obsessives on phenothiazine regimens, probably reflecting obsessives with an underlying schizophrenic process. Here, the phenothiazines would modify the underlying schizophrenic process and hence the obsessive symptomatology, which was a defense against the underlying schizophrenic disorganization. It is important to realize that obsessive-compulsive symptomatology appears in the schizophrenic long before overt schizophrenic symptoms develop; seldom, if ever, does an overtly schizophrenic patient suddenly develop obsessive-compulsive symptoms. The obsessive-compulsive schizophrenic soon loses his insight into the meaninglessness of his obsessions. His behavior becomes increasingly disorganized and delusional, so that perhaps bills go unpaid, while his paychecks are hidden in drawers because of persecutory ideas; the house becomes a shambles, and despite compulsive washing, bed linen and clothes remain unchanged for months. With the final disorganization, one can see such extreme behavior as an individual who fears contamination standing in a pan of Lysol, while smearing feces on the wall. By the time such behavior develops, there is usually no question of the underlying

schizophrenia, as there are accompanying hallucinations, delusions, and disorganization in cognitive functioning.

Obsessions and Chronic Brain Syndrome

Obsessive-compulsive symptoms are also defenses utilized in the chronic organic brain syndrome as an attempt to deny illness or intellectual deficits. For instance, if such an individual is asked to perform beyond his diminishing capacity, his behavior becomes abnormally rigid, stereotyped, and compulsive. He prefers to remain in a familiar environment with a familiar life style, preoccupied with mundane activities. Such defensive obsessiveness is also seen in some impulsive patients who control their unacceptable impulses, although often unsuccessfully, by being rigid, conventional, cold, calculating, pedantic, and meticulous; and in some patients with underlying epileptic mechanisms, who likewise have difficulty in controlling their emotions and impulsive aggressiveness, except through obsessive mechanisms. In most instances, such patients show little resistance to their obsessive behavior. Thus, their behavior is not felt as being forced to do something against their will, but they accept their rituals as natural behavior which strengthens their weak control mechanisms. In these individuals, the obsessive behavior is egosyntonic, as in the obsessive personality disorder, whereas in the obsessive neurotic the behavior is ego-alien.[19]

Obsessions in Childhood

Frequently the first attack of obsessive symptoms occurs in childhood or adolescence. The behavior is in no way different from that of the adult obsessive-compulsive neurotic. However, Anna Freud[4] and other psychoanalysts point out that children usually show symptoms that resemble those of the obsessional neurosis. These occur during the anal phase of development and are not strictly speaking neurotic, because they occur during the course of progressive development rather than as a consequence of regression. Such symptoms, during the first five years of life, occur more as a pleasant game than as a compelling activity to avoid anxiety. Anna Freud, in commenting on children who develop a true obsessional neurosis, suggests that such symptoms during childhood and adolescence (6-15 years of age) seem to be related to a precocious ego development with "distancing" of the ego functions from the drives; that is, there appears to be a premature intellectuality that leads to a particular perceptual and cognitive style.[25] The regression in ego function which occurs in the childhood obsessive neurosis is not the type seen in childhood psychoses; that is, what the psychoanalysts call a "structural" ego regression. However, both the concepts of functional ego regression and premature intellectuality need considerable elaboration if they are to have heuristic value in explaining the development of the obsessional neuroses.

❲ The Genetics of Obsessive Behavior

One way to establish that a psychiatric syndrome is best understood within the disease model is to identify a genetic predisposition for the syndrome. This now seems relatively well established for schizophrenia, manic-depressive psychosis, epilepsy, and some of the episodic behavioral disorders associated with epilepsy. It is a frequent clinical observation that one of the parents, usually the mother of the obsessive-compulsive neurotic, has had obsessive-compulsive personality traits, but it is not surprising that a mother preoccupied with cleanliness should exaggerate what Rado calls the "battle of the chamber pot." One way to resolve the nature-nurture complexities of the family relationship is to express the heritability of the syndrome in terms of the monozygotic–dizygotic twin concordance ratios. For instance, in schizophrenia, this ratio ranges from 6.1 to 3.1 and relatively high ratios have been established for

personality disorders (3.6) and psychophysiologic disorders (3.5). The importance of genetic factors in psychoneurotic disease is low, with a monozygotic–dizygotic ratio of only 1.3, similar to the ratios found in bacterial pneumonia (1.7) and fractures (1.5).[21] Of all the psychoneurotic disorders, it is more frequently reported that obsessive behavior has a significant genetic determinant. Other studies seem to contradict these findings, which may be due to their failure to strictly differentiate the obsessive-compulsive neurosis from the obsessive symptoms in schizophrenia or depressive reactions, both diseases with important genetic factors.

In a family study of 144 cases of strictly defined obsessional neurotics, Rosenberg[23] evaluated 574 first-degree relatives and found only two instances of obsessional neuroses among the relatives, even though there was a prevalence of varied psychiatric illness among the first-degree relatives of 9.3 percent. Consequently, Rosenberg felt that this study did not support the view that the obsessional personality or classic obsessional neurosis had significant genetic determinants. Sakai[24] investigated family pedigrees of a number of pathological conditions and came to the conclusion that in uncomplicated obsessions, that is, clear-cut obsessional neuroses, there was no hereditary predisposition, but in the complicated group where it was not clear whether it was a pure obsessional neurosis, there was often a family history of either epilepsy, manic-depressive psychosis, or schizophrenia. This probably reflects the fact that the obsessive symptoms were a pathological variation of the basic disorder.

In two in-depth studies of two pairs of monozygotic twins concordant for obsessive neurosis,[20,31] the twins were concordant not only for the type of symptoms but also for severity of symptoms and course of illness. All had early onset, fluctuating course, as well as exacerbation and remission of symptoms. They recognized that the obsessions were silly, but demonstrated endless ruminations, checking and rechecking, multiple phobias, and minimal feelings of depersonalization and derealization, which would have suggested a basic schizophrenic process. Even the investigators, however, doubted that this was adequate evidence for a hereditary predisposition in obsessive illness, and if there was a genetic factor, it was complex "which did not admit to present analysis."

(Course of Illness

It is frequently said that the obsessive-compulsive individual has a poor prognosis, particularly if therapy is initiated may years after the appearance of the first symptoms. However, the few long-term studies available suggest that this is not true if one carefully distinguishes between the obsessive neurotic and other disorders with obsessive symptoms. The over-all improvement rates for the true obsessional neurotic are 60 to 70 percent, a rate similar to that of other neuroses.

Pollit[22] studied a group of classical obsessive neurotics after excluding patients with obsessional personality disorders, with other neurotic reactions such as anxiety states, as well as those patients with obsessional symptoms occurring in the course of depression or schizophrenia. Meeting these criteria were 150 patients, representing fewer than 2 percent of those seen either as inpatients or outpatients. In two-thirds of these individuals the course was episodic, with most attacks lasting for less than one year. Symptoms were more likely to appear between the ages of six and twenty-five years of age (68 percent), with only 4 of the 150 developing symptoms for the first time after age forty-five. Thus, there appeared to be decreasing risk with increasing age. The symptoms were often precipitated by environmental events, particularly sexual traumata.

Grimshaw,[10] in a study of 100 cases seen six to fourteen years after the original diagnoses, found that 64 percent of this group improved both in terms of symptom disappearance and social functioning. Of the group, 40 percent were considered recovered or very considerably improved, and 77 percent maintained their pre-illness adjustment in that they were

working at their normal level. Of the patients who recovered socially, 13 percent remained symptomatically unchanged or even worse.

(Treatment

There have been enthusiastic reports on the treatment of obsessive-compulsive symptoms utilizing psychoanalysis, briefer forms of insight therapy, supportive therapy, electroconvulsive therapy, both major and minor tranquilizers, and even lobotomy. However, in Grimshaw's study, where 31 patients received electro-shock treatment, 14 insight psychotherapy, 36 supportive psychotherapy often reinforced with medication, 3 lobotomy, and 16 no treatment, there appeared to be no significant difference in the recovery rates among these groups, nor were their recovery rates significantly different from those found in the literature supporting one or another specific therapy. In those patients who spontaneously improved without treatment, the author usually noted some significant environmental change. In view of the episodic nature of the neurotic obsessive, as well as the high spontaneous recovery rate, it would appear that drastic therapies are not indicated unless these rest on the diagnosis of an underlying mental illness with superimposed obsessive symptoms. Antidepressant drugs or ECT might be considered if the obsessive symptoms are significantly associated with depressive reactions; the major tranquilizers or even lobotomy indicated if the underlying process is schizophrenic. For the obsessive neurotic in his first episode, it would seem that supportive psychotherapy would be the treatment of choice, with more intensive psychotherapy if the symptoms failed to respond within one year.

It is the impression of older psychiatrists that obsessive-compulsive neurosis, as well as other structured neuroses, such as conversion and phobias, are now seen considerably less often than in the first half of this century, although there are no rigorous data to support this observation. If our psychodynamic concepts are correct, this should be the case, as the residuals of Victorian child-rearing practices have been replaced by more permissive methods. Perhaps the price one pays for less neurosis is more delinquency and drug dependency. The ideal preventive child-rearing practice would be avoiding extreme permissiveness on the one hand, and authoritative attempts to enforce behavioral controls before the child's neuromuscular and intellectual development is capable of responding to these attempts on the other. We now have considerable data establishing maturational levels, so that we can delay toilet training until the lower bowel is capable of responding to enforced discipline from parents, and such discipline can be initiated after the height of the normal negativistic phase in the child's development. Whether there is a genotypical excessive fear-rage pattern associated with a deficit in pleasure responses that make an individual highly susceptible to the development of obsessive behavior, regardless of an enlightened child-rearing practice, is not clear, but this has been proposed by both Straus[28] and Rado (Part A). If so, perhaps the best solution would be specific psychopharmacologic agents which would reduce fear-rage affects or increase pleasurable ones, thus reducing the risk of subsequent obsessive symptoms. In fact, Straus makes the interesting suggestion that a substance such as marijuana might increase what he calls the "sympathetic" emotions of warmth, growth, peace, and love. Now, that the active tetrahydrocannabinols have been identified and pharmacologic activity correlated with specific molecular structure, this hypothesis could be systematically investigated.

It is reported that between 60 to 80 percent of obsessives respond well to psychoanalysis or insight psychotherapy. This would not be impressive in view of the reported spontaneous improvement rates, except that where detailed clinical data are given, one has the impression that the psychoanalytic patients were much more severe obsessive neurotics than those in the general sample of patients attending outpatient clinics. However, even the psychoanalyst recognizes that the obsessive patient presents unusual resistances to classical psychoanalytic techniques, due to several factors: First, the routine of therapy itself becomes just another ritual for the obsessive; second, the emphasis on insight in the psychoanalytic setting can be distorted by the obsessive's defenses of intellectualization and rationalization. To circumvent this, Rado suggests facilitating cathartic expression of rage and fear in "the memory content of the original cast and experiences that provoked them," and then once composure has been regained, show why the patient behaved as he did and how healthy people would have behaved in similar circumstances. Rado suggests that to help control the rage and fear once uncovered, one should teach the patient simple hypnoidal relaxation techniques. In this way, the patient first faces his fear and rage, learns from where they derive, and then conquers them through relaxation rather than through suppression. One technique I have found useful for facilitating this cathartic expression of fear and rage is a simple variation in the treatment setting. The therapist's behavior, unlike that in the usual psychoanalytic setting, should not be consistent or neutral, but varied. One day the therapist can be verbally active, on another silent. Still another time, one rushes to the patient and shakes his hand in greeting, the next time one remains taciturn and aloof upon the patient's arrival. One can rearrange the furniture, utilize varied seating arrangements, or sometimes seat the patient vis-à-vis, other times put the patient on the couch. This is particularly useful when one is treating an obsessive-compulsive personality disorder; that is, when the obsessive's behavior is egosyntonic. Such techniques seem drastic by usual psychoanalytic standards, but are far less drastic than ECT or lobotomy now utilized in chronic, severe obsessive-compulsive neurotics who are not responding to psychotherapy.

(Bibliography

1. Boss, M. *Psychoanalysis and Daseinanalysis.* New York: Basic Books. 1963.
2. BROCK, W., ed. *Existence and Being.* Chicago: Henry Regnery Co., 1949.

3. FENICHEL, O. *The Psychoanalytic Theory of Neurosis.* New York: W. W. Norton, 1945.

4. FREUD, A. *Normality and Pathology in Childhood.* New York: International Universities Press, 1965.

5. ———. "Obsessive Compulsive Neurosis," *International Journal of Psycho-Analysis,* 47 (1965), 230–235.

6. FREUD, S. *A General Introduction to Psychoanalysis.* New York: Liveright, 1935.

7. GABE, S. "Genetic Terminance of Compulsive Phenomena in Character Formation," *Journal of American Psychoanalytic Association,* 13 (1965), 591.

8. GEBSATTEL, V. E. VON. "The World of the Compulsive," in R. May, E. Angel, and H. F. Ellenberger, eds., *Existence: A New Dimension in Psychiatry and Psychology.* New York: Basic Books, 1958.

9. GITTLESON, N. L. "Phenomenology of Obsessions in Depressive Psychosis," *British Journal of Psychiatry,* 112 (1966), 253–259, 261–264, 705–708, 883–887.

10. GRIMSHAW, L. "The Outcome of Obsessional Disorder: Follow-up Study of 100 Cases," *British Journal of Psychiatry,* 111 (1965), 1051–1056.

11. HEIDEGGER, M. "What is Metaphysics?" in W. Brock, ed., *Existence and Being.* Chicago: Henry Regnery Co., 1949.

12. ———. *Being and Time.* New York: Harper's, 1962.

13. HENDERSON, D., and I. R. C. BATCHELOR. *Textbook of Psychiatry.* New York: Oxford University Press, 1962.

14. JASPERS, K. *General Psychopathology.* Chicago: University of Chicago Press, 1963.

15. KARDINER, A., A. KARUSH, and L. OVERSEY. "A Methodological Study of Freudian Theory: IV. The Structural Hypothesis, The Problem of Anxiety, and Post-Freudian Ego Psychology," *Journal of Nervous and Mental Disease,* 129 (1959), 341–356.

16. LAUGHLIN, H. P. *The Neuroses.* Washington: Butterworths, 1967.

17. MACKINNON, R. A., and R. MICHELS. *The Psychiatric Interview in Clinical Practice.* Philadelphia: W. B. Saunders Co., 1971.

18. MONROE, R. R. "The Compulsive," in E. W. Straus, and R. M. Griffith, eds., *Phenomenology of Will and Action.* Pittsburgh: Duquesne University Press, 1968.

19. ———. *Episodic Behavioral Disorders: A Psychodynamic and Neurophysiologic Analysis.* Cambridge: Harvard University Press, 1970.

20. PARKER, N. "Close Identification in Twins Discordant for Obsessional Neurosis," *British Journal of Psychiatry,* 110 (1964), 181–182.

21. POLLIN, W., G. MARTIN, A. HOFFER, J. R. STABENAU, and Z. HRUBEC. "Psychopathology in 15,909 Pairs of Veteran Twins: Evidence for a Genetic Factor in the Pathogenesis of Schizophrenia and Its Relative Absence in Psychoneurosis," *The American Journal of Psychiatry,* 126 (1969), 597–611.

22. POLLIT, J. "Natural History of Obsessional States: A Study of 150 Cases," *British Medical Journal,* 1 (1957), 194–198.

23. ROSENBERG, C. M. "Familial Aspects of Obsessional Neurosis," *British Journal of Psychiatry,* 113 (1967), 405–413.

24. SAKAI, T. "Clinical Genetic Study on Obsessive Compulsive Neurosis," in H. Mitsuda, ed., *Clinical Genetics in Psychiatry.* Tokyo: Igaku Shoin, 1967.

25. SANDLER, J., and W. G. JOFFE. "Note on Obsessional Manifestations in Children," *The Psychoanalytic Study of the Child,* 20 (1965), 425–438.

26. SPIEGELBERG, H. *The Phenomenological Movement.* The Hague: Martinus Nijhoff, 1960.

27. STRASSER, S. *Phenomenology and the Human Sciences.* Pittsburgh: Duquesne University Press, 1963.

28. STRAUS, E. W. *On Obsessions: A Clinical and Methodological Study.* New York: Nervous and Mental Disease Monographs, 1948.

29. TILLICH, P. *The Courage To Be.* New Haven: Yale University Press, 1952.

30. TOKES, E. "Recurrent Obsessional Episodes as a Symptom of Underlying Depression," *Psychiatric Quarterly,* 42 (1968), 352.

31. WOODRUFF, R., and F. N. PITTS. "Monozygotic Twins with Obsessional Neurosis," *The American Journal of Psychiatry,* 120 (1964), 1075–1080.

CHAPTER 10

OTHER CHARACTER-PERSONALITY SYNDROMES: SCHIZOID, INADEQUATE, PASSIVE–AGGRESSIVE, PARANOID, DEPENDENT

Leon Salzman

THIS GROUP OF DISORDERS is characterized by maladaptive patterns of behavior that are not sufficiently definite or severe to be considered neurotic or psychotic syndromes. While there are generally no particular symptoms associated with each of these syndromes, the disorders involve an exaggeration or accentuation of the individual's personality structure, so that they may be incapacitating or so extreme as to focus attention on these character traits and thereby create anxiety. In contrast to the neuroses where the symptoms are ego-alien, in the character disorders the behavior or character traits are in general ego-syntonic and only occasionally maladaptive.

In recent years, this type of problem has constituted the major bulk of the psychotherapeutic practice of psychiatrists and psychologists, in spite of the fact that these character traits can be assets. The absence of crises or severe anxiety makes the seeking-out and follow-through in psychotherapy more difficult. In therapy, the character traits themselves constitute the resistance to the elaboration, clarification, and alteration of the character disorders. This observation was a major contribution of Wilhelm Reich to psychoanalytic theory and practice.

In general, the diagnostic categories that delineate these patients are defined by the characteristic ways in which the individual functions and deals with his anxiety. While these patterns may not constitute the total personality structure, the label generally applies to the predominant defense mechanism which characterizes the individual's functioning and which is producing difficulties in his living sufficient to require psychiatric assistance. Consequently, the labels refer not to any disorder as such, but to the prevailing technique that the individual uses to deal with his anxieties.

The Diagnostic and Statistical Manual of the American Psychiatric Association describes this category as follows:

V. Personality Disorders and Certain Other Non-Psychotic Mental Disorders (301–304) 201— Personality Disorders

This group of disorders is characterized by deeply ingrained maladaptive patterns of behavior that are perceptibly different in quality from psychotic and neurotic symptoms. Generally, these are life-long patterns, often recognizable by the time of adolescence or earlier. Sometimes the pattern is determined primarily by malfunctioning of the brain, but such cases should be classified under one of the non-psychotic organic brain syndromes rather than here.

(Character Disorder Syndromes

It is useful to conceive of these syndromes as part of a spectrum ranging from the normal to the psychotic. The characteristic or enduring pattern which becomes involved in the character disorder is often the typical technique that the individual uses to deal with stress. A variety of other mechanisms may also be employed, but these disorders are labeled by the major defense pattern that is utilized. Therefore, these syndromes are not pure instances of a particular character structure, but generally do contain defense techniques of a wide variety. In addition, the syndromes represent

disorders of functioning where the particular patterns of behavior have become more pronounced and intrusive than they might be in a more healthy adaptation, but less extreme and disruptive than they might be in a neurotic or psychotic disorganization of functioning.

This situation can be exemplified in examining the range of obsessional functioning extending from the normal to the neurotic. At one extreme is a minimum of obsessional patterns, such as minor rituals or rigid prescribed modes of behaving that are barely noticeable under ordinary circumstances. At the other extreme, the patterns are so pervasive and intrusive, such as extreme doubting, procrastination, or indecision, as to interfere with productive living. In the first instance, which we might view as normal, these obsessional defenses may even enhance one's performance. At the opposite extreme, they may produce neurotic or psychotic behavior and may seriously impair one's capacity for living. Between these two extremes are the more or less obsessional defenses, which can be identified as the cluster of behavioral patterns we call the obsessional personality.

Differentiating between manifestations of obsessional traits of behavior and an obsessional personality is a matter of consistency and the extent of the pattern's involvement with the individual's total life. While admittedly such a distinction is extremely difficult to make, it is important in our concerns about managing such problems. The label "obsessional personality" refers to a widespread, fairly cohesive set of obsessional traits in a person whose behavior patterns are fixed and durable, and can be predicted with some degree of accuracy. The consistency and durability of such behavior involves a more integrated and pervasive use of obsessional mechanisms than is generally found in the occasional bits of obsessional behavior that might occur in all personality structures.

The distinction between the obsessional personality and the obsessional neurotic is in the area of differing functional capacity. As long as an individual remains productive, even though he might be involved in extensive rituals or other obsessive behavior, he would not be considered neurotic. The label "neurotic" refers not only to a clinical syndrome characterized by specific, definable limits, but also to behavior that becomes maladaptive or runs counter to the community's standard for what is acceptable. The individual might behave strangely or impress some people as being odd, but as long as he is integrated and functioning effectively he need not be considered neurotic.

It is common to find even severe character-disordered individuals functioning effectively in settings in which their "queerness" and unconventional attitudes may be noticed by all. Either because of the sympathetic good will of the community or colleagues, or because of their contributions or value to the community, since they are generally regarded as good workers, they may be retained on the job. It is only when some untoward event or personal crisis occurs and aggravates their characterological patterns that these individuals require psychiatric assistance.

Such an instance was true in the case of an electronics engineer who was a totally undisciplined worker. He would arrive at and depart from his plant according to his own schedule, and on many occasions he would work through the night. He was meticulously precise, and had some hand-washing compulsions, as well as a total inability to settle for anything less than a perfect performance at the job. While his lack of discipline tended to disrupt the laboratory routine, the management was extremely sympathetic and even increased his hourly pay. Periodically, his preciseness and passion for order would resolve some hitherto unsolvable circuitry problem.

Shortly after his marriage, his performance became more erratic and unreliable. As his professional behavior became more extreme and undisciplined, his performance on the job became markedly disruptive. What had been considered merely odd and queer was now labeled as a character disorder that required therapy.

Another instance is that of a mathematician whose job did not require him to punch a timeclock or to follow a set routine. However, he was expected periodically to file a report on the current status of his project. He worked in a large "think tank" with a great number of brilliant scientists and technicians. While he was unusually talented and respected by his superiors, his character structure and typical personality tendencies soon became apparent and disruptive. His indecisiveness, procrastination, and anxiety about perfect performance made it impossible for him to complete any task. While such difficulties were evident in every aspect of his life, he had managed a fairly successful career until he was hired by this high-level scientific laboratory that made concrete demands on him. He came to therapy on his own volition, finally acknowledging that his indecisiveness was too extreme to be rationalized even as scientific caution. Thus, what were for a long time only personality traits congealed into a typical character structure produced sufficient complications in his living to require therapy, even though no particular neurotic or psychotic development could be identified.

While most of the existing categories of character-personality syndromes are of this order, that is, the less extreme manifestations of defined neurotic or psychotic disorders, some are not. The paranoid, cyclothymic, schizoid, obsessive-compulsive, or hysteric personality character syndromes are examples of the above. However, other personality character syndromes are merely descriptive entities unrelated to specific neurotic or psychotic disorders. Such categories as the explosive-asthenic, antisocial, or passive-aggressive character disorders are recognizable entities by virtue of the prevailing techniques and ways of orienting the individual in satisfying his needs.

Personality types are therefore defined either in terms of the underlying psychodynamics or the persistence and intrusiveness of the major integrating trait of the individual. At other times, the personality may be delineated by the community's reaction to such behavior, such as in the antisocial or psychopathic personality. It is apparent that these categories do not represent disease entities of illness as defined by a medical model of cause, pathology, and specific treatment. The cluster of traits that have a dynamic relationship to one another can often be ascribed to particular developmental experiences or to somatic origins, but our diagnostic manual does not limit its categories to such personalities.

(Personality Character Syndromes

Schizoid Personality

The behavior pattern of such individuals is described in the APA Diagnostic Manual as follows:

This behavior pattern manifests shyness, oversensitivity, seclusiveness, avoidance of close or competitive relationships, and often eccentricity. Autistic thinking without loss of capacity to recognize reality is common, as is daydreaming and the inability to express hostility and ordinary aggressive feelings. These patients react to disturbing experiences and conflicts with apparent detachment.

These individuals have a tendency to avoid close or long-term relationships. They have a limited repertory of adaptive techniques and their typical maneuver for adaptation is withdrawal, both interpersonally and psychically. Such personalities may have genetic and constitutional ingredients as an integral part of the syndrome, and this disposition may account for the experiential effects which are manifested so early in their lives. The beginnings may be noted in infancy where individual variations, such as autism, may be noted, and the tendency to move away from any difficulties rather than meeting them. In the developmental years, they tend to avoid socializing with peers and other children, as well as adults, or else tend to limit their contacts to known members of their immediate family. This type of schizoid personality is called the "shut-in personality," and while it does not necessarily precede schizophrenia, it frequently does. Those who become schizoid are shy, well-behaved, and easily managed children, although they are markedly sensitive to rejection or displeasure. They are rarely aggressive or assertive, but can easily imagine real or fantasied assaults on themselves. There is a tendency towards some grandiose feelings of omnipotence, which may be expressed or remain detached and aloof, and they give the appearance of being disinterested, isolated, and resigned to their state. In childhood and adolescence, this type of individual appears to be the outsider; a noncompetitor who does not make physical contact and remains distinct and isolated from his group. He may be talented and very bright in school, and have a large number of hobbies that separate and distinguish him from his peers. Emotionally, such individuals appear to be detached, cold, and uninvolved in people, although they may be intensely committed or involved in intellectual projects or pursuits. Such intensity may result in considerable personal success and achievement, yet they remain odd and isolated in spite of it. They generally find some kind of solace in philosophical movements or in idealistic enterprises that do not require involvement with other people, only with ideas. Mature sexuality is postponed because of their inability to form any kind of intimate relationship, particularly with the opposite sex. Consequently, they often limit their nonsexual intimacies to people of the same sex, and often set up homosexual relations when the gonadal pressures push for some sexual outlet. They are not necessarily homosexual, even though they may limit their activity, being unable to initiate heterosexual relationships. These difficulties are aggravated by the disturbed relations within the family, which also prevent the resolution of their adolescent ties to the family, and they therefore have difficulty in making moves towards separation and individuation. If they marry, they tend to remain uninvolved, and the communication with the partners is limited. Such marriages may be successful if the partners do not make excessive demands on each other, both socially or sexually. The best relationships under these circumstances are those in which the marital partners live separate lives while sharing some mutual activities. Schizoid characters seek out therapy generally because some crisis disrupts what are their minimal patterns of functioning. Whether it is the death of a person involved in their integration in the real world, or the disruption or interruption of a fragile or tenuous intimacy, it is an event that prevents the individual from functioning.

Treatment is therefore difficult since the ego resources are limited. The danger of a schizophrenic disintegration is always present, so that caution and concern must be an integral part of the treatment process.

Inadequate Personality

This type of personality is not directly related to any psychiatric syndrome or mental disorder, and describes a type of individual who cannot meet or cope with life's demands and requirements. He is unable to meet the challenges of living, either on social or professional terms, and therefore represents a description of an immature development without any particular psychopathology. The APA Diagnostic Manual describes the category as follows:

This behavior pattern is characterized by ineffectual responses to emotional, social, intellectual and physical demands. While the patient seems neither physically nor mentally deficient, he does manifest inadaptability, ineptness, poor judgment, social instability and lack of physical and emotional stamina.

This description could be applied to the diagnosis of simple schizophrenia and in fact is often confused with it. However, the capacity to relate and to be motivated is available in these individuals and, even though their personal resources are few, they are more amenable to individual psychotherapy than the schizophrenic. In addition, their relationships are more involved and intense, and while they appear to have little drive or interest, they do not energetically pursue isolation and noninvolvement as the schizoid individual does.

The assignment of this label to a particular individual is often a reflection of a value judgment of the interviewer. His standards and goals for successful living will play an essential role in the determination of such a character syndrome. The highly motivated, ambitious, and active psychiatrist might label

as an "inadequate personality" the less energetic and less competitive adolescent or adult who seems content to remain at a minimum level of functioning. The psychiatrist who adopts the cultural norms for achievement, success, work, and participation as psychiatric norms may confuse prejudice with scientific judgment, since his unneurotic, unambitious patient may be a healthy, uncompetitive individual rather than one who has neurotic fears of failure. What appears to be inadequate in the West may be appropriately healthy in the East. Consequently, this category has many cultural issues and may reflect the parental concern for a child who does not conform. This discrepancy is often the reason for the referral of these individuals for therapy. Unless the patient can accept his behavior as maladaptive for him, and not merely an instance of not conforming to the existing "system" or establishment, no change or movement can occur.

Clinically and objectively, the inadequate personality is generally deficient in emotional and physical energy, and at times resembles the classical descriptions of neurasthenia. He is socially inept, incapable, and disinterested in planning and carrying out activities of any kind. He lacks the push and the incentive to pursue even minor activities, and has an overly optimistic expectation that things will work out well without any effort or participation on his part. In this regard, he resembles the oral receptive character described by Freud, or the receptive character of Fromm, who is carefree, indifferent, and permanently optimistic. He expects to be nourished by some magical helper, and therefore feels no need for activity towards pursuing independent goals or establishing a base for future financial security. He has an expectation of an eternal, never-ending source of nourishment and care.

Consequently, his responses to all sorts of stimuli are weak, and his social adjustment is marginal. He tends to drift from job to job, unable to set up strong, meaningful relationships, and tends to be overlooked in the crowd since he makes no particular impact on anything or anyone. The diagnosis is generally made in terms of his inability to make proper and adequate social relationships or to make any occupational adjustments. Being affectively shallow, he displays little enthusiasm, interest, or drive in any direction, which conveys the impression of a mental defective or a simple schizophrenic.

The onset and development of such restricted personality structure seem to be related to deprivation of a realistic nature involved in poverty, and social disadvantage or sensory deprivation at all levels of social and financial status. There is a widespread inhibitory process that seems to dampen even the minimal thrusts and drives towards fulfillment. Even the pleasure-seeking activities are reduced in the overriding inhibitory restraints on effective and assertive action. A vicious circle is initiated, sustained, and enlarged when inability to achieve and obtain gratification from activities maintains the state of inadequacy. This leads to a widening circle of inaction, which interferes with further learning and maturation.

Passive-Aggressive Personality

This personality structure is frequently applied to individuals who attempt to fulfill their needs by controlling and manipulating others through a passive, nondoing kind of behavior. Such passivity is experienced by others as pushing and maneuvering, and therefore the totality of their behavior is described as aggressive. In this connection, aggression should not be confused with hostility, even though aggression is associated with hostility manifested covertly or overtly. These individuals may be hostile, but the label "passive-aggressive" must be understood as a way of achieving, fulfilling, or experiencing, in which passivity or nondoing mobilizes others into action. They generally are not hostile, although this group can be subdivided into subtypes in which hostility or extreme dependency is present, or where the expansive driving elements are in preponderance.

Characteristically, however, such individuals attempt to achieve their goals by achieving good will and acceptance through their pas-

sive, noncompetitive strivings. In this regard, they resemble the self-effacing personality described by Horney.

The APA Diagnostic Manual describes them as follows:

This behavior pattern is characterized by both passivity and aggressiveness. The aggressiveness may be expressed passively for example by obstructionism, pouting, procrastination, intentional inefficiency, or stubbornness. This behavior commonly reflects hostility which the individual feels he dare not express openly. Often the behavior is one expression of the patient's resentment at failing to find gratification in a relationship with an individual or institution upon which he is overdependent.

This personality type also resembles the oral and anal aggressive character types, who resent the demands made upon them and respond by active and willful refusal. There is an ease in regressing to a dependent state if their demands are unmet. At times, they resemble the stubborn, defiant anal aggressive tendencies in which one's needs are met by a tug of war whereby the other person is forced to yield. In this sense, this personality type is an exaggeration of a developmental trait that was the major way of fulfilling needs in early childhood. They could force action by their passive, defiant, and resistant behavior.

The personality type is closely related to the dependent personality, and his behavior is often explained as compliant and passive, because he is dependent and afraid to lose or destroy his benefactors. He cannot irritate or antagonize those individuals upon whom his sources of emotional and physical needs depend. Yet, his passive behavior often does precisely that, because of his cringing, spineless behavior. Under such circumstances, a crisis may occur, and these relationships may produce regressive reactions of a more infantile, passive, demanding kind. There may be passive threats of personal injury if their needs are not met.

At other times, if fulfillment is difficult, they become obstinate and petulant, and attempt to press their advantage by displays of childish pouting and complaining.

Generally, they appear to accept their life

situations, but privately they are very dissatisfied, and they accumulate grievances to demonstrate their unfulfilled and unrequited demands for love and acceptance. At these times, they may passively and covertly sabotage a job or relationship by their procrastinating, obstructionistic behavior. Unable to directly assert their needs or feelings, they covertly blame others. In therapy, unless this issue is resolved, it will result in a typical impasse in which to fulfill their demands is to accede to their pathology, while to refuse it is to reject them. This is the double-bind which often presents itself in treating this syndrome. Sometimes, the aggressive features of these individuals predominate, and they will be aggressively critical, hostile, demanding, and obnoxious. They relate almost exclusively in a contentious and contrary manner, which is rationalized in terms of a need to defend themselves against an unfriendly world. This tendency to overpower the environment is a way of providing some measure of security and self-esteem in the face of expected rejection and derogation. The passive quality in such aggressive behavior is often manifested by their reluctance to confront situations directly, but rather to achieve some dominance and authority by covert maneuvers under conditions where their aggressiveness has little chance of being challenged.

Dependent Personality

This type of individual relates to others by the plea of total helplessness and powerlessness. He strongly resembles the oral characters of Freud, the receptive characters described by Fromm, and fits into Horney's classification of the self-effacing character structure. Individuals of this type are unwilling, and ultimately become incapable of any independent judgment or decision. Rather than threaten their dependent relationships, they eschew any choice, decision, or judgment that does not arise from or is supported by their mainstay.

While it is often clear that their dependency is a way of controlling and manipulating others, overtly they appear to be powerless and incapable of sustaining themselves without the presence and active support of others. They tend to derive their significance and meaning as individuals only when they identify themselves with a person who is overvalued, or a cause that is generally overly idealized. They therefore go through life with a "clinging vine" adaptation. A parallel situation probably prevailed in the household during their formative years, where the one dominating member of the household supported the dependent parent and set a pattern for such a maneuver. Under these circumstances, the stronger member took on all the decisions, and permitted the dependent member a pseudosecurity through inaction and passivity. This model would be most effectively followed if the dependent parent maintained the position through reasonable and defensible rationalizations.

Such dependent attachments may be rewarding when they stimulate a benevolent response in others, but inevitably this attitude stirs up resentment and anger towards themselves.

While there is some cultural support for such dependencies, it is not experienced by the receiver as a productive or creative relationship. The dependent person covertly resents being dependent, and sometimes belittles and derogates the weakness of those he may be exploiting. Since such feelings may threaten the relationship, they are rarely expressed openly, but reveal themselves in many covert, subtle, and unconscious ways, such as slips of the tongue, accidental encounters, or simply by immobilizing others. There is a marked tendency towards the use of "magical helpers," either in the form of people or drugs. The typical alcohol or drug addict fits this personality configuration. His willingness to placate and accept a secondary role in living, prevents him from a full assertion of capacities and talents. This awareness is crucial in order to interest him in the therapy of his dependent personality. His greedy, insatiable, taking orientation leads to much guilt and self-derogation, which can also be utilized as motivating forces in initiating and sustaining the therapeutic process.

The Paranoid Personality

In this syndrome, the patient is characteristically suspicious, argumentative, and hypersensitive in interpersonal relations. He remains completely defensive, and in his defensiveness becomes overaggressive. Interpersonal distance is his usual stance and he may explode with anger and assaultiveness, or disintegrate if situations and relationships are pressed on him. There is great rigidity in his personality structure in order to maintain distance and constancy in his relations with others. When this becomes threatened, he becomes very angry and moves off. His tension and tightness are generally apparent to others, who respond by maintaining distance, both verbal and geographic. Frequently, his intellectual capacities are above average, and he appears to have a heightened memory for all events that he has interpreted as pieces of the malevolent atmosphere that surrounds him. Generally, his orientation is intact and his cognitive capacities unimpaired.

While paranoid personalities may have no delusions, they are constantly involved in referential thinking, which tends to view all life experiences as being imposed on them. They deal with the world as if there were a pattern and prevailing atmosphere of malevolence towards them. Because of their inability to accept any responsibility for their own feelings or behavior, they tend to externalize or project these feelings and respond as if others were accusing them of the very deficiencies and weaknesses they are trying to avoid recognizing. Generally, the accusations are attributed to individuals or groups that are significantly involved in the defensive attitudes or derogatory feelings in the first place.

These attitudes put them on the defensive, and they are constantly on the alert and easily translate external stimuli into personal references. Such perceptions may be visual, auditory, or kinesthetic, and may be real or imagined, or a misinterpretation of an incidental, accidental, or coincidental event.

Their suspiciousness extends to all areas of living but is particularly notable in their interpersonal relationships, which tend to be fragile and highly inflammable. Emotionally, they appear to be restrained, humorless, with an unwillingness to allow enough flexibility to view any phenomenon in an objective way. Rather, they insist on their views, and stubbornly resist giving up control or expressing minimal doubts and uneasiness. They store up abused feelings, which may explode in angry outbursts at unexpected times or places.

The frequent presence of jealousy protects them from any close involvements. While they may have many superficial relationships, they manage very few close ones. Characteristically, they work hard and are effective at their jobs, even though they may change jobs often because of their paranoid ideas. While there may be gradual personality deterioration, this does not necessarily occur, because the paranoid defensive structure is able to maintain distance and prevent closer involvements that threaten the fragile adaptation. Associated with their paranoid feelings, they may also have grandiose or exaggerated views of their importance or competence. This process of enhancement of self is directly related to the overwhelming sense of inferiority, worthlessness, incompetence, and incapacity. This grandiosity is a rationalization that is called upon to explain the exaggerated interest they feel is focused on them. This suggests and later becomes a conviction that they are of special importance or significance. The grandiose feelings most often precede the development of paranoid ideas and are restrained until the nonrecognition of their significance demands explanations, which are easily understood as jealous, hostile, or malevolent orientations towards them. Often the grandiosities are concomitant with and occur side by side with the paranoid feelings, and sometimes seem to follow the paranoid developments.

The development of this personality structure is closely related to the developmental mode of thinking, in which cause is related exclusively to the element of time relationships rather than to the causal agent. In this mode, which Sullivan called "parataxic," events are related because of their serial connection rather than any logical relationship.

Events that follow one another are thought to be related, regardless of their true relationship. If the thunder occurs when the door is shut, then the closing of the door is experienced as having produced the thunder. Similarly, if people laugh when one enters a room, the laughing is experienced as being related to one's entry into the room. The serial relationship in the parataxic mode of thinking establishes the relationship, not the examination of the true connection between the events. This mode of experiencing is common in human behavior, and it characterizes the distorted experiencing of the paranoid.

Developmentally, the paranoid personality occurs because of marked doubts, insecurities, and uncertainties in a family constellation where firm attachments, identifications, and the ability to separate oneself from the new environment, were most confused and incomplete. The atmosphere tended to reinforce any tendencies to blame others and deny one's own angry frustration or dependency. The tendency to externalize may be encouraged, and deficiencies and failure attributed to the malevolence of others, while the exaggerated, omnipotent, and grandiose conceptions of oneself are developed covertly. The prevailing doubts lend themselves in later years to the paranoid elaborations based on the feelings of uncertain acceptance of others. Some theories relate the presence of paranoid feelings to homosexual or latent homosexual patterns. However, in recent years, the difficulty in developing a clear gender identity is viewed as only one part of the massive over-all doubts about oneself. The aggressive assaults and suspicious accusations against others tend to sustain and nourish these doubts since they encourage actual rejection.

These individuals rarely need to come to therapy, except when some outburst takes place. In therapy, the extreme rigidity produces very little ability to correct any distortions. Since they fear and desire close relationships, a therapeutic alliance is extremely difficult to develop, and the presence of distrust and suspicion must be overcome by first raising some doubts about their point of view. When this occurs, then there is some hope of penetrating this rigid system. Since they expect derogatory responses, the therapist must be cautious in offering any tenderness. A straightforward, direct attitude must be adopted and followed.

(Treatment

The treatment of the character disorders does not differ essentially from the psychotherapeutic or psychoanalytic treatment of the neuroses. The nature of the character trait which may produce special issues in transference or countertransference phenomena must be taken into account. For example, the paranoid personality presents special difficulties in the area of trust, while the dependent personality will tend to parentify the transference immediately and throw the burden of the therapy on the therapist. Each personality will present particular issues that will need to be handled according to their manifest or covert presence in the therapeutic work.

In general, the therapy attempts to comprehend the character structure and elucidate its origins and functions. The tendency to establish simple causal relationships between character traits and certain childhood experiences, however, can be very misleading and not conducive to change. The initial impact of the development of character analysis was to alter the stress from the reconstruction of the past to the elucidation of the present modes of behavior of the individual. Although it does not obviate the need for genetic reconstruction, it is primarily concerned with the analysis of the structure of the defenses.

In elaborating the character structure of an individual, it is necessary to get a comprehensive view of how he functions and adapts in the present. This calls for a detailed presentation of his current experiencing in order to identify areas of anxiety and the ways the individual deals with these anxieties. Consequently, therapy proceeds in a more directed fashion, with immediate goals that are clear to the patient. The therapist is generally more active and may direct the patient to areas which he feels might be illuminating. Such activity is manifested by more frequent questions and interpretations, and a variety of devices, both verbal and nonverbal, designed to encourage the patient to see how his present patterns of behavior are contributing to his difficulties in living. The therapist's role becomes more than a mere facilitant to reliving the past; he becomes a collaborating partner.

In this give-and-take framework, transference becomes more than a mere revival of infant-parent relationship. It is viewed as a collection of distortions or characteristic attitudes toward a variety of people who have played meaningful and determining roles in one's life. Irrational attitudes can thus be explored through an understanding of their current adaptive value. Transference in this approach is also a major tool for therapy, since it allows for the most direct observation of the distorted attitudes that are developed in the course of maturing. In the relationship of the "here-and-now," the patient is forced to acknowledge that some of his attitudes toward the therapist do not arise out of a response to the therapist as he is, but to the therapist as the patient personifies him. Such an observation can open the way for a clarification of the distortion. The more current views on transference involve the recognition that many individuals besides the parents share in the development of these distortions. A patient's irrational hatred of the therapist arises not only from a hatred of his father, for example, but probably because of a series of relationships in which the patient has been abused and mistreated by authority figures. This leads him to expect malevolence from the analyst. In the intimacy of the therapeutic relationship, many opportunities will occur to produce this resentment. Transference would then be more than a mere repetition or transferring of feeling; it would be a dynamic process that represents and reproduces the effect of early experiencing on present behavior. The activity and lack of anonymity that characterize this type of therapeutic approach arise out of the theoretical conception that transference attitudes are more meaningful and revealing when they are produced through contact and experiencing than when they occur in a vacuum of pure fantasy.

Thus, the present tendency is not to limit or inhibit the therapist's activity or to prevent him from revealing facets of his own personality. Face to face encounters in terms of patients sitting up are more frequent and there is not such a strong taboo against activities outside the analytic hour. The role of activity may also involve a limitation of the free association technique which, while undoubtedly useful, can be abused by the patient and the therapist, thus destroying its value as an uncovering instrument. This notion has been supported by most ego analysts who use the free association technique with caution and judgment rather than as a required routine.

When the therapist takes a more active position and role, it becomes apparent that not all the patient's attitudes toward the therapist are irrational. Some of the patient's responses are realistic and rational attitudes toward the therapist, in terms of the kind of person he really is. While this was considered an artifact in orthodox analytic therapy, it has become apparent that the most stringent efforts of the analyst to remain incognito are largely impossible to achieve. In spite of all the safeguards, patients are able to discover many important pieces of data regarding their analyst through contact with him. There is a current tendency to distinguish transference responses from realistic responses. Such a distinction can serve the important function of increasing the patient's convictions regarding the significance of the transference reactions. It avoids the difficult task of convincing the patient that his attitude is irrational, when objective factors prove otherwise. Indirectly, it has lessened the authoritative atmosphere of the analytic situation and has permitted a realistic appraisal of the analyst, which is a vital need for someone who is already overburdened with distorted conceptions about others.

A most important outgrowth of the increase in activity of the therapist was the recognition and exploration of the role of countertransference in the therapeutic process.

The attitude of the therapist toward the patient can be a very powerful tool in elucidating the character structure of the patient. When the therapist is free, flexible, and willing to become involved and committed to the therapy, his reactions to the patient can illuminate character trends that would go unnoticed otherwise. Such reactions are most helpful in learning about the subtleties of the patient's activities.

When the goal of therapy extended beyond symptomatic relief to an attempt to reorganize the total character structure, the significance of the current functioning of the individual in his cultural setting became most important. From a characterological point of view, a patient is ill not because of experiences that occurred in childhood, but because such experiences still operate in the present to affect his personality and character structure. A patient may be dependent passive-aggresssive or paranoid, for example, or insecure or compulsive, not because he was unloved in childhood or infancy, but because his early experiences had so shaped his personality that in the present he is unable to be independent or to trust others. Consequently, the index of cure is not the degree of recall of early experience or certain traumatic events, but the capacity to function adequately in the present. Some theorists express this capacity in terms of an ability to relate to others without serious perceptual or conceptual distortions. Sullivan described this end state as the capacity to relate with a minimum of parataxic distortions where there is consensual validation of the patient's perceptions. Others describe health as the capacity to love and be loved, or the expression of the full potentialities of the individual. Such goals reflect a value system that conceives of man as capable of fulfilling the potentialities of a humanistic philosophical view of man's capabilities. Consequently, therapy can no longer evade the issue of values but must recognize its significance in the life of every human being. In addition, the current theoretical formulations recognize that the therapist, himself a product of the established mores and standards, cannot erase them from his own personality, nor should he attempt to do so. This accounts for our current extensive interest in countertransference phenomena. The therapist, being aware of these reactions, can refrain from imposing them on his patients.

The goals of therapy with individuals with personality-character disorders are to elucidate the functions of their particular personality structure, to free them to achieve their potentialities in a more mature and productive fashion. In each instance, the thwarting consequences of their earlier development must be viewed in the present, not only as an academic matter of insight, but also as a basis for a change in their behavior, which will be additional impetus to reconstruct their entire personality.

(Bibliography

1. *Diagnostic and Statistical Manual of Mental Disorders*, American Psychiatric Association, 2nd Edition.

2. FREUD, S. *Standard Edition, Complete Psychological Works of S. Freud.* London: Hogarth Press, 1959.

3. FROMM, E. *Man for Himself.* New York: Rinehart and Company, 1955.

4. HORNEY, K. *Neurosis and Human Growth.* New York: W. W. Norton and Company, 1950.

5. REICH, W. *Character Analysis.* New York: Orgone Institute Press, 1949.

6. SALZMAN, L. *Developments in Psychoanalysis.* New York: Grune and Stratton, 1962.

7. ————. *The Obsessive Personality.* New York: Science House, 1968.

8. SHAPIRO, D. *Neurotic Styles.* New York: Basic Books, 1965.

9. SULLIVAN, H. S. *Conceptions of Modern Psychiatry.* Washington, D.C.: William A. White Psychiatric Foundation, 1947.

PART THREE

Syndromes Associated with Action Directed Against the Environment

CHAPTER 11

EPISODIC BEHAVIORAL DISORDERS: AN UNCLASSIFIED SYNDROME

Russell R. Monroe

CLASSIFICATION OF SYNDROMES, which has had heuristic value for the general physician, is in current disrepute among psychiatrists and behavioral scientists. Even in general medicine, classifications have been devalued; for example, there are those who consider diabetes as an abstraction, since the physician is confronted with a diabetic patient rather than the disease "diabetes." Nevertheless, this abstraction is useful both to the physician in treating his diabetic patient, and to the patient who is thereby allowed certain attentions, without being labeled lazy, a malingerer, or hypochondriacal.

In psychiatry, labels have been less useful, and sometimes merely for social or political reasons, they are assigned to establish the social role "sick," without benefit to the person so labeled. Among professionals, there are two reactions to this: either to do away with labels

entirely, or to strive for a classification of behavior with precise etiologic, prognostic, and therapeutic implications. Such a pragmatic classification depends upon careful phenomenological analyses of symptoms and signs over a period of time, with a syndrome ultimately verifiable by precise laboratory methods. It is my contention that for most deviate behavior this disease model should not be discarded but, instead, refined and developed.

Many of our past failures in establishing a clinically useful classification result from neglect of the course of illness. Identifying the syndrome here discussed, episodic behavioral disorders, depends less on the manifest symptoms, but rather on the illness course—the symptoms occurring episodically with equally precipitous appearance and remission. I suggest that this characteristic course often reflects a neurophysiologic mechanism which has specific etiologic, prognostic, and therapeutic implications, despite the otherwise diverse manifestations of the syndrome. Episodic behavioral disorders should be considered as generically equivalent to such currently utilized diagnostic terms as organic brain syndrome, neurosis, personality disorder, "functional" psychosis, etc.[15]

The episodic behavioral disorders include subgroups: (1) those patients demonstrating disordered acts, referred to in the literature as "acting on impulse," "impulse neurosis," "irresistible impulse," or "acting out," which I designate *episodic dyscontrol*; and (2) episodic, psychotic, sociopathic, neurotic, and certain physiologic reactions, which I designate *episodic reactions*. The varied psychopathology covered by these previously poorly defined syndromes has been repeatedly described in the literature, although never officially labeled or included in the standard diagnostic manuals. However, the international classification (ICD-8) uses such labels as "reactive excitation," "reactive confusion," "reactive psychosis unspecified," "acute schizophrenic episodes," "depersonalization neurosis," "explosive personality," and "episodic drinking"; these probably concord with what I designate *episodic behavioral disorders*.

The common features of such diverse psychopathology are precipitous onset of symptoms, equally abrupt remission, as well as the tendency for frequent recurrences. These episodes represent interruptions in the life style and life flow of the individual, and involve either a single act or short series of acts with a single intention (episodic dyscontrol), or more prolonged behavioral disturbances with complex psychopathology and multiple dyscontrol acts (episodic reactions). The value in identifying these syndromes is the possibility of providing more effective treatment.

A brief discussion of psychopathology in general may clarify this point. During the course of human development, the individual's interaction with both his external and internal environments elicits an increasingly complex repertoire of behavioral responses, some successful, others not. Through this trial and error, aided by parental guidance and societal attitudes, the maturing individual learns that certain behavioral patterns are more successful than others; that is, more likely to be rewarded or reinforced, or at least more effective in avoiding pain and punishment. These patterns tend to be used repeatedly in similar or related situations until characteristic response patterns become established; these give the individual a unique "personality" or "character" and provide coherency and predictability to his "life style." Thus, close associates can usually predict how an individual will respond in a given situation. These consistent established patterns of psychological adaptation may be adaptive (healthy or normal) or maladaptive (disordered behavior, disease, or illness). Maladaptive patterns, identified as personality disorders, neuroses, or psychoses, all have an insidious development, a monotonous repetition in life patterns, as well as a persistence which often defies even heroic therapeutic efforts towards change. Even when acute exacerbations occur under stress, the symptoms are congruent with the previous life style and life history of the individual. For example, the obsessive character develops obsessive symptoms, the cyclothymic individual develops a depression or hypomania.

In episodic behavioral disorders the symptoms abruptly interrupt both the life style and life flow of the individual, with the disturbed behavior appearing as a break between the past and the future. The behavior is both out of context for the situation and out of character for the individual. Occasionally, episodic acts are adaptive; for example, the spontaneous act that may represent the unique contribution of the genius or the man of action. Usually, however, the abrupt precipitous acts are based on primitive emotions of fear, rage, or sensuous feelings, without concern for the effect on the immediate environment or the long-term consequences to the actor or society, and are either self- or socially destructive. These acts are often disinhibitions of behavior (in the motor sense), although there are also abrupt maladaptive responses that are inhibitions of action when action is necessary. Identifying and treating individuals with these disorders has particular social relevance, especially when episodic behaviors are sadistic or bizarre crimes, suicidal attempts, and aggressive or sexual acting out. Figure 11–1 summarizes these generalizations.

As mentioned previously, episodic disinhibition is further divided into two classes: episodic dyscontrol representing an abrupt single

the pragmatic implication that anticonvulsant medication may aid in the treatment of such patients.

A careful phenomenological analysis, with a detailed history, is usually sufficient to distinguish the characteristic episodic behavioral disorders from chronic, insidiously developing behavioral deviations. However, at times it

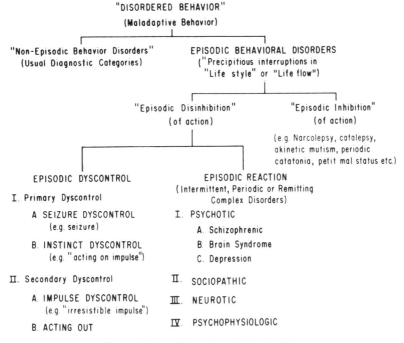

Figure 11–1. "Disordered behavior."

act or short series of acts with a common intention carried through to completion, with at least partial relief of tension or gratification of a specific need; and episodic reactions representing a more prolonged interruption in the life style and life flow of the individual, but also characterized by a precipitous onset and abrupt remission, as well as a tendency to recur. While episodic behavioral disorders may be superimposed on chronic, persisting psychopathology in other cases, behavior between episodes is relatively normal. The abruptness of appearance of symptoms, particularly when of short duration and accompanied by confusion and other signs of clouding of sensorium, strongly suggests a basic epileptoid mechanism involving circumscribed areas of excessive neuronal discharge. Neurophysiologic data support this hypothesis with

may be difficult to differentiate episodic behavioral disorders from the occasional acute "decompensation" to stress, or a persistent, impulsive life style. When differentiation is difficult, supplementary psychodynamic and neurophysiologic analyses may aid in making this discrimination. First, we will consider in detail the phenomenologic and psychodynamic aspects of episodic dyscontrol and reactions, and then we will consider the neurophysiologic differentiation.

(Episodic Dyscontrol

It is important in evaluating dyscontrol acts to establish the specificity of the drives or urges behind the act, the co-ordination and complexity of the motor behavior during the act, and the appropriateness of the motives or goals of the act. In doing so, one can identify more primitive dyscontrol acts (primary dyscontrol), and more sophisticated or complex dyscontrol acts (secondary dyscontrol). Primary dyscontrol is further divided into two levels, those of seizure dyscontrol and instinct dyscontrol, while secondary dyscontrol is divided into impulsive dyscontrol and acting-out dyscontrol.

Primary Dyscontrol—Seizure Dyscontrol

This is the most primitive dyscontrol act and is characterized by intense, indiscriminate affects, chaotic and unco-ordinated motor patterns, and indiscriminate selection of the object acted upon, often the person closest at hand. Little specific need gratification is apparent, although there is usually tension reduction. Often the intention of the act is completely lost and the effectiveness of the act very limited; in this way, seizure dyscontrol can be used consciously or unconsciously to abort higher level dyscontrol acts, where the intentions are obvious and at the same time unacceptable to the actor. A typical example of seizure dyscontrol is the post ictal confusional state often manifested by a mixture of fright-fight responses, as well as demands for closeness.

A fourteen-year-old boy patient had grand mal epilepsy since the age of eight months. The attacks most often occurred at night. When they occurred during the day, they were associated with extremely aggressive outbursts. Rarely were there aggressive episodes without a prior seizure. Typically, the person attacked was the individual closest at hand, who in some way had physical contact with the patient. For instance, the father trying to loosen the patient's belt following a grand mal seizure was assaulted by the boy who the moment before appeared unconscious. The boy, despite his small size, picked up his much larger father, threw him against the wall and then beat him unmercifully. This was sometimes accompanied by the indiscrim-

inate breaking of furniture. The boy's behavior was so frightening that it lead to hospitalization, where the aggressive outbursts continued, terrorizing other patients and ward personnel. The boy himself would say, following such episodes, "I cannot understand why I become so destructive, I don't know what gets into me." When asked as a young child by a psychiatrist what three wishes he would like, the last wish was "to be a good boy and not lose control."

Primary Dyscontrol—Instinctual Dyscontrol

This is a higher level of dyscontrol act in which the affects are more clearly differentiated (e.g., fear, rage, sensuality), and more effectively gratified. The motor pattern, although lacking in subtlety, is nonetheless efficient and co-ordinated. The object acted upon has at least simple associative links with past experiences; therefore, it is selected with some degree of appropriateness.

In both instinct and seizure dyscontrol, the behavior is characterized by an explosive, immediate response to an environmental stimulus that represents a "short circuit" between stimulus and action. The onlooker is startled at the individual's behavior, and the individual may be equally surprised, saying, "I just did it, I don't know why." There is the experience of "having executed a significant action . . . without a clear and complete sense of motivation, decision or sustained wish, so that it does not feel completely deliberate or willfully intended." The behavior is usually described by the actor as a whim, impulse, or sudden urge. Judgment during such acts is reckless or arbitrary, and the act more concerned with the actor's need for gratification than the characteristics of the object acted upon.[18] As an example, another patient would aggressively attack people. However, unlike the previous patient, she was not particularly confused nor amnesic for the attack itself, and the person involved was not necessarily the individual closest at hand, nor was the attack precipitated by physical contact. Instead, the object of her aggression was always male and, in retrospect, the person had mannerisms of speech reminiscent of her father. Further confirmation of the associative link with her father occurred during projective testing where, whenever the stimulus card elicited associations related to her father, she would jump up, tear up the card that had provoked her, and then be at a loss to explain this pre-

if an immediate precipitating event exists, it seems spurious or unimportant, and the motivational aspects of the behavior are hidden or bizarrely elaborated. For this reason, impulse dyscontrol and acting-out dyscontrol can be better characterized at the psychodynamic level. To do this, we must first understand the short circuit between the impulse and the act

EPISODIC DYSCONTROL

PRIMARY DYSCONTROL		SECONDARY DYSCONTROL		
SEIZURE	INSTINCT	IMPULSE	ACTING-OUT	
PHENOMENOLOGIC DIFFERENTIATION	NO DELAY BETWEEN STIMULUS AND RESPONSE		DELAY BETWEEN STIMULUS AND RESPONSE	PHENOMENOLOGIC DIFFERENTIATION
	—UNINHIBITED ACTION—		---TRANSITION---•—INHIBITED ACTION—	
	UNCOORDINATED ACT•—--- TRANSITION---•—		SOPHISTICATED COORDINATED ACT—	
PSYCHODYNAMIC DIFFERENTIATION	•— TENSION RELIEF —•——DIRECT NEED GRATIFICATION—		INDIRECT GRATIFICATION	PSYCHODYNAMIC DIFFERENTIATION
	—INHIBITED REFLECTION—		—EXCESSIVE REFLECTION—	
	INHIBITED INTENTION	---TRANSITION--•	CONSCIOUS INTENTION	UNCONSCIOUS INTENTION

Figure 11–2.   Episodic dyscontrol.

cipitous act. There was no evidence for altered consciousness, except for the misidentification of the object attacked. Her response was stereotyped, as was her characteristic pattern for controlling urges; that is, obsessive-compulsive behavior.

Figure 11–2 summarizes the phenomenological characteristics of the primary dyscontrols where there is little or no delay between the impulse and act and undisguised, primitive motives. The two levels of primary dyscontrol can be differentiated by the uncoordinated motor behavior and the simple relief of tension apparent in seizure dyscontrol while instinctual dyscontrol is more coordinated with direct need gratification.

Secondary Dyscontrol—Impulsive Dyscontrol

Secondary dyscontrol, that is, impulse dyscontrol and acting-out dyscontrol, are difficult to differentiate phenomenologically from instinct dyscontrol. But in secondary dyscontrol,

characteristic of primary dyscontrol but not characteristic of secondary dyscontrol.

It is precisely the short circuit, or action without premeditation, that results in the maladaptive quality of the seizural and instinctual acts described above. Such precipitous behaviors usually mean that the action has not been corrected by reflection on past experiences or anticipation of future consequences. Because of this, the act is usually self-destructive or self-defeating for the individual, or appears antisocial to the onlooker. However, careful evaluation of some precipitous acts, which appear unpremeditated and otherwise indistinguishable from the instinctual acts, reveals considerable premeditation. This is obvious if the premeditation is conscious and willingly reported by the patient (impulse dyscontrol), but at other times the premeditation remains unconscious and can only be inferred on the basis of other data (acting-out dyscontrol). When the premeditation is conscious, the patient usually reports long periods of wavering and doubt about whether he should act or not, with mounting tension, as well as conscious attempts, often bizarre, to resist the impulse to act. Hence, in legal jargon this has been labeled the "irresistible impulse." As an example:

In one patient, impulse dyscontrol occurred following real or imagined rejection. She would become increasingly irritable and hyperactive, and report mounting tension with waves of hopelessness followed by conscious urges to be aggressive, and then attempts to control it. However, such periods almost always culminated in an explosive act, even though during the act itself she might deflect her behavior. For example, following rejection by her mother, she began ruminating about choking her infant sister. She attempted to resist this by locking herself in her room, but the tension became unbearable. She described this tension as a sensation of warmth or flushes traveling over her face and head with a "sense that everything was closing in on me." She then suddenly broke out of the room, grabbed her sister around the neck and began furiously choking her. In the middle of the act, she dropped the child and ran to her mother to confess. Other times, the act was carried through to completion; for instance, she would drown, torture, or otherwise harm animals, destroy furniture, or occasionally indulge in self-mutilative acts. In each instance, however, there was considerable conscious premeditation as to whether she should succumb to the impulse, with attempts to resist the impulse through bizarre control mechanisms.

Secondary Dyscontrol—Acting-Out Dyscontrol

In acting out, despite careful evaluation, the individual denies any awareness of premeditation, yet the objective observer can only assume that the eliciting event has been separated by considerable time from the dyscontrol act. The act itself is so patently inappropriate for the situation, so out of character and so inadequately explained by the actor, one can only conclude that the act is largely determined by unconscious motives to solve repressed conflicts; this I call acting-out dys-

control. As an example, one patient was a docile adolescent girl very much attached to her father. Without any conscious goal to her behavior, she began to pawn her belongings and save money several months before acting out. Supposedly on impulse, she flew to Puerto Rico and upon her arrival at the airport met a policeman whom she married three days later. The precipitating event preceded this act by considerable time. Her father and she had become estranged. The father, obviously jealous of her adolescent boyfriends, had become harshly punitive and restrictive of her freedom. Disconcerted by angry confrontations with her father, she would retreat to her bedroom and lock herself in. Several weeks before she ran away, the father had broken down her door and refused to let her replace the lock. Therapeutic sessions revealed that she was running from a threatened incestuous encounter with her father. On her trip, she found her own sexual partner, an older policeman who, as was revealed through her associations, was a father substitute.

In summary, then, the differentiation between primary and secondary dyscontrol is the lack of premeditation in the former, and presence of this premeditation, either conscious or unconscious, in the latter. The acts themselves may appear equally explosive or precipitous to the casual observer, but only in the primary dyscontrol is there a true short circuit between the impulse and the act.

Psychodynamics of Primary and Secondary Dyscontrol

It will elucidate other dynamic differences between primary and secondary dyscontrol if we examine the mechanisms of delay between a stimulus and the response. We can identify two facets to this delay. The first is designated "reflective delay" (often referred to in the psychoanalytic literature as "thought as trial action"), which is the time necessary for establishing the uniqueness or familiarity of the stimulus by associative connections with past experiences; the time necessary to contemplate alternative courses of action; the time necessary to project into the future and predict the outcome of alternative actions. The second facet is "choice delay," which is only possible following the reflective delay. Choice delay is a decision to postpone immediate action or gratification for long-term rewards; that is, "biding one's time." This choice delay is absent in the extractive sociopathic individual who gives in to his urges in seeking immediate gratification, consequences be damned, even though there may have been careful appraisal of the situation and realization of the possible long-term consequences. This sociopathic individual has often been labeled in the literature as an "actor outer," but by the definition here proposed would not exemplify episodic dyscontrol. To fit our definition, the reflective delay either must be absent (with the associated absence of choice delay), as occurs in primary dyscontrol, or the reflective delay must be severely distorted, as in secondary dyscontrol. The reflective delay depends upon a complex interaction between affects, hindsight and foresight, reason, discrimination and appropriate generalizations, as well as conscience mechanisms. If any of these is significantly deficient or inappropriately dominant, the whole process may fail, resulting in a total absence of reflective delay, leading to primary dyscontrol and a concomitant absence of choice delay, resulting in action that seeks immediate need gratification, with no concept that there is even an alternative. This is a true short circuit between stimulus and response, characteristic of primary dyscontrol.

On the other hand, in secondary dyscontrol, the conscious or unconscious premeditation and the delay between the true stimulus and the act indicate the extent of reflection, as well as the ambivalent vacillating attitudes towards the choice of either succumbing to or restraining the impulse. By and large, individuals showing secondary dyscontrol are, in their general life style, overly inhibited and at some level aware of the true, even though neurotic, intentions of their action. The act itself then, is more likely to represent a rebellion against overly strict conscience mechanisms or a devious substitute gratification of forbidden, unacceptable impulses, such as the explosive act in the overly controlled obsessive character or

the hysterical patient's extramarital affair during her analyst's vacation.

Another dynamic consideration of episodic dyscontrol is that "urges overwhelm controls," but this has operational value only if we can determine where an individual falls between the extremes of excessively strong urges overwhelming normal control mechanisms on one hand, and normal urges uncontrolled by weak or deficient inhibitory mechanisms on the other. The traditional psychiatric view stresses weak control mechanisms. However, my view, supported by growing neurophysiologic evidence, is that sometimes intense dysphoric affects associated with excessive neuronal discharges in the limbic system overwhelm even normal control mechanisms. To identify this group where "urges overwhelm normal controls" is particularly important for planning an appropriate therapeutic regimen, because the goal becomes not so much to develop stronger inhibitory mechanisms, but in some way to blunt or neutralize the intense dysphoria. As discussed later, perhaps the most effective way to do this is with drugs.

Another very important dynamic consideration in planning treatment depends upon the patient's "retrospective self-evaluation." In episodic dyscontrol, during the act itself, the behavior is ego-syntonic, in that it is an abrupt, often explosively quick act, carried through to completion with relief of tension or need gratification. There is no procrastination or doubt about the action. However, in retrospect, often the actor sees the act as ego-alien. This is particularly true if the behavior represents an underlying epileptoid rather than a motivated mechanism. The individual's retrospective recognition of the act as ego-alien considerably facilitates any psychotherapeutic endeavor.

However, in other instances, responsibility for the dyscontrol act is defensively denied (e.g., amnesias), projected, or rationalized so that one can only assume the behavior is recognized as ego-alien at the unconscious level. This defensive behavior, of course, further complicates psychotherapy. Occasionally, one sees a patient who is completely unconcerned by the dyscontrol acts, no matter how much anguish such acts cause others. In these instances, the acts are truly ego-syntonic, both at the time the act is committed and also in retrospect. Even in this instance, if the acts were truly episodic and not just a way of life, this patient would represent an example of episodic dyscontrol. This group presents the most difficult psychotherapeutic problem, because their deviant behavior causes so little personal discomfort. Nevertheless, if the truly ego-syntonic dyscontrol acts are also episodic, that is, an interruption in the usual life style and life flow of the individual, and not just a "dyscontrol way of life," appropriate therapeutic motivation can be developed.

The "dyscontrol way of life" has been described by Shapiro.[18] These individuals truly demonstrate the "alloplastic readiness to act," and may have the appearance of episodic dyscontrol, but closer scrutiny reveals such behavior as a waxing and waning of a persisting pattern, the intermittent quality representing need arousal alternating with satiation. This group represents a failure in choice rather than reflective delay, and is not truly an example of episodic dyscontrol.

Finally, one must consider the intentions of the act (Figure 11–2). In acting-out dyscontrol, the intention is throughly disguised, usually representing the symbolic fulfillment of a forbidden impulse. On the other hand, in impulse dyscontrol and instinct dyscontrol, the true intention is either directly expressed or only superficially disguised and rationalized. For example, the adolescent boy in the throes of an oedipal renunciation kills his mother's lover.

At the most primitive level of episodic dyscontrol (seizure dyscontrol), the act is so diffuse and unco-ordinated that it becomes totally ineffective, hence any unacceptable intentions are blocked. Some patients seem to use this regressive seizural act as a substitute for more effective but unacceptable intentional acts, substituting tension reduction for a more specific (but unacceptable) need gratification. This is one explanation for the frequently reported clinical observation that with an increase in seizures there is a decrease in other dyscontrol acts. Likewise, patients mani-

festing the episodic disinhibitions discussed in this chapter frequently show episodic inhibitions of actions (Figure 11–1). These, too, protect them from the self-destructive consequences of the dyscontrol acts.

❲ Episodic Reactions

Before turning to the possible neurophysiologic mechanisms behind the episodic behavioral disorders, we must consider the second large subgroup, the episodic reactions, which were defined as more prolonged interruptions of the life style and life flow of the individual, characterized by multiple dyscontrol acts, as well as other psychotic, neurotic, sociopathic, or physiologic symptoms. What the episodic reactions share in common with episodic dyscontrol is the precipitous onset and equally abrupt remission of symptoms, which in turn reflect a common etiologic (epileptoid) mechanism in many of the patients suffering from these disorders. Even though the symptoms in the episodic reactions may be prolonged for weeks or months, the possibility of epileptoid mechanisms in these more prolonged disorders should be considered. Data available on subcortical recordings in man have demonstrated prolonged but circumscribed excessive neuronal discharges in the limbic system, associated with diverse psychiatric symptomatology.[15] It is for this reason that both episodic dyscontrol and episodic reactions are grouped under episodic behavioral disorders.

Episodic Psychotic Reactions

Many patients showing episodic reactions manifest symptoms that are characteristic of schizophrenia. Most patients labeled as having remitting, intermittent, atypical, or reactive schizophrenia are examples of this episodic psychotic reaction. Some of these patients show clouding of sensorium, difficulties in orientation or identification, and a partial memory loss for the episode—symptoms suggestive of an acute brain syndrome rather than schizophrenia. However, their schizophrenic behavior so overshadows these sensorial defects that the possibility of a toxic reaction is either overlooked or disregarded, particularly in the absence of an obvious exogenous toxin. This disturbance in awareness undoubtedly reflects an underlying excessive neuronal discharge or epileptoid mechanism. It is this group of atypical psychotic patients with clouding of sensorium that Meduna[11] designated as "oneirophrenia" and Mitsuda[12] as "atypical" psychosis. Rodin[17] discussed such a syndrome which, although phenomenologically related to schizophrenia, seemed etiologically closer to epilepsy, and proposed the term "symptomatic" schizophrenia. Vaillant[21] emphasized the recurrent quality of the disturbance and the frequent shift in diagnosis from schizophrenia to manic-depressive psychosis in an eighty-five-year retrospective study of remitting schizophrenias. Although this group of patients ultimately become chronic, for long periods they managed independent successful lives. Altschule[2] and Williams[23] observed that episodic schizophrenic symptoms with confusion occur with regular periodicity associated with the menstrual cycle in some women.

The epileptoid mechanism behind many of these episodic psychotic reactions is further emphasized by studies where extensive clinical EEG's were obtained on patients before, during, and after psychotic episodes.[4,10] These studies suggested at least two types of epileptoid psychotic reactions—one correlated with centrencephalic epilepsy, either petit mal status in children or a prolonged post ictal response in adults, characterized by torpor, apathy, confusion with minimal hallucinations and delusions. A second type of psychotic reaction was correlated with focal, particularly temporal lobe, abnormalities, and characterized by florid psychotic behavior with mixed manic-depressive or schizophrenic symptoms and varying degrees of clouding of sensorium. It has also been observed that these atypical psychotic patients often have a history of epilepsy, a low convulsive threshold, and activated EEG abnormalities.[7,15,20] Because these patients show the clouding of sensorium and disorientation characteristic of the acute brain syndrome, I chose to designate them as manifesting an episodic brain syndrome rather than episodic schizophrenia.

Undoubtedly some episodic psychotic reactions are not determined by epileptoid mechanisms. Experience during World War II suggests that the "three-day schizophrenia" represents an individual's adaptive potential to protect himself against extreme external stress. Such behavior is seen following natural catastrophes, such as earthquakes, floods, fires, etc., and under the official nomenclature would be designated as disassociative states. Although there is usually complete amnesia for these episodes and, in fact, during the episode the individual may be confused about his own personal identity, this disorientation can be readily differentiated from the clouded sensorium of the episodic brain syndrome. If the individual shows typical schizophrenic symptoms with a clear sensorium, I chose to designate the syndrome as an episodic schizophrenic reaction. The dual personality or split in orientation that occurs in hysterical disassociative states is distinguished from both the episodic brain syndrome and the episodic schizophrenic reaction.

One patient showed a true episodic schizophrenic reaction without any clouding of sensorium. She had a change in personality two weeks before admission to the hospital. Previously a devoted mother, she suddenly wanted to give up her children for adoption, and became so physically abusive towards them that she was hospitalized for the children's safety. At the time of hospitalization, she showed press of speech, incoherency, and poorly organized delusions that she was under some mysterious control from the outside and that unidentified enemies were going to destroy her family. She had auditory hallucinations of a sexually accusatory nature. The delusions and hallucinations disappeared within four days and within a week she had full insight regarding her bizarre behavior and illogical ideas, remembering clearly all that transpired during this episode.

Another patient on the other hand showed considerable clouding of sensorium during her acute psychotic episodes. Problems had been building up from the preceding year; the patient reported that at times "thoughts were racing through my mind and I couldn't control them." The family noted mild referential ideas. Two weeks before admission, her symptoms became florid. She was confused, disoriented, believed she was being influenced by mental telepathy, changed into a mulatto and that her husband was Eichmann. She identified the hospital personnel as persecutors, thought the hospital itself was a concentration camp, was disoriented as to date, time, place, and situation, and otherwise gave evidence of an acute brain syndrome. However, even at the height of the disorder, there were periods when she paused with considerable perplexity asking, "Why is everything so different?" At other times, she had a fleeting recognition that something was wrong with her. Two weeks after hospitalization, her sensorium was clear and she spontaneously said, "I haven't imagined anything for the past four days."

Episodic Psychotic Depressions

In this group of disorders, intense depression occurs and remits precipitously and unexplainedly, sometimes lasting for only a few hours, but often lasting for days or weeks. It is distinguishable from the usual psychotic depression, not only by the abruptness of onset, but also by less motor retardation, less conceptual elaboration of guilt and inferiority feelings, and more anxiety.[22,24] The patient often refers to these episodes as "attacks," and describes the depression as coming in waves, as if being engulfed in the ocean, or smothered in a cave, or surrounded by flames, sensations which occasionally occur as auras of typical epileptic seizures. In fact, some patients who develop epilepsy late in life have had such depressive episodes before the appearance of seizures, suggesting the likelihood that such depressions were prodromal symptoms of typical epilepsy, which preceded the appearance of convulsions by months or even years.

A patient would describe depressive episodes as if they were auras, saying that the sensation was like a wave overwhelming him.

This would be so intense that he would have the visual sensation of being engulfed by flames or swallowed by the sea. At the same time, he would develop somatic preoccupations that he had a brain tumor, liver disease, heart trouble, or arthritis, all of which had some basis in reality. The sensations were so overwhelming that he contemplated suicide and made dramatic appeals for hospitalization. Some months later, at the age of forty-four, he had his first grand mal seizure. After a second seizure and EEG evidence suggesting temporal lobe epilepsy, he was placed on a Dilantin-Mysoline combination, which controlled his seizures as well as the severe depressive episodes.

Episodic Physiologic Reactions

In view of the association of disturbing somatic sensations as an aura to typical epileptic seizures, it is not surprising that many of the episodic reactions are characterized by episodic hypochondriasis. In fact, Ging et al.[6] report a significant relationship between paroxysmal EEG abnormalities and multiple physical complaints as scored on the MMPI; this supports Ervin et al.'s[5] hypothesis that the frequency of hypochondriasis found in temporal lobe epilepsy patients might be a consequence of ictal visceral sensations these individuals experience. Often these episodic complaints are not hypochondriacal but a manifestation of true physiologic disturbances. Shimoda[19] studied 2,500 patients with episodic somatic disturbances and found a high incidence of paroxysmal EEG abnormalities, which suggests the importance of an unrecognized group of disorders associated with an ictal phenomenon, the episodic physiologic reactions. Such disorders may involve almost any system and may lead, for example, to multiple laparotomies. From the clinical description of Shimoda's patients, many appear similar to what Reiman[16] labeled "periodic disease." Also, the controversial "14 and 6 positive spike" syndrome[9] manifests both episodic physiologic reactions and occasional impulsive, aggressive acts. Deutsch's[3] fifty-year follow-up of Freud's "Dora," the patient to whom Freud first applied the concept of "acting out," indicates that she apparently suffered from an episodic physiologic reaction, including migraine, coughing spells, hoarseness, palpitations, and multiple gynecological complaints, which kept "everyone in the environment in continual alarm."

A thirty-three-year-old single female patient has had literally over one hundred hospitalizations starting at age five, and had undergone five medical hospitalizations during the three years prior to her present admission. Always, her complaints were severe, but the cause of the disability unclear. The first two times she was hospitalized for urinary retention, double vision, puffiness of the face, recurrent fever, and headaches. The third time she was admitted in an unresponsive state, supposedly having taken an overdose of barbiturates. However, the blood barbiturate levels were not significant and the patient denied any suicidal attempt. The coma was never adequately explained. Two months following this, she was again admitted, but this time for an actual suicide attempt wherein she had taken an overdose of barbiturates. Followed carefully on an outpatient basis, it was noted that she not only had transitory episodes of confusion, agitation, and depression, but also marked fluctuations in weight, dyplopia, transitory slurring of speech, and unsteady gait. She improved considerably when on a carefully controlled regimen of Dilantin.

Episodic Neurotic Reactions

In discussing episodic dyscontrol, we have mentioned the dysphoric affects that accompany the dyscontrol acts. At times, this dysphoria, although appearing precipitously and remitting in the same way, persists for a significant period of time, either without dyscontrol acts or with multiple dyscontrol acts which do not relieve the tension. We have already described such depressive episodes, but there also may be typical attacks of anxiety, acute rages, and even sexual excitement with neurotic defense mechanisms. The pragmatic value of making these observations is the possibility that these, too, may be epileptoid phenomena that will respond to a specific therapeutic regimen, including the use of anticonvulsants.

An adolescent chronic schizophrenic boy patient would be suddenly overwhelmed by phobias, particularly fear of the dark, being alone, being on the street or among crowds, without any particular change in his schizophrenic symptoms. At such time, he would come to the hospital begging for admission. These experiences would be transitory, sometimes lasting only a few hours or at most a few days, clearing up again with no particular change in the underlying chronic schizophrenia.

Another patient was admitted to the neurological service in status epilepticus. After this terminated, she was transferred to the psychiatric service, because she developed blindness, hemiparesis, hemianesthesia, and aphonia. These symptoms cleared rapidly under minimal reassurance. However, she was considered to be representative of an episodic conversion syndrome, because these symptoms occurred repeatedly when she was under stress, with the varied conversion symptoms either occurring simultaneously or in rapid sequence.

A third patient, a very conscientious, prudish mother and respected member of the community, would periodically experience fugue states during which time she adopted a new name and the identity of a wild, promiscuous single girl. These changes in personality were sometimes transitory, occurring several times a day, and at other times persisted for two to three days. They occurred in clusters, sometimes following obvious external stress, and at other times seemingly unexplained. She also manifested episodic physiologic symptoms.

Episodic Sociopathic Reactions

Social values, to have meaning, depend on a stability and continuity in the world,[18] so that antisocial behavior, in the broadest sense, is typical of most episodic behavioral disorders, because frequent breaks in life style and life flow leave the patient's world discontinuous and inconstant. For this reason, the diagnosis of the episodic sociopathic reaction must be made carefully, and should be limited to the occasional patient who shows "bursts" of sociopathic behavior which completely overshadows other episodic behavior, such behavior being totally out of character for the individual, except for brief and infrequent intervals, yet sustained enough so that we cannot consider it as merely a dyscontrol act.

One patient, a twenty-seven-year-old married housewife, demonstrated momentary blackouts, periods of slow, hesitant speech, and episodes where she would impulsively break up furniture or destroy her belongings. The sociopathic episodes involved a period of mounting tension followed by sustained promiscuity, lasting for weeks or months, where she actively solicited favors from young men, often having sexual contacts with many men during the same evening. Such periods resulted in several pregnancies and at least two illegitimate children. However, these promiscuous periods alternated with long intervals of marital fidelity and even periods of complete sexual abstinence.

⟮ Episodic Behavior Associated with Chronic Psychopathology

Although behavioral characteristics of episodic dyscontrol or episodic reactions may be the presenting difficulty, perhaps serious enough to precipitate hospitalization, this may not be the primary problem. Careful scrutiny may reveal that the episodic disorder is but a minor aspect of the total psychopathology, exploited for its secondary gains. For example, a dyscontrol act may be a cry for help (such as the impulsive suicidal attempt), rebellion against phobic or obsessive inhibitions, or an attempt to differentiate one's self from others in chronic schizophrenic patients. It is important to distinguish between the dynamic and etiologic mechanisms of the underlying persistent nonepisodic psychopathology and the superimposed episodic dyscontrol or reactions.

A comparative evaluation between the level of regression of dyscontrol behavior and the regression of the basic chronic psychopathology gives significant diagnostic and prognostic clues. Usually, the more regressive the basic psychopathology, the more regressive will be the episodic behavioral disorder. If there is a marked disparity between the level of regression of the chronic psychopathology and the episodic behavior, the more complicated will be the dynamic and the etiologic interpretation. For instance, if the patient has a well-organized defense neurosis, yet manifests episodic dyscontrol at the level of seizural or instinctual acts, one would have to investigate several alternatives to explain this disparity: (1) Does the current reality have an overwhelming traumatic implication? (2) Was the structured neurosis really covering a more regressive psychotic potential? (3) Was the seizural or instinctual act epileptoid rather than motivated?

Where the superimposed episodic behavior is used in the service of the basic psychopathology, or has attained value because of the secondary gains received by the patient, symptomatic improvement of the episodic behavior will lead to an exacerbation of the basic psychopathology. This may in part explain the frequent observation that successful treatment of typical epileptic seizures leads to overt psychosis. Of course, the presence of severe chronic psychopathology alters considerably the prognosis and therapeutic regimen of these patients.

⟮ Neurophysiologic Mechanisms

Man's capacity to respond appropriately to environmental demands depends on two factors: the individual's endowment or the functional integrity of the equipment he possesses, and the appropriateness and extent of his learned behavior. It is difficult to evaluate how much of a maladaptive response is due to "faulty equipment," and how much is due to "faulty learning." In clinical practice, a patient seldom falls at one or the other of these extremes. Rather, the maladaptive behavior results from some mixture of faulty equipment and faulty learning. Nevertheless, it becomes important for the clinician to evaluate the extent each deficit contributes to the maladaptive behavior, in order to make an accurate prognosis and to establish appropriate therapeutic goals. The possible epileptoid nature of many episodic behavioral disorders is suggested by the frequent concurrence of more typical epileptic phenomena (e.g., grand mal, petit mal, or simple automatisms).

Unfortunately, there is no reliable laboratory procedure to measure neurophysiologic deficits, not even the clinical EEG, which does not reveal the excessive subcortical neuronal discharges that are most likely correlated with dyscontrol behavior.[8] Statistically, clinical EEG's with sleep recordings may indicate a higher number of abnormalities among these patients than would be expected in the normal population, or for that matter in a population of chronic psychotic patients. However, this is of little help in diagnosing a given patient who has had one routine electroencephalogram which is read as within normal range.[15] In fact, typical epileptic behavior can occur in proven epileptics with known pathophysiologic dysfunction without EEG abnormalities, in the scalp recordings during the aura, the seizure itself, or the post-ictal period.[1] For this reason, the routine scalp EEG is no absolute measure of whether epileptoid phenomena play a significant role in episodic dyscontrol or episodic reactions.[13]

Also, excessive neuronal discharges in subcortical structures may be sustained for considerable periods of time, that is, weeks or months, without spread to the cortex and without typical epileptic seizures. Often, such limited excessive neuronal discharges are accompanied by marked behavioral changes not usually identified as epileptic. These include dysphoria, depression, mounting irritability, altered levels of awareness, impulsivity, depersonalization, and even hallucinations or delusions.[15] The only common characteristic of these varied symptoms with that of typical centrencephalic or temporal lobe epilepsy is a precipitous onset and equally precipitous remission.

An EEG technique that would significantly reduce the number of false negatives without an excessive increase in false positives is needed. If one uses a combination of activation techniques, such as sleep, hyperventilation, and drugs, such as Alpha-chloralose, false negatives are virtually nil in classic epileptic patients and rare in the group of episodic behavioral disorders that on other criteria seem to be epileptoid.[14] However, there is an increase in the number of false positives (up to 20 percent in nonpatient groups). I have preferred to use Alpha-chloralose rather than Metrazol, or other drugs, because of its effectiveness in activating latent abnormalities, as well as the patient's acceptance of the subjective concomitants of this drug. Alpha-chloralose gives one a feeling of pleasant, mild intoxication, in contrast, for instance, to Metrazol which induces unpleasant anxiety. There are two drawbacks to Alpha-chloralose; namely, while it has been used in Europe for many years as a sedative, it has never been marketed in this country, therefore, it is considered an experimental drug requiring a Federal Drug Administration IND number. The other practical disadvantage is that Alpha-chloralose is not readily soluble and must be given orally. This means an unpredictable response appearing from fifteen to sixty minutes after ingestion, with the duration of pharmacological action from two to five hours, during which time the patient should be under medical observation. Thus, this activation procedure requires from three to five hours, an excessive amount of time for most busy clinical EEG laboratories.[14] However, for the psychiatric hospital with a clinical EEG laboratory, the effort and time would be rewarded by affording more accurate diagnoses and more effective therapeutic planning.

"Positive activation" induced by Alpha-chloralose or other drugs can be seen as representing two types of EEG responses. The first pattern is "specific," characterized by the focal appearance of hypersynchrony and/or slow waves or typical generalized patterns of centrencephalic epilepsy. If this pattern occurs in the resting baseline, it is augmented by the activation procedure. The second type of EEG activation pattern is "aspecific" and characterized by high amplitude, paroxysmal slow waves (three–seven per second) that are generalized and bilaterally synchronous, sometimes with intermixed hypersynchronous wave forms in the same distribution. According to the literature, the prevalence of such "aspecific" patterns is high in uncomplicated epilepsy, and my findings indicate it is almost equally high in patients showing episodic behavioral disorders.[15]

Most patients who show activated "aspecific" EEG patterns, as well as episodic dyscontrol or episodic reactions, also have a clear-cut history of a psychologically traumatic past, underlining the fact that the excessive neuronal discharges probably are not sufficient causes of episodic behavior. Studies have consistently reported that dyscontrol patients were usually subjected to intense overstimulation during the first several years of life; that is, exposure to extreme aggression in parents, siblings, or other significant adults in the environment, or exposed to severe panic reactions, or to persistent sensual and often overtly sexual stimulation. Thus, it may be conservatively generalized that if a person, for whatever reason, is destined to become neurotic, psychotic, or sociopathic, he will likely manifest this as an episodic disorder if there is an associated epileptoid mechanism (epileptoid meaning periods of circumscribed excessive neuronal discharges within the central nervous system). This underlying epileptoid mechanism can usually be demonstrated by special EEG activating techniques, which, if positive, suggest that anticonvulsant medication will significantly facilitate an effective therapeutic regimen.[15]

Certain phenomenological characteristics give us further clues regarding whether the prominent mechanism is epileptoid or learned. Epileptoid mechanisms are probable if the dyscontrol acts are primitive and diffuse (primary dyscontrol), the eliciting situation neutral or ambiguous, and the secondary gains slight or absent. Although these statements have common sense obviousness, the complexities of coming to such conclusions on the basis of clinical data can be surprisingly diffi-

cult. Another distinguishing characteristic between epileptoid or motivated episodic dyscontrol is the disparity between the hierarchical levels of dyscontrol behavior and the behavior between episodes. This is greater in the epileptoid patient. For instance, in a sophisticated, intelligent man whose episodic dyscontrol is primary dyscontrol, that is, a seizural or instinctual act, one must assume that there is a likelihood of an epileptoid element, particularly if there is a stereotyped repetitive quality to the dyscontrol acts. On the other hand, this would not necessarily be true if the patient were a mental defective showing organic perseveration and obsessive-compulsive traits.

At the phenomenological level, there are several other criteria for differentiating between epileptoid or motivated episodic dyscontrol. If there is clouding of sensorium during the episodic act, it is more likely epileptoid. Because it is usually impossible to evaluate the clouding of sensorium during the dyscontrol act itself, we are forced to rely on a history of amnesia to determine the likelihood of such clouding. Contrary to what is usually thought, it is the epileptoid patient who is more likely to have partial recall for the episode (except during a grand mal seizure or simple automatism). Also, he is more willing to accept the responsibility for this behavior. He feels his behavior is "driven," is perplexed by both the quality and intensity of the act, and is willing to be confronted with his behavior in the hope of excising the "foreign body." He sees his act as truly ego-alien. On the other hand, the motivated or so-called hysterical patient often has complete amnesia for the episodic behavior, because he recognizes unconsciously the unacceptable intentions of his act and, therefore, denies responsibility for his behavior.

(Treatment

The concept of episodic behavioral disorders aids in planning an effective therapeutic regimen for a group of patients who are otherwise difficult therapeutic problems.[15] Some of the difficulties are enumerated below.

1. Although these patients episodically may be seriously dangerous to both themselves and society, they have relatively long periods of quiescence or normality, making it difficult to insist upon long-term hospitalization for the protection of the patient or society. The symptoms often abate within a few days after hospitalization; on the other hand, they may recur a few days after discharge, following months of intensive milieu therapy within the hospital.

2. Outpatient therapy is complicated by the tendency of these patients to precipitously terminate therapy as a dyscontrol act, or to otherwise manipulate the therapist with their dyscontrol behavior.

3. Dyscontrol patients with episodic physiologic reactions or abnormal EEG's are likely to have multiple physicians, hence multiple, often conflicting, therapeutic regimens. The corollary is that an adequate therapeutic program often requires combined pharmacologic and re-educational techniques; this complicates the delegation of responsibility for "change" to the various physicians on the one hand, and to the physician and the patient on the other.

4. Often, these patients misuse drugs, either frantically trying to control their dysphoria by indiscriminate drug use, with habituation to drugs or alcohol becoming an additional problem, or they may not remember to take the prescribed medication because of the clouded sensorium. Furthermore, toxic symptoms of drug overdose and the episodic symptoms themselves are often similar, so that the differential between too much or too little medication cannot be easily determined.

On the positive side, patients with episodic behavioral disorders often have long periods of relative rationality, during which they can examine the episodic disturbances with realistic concern. Thus, there is the "split in the ego" which is so necessary for any re-educational insight psychotherapy.

The first prerequisite in the therapy of episodic behavioral disorders is that the therapist must be willing to take chances. If he becomes overly concerned about his patients' behavior, they will unmercifully manipulate and punish him. The second prerequisite for effective therapy is to anticipate the type of dyscontrol acts and make preparatory plans (discussed with the patient) for handling such behavior. This may require the aid of responsible family, peers, or co-operating professionals. A third requirement is that as soon as there is a quiescent period after any episodic behavior, the therapist should relentlessly confront the patient with his behavior, particularly those patients most reluctant to reconsider it. Fourth, the therapist must be willing to combine drug and re-educational (psychotherapeutic) techniques, but on the other hand, he must be prepared to withhold all medication, even though it might otherwise be indicated, if the patient will not follow carefully the prescribed drug regimen. Fifth, the therapist must be flexible within the therapeutic setting itself, so that dyscontrol acts will occur in the office and can be microscopically scrutinized by the patient and therapist together. Conjoint sessions with patient and significant peers are sometimes beneficial, particularly in confronting the patient with dyscontrol behavior which he is defensively rationalizing. This flexibility, however, does not apply to the frequency, time, or setting of the therapeutic sessions. A schedule must be rigidly adhered to if the therapist is to resist manipulation. Sixth, it is desirable to have one clinician responsible for the total medical management; he may utilize consultants, but he should interpret the consultants' findings and dispense recommended medications himself. These aspects of therapy are discussed in greater detail elsewhere.[15]

It is particularly important to develop a therapeutic motivation in those dyscontrol patients who lack it, by twenty-four-hour control of environment with immediate, inescapable punishment for failures and equally immediate and appropriate reward for successes. Hopefully, the frustration and anxieties caused by such an environment will instil an appropriate motivation for change. This disciplined environment rarely can be provided by the same individual who is responsible for the re-educational or insight therapy.

Procedures must be established for preventing acting out in the form of termination or avoidance of effective therapeutic sessions. Also, one must insist that the sole responsibility for the patient's behavior lies with the patient himself, no matter what neurophysiologic deficits there may be, or how capricious the environment.

Insight can be developed in these patients by making the dyscontrol acts ego-alien and then examining the full implications of the act itself. Resistance can be minimized by utilizing first the patient's narcissism rather than confronting it head on, avoiding disapproval of the patient's behavior by emphasizing alternative and more effective ways for meeting his needs. Understanding the dyscontrol acts is more rapidly accomplished by focusing on why the patient committed himself to action at a given time and place. Later, one examines the behavioral pattern itself; that is, the associational connections with and consequences of the act. This is particularly true for secondary dyscontrol, which occurs in patients whose lives are generally characterized by a neurotic inhibition of action rather than an "alloplastic readiness to act." In fact, dyscontrol acts may be the first sign of improvement in neurotically inhibited patients, an indication that the patient is ready to overcome his inhibitory fears of action.

Medication, as an adjunct to, and sometimes as a primary form of, therapy, can be recommended in the following manner: If epileptoid etiologic mechanisms are presumed, or have been demonstrated by EEG activation techniques, anticonvulsants should be used, keeping in mind several limitations. Anticonvulsants are not universally effective, even in typical epilepsy; and sometimes one will work when another fails. Also, there is little range between effective therapeutic dose and toxic level. The therapeutic index can often be increased by combining several synergistically acting drugs. In episodic dyscontrol, this is best obtained by using the benzodiazepines, either alone or in combination with the usual anticonvulsants.

If control of the dyscontrol acts results in other disordered behavior, close scrutiny usually reveals that inadequate attention has been given to the re-educational psychotherapeutic program; or the importance of secondary gains of the dyscontrol behavior has been overlooked; or no opportunity has been provided for the realistic expression of affects and the gratification of needs. Phenothiazines, if used to control episodic psychotic reactions and not to treat a chronic, persistent psychosis underlying the episodic disorder, need not be maintained beyond clinical improvement. In fact, maintenance medication may be contraindicated. If at all possible, phenothiazines should be avoided, as they may aggravate dyscontrol acts. If they are needed, they should be combined with anticonvulsants and/or benzodiazepines. Patients with episodic depressions may respond well to benzodiazepines, or even to anticonvulsants, whereas they may be untouched or perhaps aggravated by the usual antidepressants. The fact that such a complicated pharmacologic combination may be necessary, indicates that the ideal pharmacologic agent has not been found.

Long-term follow-up suggests that contrary to the usually expressed pessimism regarding therapy with these patients, they respond well to an appropriate regimen and may contribute significantly to society. Despite the turmoil of the treatment process itself, the most gratifying therapeutic results, both for the patient and the therapist, occur with this group. A top executive who had been incapacitated for five years, drank heavily, completely neglected his family, and whimpered childishly for help, is now abstinent, authoritatively assuming his role as head of the household, and functioning well in his executive position. A mother whose fugue states were so prolonged and irresponsible that she lost her husband and control of her children, becoming utterly dependent on elderly parents, has finished her professional training, is gainfully employed, and has resumed caring for her children. Another woman whose life was so totally chaotic that she, too, gave up caring for her children and divorced her husband, is now working in a highly competent professional position and at the same time caring for her children and household. A man who could function only at a menial clerical level because of his impulsiveness and frequent habituation to drugs now successfully manages his own large business. These results are typical of many patients with episodic behavioral disorders who have been treated intensively, both pharmacologically and psychotherapeutically, over a sustained period.

(Bibliography

1. AJMONE-MARSAN, C., and B. L. RALSTON. *The Epileptic Seizure: Its Functional Morphology and Diagnostic Significance: A Clinical Electroencephalographic Analysis of Metrazol-Induced Attacks.* Springfield: Charles C. Thomas, 1957.

2. ALTSCHULE, M. D., and J. BREM. "Periodic Psychosis of Puberty," *The American Journal of Psychiatry,* 119 (1963), 1, 176.

3. DEUTSCH, F. "A Footnote to Freud's 'Fragment of an Analysis of a Case of Hysteria,'" *Psychoanalytic Quarterly,* 26 (1957), 159.

4. DONGIER, S. "Statistical Study of Clinical and Electroencephalographic Manifestations of 536 Psychotic Episodes Occurring in 516 Epileptics Between Clinical Seizures," *Epilepsia,* 1 (1959), 117.

5. ERVIN, F., A. W. EPSTEIN, and H. E. KING. "Behavior of Epileptic and Nonepileptic Patients with 'Temporal Spikes,'" *Archives of Neurology and Psychiatry,* 74 (1955), 488.

6. GING, R. J., E. JONES, and M. MANIS. "Correlation of Electroencephalograms and Multiple Physical Symptoms," *Journal of the AMA,* 187 (1964), 579.

7. GLASER, G., R. NEWMAN, and R. SCHAFER. "Interictal Psychosis in Psychomotor-Temporal Lobe Epilepsy: An EEG Psychological Study," in G. H. Glaser, ed., *EEG and Behavior.* New York: Basic Books, 1963.

8. HEATH, R. G., W. A. MICKLE, and R. R.

9. HUGHES, J. R. "A Review of the Positive Spike Phenomenon," in W. P. Wilson, ed., *Applications of Electroencephalography in Psychiatry.* Durham: Duke University Press, 1965.

10. LANDOLT, H. "Serial Electroencephalographic Investigations During Psychotic Episodes in Epileptic Patients and During Schizophrenic Attacks," in A. M. Lorentz De Has, ed., *Lectures on Epilepsy.* Amsterdam: Elsevier Publishing Co., 1958.

11. MEDUNA, L. J. *Oneirophrenia, "The Confused State."* Urbana: University of Illinois Press, 1950.

12. MITSUDA, H., ed. *Clinical Genetics in Psychiatry: Problems in Nosological Classification.* Tokyo: Igaku Shoin, 1967.

13. ———. "The Comprehensive Approach to Patient Care: The Electroencephalogram as a Diagnostic Aid," in Tice's *Practice of Medicine,* 10 (1969), 43–47.

14. MONROE, R. R., et al. "EEG Activation with Chloralosane," *Electroencephalography and Clinical Neurophysiology,* 8 (1956), 279.

15. ———. *Episodic Behavioral Disorders.* Cambridge: Harvard University Press, 1970.

16. REIMAN, H. H. *Periodic Disease.* Philadelphia: F. A. Davis Co., 1963.

17. RODIN, E. A., et al. "Relationship Between Certain Forms of Psychomotor Epilepsy and Schizophrenia," *Archives of Neurology and Psychiatry,* 77 (1957), 449.

18. SHAPIRO, D. *Neurotic Styles.* New York: Basic Books, 1965.

19. SHIMODA, Y. "The Clinical and Electroencephalographic Study of the Primary Diencephalic Epilepsy or Epilepsy of the Brain Stem," *Acta Neurovegetativa,* 23 (1961), 181.

20. SLATER, E., A. W. BEARD, and E. GLITHERO. "The Schizophrenic-Like Psychoses of Epilepsy," *British Journal of Psychiatry,* 74 (1955), 488.

21. VAILLANT, G. E. "The Natural History of the Remitting Schizophrenias," *The American Journal of Psychiatry,* 120 (1963), 367.

22. WEIL, A. A. "Ictal Emotions Occurring in

MONROE. "Characteristic Recording from Various Specific Subcortical Nuclear Masses in the Brains of Psychiatric and Non-Psychiatric Patients," *Transactions of the American Neurological Association,* 80 (1955), 17.

Temporal Lobe Dysfunction," *Archives of Neurology*, 1 (1959), 87.

23. WILLIAMS, E., and L. WEEKES. "Premenstrual Tension Associated with Psychotic Episodes," *Journal of Nervous and* *Mental Disease*, 116 (1952), 321.

24. YAMADA, T. "A Clinico-Electroencephalographic Study of Ictal Depression," in H. Mitsuda, ed., *Clinical Genetics in Psychiatry*. Tokyo: Igaku Shoin, 1967.

CHAPTER 12

ANTISOCIAL BEHAVIOR

Jonas R. Rappeport

THERE IS A GROUP of individuals in our society whose behavior, at times, defies belief. For many years, they have intrigued judges, lawyers, penologists, and psychiatrists. Most recently, the terms "psychopath," "sociopath," or "antisocial personality," have been used to describe their behavior. However, before we can effectively describe the so-called psychopathic personality, we should attempt to delineate the differences between the "true" antisocial personality and "others" who exhibit behavior of an antisocial nature, i.e., behavior which proves to be, upon closer observation, actually symptomatic of underlying causes connected with economic, cultural, and physical factors, as well as other emotional illnesses.

It would seem appropriate at this point to juxtapose various examples of behavior that cannot be classified as truly psychopathic in terms of a primary diagnosis. All have components of psychopathic behavior but, in fact, do not fulfill the definition of the specific disease entity of the antisocial personality.

Today, there is evidence that "acting out against the environment" has increased as a means of managing inner conflicts, as an expression of individual and group behavior, and as a form of political action.

For example, a man who seeks out and shoots five fellow workers without apparent cause and then holds off the police until seriously wounded, may be seen as suffering from an emotional illness, such as a paranoid psychosis. On the other hand, the man who shoots a guard while escaping from an attempted robbery may not be seen by society as suffering from a psychiatric illness. He may, in fact, represent an example of the true antisocial personality for whom crime is a way of life and his business.

A teenager who shoplifts may just be rebelling while attempting the resolution of an identity crisis. In contrast to this, the wealthy, middle-aged matron who is caught stealing a screwdriver is behaving entirely out of character and probably is acting out, in order to defend against a severe involutional depression.

Society would certainly tend to take a different view toward a man who steals food to provide a Christmas dinner for his wife and children than toward the professional thief.

And, in the realm of more socially acceptable but nonetheless aggressive acts toward society in general, let us consider the so-called white-collar crimes. It is a fact that well over a billion dollars' worth of office supplies are stolen from employers annually. Individual cheating on personal income tax and corporate maneuverings in the world of big business are widespread enough to have prompted the government to establish stiff legal penalties to deal with such acts. There are those who feel that such white-collar crimes merely reflect our "sick" society. We could cite the example of the bookie or the football pool operator and their customers, as well as many other forms of petty but illegal gambling, some of which may be considered as acceptable actions within a community or subculture. However, regardless of how severely or benignly society views these various crimes, all are, in effect, aggressive actions directed against the environment, whether the environment be another person, the state, or a bank.

In addition to the above examples of behavior containing antisocial components, but not necessarily fulfilling the conditions for a diagnosis of the true psychopathic personality, we must add the following group. That is, we must distinguish between true psychopathic states and other types of psychiatric disorders that contain antisocial elements. Seen in terms of currently accepted psychiatric disorders, we know that any patient, regardless of his basic diagnosis, may also exhibit symptoms of antisocial behavior. Examples of this would include the patient suffering from a post-partum psychosis who murders her child, the excited catatonic whose violence may be almost indescribable, the manic depressive who buys Cadillacs and writes checks without sufficient funds, the man who commits a murder in a disassociative state.

As for the gambler, bookie, and prostitute mentioned above, DSM II[22] considers them not to have a psychiatric disorder. Their behavior is called dyssocial behavior: "This category is for individuals who are not classifiable as antisocial personalities, but who are predatory and follow more or less criminal pursuits, such as racketeers, dishonest gamblers, prostitutes, and dope peddlers."

We know that antisocial behavior can be present regardless of whether one is considered to be psychiatrically ill or not. It is my belief that the majority of antisocial behavior (crime) is not simply the result of psychiatric illness, but is, in fact, the result of a complex social, moral, psychologic, and economic milieu beyond the scope of this article. There are some excellent discussions of these factors and their relationship to criminal behavior in articles and texts in the criminologic literature.[85,80,42]

In the above examples we have seen how antisocial behavior can result from a complexity of causes and at times represent just the tip of an iceberg of serious psychiatric or sociocultural problems. There is, however, a group whose antisocial behavior does not seem to be symptomatic of something else—a group whose antisocial behavior is not just a component of another problem but the primary expression of the illness. Now we come face to face with the true psychopathic personality. We find ourselves in the presence of a group of antisocial specialists, so to speak. These are individuals who seem to have no loyalty, no guilt or conscience; who care only for themselves, and do generally as they want. They appear to be of superior intelligence, but are not, and, in fact, get caught easily. They make promises they never keep; they are so brazen that we are regularly taken in by them. As a group, they have defied sharp delineation or definition until relatively recently, despite the recognition of their existence for many years.

(History

Over thousands of years, behavior that strays from the usual or ordinary has been labeled the product of the "mad," "bewitched," and "bad," to mention only a few of the attempts to explain it. In 1800, the phrenologist Franz

Gall explained criminal behavior on the basis of "head bumps," supposedly the external representation of over– or underdeveloped parts of the brain containing centers of love, hate, fear, meanness, etc. Throughout history we see two forces operating. One is an attempt to explain aberrant (antisocial) human behavior via a mental health model, and the other, a sociomoral model.

Pinel tells of a patient who was so "enraged at a woman who had used offensive language to him, he precipitated her into a well."[51] Despite this violent behavior, the patient displayed none of the usual symptoms of psychiatric classification, so Pinel described the case as *"manie sans délire."* Although it is probable that he included in the group other patients besides the psychopath, this appears to be the first recognition of the specific symptom of the antisocial personality.

In 1835, J. C. Prichard[68] coined the phrase "moral insanity," in which, however, he still included such disorders as manic-depressive psychosis. In what is considered the first scientific treatise on criminality, published in 1876, Lombroso,[58] an Italian psychiatrist, presented a classification he called "the born criminal." This classification was later defined by Gouster[32] as those suffering from moral insanity. This label suited most medical men of the late nineteenth century, since an impaired moral sense seemed to explain the behavior of this large group of individuals who broke the law in various ways, despite the fact they knew such behavior was wrong. The concept of moral insanity did, however, upset lawyers and clergymen for fear that we were saying these persons were insane and therefore not responsible. Because of this concern, Koch suggested in 1888 that the name "constitutional psychopathic inferiority" be used. The syndrome was further delineated by Meyer who excluded neurotics, and by Birnbaum who pointed out that psychopaths were not all intellectually defective, nor were all criminals psychopaths.

Glueck,[30] in his famous Sing Sing study of 1918, is considered to be the first to conduct an empirical study of such individuals. He pointed out their recidivism and early onset of antisocial behavior. The group, however, was still quite broad and included sexual offenders, addicts, alcoholics, etc. The McCords[62] inform us that in 1922 John Visher presented an almost modern picture of the psychopath's character traits: "Extreme impulsivity, lack of concentration, marked egotism, and abnormal projection. The most critical disability of the patients centered around a guiltless, uninhibited social nihilism."

The organic basis of our syndrome received impetus in 1924 with Bolsi's discovery of encephalitis as a contributing cause of psychopathic behavior. Countering this, however, was the psychoanalytic movement which saw such behavior in many patients related to unresolved oedipal conflicts or earlier developmental problems.

Alexander[4] influenced the entire field of criminology in 1930 with his paper on the neurotic character, which described patients as "living out their impulses," acting out in order to solve conflicts, being self-destructive, etc. However, time has led us to consider Alexander's description to apply to the acting-out neurotic who becomes antisocial as a means of attempting to deal with his inner conflicts.

Another group who attempted to explain this behavior were the classifiers such as Kraepelin and Kahn.[47] They divided the psychopathic personality into many subcategories, most of which included many mixtures of other illnesses.

In 1939, Sir David Henderson[43] stirred much discussion since he included such persons as Lawrence of Arabia and was felt in general to have overextended the concept. Nevertheless, this represented the emergence of a discrete syndrome, which could no longer be challenged as contributing a diagnostic entity. Cleckley more closely defined the concept and argued to change the name to "semantic dementia," which he felt described the syndrome more precisely. In 1941, Karpman[49] drew attention to his idea of two types of antisocial personality—idiopathic and symptomatic. The latter, he said, were actually neurotics, and the former the result of constitutional factors. Lindner[57] disagreed and presented numerous Rorschach protocols and other data indicating a psychological basis for the illness.

Further changes occurred, so that with the publication of DSM I[21] in 1952 the name was changed to the "sociopathic personality disturbance," under which there were several "reactions:" antisocial, dyssocial, sexual deviation, and addiction. In 1956, the McCords[62] set forth, with good evidence, the idea that psychopathy was a clear and discernible clinical entity which could be separated from other diagnostic groupings. At present, there are very few[13] who do not accept the concept of the antisocial personality as an absolute condition, although there is some disagreement about separating off dyssocial behavior.[78]

(Diagnosis

Cleckley's *The Mask of Sanity*[16] is perhaps the clearest and most precise treatise on the subject to date. While many of his thoughts as to causation and treatment have not been fully accepted, his case descriptions are unparalleled for clarity and beauty of prose. He lists the characteristic symptoms as:

1. Superficial charm and good intelligence
2. Absence of delusions and other signs of irrational thinking
3. Absence of "nervousness" or psychoneurotic manifestations
4. Unreliability
5. Untruthfulness and insincerity
6. Lack of remorse or shame
7. Inadequately motivated antisocial behavior
8. Poor judgment and failure to learn by experience
9. Pathologic egocentricity and incapacity for love
10. General poverty in major affective reactions
11. Specific loss of insight
12. Unresponsiveness in general interpersonal relations

13. Fantastic and uninviting behavior with drink and sometimes without
14. Suicide rarely carried out
15. Sex life impersonal, trivial, and poorly integrated
16. Failure to follow any life plan

The McCords[62] stress, "The psychopath's underdeveloped conscience and his inability to identify with others differentiate him from other deviants."

In a survey of psychiatrists in Canada,[33] the following features were considered most significant in diagnosing psychopathy:

1. Does not profit from experience
2. Lacks a sense of responsibility
3. Unable to form meaningful relationships
4. Lacks control over impulses
5. Lacks moral sense
6. Chronically or recurrently antisocial
7. Punishment does not alter behavior
8. Emotionally immature
9. Unable to experience guilt
10. Self-centered

Craft[19] emphasizes the psychopath's inability to love and feel affection, as well as "a liability to act on impulse without forethought." He further speaks of aggression, lack of shame or remorse, an inability to learn from experience, and lack of motivation. In addition, he feels there must be no psychosis or neurosis present, nor should the patient be handicapped by severe intellectual limits.

DSM II[22] says of the antisocial personality:

This term is reserved for individuals who are basically unsocialized and whose behavior pattern brings them repeatedly into conflict with society. They are incapable of significant loyalty to individuals, groups, or social values. They are grossly selfish, callous, irresponsible, impulsive, and unable to feel guilt or to learn from experience and punishment. Frustration tolerance is low. They tend to blame others or offer plausible rationalizations for their behavior. A mere history of repeated legal or social offenses is not sufficient to justify this diagnosis.

The consistency of these criteria or definitions is amazing and lends further support to our seeing these patients as a specific group.

Many clinicians believe that some features of the antisocial personality should be evident in the earlier years. Robins[71] has shown a very high incidence of adult antisocial personalities who as children were referred to a clinic for delinquent behavior. School failures, cheating, truancy, petty larceny, cruelty to animals, etc., should be seen in childhood with similar behavior in adolescence. Guze[38] offers support of this in his study of adult offenders. Those who do not show evidence of antisocial behavior until they are adults probably should be considered symptomatic and not true antisocial personalities.

The psychopathic personality shows no response to being caught or incarcerated. He presents himself well and does not convince us that he is remorseful, despite his statements to the contrary. He has no real loyalty to any individual or group. An aura of superior intelligence surrounds the antisocial personality. At first glance, one has the impression that he is at least a college graduate. However, if observed closely, words are not used correctly and his knowledge is actually quite superficial. (Close observation is, however, not easy, as the psychopath is quite skillful at dodging detection.)

He is egocentric and primarily incapable of loving, that is, he seems only to care for himself. Upon being asked by a judge how he (a psychopathic defendant) could so readily cheat people who trusted him, the defendant replied that it was very difficult to cheat people unless they did trust him. Although he becomes involved in many relationships, he appears able to disengage himself with impunity for both the hurt feelings of others and any of his incurred responsibilities. He does not really seem to experience guilt. He will admit errors and failures willingly, but seems unable to comprehend the significance of his actions. Hare[40] says of these patients: "He knows the words, but not the music." Equally descriptive is Miller's[64] definition of the psychopath as one who "can walk through snow without leaving footprints."

He may be self-destructive or at least appear to be. Somehow, he always seems to get caught when it is apparent that he has the ability to avoid such detection. It is as if he did not really care.

There is also Greenacre's[36] concept that the psychopath has such an overwhelming superego (guilt) that he repeatedly sets up situations resulting in his punishment. We do know that despite his intelligence and sometimes careful preparation, he seems to leave something undone, so that he is readily apprehended. Alexander[4] speaks of the neurotic who displays antisocial behavior, yet this is qualitatively different from Greenacre's concept of this superego defect. It may seem curious to speak of such seemingly guilt-free persons as guilt-driven, yet clinically one is frequently impressed with such theoretical concepts.

The use of words in a manner apparently different from the rest of us requires special mention. This is part of a feature Cleckley so aptly named the "semantic psychosis." Although he uses this term to explain his theory of an organic causation, I feel it offers a great deal to our understanding of a particular part of the antisocial personality. These people use words in a way so unreal as to warrant the appellation "semantic psychosis." "I am sorry," seems to mean, "That is what he [the listener] wants to hear and then he will let me go." Or, "I like you, doc. I think you understand me. Of all the psychiatrists I've seen [usually a lot] you understand me better than any of them. If I make probation and get that good job, could I see you regularly?" What the patient, however, is saying is: "I've only known this doctor for five minutes, but I need to butter him up. He'll fall for my line, just like everyone else. . . ."

Cleckley describes one case as follows:

A man in his twenties, who has been arrested seventy or eighty times, as a child was often truant from school. Occasionally, he stole from his parents some object such as a watch or a piece of table silver. These acts never seemed prompted by a keen desire or ordinary temptation. He often sold for a pittance the object he had stolen. When truant from school, he did not engage in anything that the ordinary boy might regard as high adventure. He wandered about, engaging, apparently without enthusiasm, in petty mischief such as setting fire to a privy at the edge of town or shooting at chickens with an air gun. Often he hung idly about a drugstore and, vaguely bored, read comic books. During his teens he bought many articles for which he had no particular use and, without asking permission, charged them to his father. Neither punishment nor reasoning influenced his conduct.

Always this young man seemed to understand that he had done wrong, and he solemnly agreed never to repeat the errors that were causing his family so much sorrow. His appearance of sincerity at such times was impressive. After being apprehended, he freely discussed the gravity of his misdeeds and the importance of avoiding anything similar in the future. His stated resolutions did not seem perfunctory or sullen but rather reflected good judgment, insight, and the utmost candor. Despite this, his maladjustment continued. In the late teens he several times drove off the automobile of some neighbor or in one he found parked downtown. His father, who had considerable financial means and who was influential in the community, faithfully made restitution for his thefts and other damaging acts. His schoolteachers and the minister joined his parents in efforts to influence him.

Those who dealt with him came, in time, to feel that such a continual pattern of misbehavior must differ profoundly from ordinarily motivated rebellion. After he became old enough to obtain a driver's license, his father, thinking that he might have some strong and specific desire to possess an automobile, bought one for him in the hope that it would influence him favorably. Not long afterward, while out driving, he parked the new car, crossed the street, and took possession of a battered and inferior vehicle which he later abandoned in the country after a minor accident. Subsequently, after driving another stolen car across a state line, he fell into the hands of the federal authorities.

After months of imprisonment he was granted parole. He appeared to have gained real maturity and expressed the most appropriate intentions about his future. For a while he seemed industrious, confident, and happy in work that he had obtained. Then, without warning to his parents (with whom he was living), he disappeared. Approximately a week later his father received a telephone call from a city on the other side of the state, informing him that his son was in jail. Numerous forgeries and swindlings now came to light, as well as an episode of disorderly conduct in a low dance hall. Our subject had there provoked a quarrel and, after a deplorably unpleasant scene in public, had inflicted a minor injury on one of the waitresses who was trying to restore order.

This habit of casually leaving his parents' home at the behest of any whim persisted over the years. He expressed strong natural affection for both father and mother and was most convincing when he spoke of being willing to do anything to avoid causing them sorrow or distress. Nevertheless, after saying he was going down to the drugstore or perhaps to a moving picture, he would sometimes not return that night or be heard from for many days.

Once a friend of the family, who was thought to be very influential with younger people, set out to counsel him about his problems. The older man was astonished, and also gratified at what appeared to be the frankness and courage with which the younger man faced every issue. So impressed was he with the attitude of our subject that he could not restrain admiration. As plans for the future were discussed, the counselor found himself increasingly influenced by the other's expressed aims and his wise analysis of life and its potential values. In fact, he found himself beginning to give thought to his own status and to possible changes that might enable him to live more meaningfully. After this heartening interview the older man drove the younger to his parent's home. Full of confidence, he departed as his new disciple walked in the front gate. The latter did not, however, enter the house. Strolling casually around it, he went out of the back gate and sent no word to his parents until he was again in the hands of the authorities.

Truman Capote[15] in *In Cold Blood* describes Richard Hickock and Perry Smith, both of whom might be classified as antisocial personalities. Numerous other excellent descriptions have been published.[3,9,16,18,40,57,63]

Various clinicians have delineated the antisocial personality into subgroups, which should make it easier for us to understand and classify individual variations. Unfortunately, none of these have acquired universal or even general acceptance. Karpman[49] speaks of the "aggressive-predatory type" or the "passive-parasitic type," as well as other groupings.[48] Arieti[6] speaks of a "simple type," and a "complex type." The former tends to act on pure impulse, while the latter may plan his schemes in the manner of the professional bank robber or swindler. We tend to see various types of behavior from our sociopath. Some are violent, dangerous persons who rob, rape, and shoot without a second thought. Others seem to be keen and shrewd confidence men or swindlers who would not use physical force unless absolutely necessary. Rather than separating the antisocial personality into classifications on the basis of his specific behavior, most clinicians tend to view all of these patients simply as antisocial personalities.

(Differential Diagnosis

Antisocial Behavior

The difficulties one encounters in correctly diagnosing a patient as an antisocial personality are many and varied. For example, we often come into contact with a person who has made a good adjustment through childhood and adolescence and who appears to have developed meaningful adult relationships, but who then suddenly, begins to cheat and lie, and exhibit other features of antisocial behavior. Such cases are frequently seen in professional people or previously competent businessmen who begin to gamble, embezzle funds, desert their families for showgirls, etc. Such individuals are not true antisocial personalities, but neurotic or character problems who utilize antisocial behavior to deal with their problems. Unless we make this type of differentiation, our diagnosis becomes useless. A careful diagnosis is important because of the treatment and prognostic implications, as well as the social and legal problems. Kernberg[52] has recently written about prognostic considerations and he points out the significance of the degree and quality of ego weakness, superego pathology, and object relationships, as important factors in evaluating the patient.

I doubt if any true antisocial personality ever graduated from college and practiced a profession, or remained married and reasonably faithful for any length of time. Such determination and loyalty are not characteristic of the antisocial personality. The patient who has accomplished the above and begins to act out is only utilizing antisocial behavior. Beneath such behavior lies a neurosis or some form of character disorder other than the antisocial personality. Some believe that the antisocial personality never becomes an alcoholic or addict because his high degree of narcissism will not allow him to lose control to that degree. Such a statement may sound unusual considering our patient's impulsivity, but in this case the narcissism seems to take precedence over the impulsivity. Antisocial personalities are polymorphous perverse in their sexuality. They have their sex on impulse with little regard as to the propriety of the partner or place, so that many feel that the homosexual does not belong in this group.

Are there female antisocial personalities? They certainly exist, although they are rare and generally not in pure form. (For example, Bonnie of "Bonnie and Clyde" fame.) However, perhaps this is further proof of the different psychologic structure of the female. Guze et al.[37] have produced evidence which indicates that the family that produces an antisocial male will produce a hysteric female.

In my experience, there is another related group of individuals who may not be ill at all but consist of people who adopt many of the features discussed by Cleckley and others as a way of adapting to life. I refer here to individuals who never clearly break the law but who are exceptionally opportunistic and not particularly careful with the truth. They seem to relate to those close to them, but in a minimal way. Examples of this group might be certain politicians and businessmen, like the "used car salesman." We might say that these people evidence some psychopathic-like behavior.

Neurosis and Psychosis

When a patient shows primary features of neurosis or psychosis, his primary diagnosis should not be that of an antisocial personality, regardless of how antisocial his behavior has been. In such cases, the diagnosis should center on the specific neurosis or psychosis involved. One must remember, particularly in forensic work, to be on the alert for the patient who will feign psychosis or neurosis in order to cover up his basic antisocial personality. We see this more frequently today, with an increased utilization of the insanity plea. To complicate matters further, when placed under sufficient stress (limiting the opportunity to act out), many antisocial personalities appear to regress into a full-blown paranoid psychosis resembling a schizophrenic illness. Upon recovery, they appear antisocial again. This would seem to supply further evidence for a "continuum" theory of mental illness.[8]

(Causation

There are almost as many theories as to causation as there are patients, which tells us that no one has a good explanation, and that the causes are really multiple. The major theories of causation of the antisocial personality include genetics, brain damage, and environmental or psychogenic influences.

Genetics

Many studies of twins have pointed to evidence that two-thirds of monozygotic twins observed were concordant for criminal behavior. With reference to genetic implications, Eysenck[25] says:

Since the evidence is so conclusive and reproduced by so many different investigators in different countries, and since it agrees so much with what might be called the common wisdom of the ages, one might expect that common acceptance had been accorded to it, and that any textbook of criminality would give pride of place to these findings. This is not so, however, and it is interesting

to consider for a moment why these findings have been largely disregarded. One reason for this may lie in the climate of opinion which prevails, particularly in the United States and in the Soviet Union. In both these countries there is a strong belief in what one might call the technological or manipulative outlook on life. In both countries, there is a widespread belief that almost anything is possible to the person with technical knowledge who is determined to effect certain changes.

Frankenstein[27] also feels there may be congenital factors. On the other hand, McCord and McCord[62] say, "Heredity cannot yet be excluded as a causal factor. . . . Given our current knowledge, however, the extravagant claims of the geneticists must be questioned." Halleck[39] and others strongly support this statement. There has also been some work done by Sheldon[77] with somatotypes, indicating that delinquents are more muscular than nondelinquents. However, this has failed to produce any convincing evidence of a criminal or antisocial body type. Recently,[67,14] the XYY ("supermale") factor had been noted as occurring as a genetic variant in many mentally deficient prisoners. This suddenly became the antisocial factor. However, more recent articles[1,61] have tended to question a clear-cut relationship between XYY and antisocial behavior. In fact, one report[7] indicates that there may be the same incidence of antisocial behavior in the XXY, the "female-male," as in the "supermale."

Brain Damage

Many clinicians[82] have been convinced that the antisocial personality must suffer from some intracranial damage, which would account for their impulsivity, aggressiveness, etc. However, their ability to use language and limited information for a maximum effect suggests very discrete or specific brain damage, if any.

Hare[40] points out, "A large number of studies with various forms of the Wechsler-Bellevue Intelligence Scale strongly supports the clinical impression that psychopaths as a group have at least average global intelligence." There have been claims that the anti-social personality scores higher on the performance scales than on the verbal scales, but results have been inconsistent. Wechsler[84] and Manne[60] support this, while Craddick[17] and Gurvitz[37] do not. Unfortunately, this does not help us to understand the clinical impression these patients give of superior intelligence.

As for EEG findings, Hare[40] says:

In spite of their limitations, the EEG studies of psychopathy have produced rather consistent results. One finding—the widespread slow-wave activity often found in psychopaths bears a certain resemblance to the EEG patterns usually found in children—has led to a cortical immaturity hypothesis of psychopathy. A second hypothesis, based on the presence of localized EEG abnormalities, is that psychopathy is associated with a defect or malfunction of certain brain mechanisms concerned with emotional activity and the regulation of behavior. Finally, it has been suggested that psychopathy may be related to a lowered state of cortical excitability and to the attentuation of sensory input, particularly input that would ordinarily have disturbing consequences.

On the other hand, a prison study[66] found a higher percentage of abnormal EEG's in conscientious objectors than in psychopaths. However, Kurland et al.[54] found abnormal EEG's in two-thirds of ninety men in the Navy and Marine Corps who had such severe character disorders that they received unsuitability discharges. Thompson[82] felt there was a relationship between EEG signs of psychomotor epilepsy and psychopathy. He also felt that these patients exhibited a lot of "minor" neurologic deviations. There has been an increasing interest in the autonomic nervous system and behavior, both in terms of causation and treatment possibilities. Three studies[55,31,5] have separated a hostile and simple sociopath on the basis of cardiac response to epinephrine, and feel that this may represent some basic physiologic difference of a neuro-hormonal type. Abrahamsen[2] found a high incidence of psychosomatic disorders in his delinquent population.

Eysenck[25] believes, as does Hare,[40] that there are inherited autonomic nervous system differences, and bases treatment suggestions on these theoretical constructs.

Environmental-Psychogenic Influences

While there has been no conclusive statistical evidence that environment plays a controlling role in the development of the sociopathic personality, individual case reports have exemplified such an influence. Lindner's[56] *Rebel Without a Cause* is a detailed example, as are cases presented by Craft,[18] McCord and McCord,[62] Sturup,[79] and others. A most thorough follow-up study of a child outpatient clinic by Robins[71] has shown that a very high incidence of adult antisocial personalities come from homes in which the father was himself an antisocial personality or alcoholic. Guze[37] has evaluated a large number of criminals and found that their female relatives show a high incidence of hysteria, prompting him to consider hysteria the female equivalent of antisocial behavior. Other theories have dealt with early parental death or separation,[12] severe rejection by the parents, or in some cases, a constant seesawing back and forth between indulgence and rejection. Where there is question as to the specific influence any of these extreme experiences might have on the given individual, most behavioral scientists agree that there is going to be some unfavorable effect. Usdin's[83] statement, "It is better to be wanted by the police than no one at all," may reflect the total feeling of rejection to which some psychopaths have been exposed. Manne[59] presents "a theory of sociopathic behavior based on action-oriented, often nonverbal, communications between the sociopath and the important figures in his life. Attempts to explain the serious ego and superego defect in the psychopath have been numerous and varied.[28,29] Johnson and Szurek[45] have spoken of the unconscious push by the parents in a vicarious "I can't do it, you do it for me."

⟮ Medicolegal Status

Although we speak of the antisocial personality as suffering from a mental illness, he is generally considered responsible in the eyes of the law, regardless of which test of criminal responsibility is used. This may seem unusual when we have said that these patients suffer with severe ego and superego defects, cannot seem to control their impulses, feel no guilt, etc. There are several important factors that must be taken into account. The first is whether or not the antisocial personality is to be considered as a mental illness or merely a personality disorder. This is primary since all tests of criminal responsibility have as their first requirement that the person be suffering from a "mental disorder" (or mental disease or defect). We might answer this by saying that the official diagnostic manuals throughout the world recognize this group of patients as suffering from a mental illness, although there are some variations as to who might be included. Nevertheless, many psychiatrists and legal systems continue to feel that these patients are not mentally ill.

In my opinion, no diagnostic label alone should determine criminal responsibility. For example, there are many severe schizophrenics who are legally responsible for the crimes they commit. The important factor is not the diagnosis alone but the relationship between the illness and the offense. This relationship is what must determine the psychiatrist's medical opinion and is what he must explain to the judge or jury so they may arrive at their legal decision. In some cases, they will find an antisocial personality not responsible.

The Durham Rule[24] which considers the defendant not responsible if his crime was the product of a mental disease or defect, caused some difficulty, since many psychiatrists felt that the designation of antisocial personality as a mental disease meant that the individual could not be held responsible for his offense. Such a simplistic use of diagnostic labels was not acceptable to Judge Bazelon, the framer

of the Durham decision, so that the court in the McDonald case[63] found:

Our eight-year experience under Durham suggests a judicial definition, however broad and general, of what is included in the terms "disease" and "defect." In Durham, rather than define either term, we simply sought to distinguish disease from defect. Our purpose now is to make it very clear that neither the court nor the jury is bound by ad hoc definitions or conclusions as to what experts state is a disease or defect. What psychiatrists may consider a "mental disease or defect" for clinical purposes, where their concern is treatment, may or may not be the same as mental disease or defect for the jury's purpose in determining criminal responsibility.

When the framers of the Model Penal Code[65] devised their test, they included a third section: "As used in this Section, the term 'mental disorder' does not include an abnormality manifested only by repeated criminal or otherwise antisocial conduct." Thereby, the antisocial personality was excluded. Birnbaum[10] quotes Professor Wechsler of the Columbia Law School: "The problem is to differentiate between cases which, in the division of function that our society and culture have established, belong exclusively to mental health and those which may be reviewed as cases for correction." Kozol[53] feels the antisocial personality should be found not responsible and should be hospitalized. The opposite point of view, with which I am in agreement, is presented by Birnbaum, a lawyer-physician. He feels that for many practical reasons we must consider the antisocial personality legally responsible. He points out, most convincingly, that such patients may fare no better if placed in mental hospitals, and possibly the public may be less well protected under this system. Certainly, neither our knowledge, understanding, ability to treat, or facilities, are adequate enough for us to suggest that mental health professionals accept full responsibility for these patients, although the courts and the community might like us to do this. On the other hand, we have made sufficient progress in the above items, so that we should be involved in the management of these patients in correctional or special facilities. It is in the latter that we have made some meaningful progress.

❨ Treatment

The search for a treatment for the antisocial personality has not revealed any single treatment for this disease any more than have similar efforts in search of a single treatment for schizophrenia or other mental illnesses. The treatment prescribed will be obviously dependent upon the theory of causation to which one subscribes.. Therefore, Thompson[82] recommended electroshock treatment and Eysenck[2] recommends conditioning by various techniques. McCord and McCord[62] recommend milieu therapy as do others,[46] each with his own variation. One factor that we must constantly keep in mind when speaking of the treatment of this group of patients is whether or not we are speaking of the real antisocial personality or the borderline or neurotic personality who shows antisocial behavior. I have no doubt that many of the various treatments recommended will help those who display antisocial behavior; however, the antisocial personality probably always requires special inpatient facilities.[52,20]

There are several of these special institutions in the world, all of which have produced astounding results,[20] if we are to accept their cases as true antisocial personalities. The results coming from institutions such as Herstevester, Denmark,[79] the Van der Hooven Clinic in Utrecht, Holland,[72] Balderton Hospital, Newark, England,[19] and Patuxent Institution in Jessup, Maryland,[11,44,36] would support the view that one needs a secure institution, long (indeterminate) sentences, a devoted and well-trained staff, and varying mixtures of group and individual therapy. In addition, one must provide a therapeutic and behavioristic milieu, job training, and social re-education, all based on a scheme of "It's not what you say, but what you do that counts." Many who have worked with antisocial personalities of the most incorrigible and dangerous type have reported good results under ideal circumstances, but at great expense.[11,44,79,72,18]

I am personally acquainted with the Patuxent Institution at Jessup, Maryland. Recent data[44] would indicate that recidivism occurred in 81% of the untreated group, 46% of the minimally treated group, 39% with more treatment, and in only 7% of the fully treated group.* Similar results have been reported by others. Herestevester is similar to Patuxent in its structure and program while the Van der Hooven Clinic[72] is more open and operated on the principle of a therapeutic community, as originally described by Jones.[46] An approach such as the one used in these institutions would appear to be the current choice. Besides the security and the indeterminate sentence, there is sufficient individualization and flexibility in their programs. Privileges are given on the basis of "ability to accept responsibility," which seems to allow for the development and growth of ego and superego assets. All patients are released slowly and followed up closely in the community.

As a result of these institutional successes, the prognosis for the antisocial personality may not be as bad as previously thought, although some, such as Kernberg,[52] continue to feel that no real psychological insights or changes are made. While the changes may not appear deep, they nevertheless occur. When we consider that these institutions have treated the most serious cases, any good result seems excellent, particularly when we discover that the average time for successful treatment is three to five years.[11,79]

Future developments in the treatment of such patients should certainly bring better results, although at the moment no newer ideas have taken hold. Conditioning may have some hope, as Eysenck[25] has proposed, but Hare[40,41] believes it is of limited value with the antisocial personality. Conditioning experiments have produced results in some antisocial obsessive disorders, such as gambling,[76] and in homosexuality,[26] etc.

* *Maryland Defective Delinquent Statute: A Progress Report*, Patuxent Institution, Jessup, Maryland, 1973.

There are patients who appear to be seriously antisocial and who have been successfully treated by other methods, such as the milieu therapy at Wiltwych described by McCord and McCord.[62] Milieu therapy has been tried with some of Karpman's[50] patients also, but Karpman felt that no true antisocial personality could be treated. Donnelly[23] describes some of the necessary treatment variations for treating those with antisocial behavior problems in regular psychiatric hospitals. Classical psychoanalytic treatment is rarely considered as a technique useful for these patients in view of their ego and superego structure. Lindner[56] successfully treated a patient in prison with hypnotherapy. Others [28,81,69,70] report successful use of psychoanalytic treatment with delinquent children. However, these seem to be selected cases who might more properly be classified as neurotic patients with antisocial behavior, and not true antisocial personalities.

The patients treated by Schmideberg[73,74,75] and others[62,50,23] represent an interesting challenge for the psychiatrist. These are the neurotic antisocial offenders. They are seen regularly in court and frequently in the consultation room. They want help if you can make them hold still long enough to get it. Most therapists have been tricked and cheated by such patients and then tend to shy away from them. Yet we see more and more of such people who need help. In dealing with such borderline personalities or character disorders, it is obvious that special techniques must be utilized, as described. These techniques include close co-operation between doctor and probation officer, strong reality orientation, support and guidance, allowing the ego and superego to develop, and dealing with the neurosis slowly. Although quite frustrating and challenging as patients, they can add a change to the regular office routine.

It is hoped that the lessons learned at Herstevester and Patuxent, as well as that of Schmideberg and others, can be transferred to our correctional institutions. The application of these lessons, however, will require a greater involvement of psychiatrists in correctional institutions, and a willingness of the community to support such efforts. With crime and violence on the increase all over the world, such efforts are sorely needed.

(Bibliography

1. Abdullah, S., L. F. Jarvik, T. Koto, et al. "Extra Y Chromosome and Its Psychiatric Implications," Archives of General Psychiatry, 21 (1969), 497–501.
2. Abrahamsen, D. The Psychology of Crime. New York: Columbia University Press, 1960.
3. Aichhorn, A. Wayward Youth. New York: Viking Press, 1935.
4. Alexander, F. "The Neurotic Character," International Journal of Psycho-Analysis, 11 (1930), 292–311.
5. Allen, H., L. Lindner, H. Goldman et al. "Hostile and Simple Sociopaths: An Empirical Typology," Criminology, 9 (1971), 27–47.
6. Arieti, S. The Intrapsychic Self. New York: Basic Books, 1967.
7. Baker, D., M. A. Telfer, C. E. Richardson et al. "Chromosome Errors in Men With Antisocial Behavior," Journal of the AMA, 214 (1970), 869–878.
8. Bellak, E., ed. Schizophrenia. New York: Logos Press, 1958.
9. Bergman, R. E. The Sociopath. New York: Exposition Press, 1968.
10. Birnbaum, M. "Medicine and the Law," New England Journal of Medicine, 261 (1959), 1220–1225.
11. Boslow, H. M., and W. Kohlmeyer. "The Maryland Defective Delinquency Law," The American Journal of Psychiatry, 120 (1963), 118–124.
12. Bowlby, J. "Maternal Care and Mental Health," Monograph Series No. 2, Geneva: World Health Organization, 1951.
13. Bromberg, W. "Psychopathic Personality Concept Evaluated and Reevaluated," Archives of General Psychiatry, 17 (1967) 641–645.
14. Brown, W. M. C. "Males With An XYY Sex Chromosome Complement," Journal of Medical Genetics, 5 (1968), 341–359.
15. Capote, T. In Cold Blood. New York: Random House, 1965.
16. Cleckley, H. The Mask of Sanity. St. Louis: C. V. Mosby Co., 1964.

17. CRADDICK, R. A. "Wechsler-Bellevue I. Q. Scores of Psychopathic and Non-psychopathic Prisoners," *Journal of Psychological Studies*, 12 (1961), 167–172.

18. CRAFT, M. *Ten Studies Into Psychopathic Personality*. Bristol: John Wright & Sons Ltd., 1965.

19. ———. *Psychopathic Disorders and Their Assessment*. New York: Pergamon Press, 1966.

20. ———. "The Natural History of Psychopathic Disorder," *British Journal of Psychiatry*, 115 (1969), 39–44.

21. *Diagnostic and Statistical Manual, Mental Disorders* (DSM I), American Psychiatric Association, Mental Hospital Service, Washington, D.C., 1968.

22. *Diagnostic and Statistical Manual, Mental Disorders* (DSM II), American Psychiatric Association, Mental Hospital Service, Washington, D.C., 1968.

23. DONNELLY, J. "Aspects of the Treatment of Character Disorders," *Archives of General Psychiatry*, 15 (1966), 22–28.

24. DURHAM VS. UNITED STATES, 1954, U. S. Court of Appeals, Washington, D. C., 214 F. 2d., 862, *Federal Reporter*.

25. EYSENCK, H. J. *Crime and Personality*. Boston: Houghton Mifflin Company, 1964.

26. FELDMAN, M. P., and M. T. MacCULLOCH. *Homosexual Behavior, Therapy and Assessment*. New York: Pergamon Press, 1971.

27. FRANKENSTEIN, C. *Psychopathy*. New York: Grune & Stratton, 1959.

28. FRIEDLANDER, K. "Formation of the Antisocial Character," in *The Psychoanalytic Study of the Child*, I. New York: International Universities Press, 1945.

29. ———. "Latent Delinquency and Ego Development," in K. R. Eissler, *Searchlights on Delinquency*. New York: International Universities Press, 1949.

30. GLUECK, B. "A Study of 608 Admissions to Sing Sing Prison," *Mental Hygiene*, II (1918), 85–151.

31. GOLDMAN, H., L. A. LINDNER, S. DINITZ et al. "The Simple Sociopath: Physiologic and Sociologic Characteristics," *Biological Psychiatry*, 3 (1971), 77–83.

32. GOUSTER, M. "Moral Insanity," *Revue des Sciences Médicaux* (abstracted in *Journal of Nervous and Mental Disease*, 5 [1878], 181–182).

33. GRAY, K. C., ad H. C. HUTCHISON. "The Psychopathic Personality: A Survey of Canadian Psychiatrists' Opinions," *Canadian Psychiatric Association Journal*, 9 (1964), 452–461.

34. GREENACRE, P. *Trauma, Growth and Personality*. New York: International Universities Press, Inc., 1952.

35. GURVITZ, M. "Wechsler-Bellevue Test and the Diagnosis of Psychopathic Personality," *Journal of Clinical Psychology*, 6 (1950), 397–401.

36. GUTTMACHER, M. S. *The Role of Psychiatry in Law*. Springfield: Charles C. Thomas, 1968.

37. GUZE, S. B., R. A. WOODRUFF, JR., and P. J. CLAYTON. "Hysteria and Antisocial Behavior: Further Evidence of an Association," *American Journal of Psychiatry*, 127 (1971), 957–960.

38. GUZE, S. B. "Diagnostic Consistency in Antisocial Personality," *The American Journal of Psychiatry*, 128 (1971) 360–361.

39. HALLECK, S. L. *Psychiatry and the Dilemmas of Crime*. New York: Harper and Row, 1967.

40. HARE, R. D. *Psychopathy: Theory and Research*, New York: John Wiley & Sons, Inc., 1970.

41. ———. "Autonomic Activity and Conditioning in Psychopaths." Symposium on Psychophysiological Responses in Sociopaths, Society for Psychophysiological Research, New Orleans, La., Nov. 19–22, 1970.

42. HARTUNG, F. E. *Crime, Law and Society*. Detroit: Wayne State University Press, 1965.

43. HENDERSON, D. K. *Psychopathic States*. New York: W. W. Norton & Co., Inc., 1939.

44. HODGES, E. F. "Crime Prevention by the Indeterminate Sentence Law," *The American Journal of Psychiatry*, 128 (1971), 291–295.

45. JOHNSON, A. M., and S. A. SZUREK. "The Genesis of Antisocial Acting Out in Children and Adults," *Psychoanalytic Quarterly*, 21 (1952), 323–343.

46. JONES, M. *The Therapeutic Community*. New York: Basic Books, 1953.

47. KAHN, E. *Psychopathic Personalities*. New Haven: Yale University Press, 1931.

48. KARPMAN, B. "Myth of Psychopathic Personality," *The American Journal of Psychiatry*, 104 (1948), 523–534.

49. ———. "On the Need for Separating Psychopathy Into 2 Distinct Clinical Types:

Symptomatic and Idiopathic," *Journal of Clinical Psychopathology*, 3 (1941), 112–137.

50. ———. *Case Studies in the Psychopathology of Crime*. Vols. 1–4. Washington: Medical Science Press, 1947.

51. KAVKA, J. "Pinel's Conception of the Psychopathic State: An Historical Critique," *Bulletin of the History of Medicine*, 23 (1949), 461–468.

52. KERNBERG, O. F. "Prognostic Considerations Regarding Borderline Personality Organization," *Journal of American Psychoanalytic Association*, 19 (1971), 595–635.

53. KOZOL, H. "The Psychopath Before the Law," *New England Journal of Medicine*, 260 (1959), 637–644.

54. KURLAND, H. D., C. T. YEAGER, and R. J. ARTHUR. "Psychophysiologic Aspects of Severe Behavior Disorders," *Archives of General Psychiatry*, 8 (1963), 599–604.

55. LINDNER, L. A., H. GOLDMAN, S. DINITZ, et al. "Antisocial Personality Type With Cardiac Lability," *Archives of General Psychiatry*, 23 (1970), 260–267.

56. LINDNER, R. M. *Rebel Without a Cause*. New York: Grune & Stratton, 1944.

57. ———. "Experimental Studies in Constitutional Psychopathic Inferiority," *Journal of Criminal Psychopathology*, 4 (1942–1943), 252–484.

58. LOMBROSO, C. *Crime, Its Causes and Remedies*. H. P. Horton, transl. Boston: Little Brown, 1911.

59. MANNE, S. H. "A Communication Theory of Sociopathic Personality," *American Journal of Psychotherapy*, XXI (1967), 797–807.

60. MANNE, S. H. et al. "Differences Between Performance I. Q. and Verbal I. Q. in a Severely Sociopathic Population," *Journal of Clinical Psychology*, 18 (1962), 73–77.

61. MARINELLO, M. J., R. A. BERKSON, J. A. EDWARDS et al. "A Study of the XYY Syndrome in Tall Men and Juvenile Delinquents," *Journal of the AMA*, 208 (1969), 321–325.

62. McCORD, W. and McCORD, J. *Psychopathy and Delinquency*. New York: Grune & Stratton, 1956.

63. MCDONALD vs. UNITED STATES, 1962. U.S. Court of Appeals, Washington, D.C., 312 F 2d., 847, *Federal Reporter*.

64. MILLER, M. "Time and The Character Disorder," *Journal of Nervous and Mental Disease*, 138 (1964), 535–540.

65. MODEL PENAL CODE. *The American Law Institute*. Article 4, Section 4.01, 1962.

66. OSTROW, M., and OSTROW, M. "Bilaterally Synchronous Paroxysmal Slow Activity in the Electroencephalogram of Non-Epileptics," *Journal of Nervous and Mental Disease*, 103 (1946), 346–358.

67. PRICE, W. H., and P. B. WATMORE. "Behavior Disorders and Pattern of Crime Among XYY Males Identified at a Maximum Security Hospital," *British Medical Journal*, 1 (1967), 533–536.

68. PRICHARD, J. C. *Treatise on Insanity*. London: Sherwood Gilbert and Piper, 1835.

69. REDL, F., and D. WINEMAN, *Controls from Within: Techniques for the Treatment of the Aggressive Child*. Glencoe: Free Press, 1954.

70. REDL, F. *Children Who Hate*. Glencoe: Free Press, 1951.

71. ROBINS, L. N. *Deviant Children Grown Up*. Baltimore: Williams & Wilkins Co., 1966.

72. ROOSENBERG, A. M. "The Therapeutic Community in the Rehabilition of Delinquents." Presented at 122nd APA Meeting, Miami, Florida, 1969.

73. SCHMIDEBERG, M. "The Treatment of Psychopaths and Borderline Patients," *International Journal of Psychotherapy*, 1 (1947), 45–65.

74. ———. "The Analytic Treatment of Major Criminals: Therapeutic Results and Technical Problems," in K. R. Eissler, ed., *Searchlights on Delinquency*. New York: International Universities Press, 1949.

75. ———. Editor-in-Chief, *International Journal of Offender Therapy*, London, England. (See any recent issue for appropriate articles.)

76. SEAGER, C. P. "Treatment of Compulsive Gamblers by Electrical Aversion," *British Journal of Psychiatry*, 117 (1970), 545–553.

77. SHELDON, W. H. *Varieties of Delinquent Youth*. New York: Harper & Bros., 1956.

78. STOJANOVICH, K. "Antisocial and Dyssocial," *Archives of General Psychiatry*, 21 (1969), 561–567.

79. STURUP, G. K. *Treating the "Untreatable"*. Baltimore: The Johns Hopkins Press, 1968.

80. SUTHERLAND, E. H., and D. R. CRESSEY. *Principles of Criminology*. Philadelphia: J. B. Lippincott Co., 1966.

81. SZUREK, S. A. "Some Impressions from Clinical Experience With Delinquents," in

K. R. Eissler, ed., *Searchlights on Delinquency*. New York: International Universities Press, 1949.

82. THOMPSON, G. N. *The Psychopathic Delinquent and Criminal*. Springfield: Charles C. Thomas, 1953.

83. USDIN, G. L. "Broader Aspects of Dangerousness," in J. R. Rappeport, ed., *The Clinical Evaluation of the Dangerousness*

of the Mentally Ill. Springfield: Charles C. Thomas, 1967.

84. WECHSLER, D. *The Measurement and Appraisal of Adult Intelligence*. 4th ed. Baltimore: Williams & Wilkins, 1958.

85. WOLFGANG, M. E., L. SAVITZ, and N. JOHNSON, *The Sociology of Crime and Delinquency*. New York: John Wiley & Sons, 1962.

CHAPTER 13

MALINGERING AND ASSOCIATED SYNDROMES

David Davis and James M. A. Weiss

WEBSTER'S NEW WORLD DICTIONARY gives a very limited definition of "malinger" as "to pretend to be ill or otherwise incapacitated in order to escape duty or work; shirk." DeJong[23] in *The Neurologic Examination* defines "malingering" as "a willful, deliberate, and fraudulent imitation or exaggeration of illness, usually intended to deceive others, and under most circumstances, conceived for the purpose of gaining a consciously desired end." Present-day historical and psychiatric works tend to neglect the subject. The *Encyclopaedia Britannica* contains no article pertaining to it. Garrison's *An Introduction to the History of Medicine*[33] contains no reference to malingering in its index of thirty pages. Nor does the *Diagnostic and Statistical Manual of Mental Disorders* of the American Psychiatric Association[25] list the term, and no standard modern psychiatric textbook includes any comprehensive survey. Yet, almost every physician, almost every psychiatrist, can relate some experience with patients presenting a problem in this area, and personnel in the armed services, the courts, the prisons, and the large hospitals, find it a behavioral manifestation of concern and mystery.

Nevertheless, there are a great many articles in the literature related to malingering and associated syndromes, and numerous authors have devised complicated classifications of these phenomena based on a variety of dimensions. Such parameters include (1) the kind of organ system supposedly involved, (2) the nature of secondary gain, (3) the degree of suffering involved, (4) whether the symptoms are invented, exaggerated, based on genuine disorder or injury which has ceased but is alleged to continue, or genuine symptoms are attributed to a cause other than the cause in fact, (5) the psychological setting in which the malingering occurs, and (6) basic motives, and whether these motives and the production of symptoms are conscious or unconscious. Such taxonomic systems are theoretically intriguing but seem to have little practical application in clinical psychiatry. The basic common behavioral pattern subsumed under the term "malingering and related syndromes" may be conveniently assigned to not more than five or six categories.

⟮ Definitions

A number of terms relating to the concept of malingering are commonly found in the literature. "Imitation" is used in a good or indifferent sense as the general term meaning "copy." "Simulation" is used most often in a pejorative sense as a specific form of imitation in which the person acts or appears to be what he really is not (e.g., the simulation of poverty). Simulation of disease is considered as factitious illness or malingering. "Factitious illness" occurs when the person knows that he is acting out a disability, yet is unable to stop. Spiro[80] described what he termed "chronic factitious disease," in which there is simulation of a disorder with the subject allowing painful and dangerous diagnostic procedures to be carried out on himself.

"Malingering" is the simulation of disease or disability, in which a measure of conscious control is exercised, and the subject knows that he is acting and can stop. This is a specific form of simulation. Malingering or factitious illness occurs usually to avoid responsibility, to avoid punishment, to avoid difficult or dangerous duties, or to receive compensation. The term "malingering" appeared first in Grose's *Classical Dictionary of the Vulgar Tongue*[40] in 1785, originating from the French *malingré* meaning sickly or ailing, and from the Latin *malus aeger*, meaning an evil or base disposition.[*] Szasz[82] holds that malingering does not meet the usual criteria of diagnoses and is considered more as the violation of a set of social rules, akin to cheating, with the term really expressing the physician's moral condemnation of a patient and his behavior, and therefore without rational meaning as a psychopathological syndrome.

Some special forms of malingering include

[*] "Malinger" is pronounced with a hard "g" sound to rhyme with "singer."

self-inflicted injury, Munchausen's Syndrome (which involves the usually elaborate simulation of disease by persons who tend to wander from hospital to hospital), and the Ganser Syndrome of absurd or approximate answers.

Use of the Term "Malingering"

According to Schroeder,[75] many doctors refuse to use the term "malingering" because (1) it tends to alienate the patient, since its use does not convey a proper diagnostic impression; (2) physicians seem to be naturally cautious insofar as there is only one thing more painful than failing to discover apparent deceit, and that is to deny the existence of disease in a patient in whom a better informed physician would have diagnosed it; and (3) the fear that the patient may bring a defamation suit. Physicians who have used the term may have done so consciously to punish the patient for a perceived antisocial act, under the guise of establishing a "diagnosis" or in attempting to demonstrate lack of ill health. The same malingering behaviors, however, at one instance may be regarded with condemnation, and at another with praise (for example, in the feigning of illness to escape from a prisoner of war camp). The term "malingering" has tended to involve an emotionally loaded connotation implying that the doctor is being duped by the patient, his time being wasted, and his diagnostic and therapeutic skills being ridiculed. Many articles on the subject in the medical literature have included such pejorative words as liar, scoundrel, wretch, knave, rascal, unscrupulous, and cowardly. This probably represents a general social attitude, at least in part, since Weiss and Perry[90] found that lying and deception are regarded as fairly serious crimes in a variety of cultural loci.

⟮ Historical Aspects

The idea that people would feign or produce illness or disability to avoid duty, or for gain, has been noted since antiquity. The Greeks ranked malingering in military service with forgery, a crime punishable by death. (The punishment was later mitigated to exposure to the public gaze in female attire for three days.)

Galen,[1] in the second century, wrote a treatise entitled "On Feigned Diseases and the Detection of Them," describing Roman conscripts who cut off thumbs or fingers to render themselves unfit for military service, and a servant who inflamed his knee by application of juice of thapsia. Galen coined the term "pathomimes" for such people.

Montaigne[63] gave an account of the avoidance of military service by the Romans in an essay entitled "Of Thumbs," and in "How A Man Should Not Counterfeit To Be Sicke" discussed the possible consequences of malingering. Temkin[84] described the imitation of epileptic attacks as originally detailed by Ambroise Paré[53] in which beggars would put soap into their mouths in order to produce foam, and Mayhew[57] described in detail methods used to simulate illness for the purpose of begging in nineteenth-century London.

However, in general there has been a relative paucity of historical information concerning malingering. Murphy[64] pointed out that up until one hundred fifty years ago there was a lack of medical journals (initial description of diseases was usually published in book form), that in England there were no physicians of commissioned rank in the Royal Navy until well into the nineteenth century, and that at that time there seemed to be a fear of publishing works on malingering since it was associated with the shirking of military service and thus might have an adverse effect on morale. He noticed the tendency to ascribe socially undesirable conditions to other than one's own national source; syphilis was known in Italy as "the French evil," while in France, the sufferers were assumed to be afflicted with the "Italian pox." In the case of malingering, Jones and Llewellyn[50] wrote in 1917 that the German literature stressed that Poles, Alsatians, and Lorrainers were addicted to simulation more than Germans proper, and Austrian military surgeons found that most of their malingerers

hailed from Bohemia. Gavin[34] in 1845 remarked that the Irish seemed to be most numerous and expert in counterfeiting disease, with lowland Scotchmen being next.

Interest in malingering has usually been kindled by wars, the introduction of social reforms (e.g., the medieval religious interest in the sick), and by the introduction of medical and social insurance, as in France, Germany, and Great Britain in the latter half of the nineteenth and the earlier part of the twentieth centuries.

Hutchison,[46,47] who was surgeon to the Royal Naval Hospital in England, wrote "Some Observations on Simulated or Feigned Diseases" in 1824 and 1825, stimulated by the Revolutionary War of 1793–1815 which involved long, dreary naval voyages resulting in extremely poor morale. Cheyne, a military physician, in 1827 wrote his "Medical Report on the Feigned Diseases of Soldiers" (which he called "The English Malady"), published in the *Dublin Hospital Reports*.[14]

Later French and German works around the turn of the century, as well as those of Collie[17] in 1913 and Jones and Llewellyn[50] in 1917, were stimulated by Employer's Liability, Workmen's Compensation, and National Insurance Acts in their respective countries. In 1894, for example, studies on malingering formed the major content of the *Monatschrift für Unfallheilkunde*, and about this time the journal *La Médicine des Accidents du Travail* began publication.

Punton[70] provided an interesting example of deception of insurance and railroad companies. A man named Moffett described his "cane and screw" racket, in which he used a specially prepared cane to loosen the floor screws on streetcars and railroad cars, over which he would then pretend to stumble and then institute a claim for injuries sustained. He stated that he made it a universal rule to employ the very best doctors, as he found, by experience, that they were the most easily fooled, while the companies he fleeced were better satisfied with their opinions. In this connection, he noted that he paid the doctors' bills promptly and willingly, even though at times he thought they were exorbitant, but this was done, he said, in order to impress them with the honesty of his actions.

(Normal Occurrences

Complaints of illness without a physical basis are not uncommon in some children as an attempt to avoid a potentially unpleasant situation, such as school. These are more in the nature of hypochondriacal desires, which are usually easily dispelled by firm action on the part of the parent.

Simulation can be seen as a means of self-preservation in animals that may feign death, for example, and Shapiro[77] has pointed out that people may malinger as a "protective reflex" as a result of anxiety. Malingering may also occur in a normal situation in the prison camp, where one may feign illness or injury as as means to effect escape. Flicker[30] has estimated that about one-tenth of the malingering he has seen in the military has been in men without any other display of psychopathology.

(Prevalence and Epidemiology

Sund[81] in a study of prognoses of psychiatric disorders in Norwegian men who had been in compulsory military service between 1949–1959 found an incidence of malingering of 3 percent. During World War II, the incidence among American soldiers was variously estimated at between 2 and 7 percent. Flicker,[30] for example, estimated that about 5 percent of all inductees malingered. He stated, however, that in apparent refutation of this concept, in one station hospital, at a time when sixty thousand patients were listed in the registrar's office, there were but seventeen who were diagnosed as malingerers, which is 0.028 percent. On intensive questioning of the medical officers it was revealed that they believed there were more cases than were diagnosed, but they were deterred from making such a diagnosis because of the administrative difficulties of proving it at a court martial.

Brussell and Hitch[10] reported that 2 to 7 percent of the cases referred for military neuropsychiatric consultation were diagnosed as malingering. It has been noticed that the less psychiatric knowledge the doctor has, the greater the proclivity for making the diagnosis of malingering, and the greater the doctor's psychiatric experience, the less he is ready to use the diagnosis.

Jung,[51] for example, reported that malingering was diagnosed in only 0.13 percent of 8,430 admissions to the Swiss Mental Hospital of Burghölzli. In general, estimates of prevalence or epidemiology of malingering are extremely difficult to achieve because the diagnosis of the condition depends on the knowledge and experience of the physician, his attitude towards the person he is examining, and whether he accepts the use of the term as a diagnostic entity. Apparently, however, malingering is not concentrated in any particular age group and may occur equally among males and females.

(Etiology and Psychodynamics

It is clear from the literature that malingering is not a single entity and is not independent of the underlying personality. Indeed, Flicker[30] noted that most instances of feigned psychosis occur in persons who are already of unsound mind and that it is most frequently the oligophrenic who feigns feeblemindedness. It is presumed to occur where there is danger of an examination, criminal charges, or imprisonment, or associated with military conscription, especially when morale is low or during an unpopular war, and particularly with the danger of becoming a front-line soldier. Other reasons postulated include monetary gain in association with insurance and compensation, the need to be the center of interest and attention, a grudge against doctors and hospitals related to revenge, the desire for free board and lodging in hospital, the need for a haven from the police, as a method of obtaining drugs, and as a result of prolonged idleness leading to introspection.

Taylor[83] described what he calls "disease-rewarding situations," which are situations that are unpleasant, threatening, or stressful, and which may be avoided, terminated, or mitigated by falling ill. This allows a member in a family to avoid responsibilities, escape disliked duties, claim the special privileges accorded to invalids, and perhaps achieve the emotional subjugation of relatives. These also occur outside the family as in insurance claims, the military, and in prison. Taylor points out that "hypochondriacal desires," that is, the desires to be ill, are distinguished by the common characteristic of being disease-rewarding. The hypochondriacal desire may lead at most to a malingered disease or to the particular form known as Munchausen's Syndrome. If, however, there is an autosuggestive capacity of sufficient strength, then the hypochondriacal desire may be converted into a "hypochondriacal conviction" of being ill, which may lead to classical hypochondriasis. Hypochondriacal patients are so convinced autosuggestively that they are ill, that they succeed in repressing all knowledge of their hypochondriacal desires. Their illness is a reality for which they feel in no sense responsible, and yet the subjective suffering of the typical hypochondriac is not confirmed by evidence of objective symptoms. In this way, they differ from malingerers who often go to great lengths to simulate objective symptoms.

Taylor further goes on to state that people who are not only strongly autosuggestible but also have a strong dissociative capacity may succeed in transforming the hypochondriacal desires into hypochondriacal convictions which are self-verifying, both subjectively and objectively. They then suffer from a "hysterical illness." They are like malingerers, because they exhibit both subjective and objective symptoms, and are like hypochondriacs, because they have no memory of their hypochondriacal desires. In such cases, however, the autosuggestive and dissociative capacities of most people are insufficient to maintain a hysterical illness for a long time. As a result, the patient may become conscious of his hypochondriacal desires and may then deliberately aggravate whatever hysterical symp-

toms he still has, and thus may resort to the tricks of the malingerer. The whole malingered-hysterical mixture is then exhibited with histrionic ostentation, so that it becomes difficult if not impossible for the psychiatrist to decide where hysteria ends and where malingering begins (see Figure 13–1). Hawkings et al.[42] have interestingly drawn attention to the similarity between some cases of anorexia nervosa and malingering.

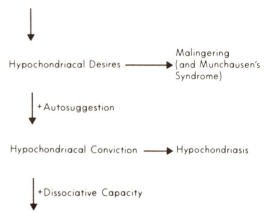

Figure 13–1.   Psychosocial development of "malingering" and related behavior (after F. Kraüpl Taylor).

Rome[73] took the point of view that like suicide and imposture, malingering is an attempt to cancel out the self, specifically through loss of ability or responsibility. In the extended sense of the term, all instances of malingering are also instances of cryptosuicide, that is, of hidden self-destructive action. Rome pointed to the malingerer's remarkable tolerance for pain, the singular absence of such affects as guilt and depression, and suggested that an undifferentiated ego lying at the base of repeated self-injury, with the plea for help based on a symbolic confusion that is the result of a failure in communication, is an essential part of the condition. He further noted the necessity of the reaction of the examiner, one usually constituted of both revulsion and compassion, and described as the primary site of psychopathology the area of interpersonal relationships between the patient and the parent with whom his identification had been hostile. Rome's data demonstrated that such patients often have experienced repeated brutality which resulted in actual physical injury. Weiss[87] has also described cases of suicidal attempts that indicate that an element of malingering may be involved.

Grinker[39] described imposture as a form of mastery over early traumata. There is usually a history of early deprivation and a discrepancy between the ego ideal and the self-image. He suggested that by imposturing, the impostor seeks love and approval from new objects, and in addition seeks revenge for past disappointments through the superiority and hostility expressed in his own secret knowledge of his deceit, thus avoiding conscious shame and the feeling of ego incompleteness.

Spiro[80] found that impostors, functional pain patients, wanderers, and masochists show phenomenologic and psychodynamic similarities to patients with chronic factitious symptoms. Early childhood deprivation and difficult relationships with aloof, absent, or sadistic parents may have sensitized the latter patients to distorted learning stemming from traumatic early illness or hospitalization. Spiro emphasized that the concept of mastery as applied by Grinker to impostors offers the most useful explanation for the subject's subsequent behavior.

❲ Role-Playing and Szasz's Point of View

Szasz[82] in a thoughtful and provocative paper discussed the relationship of the term "malingering" to diagnosis and its social connotation. He pointed out the communicative aspect of diagnosis between the physician and other physicians, and in military life between the physician and his military superiors, and suggested that the diagnosis of malingering implies the covert command from the physician to the military judicial authorities to punish the patient.

Szasz viewed malingering as part of life as a game, implying to the observer that the malingerer is getting away with something and, therefore, malingering is the same as cheating. The term "malingering" is reserved for those actions that result in the avoidance of an unpleasant duty by some motor behavior expressly disallowed by society, and the physician acts as an expert arbiter who must decide whether a person is ill within the rules that society sets for illness.

Szasz added that psychiatrists have accepted "malingering" as an entity and therefore have proceeded to describe its characteristic psychopathological features, but by so doing have substituted the concept of mental illness for other problems, and thus as a self-fulfilling prophecy find that which they are most interested in finding. He drew attention to the social context in which malingering may occur and wrote that the notion of malingering does not and cannot serve as a description of either a psychopathological syndrome or a particular psychological mechanism, in view of the fact that the term is used only in connection with a person's intention of getting out of the service or some similar aim, whereas there are many persons, for example, who enlist in the armed forces in order to get away from painful situations in their civilian and home life. This latter form of malingering called "fraudulent enlistment" is not known or regarded as true malingering, and the feigning of health by applicants for life insurance or victims of Nazi concentration camps, although termed dissimulation, may still be considered healthy, if the psychiatrist happens to side with the patient's value judgment. From the point of view of the Nazis, however, it would be considered malingering and, therefore, "the notion of malingering tells more about the observer's agreement or disagreement with the value of the social structure in which he and the patient live than it does about the latter's behavior." Thus, wrote Szasz, one can distinguish malingering as (1) a diagnosis, (2) a violation of a set of social rules, and (3) a psychopathological syndrome characterized by special psychological features. To Szasz, malingering is not a diagnosis in the usual sense of the word, but rather it expresses the physician's condemnation of behavior, and no rational meaning can be given to malingering as an alleged psychopathological syndrome; the phenomenon is best viewed in the framework of the sociopsychology of games.

❰ Symptomatology

The signs and symptoms of malingering obviously depend on the clinical picture chosen by the patient, and such clinical pictures can involve almost any system in the body. When Asher[3] originally classified Munchausen's Syndrome, he described the acute abdominal form, the hemorrhagic form with self-inflicted wounds, cranial trauma, hematuria, hematemesis, and hemoptysis, and a neurological form with headaches, syncope, meningitis, or seizures. Chapman[12] added a dermatological form involving contact dermatitis, and Cookson[18] subsequently added pulmonary edema, produced by aspirating water. More commonly, one encounters those who have ingested oral anticoagulants[38] (known as the dicoumarol eaters), those producing anemia due to voluntarily induced hemorrhage,[7] those with orthopedic problems involving low back pain,[67,32,76] those with ophthalmological conditions[79,24,59] seen sufficiently frequently for the term "Oedipism"[93] to be coined for self-inflicted injury to the eye, those with metabolic conditions[36] produced by the use of insulin or thyroid extract, and those with complaints of hearing difficulties.[49]

In a short article entitled "Artifices of War," Liddle[56] described the various methods used to simulate illness, including castor oil dysentery and the use of digitalis to produce cardiac arrhythmias. He quoted three general principles which were offered by the Germans who during World War II dropped leaflets containing advice on how to feign illness on the United States soldiers in Italy. It was suggested that the subject give the impression the feigned illness was hated, that the subject should stick to one kind of disease, and that the doctor should not be told too much.

Blinder[8] has described characteristics that he considers typical of the malingerer, such as an overriding preoccupation with "cash rather than cure" and ability to "know the law and the precedents pertinent to the patient's claim"; constant complaints about feeling miserable, with no accompanying signs or symptoms of depressive illness; symptoms that come and go; a long history of drifting about with spotty employment, as well as a history of alcoholism, drug abuse, desertion, or a criminal record. As there are many symptoms that can be produced using a variety of noxious agents, so there are methods for detecting the malingered act. These have varied from Wagner's use of ether[86] to detect feigned insanity, to the testing of urine temperature as an indication of factitial fever (as described occurring in the military forces in Vietnam by Ellenbogen and Nord).[27] In regard to using medication to verify malingering, President John Quincy Adams commented, "A medicine of violent operation, administered by a physician to a man whom he believes to be in full health but who is taking his professional advice, is a very improper test of the sincerity of the patient's complaints, and the avowal of it as a transaction justifiable in itself discloses a mind warped by ill-will."[29]

Thus, the symptomatology varies with the method employed and the literature is replete with methods for detection. One should be aware of the dictum of Charcot[13] who said, "I am forced to say and repeat that in my opinion the idea of malingering is only too often based upon the ignorance of the doctor." At an earlier time, Marines who complained of dull pains in the chest on exercise were dubbed malingerers if no signs were found by stethoscope, at another time, night blindness was regarded as a cause for dishonorable discharge, and at yet another time, it was thought that if stammerers could sing easily they must be malingering. As conditions have improved and more diagnostic tools have become available, the diagnosis of malingering has tended to decrease. "Goldbricking," a U.S. Army slang term which originally referred to simulation of minor disability or illness with the purpose of obtaining relief from arduous or unpleasant duties for a short period, is found in almost every variety of military service (and where there is gross exaggeration of genuine minor symptoms, British soldiers call it "scrimshanking"). The American term has now come to be in common usage for any shirking of responsibility.

The differential diagnosis of malingering must include such conditions as hypochondriasis, hysteria, sociopathy, compensation neurosis, and true psychosis, as well as the self-mutilator and the polysurgical patient. In terms of differentiation from hysteria, Layden[55] has stated that the hysterical person's unconscious goal is to salvage his self-esteem. The malingerer's self-esteem is of sufficient proportion that he can tolerate a reduction consequent to the act of malingering. The hysteric is seen to be not consciously simulating illness, is usually honest about his symptoms, and has a marked degree of inferiority. He deceives himself and makes no conscious efforts to produce the symptoms. However, differences between malingerers and hysterics are not absolute, and one often finds many hysterical traits in malingerers, and some near-conscious dramatic play-acting in the hysterical patient.[72]

Bachelor[4] wrote that the differentiation of hysteria and simulation is in fact arbitrary. Simulation is a voluntary production of symptoms by an individual who has full knowledge of their voluntary origin; in hysteria there is typically no such knowledge and the production of symptoms is the result of processes that are not fully conscious. He said that Kretschmer rightly pointed out, however, that the criterion of conscious or unconscious will not serve to distinguish simulation from hysteria, for not all motives of the healthy mind are conscious and not all hysterical ones are unconscious, and there appear to be gradations between hysteria and simulation. Schroeder[75] stated that the basic difference between neurosis and malingering is the degree to which the mental mechanisms of the deception are unconscious and not within the patient's awareness. The malingerer may be unaware of his motives but conscious of his deception and his pretense of symptoms. The neurotic, on the other hand, consciously believes the existence of what he feels to be his afflictions. Spaeth[79] described a variety of difficulties of differential diagnosis between neurosis and malingering and pointed out that in many cases only by confession can the differential diagnosis finally be made.

(The Malingering of Mental Illness

The kinds of psychiatric disorders that are likely to be malingered are amnesias, psychotic-like symptoms or behavior, neurotic-like symptoms or behavior, and mental defect. There are certain general principles to be followed in considering malingered psychiatric illness. The first step should be to consider the possibility of its existence. The second should be to pay attention to the setting and life history of the patient. Finally, one must determine the clinical diagnosis and the positive aspects thereof.

Jones and Llewellyn[50] pointed out that the malingerer tends to overact his part and is likely to believe that the more bizarre his behavior, the more psychotic he will be considered. It is apparently difficult for a subject to maintain a pretended symptom or behavior for a long period of time, so that hospital observation for a month or so may aid in establishing the diagnosis.

In the case of amnesia, Davidson[20] considered the following as explanations to be taken into account in the differential diagnosis: hysteria, psychosis, alcoholism, head injury, epilepsy, and malingering. Amnesia is thought to be the most common malingered psychiatric symptom, but the cause cannot be determined until all possibilities have been seriously considered and appropriate investigations performed. As good a history as possible is essential. A malingered amnesia tends to be somewhat patchy and self-selective. According to Davidson, a defendant who is pretending amnesia rarely alleges loss of his own identity. There are often inconsistencies in the memories which are claimed but, as McDonald[58] has pointed out, clear-cut amnesia which does not expand or contract from day to day may also be seen in malingering. However, in genuine amnesia, the beginning and the end of the amnesia are usually found to be somewhat blurred. The differentiation between hysterical and malingered amnesia is still a difficult one to make.

McDonald also noted that although narcoanalysis is frequently successful in resolving hysterical amnesia, it is less likely to be of value and should not be employed in suspected malingered amnesia. A simulated restoration of memory under narcoanalysis may later form a basis, however unjustified, for an insanity plea, and introduce difficult medical-legal complications at a subsequent court trial. Davidson,[20] on the other hand, did point out that because it tends to have little effect on the defendant's responsibility, the appraisal of genuineness of an amnesia is forensically less important than it might seem, and even though the emotional trauma of committing a crime might induce a hysterical amnesia, it does not necessarily absolve the defendant. This probably would be true also of the amnesia of pathologic intoxication.

With malingered psychosis, one certainly must consider the clinical picture and correlation between that and known clinical pictures and natural history of the illness. In both malingerers and genuine psychotics, the reasons given for delusions of persecution seem to be common. However, the malingerer does often find it necessary to remind the examiner that he does have delusions. Usually, well-organized delusional systems develop over a period of time, and if the malingerer has committed a crime and had no delusions prior to that crime, he may need to develop them rapidly. As Davidson wrote, a malingered persecutory delusion has no historical roots. He also pointed out that delusions of unworthiness are seldom malingered, and that since genuine delusions of unworthiness are found chiefly in depression, the accompanying signs and symptoms should establish the diagnosis. Delusions as an isolated symptom without consistent behavioral and affective changes are rare in genuine psychosis.

Ossipov,[66] in discussing the malingering of psychosis in the military, pointed out that a good objective history is basic. Also, the behavior of the malingerer after the case is settled is of significance. It is important as well to know the setting in which the malingering begins and the time of onset. Malingerers, he wrote, tend to portray a "state" or an episode but not a disease, and so one has to evaluate the whole clinical picture.

The malingered grandiose delusion seems to be either an isolated symptom or part of a bizarre overdramatized constellation of behavior that does not fit any psychosis. When excitement occurs, it is rather difficult for a sane person to keep up the hyperactivity which, therefore, usually occurs only when the subject believes that he is being observed. It is unlikely to be accompanied by elated mood and flight of ideas. Repeating the same phrase or gesture over and over is not likely to occur as an isolated symptom; when it does, one should be suspicious of malingering. Usually, very bizarre behavior in general tends to reflect a certain amount of malingering, as do ideas or behavior which conform to the subject's idea of psychosis but do not conform to the usual picture that one sees in psychiatric illness. However, Eissler[26] pointed out that malingering may be a defense against the onset of loss of ego control and that where there is such a threat of personality disintegration, the patient may feel, "I am not submitting to it but performing it." Where hallucinations and delusions are put forward, the malingerer often becomes very evasive, as he thinks that the examination is for the purpose of testing the genuineness of the symptoms.

Psychotic depression is perhaps more difficult to simulate insofar as the self-reproachful ideas are not often exhibited and the signs of insomnia and constipation may also be very difficult to simulate. Signs of lowered metabolism, subnormal temperature, lowered red blood count, and the general attitude of the depressed patient, are also rather difficult for the malingerer to keep up consistently. In the case of mutism, one has to consider the other possible causes, such as depression, mania, catatonia, epilepsy, and delirium, and again to review the history obtained from others that may suggest an alternate diagnosis. It may be difficult for the subject to maintain consistent mutism and he may slip up if awakened out of a sound sleep, or during narcoanalysis.

Davidson[20] has noted that psychosis malingered in personal injury claims differs from that feigned in criminal actions in two ways, namely, motivation and opportunities for observation. Motivation tends to be weaker in injury claimants, so they generally confine their psychotic symptoms to the kinds of feigned dementia, "harmless" delusions, and depression that would not result in their being committed to a mental hospital. A Ganser type of reaction is not uncommon in this kind of malingering. The fraudulent injury claimant is seldom under twenty-four-hour observation, so that the malingering of psychosis in this instance tends to be relatively rare with more frequency of feigning neurosis or some kind of "organic" symptom.

Since neurosis does not impair responsibility, it is not often malingered in criminal cases. Baro[6] suggested that malingering is the most common picture seen after industrial injuries. Davidson listed ten criteria by which one may be able to differentiate a true psychoneurosis from a malingered one:

1. Inability to work combined with retention of the capacity for play suggests the possibility of malingering.
2. Faithfulness in swallowing medicines, submitting to prescribed injections and other treatments, and attending clinics is common in neurotics but rare in malingerers.
3. If the patient fits into the responsible-honest-adequate class he is probably not a malingerer.
4. If the content of the patient's thinking, dreaming, and talking involves details of the (frightening) accident, he is probably neurotic.
5. Evidence that the patient carries on allegedly lost functions when he thinks he is not being observed may point to malingering; neurotics frequently are unable to carry out certain functions under emotional stress.

6. Malingerers, in contrast to neurotics, are not likely to copy symptoms they have seen in others during hospitalization.
7. Psychological testing may help discriminate.
8. Willingness to submit to surgical operation or to mental hospitalization may indicate that the patient is not malingering.
9. If the patient refuses an offer of employment in which he would have to use abilities or skills associated with unimpaired areas, he probably is malingering.
10. Obvious satisfaction with and eagerness for re-examination particularly by groups of doctors is more consistent with neurosis.

(The Ganser Syndrome

In 1898, Ganser[31] described a condition, the chief characteristic of which he called "*vorbeigehen*," meaning to pass by. The essence of this was to reply to a question with an answer that would be absurd in content (or "*vorbeireden*," meaning talking past or beside the point at which an approximately correct answer might be given). The symptom of "*vorbeireden*" was first described by Moeli[62] in 1888. Because of this characteristic, the condition has also been referred to as "the syndrome of approximate answers." The original description included not only such peculiar verbal responses but also visual and auditory hallucinations, clouding of consciousness, disturbed sensory perception, and occasional confused-anxious-perplexed state, changing from day to day and with total disappearance in a few days, leaving the patient with amnesia for the episode. Since the original observations were made in four criminals awaiting trial, the Ganser Syndrome has often been associated with such circumstances, although the condition has also been shown to occur in a civilian population under conditions of anxiety or stress. There is no real agreement as to whether the syndrome is in fact a neurosis or a psychosis or a manifestation of malingering. Wertham[91] considers it to be hysterical pseudostupidity occurring almost exclusively in jails and old-fashioned German textbooks. Other authors have suggested that there is a resemblance between *vorbeireden* and schizophrenic thought disorder, and have noted that some cases of Ganser Syndrome later are diagnosed as chronic schizophrenia.

A useful summary of *vorbeireden* is to be found in the papers by Anderson,[2] Trethowan,[85] and Kenna.[52] The main feature of the Ganser Syndrome is inconsistency, the subject failing to answer simple questions, and yet answering difficult questions with ease. Sometimes random answers are given rather than approximate or absurd replies. Tasks may be handled in the same way. Another feature is that no matter how idiotic the question asked, the subject most often seems to struggle to arrive at a correct answer, only to give an absurd kind of reply. Physical or conversion-like symptoms, such as headache, paralysis, disturbances in gait, rigidity, anesthesia, tremor, and convulsions, may also be present.

Davidson[20] suggested that it is unwise and unnecessary for the examiner of a prisoner to cite a Ganser reaction as evidence of malingering, since it is considered by some to be a genuine psychosis and since it may well be the result of the defendant's confinement. In any case, the distinction between simulation and the Ganser Syndrome may be difficult to make, but it is seldom important with regard to the question of criminal responsibility at the time of a crime.

❰ Munchausen's Syndrome

This is the name generally applied to the disorder manifested by the person who in the absence of appropriate medical or surgical need tends to wander from hopsital to hospital, to which he is admitted putatively with what appears to be an acute illness supported by a plausible, dramatic, and often elaborate history which turns out to be untrue, after which he discharges himself against advice (usually after quarreling with the doctors and nurses). Such patients were perhaps first described by Menninger[60,61] who drew attention to their masochism, but it was Asher[3] who coined the term "Munchausen's Syndrome" to describe the characteristic behavior of such wanderers and often polysurgical addicts. The name of the syndrome is derived from the book of fanciful and absurd adventures and travels attributed to Baron Hieronymous Karl Friedrich Munchausen. The real Baron Munchausen (1720–1791) of Hanover, Germany, enjoyed an established reputation as a teller of exaggerated tales related to his experiences as a cavalry officer in the German-Turkish campaigns of 1737 to 1739. In 1785, Rudolph Eric Raspe[71] published a book in London entitled *Singular Travels, Campaigns, and Adventures of Baron Munchausen*. The book, however, was a hoax derived from Raspe's imagination. He had met the Baron only briefly and did considerable elaboration upon his stories which rapidly established the Baron as a preposterous liar. It was because of the fanciful stories, which were both dramatic and untrue, that Asher decided to choose the name "Munchausen" for the patients who traveled from hospital to hospital as described, although the original character never submitted to any surgical operation. Other names given to this syndrome include *Maladie de Lucy* (after a poem by Wordsworth) and *Pathomimie de Dieulafoy*.

The characteristic features of the syndrome originally described by Asher included (1) feigned severe illness of a dramatic and emergency nature, the symptoms of which may or may not be corroborated by signs on physical examination; (2) evidence of many previous hospital procedures, particularly laparotomy scars and cranial burr holes; (3) aggressive, unruly behavior and a mixture of truculence and evasiveness in manner; and (4) a background of multiple hospitalizations and extensive travel, evidenced by "a wallet or handbag stuffed with hospital attendance cards, insurance claim forms and litigious correspondence."

Ireland et al.,[48] after an extensive review of

the literature, added the following four characteristics: (1) factitious evidence of disease surreptitiously produced by interference with diagnostic procedures or by self-mutilation; (2) departure from the hospital against medical advice; (3) pathological lying; and (4) the absence of any readily discernible ulterior motive.

Barker,[5] Chapman,[12] and Ireland et al.[48] further described such patients as follows: They tend to be aggressive in their relationships, indulging in frequent arguments with hospital staff and other patients; they are flamboyant and elaborate falsely on their past (pseudologia); they often seem to have considerable medical knowledge, are egocentric, and attempt to gain sympathy for their condition.

Barker also observed wide fluctuations of mood in these patients and pointed out that they often show considerable confidence towards physicians, although they tend to be wary with psychiatrists, and if admitted to psychiatric wards tend to leave against advice or to escape if committed. If confronted with knowledge of their past or if the validity of their condition is at all questioned, they will attempt to leave the hospital. Barker has found, however, that such confrontation tends to result in a depressive reaction and that such patients are prone to suicidal attempts. They usually tend to be socially isolated, and may have a history of petty theft or disorderly conduct. Considerable travel is a characteristic feature and they have the ability to withstand great amounts of discomfort associated with diagnostic procedures that may be initiated.

Impostorship is not uncommon among such patients, with claims of being a war hero or a member of a profession. In some instances, they may have a medically related background with a sibling or parent who was a physician or nurse. They may have a conspicuous physical appearance, such as being obese or tattooed. They also tend to be young and to appear more frequently in countries where hospitalization is free. There are many reviews of the syndrome in the literature, with those by Ireland et al.,[45] Spiro,[80] and Barker[5] being of special interest.

(Psychological Tests

A useful review of psychological tests in relation to malingering is included in McDonald's book, *Psychiatry and the Criminal.*[58] Some work has been done in an attempt to distinguish the person who appears to be less intelligent on his test scores than he may in fact be. Hunt[44,45] described a predictable test pattern for the mental defective, which is different from that of the malingerer. An example was found in responses to the question, "If eight boys clubbed together and paid two dollars for the use of a room, how much should each boy pay?" Apparently, the two most common answers given by retarded persons are four dollars and sixteen dollars. This seemingly occurs because the defective is unable to manipulate the numbers appropriately and might either divide or multiply eight by two. The malingerer, however, works the problem correctly, but then deliberately distorts the results by a small amount, to produce an answer such as twenty-three or twenty-six cents.

Davidson[20] pointed out that malingering should be suspected when the subject can do all the nine-year-old tests, but consistently fails at the six-year level, or where a wild and wide scatter of passed and failed tests occurs without the pattern of normal age-grade development. Crowley,[19] using the Kent EGY, attempted to distinguish differences between the test performance of truly feebleminded women and women who were asked to feign mental deficiency. The mean scores of the malingering groups were significantly lower than those of the truly feebleminded group, although it was impossible to identify individual malingerers from the total scores unless they were extremely low.

Pollaczek[69] studied the possibility of detecting malingering on the CVS abbreviated intelligence scale, consisting of the comprehension and similarities subtests of the WAIS, together with a vocabulary test selected from items of the Stanford-Binet, in which experimental groups were requested to simulate mental deficiency on the test, while genuine mental defectives were given the test in the usual manner. Although it was again not possible to detect malingering using the total test scores, there were enough significant differences between the experimental and control groups on individual items to make a key for malingering. Using this key, it was possible to distinguish about 90 percent of the malingerers, with only 10 percent of the mental defectives being falsely identified as malingerers.

Goldstein[35] also developed a key for the detection of malingering of mental deficiency. On the basis of experiments involving the use of a good group who passed the examination, a failure group who failed the examination, and a simulated malingerer group, he developed an instrument specifically adapted to the Army's Visual Classification Test. The key which he evolved was successful in identifying 97 percent of simulated malingerers and 85 percent of presumed genuine failures. He suggested that for optimum results such a test should probably have the following characteristics: (1) a liberal sprinkling of easy items, (2) items of varying difficulty, and (3) a scrambled sequence.

Davidson noted the importance of the life history in relating the genuineness of alleged mental defect. If the subject is a high school graduate, genuine defect is unlikely. He suggested adding five to the last successfully completed school grade to obtain a quick approximation of true mental age (i.e., if the subject successfully completed the ninth grade and dropped out of school in the tenth, one would expect to find a mental age of about fourteen). Davidson stated that this formula is seldom more than two or three years out of line.

Rosenberg and Feldman[74] used the Rorschach to study 93 malingering soldiers, and described eleven Rorschach signs and four behavioral signs produced as a result of evasion due to the subjects' conscious fear that the test might be too revealing. The Rorschach signs included (1) few responses, less than five or six, mostly of the nature of "I don't know" or "It's an inkblot"; (2) mostly popular responses; (3) other responses of vague indefinite form, such as maps or clouds;

(4) inconsistencies of response with recognition of difficult forms and rejection of easy forms, and refusal to see new responses on testing limits; (5) perseveration with the same response being given on ten different cards; (6) description and color-naming which is usually an explanation of how the inkblots are formed; (7) delayed responses and excessive turnings of the cards; (8) partial rejection of responses, usually asked as a question or qualified by "It might be," etc.; (9) rejections in inquiry; (10) marked lack of additional responses; and (11) often one response per card. The behavioral patterns involved misunderstanding of directions, attempts to impress the examiner with exaggerated furrowing of the brow and overconcentration on the cards, frequent questions, such as "What's all this for?" and increased complaints such as pains, headaches, and dizziness during testing (as compared to neurotics who usually do not complain during the test). They also observed that malingering subjects were more likely to describe animals as dead than alive when the subject was pushed. In general, the unstructured nature of the Rorschach Test appeared to be helpful in differentiating malingerers from nonmalingerers. The Thematic Apperception Test has also been used in an effort to detect malingering, but it appears that because of the more obvious nature of the stimuli, deception is more easily possible.

The Minnesota Multiphasic Personality Inventory has been studied extensively in this regard. An excellent review of the relevant MMPI literature appears in a paper by Exner et al.,[28] in which they discuss the value of four validity scales on the MMPI. Cofer et al.[15] found that college students attempting to fake "normal" performance could be detected by an additive combination of the L and K scores. Calvin and McDonnell[11] noted eight studies in which faking on the MMPI could be detected at a statistically significant level, again using the validity scales. Recently, however, other studies have suggested that a high score on a single validity scale does not necessarily invalidate the diagnostic patterning.

Gough[37] also found that there are 74 items in the MMPI to which persons attempting to malinger respond significantly differently than do diagnosed psychoneurotics. Gough termed this group of items a "Dissimulation Scale" (DS). Exner et al.[28] pointed to the usefulness of Gough's DS and the F-K dissimulation index as valid methods for detecting malingering. He also supported Cofer's original findings that the F scale taken alone can be useful for the detection of malingered records.

Management of Malingering

The physician is likely to come into contact with the malingerer either in the military, in prison, in the general or mental hospital, or in connection with compensation. It is not unusual for the response of the physician to the malingerer to be a hostile one. The physician usually sees the role of the patient carrying with it certain built-in expectations, including the motivation to accept therapeutic help. When he suspects that a patient may not fit the traditional mold, he attempts to resolve his shaken professional role by controlling the situation in which he feels he has been controlled or duped, by attempting to expose the individual.[21] The diagnostic procedure in such instances becomes confused with the management of the case, and may become more of a punishment than actual diagnostic aide. In this connection, Layden[55] has described the necessity for the physician to understand the dynamics of how he and the patient may become hostile in order to avoid the tendency to blame. He suggested that the malingerer may reduce his deception as an unconscious means of insuring the continuance of the physician's esteem, and that attempts through therapy to reduce the malingerer's hostility to significant persons in his environment may induce him to give up his symptoms.

Hollender and Hersh[43] described a situation where the psychiatrist as consultant is asked to see a patient suspected of or known to be inducing a medical illness by ingesting pills or injecting pathogens. They noted the paradox of the psychiatrist behaving first as

detective or prosecutor to determine whether the patient is in fact malingering, and then expecting to be accepted as ally or helper by the patient to resolve the dilemma. They suggested that the psychiatrist meet first with the referring physician and persuade him to confront the patient with the facts. Once this has been done, then psychiatric help can be offered, and when the patient can acknowledge that he is not medically ill and will redefine himself as being psychiatrically ill, it may be possible to institute psychiatric treatment. In this way, the psychiatrist is seen as a helper rather than as an adversary. The variables involved in the management obviously are dependent on the examiner's skill and knowledge and time available, the type of malingerer and his skill and knowledge, and the injury or illness feigned. Where compensation is involved, it is probably wiser to settle all compensation claims either by their outright rejection or by a lump sum payment.

Earlier, Shaw[78] also found that confrontation by the physician was not effective because of the threat of disgrace for the patient. He, therefore, allowed the malingerer to save face by employing an intensive therapeutic regimen that would have been used if the patient's pain, for example, had been real. Group therapy was used with some success by Brody,[9] mainly for the treatment of so-called polysurgery addicts, and Ireland et al.[48] suggested that some patients with Munchausen's Syndrome might be committed to a mental hospital, where long-term psychotherapy to eliminate the expressed motive may be the best approach.

Brussel and Hitch[10] suggested that in dealing with the military malingerer, the examiner maintain himself on the alert, refrain from asking leading questions or showing his own suspicious attitude, and avoid any display of surprise or sarcasm. They pointed out that while the diagnosis of malingering may be the first one contemplated, it should be the last one to be accepted. They suggested that persons who malinger rarely do well in military service and should be returned to civilian status. This concept was substantiated by the work of Weiss et al.,[89] who found in a blind follow-up study that "pathological personality types" (in which category most malingerers were placed) were among the poorest adjustment risks in Army service.

Cheyne[14] in 1827 detailed his prescription for dealing with malingerers in the military. He wrote:

> The medical officer must not allow even flagrant imposition to deprive him of the command of his temper; he must listen to the most contradictory statement, not really with patience, but without evincing the slightest distrust; in short, his manner must be the same to a soldier laboring under strong suspicion of fraud, as it would be to the best man in the regiment, and he will in general find that complete ignorance of his sentiments will, more than anything, disconcert the malingerer. Secondly, if the case is evidently feigned, he ought to take the malingerer aside, mildly expostulate with him on his folly, or if necessary, threaten to report him to the commanding officer if he should persist in his misconduct, or again attempt to feign sickness. By such means, many a good soldier has been reclaimed, who had he been exposed to shame, would have become a callous profligate.
>
> Thirdly, if he should fail by means of persuasion, and if the thought be palpable, he ought to take the malingerer into hospital and without prescribing for his pretended complaints, lay the case before the commanding officer.
>
> Fourthly, but if the grounds of his suspicion cannot be convincingly stated, he must cautiously conceal his sentiments, until by patient investigation, his doubts are removed, and a satisfactory report of the case can be prepared.
>
> Fifthly, in this stage of the inquiry, he must employ no means but such as would be applicable to the case were it genuine. He must not, on his own authority, employ any coercive or penal measures, or even irritating applications or nauseating medicines, nor spare diet unless such would be proper if the disease were real.
>
> Sixthly, when after the calmest inquiry, he is convinced that the complaint is unfounded, or the disease fabricated, and shall have reported accordingly to the commanding officer, the case is no longer in his hands; he ought not to prescribe for the malingerer, but ought to pass him in going through the wards. Neglect will often bring him to resume his duty. . . .

Because of sociocultural taboos about lying and deception, especially to achieve unfair or undeserved gains or to escape duty or punishment, and because of the physician's own self-image and fears of being manipulated, malingering has been a phenomenon of medical, legal, penal, military, and general social interest for centuries. It is now clear, however, that this and related behaviors do not represent a disease per se, but rather a mode of adaptation influenced by environmental and developmental patterns, as well as being an immediate and sometimes ongoing reaction to stress. Such behavior may be related to a variety of psychiatric disorders, including personality disorder, neurosis, psychosis, and mental retardation. Obviously, it is important for the psychiatrist to establish the fact that malingering may be present, but more important is the investigation of the relevant etiologic and dynamic factors involved, and the diagnosis and treatment of the basic disorder in which malingering, imposture, factitious illness, or even the Ganser or Munchausen Syndromes may occur.

(Bibliography

1. ADAMS, F. The Seven Books of Paulus Aegineta. London: Sydenham Society, 1846.
2. ANDERSON, E. W. "An Experimental Approach to the Problem of Simulation in Mental Disorders," Proceedings of the Royal Society of Medicine, 49 (1956), 513–515.
3. ASHER, R. "Munchausen's Syndrome," Lancet, 1 (1951), 339–341.
4. BACHELOR, I. R. C., ed. Henderson and Gillespie's Textbook of Psychiatry, 10th ed. New York: Oxford University Press, 1969.
5. BARKER, J. C. "The Syndrome of Hospital Addiction (Munchausen Syndrome)," Journal of Mental Science, 108 (1962), 167–182.
6. BARO, W. Z. "Industrial Head and Back Injuries," Indust. Med., 19 (1950) 69–71.
7. BERNARD, J., et al. "Hypochromic Anemias Due to Voluntarily Induced Hemorrhages (L'Asthénie de Ferjol's Syndrome)," Press Med., 75 (1967), 2087–2090.

8. BLINDER, M. "Composite Picture of the Malingering Patient," *Medical World News*, 1970.

9. BRODY, S. "Value of Group Psychotherapy in Patients with 'Polysurgery Addiction,'" *Psychiatric Quarterly*, 33 (1959), 260–283.

10. BRUSSELL, J. A., and K. S. HITCH. "Military Malingerer," *Military Surgeon*, 93 (1953), 33–44.

11. CALVIN, A., and J. E. McDONNELL. "Ellis on Personality Inventories," *Journal of Consulting Psychology*, 17 (1953), 462–464.

12. CHAPMAN, J. S. "Peregrinating Problem Patients—Munchausen's Syndrome," *Journal of the AMA*, 165 (1957), 927–933.

13. CHARCOT, J-M. Quoted in Jones and Llewellyn, Ref. #47.

14. CHEYNE, J. "Medical Report on the Feigned Diseases of Soldiers," *Dublin Hospital Reports*, 4 (1827), 123–181.

15. COFER, C., J. CHANCE, and A. JUDSON. "A Study of Malingering on the MMPI," *Journal of Psychology*, 27 (1949), 491–499.

16. COLLIE, SIR J. "Malingering," in W. R. Bett, ed., *Short History of Some Common Diseases*. London: Oxford University Press, 1934.

17. ———. *Malingering and Feigned Sickness*. London: Edward Arnold, 1913.

18. COOKSON, H. "Correspondence," *British Medical Journal*, 2 (1955), 1330.

19. CROWLEY, M. E. "The Use of the Kent EGY for the Detection of Malingering," *Journal of Clinical Psychology*, 8 (1952), 332–337.

20. DAVIDSON, H. A. *Forensic Psychiatry*, 2nd. ed. New York: The Ronald Press, 1965.

21. DAVIS, D. "The Physician-Patient Relationship: Involvement Versus Insight," *Missouri Medicine*, 58 (1961), 569–571.

22. ———. "They Were Fain to Feign," in preparation.

23. DEJONG, R. N. *The Neurologic Examination*, 3rd ed. New York: Hoeber-Harper, 1967.

24. DEUTSCH, A. R. "Malingering and Conversion Reactions in Ophthalmology," *Journal of Tennessee Medical Association*, 61 (1968), 694–698.

25. *Diagnostic and Statistical Manual of Mental Disorders*, 2nd ed. (*DSM II*). Washington: American Psychiatric Association, 1968.

26. EISSLER, K. R. "Malingering," in G. B. Wilbur, and W. Muenstenberger, eds., *Psychoanalysis and Culture*. New York: International Universities Press, 1951.

27. ELLENBOGEN, C., and B. M. NORD. "Freshly Voided Urine Temperature: A Test for Factitial Fever," *Journal of the AMA*, 219 (1972), 912.

28. EXNER, J. E., JR., et al. "On the Detection of Willful Falsifications in the MMPI," *Journal of Counseling Psychology*, 27 (1963), 91–94.

29. FLEXNER, J. T. *Doctors on Horseback—Pioneers of American Medicine*. New York: Dover Publications Inc., 1969.

30. FLICKER, D. "Malingering, a Symptom," *Journal of Nervous and Mental Disease*, 123 (1956), 23–31.

31. GANSER, S. J. "*Über einen eigenartigen Dämmerzustand*," *Arch. für Psychiat. Nerventk.*, 30 (1898), 633.

32. GARDNER, R. C. "Malingering Test for Low Back Pain," *New England Journal of Medicine*, 282 (1970), 1050.

33. GARRISON, F. H. *An Introduction to the History of Medicine*, 4th. ed. Philadelphia: W. B. Saunders, 1929.

34. GAVIN, H. *On the Feigned and Factitious Diseases of Soldiers and Seamen*. Edinburg: University Press, 1838.

35. GOLDSTEIN, H. "A Malingering Key for Mental Tests," *Psychology Bulletin*, 42 (1945), 104–118.

36. GORMAN, C. A., et al. "Metabolic Malingerers," *American Journal of Medicine*, 48 (1970), 708–714.

37. GOUGH, H. "The F Minus K Dissimulation Index for the MMPI," *Journal of Consulting Psychology*, 14 (1950), 408–413.

38. GREIDANHUS, T. H., et al. "Surreptitious Ingestion of Oral Anticoagulants," *Henry Ford Hospital Medical Journal*, 18 (1970), 99–106.

39. GRINKER, R., JR. "Imposture as a Form of Mastery," *Archives of General Psychiatry*, 5 (1961), 449–452.

40. *Grose F. Classical Dictionary of the Vulgar Tongue*. London: Printed for S. Hooper, 1785.

41. GUTTMACHER, M. S. "Lie Detection and Narcoinvestigation," in *The Role of Psychiatry in Law*. Springfield, Ill.: Charles C. Thomas, 1968.

42. HAWKINGS, J. R., et al. "Deliberate Disability," *Brit. Med. J.*, 1 (1956), 361–367.

43. HOLLENDER, M. H., and S. P. HERSH. "Impossible Consultation Made Possible," *Archives of General Psychiatry*, 23 (1970), 343–345.

44. HUNT, W. A. "The Uses and Abuses of Psychometric Tests," *Kentucky Law Journal*, 35 (1946), 38.

45. ———, and H. J. OLDER. "Detection of Malingering Through Psychometric Tests," *U.S. Naval Medicine Bulletin*, 41 (1943), 1318–1323.

46. HUTCHISON, A. C. "Some Observations on Simulated or Feigned Diseases," *London Med. & Phys. J.*, 51 (1824), 87–99.

47. ———. "On Simulated or Feigned Diseases," *London Med. & Phys. J.*, 54 (1825), 87–93.

48. IRELAND, P., J. D. SAPIRA, and B. TEMPLETON. "Munchausen's Syndrome: Review and Report of an Additional Case," *American Journal of Medicine*, 43 (1967), 579–592.

49. ISTRE, C. O., et al. "Automatic Audiometry for Detecting Malingering," *Arch. Otolaryng.*, 90 (1969), 326–333.

50. JONES, A. BASSETT, and J. L. LLEWELLYN. *Malingering or the Simulation of Disease*. Philadelphia: P. Blakison's Son and Co., 1917.

51. JUNG, C. G. "On Simulated Insanity (1903)," in *Collected Works*. London: Routledge and Kegan Paul, 1 (1959), 159.

52. KENNA, J. C. "An Experimental Approach to the Problem of Simulation in Mental Disorders: III. Psychological Aspects," *Proceedings of the Royal Society of Medicine*, 49 (1956), 519–520.

53. KEYNES, G., ed. *The Apologie and Treatise of Ambroise Paré*. London: Falcon Educational Books, 1951.

54. KINGSLEY, H. J. "Pecularities in Dermatology: A Case of Dermatitis Artefacta," *Central African Journal of Medicine*, 13 (1967), 264.

55. LAYDEN, M. "Psychiatric Aspects of Malingering," *Southern Medical Journal*, 60 (1967), 1237–1239.

56. LIDDLE, G. G. "An Artifice of War," *Journal of the AMA*, 212 (1970), 785.

57. MAYHEW, H. *London's Underworld: Selections from London Labor and the London Poor*. London: William Kimber, 1950.

58. McDONALD, J. M. *Psychiatry and the Criminal*. Springfield, Ill.: Charles C. Thomas, 1958.

59. MEHRA, K. S., and B. B. KHARE. "Sub-conjunctival Saline as Test and Treatment for Ocular Malingering," *Journal of All-India Ophthalmologic Society*, 15 (1967), 77.

60. MENNINGER, K. A. *Man Against Himself*. New York: Harcourt, Brace and Co., 1938.

61. ———. "Psychology of a Certain Type of Malingering," *Archives of Neurology and Psychiatry*, 33 (1935), 507–515.

62. MOELI, C. *Über irre Verbrecher*. Berlin, 1888.

63. MONTAIGNE, M. DE. *The Essays of Montaigne*, J. Florio, transl. New York: Random House, 1933.

64. MURPHY, E. L. "Malingering," in W. R. Bett, ed., *The History and Conquest of Common Diseases*. Normans: University of Oklahoma Press, 1954.

65. ———. "Skulkers Unveiled: Or Further Notes on Malingering," *Irish Medical Association Journal*, 32 (1953), 9–17.

66. OSSIPOV, V. P. "Malingering, the Simulation of Psychosis," *Bulletin of the Menninger Clinic*, 8 (1944), 39–42.

67. PACKARD, A. J., JR. "Orthopedic Detection of Malingering," *Southern Medical Journal*, 60 (1967), 1233–1237.

68. PINEL, P., "Feigned Mania: The Method of Ascertaining It," in *A Treatise on Insanity*. New York: Hafner Publishing Co., 1962.

69. POLLACZEK, P. P. "A Study of Malingering on the CVS Abbreviated Individual Intelligence Scale," *Journal of Clinical Psychology*, 8 (1952), 77–81.

70. PUNTON, J. "Medical Malingering and International Fraud," *Kansas City Medical Index-Lancet*, 24 (1903), 273–280.

71. RASPE, R. E., et al. *Singular Travels, Campaigns, and Adventures of Baron Munchausen*. New York: Dover Publications, Inc., 1960.

72. REDLICH, F. C., and D. X. FREEDMAN, *The Theory and Practice of Psychiatry*. New York: Basic Books, Inc., 1966.

73. ROME, H. P. "Malingering as Crypto-Suicide," in A. W. R. Sipe, ed., *Hope, Psychiatry's Commitment*. New York: Brunner/Mazel, 1970.

74. ROSENBERG, S. J., and T. M. FELDMAN. "Rorschach Characteristics of a Group of Malingerers," *Rorschach Research Exchange*, 8 (1944), 141–158.

75. SCHROEDER, O. D., JR., et al. "Malingering: Fact or Fiction," *Post-Graduate Medicine*, 40 (1966), A22–A28, A58–A64.

76. SEGARRA, J. M. "Test for Malingering," *New England Journal of Medicine*, 283 (1970), 375.

77. SHAPIRO, S. L. "Malingering with Reference to the Eye, Ear, Nose, and Throat," *Industrial Medicine and Surgery*, 22 (1953), 65–68.

78. SHAW, R. S. "Pathologic Malingering. The Painful Disabled Extremity," *New England Journal of Medicine*, 271 (1964), 22–26.

79. SPAETH, E. B. "The Differentiation of the Ocular Manifestations of Hysteria and of Ocular Malingering," *Archives of Ophthalmology*, 4 (1939), 911.

80. SPIRO, H. R. "Chronic Factitious Illness: Munchausen's Syndrome," *Archives of General Psychiatry*, 18 (1968), 569–579.

81. SUND, A. "Prognosis of Psychiatric Disorders in Norwegian Men in Military Service," *Norwegian Medicine*, 84 (1970), 843–849.

82. SZASZ, T. S. "Malingering: 'Diagnosis' or Social Condemnation?" *Archives of Neurology and Psychiatry*, 195 (1957), 432–443.

83. TAYLOR, F. KRAÜPL. *Psychopathology*. Washington: Butterworths, 1966.

84. TEMKIN, O. *The Falling Sickness: A History of Epilepsy from the Greeks to the Beginning of Modern Neurology*. Baltimore: Johns Hopkins Press, 1945.

85. TRETHOWAN, W. H. "An Experimental Approach to the Problem of Simulations in Mental Disorders: II. Experimental Data," *Proceedings of the Royal Society of Medicine*, 49 (1956), 515–519.

86. WAGNER, C. G. "Feigned Insanity: Malingering Revealed by the Use of Ether," *American Journal of Insanity*, 61 (1904), 193–198.

87. WEISS, J. M. A. "The Gamble With Death in Attempted Suicide," *Psychiatry*, 20 (1957), 17–25.

88. ———. "The Role of the Psychotherapist in Military Training Centers," *Military Medicine*, 118 (1956), 95–108.

89. ———, W. G. HILL, and J. L. BOYER. "Subsequent Military Performance of Soldiers Treated at a Mental Hygiene Consultation Service," *Mental Hygiene*, 38 (1954), 604–612.

90. ———, and M. E. PERRY. "Transcultural Attitudes toward Crime," in preparation.

91. WERTHAM, F. *The Show of Violence*. New York: Doubleday and Co., Inc., 1949.

92. WHITLOCK, F. A. "The Ganser Syndrome," *British Journal of Psychiatry*, 113 (1967), 19–29.

93. WILSON, W. A. "Oedipism," *American Journal of Ophthalmology*, 40 (1955), 563–567.

PART FOUR

Sexual Behavior and Syndromes

CHAPTER 14

HOMOSEXUALITY

Charles W. Socarides

THE DEFINITION OF HOMOSEXUAL and homosexuality can well be preceded by definitions of sexual, heterosexual, and heterosexuality.

Sexual reproduction was antedated by asexual reproduction or fission, that is, one cell splitting into two identical cells. The word *sexual* is derived from biology and refers to a form of reproduction occurring between two cells which are different from each other. Their combined nuclear material resulted in a completely new individual cell and this became the basis of all evolutionary development. Sexual development began solely as reproductive activity. It was later enlarged to include sexual pleasure activity with or without reproduction.

Heterosexual object choice is determined by two-and-a-half billion years of human evolution, a product of sexual differentiation. At first based solely on reproduction, it later widened to include sexual gratification: from one-celled nonsexual fission to the development of two-celled sexual reproduction, to organ differentiation, and finally to the development of two separate individuals reciprocally adapted to each other anatomically, endocrinologically, psychologically, and in many other ways.

In man, heterosexual object choice is not innate or instinctual, nor is homosexual object choice; both are learned behavior. The choice of sexual object is not predetermined by chromosomal tagging. However, most significantly, heterosexual object choice is outlined from birth by anatomy and then reinforced by cultural and environmental indoctrination. It is supported by universal human concepts of mating and the tradition of the family unit, together with the complementariness and contrast between the two sexes.[73]

Everything from birth to death is designed to perpetuate the male-female combination. This pattern is not only culturally ingrained but anatomically outlined and fostered by all the institutions of marriage, society, and the deep roots of the family unit. The term "anatomically outlined" does not mean that it is instinctual to choose a person of the opposite sex (heterosexuality). The human being is a biological emergent entity derived from evolution, favoring survival.

In man, due to the tremendous development of the cerebral cortex, motivation—both conscious and unconscious—plays a crucial role in the selection of individuals and/or objects that will produce sexual arousal and orgastic release. Where massive childhood fears have damaged and disrupted the standard male-female pattern, the roundabout method of achieving orgastic release is through instituting male-male or female-female pairs (homosexuality). Such early unconscious fears are responsible not only for the later development of homosexuality but of all other modified sexual patterns of the obligatory type.

The term "standard pattern" was originated by Rado[73] to signify penetration of the male organ into the female at some point before orgasm and, of course, carries with it the potential for reproduction. Within the standard pattern, from which the foregoing characteristics are never absent, there are innumerable variations dependent upon individual preference. Homosexuality is a modified pattern because it does not conform to the essential characteristics of the standard pattern. Other modified sexual patterns, also referred to as perversions or deviations, are fetishism, voyeurism, exhibitionism, pedophilia, etc. Individuals suffering from these conditions have in common the inability to perform in the standard male-female design and, as one of their aims, attempt to achieve orgastic release in a substitutive way. A homosexual is an individual who engages repetitively or episodically in sexual relations with a partner of the same sex or experiences the recurrent desire to do so, as explained in the section on classification. If required to function sexually with a partner of the opposite sex, he can do so, if at all, only with very little or no pleasure.

(Biological Studies

There have been numerous chemical, genetic, and somatic studies over the past century in an effort to establish that homosexuality has an organic or nonpsychogenetic origin.

In 1896, Krafft-Ebing[61] suggested that homosexuality is an inborn characteristic due to large amounts of male and/or female substances in the hereditary composition of the brain. Mantegazza,[67] in 1914, explained homosexuality as a genital malformation caused by the fact that sensory nerves, normally originating in the penis, are displaced to the rectum and the erogenous zone is correspondingly shifted. Hirschfeld[49] stated that "Homosexuality is always an inborn state, conditioned by a specific homosexual constitution of the brain." In 1940, Glass et al.[41] cited hormonal or endocrine factors. H. Ellis[20] agreed with Krafft-Ebing's theory of hereditary composition.

Contemporary scientific findings clearly establish that homosexuals can have endocrine dysfunction, as can any individual, but that the androgen-estrogen ratio among male homosexuals usually falls within normal limits. Large doses of androgens or estrogens influence the strength of the sexual drive but cannot change the sexual object choice.

In 1941, Henry[48] studied 250 adult patients grouped according to the predominance of heterosexual or homosexual tendencies. He observed that homosexuals had considerably greater constitutional somatic deviations on average than had heterosexuals, but could not conclude from this finding that homosexuality was organically determined. In fact, he tended to the opposite point of view. Parenthetically, it is of interest that he found when personality disorders do occur, heterosexuals tend to develop "benign" psychoses, while homosexuals are prone to paranoiac and schizophrenic illnesses.

Kallman's[52] studies on the genetic predetermination of homosexuality in identical twins show "concordance as to the overt *practices* of homosexual behavior after adolescence." However, these statistical studies must be viewed with caution. The behavior may be due to the temperamental similarity of identical twins and their reacting similarly to environmental influences. More revealing would be studies made on identical twins who have been separated at birth and brought up in divergent environments. Kallman himself, in the same paper, states that the "project was extremely difficult. . . . It is fair to admit that the question of the possible significance of a genetic mechanism in the development of overt homosexuality may still be regarded as entirely unsettled."

Rainer and co-workers[75] described seven cases of monozygotic twins without concordance. It would seem that concordance does not prove a biogenetic etiology since the developmental history of monozygotic twins is uniquely different from that of other individuals.

Assumptions as to the origin of human homosexuality cannot be based on the study of lower primates, because in man the enormous evolutionary development of the cerebral cortex has made motivation, both conscious and unconscious, of overwhelming central significance in sexual patterning. Below the level of the chimpanzee, sexual arousal patterns are completely automatic and reflex. One of the world's outstanding experts on animal behavior, Beach,[55] commented in a 1971 interview: "I don't know any authenticated instance of males or females in the animal world preferring a homosexual partner —if by homosexual you mean complete sexual relations, including climax. . . . It's questionable that mounting in itself can properly be called sexual."

A. Ellis[19] studied forty-eight cases of hermaphrodites from the medical literature. He reported that heterosexuality or homosexuality in hermaphrodites is caused primarily by environmental rather than hormonal or physiological factors. Since, however, the hermaphrodite's environment conspicuously includes the somatic anomalies, he concluded that the problem of "normal" and "abnormal" sexual behavior among hermaphrodites is a psychosomatic one, as is true of psychosexuality in normal human beings.

Kolodny et al.[60] reported that thirty-five exclusively homosexual subjects had a lower amount of testosterone in the bloodstream than would be found in heterosexual males. Evidence of the inconclusiveness of this finding is seen by the authors' statement in the same paper: "There is no suggestion that en-

docrine abnormalities will be found in the great majority of homosexuals, or that endocrine dysfunction is a major factor in the pathogenesis of male homosexuality."

Various objections were raised in connection with the Kolodny material. For example, Barry and Barry[3] wrote: "Their data showed that most of their subjects whose homosexuality had been rated as moderate to predominant had plasma testosterone levels within normal limits. Subjects with extreme degrees of homosexuality did have significant decreases in testosterone levels. . . ." The relation between decreased testosterone levels and decreased libido in heterosexual males is well known, the objection continues, so that it is not necessary to attribute any of these endocrine findings to homosexuality.

Commenting on Kolodny's alternative theory—that decreased testosterone levels could be a result of homosexuality rather than a cause and could be mediated through hypothalamic mechanisms—Barry and Barry point out that the life style of persons with "obsessive-compulsive" homosexual activity could also be involved. Many such subjects have said that while "cruising" and patronizing "gay" bars, they frequently averaged less than four hours of sleep. Testosterone levels normally decrease during the day by some 30 percent, and the high early morning levels are presumably restored during sleep. "Might not the result reported have been due to the cumulative effects of sleep deficits? . . . Kolodny et al. did not mention any alcohol consumption . . . although an association between heavy alcoholic consumption and homosexuality is not uncommon, and alcohol is believed to have adverse effects on the testes and male sexual activity. In view of the lability of testosterone level and their wide variations owing to environmental factors, the reported decrease among adult males is more likely to be a result than a cause of homosexuality."

The entire issue was succinctly resolved by Rado:[73] "If a person of the opposite sex is available, why should a male choose another male or a female another female . . . or even, sometimes, a lock of hair or a piece of under-clothing?" The answer is to be found in the history of the individual's psychic development.

(Cultural Studies

Homosexuality, present throughout the ages, can be found in almost all cultures. It has been treated in ways ranging from acceptance to hostile rejection. Efforts to deal with it can be traced to some of the earliest writings, for example, to the laws of Hammurabi (second century B.C.) in Babylon, to Egyptian papyri, in which it is referred to as an ancient custom of the gods, to the Old Testament, where it is described as a "sin and scourge," e.g., Sodom and Gomorrah. Under Roman law, many aspects of homosexuality were ignored, especially female homosexuality. Early Anglo-Saxon laws were not as lenient, but it has been inaccurate to regard taboos against homosexuality as deriving entirely from the Judaeo-Christian code. During the Dark Ages, homosexuality was regarded as a form of heresy and those "afflicted" were burnt at the stake.

Fisher[25] states that physical relations were definitely a part of the homosexuality of the Greeks (Athenians). "The evidence is strong that homosexuality in the form of pederasty came later and flourished in the historic period from the 6th century B.C. on, coinciding with the development of a monetary, commercial, enslaved form of society."

In the Homeric period, the absence of pederasty coincided with the more elevated status of women, whereas in the historic period, the presence of pederasty coincided with the degraded status of women. According to Fisher, "This pattern suggests that in approaching the problem of homosexuality today, it is not enough to deal with the so-called 'instinctual' and interpersonal factors; social factors must be taken into account as well."

A most comprehensive and scholarly examination of family life in ancient Greece was published by the brilliant Cambridge investigator, W. K. Lacey.[62] He writes:

We are sometimes told that the Greeks were fully bisexual, enjoying both homosexual and heterosexual intercourse, and that romantic love in Greece was associated with attachments to boys and not to girls. Whatever the truth of the latter statement, there can be no doubt that, while the Greeks had a deep admiration for the physical beauty of the young male, in Athens the practice of sodomy was strictly circumscribed by the law.

Boys still at school were protected against sexual assaults by a law (said to go as far back as Dracon and Solon), and we hear of strict regulations about schools with this in mind; schoolboys always had a *paidagogos* escorting them; in art the *paidagogos* is always depicted as carrying a long and heavy stick; what was this for if not to protect their charges?

Sodomy was thought reprehensible for older men even when the catamite was not a citizen, as is clear from the speech of Lysias, but it was not illegal; it may be thought that the law in this field is likely to have been similar to that about adultery; what was quite legal with slaves and other non-citizens was illegal with citizens, and the law took notice of the private morals of individuals, and punished offenders.

Pederasty was expensive; whether this was because the youths' admirers wanted to compete in generosity for favours or the youths were able to use the law virtually to blackmail their admirers no doubt varied in individual cases, but the result of the expense was to make paederasty a habit of the upper class and of those who imitated them, and hence suspect to the common people and a means of arousing prejudice in legal cases. Plato's attack on sodomy, especially in the *Laws*, reveals that the practice was not unknown to him, and that it was more repugnant to his ideals than heterosexual intercourse outside marriage, since this latter (if secret) was tolerated in the *Laws* as a second-best to the ideal of virginity till marriage and sexual intercourse only within marriage for the purpose of breeding children.

Opler[69] concludes from anthropological and cross-cultural studies that "Actually, no society, save perhaps ancient Greece, pre-Meiji Japan, certain top echelons in Nazi Germany, and the scattered examples of such special status groups as the berdaches, Nata slaves, and one category of Chukchee shamans, has lent sanction in any real sense to homosexuality. Regardless of what may be said concerning all the factors—social, legal, and psychodynamic—entering into homosexual behavior, one thing is clear: in the absence of an organic or hormonal basis, homosexuality in practically all cultures is regarded as a deviation from the major values and norms of conduct." He points out that in nonliterate hunting and gathering societies homosexuality is generally rare and in some instances virtually non-existent, e.g., the Mescalero and Chiricahua Apache.

Kardiner,[54] in a psychoanalytic study of anthropology, has shown that in the Comanche tribes of the midwestern United States there was no homosexuality; an occasional transvestite was treated like a foolish old woman. It was completely unadaptive for a young man to be homosexual in the Comanche tribe. The tribe was geared for warfare and for hunting. All children were bound physically close to the mother for the first year or two of life. Boys were thereafter turned over to the father and the other men to begin training and cultivation of those attributes and skills leading to being successful warriors and hunters.

Observers of kibbutz-reared children in Israel have reported that there was no evidence of homosexuality in adulthood.[7]

❨ Developmental Factors

The experientially derived nature of homosexuality was explicated in 1905 by Freud.[38] He, Sadger,[78] and Ferenczi[24] had penetrated the interconnection between infantile sexuality, perversions, and neurosis, and arrived at the conclusion that the latter represents the negative of perversion. A formulation of the essential psychological developmental factors in homosexuality was described by these foremost psychoanalytic investigators of their time, circa 1910. For example, they stated that the homosexual has experienced an excessively intense mother fixation during the first three years of life. He continues thereafter to identify with the mother, taking himself narcissistically as a sexual object. Consequently, starting in adolescence, he searches for a male

resembling himself whom he attempts to love as he wished his mother had loved him. In addition, an unloving, cruel, or absent father increases the difficulties in the formation of male identification.

The clinical papers of the era focused almost exclusively on the failure to resolve the Oedipus complex as the causative factor in homosexuality. Freud himself was not content with this application of the oedipal theory as the definitive answer and stressed the necessity to seek out other determinants, namely, the psychic mechanism responsible for homosexuality and an explanation of what determines this particular outcome rather than another. He concluded that homosexuality represents an inhibition and dissociation of the psychosexual development, one of the pathological outcomes of the oedipal period.

Freud stated that in cases where exclusiveness of fixation (obligatoriness) was present, we are justified in calling homosexuality a pathological symptom. He maintained that constitutional factors played a part in sexual perversions, but that they played a similar role in all mental disorders. This in no way indicated any repudiation of psychological factors, which are responsible for a predisposition to homosexuality. In actuality, he was thereby emphasizing precisely the psychological developmental factors which remain. (For a complete summary of Freud's contributions to the subject of homosexuality see *The Overt Homosexual*, Chapter III.[80])

Castration fear is of major importance in the development of homosexuality. However, in this writer's view, it is a nonspecific agent, being present as well in neurotic or other types of deviant sexual development. In male homosexuality, the hated rival appears to be transformed into the love object, in contrast, for instance, with the paranoiac whose male love object becomes the unconscious persecutor.

In a 1915 footnote to the *Three Essays*, Freud[38] added an observation of paramount importance: "The connection between the sexual instinct and the sexual object" is not as intimate as one would surmise. They are merely "soldered together." He warned that we must loosen the conceptual bonds which exist between instinct and object. "It seems probable that the sexual instinct is in the first instance independent of its object, nor is its origin likely to be due to the object's attraction." These conclusions have been largely ignored by research investigators as regards the independence between the sexual instinct and sexual object, which further clarifies the etiology of homosexuality.

Those who stress a basic biological tendency toward heterosexuality commit the same error as advocates of the theory of constitutional bisexuality. Rado[74] puts "constitutional bisexuality" in its proper place.

In both lines of experimental study, the available evidence points to the same conclusion: the human male and female do not inherit an organized neuro-hormonal machinery of courtship and mating. Nor do they inherit any organized component mechanism that would—or could—direct them to such goals as mating or choice of mate. In the light of this evidence, the psychoanalytic theory of sexual instincts evolved in the first decades of this century has become an historical expedient that has outlived its scientific usefulness. Each of the sexes has an innate capacity for learning, and is equipped with a specific power plant and tools. But in sharp contrast to the lower vertebrates, and as a consequence of the encephalization of certain functions first organized at lower evolutionary levels of the central nervous system, they inherit no organized information.

In Anna Freud's[28] opinion, the crucial factor in homosexual behavior is the search for male identity through identification with the partner of the same sex in sexual contacts.

Documentation as to the experientially derived origin of homosexuality has been provided by numerous clinicians. Bychowski[15] cited similarities between homosexuals and schizophrenics in terms of psychic structure, especially "infantilisms in the libidinal organization and certain primitive features of the ego." The boundaries of the homosexual ego lack firmness, which makes possible fleeting identifications.

Most cases of homosexuality reveal a basic structural psychological pattern. The intense attachment, fear, and guilt in the boy's relationship with his mother bring about certain major psychic transformations which are effective through the mechanism of the repressive compromise. It is a solution by division, whereby one piece of infantile sexuality enters the service of repression (that is, is helpful in promoting repression through displacement, substitution, and other defense mechanisms). Pregenital pleasure is thereby carried over into the ego, while the rest is repressed. This is one of the major mechanisms in the development of homosexuality and is known as the "Sachs mechanism."[77]

The breast-penis equation is utilized against the positive Oedipus complex.[6,21,23] Because of his attachment to his mother, and hatred for his father, and punitive aggressive-destructive drives toward the body of his mother, he substitutes the partner's penis for the mother's breast. Other mechanisms are psychic masochism and, of crucial importance, identification with the male partner, his penis, and his body in the sexual act.

This writer introduced the concept that in all obligatory homosexuals there has been an inability to make the psychological progression from the mother-child unity of earliest infancy to individuation (preoedipal theory of causation).[83] As a result, there exists in homosexuals of the preoedipal type a partial fixation, with the concomitant tendency to regression to the earliest mother-child relationship. This is experienced and manifested by the homosexual as a threat of personal annihilation, loss of ego boundaries, and sense of fragmentation. This position was documented by a substantially large number of cases of obligatory homosexual patients who had undergone psychoanalysis with this therapist.

To assume that homosexuality is experientially derived means that once the anxiety which originally caused the inhibition of development and the later appearance of homosexuality is removed through suitable psychological measures, the attainment of heterosexuality and heterosexual object love is possible. This has been verified in approximately one-third to one-half of all such patients who were motivated to undergo depth therapy and to seek change.[8,18,47,82]

Bieber et al.[8] presented a systematic study of 106 male homosexuals and 100 male heterosexuals in psychoanalytic treatment with 77 members of the Society of Medical Psychoanalysts in New York. Of the homosexual patients treated, 60 were in analysis less than 200 hours and 46 received 20 treament hours. In the control group of heterosexual cases, 40 had less than 200 treatment hours and 60 were in treatment for at least 200 treatment hours.

According to this report, the outstanding behavior of mothers of homosexuals was an excessive intimacy with their sons. These mothers exerted a binding influence through preferential treatment and seductiveness on the one hand, and inhibiting, overcontrolling attitudes on the other. In many instances, the son was the most significant individual in their lives. Their husbands were usually replaced by the sons as the primary object for libidinal investment. These findings are consistent with those of other psychoanalysts and psychiatrists treating homosexual patients in depth. The son often felt that he had usurped his father's position, and consequently felt guilty and uncomfortable with him.

The Bieber study also found a seriously defective father-son relationship; detachment and rejection by the father, as well as reciprocal hostility. This contrasted markedly with the close-binding maternal intimacy. The father had discontinuous contact with his son, which represented a fear of closeness on the father's part to his own family.

❲ Classifications

Nearly seventy years ago, Freud[38] proposed a classification based on both conscious and unconscious motivation:

1. Absolute inverts whose sexual objects are exclusively of their own sex and who are incapable of carrying out the sexual act with a person of the opposite sex or derive any enjoyment from it.
2. Amphigenic inverts whose sexual objects may equally well be of their own sex or of the opposite sex because this type of inversion lacks the characteristic of exclusiveness.
3. Contingent inverts, whose circumstances preclude accessibility to partners of the opposite sex, may take as their sexual objects those of their own sex.

Current research has prompted the present author to outline five major types of homosexuality as follows.*

1. PREOEDIPAL TYPE

(a) This type is due to a *fixation* to the preoedipal phase of development (age, birth to three).

(b) It is unconsciously motivated and arises from anxiety. Because nonengagement in homosexual practices results in intolerable anxiety, and because the partner must be of the same sex, it may be termed obligatory homosexuality. This sexual pattern is inflexible and stereotyped.

(c) Severe gender identity disturbance is present: in the male, a faulty and weak masculine identity; in the female, a faulty, distorted, and unacceptable feminine identity derived from the mother who is felt to be hateful and hated.

(d) Sexual identity disturbance is due to a persistence of the *primary feminine identification*, as a result of the inability to traverse the separation-individuation phase (age, one-and-a-half to three) and develop a separate and independent identity from the mother. In the female, there persists an identification with the hated mother which she must reject. It is essential here to differentiate between primary and secondary feminine identification. Following the birth of the child, the biological oneness with the mother is replaced by a primitive identification with her. The child must proceed from the security of identification and oneness with the mother to active competent separateness; in the boy, toward active male (phallic) strivings; in the female, to active feminine strivings. If this

* Acknowledgment is made here of this author's indebtedness to Rado[73] for his original concepts of reparative, situational, and variational homosexuality.

task proves too difficult, pathological defenses, especially an increased aggressiveness, may result. These developments are of the greatest importance for the solution of conflicts appearing in the oedipal phase and in later life. In the boy's oedipal phase, under the pressure of the castration fear, an additional type of identification, secondary identification, with the mother in a form of *passive* feminine wishes for the father is likely to take place. However, beneath this feminine position in relation to the father one may often uncover the original passive relation with the mother, i.e., an active feminine preoedipal primary identification. In the oedipal phase of the girl, fear emanating from both parents—a conviction of rejection by the father because she is a female, and by the mother because the latter is hateful and hated—leads to a secondary identification. This results in *passive* feminine wishes for the mother and in a masculine identification superimposed on the girl's deeper, hated feminine identification, in order to secure the "good" mother (the female homosexual partner later in life).

(e) The anxieties which beset persons of this type are of an insistent and intractable nature, leading to an overriding, almost continual search for sexual partners.

(f) Persistence of primitive and archaic mental mechanisms, leading to an abundance of incorporation and projection anxieties.

(g) The anxiety which develops is due to fears of engulfment, ego dissolution, loss of self and ego boundaries. The homosexual act is needed to insure ego survival and transiently stabilize the sense of self. Consequently, the act must be repeated frequently and out of inner necessity to ward off paranoidal and incorporative fears. (The rare exceptions in this type, who cannot consciously accept the homosexual act, struggle mightily against it and, therefore, the symptom remains latent, as explained in Type 5.)

(h) The homosexual symptom is *ego-syntonic*, as the nuclear conflicts, e.g., fears of engulfment, loss of ego boundaries, loss of self, have undergone a transformation and disguise through the mechanism of the repressive compromise, allowing the more acceptable part of infantile sexuality to remain in consciousness. (See Sachs mechanism in section on Developmental Factors).

(i) There is a predominance of pregenital characteristics of the ego; remembering is often replaced by acting out.

(j) Aim of the homosexual act: ego survival and a reconstitution of a sense of sexual identity in accordance wih anatomy. The male achieves "masculinity" through identification with the male sexual partner; reassures against and lessens castration fear. The female achieves "resonance" identification with the woman partner; reassures against and lessens castration fears. She also creates the "good" mother-child relationship.

2. OEDIPAL TYPE

(a) This type is due to a failure of resolution of the Oedipus complex and to castration fears, leading to the adoption of a negative oedipal position and a *regression* in part to anal and oral conflicts (a partial preoedipal regression). The male assumes the role of the female with the father (other men); the female the role of the male to the mother (other women).

(b) Homosexual wishes in this type are unconsciously motivated and dreaded; engagement in homosexual practices is not obligatory. The sexual pattern is flexible in that heterosexuality can be carried out and is usually the conscious choice.

(c) Gender identity disturbances of masculine sexual identity in the male (or deficient feminine sexual identity in the female) are due to a *secondary identification* with a person (parent) of the opposite sex in this type. (This is simply a reversal of normal sexual identification in the direction of the same-sex parent.)

(d) The anxiety which develops in the male is due to fears of penetration by the more powerful male (father); the female fears rejection by the more powerful female (mother). Common to both are shame and guilt arising from superego and ego conflicts, conscious and unconscious, attendant to engaging in homosexual acts in dreams and fantasies and, occasionally, in actuality, under special circumstances of stress. Homosexual acts in this type are attempts to insure dependency and attain power through the seduction of the more powerful partner.

(e) Primitive and archaic psychic mechanisms may appear due to *regression*. These are intermittent and do not lend a stamp of pregenitality to the character traits of the individual, as they do in the preoedipal type.

(f) The homosexual symptom is *ego-alien*. Although unconsciously determined, it is not the outcome of the repressive compromise (Sachs mechanism), as described in Type 1 above. The symptom may remain at the level of unconscious thoughts, dreams, and fantasies, as it is not a disguised, acceptable representation of a deeper conflict. When it threatens to break into awareness, anxiety develops. However, under certain conditions, e.g., defiant rage overriding the restraining mechanism of conscience, periods of intense depression secondary to loss, with resultant needs for love, admiration, and strength from a person of the same sex, homosexual acts may take place. Such acts, however, do not achieve the magical symbolic restitution of the preoedipal type. They may exacerbate the situation through loss of pride and self-esteem.

(g) Aim of the homosexual act: to experience dependency on and security from "powerful" figures of the same sex. The sexual pattern of the negative oedipal type is not as inflexible or stereotyped as in the preoedipal type. There are exacerbations and remissions in the sense of masculine identity (in the female, in the sense of pride and achievement in feminine identity) secondary to successful performance in other (non-sexual) areas of life. Such feelings of success diminish any fantasied or actual need for sexual relations with persons of the same sex.

3. SITUATIONAL TYPE

(a) Environmental inaccessibility to partners of the opposite sex.

(b) The behavior is consciously motivated.

(c) Homosexual acts are not fear-induced but arise out of conscious deliberation and choice.

(d) The person is able to function with a partner of the opposite sex.

(e) The sexual pattern is flexible and these individuals do return to opposite sex partners when they are available.

4. VARIATIONAL TYPE

(a) The motivations underlying this form of homosexual behavior are as varied as the motivations which drive men and women to pursue power, gain protection, assure dependency, seek security, wreak vengeance, or experience specialized sensations. In some cultures, such surplus activity is a part of the established social order; in others, entirely a product of individual enterprise, contrary to the general social order. The homosexuality practiced in ancient Greece was in all probability variational in type. There were strict laws against it (except for its practice during a brief period in late adolescence). Penalties included disenfranchisement of those engaged in catamite activities (anal intercourse). Sentiments expressing admiration and affection for youth (so-called homosexual sentiments), short of homosexual relations, were allowed.[62] In ancient Sparta, homosexuality could be punished by death.

(b) The behavior is consciously motivated.

(c) Homosexual acts are not fear-induced, but arise out of conscious deliberation and choice.

(d) The person is able to function with a partner of the opposite sex.

(e) The sexual pattern is flexible, and these individuals do return to opposite sex partners when they so prefer.

5. LATENT TYPE

(a) This type has the underlying psychic structure of either the preoedipal or oedipal type, without homosexual practices.

(b) There is much confusion in the use of the term "latent homosexuality," due to the erroneous and outmoded concept of constitutional bisexuality, which implies that side-by-side with an innate desire for opposite-sex partners there exists an inborn or innate desire for same-sex partners. Correctly, latent homosexuality means the presence in an individual of the underlying psychic structure of either the preoedipal or oedipal type, without overt orgastic activity with a person of the same sex.

(c) The shift from latent to overt and the reverse is dependent on several factors:

(i) The strength of the fixation at the preoedipal level (quantitative factor), severity of anxiety, and the intensity of regression from the later oedipal conflict.

(ii) The acceptability of the homosexuality to the ego (self), the superego (conscience mechanism), and the ego ideal.

(iii) The strength of the instinctual drives, i.e., libido and aggression.

These individuals may never or rarely engage in overt homosexual activities.

(d) The latent homosexual may or may not have any conscious knowledge of his preference for individuals of the same sex for orgastic fulfillment. On the other hand, there may be a high degree of elaboration of unconscious homosexual fantasies and homosexual dream material, with or without conscious denial of its significance. They may live an entire lifetime without realizing their homosexual propensities, managing to function marginally on a heterosexual level, sometimes married and having children.

(e) Another pattern is that of the individual who, fully aware of his homosexual preference, abstains from all homosexual acts. Others, as a result of severe stress, infrequently and transiently do engage in overt homosexual acts, living the major portion of their lives, however, as latent homosexuals. In the latent phase, they may maintain a limited heterosexual functioning, albeit unrewarding, meager, and usually based on homosexual fantasies. Or, they may utilize homosexual fantasy for masturbatory practices or may abstain from sexual activity altogether. These individuals are, of course, truly homosexual at all times; the shift between latent and overt and the reverse constitutes an alternating form of latent homosexuality.

(f) All forms of latent homosexuality are potentially overt. Social imbalance—where severe inequities exist between one's survival needs due to the failure of society to ensure their adequate satisfaction—has a precipitating effect in some borderline and/or latent cases of both preoedipal and oedipal homosexuality. Such imbalance also brings a flight from the female on the part of the male, a flight from all aspects of masculine endeavor, and a retreat to a less demanding role.[53] This is a possible explanation of the apparent rise in the incidence of male homosexuality during periods of social turbulence when many traditional roles, privileges, and responsibilities are overturned. The same factors may cause an increase in female homosexuality.

Discussion

Preoedipal and oedipal homosexuality are reparative in nature, and "ushered in by the inhibition of standard performance through early [childhood] fears."[73] Preoedipal homosexuality may be compared to the narcotic addict's need for a "fix." The purpose of the homosexual act is to maintain the equilibrium of a highly disturbed individual.

In connection with the situational type, Bieber reported that men who had not been homosexual prior to military service were found not to have engaged in homosexual activity throughout their tour of duty, despite the absence of female partners, with rare exceptions.[7] This finding suggests a possible revision of the concept of situational homosexuality in instances where the coercive factor is absent. Much of the so-called situational factor in prisons is an outcome of the struggle for dominance and is, in fact, rape. The infrequency of validated situations in which heterosexuals engage in homosexual relations reaffirms the strength of the male-female design, once it has been established in the human psyche; parenthetically, it explains the popularity of the "pin-up" during World War II. Undoubtedly, sexual outlet was achieved under those trying conditions of sexual deprivation via masturbation, within the fantasy twosome of heterosexual relations abetted by photographs of artistically posed semi-nude females.

Variational homosexuality may occur in individuals who seek to gratify the desire for an alternation of sexual excitation, often for reasons of impotence or near-impotence in the male partner of the heterosexual pair. Much of the heterosexual group sex activity currently reported includes homosexual behavior between male and female participants, and is of this type. In some instances, individuals with unconsciously derived homosexual conflicts take part in such group activities, in order to act out their homosexual wishes and simultaneously to deny their homosexual problem.

Variational homosexuality may also be seen in the neurotic, psychotic, and sociopath. It frequently occurs in those suffering from alcoholism, as well as in depressive states.

(Psychopathology

Pathology, whether somatic or psychic, is defined as failure of function with concomitant pain and/or suffering. It is this failure, its significance and manifold consequences, which is so obvious in obligatory preoedipal homosexuality—a failure in functioning which, if carried to its extreme, would mean the death of the species.

A number of items serve as indicators of psychic pathology in the obligatory homosexual.[81] They may not appear in all cases, and they may differ qualitatively and quantitatively from patient to patient:

1. A lifelong persistence of the original primary feminine identification with the mother, and a consequent sense of deficiency as regards one's masculine identity. The end result is a pervasive feeling of femininity or a deficient sense of masculinity.[88]

2. A fear of engulfment and consequent extreme anxiety whenever an obligatory homosexual attempts to establish any sexual relatedness to a woman.[46,50]

3. A persistence of archaic and primitive psychic mechanisms, e.g., the presence of incorporative and projective anxieties.[38]

4. There is often present a deficit in the body ego boundaries, with fears of bodily disintegration[83] and unusual sensitivity to threats of bodily damage by external objects.

5. In the dream life of all obligatory homosexuals lies the fear of engulfment. This is commonly symbolically represented by fears of encasement in caves, tunnels, whirlpools, deep immersion into bodies of water, etc. with a threat of personal annihilation and loss of self.[26] These derive from the fear of engulfment by the body of the female.

6. Sexual acts can be carried out only with a person of the same sex or through the combined use of other perversions.

7. Beneath the surface rationalizations of "love and affection," severe, damaging, disruptive, aggressive impulses threaten to destroy both the relationship and the partner.

8. Homosexual acts are sometimes carried out to avoid a paranoid development or a paranoid psychosis.

9. The homosexual act itself may be likened to the effects of the opium alkaloids in their magical restorative powers: the optimum "fix," reinstating the body ego and sense of self against a threat of disruption, and in severe cases, imminent disintegration of the personality. Homosexual acts, therefore, are intense, impulsive, their urgency deriving from the emergency need of survival for the ego of the homosexual.

10. Beneath the male homosexual's apparent affection for men lies the search for love from the father or father-surrogate and a concomitant wish to wreak vengeance upon him, the son's wish for masculine identification having been frustrated by the father's absence, coldness, apathy, or disdain. Furthermore, the father fears his phallic, castrating wife and does not interfere with her domination of the child. The son harbors deep distrust, rage and resentment toward men, because the father failed to protect him from the engulfing mother.

11. All obligatory homosexuals suffer from a deep sense of inferiority, worthlessness, and

guilt because of their inability to function in the male role. These feelings are not caused by societal attitudes but are aggravated by them.[42]

12. Most homosexuals suffer from a considerable degree of psychic masochism.[5,35,79] The aggressive assault toward the mother and secondarily toward the father is drained off into a psychic masochistic state. All homosexuals deeply fear the knowledge that their homosexual behavior constitutes an eroticized defense against this more threatening masochistic state.[36] The masochism seeks discharge through homosexual activity.

13. In most homosexuals, anxiety derived from preoedipal and oedipal conflicts undergoes an eroticization or libidinization.[23]

14. Homosexuals tend to suffer from concomitant psychiatric conditions. For example, a large number of paranoid schizophrenics, paranoiacs, and pseudo-neurotic schizophrenics have a homosexual conflict, and many manifest homosexual behavior. Freud[37] first called attention to the possibility that certain neurotic and psychotic symptoms were the expression of an underlying homosexual conflict. In the schizophrenic, homosexuality may be an outgrowth of a confused, chaotic, and fragmented psychic organization. The desperate need to make human contact on any basis leads the individual to engage in all forms of sexual activity, including homosexual acts. These may be spasmodic attempts to experience relatedness, and there is often no consistency or specific quality to these episodes.[73]

15. It is characteristic that upon attempting interruption of homosexual activities, severe anxiety, tension, depression, and other symptomatology will make a dramatic appearance, therefore underscoring a function of the homosexual symptom, namely, that it is a compromise formation against deep anxieties.[40] This outcome of such interruption is consistently seen in the course of treating homosexuals in depth.

16. A frequent finding is that additional sexual deviations occur simultaneously, or sometimes alternate, with homosexuality; the most common are fetishism,[32] transvestitism,[2,22] and exhibitionism.

Clinical Symptoms

To ensure completeness, in addition to the items set forth in the preceding section on psychopathology, a comprehensive listing of the symptomatology of obligatory preoedipal homosexuality is outlined below:

(a) Symptoms arising out of the failure to make the intrapsychic separation from the mother:[65,66]

(i) Excessive clinging to the mother in infancy and early childhood.

(ii) Severe anxiety upon separation from her, noticeable from earliest childhood ("screaming phenomenon"[80]), and continuing throughout life.

(iii) Merging and fusion phenomena;[26] fear of the engulfing mother; faulty body ego image because of the failure to separate, and the lack of delineation of one's own body from that of the mother; there may be a consequent inability to appreciate body-space relationships.

(iv) Intensification of primary feminine identification.

(b) Symptoms arising from the predominance of archaic, primitive psychic mechanisms:

(i) Incorporative anxieties (fears of swallowng parts of one's own body, fears of internalized harmful objects, etc.).[13,58,59]

(ii) Projective anxieties (paranoidal anxieties, e.g., fears of poisoning, bodily attack, and persecution).[58,59]

(c) Symptoms arising from faulty gender identity:

(i) Continuation of the persistence of primary feminine identification with the mother (inner feelings of femininity).

(ii) Corresponding feelings of a deficit in masculinity with anxiety appearing when faced with attempted performance in the appropriate gender role.

(d) Symptoms which are manifestations of the negative Oedipus complex:

(i) Wishes to replace the mother in sexual relations with the father by vaginalizing the anus.

(ii) The sexual wish for intercourse with the father is realized in fantasy or is enacted vicariously in the homosexual act with another male.

(e) Symptoms representing castration anxiety:

(i) Fears of penetrating objects, accidents, open wounds, haircuts.

(ii) Other symbolic representations of the forceful removal of the penis.

(f) Symptoms arising from the wish for and fear of extreme closeness to the mother, the intense dependency on her for a feeling of well-being and survival, and the intense identification with her:

(i) Intense oral-sadistic relationship with the mother (intense sadism toward her is disguised by its opposite, a masochistic attitude toward her).

(ii) Passive homosexual feelings toward the father, often repressed (taking the place of the mother in sexual intercourse, both to protect and supplant her and to wreak vengeance on the father through appropriating his penis).

(iii) Maintenance of a position of optimal distance from and/or

closeness to the mother and other women.[83]

(iv) Fear of the sudden approach of the mother, as if she would devour, engulf, and incorporate him. (This fear of the mother's engulfment and control, which in part reflects his wish for and dread of her domination, is then generalized to a fear of all women and engulfment by them, especially by the female genitalia and pubic hair.)

(g) Symptoms relating to the father, arising from persistent primary feminine identification and the father's failure to provide appropriate masculine identity and protection from the mother:

(i) Hostile, contemptuous attitude toward the father.

(ii) Yearning for lost masculinity and attempts to find it by soliciting affection and admiration from other boys during childhood.

(iii) Development of unconscious wishes to control older boys (the father) through feminine-like seductiveness and sexual fantasy.

(h) At puberty and in early adolescence, the response to hormonal stimulation and anatomic growth is an intensification of anxiety due to a deficient masculine identity and inability to perform in the masculine anatomic, physiological, and psychological roles:

(i) Powerful feelings of inferiority, shame, and guilt.

(ii) Hostility toward his penis and masculinity, which reinforces aspects of his feminine identification (mood, manner, stance, posture, dress, voice, facial expression, hand gestures, areas of interest—a psychophysiological "molding" of appearance or "psychosomatic compliance").

(iii) Sensing of defect in masculinity; may engage in a compensatory "masculinization" through weight-lifting, body-building, and a heightened narcissistic overvaluation of the body.

(iv) Onset of experiencing the insistent internal need for "filling up" the emptiness of his masculine ego (self) through the incorporation of the body of a male partner, especially of the latter's penis; full-scale homosexual activity usually begins in adolescence to alleviate the defects of the masculine ego and to acquire a sense of masculine self in accordance with anatomy.

(i) Symptoms present in adulthood:

(i) Constant yearning and search for masculinity; by engaging in homosexual acts, he incorporates the male partner and his penis, thus strengthening himself.

(ii) Every homosexual encounter first concerns itself with disarming the partner through one's seductiveness, appeal, power, prestige, effeminacy, or "masculinity." This simulation of the male-female pattern (active vs. passive, the one who penetrates vs. the one who is penetrated) should not lead to the conclusion that the motivation of either partner is to achieve femininity; both partners are intent upon acquiring masculinity from each other. To disarm in order to defeat is the motif, and if one submits in "defeat," gratification is nevertheless obtained by the victim vicariously, through identification with the victor.

Despite any surface manifestations to the contrary, *to disarm and defeat* invariably characterizes all encounters between homosexuals.

(iii) Many homosexual acts are purely egocentric. Tender, affective reciprocity, when present, is frequently based on the need for parental care, economic security, or magical fulfillment. Quite commonly, some homosexuals prefer to achieve contact anonymously, even to the use of an aperture in a toilet stall wall, extending one's own penis and/or grasping the other's penis without face-to-face encounter. This is the enactment of the fundamental nature of their object relationships, namely, relating to part objects, not whole objects.

(iv) Both one-to-one as well as multiple homosexual contacts between a variety of partners assembled in a group have as their aim the immediate gratification and alleviation of urgent destructive feelings threatening extinction to the self, were they to be contained; other individuals are the instruments through which the homosexual seeks expression of and release from oppressive and importunate anxieties, guilts, incestuous feelings, and feelings of aggression.

(v) This stereotyped compulsive searching for sexual gratification with individuals of the same sex may completely dominate the life of the homosexual, not allowing him to invest his interest in other important activities, a realization which is often the source of great personal anguish to him.

(vi) Chronic psychic masochism.

(vii) Whenever homosexuality is not engaged in for any reason, including self-denial or lack of opportunity, there is a mounting tension, anxiety, and depression. If the homosexual act does not take place, severe anxiety will result, other perverse activities may be pressed into service, and other signs of neurotic conflict may appear, e.g., psychosomatic symptoms.

(viii) Deep, unconscious sense of worthlessness and consequent inability to function well in other major life areas.

(ix) Chronic paranoid anxiety of mild to severe degree is often present.

(x) Deep-rooted sense of guilt and shame derived from aggressive impulses toward parents and from inability to fulfill biological gender role; societal guilt may be superimposed.

(xi) Premature attempts at sexual relations with women may result in severe anxiety, fears of engulfment, a sense of bodily disintegration, other regressive symptomatology. It must be remembered that the homosexual act "magically" produces a psychic equilibrium in order to temporarily withstand the multiple anxieties which beset the homosexual.

❨ Female Homosexuality

Kinsey's statistical compilations show that among females the cumulative evidence of homosexual responses was 28 percent, and those to the point of orgasm, 13 percent. He reported that homosexual responses occurred in about only one-half as many females as males, and homosexual contacts between women to the point of orgasm in about one-third as many females as males. Compared to males, there were only about one-half to one-third as many females who at any age were primarily or exclusively homosexual.[56,57]

To the present author, these statistics are of questionable validity, as female homosexuality may exist largely unnoticed. The changing psychoanalytic concepts of male and female homosexuality have been summarized by Wiedeman[90] and Socarides.[85] In these reports, it was pointed out that while the literature on male homosexuality has been rather extensive, that on female homosexuality has been relatively neglected. Its literature is meager both quantitatively and qualitatively, with some notable exceptions.

Many scientific writers prefer to use the term "Lesbianism" to describe the clinical condition of female homosexuality. This reflects an attempt to romanticize and minimize it. In most instances, female homosexuality is pictured as either a psychosis or a case of "perverse morality" which ultimately becomes good morality through the love of a man. An alternative depiction is that of the unfortunate woman virtuously fighting off her homosexual desires but remaining emotionally unfulfilled. Men themselves generally consider homosexual relations between women as providing only superficial pleasure at best, and some do not even consider female homosexual contacts as sexual at all, despite intense orgastic experiences between the women involved.

In contrast to the frequent interest of the male homosexual in young adolescents, the female homosexual is seldom attracted to early postpubertal girls to the point of actual seduction.

Very often, a homosexual woman will view her future with more anxiety than will the heterosexual woman. She will, therefore, undertake marriage for the sake of economic security, to overcome a sense of inner and social isolation, and to satisfy the expectations of family and society. Once married, her sexual life with a partner of the same sex may of necessity become a highly clandestine one. A wife may have a female lover completely without her husband's knowledge. Many homosexual women marry and are regarded as heterosexual, although they remain sexually unresponsive to their husbands.

It is difficult to ascertain how many marriages are ultimately dissolved because the female partner is an overt or latent homosexual. Occasionally, a homosexual woman may marry simply to have a child whom she then treats as she wished to have been treated during her childhood. She will divorce the husband and thereafter lead a completely homosexual life. In general, homosexual men do not ordinarily view marriage as a social or economic solution, nor feel impelled to it in order to achieve fatherhood.

Of crucial importance is the fact that women can have sexual intercourse without desire. This aids in both the conscious or unconscious self-deception on the part of the woman as to her homosexual feelings and wishes. She may not even know that her resentment and lack of love for her husband are due to her homosexual conflict. A man, however, requires the preliminary presence of desire in order to achieve erection; in its absence, he must perforce appear inadequate and face the loss of sexual pride and the esteem of the partner. Women may successfully submit to a sexual life which they find meaningless and even distasteful, and still manage to hide their narcissistic mortification, humiliation, and resentment, living out a masquerade of womanliness.[43]

Female homosexuality has important and significant social and psychological effects. It is severely disruptive of the family unit. Any child of an overtly homosexual mother is exposed to a variety of psychological traumata of intense proportions.

Psychodynamics of Female Homosexuality

Obligatory female homosexuality is always reparative in function, as already explained in the discussion on obligatory homosexuality in the male. In female homosexuality, only the organs of the female partner are desired, while those of the male are abhorred and feared. These women react to penetration by,

at best, little or no sensation; at worst, with pain and fantasies of invasion.

In the female, preoedipal and oedipal phase conflict (age, birth to five) may be reanimated and has to be overcome every time a new sexual stage, such as puberty, menstruation, sexual intercourse, pregnancy, childbirth, occurs. This is a tremendous complication, and in those women whose sexual functioning has already been weakened by infantile conflicts, female homosexuality may be activated at any point.[11,12,17]

Female sexuality is further complicated by the fact that girls do not develop directly toward femininity; they make a roundabout detour through masculine attitudes, not only in childhood but often in puberty.

A still further complication is the fact that the little boy can inspect his genital to see if any consequences of masturbation or castration fear have occurred, whereas the little girl cannot thus reassure herself. Her anxiety and guilt may cause her to assume a fictitious male role for varying periods of time.

In 1931, in his article on female sexuality, Freud[31] stated that if the girl clings in obstinate self-assertion to masculinity, we may see that the hope of acquiring a penis is prolonged to an incredible age and may become the aim of her life. The fantasy of really being a man in spite of everything may dominate her, and may result in a homosexual object choice.

Clinical Picture

A female homosexual usually does not seek treatment because of homosexuality. She may have been forced into therapy by pressure from her family, by depression over the loss of a love partner, or a concomitant neurosis and/or psychosis. The homosexuality itself may be a partial expression of the underlying neurosis and/or psychosis which may have been temporarily warded off through homosexual activities.

Usually, she suffers from feelings of depression or anxiety, arising from insecurity about the loyalty of her partner. Often, she suffers from suicidal ideas. In many instances, therapy reveals an unconscious aggressive, murderous hatred against her mother. Sexual excitement is bound up with maternal prohibition. Aggressive impulses are resisted, and as a reaction to them an intense sense of guilt toward the mother appears. This leads to the transformation of hate into a masochistic libidinal attitude. This libidinal relationship, although masochistic, appears in place of the anxiety and hostility which would have caused openly neurotic symptoms. In later life, the mother-substitute (homosexual partner) pays off the infantile grievances by granting sexual satisfaction.

Some overtly homosexual women recognize the mother-child relationship implicit in their partnerships. In all of them, sexual satisfaction is obtained from close embrace, sucking of the nipples and genitals, anal practices, mutual cunnilingus, or the use of phallic devices. Often, there is a double role casting for both partners, one now playing the male and the other playing the female. In other pairs, there can be a consistent male or female role for each partner.

In those cases of overt female homosexuals who are borderline schizophrenics, conscious or nearly conscious thoughts of killing the mother and the siblings are present.

During sexual experiences between women, both partners are able to transform the hate of the mother into love, while simultaneously receiving the "good" mother's (partner's) breast. Each of them thereby obtains what she wished so much to have had—the "good" mother—during the early years of life.

Almost always, there is an intense conflict over childhood masturbation. In the sexual act, the "mother" sanctions masturbation through a mutuality of action and sharing of guilt by the partners.

The homosexual woman is in flight from the man. The reasons for this flight are childhood feelings of guilt toward the mother, and fears of disappointment and rejection by the father if she dared to turn to him for love and support. On the other hand, she may expect that he would even gratify her infantile sexual wishes, thus incurring for her a masochistic danger. If he refuses her, it would constitute a narcissistic injury. The resolution of these dangers is to turn to the earlier love object, the mother, in the form of a homosexual partner. It is a reversion to a fantasied previous pleasure. "The economic advantage of this new turning to the mother lies in the release from a feeling of guilt. But it seems to me that its most important accomplishment lies in the protection from a threatened loss of object: 'If my father won't have me and my self-respect is so undermined, who will love me, if not my mother?' "[17]

In other cases of female homosexuality seen by the present author,[80] preoedipal fears of the primitive type described by Melanie Klein appear,[59] especially when a threat of rejection by the partner occurs. Fears of being poisoned, devoured, attacked, contaminated, or dismembered by the partner (preoedipal mother) are evident in dreams and in the waking state. In childhood, the original flight to the mother was an attempt to gain her love ("buy protection"), alleviate feelings of murderous aggression toward her, and to protect the self against the assumed murderous impulses of the mother. This is what is reenacted in the adult female homosexual relationship.

The homosexual woman is prone to experience a crisis state first described by Jones in 1927 as "aphanisis."[51] While castration is a partial threat, aphanisis is a total threat—a threat to survival, involving total extinction and abandonment. Having renounced all interest in men and believing themselves hated by women, female homosexuals very often become suicidal if faced with loss of the love object.

Homosexual women who do retain any interest in men have as their underlying goal to be accepted by men as one of them.* These are the women who often complain of the unfairness of their lot, and of unjust and ill treatment meted out to them by men. Others, with little or no interest in men, vicariously enjoy femininity via their women partners.

Those who desire penetration by the tongue

---

* Acknowledgment is made here to the two major studies on the clinical varieties of homosexual women, which contributed substantially to the present author's formulations.[10,16]

or finger (some female homosexuals object to any form of penetration) require that this be done only by a woman. Seemingly the "most homosexual," these patients have the best prognosis of all female homosexuals. Quite commonly, the identification with the father is present, which serves to keep feminine wishes in repression. This identification is also for the unconscious purpose of giving a child to the mother.

The female homosexual projects her femininity onto the mother, and then onto other women who continue to represent the mother. She may see herself mirrored in other women who have a high degree of feminine narcissism. In effect, she has projected her femininity onto others and enjoys an identification with herself. This femininity sometimes is projected only onto women who are known by her to cause men to suffer and refuse them satisfaction; with them she has an "ideal" partner.

Homosexual women play a "mother and child" relationship to the exclusion of the intruding father. Those who identify themselves with the active mother may be attracted to very young girls, although they do not attempt to actively seduce them. Conversely, those who continue to act the child are attracted chiefly to older, maternal, protective women, toward whom they are very passive. On occasion, both active and passive attitudes are evident in the same person or alternate between the partners. It is striking in those who identify as the child that any device substituting for the penis is abhorred, and no masculine clothing is worn at any time by either individual of this pair.

Other homosexual women wear masculine clothing, including ties, and strive to act the man in relation to the partner. These women have double identifications, one superimposed upon the other. They identify with the father and with the "good" mother who cares for the child. They find it extremely difficult to admit to any passivity or wish to be caressed themselves.

The most difficult of all women to treat are those who ostensibly give up "loving" mother

(other women), and take the father as their love object. They cannot tolerate any love object without a penis, perceiving this as a severe inferiority. They unconsciously cling tenaciously to the idea that they themselves possess a fictive penis; at times, this may become a conscious fantasy. Although they may engage in heterosexual intercourse, they are ambivalent in the extreme in their relationship to their male partners and experience intermittent intense unconscious and conscious homosexual wishes. On occasion, when tense and depressed following a rejection or failure, they may briefly engage in an actual homosexual encounter.

It is important to note that some female homosexuals may appear extremely feminine. These women choose the opposite extreme of masculine-appearing homosexual women for their partners, seeking from them the attention they wished to have had from their fathers.

⟨ Therapeutic Considerations

Psychoanalytic Therapy

In 1905, Freud[38] wrote that the only possibility of helping homosexual patients was to demand a suppression of their symptoms through hypnotic suggestion. By 1920, he believed that psychoanalysis itself was applicable to the treatment of perversions, including homosexuality, but later expressed caution about the possibility of complete cure. His criterion of cure was not only a detachment of cathexis from the homosexual object but also the ability to cathect the opposite sex.[34]

In 1950, Anna Freud lectured in New York on the recent advances in treatment of homosexuals, stating that many of her patients lost their inversion as a result of analysis. This occurred even in those who had proclaimed their wish to remain homosexual when entering treatment, having started only to obtain relief from their neurotic symptoms.[29]

It subsequently became the consensus that

homosexuals could be treated for the most part like phobics. However, this presented considerable difficulty, including the probability of premature termination of treatment and the production of excessive anxiety. The major challenge in treating homosexuality from the point of view of the patient's resistance has, of course, been the misconception that the disorder is innate or inborn.

It is now widely agreed that to achieve therapeutic success it is necessary to interpret to the patient his fear of castration; his fear of oral dependence; his distrust of the opposite sex; and his fear of his own destructiveness and sadism. However, in this writer's experience, the interpretation that most effectively achieves a relaxation of the patient's resistance is that of the attempt to acquire masculinity through identification with the partner and his penis in the homosexual act.[30] After this interpretation is worked through, the patient may be able to function heterosexually, going through a strong narcissistic-phallic phase, women serving only the "grandeur" of his penis.

Detailed reports of successful resolution of cases of overt homosexuality have been published by Flournoy,[27] Lagache,[63] Poe,[71] Socarides,[82] Vinchon and Nacht,[89] and Wulff.[91] In addition, important insights are offered by Bergler,[4,5] Bychowski,[14,15] Anna Freud,[30] Freud,[33,34] Glover,[42] Lorand,[64] Nunberg,[68] Ovesey,[70] Rosenfeld,[76] Socarides,[80,86,87] and Sachs.[77]

Data on positive therapeutic outcome have been collected in surveys by the American Psychoanalytic Association,[1] and by the Bieber study[8] conducted by the Society of Medical Psychoanalysts, the former presented in statistical format.

The central issues which must be uncovered and worked through by both patient and therapist are the following:

1. While the analysis of oedipal fears of incest and aggression is of paramount importance in the course of treatment, it is vital to the understanding and successful resolution of homosexuality that the nuclear preoedipal anxieties be revealed. These consist of primitive fears of incorporation, threatened loss of personal identity, engulfment by the mother, and personal dissolution which would accompany any attempt to separate from her.

2. The homosexual makes an identification with his partner in the sexual act. Homosexual contact promotes a transient, pseudo-strengthening of his own masculinity and identity, which must be constantly repeated or a psychic decompensation occurs. The homosexual seeks masculinity, not femininity, and knowledge of this unconscious motivation becomes a potent source of strength, reassurance, and determination for change in the direction of heterosexual functioning.

3. The conditions under which the imperative need for homosexual relief occurs include mounting anxiety, depression, and paranoid-type fears.

4. The ubiquitous presence of a distorted body ego is manifest.

5. The penis of the partner is revealed to be a substitute for the feeding breast of the sought-after "good" mother (breast-penis equation). The homosexual thereby escapes the frustrating cruel mother and makes up for the oral deprivation suffered at her hands.

6. There is a characteristic demeaning and degrading of the father, often quite openly. The patient identifies with the aggressor (mother). This hatred of the father produces guilt, and in therapy is an impediment to his feeling entitled to be a man.

7. At unconscious levels, there exists an intense yearning for the father's love and protection. This deprivation is a further frustration of the need for masculine identification. The homosexual act dramatizes the yearning as well as the frustration-derived aggression toward all men as a consequence.

8. Heterosexual interest and strivings are continually subject to suppression and repression in the course of therapy. This is due to unconscious guilt feelings toward the mother because of intense incestuous and aggressive impulses.

9. The careful maintenance of the positive therapeutic alliance is a considerable source of strength to the patient in his attempts to con-

trol and finally triumph over his fears of murderous retaliation on the part of the mother, as he gradually moves toward his long sought-for masculine identity.

Group Therapy

Because the exploration of conscious and unconscious fantasies, feelings, and actions are limited in group therapy, it is wise to combine it with individual therapy. Successful results utilizing group therapy have been reported by Gershman,[39] Hadden,[44,45] and T. Bieber.[9]

Gershman has provided a clear description of the group process. He has conducted a combined program of simultaneous group and individual therapy for the past twelve years. He shows that healthy and unhealthy interplay between a patient and seven or eight of his peers brings issues sharply into focus. The therapist along with others in the group assists in promoting awareness of healthy interactions, neurotic defenses, and conflicted feelings toward oneself and others. The groups are composed entirely of homosexuals, generally five men and four or five women.

It was found that such homogeneous groups go far toward minimizing competitiveness, feelings of inferiority, and secretiveness. Because of their common sexual orientation, mutual interest and concern are evident; sometimes, their feelings are acted out homosexually outside the sessions. The attitude of the group to such liaisons is generally empathic, but sceptical as to the motivation and durability of such a relationship. During the ordinarily brief duration of the liaison, the partners involved are generally reticent about discussing it. But upon its termination, much material emerges in retrospect regarding the underlying anxieties that drove one to the other.

Thus, an atmosphere of mutual acceptance and dedication to a common goal of trying to understand the source, nature, dynamics, and tenacity of the homosexual symptom is established. Although homosexuality is the common basis of the group, the emotional difficulties from which each member suffers in his own life are unique to that individual. Anxiety,

either conscious or unconscious, provides valuable therapeutic material. The advantage of group examination of the material stems from the fact that resistance is lowered through the contributions of additional personal insights offered by all members of the group and heightened by the special psychodynamic knowledge of the therapist.

The predominant attitude toward fellow-group members is generally sympathetic, encouraging, and growth-promoting. Inasmuch as the group meets only for one-and-a-half to two hours weekly, it would seem that not enough time is available for each participant to investigate his life situation in depth. That, however, is not true. Customarily, one or two members dominate any given session, as a result of the intensity of the conflicts that have erupted within them. As that material unfolds, each member identifies with it and often brings in correlative material that stems from his own life, to help to explain and expand the significance of the material brought out by the presenting member. As a consequence, each learns the nature, application, and efficacy of expressing and communicating his thoughts and feelings as freely as possible. Similarly, dream material, emotional responses, changes in mood, sudden blocks to verbalization, and other phenomena, are understood in terms of intrapsychic processes by each member through memory or through identification with other members.

The consequences of such experiences are often dramatic. This is in part due to the intense interaction, clarification, and understanding of various events that come under group scrutiny. Members gradually learn the dynamics of their unconscious and the correlation of their present manner of living to the conditioning factors of their early life. More than that, they learn to recognize the psychodynamic forces that gave rise to homosexuality.

The position of the group as to the question of changing from homosexuality to heterosexuality becomes in time a belief that such change is possible, depending upon the strength of motivation and the willingness to withstand the anxiety entailed in such progress. From many years of experience with group therapy with homosexuals, Gershman reports that he has yet to see a patient whose degree of anxiety at least has ultimately not diminished. About 20 percent, he estimates, have been able to change to active heterosexual functioning as a result of combined individual and group therapy.

Discussion

The general pessimism as to the outcome of treatment of homosexuality is diminishing. The unpublished informal report of the Central Fact Gathering Committee of the American Psychoanalytic Association was one of the first surveys to be made available on this issue.[1] Out of 46 cases, 8 in the completed group (which totaled 22) were described as cured, 13 as improved, and 1 as unimproved. This constituted one-third of all cases reported. Of this group, those that did not complete treatment (24), 16 were described as improved, 3 as untreatable, 5 as transferred. In all reported cures, follow-up communications verified assumption of full heterosxeual role and function.

Out of the 106 homosexuals studied by Bieber[8] et al., 29 (27 percent) became exclusively heterosexual.

This writer noted in 1968 that over 50 percent of the obligatory homosexuals whom he has seen (over a seventeen-year period), strongly motivated for change and undergoing depth therapy, have not only shown full heterosexual functioning but have been able to develop love feelings for their heterosexual partners.[80]

In addition to the uncovering techniques of depth psychotherapy and psychoanalysis, treatment requires educational and retraining measures, interventions and modifications in the handling of transference, resistance, and regression.[80]

In 1953, the Portman Clinic survey in England reached the following conclusions:[42] "Psychotherapy appears to be unsuccessful in only a small number of patients of any age in whom a long habit is combined with . . . lack of desire to change." The Portman Clinic, under the direction of E. Glover, divided the degrees of improvement into three categories: (a) Cure, i.e., abolition of conscious homosexual impulse, and development of full extension of heterosexual impulse. (b) Much improved, i.e., the abolition of conscious homosexual impulse, without development of full extension of heterosexual impulse. (c) Improved, i.e., increased ego integration and capacity to control the homosexual impulse.

In conducting *focal treatment* (brief therapy aimed at the relief of the homosexual symptom), Glover states that the degree of social anxiety that prevails, particularly among patients seen in private, is based on a projected form of unconscious guilt. He is of the opinion that the punitive attitude of the law and society enables the patient to project concealed superego reactions onto society or the law.

A therapist must decide whether to treat homosexuality through the regular course of depth therapy, or whether he and the patient will be satisfied with focal relief. In any case, according to Glover, the therapist must deal with both conscious and unconscious guilt, severe anxiety upon the patient's attempting heterosexual relations, and, of course, oedipal conflict and castration anxiety.

It is necessary to demonstrate to the patient the defensive aspects of homosexual relationships. Only by uncovering the positive aspects of his original relationships to women (mother, sister), and by revealing their associated anxieties or guilts (real or fantasied) derived from the hostile aspects of these early experiences, can heterosexuality be attained.

The question of prohibiting homosexual activity in therapy should be decided on the basis of its unconscious meaning to the patient. Outbursts of hostility and anxiety may threaten continuation of therapy if the therapist prohibits activities that the patient considers necessary for survival.

In my experience, it is vital that the depth of regression be controlled, in order to offset its utilization as resistance in the transference relationship. It must be stressed to the patient that the resolution of his problems will have to take place outside the psychiatrist's office in attempting heterosexual functioning.

The following are important criteria for the selection of patients:

1. A feeling of guilt on the part of the patient for the unconscious wishes underlying homosexuality. The absence of conscious guilt does not mean that the patient does not suffer guilt, but instead this may be experienced by him as a need for punishment and for engaging in self-damaging behavior. The presence of unconscious guilt arising from infantile fears and wishes lifts the problem out of its externalized context into an internal conflict. Once seen as an internal psychic conflict, the patient is at last on the path toward resolution of his homosexuality, and no longer can view himself solely as a victim of society's attitudes and judgments, should he have been so inclined.

2. Treatment must be voluntarily undertaken by the patient. Ideally, homosexual patients should not seek treatment under duress from parents or other authority figures because of the hostility they already feel toward their parents.

The patient's turning to heterosexual relationships often coincides with a strong positive transference. In the positive transference, the patient is able to identify himself with the "good" father (the therapist) and thus achieve in the transference what he has been unsuccessfully trying to achieve in homosexual relationships, namely, to become strengthened through the masculinity of the therapist. He can thereby begin to free himself from his enslavement to the mother.

When homosexual contacts become less frequent and lose their imperativeness, the patient is no longer so anxiety-ridden. Awareness of all feelings becomes much greater and he is more potentially capable of object love. He becomes aware, too, that in reality his main competition in life is with men; that love and comfort are to be found with women in a complementary relationship.

While neither the hard work and resoluteness required of the therapist nor the courage and endurance required of the patient can be minimized in treating this serious disorder, in time both find the challenge and fulfillment to be equal in measure.

❡ Bibliography

1. AMERICAN PSYCHOANALYTIC ASSOCIATION. *Report of the Central Fact Gathering Committee.* New York, 1956 (unpublished).

2. BARAHAL, H. S. "Female Transvestitism and Homosexuality," *Psychiatric Quarterly,* 27 (1953), 390–438.

3. BARRY, H., JR., and H. BARRY, III. "Homosexuality and Testosterone," *New England Journal of Medicine,* 286 (1972), 380–381.

4. BERGLER, E. *Homosexuality: Disease or Way of Life?* New York: Hill & Wang, 1956.

5. ———. *Counterfeit Sex.* New York: Grune & Stratton, 1951.

6. ———, and L. EIDELBERG. "The Breast Complex in Men," *Internazionale Zeitschrift für Psychoanalyse,* 19 (1933), 547–583.

7. BIEBER, I. Personal Communication, 1972.

8. ———, et al. *Homosexuality: A Psychoanalytic Study of Male Homosexuals.* New York: Basic Books, 1962.

9. BIEBER, T. B. "Group Therapy with Homosexuals," in H. I. Kaplan, and B. S. Sadock, eds., *Comprehensive Group Therapy.* Baltimore: Williams and Wilkins, 1971.

10. BONAPARTE, M. *Female Sexuality.* New York: International Universities Press, 1953.

11. BRIERLEY, M. "Specific Determinants in Feminine Development," *International Journal of Psycho-Analysis,* 17 (1935), 163–180.

12. ———. "Problems of Integration in Women," *International Journal of Psycho-Analysis,* 13 (1932), 433–448.

13. BYCHOWSKI, G. "The Ego and the Introjects," *Psychoanalytic Quarterly,* 25 (1956), 11–36.

14. ———. "The Structure of Homosexual Acting Out," *Psychoanalytic Quarterly,* 23 (1954), 48–61.

15. ———. "The Ego of Homosexuals," *International Journal of Psycho-Analysis,* 26 (1945), 114–127.

16. DE SAUSSURE, R. "Homosexual Fixations in Neurotic Women," *Revue Française de Psychanalyse*, 3 (1929) 50–91. (Translation by Hella Freud Bernays, 1961; New York Psychoanalytic Institute Library.)

17. DEUTSCH, H. "On Female Homosexuality," *Psychoanalytic Quarterly*, 1 (1932), 484–510.

18. ELLIS, A. "The Effectiveness of Psychotherapy in Individuals Who Had Severe Homosexual Problems," *Journal of Consulting Psychology*, 20 (1956), 191–200.

19. ———. "The Sexual Psychology of Human Hermaphrodites," *Psychosomatic Medicine*, 7 (1945), 108--125.

20. ELLIS, H. *Studies in the Psychology of Sex.* New York: Random House, 1940.

21. FAIRBAIRN, W. R. D. "A Note on the Origin of Male Homosexuality," *British Journal of Medical Psychology*, 37 (1964), 31–32.

22. FENICHEL, O. "The Psychology of Transvestitism," in *Collected Papers*, Vol. 1. New York: W. W. Norton, 1953.

23. ———. *The Psychoanalytic Theory of Neurosis.* New York: W. W. Norton, 1945.

24. FERENCZI, S. "More About Homosexuality," in *Final Contributions to the Problems and Methods of Psychoanalysis.* New York: Basic Books, 1955.

25. FISCHER, S. H. "A Note on Male Homosexuality and the Role of Women in Ancient Greece," in J. Marmor, ed., *Sexual Inversion: The Multiple Roots of Homosexuality.* New York: Basic Books, 1965.

26. FLEISCHMANN, O. "Choice of Homosexuality in Males," in panel report on Theoretical and Clinical Aspects of Overt Male Homosexuality, *Journal of American Psychoanalytic Association*, 8 (1960), 552–566.

27. FLOURNOY, H. "An Analytic Session in a Case of Male Homosexuality," in R. M. Loewenstein, ed., *Drives, Affects, Behavior.* New York: International Universities Press, 1953.

28. FREUD, A. "Problems of Technique in Adult Analysis," *Bulletin of Philadelphia Association of Psychoanalysts*, 4 (1954), 44–70.

29. ———. "Homosexuality," *Bulletin of American Psychoanalytic Association*, 7 (1951), 117–118.

30. ———. "Some Clinical Remarks Concerning the Treatment of Cases of Male Homosexuality," *International Journal of Psycho-Analysis*, 30 (1949), 195.

31. FREUD, S. "Female Sexuality," in Standard Edition, Vol. 21, pp. 223–247. London: Hogarth Press, 1961.

32. ———. "Fetishism," in *Collected Papers*, Vol. 5, pp. 198–204. London: Hogarth Press, 1950.

33. ———. "Some Neurotic Mechanisms in Jealousy, Paranoia and Homosexuality," in Standard Edition, Vol. 18, pp. 221–235. London: Hogarth Press, 1955.

34. ———. "Psychogenesis of a Case of Homosexuality in a Woman," in Standard Edition, Vol. 18, pp. 145–175. London: Hogarth Press, 1955.

35. ———. "A Child Is Being Beaten," in Standard Edition, Vol. 17, pp. 175–204. London: Hogarth Press, 1955.

36. ———. "From the History of an Infantile Neurosis," in Standard Edition, Vol. 17, pp. 3–104. London: Hogarth Press, 1955.

37. ———. "Psychoanalytic Notes on an Autobiographical Account of a Case of Paranoia," in Standard Edition, Vol. 12, pp. 3–82. London: Hogarth Press, 1958.

38. ———. "Three Essays on the Theory of Sexuality," in Standard Edition, Vol. 7, pp. 125–145. London: Hogarth Press, 1953.

39. GERSHMAN, H. "The Evolution of Gender Identity," *American Journal of Psychoanalysis*, 28 (1967), 80–91.

40. GILLESPIE, W. H. "The General Theory of Sexual Perversions," *International Journal of Psycho-Analysis*, 37 (1956), 396–403.

41. GLASS, A. J., et al. "Sex Hormone Studies in Male Homosexuality," *Endocrinology*, 26 (1940), 590–599.

42. GLOVER, E. *The Roots of Crime: Selected Papers on Psychoanalysis*, Vol. 2. London: Imago Publishing, 1960.

43. ———. "The Relation of Perversion Formation to the Development of Reality Sense," *International Journal of Psycho-Analysis*, 14 (1933), 486–504.

44. HADDEN, S. B. "Treatment of Male Homosexuals in Groups," *International Journal of Group Psychotherapy*, 16 (1966), 13–21.

45. ———. "Treatment of Homosexuality by Individual and Group Psychotherapy," *The American Journal of Psychiatry*, 114 (1958), 810–821.

46. HANDELSMAN, I. "The Effects of Early Object

Relationships on Sexual Development: Autistic and Symbiotic Modes of Adaptation," in *The Psychoanalytic Study of the Child*, 20. New York: International Universities Press, 1965.

47. HATTERER, L. J. *Changing Homosexuality in the Male*. New York: McGraw-Hill, 1971.

48. HENRY, G. W. *Sex Variants: A Study of Homosexual Patterns*. New York: Hoeber, 1941.

49. HIRSCHFELD, M. *Sexual Anomalies and Perversions*. London: Encyclopaedia Press, 1938.

50. JACOBSON, E. *The Self and the Object World*. New York: International Universities Press, 1964.

51. JONES, E. "Early Development of Female Homosexuality," *International Journal of Psycho-Analysis*, 8 (1927), 459–472.

52. KALLMAN, F. J. "Comparative Twin Studies of the Genetic Aspects of Male Homosexuality," *Journal of Nervous and Mental Disease*, 115 (1952), 286–294.

53. KARDINER, A. "The Flight From Masculinity," in H. M. Ruitenbeek, ed., *The Problem of Homosexuality in Modern Society*. New York: Dutton, 1963.

54. ———. *The Individual and His Society: The Psychodynamics of Primitive Social Organization*. New York: Columbia University Press, 1939.

55. KARLEN, A. *Sexuality and Homosexuality*, p. 399. New York: W. W. Norton, 1971.

56. KINSEY, A. C., W. B. POMEROY, C. E. MARTIN, and P. H. GEBHARD. *Sexual Behavior in the Human Female*. Philadelphia: W. B. Saunders Co., 1953.

57. ———. *Sexual Behavior in the Human Male*. Philadelphia: W. B. Saunders Co., 1948.

58. KLEIN, M., et al. "Notes on Some Schizoid Mechanisms," in *Developments in Psycho-Analysis*. London: Hogarth Press, 1952.

59. ———, et al. *Developments in Psycho-Analysis*. London: Hogarth Press, 1952.

60. KOLODNY, R. C., W. H. MASTERS, J. HENDRIX, and G. TORO. "Plasma Testosterone and Semen Analysis in Male Homosexuals," *New England Journal of Medicine*, 285 (1971), 1170–1178.

61. KRAFFT-EBING, R. VON. *Psychopathia Sexualis*. Brooklyn: Physicians and Surgeons Book Co., 1922.

62. LACEY, W. K. *The Family in Classical Greece*. New York: Cornell University Press, 1968.

63. LAGACHE, D. "De l'Homosexualité à la Jalou-

sie," *Revue Française de Psychanalyse*, 13 (1953), 351–366.

64. LORAND, S. "The Therapy of Perversions," in S. Lorand and M. Balint, eds., *Perversions: Psychodynamics and Therapy*. New York: Random House, 1956.

65. MAHLER, M. S. "On Human Symbiosis and the Vicissitudes of Individuation," *Journal of American Psychoanalytic Association*, 15 (1967), 740–764.

66. ———, and B. J. GOSLINER. "On Symbiotic Child Psychosis: Genetic, Dynamic and Restitutive Aspects," in *The Psychoanalytic Study of the Child*, 10. New York: International Universities Press, 1955.

67. MANTEGAZZA, P. *Sexual Relations of Mankind*. New York: Anthropological Press, 1932.

68. NUNBERG, H. "Homosexuality, Magic and Aggression," *International Journal of Psycho-Analysis*, 19 (1938), 1–16.

69. OPLER, M. K. "Anthropological and Cross-Cultural Aspects of Homosexuality," in J. Marmor, ed., *Sexual Inversion: The Multiple Roots of Homosexuality*. New York: Basic Books, 1965.

70. OVESEY, L. *Homosexuality and Pseudohomosexuality*. New York: Science House, 1969.

71. POE, J. S. "The Successful Treatment of a Forty-Year-Old Passive Homosexual Based on an Adaptational View of Sexual Behavior," *Psychoanalytic Review*, 39 (1952), 23–33.

72. RADO, S. "Evolutionary Basis of Sexual Adaptation," *Journal of Nervous and Mental Disease*, 121 (1955), 389–401.

73. ———. "An Adaptational View of Sexual Behavior," in P. H. Hoch, and J. Zubin, eds., *Psychosexual Development in Health and Disease*. New York: Grune & Stratton, 1949.

74. ———. "A Critical Examination of the Concept of Bisexuality," *Psychosomatic Medicine*, 2 (1940), 459–467.

75. RAINER, J. D., A. MESNIKOFF, L. C. KOLB, and A. CARR. "Homosexuality and Heterosexuality in Identical Twins," *Psychosomatic Medicine*, 22 (1960), 251–259.

76. ROSENFELD, H. A. *Psychotic States*. New York: International Universities Press, 1965.

77. SACHS, H. "On the Genesis of Sexual Perversion," *Internazionale Zeitschrift für Psychoanalyse*, 9 (1923), 172–182. (Translation by Hella Freud Bernays, 1964; New

York Psychoanalytic Institute Library.)

78. SADGER, J. *"Zur Aetiologie der conträren Sexualempfindungen,"* Medizinische Klinik, 1909.

79. SHERMAN, M., and T. SHERMAN. "The Factor of Parental Attachment in Homosexuality," *Psychoanalytic Review*, 13 (1926), 32–37.

80. SOCARIDES, C. W. *The Overt Homosexual.* New York: Grune & Stratton, 1968.

81. ———. "Homosexuality and Medicine," *Journal of the AMA*, 212 (1970), 1199–1202.

82. ———. "Psychoanalytic Therapy of a Male Homosexual," *Psychoanalytic Quarterly*, 38 (1969), 173–190.

83. ———. "A Provisional Theory of Etiology in Male Homosexuality: A Case of Preoedipal Origin," *International Journal of Psycho-Analysis*, 49 (1968), 27–37.

84. ———. "Female Homosexuality," in R. Slovenko, ed., *Sexual Behavior and the Law.* Springfield: Charles C. Thomas Co., 1965.

85. ———. "The Historical Development of Theoretical and Clinical Concepts of Overt Female Homosexuality," *Journal of American Psychoanalytic Association*, 11 (1963), 386–414.

86. ———. "Theoretical and Clinical Aspects of Overt Female Homosexuality" (Panel Report), *Journal of American Psychoanalytic Association*, 10 (1962), 579–592.

87. ———. "Theoretical and Clinical Aspects of Overt Male Homosexuality" (Panel Report), *Journal of American Psychoanalytic Association*, 8 (1960), 552–566.

88. VAN DER LEEUW, P. J. "The Preoedipal Phase of the Male," in *The Psychoanalytic Study of the Child*, 13. New York: International Universities Press, 1958.

89. VINCHON, J., and S. NACHT. *"Considerations sur la Cure Psychanalytique d'une Névrose Homosexuelle,"* Revue Française de Psychanalyse, 4 (1931), 677–709.

90. WIEDEMAN, G. H. "Survey of Psychoanalytic Literature on Overt Male Homosexuality," *Journal of American Psychoanalytic Association*, 10 (1962), 386–409.

91. WULFF, M. *"Über einen Fall von Männlicher Homosexualität,"* Internazionale Zeitschrift für Psychoanalyse, 26 (1941), 105–121.

CHAPTER 15

SADISM AND MASOCHISM: PHENOMENOLOGY AND PSYCHODYNAMICS

Irving Bieber

Sadism and masochism were introduced as syndromes into the psychiatric literature by Krafft-Ebing[15] in 1882 in his now classic work, *Psychopathia Sexualis*. This volume contains the most extensive and probably best collection of illustrative clinical cases. The author derived some of his data from his consultation practice, some from the reports of physicians, but most were obtained from prostitutes who had first-hand experience with sadomasochistic clients.

⟨ Sadism

Krafft-Ebing borrowed the term "sadism" from the French novelists of his time who had come to use it to describe the association of sex and cruelty, a theme made prominent by the Marquis de Sade in his autobiographical writings on the subject. Krafft-Ebing defines sadism as,

The experience of sexually pleasurable sensations (including orgasm) produced by acts of cruelty, bodily punishment, inflicted by one's own person, or when witnessed in others, be they animals or human beings. It may also consist of an innate desire to humiliate, hurt, wound, or even destroy others in order thereby to create sexual pleasure in oneself.

He identified three categories: (a) sadistic acts following coitus that gave inadequate gratification; (b) sadistic acts by individuals with diminished virility in attempts to enhance sexual desire; (c) sadistic acts calculated to induce orgasm without intercourse in cases of total impotence.

The spectrum of described sadistic behaviors ranged from the infliction of pain and injury during the height of sexual excitation to cases where victims were mutilated and murdered. Only men participated in sadistic violence; they derived sexual pleasure through strangling their victims, disemboweling them, hacking them to pieces, and cutting off breasts and genitals. In several instances, the sadists reached a high pitch of excitement by the odor of the body and by the odor and taste of blood. In most, though not all, instances, the victims were women; ages varied from young children to old people; appearances varied from the beautiful to the ugly. A particularly gruesome case was that of Maréchal Gilles de Rez who was executed in 1440 "on account of mutilation and murder which he had practiced for eight years on more than 800 children. . . . This inhuman wretch confessed that in the commission of these acts he enjoyed inexpressible pleasure." Krafft-Ebing noted that sexual sadism occurred far less frequently in women and he described only two such cases.

In a subcategory, "Injury to Women (Stabbing, Flagellation, etc.)" the author noted a special group of cases where the erotic cue was the blood of the victim. As to the Marquis de Sade, "Coitus only excited him when he could prick the object of his desire until blood came. His greatest pleasure was to injure naked prostitutes and dress their wounds." In another subcategory, "Defilement of Women," cases of men are described who have the need to defecate or urinate on women or in other ways to defile their persons. Of special interest, because of Freud's[9] well-known paper, "A Child Is Being Beaten," are Krafft-Ebing's cases under the heading, "Sadism with Any Other Object—the Whipping of Boys." One case is of a twenty-five-year-old man. "At the age of eight while at school, he saw the teacher punish the boys by taking their heads between his thighs and spanking them with a ferule." The sight promoted lustful excitement in the boy. "From that time on until the age of twenty, this man masturbated with a fantasy of a boy being punished." In a second case, there was a history of sexual excitation from the age of six on, when the subject saw his father whip the other children and later when

his teacher whipped his classmates. He masturbated from then on with the fantasy of seeing children whipped. When he was twelve, he convinced a companion to permit himself to be whipped by the patient who reported sexual excitement during the incident.

Krafft-Ebing explained sadism in two ways; the first applied to both sexes.

> At the moment of most intense lust, very excitable individuals who are otherwise normal, commit such acts as biting and scratching which are usually due to anger. It must further be remembered that love and anger are not only the most intense emotion but also they are the only two forms of robust emotion.

The idea that sex and anger are the only two forms of "robust emotion" is original and prophetic; it is a forerunner of Freud's[10] theory that there are two basic instincts, sex and aggression. The concept that one excitatory organization—sexuality—can lock into and use behavioral components of another excitatory organization—anger and rage—gains support from the observations of ethologists who demonstrated that components of the attack constellation of behavior are incorporated into the sexual organization.[17]

Krafft-Ebing's second explanation centered around the concept of power, specifically, masculine power.

> In the intercourse of the sexes, the active or aggressive role belongs to the man; woman remains passive-defensive. It affords a man great pleasure to win a woman, to conquer her; and in the art of love making the modesty of a woman who keeps herself on the defensive until the moment of surrender, is an element of great psychological significance and importance. Under normal conditions, man meets obstacles which it is his part to overcome, and for which his nature has given him an aggressive character. This aggressive character, however, under pathological conditions may likewise be excessively developed, and express itself in an impulse to subdue absolutely the object of desire, either to destroy it or kill it.

Power was the central idea in Krafft-Ebing's view of sadism and masochism. It was conceived to be a biological component of sexuality. In sadism, power was biologically rooted and masculine; its function was to overcome

feminine resistance in the service of propaga-
tion. Masochism was conceptualized as feminine, since the masochist was acted upon and
submitted to the power of the other; the male
masochist was thought to have feminine traits.
Krafft-Ebing's explanation of sadism reappeared in Freud's[7] discussion of it:

As regards active algolagnia, sadism, the roots
are easy to detect in the normal. The sexuality of
most male human beings contains an element of
aggressiveness—a desire to subjugate; the biological significance of it seems to lie in the needs for
overcoming the resistance of the sexual object by
means other than the process of wooing. Thus,
sadism would correspond to an aggressive component of the sexual instinct which has become
independent and exaggerated and by displacement
has usurped the leading position.

Freud equated sadism with aggression, activity, masculinity; masochism with passivity
and femininity. When he expanded his concepts of sexuality to include the pregenital
phases—oral and anal (genetic theory)—he
assigned active and passive components to
each phase. The oral active component included all activities in which the mouth acted
on objects, as in eating, biting, and so forth.
This active component was termed the sadistic
component where he again equated action
and sadism. The receptive component was
conceived of as the oral passive one. In the
anal phase, the rectal and perianal musculature was thought to mediate the activities of
the active phase, such as in the expulsion of
feces. The erotogenic anal mucosa, which was
eroticized by objects, including feces acting on
it, was the passive component. Note that again
the active component was identified with
sadism, a formulation that became the basis
for theorizing an anal sadistic libidinal phase.
It must be remembered that Freud's formulations on sadism and libidinal phases were
highly speculative; they had no foundation in
observed behavior nor any relation to the syndrome of sadism described by Krafft-Ebing.

The term "sadistic" has come to be used to
describe various types of cruel and destructive
behavior, particularly where the perpetrator
derives pleasure from it. In a literal sense, the
term should be restricted to acts of cruelty

that are sexually arousing. In my view, sadism
is a maladaptive response to threat; it is a
paranoid constellation in which the victim is a
personified representative of a variety of irrationally perceived threats. The victims may
represent a parent, or an authority who
threatens to punish or prohibit sexual activity;
or the person who arouses dangerous sexual
feelings; or one who personifies submission,
masochism, or other unacceptable attitudes.
The victim must then be dominated, injured,
neutralized, or destroyed. The affect operant
in sadistic sexual behavior is a complex of
rage, anxiety, relief, vengeance, and frenetic
ecstasy accompanying a sense of triumph in
subjugating an enemy or otherwise extinguishing a threat. The sexual sadist confuses this
affect complex with sexual arousal, most particularly because sexual excitation is actually a
component part of the complex.

Cases of sexual sadism are rarely encountered in psychiatric practice today. The actual
frequency of such behavior is not known.
Most of the reported case material has been
anecdotal and derived largely from prostitutes. An index listing under sadism for either
men or women is even absent from Kinsey's[13,14] studies.

❨ Masochism

Krafft-Ebing introduced the term "masochism" to define a syndrome described in the
writings of Sacher-Masoch, a nineteenth-
century novelist who was himself a masochist.
Krafft-Ebing defined masochism as the opposite of sadism:

While the latter is the desire to cause pain and
use force, the former is the wish to suffer pain and
to be subjected to force. By masochism, I understand a peculiar perversion of the psychical sexual
life in which the individual affected in sexual feeling and thought is controlled by the idea of being
completely and unconditionally subject to the will
of a person of the opposite sex; of being treated
by this person as by a master, humiliated and
abused. This idea is colored by lustful feelings . . .
from the psychopathological point of view, the
essential and common element in all these cases *is*

the fact that the sexual instinct is directed to ideas of *subjugation and abuse by the opposite sex.*

In defining and describing masochism, Krafft-Ebing repeatedly stressed power rather than the pain motif. The emphasis was on subjugation and abuse, not on being physically pained, whereas in sadism he stressed both the subjugation of the victim and the infliction of pain and injury. In some instances, the masochistic activity was a prerequisite for coitus; in others, it replaced coitus and resulted in orgasm without intercourse. Krafft-Ebing's case material still has heuristic value and remains didactically useful as the following cases illustrate:

Case #50. A twenty-nine-year-old male from the age of five became sexually aroused by whipping himself or fantasying other boys being whipped. He masturbated with fantasies of whipping. On the first occasion that he visited a prostitute, he was flagellated by a pretty girl but this did not produce arousal. The second time, he fantasied the idea of subjection to the woman's will and he became sexually aroused. He would also derive pleasure from the fantasy that he was a page to a beautiful girl. The patient was also fetishistic and was aroused by women wearing high heels and short jackets.

Case #51. A twenty-six-year-old male whose masochistic pattern first surfaced at the age of seven when he took part in a fight between the pupils of his school. "[Afterwards] the victors rode on the backs of the vanquished. He thought the position of the prostrate boys a pleasant one, wanted to put himself in their place, imagining how by repeated efforts he could move the boy on his back near his face so that he might inhale the odor of the boy's genitals."[*] When he reached puberty, he began to fantasy being straddled by young women who would urinate on his face and in his mouth. He never activated his masochistic fantasies and remained totally impotent and abstinent.

Case #52. A male aged twenty-eight who at

[*] In this sequence, a power figure, the victor, is eroticized—a dynamic commonly observed among male homosexuals. The emphasis on odor also illustrates the mediating role of olfaction in sexuality.[3,12]

the age of six had dreams of being whipped on the buttocks by women. When he became sexually active, coitus was possible only if his partner told him how she had flagellated other impotent men and threatened to give him the same treatment. At times, it was necessary for him to either fantasy himself bound or to be, in fact, bound. "The only thing in women that interested him were the hands. Powerful women with big fists were his preference."

Case #55. A thirty-four-year-old male had strong homosexual impulses but never acted them out. "Occasionally he would obtain a prostitute, undress himself completely (while she did not), and have her tread upon, whip and beat him. He was filled with the greatest pleasure while this was being done, and would lick the woman's foot which was the only thing that could increase his passion and he then achieved ejaculation."

Case #56. A twenty-eight-year-old male who visited a brothel once a month, "would always announce his coming with a note reading thus: 'Dear Peggy, I shall be with you tomorrow evening between eight and nine o'clock—Whip and Knout! Kindest regards.' He always arrived at the appointed hour carrying a whip, a knout and a leather strap. After undressing, he had himself bound hand and foot and was then flogged by the girl on the soles of his feet, calves and buttocks until ejaculation ensued."

Case #57. This case of a thirty-five-year-old man most clearly illuminates the psychodynamics of masochism. "Even in my early childhood I loved to revel in the ideas about the absolute mastery of one man over others. The thought of slavery had something exciting in it for me, alike whether from the standpoint of master or servant. That one man could possess, sell, or whip another caused in me intense excitement and in reading *Uncle Tom's Cabin* which I read about the beginning of puberty, I had erections. Particularly exciting for me was the thought of a man being hitched to a wagon in which another man sat with a whip driving and whipping him." After the age of twenty-one, the fantasy of a powerful figure became exclusively that of a woman. "From this time I was always in my fantasies the subject; the mistress was a rough woman who made use of me in every way, also sexually, who harnessed me to a carriage and made me take her for a drive, whom I must follow like a dog, at whose feet I must lie naked and be punished, that is, be whipped, by her."

Krafft-Ebing's emphasis on a feeling of being subjugated as the primary motif in masochism, rather than the experience of pain, is well illustrated in the above case. The power interplay initially took place between males. It was only after the patient reached the age of twenty-one that a woman who seemed powerful became a stand-in for the feared and admired powerful man. The substitutive role of the woman is further substantiated by the patient's remarks, "I remember that when I was a boy it affected me intensely when an older boy addressed me in the second person (*du*) while I spoke to him in the third (*sie*). I would keep up a conversation with him and have this change of address (*du* and *sie*) take place as often as possible. Later, when I became more mature sexually, such things affected me only when they occurred in a woman, and one relatively older than myself."

In all, Krafft-Ebing described thirty-three cases of masochism in men. Among them were those whose initial masochistic pattern could be traced to an actual spanking on the buttocks administered more often than not by a woman, though in some instances by a man. Several of the cases were examples of what was termed "ideal" masochism, by which the author meant that fantasies of masochism were indulged in but never acted out.

These cases of ideal masochism plainly demonstrate that the persons afflicted with this anomaly do not aim at actually suffering pain. The term *algolagnia*, therefore, as applied by Schrenk-Notzing and by v. Eulenburg to this anomaly, does not signify the essence, that is, the psychical nucleus of the element of masochistic sentiment and imagination. This essence consists rather of the lustfully colored consciousness of being subject to the power of another person. The ideal of even actual enactment of violence on the part of the controlling person is only the means to the end, that is, the realization of the feeling.

Clearly, the power motif was put forward as the primary theme in both sadism and masochism.

In another group of cases, fantasies about masochistic behavior were associated with foot and shoe fetishism. In some individuals, smelling and licking sweaty or dirty feet or soiled shoes were the central fetishistic elements; in others, sexual excitement occurred when a woman urinated or defecated on the subjects' bodies.

Krafft-Ebing described only three cases of sexual masochism in women: the first became sexually excited by the fantasy of being beaten on the buttocks with a rattan cane by a man. The origin of the fantasy was traced to an experience at the age of five when a friend of her father's "took her for fun across his knee pretending to whip her." The second fantasied being whipped by another woman, the fantasy being accompanied by feelings of delight. The third involved a woman who would attend medical clinics so that a gynecologist would examine her against pretended resistance.

Krafft-Ebing's statements on masochism in women are especially noteworthy when compared to Freud's concepts which were identical in all major details. Krafft-Ebing stated:

In woman, voluntary subjection to the opposite sex is a physiological phenomenon. Owing to her passive role in procreation and long existent social conditions, ideas of subjection are, in woman, normally connected with the ideas of sexual relations. They form, so to speak, the harmonics which determine the tone quality of feminine feeling . . . thus, it is easy to regard masochism in general as a pathological growth of specific feminine elements—as an abnormal intensification of certain features of the psychosexual character of woman—and to seek its primary origin in this sex. It may, however, be held to be established, that, in woman an inclination to subordination to man (which may be regarded as an acquired, purposeful arrangement, a phenomenon of adaptation to social requirements) is to a certain extent a normal manifestation.

In Freud's formulations, femininity was equated with passivity and the notion of submission as a normal concomitant of feminine sexuality on biological and social grounds reappeared.

Krafft-Ebing offered two theoretical explanations to account for sadism and masochism. Firstly, he conceptualized sadism as a pathological intensification of the masculine sexual character; masochism was seen as "a pathological degeneration of the distinctive psychical peculiarities of woman." Secondly, he thought that sexual stimuli emanating from the love object, including all that are ordinarily painful, such as being bitten, are perceived as excitatory and reinforcing. He further hypothesized that masochism resulted from an unusually intense dependence on the love object, which he termed "sexual bondage."* He accounted for excessive sexual dependence as a combination of strong love and weak character in individuals whose fear of loss of the love object drove them to submission. Yet, he did not consider sexual bondage to be pathological, despite the fact that masochism had its roots in it.

Krafft-Ebing did not provide an adequate explanation for the masochist's fear of power or for his subjection and self-injury, although he pointed out that during flagellation the masochist did not experience pain as such.

The person in a state of masochistic ecstasy feels no pain, either because, by reason of his emotional state (like that of a soldier in battle) the physical effect on the cutaneous nerves is not apperceived or because (as with religious martyrs and enthusiasts) in the preoccupation or consciousness with lustful emotions, the idea of maltreatment remains merely a symbol without the quality of pain.

Kinsey[11] described the same phenomenon:

Specific observation and experimental data indicate that the whole body of the individual who is sexually aroused becomes increasingly insensitive to tactile stimulation and even to sharp blows and severe injury. . . . Toward the peak of sexual arousal there may be considerable slapping and heavier blows, biting and scratching and other activities which the recipient never remembers and

* Somerset Maugham described a classic situation of sexual bondage in his novel, *Of Human Bondage*. It is likely that he drew inspiration from Krafft-Ebing's work.

which appear to have a minimal, if any, effect upon him at the time they occur. Not only does the sense of touch diminish but the sense of pain is largely lost. If the blows begin mildly and do not become severe until there is a definite erotic response, the recipient in flagellation or other types of sadomasochistic behavior may receive extreme punishment without being aware that he is being subjected to more than mild tactile stimulation.

My own observations accord with those of Krafft-Ebing and Kinsey. The threshold for pain during sexual excitation rises markedly and masochists have reported to me that they do not experience pain. I have noted that should pain actually be experienced, sexual excitation rapidly terminates, as does the masochistic behavior.

Masochism appears to have been an enigma to Freud from the beginnings of his explorations. In his formulation of the pleasure principle, he viewed unlust (unpleasure or pain) as the psychological state that triggered release or discharge. That pain was associated with an increase of sexual excitation and could even be a goal in itself, was inconsistent with the pleasure principle.[11]

The existence of the masochistic trend in the instinctual life of human beings may justly be described as mysterious from the economic point of view. For if mental processes are governed by the pleasure principle in such a way that their first aim is the avoidance of unpleasure and the obtaining of pleasure, masochism is incomprehensible. If pain and unpleasure can be, not simply warnings, but actually aims, the pleasure principle is paralyzed. It is as though the watchman over our mental life were put out of action by a drug.

In order to achieve consistency between his theory of masochism and the pleasure principle, Freud concluded that masochism was retroverted sadism; primary masochism did not exist.

In "Instincts and Their Vicissitudes" (1915), Freud[8] revealed his continued struggle with the question of whether masochism was primary or secondary to sadism, or whether sadism was primary or secondary to masochism.

Once the transformation into masochism has taken place, the pains are fitted to provide a passive masochistic aim; for we have every reason to believe that sensations of pain, like other unpleasurable sensations trench upon sexual excitation and produce a pleasurable condition for the sake of which the subject even willingly experiences the unpleasure of pain. Once feeling pain has become a masochistic aim, the sadistic aim of *causing* pain can arise also retrogressively; for while these pains are being inflicted on other people, they are enjoyed masochistically by the subject through his identification of himself with the suffering object. In both cases, of course, it is not the pain itself which is enjoyed but the accompanying sexual excitation—so that this can be done especially conveniently from the sadistic position. The enjoyment of pain would thus be an aim which was originally masochistic, but which can only become an instinctual aim in someone who was originally sadistic.

Note that the quotation also contains contradictory statements as to whether pain was or was not in itself an instinctual aim.

In his paper, "A Child Is Being Beaten," Freud[9] traced a woman's fantasy of being beaten through several phases. The first involved her father beating a hated sibling and it gave her sadistic pleasure. Freud thought that because of her guilt about experiencing this pleasure, she converted sadism into masochism and then saw herself as the one who was being beaten. It was always guilt that transformed sadism into masochism. When the fantasy of being beaten by the father took over, her oedipal wishes then became integrated into the experience. Freud interpreted the beating fantasy as punishment for the oedipal wishes which, at the same time, made up the erotic component of her relationship with her father. Since the erotic component was not a direct genital experience but was transmitted through a beating, Freud theorized that the component represented a regression to the anal sadistic level. Thus, the masochistic experience in the beating fantasy was at once a punishment and an erotic experience at the anal-sadistic libidinal level. Pressed by the oedipal component and the accompanying guilt, the fantasy was further disguised—the punishment was now meted

out, not by the father, but by a father substitute, and the object being beaten was not a woman, but a boy. In this paper, Freud conceptualized the masochistic fantasy as a synthesis of forbidden sexual wishes, guilt, and punishment. At this point, he had not yet abandoned a theoretical reliance on direct, clinical observations; his later work was completely anchored in metapsychology.

In "The Economic Problems of Masochism," Freud[11] stated:

Masochism comes under our observation in three forms: as a condition imposed on sexual excitation; as in expression of the feminine nature and as a norm of behavior. We may accordingly distinguish an erotogenic, a feminine and a moral masochism. The first, the erotogenic masochism—pleasure in pain—lies at the bottom of the other two forms as well.

Despite Krafft-Ebing's admonition and Freud's own earlier ideas, in his final position, he viewed masochism as primary and pleasure in pain as an instinctual aim. As had Krafft-Ebing, Freud, too, explained masculine sexual masochism as a feminine situation.

But if one has the opportunity of studying cases in which masochistic fantasies have been especially richly elaborated, one quickly discovers that they place the subject in a characteristically female situation. They signify that he is being castrated or copulated with or giving birth to a baby. For this reason, I have called this form of masochism the feminine form. This feminine masochism which we have been describing is entirely based on primary erotogenic masochism or pleasure in pain.

When Freud integrated masochism into his reformulated instinctual theory of libido and the death instinct,[10] the formulation became entirely speculative. He postulated that a portion of the death instinct remained within the organism and, when fused with libido, became the instinctual source of primary erotogenic masochism.

Erotogenic masochism accompanies the libido through all its developmental phases and derives from them its changing psychical coatings. The fear of being eaten up by the totem animal (the father) originates from the primitive oral organization. The wish to be beaten by the father comes from the sadistic anal phase which follows it; castration, although it is later disavowed, enters into the content of masochistic fantasies as a precipitate of the phallic stage of organization and from the final genital stage there arises, of course, the situation of being copulated with and of giving birth which are characteristic of femaleness.

In his initial statements, Freud noted the difference in Krafft-Ebing's position, which emphasized the power motif, and Schrenck-Notzing's, which emphasized the pleasure in pain. In "Three Essays on Sexuality," Freud[7] stated:

> The most common and most significant of all perversions—the desire to inflict pain upon the sexual object, and its reverse—received from Krafft-Ebing the names of 'sadism and masochism' for its active and passive forms respectively. Other writers, (Schrenck-Notzing, 1899), have preferred the narrower term 'algolagnia.' This emphasizes the pleasure in *pain*, the cruelty; whereas the names chosen by Krafft-Ebing bring into prominence the pleasure in any form of humiliation or subjection.

In explicating masochism, Freud followed the hypothesis of pleasure in pain and ultimately integrated it into his metapsychological, instinctual theories. In taking this direction, he ultimately lost the opportunity to solve the many varied problems raised by the interesting and complex phenomenon that is masochism.

Wilhelm Reich[16] was the first theorist to propose that masochism was a defensive maneuver or adaptation. He saw masochism as a way of seeking a lesser injury when a greater one was anticipated; he cited the case of a boy who felt relieved when he was spanked by his father, since the child believed it forestalled his castration, the punishment he really feared. Reich also discussed masochism as a way of compelling love by producing guilt in the one from whom love was sought. He noted the inability of masochistic characters to accept praise and to be outstanding. Following Reich, other authors contributed to the literature on masochism—Horney, Reik, Bergler, Rado, and Thompson. Although each of these authors had an adaptational view of masochism, only Rado and Thompson completely abandoned the pleasure in pain hypothesis. I have detailed their views in a previous paper on sadism and masochism.[5]

In my view, a theory of sexual masochism should be consistent with the following items of behavior: (i) the sexual masochist is either impotent or is unable to attain satisfactory arousal without masochistic maneuvers and techniques; (ii) the masochist does not experience actual pain during sexual excitation; (iii) the individual inflicting the bondage, flagellation, or humiliation is perceived as one having much greater power than the masochist himself, or he pretends that this is so. His impotence or other sexual inadequacy indicates that he is sexually inhibited.

Sexual inhibition is based upon an expectation of injury for sexual behavior, especially with a valued love object. The masochistic constellation is a defense against an expectation of injury; it permits a circumvention of sexual inhibition and allows sexual arousal to develop. Flagellation or equated behaviors are substitutes for more severe, anticipated injury. But masochism is not only a lesser punishment than feared; it locates the punishment and establishes that it has already taken place; therefore, no further punishment need be feared for the time being. The punishing individual is the stand-in for the powerful figure from whom the subject actually expects injury. In the charades of masochistic men, this power figure is usually the father or father surrogate. The "powerful" woman is a substitute for the feared father. Many elements in masochistic play-acting represent attempts at establishing a picture of the woman's power; however, the masochist does not actually fear her; he knows that the farce can be terminated at any point in the sexual encounter.

Several of Krafft-Ebing's cases demonstrate that the original figure involved in childhood masochistic experiences and fantasies is a male and that the transformation to a female occurs after puberty. The powerful female may also represent a mother figure who rejected and punished male sexuality. In many masochistic fantasies, such a woman is beautiful, powerful, and she compels the man to have sex—a type of male rape fantasy. In such instances, instead of rejecting and punishing the sexual behavior, the woman commands and demands it. A son's actual experience in childhood where his mother spanks him on the buttocks is a situation in which the mother's hand is brought into contact with the boy's perigenital area. The proximity to his genitals may be perceived as erotic and can condition sexual masochism. An erotic situation is concealed under the presumably nonsexual act of spanking. It may be compared to the childhood game of playing doctor, where the sexual behavior is concealed in the make-believe practice of medicine.

Sexual masochism may, in fact, include two different types of behavioral constellations, which share in common problems about power. In one type, the basic goal is sexual gratification. This type of masochist fears he will be punished for sexual gratification by power figures, such as parents; he incorporates the punishment by the threatening parent into the masochistic sexual constellation. By this maneuver, he locates the threatening figure and takes the punishment together with the pleasure in an inextricable combination. The second type consists of masochists who cope with a feared power figure by eroticizing that individual. In this instance, the goal of the behavior is to neutralize threatening power through sexual channels. Krafft-Ebing stated that masochism is establsihed as a perversion when the witnessing or experiencing of tyranny becomes an erotic stimulus. Some masochists are so responsive to power that they become stimulated simply by witnessing the exercise of authority. They eroticize power which they fear or wish to use in their own behalf.[6] Among male homosexuals, power themes are readily delineated. The core of their fear is aggressive, masculine power and this they eroticize, a dynamic that constitutes a basic element in a homosexual adaptation. Sexual masochism occurs frequently among male homosexuals.

Individuals of both sexes who are pathologically dependent may eroticize power. Their aim is not primarily to achieve sexual gratification; it is, rather, to use or acquire power.

Nonetheless, eroticizing power does produce sexual arousal and, if pursued, results in sexual gratification. Differentiation between these two types of sexual masochists may require the determination of the motivation for any specific sexual experience. In general, if an individual's sexual functioning is almost entirely dependent on masochistic techniques, he is likely to belong to the type whose goal is sexual gratification. Those who eroticize power are usually capable of sexual activity without masochistic techniques. This differentiation is not an absolute one, since some of the first type may go through periods of sexual activity free of masochism; or, sometimes, they may be able to have sexual activity with individuals who have little value to them, such as prostitutes, without the need for masochistic defenses.

Nonsexual Masochism

Krafft-Ebing defined a type of masochism, which he termed "moral masochism," that presumably was not associated with sexual arousal, although he thought there was some gratification in the suffering. Freud adopted the term, but stated that this type, too, was sexual; it was only on cursory examination that moral masochism appeared to have no connection with sex. He hypothesized that the superego was established through the desexualization of the oedipal figure. Through this defusion, morality was desexualized. He speculated that in moral masochism there was a regression to the sexualized phase of the superego and to a sexualization of morality. He concluded that moral masochism was rooted in sexuality.

Occurring much more frequently than sexual masochism is a category of behavior in which the individual self inflicts or invites injury, the goal being the extinction of threat, or the evocation of positive feelings in others. I mean by the term "injury" any condition or situation deemed inimical to one's integrity or safety. This may include physical injury, or such other items as humiliation, rejection, neglect, and so forth. Masochistic patterns can be identified in almost everyone, but individuals in whom they are salient are referred to as masochistic characters.

Masochistic Goals

A major goal of masochistic behavior is the prevention or extinction of hostile aggression in others, in particular, powerful others. Elsewhere,[6] I have defined power as the capability to influence, direct, or control matters of value in another's life. If this capability extends to matters of life and death, then the power is supreme. The wielder of power and the target may be an individual, group, institution, or government.

Psychoanalysis has made much of the fear of one's own aggressive impulses and acts. The fear of aggression of others has been very much underemphasized. Yet, in general, people are far more afraid of the aggression of others than of their own. When masochism is directed toward controlling the aggression of others, the behavior is a masochistic defense.

A child's first experience with power occurs within the family. The parents are all-powerful, and perceived parental power is proportional to the child's helplessness. First exposure to aggression is from parents and siblings; masochistic defenses develop and become prominent when protection is needed against their hostile aggression. I observed well established masochistic defense patterns in a three-and-a-half-year-old girl, in whom self-injury had already been obvious for one year. Since both parents were present when I examined the child, I could witness the interactions among the three. During the preceding year, whenever one parent, especially the mother, punished the girl physically, the child would inflict or threaten to inflict self-injury. She would strike her hands or head on solid objects with sufficient force to produce hematomata; or she would burn her hand on a radiator, or over an open gas flame, if she could get to it. By these maneuvers, she was largely successful in preventing physical punishment. The mother was noticeably hostile, overcontrolling, and resentful about the child's seeming victory in their power struggle; corporal punishment was not entirely renounced, despite the disturbing consequences. The child learned to extend her defensive tactics. When a physician inadvertently gagged her with a tongue depressor during pharyngeal examination, the child tore at her buccal mucuosa, drawing blood and successfully discouraging further examination. On another occasion, during aural examination, the physician apparently hurt her. She then tore at the skin of her external auditory canal, this time also drawing blood. During my interview with the child, she became playfully and affectionately related to me; the mother's irritation and displeasure were overt. In this case, a masochistic technique was discovered that partially controlled attack, particularly from the mother. It demonstrates a basic principle of masochism: self-inflicted injury wards off threats believed to be even more dangerous. The child's masochism was her defense against external threat. For the masochistic pattern to become established, it must have had adaptive value at some time, even though it is essentially maladaptive.

Physical aggression is the most primitive and obvious manifestation of the abuse of parental power. Parents may also aggress in less obvious ways. They may exploit their children in pursuit of their own needs and desires; they may compete with them; they may constrict and extinguish those areas of functioning and development that are felt to be strange, dissonant, and/or threatening. Such areas may include sexuality, creativeness, and other behavior reflecting successful enterprise. Parental aggression in such instances may be characterized by explicit negative responses or failure to relate appropriately and enthusiastically to their child's achievements.

When children are given nonambivalent parental affection only when ill, injured, or failing in some respect, it would appear quite certain that the parents are hostile and destructive, and that the victim will likely evolve masochistic coping behavior. Although the psychopathology of masochism is in most cases traceable to destructive family influences, nonetheless, the family is usually felt as a haven from the cruelties of strangers and the outside world. The family, nuclear and extended, among its many other institutionalized functions, is a human unit from which the individual draws strength for coping with life's vicissitudes, including aggression from others. Fear that the envy of others has the potential of destructive, aggressive predation, has been expressed in the culturally rooted and paranoid idea of the evil eye, a myth defended against by masochistic techniques. Valued possessions may be concealed, denied, and minimized; riches may be hidden behind a façade of poverty. In Oriental cultures, children, possessions, and self are often minimized, presumably out of humility and good manners, but actually out of an institutionalized expression of masochism.

Minority groups continue to be targets for aggression, but these days they usually fight back. Up until recently, however, masochistic stereotypes were common. Stepin Fetchit, a movie actor of a past era, was a sterotypic black masochist. He looked defective, was slow-moving, and always submissively addressed his white master as "Yassuh, boss." In the period before the Black Power movement, especially in the South, black parents inculcated submissive patterns, particularly in their sons, as life-saving devices. To what extent masochistic behavior is explicitly taught or acquired through identification with masochistic parents has yet to be determined. Among the upwardly mobile, particularly among minorities, masochistic behavior may be quite prominent. More often than not, they are a target for attack by an established power hierarchy although members of their own group may attack out of competitive resentment or fear of losing one of their number to the majority. The function of the masochistic adaptation is to permit the achievement of desired goals, sexual and other, while neutralizing or extinguishing anticipated aggression for the achievement of these goals.

Masochism and Love

In pursuit of love, acceptance, affection, a kind look, or because of a fear or reluctance to hurt the feelings of others, some individuals may injure themselves or their best interests. If one believes he is better looking, more accomplished, more successful, or more desirable than the individual whose acceptance is sought and who therefore will turn away in envy or become aggressive, then those resources thought to incite envy will be sabotaged. When one sabotages efforts, constricts maximum potential, or renounces constructive goals, on the assumption that fulfillment and gratification will alienate sought-for positive feelings in another, the motivation may be love-preserving but the behavior is masochistic and maladaptive. As noted previously, such patterns develop as a consequence of parental aggression. In these cases, one or both parents were jealous of their child, or were made anxious by his achievements. Such parents subtly communicate their displeasure, or show a lack of interest or enthusiasm. Children soon discern the parents' meaning and submissively renounce gratifications. Older siblings who are jealous and competitive may also promote masochistic behavior, especially if they are admired and respected. Peermates and significant others outside the family may set off masochistically inspired inhibitions in academic work or in occupational interests, out of fear of group rejection. Gifted students sometimes relinquish high-level performance, because peermates disparage it by such epithets as bookworm, egghead, sissy, and so forth. In adult life, beliefs about the prerequisites for love, affection, and acceptance may be derived, on the one hand, from beliefs about what others desire or demand, and, on the other, from the projections of personal responses to those situations that either evoke or inhibit positive affects in oneself. An individual may feel threatened by another who is believed to be superior in some way and whose acceptance is valued and desired. Because of fear of superseding that individual, the tendency will be to sabotage those personal attributes believed to be a threat to the power figure who then might withhold goods, services, or wished-for affection; or, worse, turn into an attacking, fearsome rival.

Masochistic techniques to evoke positive affects in others or as responses to affection by valued others constitute a psychological trap. Masochistic characters become very fearful of acceptance, much as they may wish to have it, for they hate their own masochism which they cannot control, yet fear they may act it out and lose the personal assets they wish to retain. Hence, such people fear affection and avoid closeness to others lest they become enslaved. In treatment, these patients lose such fears when they develop confidence in their ability to control masochistic, submissive behavior in situations where affection is being given or withheld.

Those who react masochistically in situations perceived as a choice between hurting themselves or others have a somewhat different problem. They choose a masochistic route even when they do not care about or desire the affection and acceptance of the individual(s) being "saved." This type of masochist cannot bear to inflict discomfort or suffering on others. The background of some such patients often reveals a childhood saddened by a parent who had undergone considerable physical or psychological suffering. Others may have had parents who used real or simulated suffering as a way of provoking guilt and as a technique of control. If the parents' suffering is perceived by the child to be the consequence of his own activities, he may then attempt to ease their distress by masochistic renunciation of his own normal wishes. The inability to tolerate the suffering of another is therefore not necessarily a reaction formation to one's own sadistic instincts, as classical theory proposes. The repression of sadistic desires is but one parameter, and one which I have been able to delineate rather infrequently.

In treating patients who respond masochistically to the hurt feelings of others, they should be led to the realization that hurt feelings are hardly fatal. The point to be emphasized is that if intent and behavior are constructive, the patient is not then responsible for possible neurotic reactions in another. A good criterion for readiness for discharge from treatment is an immunity to masochistic responses when hurt feelings are manifested by others.

Masochistic Phenomena

Masochistic maneuvers are as varied as man's inventiveness. Injury may be solicited or self-inflicted; it may be directed to one's person, to a function, to a valued possession—be it object or person. If one were to select any single type of dynamic constellation to exemplify the psychopathology of everyday life, masochism would be a good choice. Few, if any, are totally free of masochistic behavior. Accident-proneness, in and out of automobiles, is often masochistic. Car accidents, even of a trivial sort, are a way of acting out anxiety about achievement, since among its many uses, automobiles serve as symbols of achievement and luxury.

The fear of success, whether in work, romance, or other important spheres of life, may be defended against by a masochistically inspired disability. The realization of a meaningful aspiration or the start of an enterprise that promises success may be followed by an accident or illness. Certain behaviors are overtly masochistic and may directly promote accidents or illness, such as in the excessive use of alcohol, tobacco, drugs, and activities that result in getting the insufficient rest and sleep that promote exhaustion syndromes. Fending off a normal level of health and vigor compatible with the energy needed to sustain one's efforts indicates a masochistic drive to sabotage potential success. All drug abuse, be it with alcohol, marijuana, or heroin, has a masochistic motive—physical self-injury through the toxic effect; social damage through the opprobrium and degradation associated with the life of the addict.

Food abuse through overeating is similarly a masochistic syndrome. In most such cases, the masochistic orientation is toward impairing physical attractiveness, health, and vitality. There are, of course, motivational components other than masochism in drug abuse and obesity, as, for example, where the effects of intake are sought to alleviate intense anxiety and agitation.

Most patients who have developed a well-defined line of masochistic behaviors have also convinced themselves that they can control at will and reverse damaging consequences. They tend to discount the irreversible effects of long-term smoking, drinking, drug or food abuse, and they cling to the illusion that they will somehow be forgiven the injuries and destructiveness their masochistic activities cause others.

Major insults to one's security and prestige may be courted by illegal involvements where apprehension would lead to financial disaster and social disgrace. Risk-taking and brinkmanship are inspired by a masochistic orientation toward self and may include one's family.

Sometimes a child becomes the symbol of masochism, and the parents become excessively preoccupied with the masochistic focus he personifies. In such a family, the youngster's every illness, injury, or other vicissitude, no matter how minor, becomes a source of great travail. The parents believe and create the impression that were it not for their child's difficulties, life would be an idyll. The victim almost always pursues his assigned masochistic role, in part as patterned behavior, in part as a way of obtaining and preserving parental interest and love.

The dissipation of financial resources is commonly acted out in a masochistic gambit. Despite an excellent income, debts may be accumulated, in some cases as a result of compulsive gambling. One such patient was excellent at cards, but when in masochistic gear, he would pile up huge losses. Like others in this category, he had fears of success, and was driven to lose, rather than gather up the evidence of successful play. It was quite predictable that he would lose large sums just when he had almost paid up his debts, or when he had accomplished something notable in his work. Among patients whose fortunes are in alternate phases of waxing and waning, rich one period and poor the next, I have always been able to observe self-sabotage.

A mechanism similar to the need to lose money is the masochistic loss or destruction of objects of value. In the repertoire of such lost objects, some are more frequently represented because of their symbolic value—wallets, handbags, briefcases containing important papers, and so forth. The lost and found departments are the repositories for acted-out masochism. During the great depression of the 1930s, I treated a patient whose masochism reflected the stringent times. One evening, when returning from work, the patient discovered she had left her handbag on a subway train. She could ill afford to lose the twenty-dollar bill her purse contained. As she undressed later that night, she found the money in one of her shoes but had no memory of having put it there. She had a masochistic need to lose a symbol of value represented by her purse, yet she was too practical to lose her money as well.

Forgetfulness may be viewed as a variant of masochistic losing behavior. Blocking on the name of someone well known to one, particularly when performing a social introduction, forgetting information needed to pass an important examination, or forgetting theater and travel tickets—each may represent an item of forgetfulness in the psychopathology of everyday masochism. Some individuals "forget" what time it has gotten to be and manage to come late to an event they had looked forward to; sometimes, an event may be overlooked entirely, or attended a day or a week too late.

Some individuals are made anxious when they perceive that they are presenting themselves in a good light to others; they are then compelled to minimize themselves in some way. Such compulsive acts may include inappropriate remarks, socially unacceptable behavior, such as nose-picking, awkward manners at table, and so forth. A good clinical test for discerning a masochistic character is his response to a compliment; usually, a self-minimizing remark or act will follow.

Masochism and Humor

Humor, especially masochistic humor, is an effective technique for coping with aggression. If one can manage to be a target for laughter, one is not likely to be a target for hostility. Laughter extinguishes anger, hostility, and allied affects, at least for the period during which the laughter continues. Many comedians use masochistic techniques to evoke laughter, particularly when an audience is being unresponsive. Arieti[1] has clearly described masochistic wit in the following passage:

Granted that Jewish jokes originating by non-Jews are more offensive than those originating with Jews, the fact remains that even the latter may be offensive. Jews know that even mild jokes dealing with dirtiness and thriftiness may be used by anti-Semites as a disparaging weapon. I have the feeling that this habit of the Jews is paradoxically an unconscious defense against anti-Semitism. Aware as they have been in the course of centuries of the great hostility by which they were surrounded, the Jews have tried to make the Gentiles discharge their hostility by means of these not too harmful jokes. It is better to be accused of stinginess and dirtiness than of ritual murder. It is better to be laughed at than to be massacred.

Masochism and Suicide

By definition, the techniques of masochism involve self-injury as this term has been defined; however, the goals of masochism are the *preservation* of life and the attainment of maximum integrity compatible with the threat against which the masochistic defense is being used. In suicide, the goal is the *extinction* of one's life. Suicide and masochism have in common self-destructiveness, but here the similarity ends. Freud associated masochism with femininity, with passivity, with a desire to experience pain. He interpreted masochism, not as a defense against aggression, but as a manifestation of the aggressive instinct turned in against the self. Starting with this assumption, it was logical for him to conceptualize suicide as the ultimate point on a masochistic continuum. Yet, clinical observations reveal that a central motif in suicide is to relieve intolerable pain, and to escape irrevocably from a hopeless entrapment in suffering. According to Freud's concept of masochism, there is pleasure in experiencing pain; certainly not pleasure in the *relief* of pain. The confusion of suicide with masochism has resulted in theoretical and therapeutic errors. To be sure,

some masochists may commit suicide because life has become too weighed down by psychopathology and too painful to tolerate. They do not commit suicide, however, to experience the ultimate in masochistic pleasure!

A dynamic known as "riddance" is closely related to masochism. A phylogenetic analogy to riddance may be seen in the capability of some reptiles to shed a limb or tail that has been trapped or injured. Humans may also attempt to eliminate a structure or function that has become a source of pain and distress. Transsexuals seek to have themselves castrated in order to eliminate a structure to which they attribute their profound suffering and whose malfunction seems beyond repair. Riddance phenomena may be observed in other types of obsessive, masochistic patients who also seek out surgical intervention. A woman in her early thirties whom I treated some years ago was tormented by a conflict arising from an ardent desire to have a second child, yet she was prevented from becoming pregnant because of her overweening fears about it. While I was away on vacation, she located an obliging gynecologist who removed her uterus. In sum, riddance is concerned with destroying a part of oneself in order to preserve one's life, while the goal in suicide is to eliminate life itself.

Masochism and Psychiatric Syndromes

Since masochism threatens to produce or produces self-injury, it activates basic security operations, both biological and psychological. Anxiety and inhibition are the most prominent biological defenses.

The term "anxiety" connotes a constellation of perceived physiological reactions that represent a hypermobilization of somatic resources preparatory to meeting a threat. Masochistic impulses and acts almost always evoke anxiety. The compulsive gambler referred to previously was an excellent poker player, but when in a masochistic mood he would gamble recklessly and for excessively high stakes. He would, at these times, experience severe anxiety, an affective state he had long interpreted as excitement of enthusiasm, expectation, pleasure, and so forth. Anxiety is often mistaken for these types of excitement. One patient who experienced extreme anxiety during sexual activity, in a slip of the tongue coined the word, "anxirement," a composite of anxiety, desire, and excitement.[2] When masochists play a game of brinkmanship with dangerous situations, anxiety is triggered, although it may be experienced as excitement.

Inhibition is an automatic "braking" to prevent action perceived as potentially injurious. Undoubtedly, many masochistic impulses are inhibited, yet many masochistic situations are mediated through inhibition. Those who seek achievement but become inhibited because of their neurotic fears of success may masochistically have their opportunities destroyed through inhibition. This may occur among actors who forget lines when given an important role, speakers who develop stage fright, athletes who lose concentration during the crucial period of an important event, and so forth; avoidance behavior is a defense mechanism transitional between inhibition and a range of psychological defenses. Avoidance may be as automatic and unconscious as inhibition; it, too, is a way of preventing or avoiding actions or situations that threaten to be injurious. Avoidance linked to masochism manifests itself in essentially three types of situations: In the first, the individual is tempted to act out a masochistic impulse and, fearing he may arrange to humiliate or otherwise injure himself, he bypasses the situation; in the second, the individual finds himself in conflict over a wish to win, with its attendant anxieties, and a masochistic impulse to lose, also a frightening prospect. Either alternative is defended against by an avoidance maneuver. The third type of masochistic avoidance, and the most destructive, may be observed among individuals who are bent upon acting out a self-destructive impulse; they will avoid anyone who they suspect might interfere with their masochistic acting out. It must be kept in mind that masochism is a defense mechanism; it is a way of avoiding a greater injury by inviting or sustaining a lesser one. Individuals who are on a compulsively masochistic course

are actually trying to prevent a greater catastrophe from befalling them; hence, they avoid anyone who might prevent their masochistic behavior, however irrational it might appear. The avoidance of constructive figures not infrequently includes the analyst; it is during a masochistic period that patients tend to skip sessions or fail to discuss ongoing problems and decisions.

Masochism and Obsessive Symptoms

Masochism is often a core element of obsessive reactions. For example, a man may become obsessed about turning off gas jets and faucets, impelling him to turn back after leaving his home just to check out his obsessive doubts. Such doubts arise because of an unconscious masochistic impulse to burn down his home or flood it. His masochistic defense is motivated by anxiety about possessing an object of great value to him. Individuals who masochistically run themselves down physically, may become obsessively concerned with matters of health. Obsessive dread of accidents, illness, contagious diseases, and dying, may represent fears about masochistic self-injury. Such fears are sometimes projected to a loved one who becomes the focus of an overanxious parent, child, or spouse. Pregnant women may become obsessed with fear that there will be something seriously wrong with their newborn. In my clinical experience with such patients, most were expressing fears about their own masochistic impulse to injure their child in order to protect themselves from being attacked for having a wished-for baby. Homosexual obsessions may surface when an individual who fears success in work or in a relationship with a woman sabotages his efforts and brings on a masochistically inspired defeat. Psychologically, the defeat is a submission to a feared competitor (father or brother figure) who will then spare the vanquished. Whenever homosexual obsessions appear in heterosexuals, one can always identify a significant masochistic component. To reemphasize the essential point: Masochistic mechanisms are often identifiable in the dynamics of obsessions. The therapeutic gain in teasing out these mechanisms is obvious.

Phobias are closely similar to obsessions, so much so that where obsessiveness is a salient characteristic, phobias may be identified in childhood history and current functioning. As with all psychological defenses, there is no single explanation for a phobic defense; however, in acrophobia and the fear of falling, there appears to be a direct dynamic connection with masochism. Patients who are definitely not suicidal may, in a masochistic period, develop fears of walking through a window during sleep, or become panicky about falling from a height. One patient who feared he would walk to his death during sleep, tied his foot to the bed to prevent himself from leaving it.

Masochism and Depression

Some of the consequences of masochistic acting out are self-anger, self-hatred, loss of self-esteem and confidence, and a reactive depression. The depression may be consciously felt or repressed out of awareness; it may be visible or masked, evanescent or chronic. The psychodynamics of masochism may be identified in almost all depressive states. Where such dynamics are central and the patient is compulsively bent on destroying something of value to himself, the depression will be of an agitated type. The conflict between impulses toward destructive action and attempts to conserve valued objects and functions, despite fears about holding on, is often the crucial conflict in an agitated depression. When in a state of depression, patients may destroy their business or profession that took years to build; they may dissipate fortunes, break up a marriage with a beloved spouse, ruin valued friendships, and so forth. When masochism is acted out with such destructive consequences, the patient may become potentially or actually suicidal. Losses resulting from masochistic behavior are extremely painful, if only because they are self-inflicted and thus accompanied by enormous self-hatred and contempt.

Masochism and Paranoid Mechanisms

Paranoia as a description of behavior basically refers to an irrational expectation of injury from others. A discussion in depth on paranoid mechanisms is not germane to this chapter, but since its relation to masochism has a significant bearing on our subject, three types will be briefly described. The first involves victimization; mistrust, suspicion, and hostility are experientially derived and then irrationally transferred to others who may even be constructively related. This type may be termed the "transferential paranoia." The second involves being taught paranoid ideation by paranoid parents or surrogates. One who emerges from such influences might be termed the "indoctrinated paranoid." The third is the psychiatrically familiar and classical type in which the paranoia involves the projection onto others of unacceptable feelings and impulses—"projectional paranoia." In this type, sexual and aggressive wishes are usually recognized psychiatrically; however, the projection of masochistic impulses is generally overlooked or insufficiently emphasized, yet such projections are common features. The individual who masochistically loses in gambling may suspect others of cheating; a masochist who somehow destroys an opportunity for advancement may accuse his employer of keeping him down or unfairly preferring someone else. Individuals who sabotage their appearance through obesity or a bizarre style of dressing or makeup may believe that others are laughing at them, showing them contempt, deriding them, and so forth.

Masochism and Pathological Dependency

In general, masochism is a psychodynamic component in pathological dependency. Where an individual is pathologically dependent upon another, he must be prepared to please and placate the object of his dependency. This may require submissiveness, or self-demeaning, minimizing, and noncompetitive behavior. Masochistic attitudes and behavior are almost always present in individuals whose adaptation is a significantly dependent one. A common dynamic in dependency is the inflation of the image of the person depended on.[2] This enlargement effect is achieved through minimizing the self. The deflation of self is a masochistic process, since it involves damaging one's self-image and inhibiting one's own resourcefulness, in order to magically obtain hoped-for advantages from the enlarged other. These psychodynamics appear in exaggerated forms among psychotics. Their paranoid fears may derive, in part, from their irrational concept of inflated power which they ascribe to individuals seen as likely ones to be dependent upon. Because of the anxiety associated with the masochistic components inherent in pathological dependency, defensive maneuvers against becoming dependent on another may consist in avoiding those individuals with whom one would be tempted to form such a relationship, or responding to them with hostility, i.e., attempts to minimize or degrade them, or otherwise make them inaccessible for such a role.

Treatment of Masochism

Masochistic behavior may be conceptualized as an aggregation of adaptational mechanisms. Based upon this formulation, therapy may be oriented toward working out the adaptational significance of every masochistic mechanism whenever it occurs. If, for example, it is oriented toward extinguishing another's aggression, the patient is made aware that inflicting self-injury in order to prevent injury from others is maladaptive. He must learn that fear of reprisal from others for fulfilling his wishes, is, in general, unfounded, but that even where actual aggression may eventuate, the injury anticipated is almost always grossly distorted. Where real aggression is a possibility, the patient must learn to recognize and reality-test effective techniques for coping with another's aggression, and that coping behavior does not include masochistic, maladaptive defenses. Where a patient is masochistic in order to evoke love or conserve

it, he has to become convinced that those who demand masochistic behavior in exchange for affection are exacting an exorbitant price, hardly worth it.

As a general principle of therapeutic technique, I do not analyze defenses until the fears that have established and maintained them are understood.[4] Thus, if a patient fears displacement by a preferred sibling, I engage this problem before approaching his competitiveness toward the sibling. After the patient has become familiar with his underlying fears, the next phase may include the analysis of his desire to surpass or even annihilate the sibling or his transferential representatives. Exceptions to this rule concern (a) the analysis of defenses that produce analytic resistances which may interfere with treatment or threaten its continuity, and (b) the analysis of masochistic defenses. When a patient prepares to act out a masochistic impulse, the therapist should endeavor to prevent it, especially if it threatens to be significantly harmful. Insight should be given into the meaning of the masochism and its injurious consequences; even directive techniques, if they can be effective, should be employed. Despite the traditional pessimism about successfully treating masochistic characters, I have found that the maladaptive processes inherent in masochism can be significantly altered in most cases, and actually extinguished in some.

(Bibliography

1. ARIETI, S. "New Views on the Psychology and Psychopathology of Wit and of the Comic," *Psychiatry*, 13 (1950), 43.

2. BIEBER, I. "The Meaning of Masochism," *American Journal of Psychotherapy*, 7 (1953), 29.

3. ———. "Olfaction in Sexual Development and Adult Sexual Organization," *American Journal of Psychotherapy*, 13 (1959), 851.

4. ———. "A Concept of Psychopathology," in P. H. Hoch, and J. Zubin, eds., *Current Approaches to Psychoanalysis*. New York: Grune & Stratton, 1960.

5. ———. "Sadism and Masochism," in S.

Arieti, ed., *American Handbook of Psychiatry*, Vol. 3. New York: Basic Books, 1965.

6. ———. "Sex and Power," in J. Masserman, ed., *Science and Psychoanalysis*, Vol. 20. New York: Grune & Stratton, 1972.

7. FREUD, S. "Three Essays on the Theory of Sexuality" (1905), in Standard Edition, Vol. 7. London: Hogarth Press, 1953.

8. ———. "Instincts and Their Vicissitudes" (1915), in Standard Edition, Vol. 14. London: Hogarth Press, 1955.

9. ———. "A Child Is Being Beaten" (1919), in Standard Edition, London: Hogarth Press, 1955.

10. ———. "Beyond the Pleasure Principle" (1920), in Standard Edition, Vol. 18. London: Hogarth Press, 1955.

11. ———. "The Economic Problems of Masochism" (1924), in Standard Edition, Vol. 19. London: Hogarth Press, 1961.

12. KALOGERAKIS, M. "The Rose of Olfaction in Sexual Development," *Psychosomatic Medicine*, 25 (1963), 420.

13. KINSEY, A. C., W. B. POMEROY, C. E. MARTIN, and P. H. GEBHARD. *Sexual Behavior in the Human Male*. Philadelphia: W. R. Saunders, 1948.

14. ———. *Sexual Behavior in the Human Female*, p. 614. Philadelphia: W. B. Saunders, 1953.

15. KRAFFT-EBING, R. VON. *Psychopathia Sexualis*. (Translated from the 12th German Edition, by F. S. Klaf.) New York: Stein and Day, 1965.

16. REICH, W. *Character Analysis*. New York: Orgone Institute, 1949.

17. THORPE, W. A., and O. L. ZANGWILL. *Current Problems in Animal Behavior*, p. 114. London: Cambridge University Press, 1961.

CHAPTER 16

INTERSEXUAL AND TRANSEXUAL* BEHAVIOR AND SYNDROMES

John Money

INTERSEXUALITY IS OF A SIGNIFICANCE for psychiatry disproportionate to the demand it creates for psychiatric service, essential though that service is. Its significance lies in the fact that human intersexuality is the clinical complement, and the only one in human beings, of experimental animal studies into the differentiation of gender-related behavior and gender identity.

(Determinants of Gender Identity Differentiation

Studies in intersexuality show that the sex chromosomes, or indeed any of the chromosomes, do not, of and by themselves alone, have a direct line of influence on the dimorphism of gender identity and gender behavior.

The chromosomes exert their influence only indirectly, as the first link in a chain or sequence of determinants (Figure 16–1).

The second link is the fetal gonad which, from a bipotential beginning, differentiates at

* The first use of this word in print was: Caldwell D. O. (1949) Psychopathia Transexualis. *Sexology*, 16:274–280. Caldwell also used the English form, transexual, with one "s."

In ordinary English one has the parallel orthography with one "s" in transcribe, transect, transistor, transonic, etc.

In medical orthography, one has transsternal, transsacrum, etc; and transsection as an alternate to transection.

My policy is to have transsexual as an allowable alternate to the preferred spelling, transexual. This keeps the spelling as simple as possible, and also is in keeping with the fact that transexual is not specifically a medical term, but belongs to the general vocabulary.

Many books and articles (my own included) now use the preferred spelling, transexual; and the Erickson Education Foundation, sponsor of transexual research, has officially adopted that spelling.

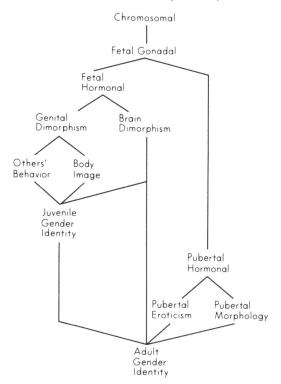

Figure 16-1.   Sequence of determinants of adult gender identity.

six weeks of gestation as a testis, when the sex chromosomes are XY, or at twelve weeks as an ovary, when the sex chromosomes are XX. It is from this stage of differentiation that the traditional nomenclature of intersexuality derives. True hermaphroditism occurs when the bipotentiality of the indifferent gonad does not resolve, but issues in ovotestis, or ovary and testis —the chromosomes are usually 46,XX, but may be mosaic or in some other way anomalous. Male hermaphroditism or pseudohermaphroditism (the "pseudo" is superfluous, for all forms of hermaphroditism are genuine) occurs when only testicular structure, even though imperfect, is present, ambiguity residing elsewhere in the reproductive anatomy. Similarly, for female hermaphroditism (pseudohermaphroditism), only ovarian tissue is present, with ambiguity elsewhere in the system. Female hermaphrodites are almost invariably 46,XX chromosomally; whereas some male hermaphrodites may be not the expected 46,XY, but a mosaic like 46,XY/45,X.

The third link in the chain of gender identity differentiation is hormonal. It is actually a bifurcated link, connecting with both the genital morphology and the central nervous system. In normal fetal development, hormonal differentiation is a function of the fetal gonad. More accurately, it is a function of the fetal testis: Whereas hormones from the fetal testis are essential for the morphologic differentiation of a male, no sex hormone whatsoever is necessary for the differentiation of a morphologic female. Nature's primary archetype is the female; the male depends on the principle of something added. There are two masculinizing substances released by the fetal testis. One, known only by its function, is the mullerian inhibiting substance. Without it, the male is born with the mullerian ducts differentiated into a uterus and fallopian tubes, as in the female. The other fetal testicular substance is androgen, the male sex hormone, essential for differentiation of the internal masculine reproductive tract, and essential also for the differentiation of the external sexual *Anlagen* into male structures, instead of their female homologues, that is the clitoris, clitoral hood plus labia minora, and labia majora, instead of, respectively, the penis, penile skin covering, and scrotum.

Fetal androgen has also an action on the central nervous system in the region of the hypothalamus. This effect has been well demonstrated experimentally in various laboratory species, especially rodents, that have estrous cycles. Androgenization of the fetal hypothalamus, during the critical developmental period, prevents subsequent cycling of the pituitary, and thus of the gonadal hormones in adulthood. This effect is independent of genetic sex. Removal of androgen from the male before the critical period permits pituitary cycling to occur subsequently, as can be demonstrated if ovarian tissue is experimentally implanted in the aqueous chamber of the animal's eye.

The neural mechanisms of cyclicity have been experimentally located with a fair degree of certainty in the posterior region of the hypothalamus. Other neural centers governing behavioral patterns associated with hormonal cycling, or noncycling, in adulthood are situated in the anterior region of the hypothalamus. There is less actual experimental certainty of an androgenizing effect on these centers, but a good deal of presumptive experimental evidence which is not confined to rodents and lower species but extends also to the primates.

Among the primates, including man, sexually dimorphic, fetally androgen-determined behavior manifests itself in juvenile play. Animal-experimental and human-clinical evidence suggests that vigorous, athletic energy expenditure (tomboyism, in girls) is one such form of play. Challenging or defending a position in the dominance hierarchy is another. Play-rehearsal of sexual, pelvic thrusting movements may be another. On the negative side, absence of maternalism in rehearsal-play is also a masculine trait, its presence being common in girls. At puberty, and in especially the beginning of adolescence, there is also a likelihood that boys more easily than girls are genitally arousable by visual and narrative materials, independently of sentimentalism and the sense of touch.

None of these androgen-dependent traits is the exclusive prerogative of boys. They can, if present, be incorporated into a feminine gender identity. Conversely, their presence is not a *sine qua non* of a masculine gender identity, though by today's cultural standards in our society it is difficult to be accepted as a "sissy" boy. By contrast, a tomboyish girl is readily acceptable.

The fourth link in the chain of gender identity differentiation is the morphology of the external genitals, itself a product of hormonal differentiation. This is also a bifurcated link, connecting with the behavior of other people and also that of the child. Dimorphism of the external genitalia is a stimulus of extraordinary potency with respect to the program of behavior that it releases from other people. As a new baby is expected, parents and others stay poised, so to speak, with two programs of behavior at the ready, only one of which will be progressively brought into action. It begins with name choice, and continues in countless activities and responses of day-to-day living.

The appearance of the genitalia also influences, eventually, the body image and the program of the child's own gender behavior by reinforcing the self-sex concept, as a boy or girl. This happens as a child discovers his or her similarity to others of the same sex, and difference from others of the opposite sex.

(Core Gender Identity

Like a loop that links together the social and, later, the personal effects of genital morphology with fetal-hormonal brain effects, personal gender identity (see Figure 16–1) begins to emerge in late infancy and early childhood, at around the same time as native language becomes established. The core gender identity, to use a recently minted term, becomes differentiated as male or female prior to the developmental phase identified in psychoanalytic doctrine as oedipal, and contemporaneously with the preceding phases, named according to that doctrine the late oral (or more literally, oral-haptic) and the anal. The core gender identity is developmentally neither psychoanalytically oral nor anal in origin, though its differentiation is vulnerable to developmental disturbances, regardless of source, that take place during those early developmental periods of life.

Evidence that postnatal development is critical in gender identity differentiation is especially clear in the case of matched pairs of hermaphrodites homogeneous for diagnosis and etiology,* but heterogeneous for sex of rearing. Then, gender identity typically differentiates in conformity with assigned sex. The predictability of this outcome is enhanced if parental anxiety and uncertainty are dispelled, and if surgical correction of the external genitalia in conformity with assigned sex is achieved as early as possible.

In the case of sex assignment as a girl, stage one of surgical feminization, the removal of a too-large phallic protuberance, can be accomplished as early as the second week of life. If

* Consult items 5, 6, 12, 18, 27, and 30 in the Bibliography for detailed information concerning etiology, diagnosis, treatment, and prognosis, of the various types of intersexuality and hermaphroditism. (The two terms are nowadays used synonymously.)

no vaginal cavity is present, the construction of one by means of plastic surgery is best postponed until after full growth has been achieved in middle-to-late teenage.

In the case of sex assignment as a boy, surgical repair of an incompletely formed phallic protuberance usually requires surgical release of the organ to make it pendulous, and the construction of a penile urethra. The procedure fails if the organ is not big enough to begin with. Consequently, many genetic and gonadal male intersexes should be assigned and surgically repaired as females.

Surgical repair as a male cannot be accomplished as early as repair as a female. Therefore, it is doubly important, when the decision is to assign an intersexed baby as a boy, to guarantee the education of the parents as to the whys and wherefores of their baby's intersexuality, and the program of its case management and prognosis. Otherwise, there is a high risk that ambiguity of genital appearance will generate ambiguity or uncertainty of rearing, as ostensibly a boy or girl, which in turn will generate ambiguity or uncertainty of gender identity in the child.

Ambiguous Gender Identity and Sex Reassignment

The intersexed child most likely to grow up with an ambiguous gender identity is one with uncorrected, ambiguous-looking genitalia, raised under a shadow of doubt as to whether the sex had been correctly declared at birth. The doubt may have emanated either indirectly from the medical profession, or directly. There are still some misinformed physicians who say, quite incorrectly, that the correct declaration cannot be made until nature plays her hand at puberty.

Statistically speaking, intersexed babies most likely to grow up to differentiate an ambiguous gender identity leading to a request for sex reassignment have a small, imperfectly formed (hypospadiac) phallus, atrophic or barely palpable gonads presumed to be testes, and an assigned sex as a provisional female. The provisional or equivocal nature of the sex of assignment, without surgical feminization, reflects lack of up-to-date criteria in the knowledge of specialist consultants at the time of birth. On the one hand, common sense dictates that a baby with little more than a clitoral-sized phallus and urogenital sinus should be a girl. On the other hand, presumed testes suggest, to the uninformed, a quasimoralistic obligation to declare the baby as a boy. A compromise, misguided though it is, is to declare the baby as a girl, while waiting to see what happens at puberty.

If, meantime, the ambiguous pendulum of the child's gender identity differentiation swings in the male direction, and if at puberty she undergoes hormonal masculinization, then she will, after a long overdue diagnostic verification as a genetic and gonadal male, almost certainly be permitted a sex reassignment if she requests it, though she may be denied the request to continue living as a girl. Here again, there is a quasi-moralistic element in the decision, on the basis of the criterion of the gonads. The case that illustrates the converse is that of a very similar but genetically female intersexed child with the precociously pubertal, adrenal virilization of the adrenogenital syndrome. It is not too common, because of lack of palpable gonads, for such a child to be assigned as a male. When the neonatal diagnostic workup is incomplete, however, assignment as a female may be left surgically unconfirmed, and also unconfirmed by corrective hormonal therapy with cortisone. In that case, the child will grow up with a masculine puberty, and premature to boot. Should her gender identity differentiation have been more masculine than feminine, leading her to request sex reassignment, the request is likely to be denied, though wrongly so. The reason for the denial is that many medical professionals have a feeling, moralistically rather than empirically based, that an individual with two ovaries, a large phallus—even though large enough to be corrected into a functional penis—and a pubertally virilized physique, should not be permitted elective rehabilitation as a man, after having been originally registered as a female. Instead, she should be required to accept surgical feminization of the external genitalia, and hormonal feminization (adequate but not total) of the physique, as a sequel to corrective hormonal therapy with cortisone. The folly of such an imposition is that it is not maximally rehabilitative: The person who would have succeeded in life as an infertile male and husband is required to fail in life as a fertile female who is, with respect to erotic responsivity, to all intents and purposes an iatrogenic lesbian, albeit inadvertently so.

The parallel of iatrogenic lesbianism, as above, occurs in a genetic male with a micropenis—hypospadiac and lacking or partially lacking corpora cavernosa—assigned as a boy and failing to masculinize at puberty, as a result of complete testicular failure. If a boy with intersexuality of this type grows up with an ambiguous gender identity, plus the conviction that he can resolve it only by sex reassignment to live as a girl, his atrophic, sterile testes and male chromosomal status are likely to prove a stumbling block. He may be required to take male hormone therapy for masculinization of the physique. It will not change his gender identity. If his only erotic attraction is toward males, then he is, on that criterion, an inadvertent iatrogenic male homosexual, who could have succeeded better in life in the role of a woman.

A boy with similar intersexual status, except that he feminizes and grows breasts at puberty, may also be placed in a similar predicament. It has in the past been easier for many physicians to reconcile themselves to removal of breasts and attempted construction of a penis that will never be capable of erection, than to reconcile themselves to removal of feminizing testes, construction of an artificial vagina, and legal sex reassignment.

Intersexuals of the above type of feminizing male hermaphroditism, assigned at birth as boys, are few. As in all types of intersexuality, their requests for sex reassignment are rare, and chiefly dependent on the element of ambiguity absorbed from their rearing. Diagnostically, their intersexuality represents an incomplete form of the androgen insensitivity, testicular-feminizing syndrome, a genetically transmitted condition in which there is a body-

wide inability at the cellular level to respond to the male sex hormone. In the complete form of the syndrome, the genital morphology is not ambiguous, but female, and puberty is exclusively feminizing, except for lack of menstruation, secondary to vestigal formation of the uterus. The breasts develop well. Requests for sex reassignment, despite the masculine genetic and gonadal status, are no more a part of the syndrome than of congenital atresia of the vagina and uterus in a genetic and gonadal female.

(Avoidance of Ambiguous Gender Identity

Differentiation of an ambiguous gender identity, with ultimate resolution of the ambiguity in favor of a sex reassignment request, is not restricted to any one form of intersexuality. It occurs in male, female, and true hermaphroditism. It occurs irrespective of status on the criteria of chromosomal, gonadal, and hormonal sex. It occurs in either direction, male-to-female, or female-to-male, in individuals otherwise homogeneous for diagnosis and prognosis. The two identifiable variables most likely to lead to ambiguous gender identity and sex reassignment as its resolution are (1) therapeutic negligence in resolving ambiguity, in the minds of parents, regarding the sexual status of their genitally deformed baby and the rationale leading to the sex of assignment, and (2) therapeutic delay, beyond the demands of good surgical practice, in correcting the appearance of the external genitalia to agree with the sex of assignment.

The latter applies especially when the decision has been to raise an infant with a large phallic organ, irrespective of chromosomal or gonadal sex, as a girl. With rare exceptions, it is possible to undertake corrective feminization of the external genitalia during the second or third week of life, or soon thereafter. Removal of the phallic structure does not remove the capacity for orgasm in adulthood, if there is a vaginal orifice, naturally formed. In the absence of a vaginal orifice, the prognosis of orgasm after phallic removal is made with less confidence, though the build-up of erotic feeling and pleasure, if the extended perineal area is intact, can always be counted on.

It is fairly standard in today's practice, provided the diagnosis is established neonatally, to assign female hermaphrodites to the female sex. This practice is justifiable, since neonatal feminizing surgery is successful, even if fetal masculinization had been so extreme as to differentiate the genital tubercle into a penis, with a penile urethra, instead of a clitoris with its hood and labia minora. Fertility as a female and the possibility of pregnancy are preserved. Alternatively, it is also feasible, when the penis is normally formed, to leave it intact, removing the internal organs, planning for a masculine hormonal puberty, which will take place spontaneously, should androgenic adrenal overactivity remain uncorrected. Otherwise, it will be induced with testosterone therapy.

In the case of male hermaphroditism, and also true hermaphroditism, it is a cardinal rule not to assign the newborn baby as a male, unless the malformed phallic organ is large enough to be repaired for efficient masculine erotic function in adulthood. It is desirable to test the phallus of borderline size for sensitivity to male sex hormone by local application of testosterone ointment for a period of a month. If the organ does not respond with increased vascularization and size, the prognosis is for future pubertal feminization. Therefore, the baby should be assigned as a girl, and treated as such surgically and hormonally, with the appropriate timing. There is no serious issue to be argued regarding castration, for the more defective the penis at birth, the greater the likelihood of testes that are infertile, defective, and subject to malignancy in young or middle adulthood.

Age, Gender Identity, and Imposed Reassignment

The ideal decision concerning sex of assignment is not invariably made, as it should be, at the time of an intersexed child's birth. If

subsequently a more extensive diagnostic workup is undertaken, it may be deemed desirable that the original decision should be changed. An imposed change of sex during the juvenile years, however, no matter how convincing the rationale, may be as catastrophic for one intersexed child, as for a morphologically normal one, whereas for another one it may be a joyous return from exile in what the child believes to have been the wrong sex. The difference lies in the unitary versus the ambiguous nature of the gender identity that has differentiated, up to the time the reassignment is imposed. Only the child who has differentiated an ambiguous gender identity in the sex of original assignment is able to make the transition of reassignment successfully. This fact has been overlooked by a few misinformed zealots who advocate changing intersexed children's assigned sex, without consideration of the child's gender identity, so as to make the sex of rearing agree with the chromosomal or gonadal sex, or, as they sometimes diffusely and inaccurately call it, the somatic sex.

Close as some cases of forced reassignment of sex come to therapeutic malpractice, they are, nonetheless, of singular scientific value for the empirical light they shed on the timing of gender-identity differentiation.

In the first few months of a child's life, if the original declaration of sex is changed, adjustment to the change is one for which the parents, but not the baby, need help and guidance. Such an early change may be called simply a re-announcement of sex, to distinguish it from a reassignment which, occurring later, involves the child's own cognizance and memory.

By the age of eighteen months to two years, a normally developing child has a concept of himself as a boy, or herself as a girl. The concept is imbedded in the very language the parents use in talking with their child, with its differentiation of the sexes by generic noun (boy-girl, man-woman, brother-sister, mother-father, etc.), by pronoun, and by proper name. The concept of sex difference in the language is supported by the child's visual experience of the difference, clothed and naked. Above all, it is supported by the contingencies of reinforcement that the parents put into action when the child reacts like the little boy, or the little girl, of their own traditions and expectations.

A two-year-old who is subjected to a sex reassignment may subsequently have explicit recall of the event, but probably will not. In the latter case, the period of living in the other sex, prior to the change is not a *tabula rasa*. It leaves its imprint in much the same way as does a native language that falls into disuse and is replaced by another at, say, the age of two. Later in life, that original language will be learned with greater facility than any other foreign language.

The success with which a child will negotiate a sex reassignment imposed at around the second year of life, or later, will depend partly on the success with which the parents, other members of the family, including siblings, and neighbors negotiate it. The older a child becomes, and the more differentiated his or her gender identity, the more arbitrary does a sex reassignment seem to him or her, defective anatomy notwithstanding. An imposed reassignment then turns out to be rehabilitatively negative, for the sense of self as a member of one sex fails to follow the would-be rehabilitative surgical and/or hormonal therapy.

possibly as ambiguous, or as marred in some way by paraphiliac distortion. The erotic status of gender identity at puberty is a product of childhood erotic rehearsal in fantasy and play, both of which will have been influenced by the erotic traditions and behavioral models to which the child has been exposed. They will also have been influenced by the inhibitions and sanctions against erotic fantasy and play to which the child has been exposed —particularly important in our cultural tradition which has a strong taboo on the normal erotic play of primate childhood.

The hormones of puberty do not determine the cognitive or imagistic content of eroticism as masculine, feminine, or otherwise. They activate or increase the frequency of activation of what is already there. More accurately, androgen does the activating, for it appears to be the libido-regulating hormone of both sexes, controlling the subjective feeling of sexual desire or urge to use the sexual organs brought to reproductive maturity at puberty. In normal males, the libidinal influence of androgen is not cyclic, as it is in women. During the phase of ovulation, when her estrogen level peaks, woman is more erotically compliant and acceptive than during the menstrual phase of her cycle. Then, she is more erotically outgoing and initiating.

❰ Puberty and Gender Identity

An intersexed child, upon reaching the normal age of puberty, typically does not develop a desire for sex reassignment, even if the hormonal changes of the body should be contradictory of the assigned sex. Thus, a boy who develops breasts and urethral bleeding, which is actually menstruation, is mortified by these "stigmata" of femininity, and wants to be rid of them. Conversely, a girl whose voice deepens and body hair masculinizes, also is mortified and wants to be rid of these unfeminine impediments.

By the normal age of puberty, the differentiation of gender identity has been well established as either masculine or feminine, or

❰ Personal Erotic Arousal Imagery

Most human beings at puberty discover that a certain content or program of imagery, perceptual and/or in fantasy, stimulates them to maximum erotic arousal and optimal sexual performance. It usually includes the appearance of the partner. The visual component is typically more important for men than for women. Woman's arousal is initiated more in relationship to sentiment and the sense of touch.

The content of personal erotic arousal imagery is remarkably persistent over the span of a lifetime. It usually declares itself at puberty, but it may be masked by erotic inertia and inhibition if it conflicts with the individual's moral conceptions of sexual activity. Then, it may declare itself only later in life, perhaps released by an intense or traumatic emotional experience.

Once having declared itself, an individual's personal erotic arousal imagery tends not to change, neither to be inhibited, nor to be supplanted by an alternative of equal erotic potency. This resistance applies both to spontaneous change and to attempted change through therapy. Change is not actually impossible, but, like the experience of religious conversion, it tends to be unpredictable in the timing of its occurrence. Thus, it is not feasible to predict whether a man with a typical heterosexual arousal imagery will undergo a change and be arousable only by typical transvestite imagery. Likewise, it is not feasible to predict whether a transvestite will change to regular heterosexual imagery, although both types of change have been recorded.

The persistence and potency of personal erotic arousal imagery at puberty are responsible for the determination of some intersexuals to refuse a sex reassignment, and of others to obtain one. In one case history, for example, a teenager with a diagnosis of male hermaphroditism, decided to agree to take estrogen tablets and to undergo surgery that would externalize an internally opening vagina, which connected with a uterus from which menstruation could be induced. She did so in the hope that, having a vagina, menses, and feminine breasts, she might finally be able to accommodate to her official assignment as a girl. It had always been an equivocal rearing at best, and the crowning uncertainty was partial amputation, at the age of five, of a large phallus, without prior warning.

After the vaginal operation which proved highly successful from the surgical viewpoint, the girl discarded her estrogen tablets as soon as she saw evidence of breast enlargement. She did so, and became determined to live the rest of her life as a man, because neither the feminizing surgery, nor the female hormones, nor the brief amount of psychotherapy received, have lessened the intensity of her erotic imagery toward females, and toward

one girlfriend and lover in particular. Subsequently, she preferred her life as a man, despite the fact that attempted plastic surgical reconstruction of a penis is always less than satisfactory. She possessed a totally adequate vagina, but the potency of her erotic imagery of only females as lovers made it useless to her.

Transexual Sex Reassignment

Psychically, there is only a thin dividing line between sex reassignment in a case of intersexuality, like the one just quoted, and a case of transexualism without congenital sex-organ defect. Both could, in fact, be called transexualism, although it is not yet customary to refer to an intersexual individual who wants a sex reassignment as a transexual. The similarity between the two is that they both feel the conviction of having a gender identity that does not agree with the sex of assignment, and both feel the incongruity of being maximally sexually aroused by personal erotic imagery, perceptually and/or in fantasy, of persons living in the same sex as that to which they feel themselves to have been wrongly assigned. They both arrive at the resolution of their predicament by means of sex reassignment.

One difference between an intersexual and a transexual resolved on sex reassignment is that the former is more likely to be embarrassed, ashamed, shy, and perhaps electively mute, whereas the latter is more brazen, insistent, manipulative, and even overtly deceitful in order to achieve his own ends. But the difference is not universal; there is some overlap. Another difference is that the transexual has no identifiable anomaly of the reproductive system. In fact, he has no identifiable genetic, anatomic, or physiologic defect or abnormality that can be measured by today's techniques. The same is true both for female and male transexuals. The most likely site where some etiologic defect might be uncovered in the future is the brain, possibly in connection with a fetal hormonal effect. To illustrate, it is now known from animal experiments that certain barbiturates and anti-biotic substances can cancel out the mas-culinizing effect of male hormone injections given to a pregnant animal for the experimen-tal purpose of masculinizing the female off-spring.

There may be lessons to learn here, by analogy, with respect to substances either in-gested by pregnant human mothers, or other-wise influencing the hormonal equilibrium of pregnancy, which may either demasculinize the fetal male brain or, conversely, masculin-ize the fetal female brain. All such analogies are, at present, in the realm of science fiction. The empirical facts are not yet forthcoming, but the possibility of their undiscovered exis-tence should not be overlooked in the attempt to understand the etiology of either transex-ualism or any of the gender identity anoma-lies.

Until new information is discovered, the most likely explanation of the etiology of transexualism is that its origins lie in the pe-riod of late infancy and early childhood when, presumably, something disturbs the normal process of gender identity differentiation. It is quite possible that gender identity differentia-tion can be disturbed only in selected, predis-posed infants. For example, boys who have the extra X chromosome (47,XXY) of Kline-felter's syndrome, constitute a population at risk for psychopathology of all types, which includes psychosexual pathology, which in-cludes, it would appear, transexualism of a frequency too high to be expected by chance alone.

For a second example, one may note the fact that a majority of male transexuals, like extremely effeminate homosexuals, lack from infancy onward the assertiveness needed to es-tablish a position in the dominance hierarchy of growing boys. This lack may be the end product of a fetal hormonal deficit resulting in an incompletely masculinized nervous system. By itself alone, such a deficit would not auto-matically lead to a transexual development— no more so than the converse of tomboyish energy expenditure in a girl would do. How-ever, the nonassertive male infant may be es-pecially prone to interact with a particular

type of parental social milieu, the outcome being transexualism. The predictable formula has not yet been discovered. It seems likely that any major emotional disturbance in the family life, including such a nonsexual distur-bance as death or dying in the household, as well as more obviously sexual problems as emotional distance between the parents, may have an adverse effect on the gender identity differentiation of some children.

Sex Reassignment: Rationale and Probationary Period

The treatment of transexualism by means of sex reassignment resembles the treatment of congenital or traumatic organ defects by means of plastic surgery and mechanical prostheses. Both treatments represent the practice of ameliorative and rehabilitative medicine, the practice of choice in the absence of curative medicine. Broadly effective, widely available, and economically accessible meth-ods of curative therapy have not yet been discovered for the gender identity disorders in general, and particularly not for the extreme forms like transexualism. It is universally agreed that transexualism is resistant to psy-chotherapy. Hence, no doubt, the reasonably widespread acceptance of sex reassignment therapy for transexuals, despite initial con-troversy. Those who are against reassignment fear that it represents playing along with psychosis. The alternative view is that the organism, following the wisdom of the body, tries to heal its own injuries and traumas, and that there are occasions when medicine, hav-ing no better technique at its disposal, does best to respect that wisdom. Empirically, it happens that in a properly selected case, sex reassignment does improve a transexual's over-all life situation.

To guarantee that a case is properly se-lected, it is best to require evidence that the person has actually lived in the sex of re-quested reassignment, establishing emotional, vocational, and financial autonomy, for a pe-riod of, preferably, two years. This is an admittedly difficult test for a transexual to be put through with genital anatomy that belies civil status, but it is a necessary safeguard against a too hasty decision with future regret. No matter how much a transexual, male or female, feels convinced about the virtue of living as a member of the other sex, and no matter how satisfying the image of that life, or the occasional impersonation in it, there is no substitute for full-time experience. The reason is quite straightforward: No one can behave convincingly as either a man, or a woman, until experienced in being treated convincingly as such by other people in society at large, and acquainted at first hand with the disadvantages as well as the advantages. While appearing publicly as a man, a person does not, for example, know what it will be like to lose freedom of movement, unaccompanied, on the streets at night, as a woman— and so on.

A two-year probationary period serves also, in effect, as a preliminary period of social and hormonal rehabilitation. Hormonal therapy, by inducing changes in visible appearance, facilitates social rehabilitation. The majority of hormonal changes are reversible, should the probationary period lead to a change of prognosis and a decision against surgery, in which instance none of the changes is permanently disabling. In addition, hormonal changes have the advantage of helping to verify the differential diagnosis in borderline cases, before the irrevocable step of surgical reassignment is undertaken.

(Differential Diagnosis

The differential diagnosis lies between transvestism, transexualism, and homosexuality of extremely effeminate type in the male, or of extremely virilistic type in the female. In each instance, the individual will dress partially or completely in the clothes of the opposite sex on at least some occasions.

The transvestite does so episodically, in response to a feeling of intense psychic urgency to relieve a pent-up inner tension from which

he cannot otherwise find respite. In this sense, he has an addiction to female clothing. His tension release is specifically related to sexual orgasm, insofar as the ideal ending to his cross-dressing episode is to have sexual intercourse while wearing items of feminine attire. Only then is he able to insure himself of the complete fulfillment of sexual abandon, or even to guarantee that he will keep an erection. With a partner whose own erotic response dies when she is trying to copulate with a man wearing female garments, his only method of success in intercourse while not cross-dressed may be to imagine himself as the woman, and his partner as the man. Unlike the effeminate male homosexual, he has no erotic resource for having sex with another male, although he probably has tried, or will try it, in a vain effort to find an alternative to his dilemma with women. His dilemma is that his erotic arousal is directed toward the female, if only she could accept him on his own transvestite terms; and that his erotic performance is not divorced from his own penis, despite the insistence of his obligation to dress in women's clothes and imagine himself as a woman. The transvestite who considers sex reassignment as a solution to his dilemma in life is rare. He is definitely a person who benefits from a probationary period of a real-life test, in order to discover his proper decision.

Transvestism of the type just described in males, addictive in quality and prerequisite to coitus and orgasm, must be extremely rare in females, if it occurs at all, for it is not reported in the sexological literature. The explanation probably lies in the fact that all of the psychopathologies of sex, especially the more exotic and bizarre ones, occur either more frequently or exclusively in the male. Here, one perhaps sees an extension of the principle of sexual differentiation, namely, that nature's archetype is the female. The male requires something added—in psychosexual differentiation, apparently, as well as in morphologic differentiation. In the final additive stage, there is evidently an increased opportunity for something to go wrong in the psychosexual status of the male.

As compared with the bivalency of a transvestite's dressing in the clothing of both sexes, the homosexual with extreme contrasexual deviancy of gender role and identity has only one preferred way of dressing, namely, as close to the style of the other sex as possible. The limit is set by the tolerance of family, community, employer, and the law. According to currently acceptable fashion, there is more latitude for a lesbian to wear masculine clothing than vice versa, although by convention she should, like any women, visibly declare her femininity, no matter how masculine her styling.

The effeminate homosexual male, regardless of his history as a female impersonator in women's clothing, differs from the transexual male in the erotic value his penis has to him. The capacity of his penis to achieve an orgasm is not inhibited, and he is not disgusted by penile orgasm as a sign of masculinity, as a transexual may frequently be. The effeminate male homosexual may be impotent during a relationship with his male partner, but able to achieve orgasm alone afterwards. He enjoys the erotic relationship as the oral or anal recipient, nonetheless. He has no coital inclination toward using his own penis to insert into a vagina—or into a mouth or anus, for that matter. His erotic imagery does not require him to fantasy a female partner as a male, for the partner always is, in fact, a male with whom he can fantasy himself as feminine counterpart. Should an extremely effeminate homosexual happen to be on the borderline of transexualism, then the two-year probationary period of living in a state of estrogenic impotence and nonorgasm will be essential to his arriving at a proper decision.

The probationary period is essential also for the virilistic lesbian on the borderline of transexualism. For her, however, the ultimate surgical decision is not of quite identical import as for her male counterpart, since it does not entail the risk of diminution of erotic response. Androgen will increase the erotic response of her clitoris, not diminish it, and reconstructive surgery will entail its preservation, not obliteration. Yet, reconstructive surgery today cannot produce a coitally serviceable penis in a female, as it can a coitally serviceable vagina in the male. The strongly virilistic lesbian fantasies herself, in her sexual relationship with a girlfriend, as having a penis as she makes the thrusting movements of a man. From stimulating her clitoris in this way, and not from having her own vagina penetrated, which is anathema to her, she is able to bring herself to orgasm. Her primary surgical decision will involve not only her own body image with respect to mastectomy, hysterectomy, and attempted penile construction, but also the erotic attractiveness of her body to a sexual partner. A lesbian partner may abhor the lack of breasts and unfeminine genitalia, whereas a nonlesbian woman may be well satisfied with a flat chest, but not with imperfect male genitalia. The issue of how to be attractive to oneself and how to attract a partner, or else to be alone, is the one that needs the probationary period, in order to be resolved.

The transexual male or female suitable for sex reassignment is, then, a person who has met the criterion of living as a member of the other sex for a probationary period of two years, more or less, before the final step of genital reconstruction is undertaken. He or she should be able to pass unnoticed in a crowd as a member of the new sex. In both cases, there will have been a history of gender identity ambiguity from an early age. This ambiguity may have shown itself overtly and consistently in childhood in the behavior of a feminized gender role in a boy, or a masculinized gender role in a girl. Alternatively, it may have been covert, as the child attempted to conform to the norm.

At puberty, acceptance of oneself as erotically different may have been overt, with no attempt to fake what seemed unnatural. Alternatively, there may have been an attempt to conform to the moral norm, punctuated by lapses into opposite-sexed behavior, in obedience to an ever-present fantasy and desire to do so permanently. The attempt to conform may have led to marriage and parenthood, neither of which, however, resolves the ambiguity of gender identity in the direction approved of by society. The female transexual can have heterosexual intercourse as a gymnastic exercise, faking her way, so to speak, without positive erotic response. The male transexual without positive erotic response cannot fake an erection, so he is less likely than his female counterpart to have had heterosexual coitus.

Both the male and the female transexuals are likely to have tried homosexual intercourse by the time they apply for sex reassignment, though not inevitably so. Some transexuals, especially males, exhibit not only an inhibition of the gender identity appropriate to their morphologic sex of birth, but also an inhibition of any erotic role associated with that identity. Thus, a male transexual may be unable to engage in any form of sexual activity with a man while he still has his own masculine genitalia. Such behavior would be morally reprehensible to him, and repulsive. Even masturbation may be impossible, so intense is the phobia of the penis. A masturbation fantasy of himself as a woman is not powerful enough to cancel out the phobia of the male organ itself. The male transexual with this extreme degree of avoidance of his genitalia views reassignment in romantic rather than coital terms, and he may actually end up in the role of a spinster.

The male transexual who does have sexual relations with a boyfriend prior to reassignment typically does not get an erection, and does not want to. He does not even want his penis to be seen by his partner, and certainly not touched. A male transexual, prior to reassignment, may live by impersonating a female prostitute. He becomes adept at hiding his penis completely, with a technique of binding it between the legs or against the abdominal wall. He can safely predict that it will not erect, as he talks a customer into oral or anal coitus, or has him sufficiently inebriated that he scarcely knows what he is doing.

The male transexual's conception of woman's sexuality is the conventional one of feminine passivity. In his feminine role, either before or after surgical reassignment, it is far more important to satisfy the partner than the self. Thus, the male transexual does not capitalize on his male orgasm while he has it,

and does not miss it when it is gone. After surgery, in the feminine role, a climactic experience may be reached; otherwise, the feeling of a diffuse, warm glow of eroticism is accepted as more than adequate compensation for the ability to love a man as a woman loves him.

A female transexual may have an extensive phobia of her female genitalia, but the clitoris is likely to be excepted, being to her a prototype penis. She is more likely to have had active love affairs as a dominant lesbian than her male counterpart is likely to have had as a submissive homosexual. She may use a strap-on prosthetic penis, but would refuse the penetration of anything into her own body. Her breasts to her are almost certainly the mortifying part of her body, corresponding to the penis of the male homosexual. Her body image, as judged from posed snapshots, is that of a male athletic model or weightlifter, posing with tightened muscles. So she binds her breasts, and does not want them seen or touched, even by her lover.

(Hormonal Reassignment: Male

For the postadolescent male, estrogen will bring about a functional castration which, while having the safeguard of being reversible, will acquaint the recipient at first hand with the subjective experience of loss of potency and reduction of libido, both of which are consistent with the male transexual's phobic avoidance of his own genitalia. Estrogen will also promote proliferation of mammary duct tissue with variable individual success. Although this effect is not totally reversible upon withdrawal of estrogen, it can be readily reversed surgically. Estrogenic therapy does not arrest the growth of body or facial hair already established, although it does retard the speed of growth and makes wiry hair more silky. Electrolysis is necessary for complete removal of facial hair. Although the larynx does not change under the influence of estrogen, vocal mechanics are so modulated in the majority of transexuals as to sound femininely husky, instead of masculinely deep-toned—and consistently so, without lapses. The surface appearance of the body becomes more femininely adipose under the influence of estrogen-induced subcutaneous fat distribution; but narrow hips do not broaden after the bone shape has been set by epiphyseal closure.

Because of the irreversibility of adolescent masculinization of bone, hair, and voice, it is highly desirable in the case of a virilizing intersexed child not to postpone reassignment therapy as a female, once the psychologic and psychiatric examination has confirmed the advisability of the decision. In similar fashion, it is desirable not to temporize in instituting feminizing therapy in the case of an intersexed child reared and living as a girl with a female gender identity, if she commences to undergo a masculinizing puberty—even if the diagnosis is one of male hermaphroditism. The day may come when this same principle of preventing pubertal masculinization will be applied to the extremely effeminate transexual boy at the age of puberty. At the present time, however, those who work with transexualism prefer to accumulate more statistics on outcome in older patients, before lowering the age of treatment. The same applies to masculinization of the transexual girl.

The most up-to-date schedule of medication for the male transexual, recommended by Claude Migeon in an unpublished personal communication, is as follows:

Diethylstilbestrol—0.25 to 0.50 mg. daily with Provera (medroxy-progesterone acetate) 2.5 to 5.0 mg. daily.

In place of Diethylstilbestrol, Estinyl (ethinyl estradiol) 0.02 to 0.05 mg. daily, or Premarin (conjugated equine estrogens) 1.25 to 2.50 mg. daily might be substituted. Before gonadectomy, the treatment would be every day for a minimum of four to eight months. Following surgery, treatment could be cyclic, for the first three weeks of each month, missing the fourth week.

An alternative to the foregoing combination of estrogen plus progestin taken separately would be a commercial product combining the two, for example:

Ortho-Novum 1 mg. (norethindrone 1 mg. and mestranol 0.05 mg.), or Norlestrin, 1 mg. (norethindrone acetate 1 mg. and ethinyl estradiol

0.05 mg.), or Provest (Provera 10 mg. and ethinyl estradiol 0.05 mg.). The dosage of these preparations is one tablet daily for the first three weeks of each month.

If the patient prefers not to accommodate to a daily oral therapy, but to an intramuscular one instead, then the following could be prescribed:

Delestrogen (estradiol valerate) 5-20 mg. plus Delalutin (hydroxy-progesterone caproate) 62.5-125 mg. every two weeks. Another intramuscular combined treatment could be: Depo-Estradiol cypionate 1-5 mg. plus Depo-Provera 25-100 mg. every two weeks.

After four to eight months of biweekly therapy, the same dosages could be given once every three or four weeks.

If in the preoperative state, the above dosages prove insufficiently effective after four to six weeks, then the dosage could be doubled. Otherwise, the rule is to use the dosage that is thought presently to be replacement therapy for normal women. For further details concerning hormonal treatment of the male, see Green and Money.[10]

❡ Hormonal Reassignment: Female

For the postadolescent transexual female given androgenic therapy during the probationary period, the first effect will be to suppress the menses. Since eventually breakthrough bleeding will occur, permanent suppression requires hysterectomy as well. Androgen will also induce deepening of the voice through lengthening of the vocal cords. This effect is not reversible, except insofar as the voice may be pitched in its higher, huskier register, instead of its deeper more resonant one. Androgen-induced growth of facial and body hair is also nonreversible, except by electrolysis. Androgen does not completely atrophy the breasts, so that the chest can be flattened only surgically, by mastectomy. The clitoris undergoes some enlargement under androgen stimulation, perhaps to three times its original size, but never to be large enough for surgical reconstruction as a penis.

In the volume by Green and Money[10] may be found details for hormonal treatment of the female transexual. Migeon recommends 100 to 300 mg. of testosterone enanthate, intramuscularly, every three or four weeks. This treatment does not prevent menopause-like symptoms following ovariectomy. Control of such symptoms requires estrogenic therapy, with gradual withdrawal over a period of three to six months.

(Psychological and Psychiatric Guidance

Sex reassignment does not, of and by itself alone, solve psychological problems over and beyond the problem of gender identity. Thus, if there is an associated problem of unresolved suicidal depression, the need for psychiatric care will continue after reassignment. Likewise, if there is an associated problem of psychopathic delinquency, lying, and stealing, continued therapy for that problem will be needed. Controversy surrounds the issue of associated schizophrenic disorder, for there are some who would see all transexualism as schizophrenia, or possibly as paranoia transexualis. To equate transexualism and schizophrenia is, however to muddy the language unnecessarily. It also confuses the issue of treatment, for there are some cases of transexualism associated with symptoms of schizophrenia and paranoia, as conventionally diagnosed. In these cases, sex reassignment does not guarantee a lifting of associated psychiatric symptoms. Sex reassignment plus assiduous psychotherapy may eventually produce a positive outcome, but there is insufficient evidence for a definitive statement at the present time.

In psychiatrically uncomplicated cases, the amount of guidance needed during the probationary period and after may be remarkably little. In those cases where more help is needed, it is wise to have it readily available, so that intervention can be undertaken on a preventive basis, keeping the troubles from multiplying.

It is good preventive therapy to involve also, wherever possible, the families. One insures thereby not only a source of additional case-history information and possible validation of the transexual's own story, but also an extra source of social support in rehabilitation.

Parents and other family members benefit from whatever help can be given them in dealing with a difficult hurdle in life, that may, nonetheless, offer them the first chance of respite in years.

(Surgical Treatment

The technical details of transexual surgery are subject to continued revision and improvement. To keep up to date, the specialist reader should consult the surgical literature. Here, it is appropriate to outline only the general principles.

In the male, the skin of the penis and of part of the scrotum is preserved for use in plastic-surgical feminization. The body of the penis is excised. The urethral tube is shortened and implanted in the feminine position. A vaginal cavity is opened up in the musculature of the perineum and fitted with a skin-graft lining made from the skin of the penis. This lining may be prepared by first amputating the penis and removing its skin like removing a condom. Alternatively, prior to excision of the body of the penis, the skin may be dissected free in the form of an apron-graft left hanging from the abdominal wall. From this apron, plus a flap from the scrotal skin, a tubular vaginal lining is sewn, augmented in size by an insert of skin grafted from the thigh.

The latter technique preserves part of the original blood supply and neural innervation, and allows greater flexibility in the deployment of scrotal skin for a more capacious artificial vagina to be formed, whereas the former dictates that the size of the vagina is more directly determined by the size of the penis. A very small penis produces a vagina too small for successful coitus. In either case, some of the scrotal skin is used for the creation of labia majora. This may be postponed until a second operation, if a period of healing from the first is needed to establish a good blood supply. Postsurgically, a form needs to be kept in place in the newly created vagina, especially during the healing period and prior to regular coital activity, to insure its patency.

Erotically, the artificial vagina supplies a

male partner with satisfying sexual feelings. The person with the artificial vagina also enjoys sexual intercourse, experiencing a pervasive warm glow of erotic feeling and, in some instances, a peak or climactic feeling that corresponds to the orgasm of former days— had such been experienced, which is not always the case—though not identical with it.

Masculinizing plastic surgery of the genitalia for the female transexual is as difficult as the same type of surgery for the boy born with no penis or the man who has suffered traumatic loss of his organ. It is a procedure not to be undertaken lightly. It requires multiple hospital admissions, the exact number being unpredictable, and may take literally years— to say nothing of expense. The end result is a soft cylinder of skin, functional for urination but too soft for intercourse. Surgical implantation of silicone stiffeners has so far not proved successful. For successful intercourse, the skin-graft penis of plastic surgery needs to be inserted in a hollow dildo made of synthetic plastic. This gives satisfaction to the female partner, as an extension of varied techniques of love play. The transexual himself receives erotic feeling and the build-up to orgasm from the tissues of the former clitoris, now imbedded in the wall of the skin-graft penis. Since the clitoris and the shell-dildo are the essential components of a mutually satisfying erotic experience, the female-to-male transexual is well advised to forego the colossal burden of surgery and to be satisfied with only a strap-on penis. Some are capable of utilizing this advice, but others are driven relentlessly to having even an imperfect organ attached permanently to their own bodies.

The surgical technique for creating this organ begins with making a tubular roll of skin on one side of the abdominal wall. At the conclusion of the first operation, this roll resembles the handle of a briefcase, since both ends remain attached to insure continuity of blood supply. After the first-stage healing is complete, the top attachment is severed, and the end of the "handle" is implanted just below the clitoris. The other end is released later. Other aspects of the surgery are the creation of a urethral tube, excision of the vagina (and, of course, panhysterectomy), and conjunction of the urinary outlet with the urinary tube in the new penis.

(Gender Identity Differentiation: Hypothesis

From transexualism it is evident that gender identity can differentiate in frank contradiction of the reproductive genitalia and postpubertal appearance of physique. From cases of intersexuality one learns that chromosomal and gonadal sex may be deliberately disregarded in deciding the sex of assignment, so that one is, in a limited and specific sense, inducing iatrogenic homosexuality, according to the chromosomal and gonadal criteria, but not the external-genital and other criteria of homosexuality. Moreover, one may pair such cases with matching ones for whom the sex of assignment was the opposite. Then, one has two individuals of matching etiology and diagnosis who differentiate opposite gender identities. Thus, both spontaneously and by iatrogenic design, one has evidence of discontinuity between gender identity and one or more other variables of sex, where normally there is continuity. Obviously, gender identity differentiation in its postnatal phase is highly malleable and not preordained. It is open to social contingencies, as is language, and as is imprinting of the type demonstrated in ethological studies.

Up until the present, it has been the theoretical fashion to consider the social contingencies of gender identity differentiation only in terms of reinforcement for copying role models of the same sex, but not for neglecting or omitting to copy models of the other sex. That both processes occur, the negative as well as the positive, is made evident in the lives of people who eventually want a sex reassignment. To catch the evidence, it is necessary to engage in longitudinal study. Then, one may be rewarded with a glimpse of a time in development when a child is able to alternate from a masculine to a feminine way of doing things, and vice versa. Later, the pendulum swings, and gender behavior, and identity with it, becomes unitary. The swinging of the pendulum can be seen and heard, and recorded on videotape, in some young transexuals. They can call on the two systems of behavior, masculine and feminine, and put them into action, at a time when their normal contemporaries cannot. Persistent availability of the two systems into adulthood can be seen particularly well in typical transvestites, who have two names, two wardrobes, and two personalities, all matching as male and female, respectively. The difference between the two personalities, and the consistency of each, the one masculine and the other feminine, is as great as the difference between two completely separate individuals of different sex.

In such cases of transvestism, one has, in fact, an equivalent of multiple personality. The possibility that the transvestite is different from the majority of people only in keeping his two personalities on call, is suggested by some rare reports in the neurosurgical literature. These are reports of transvestism and/or fetishism, in which the disturbance of gender behavior came to the fore when temporal lobe epilepsy manifested itself. Following temporal lobectomy, both the epileptic seizures and the transvestism no longer occurred. Even without seizures, it is rare for transvestism to manifest itself *de novo* in adult life, but it is known to have done so—again suggesting that a system once irretrievable from memory storage becomes retrievable and transmittable into action.

In view of the foregoing evidence, it makes good sense to postulate that gender identity differentiation is for all human beings a process constituted of coding both the masculine and the feminine systems of gender role. The double coding permits one system to be segregated from the other, negatively coded, and called upon only to verify what to exclude from the positively coded system. In other words, a boy knows how to be a boy, because he knows how not to be a girl, and vice versa for girls.

This dual system is analogous with that of two native languages. The bilingual child learns best if the carriers of the two languages

are different persons. Each language then becomes linked to a different person, or persons, with overlap minimized. So also with gender identity, the carriers of the two systems are segregated. Again, a bilingual child may use both languages throughout life, but he may also inhibit one, attaching to it a sense of shame, as in the case of an immigrant's child who is ashamed of the old-country ways of his parents.

The factors that allow one child to differentiate a unitary gender identity in the expected direction, whereas another differentiates incompletely, perhaps finally swinging in the inappropriate direction, remain a challenge to research. So also does the explanation of why gender identity, once differentiated, remains singularly immutable, when it is congruous, as well as when it is incongruous with whichever criteria of sex one may be using.

(Concluding Remarks

Intersexuality is theoretically important to psychiatry in demonstrating that the differentiation of gender identity is not preordained by genetic or chromosomal sex directly, nor by fetal hormonal sex. Fetal androgen, however, is an important contributor in that its presence induces masculinization of the external genitals and of certain hypothalamic functions, both of which otherwise differentiate as female. The external genital appearance profoundly influences the behavior of others from the time of sex assignment throughout rearing, and also the individual's own body image and self-conception. The hormone-differentiated hypothalamus probably influences such sexually dimorphic behavioral differences as energy expenditure level, pelvic thrusting movements in childhood play, and dominance assertiveness in the power hierarchy of childhood play. In human beings, postnatal differentiation of gender identity is not preordained by prenatal hormonal influences, though it may be influenced by them. Postnatal differentiation, like language acquisition, requires social interaction. It may issue in a gender identity that is congruent with its antecedents, contradictory to them, or ambiguous.

Postnatal gender identity, once differentiated, is singularly tenacious in maintaining itself. For this reason, the decision concerning an intersexed child's sex assignment should be fixed at the time of birth. If later considerations lead to a revision of diagnosis and the possibility of sex reassignment, then more attention should be given to the status of the gender identity already differentiated than to the other variables of sex. Psychological failure of sex reassignment in intersexuality is guaranteed unless gender identity has been incomplete or ambiguous in the sex of assignment. It is most successful if the intersexed child has already reached a resolution for sex change.

The success of sex reassignment in specific and highly selected cases of intersexuality is paralleled by its success also in selected cases of transexualism. The basic difference between the two cases is that the typical transexual has no visible or measurable signs of abnormality of the reproductive system. His or her condition is, if the term intersexuality is to be applied at all, one of psychic intersexuality. It is best to precede surgical sex reassignment in transexualism by a two-year probationary period of living full time in the new role.

Theoretically, the anomalies of gender identity might best be understood through the hypothesis that all human beings have both a masculine and feminine pattern of gender behavior coded in the brain, one of them usually negatively coded, the other positively. The anomalies of gender identity represent an imbalance of the usual positive-negative ratio. The process of becoming a boy is by identification on the reciprocal process of not becoming a girl, but knowing how to respond to females is by complementation, for girls the obverse holds true.

❪ Bibliography

1. BENJAMIN, H. The Transsexual Phenomenon. New York: Julian Press, 1966.

2. DAVIES, B. M., and F. S. MORGENSTERN. "A Case Of Cysticercosis, Temporal Lobe Epilespy, and Transvestism," Journal of Neurological and Neurosurgical Psychiatry, 23 (1960), 247–249.

3. EPSTEIN, A. W. "Fetishism: A Study of its Psychopathology with Particular Reference to a Proposed Disorder in Brain Mechanisms as an Etiological Factor," Journal of Nervous and Mental Disease, 130 (1960), 107–119.

4. ———. "Relationship of Fetishism and Transvestism to Brain and Particularly to Temporal Lobe Dysfunction," Journal of Nervous and Mental Disease, 133 (1961), 247–253.

5. FEDERMAN, D. D. Abnormal Sexual Development, a Genetic and Endocrine Approach to Differential Diagnosis. Philadelphia: Saunders, 1967.

6. GARDNER, L. I. Endocrine and Genetic Diseases of Childhood. Philadelphia: Saunders, 1969. (2nd ed., 1974, in press.)

7. GORSKI, R. "Gonadal Hormones and the Perinatal Development of Neuroendocrine Function," in L. Martini and W. F. Ganong, eds., Frontiers in Neuroendocrinology. New York: Oxford University Press, 1973.

8. ———. "Localization and Sexual Differentiation of the Nervous Structures which Regulate Ovulation," Journal of Reproduction and Fertility, Supplement 1 (1966), 67–88.

9. GOY, R. W. "Role of Androgens in the Establishment and Regulation of Behavioral Sex Differences in Mammals," Journal of Animal Science, 25 (1966), 21–35.

10. GREEN, R., and J. MONEY, eds. Transsexualism and Sex Reassignment, pp. 305–307, 353–354. Baltimore: Johns Hopkins Press, 1969.

11. HARRIS, G. W. "Sex Hormones, Brain Development and Brain Function," Endocrinology, 75 (1964), 627–648.

12. JONES, H. W. JR. and W. W. SCOTT. Hermaphroditism, Genital Anomalies and Related Endocrine Disorders. Baltimore: Williams and Wilkins, 1958. (2nd. ed. 1971.)

13. MITCHELL, W., M. A. FALCONER, and D. HILL. "Epilepsy with Fetishism Relieved by Temporal Lobectomy," Lancet, 2 (1954), 626–630.

14. MONEY, J. "Determinants of Human Sexual Identity and Behavior," in C. J. Sager and

H. S. Kaplan, eds., *Group and Family Therapy*, New York: Brunner/Mazel, 1972.

15. ———. "Hermaphroditism and Pseudo-hermaphroditism," in J. J. Gold, ed., *Textbook of Gynecologic Endocrinology*. New York: Harper and Row, 1968. (2nd ed., 1974, in press.)

16. ———. "Influence of Hormones on Sexual Behavior," in A. C. Degraff, ed., *Annual Review of Medicine*, Vol. 16. Palo Alto, California: Annual Reviews, Inc., 1965.

17. ———. "Matched Pairs of Hermaphrodites: Behavioral Biology of Sexual Differentiation from Chromosomes to Gender Identity," *Engineering and Science* (California Institute of Technology), 33 (1970), 34–39.

18. ———. *Sex Errors of the Body*. Baltimore: Johns Hopkins Press, 1968.

19. ———, ed. *Sex Research: New Developments*. New York: Holt, Rinehart and Winston, 1965.

20. ———. "Sexual Dimorphism and Homosexual Gender Identity," *Psychological Bulletin*, 74 (1970), 425–440.

21. ———, and A. A. EHRHARDT. Man and Woman Boy and Girl: The Differentiation and the Dymorphism of Gender Identity from Conception to Maturity. Baltimore: The Johns Hopkins Press, 1972.

22. MONEY, J. and R. GASKIN. "Sex Reassignment," *International Journal of Psychiatry*, 9 (1970–71), 249–282.

23. MONEY, J., R. POTTER and C. S. STOLL. "Sex Reannouncement in Hereditary Sex Deformity: Psychology and Sociology of Ha-bilitation," *Social Science and Medicine*, 3 (1969), 207–216.

24. NEWTON, N. *Maternal Emotions. A Study of Women's Feelings Toward Menstruation, Pregnancy, Childbirth, Breast Feeding, Infant Care, and Other Aspects of Their Femininity*. New York: Hoeber, 1955.

25. NIELSEN, J. "Klinefelter's Syndrome and the XYY Syndrome: A Genetical, Endocrinological and Psychiatric-Psychological Study of Thirty-Three Severely Hypogonadal Male Patients and Two Patients with Karyotype 47,XYY," *Acta Psychiatrica Scandinavica*, Vol. 45, Supplementum 209, Copenhagen: Munksgaard, 1969.

26. NIELSEN, J., A. SØRENSEN, A. THEILGAARD, A. FRØLAND, and S. G. JOHNSEN. "A Psychiatric-Psychological Study of 50 Severely Hypogonadal Male Patients, Including 34 with Klinefelter's Syndrome, 47,XXY," *Acta Jutlandica*, 41, No. 3. Publications of the University of Aarhus, Copenhagen, Munksgaard, 1969.

27. OVERZIER, C., ed. *Intersexuality*. New York: Academic Press, 1963.

28. STOLLER, R. J. *Sex and Gender, On the Development of Masculinity and Femininity*. New York: Science House, 1968.

29. WHALEN, R. E. "Differentiation of the Neural Mechanisms Which Control Gonadotropin Secretion and Sexual Behavior," in M. Diamond, ed., *Reproduction and Sexual Behavior*. Indiana University Press, 1968.

30. WILKINS, L. *The Diagnosis and Treatment of Endocrine Disorders in Childhood and Adolescence*. Springfield, Ill.: Charles C. Thomas, 1965.

CHAPTER 17

FETISHISM, TRANSVESTITISM, AND VOYEURISM: A PSYCHOANALYTIC APPROACH

Robert C. Bak and Walter A. Stewart

I N ORDER TO UNDERSTAND the psychoanalytic view of the perversions it is necessary to review theories of maturation and development on which this understanding is based. The term "maturation" emphasizes that aspect of growth which is primarily biologically preordained. The term "development" refers to those more incidental events and processes of growth in which environment plays the dominant role in its interaction with maturation.[11]

The distinction between maturation and development is only relative, since even in maturation of inborn functions there is no absolute autonomy from the environment;

that is to say, normal maturation is contingent on the "average expectable environment."*

From a number of such observations we can assume that an average expectable environment is essential for maturation as well as development. These environmental stimuli can be regarded as releasers of the biologically preordained functions. Both maturational and developmental growth processes should be

---

* This is illustrated in experiments by Dennis.[6] The twins raised in the first six months with almost no response from those caring for them showed at the end of the first year marked retardation in their capacity to sit up or stand. However, after a few days of being "taught" these almost autonomous functions, they soon learned them.

viewed in terms of the total interdependent unfolding of the sexual drive, the ego functions and object relations.

Some place must be allotted in our theoretical scaffolding for inborn constitutional variations in the capacity for these functions. Not all persons are endowed with equal potentiality, nor are they born with the same equipment. The variations are largely assumed under the concept of ego functions. However, there are undoubtedly constitutional factors involving the strength and nature of the drives, as well as variations in the capacity to form object relations and to react with the external world.*

The problem of developmental growth is embodied in the life history of the individual. It is in this area that psychoanalytic studies have been so richly rewarding. The analytic task can be described as the reconstruction of the interaction between maturational factors and life experiences. This genetic approach to the understanding of human behavior and motivation is not original with psychoanalysis. What was original was the discovery of the meaning and influence on the child of certain experiences. Psychoanalytic understanding enlarged and systematized the understanding of what experiences were influential in the modification of behavior. For example, the crucial timing of an experience, the so-called temporal factor, could be understood in terms of the child's specific maturational phase. The same experience at one age period might have relatively little impact, but were it to occur in another developmental phase, it could exert a quite traumatic effect. This timing of an experience was only one of a number of factors that had to be taken into account in order to understand the individual's response to an experience. Other factors, such as regression, fixation, and repression, also played a crucial role in determining the meaning of an experience.

Since the meaning and interrelationship of

these concepts have changed considerably over the last eighty years, it is desirable to review briefly those psychoanalytic concepts on which our understanding of the perversions is based.

([Psychoanalytic Theory of Drive and Ego Development

The psychoanalytic views of the beginning of psychic functioning all have what can be termed a mythological flavor. It is expressed popularly in the phrase, "In the beginning there was chaos." This first period is termed the undifferentiated phase, since there is no differentiation of the self from the nonself; also the energies are not yet differentiated into aggression and libido (i.e., the energy of sexuality); and finally, there is no structural differentiation of the personality into functional units.[11]

This beginning undifferentiated phase exists prior to birth as well as after. The birth experience is so remarkable from the point of view of the observer, that all things relevant to maturation and development seem to occur after birth. This may not be true. Ferenczi[7] emphasized the fact that the "caesura" of birth is not the beginning of life; it is to the infant a momentous change, but also a continuation, partly provided by the nurturing environment.

Rank[16] saw birth as the model or prototype for anxiety, in the sense of its being the greatest interruption of a Nirvana-like existence. It is the first and greatest example of the necessity to deal with overwhelming stimuli. Bak[1] has emphasized the problem of temperature regulation which birth imposes on the infant. Up until birth, temperature regulation was automatic and dependent on the mother. After parturition, the infant is subject to temperature fluctuations, especially cooling in the external world. The adaptation to this change is the earliest experience of the infant in self-regulation and leaves a tell-tale imprint on the sense of separation. The cooling of the infant may be the universal prototype of the vital danger of separation and castration.

---

* Bak[5] has emphasized that in the schizophrenic, for example, the capacity to invest the outside world is probably defective from the start. These biological considerations involving genetic factors are beyond the area of analytic investigation.

Greenacre[8], following some of Ferenczi's ideas, viewed the birth process as a powerful traumatic early conditioning of the infant in relation to the later impingements from the outside world. The emphasis was less on the prototypic experience of anxiety, but dealt more with the problem of the stimulus barrier. Birth was the original traumatic (overwhelming) experience, which later had to be avoided.

Developmental and maturational changes occur after birth with extraordinary rapidity. This phase of development leads from undifferentiation to the differentiation of self from object, differentiation of the drives, and the differentiation of structures.[11]

The early phases of the development of the sense of self have been studied by a number of distinguished analysts, amongst them Hoffman[14], Hermann,[12] and Hoffer.[13] However, the problem has been most systematically studied and formulated by Mahler.[15]

Mahler designates the first stage, when self and object are not differentiated, as the autistic phase. The second stage is designated as the symbiotic phase. In this period, the child and mother form a dyadic pair or unit. This is followed by the separation-individuation in which the self is aware of being a separate unit able to relate to a variety of objects.

Drive differentiation follows a different pattern. From the nondifferentiated stage of psychic energy two forms are differentiated: One is libido or sexual energy, the other the aggressive energy. These pure forms of drive energy are, however, never observable clinically. Freud hypothesized that in even the earliest months they merge and form an alloy. As a consequence of this form of fusion, each drive is modified and tamed.

Hartmann[10] suggested a different formulation to account for the taming of the drives. He saw the drives as remaining separate, even when both libido and aggression were invested in the object. Their taming was not the result of instinctual fusion, but occurred as a result of de-instinctualization, which he termed neutralization.

However the taming of the drives is thought of, whether as fusion or neutralization, it is a crucial step in development. Both the differentiation of the drives and their turning towards the outside world are dependent on good maternal care. When the mother provides trustworthy care, she is the object for the investment of the energies and brings the child out of the autistic phase, and through the symbiotic phase to the awareness of self.

At a later date, the drive differentiation is further consolidated and given greater stability. For the male child, this occurs when, most of the libido, fused with some aggression, is invested in the mother, while the father, seen as a rival, is invested primarily with aggressive energy which is also fused with some quantity of libido. The energies are not only differentiated and functionally useful, but are differently invested in outside objects. The desirable functional employment of the differentiated energies promotes the development of stable object relations and a less ambivalent tone to the sexual life.

The end result of this biological unfolding, given reasonable maternal care and fortunate constitutional endowment, is what Freud termed "genital primacy." The term does not describe the behavior in terms of sexual performance (potency, frequency, orgasm), but rather that the pregenital strivings will be present in only token amounts and will lead towards heterosexual genital union as the desired mode. If there is prolonged lingering in the pregenital forms of forepleasure, or they are the desired goals, genital primacy is undermined. Of course, if the behavior is modified by the wish to appear normal, this also does not constitute genital primacy.

Unhappily, the development is not always so fortunate, particularly in cases where there is severe maternal neglect, or severe and painful childhood illness in the first eighteen months.[9] The child is unable to master the overwhelming stimuli associated with neglect and/or pain. He experiences what can be called a helpless rage. Because the differentiation of the outside world from the inside is not yet clear or stable, the discharge consists of a raging on the inside. There can be kicking, screaming, crying, choking, but it is experienced presumably as an internal discharge, which could be characterized then as primary sadomasochism.

We emphasize these early overstimulating traumatic experiences, since they may be some of the basic factors present in all of the perversions. The marked urgency of "drivenness" of perverse needs and their acting out is in all likelihood related to these early, overwhelming, painful experiences. Since ego development is at its inception incapable of exerting any control or delay of discharge, this failure of control and poor capacity to tolerate frustration may continue into adult life.

This early damage has to be viewed also in terms of its effect on the developing capacity for object relations. The earliest form of object relation has been termed "primary identification." The infant oscillates between no objects and a dim awareness of the mother and her body, which is probably most often conceived as only an extension of himself. Good maternal care plus average frustration turn the infant's attention towards the outside world and stimulate him to differentiate between himself and the mother (self and object differentiation).

We hypothesize that overwhelming painful experiences occurring at the earliest precarious awareness of the outside world force the child to retreat to the earlier phase of no self-object differentiation. This retreat, we think, results in an undue prolongation of the primary identification. The consequences are again of major importance for an understanding of the perversions. The prolonged primary identification leads to marked fears of abandonment (separation anxiety), poor self-object differentiation (individuation), and an unclear sexual identity (bisexuality).

❨ Psychosexual Development and the Perversions

Psychoanalytic observations support the view that the child passes through a series of maturational sequences, moving from orality through anality and the phallic phase to genitality, with parallel developments in the aggressive drive, in object relations, and other ego functions.

Overindulgence, deprivation, or a combination of the two, interfere with this developmental sequence. For example, overindulgence or deprivation can result in the wish to remain at the specific phase of development at which they occur. The needs or wishes become overinvested and the energies available for further development are reduced. This failure to progress is termed "fixation." Fixation implies a weak point in the psychosexual development. It not only reduces the available energies for the full development of the psychosexual life, but remains a weak point to which, in the face of conflict or imagined threat to the genital organ, the whole progressive development can return. This threat, which occurs in an infinite number of forms, is subsumed under the term "castration anxiety." The castration fears reach their major force during the phallic phase. They represent a crystallization of the dangers of this phase. They are intimately connected with the oedipal strivings, although they can precede it.

The negative oedipal phase, involving both an aggressive and a passive relationship to the father, is a crucial factor in the genesis of the perversions. However, the intensity of the castration anxiety rising from both positive and negative oedipal strivings would not in itself appear sufficient to promote a structured perversion. The acute and overwhelming quality of the castration anxiety can only be understood if the conflicts in the pregenital phase are also taken into account. Conflicts in the oral and anal phases leading towards passivity, ambivalence, and bisexuality are important *magnifiers* of the crucial castration fears. The identification with the aphallic mother is a further illustration of the reasons for the marked intensity of the castration anxiety found in those males who suffer from a perversion.

The central point in all perversions is the height of the castration anxiety and the inhibition of genital impulses. This can then lead to several possible solutions. It has a specific dynamic role in the development of fetishism, voyeurism, transvestitism, and exhibitionism.

It is somewhat artificial to isolate one perversion from another in terms of the outstanding behavior pattern. In fact, it is usual to find a complex variety of perverse behavior in one individual. (For example, homosexuality, fetishism, transvestitism, and voyeurism can all coexist.) At the same time, there is a certain specificity in which one solution to the castration conflict dominates and becomes the main defense and discharge pattern. Also, a specific perverse pattern of behavior is often determined by certain childhood experiences.

Our approach to the perversions is that the perversion represents a symptom or mode of sexual adaptation in which the essential element is *the dramatic denial of castration*. The form or choice of the perversion is often closely linked to pregenital fixating experiences which are re-enacted in the perverse ritual.

We understand the intense castration anxiety which the perversion attempts to deny partly as the consequence of frustration and overstimulation in the undifferentiated phase. This results in heightened aggression towards the maternal object, failure in the neutralizing function of the ego, and to the establishment of a distorted discharge pattern employed prior to the development of neutralization and adequate control by the ego. The heightened and poorly controlled aggressive impulses towards the object lead to a fantasied destruction of the object. The defense against this fantasied destruction of the object results in an identification with her. The consequent marked bisexual identification results in the increased castration fears.

Other consequences follow the use of identification to overcome the unmastered aggression. The failure to achieve a clear gender identification results in a splitting of the self-representation. There are male-female, active-passive, phallic-aphallic representations.

One of the most serious consequences of the unresolved bisexuality is an uncertainty of the body image, a vagueness not only about the genitals but a lack of clear boundaries concerning the body-self. It is probably an important substratum to all of the perversions and accounts for the confusion between self and object, as well as promotes the use of primitive introjective-projective mechanisms of defense.

For example, the choice of the love object often represents an effort to heal this split in the ego representations. Because of the unclear self-object differentiation, the object choice is made on a predominantly narcissistic basis. The object chosen represents the idealized object which the patient wishes he had been, and he loves it in a fashion in which he wished his mother had been able to love him.

Another consequence of the unresolved bisexual identification is the failure of the ego to differentiate the two drives in terms of their object. The mother remains the target of both aggressive and libidinal drives. Therefore, she is also seen as the source of aggressive threats. The passive yearnings for love from the father also remain unresolved and in conflict with the natural rivalry. The child is caught in an unresolvable dilemma, in which the condition of love from both father and mother is that he should abandon his phallic strivings.

The goal of the perversion is to secure some form of sexual gratification without destroying the object or endangering the self which is identified with the object. We can examine some clinical examples that illustrate the effort to resolve this dilemma.

Fetishism

In the fetishistic perversion, as in all the perversions, the symptom represents a dramatized denial of castration.[2]

The fetishist denies a part of reality by refusing to acknowledge the lack of a penis in women. The historical core of the problem lies in the horror at the sight of the female genital. The fetish is a symbolic substitute for the maternal phallus. It may be chosen as a symbol of the penis or it may be the last object viewed, just before the woman's penislessness was observed and became frightening. While the main significance of the fetish is its value as a safeguard against accepting the penislessness of women, it also serves by condensation other functions as well. It may represent breast-skin, buttocks-feces, as well as female phallus. The fetish quite regularly is chosen in terms of its odor, its texture, and sometimes also because of its indestructibility. These aspects of the fetish reflect the patient's impulses to cling to the mother and to incorporate her through her odors.

The first clinical example represents a mixture of the homosexual and fetishistic perversions. The homosexual choice involved a preoccupation with the object's buttocks. They had to have a narrow, compact, boyish shape, and be shown off by tightly fitting trousers. The patient's sexual pleasure was based on a wish to finger the crease between the buttocks and to put his nose between the buttocks. Other fetishistic interests involved both rubber and leather boots, rubber raincoats, and riding breeches. Men dressed in these garments excited him sexually. He masturbated while dressed in this type of clothing.

The choice of these fetishistic objects was clearly related to some of the patient's experiences with his mother. In his prolonged toilet training and numerous anal accidents, the mother would wash his buttocks with a "facecloth." He fantasied how she would then use this same washrag to wash herself. This intimacy became the epitome of love. Just as his mother would put her nose to the front and back of his trousers to see if he had soiled himself, he would, when he could, smell her underwear. When he actually soiled himself, the mother would show a marked horror, undress and wash him, and end by kissing his buttocks. He obviously enjoyed his anal "accidents" and even encouraged his mother to give him enemas.

The mother would amuse the family by flatulating in their presence. As a natural extension of this "seduction," the patient would often follow his mother into the bathroom in order to enjoy the smell of her feces. He frequently saw his mother undress and particularly noted the rubber apron she wore next to her buttocks. He loved to crawl under it and to smell his mother's odor, as well as the warmed rubber apron.

In great contrast to the permissive intimacy connected to bathroom activities, his genital interests met severe prohibitions. He was warned not to play with his penis and was severely reprimanded for any interest in the genitals of little girls. It is not surprising that he was horrified to see any evidence of his growing masculinity. He despised his growing penis and hid it between his legs. The growth of pubic and body hair seemed to make him a bearded, crude ruffian, similar to his father and brother.

The fetishistic choice, rubber goods, boots, and the interest in buttocks, was clearly determined by these formative and overwhelming experiences. The rubber apron, the facecloth, and the preoccupation with odors, provided tactile substitutions for the mother's body. In dreams, the mother appeared with a "long rubber hose between her legs," and in other dreams he would be searching for something in the attic and would ejaculate when he found some rubber boots. This can be interpreted as the reparative wish that the mother's body could be completed by the presence of a penis. The preoccupation with the mother's body was fed partly from the feared separation from her, and also from the concern about her "castrated state."

The pregenital clinging, the emphasis on smell, warmth, and feeding, come in conflict with the frightening awareness of the genital differences that make the mother an object of horror. The fetish serves to deny this difference and allow the continuation of the closeness of "oneness." Dreams repeatedly concerned themselves with the effort to deny the penislessness of the mother and the sadistic role of the father's penis.

The pregenital determinants of the castration anxiety were also quite clear in this case. The patient had feeding difficulties from birth. He vomited after feeding and went through near-starvation in infancy. There were many memories of how he had to be protected because he was so "sensitive." His delicate build and smooth skin were praised by both mother and grandmother. He was in contrast to his father and four-year-older brother, and was constantly praised because, unlike them, he was nice and gentle, just like a girl.

He was not accepted by either father or

brother as a man. He was not included on hunting or fishing trips. His father tended to denigrate and ignore him, while the brother openly criticized him, bullied him, and called him a sissy.

Until the age of thirteen, the patient had passionate, shy, and unfulfilled love for girls. At fourteen, when his brother left home in elegant military attire, he suddenly switched to a homosexual object choice. Here, his hatred of the brother became reversed. It is one of the typical vicissitudes in homosexuality.

The first homosexual attraction involved a boy whose first name was the same as the brother's. The rivalry with the preferred and "masculine" brother had, because of his leaving home, changed into a love relationship. This boy and later ones represented what the patient wished he had been (idealized self) and were modeled on the admired and envied older brother. He himself acted the role of his mother. He loved his idealized self in a way in which he wished his mother had loved him.

The goal of the homosexual relation was to obtain the object's masculinity. Through the homosexual contact, the patient could vicariously enjoy the object's masculinity and maintain some semblance of a phallic self-image. The homosexuality also resolved the rivalry with and the humiliation at the hands of the brother, hiding the aggressive wishes with libidinal ones.

Finally, the homosexuality magically protected him from the mother's criticism, undid her phallic prohibitions, and protected him from castration or abandonment. The fetishistic objects all related to the mother and her body, symbolized her penis, and made the identification with her less anxiety-provoking. They also represented the adolescent image of the ambivalently loved brother and his military attire.

A second case illustrates both fetishistic and transvestite urges, and particularly clearly presents the essential role of aggression in the perversions.

The patient, a twenty-three-year-old man, came to treatment after his discharge from the army. Overseas, he related poorly to his comrades, failed in his officers' training program, and was afraid that in combat his testicles would be shot away. He had a burning ambition to be a successful army officer, and the tough General Patton was his ideal. Unfortunately, he got his feet frozen and received a neuropsychiatric discharge before he had fired a shot. This was the ultimate in failure, and he developed a depression.

This patient was also an avid horseman, preoccupied not only with riding and horses, but also with riding clothes. He was excited by women wearing jodhpurs, especially if the calves were protruding, and even more if they wore boots. The britches should have a strongly bulging appearance on the sides and the knee patches should be of suede. He bought many of these articles of clothing.

This interest had a precursor in a transitional object, as described by Winnicott.[17] As a child of two or three, he had great difficulty parting from his mother and in sleeping alone. He insisted on going to bed with a piece of velvet, which he stroked and put to his cheeks before falling asleep. His separation anxiety was made even greater when at the age of four his parents left him to go on a trip. Shortly after their return, a younger brother was born.

The change in interest from velvet to suede was understandable. The turning point occurred between the ages of five and six, during a vacation in Scandinavia. At that time, he saw his mother and aunt in the bath house, changing after a horseback ride from their riding clothes into their bathing suits. What stood out especially in his memory was the moment they shed their jodhpurs and put on their bathing suits. He would ask his aunt repeatedly what made the jodhpurs stick out at the sides. This is unquestionably an example of a choice of the fetish based on the last moment the woman could be considered phallic. Following this, he developed a fear of swimming, based on a concern that a fish would bite him. The sight of the woman's genitals, even though defended against by the fetishistic formation, was insufficient to overcome the castration anxiety. Of particular interest here is the relationship of the earlier interest in velvet, which served in part to overcome the separation from the mother, and the later interest in suede and jodhpurs, which dealt with the castration anxiety. Their similarities should not lead to conclusions about their identity. They serve different functions which, although they can be united in developmental terms, imply only a dynamic continuity. *The change in function* should be kept in the forefront of our awareness. The smelly "security blanket" is almost of universal occurrence; it attenuates the fear of separation from the mother, whereas the function of the fetish is denial of castration.

Other important clinical aspects of this case are also instructive. The patient's female ideal was a long-haired, blond, gentile "Park Avenue girl." This object choice was determined by his experiences in Scandinavia, to which he traveled with his parents frequently during the summers, by his own long, blond, silky hair, which he had as a child while he was dressed in girls' clothing, and by his interest in his mother's long hair, which he enjoyed caressing. The choice reflected narcissistic qualities, identification with his mother, and his wish to attract his father sexually. In early puberty, he had a recurrent fantasy of dancing naked, with long hair, before his father. In these fantasies, the lower part of his body was indistinct. This reflected his feminine wishes, and his own unclear body image. In effect, he left open in his fantasies some *uncertainty* about his own genitals.[4]

The castration fears also emerged at the anal level. The patient recalled a fear of using the outhouse, because of the fantasy that something might emerge from the dark hole and injure him. The smell of his feces interested him, and he was concerned when they disappeared.

This patient, in spite of his fetishistic perversion, was not able to avoid a homosexual solution as well. He would walk the streets dressed in jodhpurs until he was picked up by a man.

His heterosexual choice was finally a crippled woman, a commercial artist who was quite domineering. Her superior intellect and aggressive attitudes fulfilled his fantasies of her being phallic.

The fact that she was crippled dramatized his view of women as castrated. One might think that this is precisely what he would avoid in his object choice. In fact, he was preoccupied with and frightened by any bodily deformity.

Why then did he chose this woman? The answer is that central to the perversion is the murderous rage directed at the mother. This is followed by an overwhelming fear of separation, and a compensatory prolongation of the primary identification. This identification is threatened if the reality of the genital differences is accepted.

As a defense, two possibilities are available. The first is that both he and his mother are phallic. This fantasy draws on the pregenital identification when the mother was considered phallic. The fantasy reduces both the separation anxiety and castration fears.

Another possible fantasy is that both he and his mother are penisless. In this fantasy, the fear of separation from the mother is experienced as greater than the loss of the penis. Hidden in the fantasy of being penisless is of course the gratification of feminine wishes and the wish to obtain the father's phallus.

A follow-up on the case was most reassuring. Although the patient was diagnostically in the "borderline" category, he had made a fairly good adaptation. He had a good job, enjoyed his marriage, and was quite proud of his child. Unfortunately, he died shortly after this as a result of a gastrointestinal illness.

A final case is particularly illustrative of the role of aggression in the perversions.

The patient, a young man in his middle twenties, came to treatment because of his indecision about marrying his fiancée, to whom he had been engaged for four years. He felt uncertain of his capacity to perform sexually, and had intercourse only on a few occasions. Intercourse occurred in a furtive manner, in the dark, while he remained almost fully clothed.

His main erotic interest was focused on the female breasts. His conditions for sexual arousal consisted of large breasts sticking out prominently, not flabbily, and large erect nipples pointing upwards. Any flattening of the breast when the woman lay on her back aroused anxiety. It was clear that this interest and his conditions for sexual arousal were based on the breasts being replacements for the absent penis, for which they were a substitute by displacement. One of his highly invested pleasures was to grab the breast with force and to plop it out from behind the brassière. His feeling, "first it is hidden from sight and then it emerges," reassured him that though no penis can be seen in the woman's genitals, it is there and will appear. The same mechanism determined his impulse to press his erect penis against passengers in the subway. Even if they saw nothing, there was acknowledgment that "something" was there.

All of these activities served to reassure him that the woman possessed a hidden penis, and by his reassurance he could partly overcome his castration fears.

His masturbation fantasies led to a further understanding of his psychosexual conflicts. His nipples were highly sensitive, and during masturbation he would scratch them with a nail file until they bled. The aggressive impulses directed against the mother's body and particularly her breasts were turned back on himself.

The patient's mother had had a cardiac condition with frequent attacks of cardiac asthma at night. The mother's labored breathing, the calling of a physician at night, became confused with the primal scene and supported his view of sexual activity as an injurious and sadistic act. He keenly remembered being told not to disturb or upset the mother or come too close to her bed because he might disturb her. He felt extremely curious about her body and particularly her breasts. Later, this type of abandonment and deprivation of physical closeness would regularly lead to transvestite urges. The prohibition against touching markedly stimulated a strong scoptophilia and the exhibitionistic urges that contributed to the transvestite impulses.

From early childhood, the patient suffered from a recurrent otitis media, which required repeated punctures of the ear drum. This became the vehicle of his castration fears, and since he confused his own illness with that of his mother, further increased the feminine identification.

His character was based primarily on reaction formation. His "niceness" was a defense against the fantasy of a sadistic attack on the mother's breasts and the father's penis. The latter represented his repressed oedipal strivings. Both led to severe but unconscious feelings of guilt and a fear of retaliation.

The patient's adjustment remained fairly good and he was able to marry. However, after twelve years, his wife required a mastectomy and died of generalized cancer after two years. This unfortunate vicissitude came too close to his own aggressive impulses. His potency, which was based on a breast-penis equation, was overwhelmed, and his aggressive impulses, separation anxiety, and castration anxiety were pathologically rearoused.

The patient came back into treatment in order to deal with the feelings aroused by his wife's death. He suffered from unrecognized guilt for sadistic impulses and the rearoused castration anxiety. He had always associated his mother's cardiac failure with sexual activity, of which she was the imagined injured victim. After a year of treatment, he entered into a new courtship. Again, this produced a new wave of sadism, guilt, and masochism. He lost a considerable part of his fortune as a result of poor judgment. When he finally married, he managed to torment and provoke his wife to attack him; he used his supposed "poverty" to deprive her.

These sadomasochistic expressions of his rage, originally expressed in the attack on his own nipples, were finally worked through. He was able to take responsibility in the marriage, for the family, and his own investments.

Voyeurism, Exhibitionism

In all the perversions, the body and body image are of central importance. We have seen how true this is in the structured fetishistic perversion.

In the exhibitionist, the denial of castration employs the earlier childhood pleasure of exhibiting. Reassurance of not being castrated is obtained from the observer's shocked reaction to the sight of the penis.

At a deeper level, the exhibitionist states, in effect, "I show you what I wish you could show me (the female phallus)." This motive for exhibitionism reaches its greatest condensation when the exhibitionist sees himself as the female with a phallus exhibiting to the castrated little girl (himself). He is identified then as both the phallic and aphallic female. He reassures himself and at the same time prolongs the "uncertainty" that results from his unresolved bisexuality. One patient, for example, had the impulse to touch the genitals of little children, both boys and girls, and then ask, "What have you got there?" This patient also had a wish to be masturbated by an older man. Again, he plays both roles through a double identification: he is both the older man (father), and himself, the little child, playing with his father's penis. The strong paranoid substructure was by means of projection a defense against these homosexual impulses.

Voyeurism usually accompanies the impulses to exhibit. The "scenes" that the voyeur attempts to see are often repetitions from childhood of experiences that aroused castration anxiety. These are typically primal scenes or the sight of adult genitals. In the repetition, there is an attempt to master the anxiety, or, by changing the experience in some way that is reassuring, to disavow it.

The identification with the phallic mother in exhibitionism and the search for the female phallus in voyeurism in order to overcome castration anxiety form the central core of these perversions.

⟪ Transvestitism

A clinical vignette illustrates the dynamic determinants of this solution to the overwhelming castration anxiety.

The patient was a young man who suffered from uncontrollable urges to dress in female clothing. These urges emerged at the age of thirteen, when his five-years-older sister left home to go to college. There had been considerable sexual intimacy between them, beginning when the patient was only two and a half years old. In adolescence, the sex play stopped short of intercourse and consisted mainly of flattening out the sister's breasts.

In childhood, the sister would push the patient's penis inward and cry out, "Now you are a girl!" This decisive trauma was repressed, but reappeared in the patient's ritualistic practice of tying his bandaged penis backwards so that is disappeared from sight. At the same time, he pushed his testes back into the inguinal canal so they also would not be seen. In this state, he would dress and undress in front of a mirror with the fantasy that he was, as his sister had announced, "now a girl."

Another important determinant to this ritual was the childhood experience of watching his mother dress and undress in front of a mirror. He watched her in the mirror, and in his later rituals when he himself paraded before the mirror, the angle of the mother's mirror affixed to the wardrobe had to be reproduced exactly.

After these painful rituals, the patient would be overwhelmed wih fears that he had ruined his penis, torn the spermal duct, and that he would be sterile. This castration anxiety, based on a fear of self-damage, increased the urge to dress and appear in public in female clothing.

A further determinant for the patient's self-observation and public appearances in female clothing was based on an intense rivalry with the sister. The father partially sublimated his own scoptophilic interest in little girls by constantly photographing his daughter. The house was filled with these photographs. The patient later in life would photograph himself in female clothing, and finally more boldly would go to photographers to have his picture taken as a woman.

The irresistible impulse to pass in public as a woman fulfilled the wish, and even gave proof to it, that in reality a phallic woman did exist.

The outbreak of the symptom at the time of

the sister's leaving home for college showed that the sexual fantasies attempted to undo the separation. The patient frequently had fantasies of being dressed in a skirt and blouse and of being the sister's roommate.

The sister in fact had strong homosexual leanings involving sophisticated girls of the European type. This became his own ideal which he tried to impersonate. His feminine identification was a composite image made up of his mother, his sister, and the girls to whom his sister was attracted.

In spite of this determination of his own self-image and his goal of fusing with the female object, other object relations continued quite unimpaired outside of the area of fixation and conflict. In fact, his phallic narcissism of his sense of masculinity enabled him to excel in sports. These activities were sublimations of strong sadistic impulses toward the paternal phallus. Thus, both sides of his unresolved bisexual identification were present in his adult life.

The early determinant to this unresolved bisexual conflict was his *inability to separate from the love object*. This could be accounted for only by the early overexposure, both visual and tactile, to the mother's, father's, and sister's bodies. There was prolonged skin contact with all three in the early years of his life which, when combined with his sense of smallness and fragility, hindered his separation-individuation, promoted clinging and the wish to merge, and resulted in an overeroticization of the entire skin surface. This in turn interfered with focusing on the penis as the leading erotogenic organ. The body-skin erotogenicity weakened the phallic investment and led to a strong body-phallus confusion and identification.

From this clinical picture, we can see some of the major determinants for the perversion. The first would be the overstimulation by the mother's dressing and undressing which he watched in the mirror. The second stimulus is the rivalry with and envy of the sister's being looked at and photographed by the father. The third was the seduction by the sister and her traumatic enactment of his feared but wished-for castration that could turn him into

a girl. Becoming a girl could resolve his aggressive wishes to get his father's penis, fulfill his wishes to be loved by his father, allow him pregenital gratifications with his mother, and resolve the murderous rivalry with the sister. The patient's perversion made use of the father's scoptophilic interests as a solution to his aggressive conflicts.

It is perhaps not surprising that this patient was irresistibly drawn toward the idea of being surgically transformed into a female. It would have both fulfilled his wishes and resolved his need for punishment. As a "transformee," he could live out his homosexual wishes, but not the conventional ones. As a woman, he could reunite with his sister or her female sexual objects and act as a lesbian woman.

In fact, after many years of analysis, this patient discontinued treatment with the intention of seeking a surgical alteration. After the passage of about two years, the therapist was consulted by a team of doctors who were considering the question of transforming the patient surgically. The fact that the patient had given permission to the surgeon to raise this question and ask for information or opinion seemed like a possible wish on his part not to pursue the project further.

Only recently, the patient contacted the therapist to inform him of the birth of a son. He was, it turned out, married and now a father. One can speculate with some conviction of accuracy that the lengthy analysis in fact rescued him from his pathological feminine identification, but that the final resolution of the conflict could occur only after some separation from the analyst. Nevertheless, after many years of treatment and in the face of a potential self-destructive acting out, the patient became capable of a masculine identification which had not otherwise been available.

We see in summary how the fetishist, the exhibitionist, and the transvestite all deal with castration anxiety engendered by the lack of resolution of their bisexuality. The common solution is the insistence on the existence of the phallic female. The fetishist invents the phallic female, the exhibitionist hopes to see or be one, and the transvestite is one.

(Bibliography

1. BAK, R. C. "Regression of Ego Orientation and Libido in Schizophrenia," *International Journal of Psycho-Analysis*, 20 (1939), 64–71.
2. ———. "Fetishism," *Journal of American Psychoanalytic Association*, 1 (1953), 285–298.
3. ———. "Aggression and Perversion," in S. Lorand, and M. Balint, eds., *Perversions—Psychodynamics and Therapy*. New York: Random House, 1956.
4. ———. "The Phallic Woman: The Ubiquitous Fantasy in Perversions," *The Psychoanalytic Study of the Child*, Vol. 23. New York: International Universities Press, 1968.
5. ———. "Object Relationships in Schizophrenia and Perversion," *International Journal of Psycho-Analysis*, 52 (1971), 235–242.
6. DENNIS, W. "Infant Development Under Conditions of Restricted Practice and Minimum Social Stimulation," *Genetic Psychology Monograph*, 23 (1941), 143–189.
7. FERENCZI, S. "Stages in the Development of the Sense of Reality," in *Contributions to Psychoanalysis*. New York: Basic Books, 1950.
8. GREENACRE, P. "The Biologic Economy of Birth," *The Psychoanalytic Study of the Child*, Vol. 1. New York: International Universities Press, 1945.
9. ———. "Certain Relations Between Fetishism and Faulty Development of the Body Image," *Psychoanalytic Study of the Child*, Vol. 8. New York: International Universities Press, 1953.
10. HARTMANN, H., E. KRIS, and R. LOEWENSTEIN. "Notes on the Theory of Aggression," *The Psychoanalytic Study of the Child*, Vols. 3/4. New York: International Universities Press, 1949.
11. ———. "Comments on the Formation of Psychic Structure," *The Psychoanalytic Study of the Child*, Vol. 2. New York: International Universities Press, 1950.
12. HERMANN, I. "*Sich Anklammern—Auf Suche Gehen*," *Internazionale Zeitschrift für Psychoanalyse*, 22 (1936), 349–370.
13. HOFFER, W. "Mouth, Hand and Ego Integration," *The Psychoanalytic Study of the Child*, Vols. 3/4. New York: International Universities Press, 1949.
14. HOFFMAN, E. P. "*Projektion und Ich-Entwicklung*," *Internazionale Zeitschrift für Psychoanalyse*, 21 (1935), 342–373.
15. MAHLER, M. *On Human Symbiosis and the Vicissitudes of Individuation*. New York: International Universities Press, 1968.
16. RANK, O. *The Trauma of Birth*. New York: Harcourt, Brace, 1929.
17. WINNICOTT, D. W. "Transitional Objects and Transitional Phenomena," *International Journal of Psycho-Analysis*, 34 (1953), 89–97.

PART FIVE

Addictive Behavior and Syndromes

CHAPTER 18

ALCOHOLISM:
A POSITIVE VIEW*

Morris E. Chafetz, Marc Hertzman, and David Berenson

Lcoholism is a fascinating problem. It is a challenge. Its mysteries remain as deep as the human organism itself and as intricate as our social structure. There is only now emerging agreement among experts as to what is necessary in order to speak of someone as an alcoholic person.[38] Controversy and disagreement about the nature and the origins of alcoholism are so profound and complete that virtually every plausible explanation ranging from genetic to biochemical, from psychological to sociological, has been propounded at one time or another. To make matters even more complicated, it is possible to find research in the field that partially supports every single one of these points of view.

When it comes to treatment the situation is just as complex and confusing. Perhaps, if

anything, it is even more challenging for the sufficiently hardy and daring to undertake the treatment of those labelled "alcoholic" in our society. For many years an aura of hopelessness surrounded anybody who in one way or another acquired this diagnosis and anyone who dealt with him. It is now quite clear to those who treat alcoholic people regularly that the outcomes of treatment are very much related to the treater's expectations of them. If these expectations are high, people can be substantially restored to their former levels of function and more. A number of studies now exist which demonstrate this fact quite adequately.[29,34]

Even more surprising at first glance, the theories of causation of alcoholism often have little relation to the presentation of symptoms, and the theoretical models of development of alcoholism have only modest bearing upon the types of therapy rendered for the condition or the results achieved. No other area of psychiatry, with the possible exception of schizo-

*The authors gratefully acknowledge the assistance of National Institute on Alcohol Abuse and Alcoholism staff members Ms. Ruth Sanchez and Dr. Leonard Mitnick in the preparation of this Chapter, as well as Mrs. Lillian Light, Mrs. Anne Austin and Mrs. Katherine Schechter.

phrenia, presents so many open-ended options to the clinician, the researcher, or the programmer. And, like schizophrenia, prognosis in alcoholism is far from invariant even when no treatment is rendered at all.

We prefer to stress positive functions that alcohol use *and* alcoholism serve. Of course, we are accustomed in psychiatry to attribute positive usages to what is generally taken to be disease or illness—but not to alcoholism. There is nothing new about the notion of functions that maintain integrity. Freudian psychiatry has always stressed understanding the functions that a symptom serves. But alcoholism has always been assumed to be different from other human problems. In many clinics, hospitals, and private offices today, the alcoholic person must divest himself of his prime symptom, his drinking, before he is permitted treatment. This is somewhat akin to requiring the tuberculosis patient to stop coughing before he can receive his streptomycin.

In Ego Psychology especially during the last decade the constructive, purposeful mental processes in behavior have been newly rediscovered in relation to cognition, moral values and the like.[64,120] We propose to carry these concepts simply one step further. It is helpful, especially to the clinician, but also to people interested in other aspects of alcoholism and psychiatry, to try to recast patient and family histories in terms of what promotive functions they serve. As we shall see, this is far more than an academic exercise and is difficult to do, but quite rewarding in its consequences. This is especially true of the treatment sphere, but there are even enticing suggestions that this may be true of some research efforts as well.[62]

With so many avenues to pursue, it is necessary to conceptualize the field in a systematic way. A systems approach, the holistic concept of attempting to take into account the interrelationships among critical variables, can serve as such an organizer. Since the manifestations of alcoholism pertain to the human organism all the way from the cellular level to the network of social organization in which people live, the discussion which follows deals with a multilevel problem in exactly the same way.

Defining goals clearly is essential to both researcher and therapist. It is possible to delineate operational goals at each of the levels of system organization we are discussing. The art comes in maintaining a sense of what level is being dealt with at any given moment, while at the same time not forgetting the larger ramifications. Clues to progress in alcoholism may come from any discipline. They will be utilized only insofar as they can be articulated to others whose education and training may be quite different.

(Definitions and Criteria of Alcoholism

Current definitions of alcoholism are discussed in Volume Two of the *Handbook*, Chapter 48, by Chafetz and Demone. For purposes of this chapter we adapt the following definition of alcoholism: "Alcoholism is any drinking behavior that is associated with dysfunction in a person's life." This definition is meant to encompass all the major spheres of importance to a given person, including his or her sense of self, interpersonal relations, physical well-being, and work.

The disease model of alcoholism has been under heavy fire. In part, this is a reflection of the dissatisfaction generally in some quarters about the "mental illness" concept.[84,131] The basic argument is that such labels have been used punitively and pejoratively to single out people who are societal deviants. In the case of alcoholism, events often seem to show a time lag in relation to the discovery of similar problems in health and mental health in other areas. Thus, the disease concept was propounded in its full-blown form in a classic work by Jellinek in 1960, but is the subject of controversy a decade later.[73]

Jellinek's Forms of Alcoholism

E. M. Jellinek proposed four types of alcoholism.[73] Type *Alpha* consists of purely psychological dependency without loss of control. *Beta* alcoholism is that species in which physiological complications are present, but no physiological or psychological dependence can be demonstrated. *Gamma* alcoholism is the most clear-cut variety, and involves psychological loss of control as well as physiological evidence of tolerance. *Delta* type alcoholism is the same as *Gamma*, with the additional factor of inability to abstain from drinking. The latter was included primarily to describe the pattern most common in France.

Jellinek's views unquestionably were enormously influential. The value of his contribution in regard to the disease concepts of alcoholism was at least twofold. In the first place, he implied that there was a progression in states of alcoholism. This seems reasonable enough, unless one adopts the view that alcoholism is simply the result of drinking too much alcohol. (This latter notion formed part of the basis of the rationale of the Temperance Movement for many years.)[59]

What was more difficult for many to accept was the idea that the progression to full-blown chronic drunkenness, or physical disease and death, was inevitable. At the time that Jellinek's book was written, this was a reasonable hypothesis. However, time has not borne out the postulate of inevitability. In fact, longitudinal studies over time in the field suggest that a large number of people drift in and out of states over a period of years that by all reasonable definitions would be considered alcohol addiction.[21]

In the second place, a usable disease model was a definite advance in attitudes toward the problem *for the time* when it was formulated. The predominant American attitude toward drinking continues to be that the majority who drink alcohol—at least two-thirds of all Americans—do so in order to achieve an altered, and presumably more palatable, state of consciousness. However, Americans are profoundly ambivalent about drinking problems.[49] They look upon the "alcoholic" as the skid-row bum, despite the fact that it is increasingly clear that down-and-outers constitute only 3 to 5 percent, or less, of the total alcoholic population. The origins of the mental

hospital and the tuberculosis sanitorium are the same and both of them deal with the alcoholic person more than with any other single type of diagnostic group of people who are kept out of sight and out of mind.

The disease or illness concept thus permitted the public to reconceive of alcoholism as a problem to understand rather than to deny and penalize. "Free will," the idea that the alcoholic person could stop himself by his own efforts if only he would, has served to prevent the provision of services to the alcoholic person except *in extremis* for many years. The rationale was that help from others would compromise his efforts at self-control. By contrast, the notion of loss of control is quite consistent with psychiatric concepts of the unconscious.

There have also proved to be other uses of the disease model of alcoholism. The gatekeepers, those to whom the alcoholic person is most likely to present himself first, have traditionally been ministers, social workers, the police, and physicians.[75] The concept of illness has provided new avenues of referral that, theoretically at least, should be more likely to route the alcoholic and potentially alcoholic person toward the help he requires. The National Institute on Alcohol Abuse and Alcoholism (NIAAA), the Federal government's primary agency for dealing with alcoholism established by Public Law 91-616 in 1970, has engaged in a campaign to raise public consciousness of alcoholism problems through the media, press, and publishing. These efforts seem to be taking hold.[63] Therefore, it seems likely that the traditional gatekeepers will ultimately be affected as well. In addition, there is a movement afoot to change state laws to remove the offense of drunkenness from the criminal codes books and make alcoholism a health problem instead.

The National Council on Alcoholism Criteria for the Diagnosis of Alcoholism

The National Council on Alcoholism (NCA), the nation's largest voluntary organization dealing with alcoholism, has organized a Criteria Committee which his produced the first recent major effort at consensus in diagnostic criteria for alcoholism.[38] These criteria have now been published all over the world and are being tested for validity. The criteria are meant to be used in conjunction with the American Psychiatric Association (APA) standard psychiatric nomenclature so that the clinician makes a psychiatric diagnosis, a physical diagnosis, and then lists a category or type of alcoholism. In the Diagnostic and Statistical Manual (DSM II), in contrast to the first APA effort at standardizing diagnosis in psychiatry, in DSM I, alcoholism has been removed from the "Personality Disorders" category and given a separate listing, along with the addictions.[36,37] This was done in part to emphasize that alcoholism cuts across all standard psychiatric categories, and can be present in neurosis, schizophrenia, personality disorders, and other conditions.

The format of the NCA criteria is a double set of "tracks". Track I consists of evidence of dependency on alcohol and clinical syndromes of presentation. (For example, alcoholic hepatitis and pancreatitis are included.) Track II is the "Behavioral, Psychological, and Attitudinal" set of symptoms and signs. In each track there are major and minor criteria, and evidence for diagnosis is required from *both* tracks in order to complete a diagnostic picture.

ADVANTAGES OF THE NCA CRITERIA

The NCA criteria bring together much of the present knowledge about alcoholism in a single format, which is meant for clinicians and researchers. It is a handy reference for categorizing symptoms and signs. In addition, it should serve to alert the astute clinician, whether psychiatric or not, to the possibility that his patient is suffering from alcoholism. The criteria are in line with a long tradition in medicine, the best example of which is the Jones Criteria of Rheumatic Fever, in which, when the criteria are used methodically, clinicians in different centers can have an increased degree of confidence that their patients are like those of other physicians who have reported in the literature. The NCA criteria place alcoholism in the same rank with other chronic diseases.

DISADVANTAGES OF THE NCA CRITERIA

Although it is premature to judge the NCA criteria before they have been adequately tested, there appear to be some distinct limitations to them.[28] First, although the criteria are intended, among other things, to differentiate early- from late-stage alcoholism, the emphasis in them is quite clearly upon the later stages, where this diagnosis is more clear-cut. Possible pre-alcoholic phases do not appear at all in the tables of Major and Minor criteria (although some predisposing factors have been outlined separately by the Committee). The most significant use of the NCA criteria, therefore, may prove to be to confirm the diagnosis in those who are already likely to be known as alcoholic people. Yet, the major challenge to the alcoholism field today, from a public health standpoint, is in the *primary prevention* of alcoholism.

Incidence

(For a more complete discussion, see Chafetz and Demone, Chapter 48.) Whereas previously it was necessary to base estimates of alcoholism rates largely upon deaths by cirrhosis, multiplied by appropriate corrections factors, it is now possible to corroborate previous estimates and refine them from large-scale surveys of Americans at large. It has been found that there is a substantial group of people who apparently cure themselves of the symptoms of alcoholism.[21] Several recent studies describe a group of formerly alcoholic people who are able to go back to social drinking, with or without therapy.[21,111,123] This is contrary to the dicta of Alcoholics Anonymous, and suggests that there are subgroups of people with serious drinking problems for whom the return of functionality is quite different.

It has also been found that dysfunctional drinking behavior is normative in certain subpopulations. In the Armed Forces, the majority of men would qualify as alcoholic people by quantity-frequency indices of intake.[22,23] This is also true of some American Indian tribes and Alaskan Native villages, and is highly correlated with severe social deprivation in a number of spheres.

Women as Casualties of Alcoholism

In the past ten years, both in the United States and England, there has been a growing indication that more and more women are developing alcohol problems. The Merseyside (Liverpool) Council on Alcoholism has noted that the ratio of women to men seeking treatment for alcoholism in Britain has increased from eight to one, to four to one.[79] It is difficult to determine statistically the number of women suffering from alcoholism, as they are not as visible as male alcoholics. In the United States, Keller and Efron in 1955 showed a ratio of 5 and 6 men to one alcoholic woman,[78] while in the 1960s, as quoted in Soloman and Black, Chafetz, Demone,[32] reported a ratio of four to one.

Until recently most studies dealt with the alcoholic male and there was little interest in the alcoholic female. Data collected from the NIAAA funded programs indicates that women who come to treatment start drinking at a later age in life than men, but become alcoholic in a shorter span of time, substantiating the findings of Wanberg and Knapp.[138] NIAAA data also indicate that twice as many working women seek help for their alcoholism as do housewives.

Drinking among women is associated with anxiety and depression resulting from crisis situations such as the death of a child, children leaving the home, divorce, desertion, marital problems, menopause, menstrual pains, abortion, and demanding children. Dr. Sharon Wilsnack has found the alcoholic woman experiences chronic doubts about her adequacy as a woman, which are enhanced by acute threats to her feminine adequacy.[145] Her drinking is usually done from 9:00 A.M. to 3:00 P.M. when the children are in school, or until her husband comes home. She feels very

guilty when she is drinking alcohol and, like the alcoholic male, tries to hide her problem from her family.

Biochemistry of Alcohol and Alcoholism

The biochemistry of alcohol and its biochemical effects upon the body have been a subject of recent reviews and will be dealt with here only in passing.[16,69,81,99] Alcohol is absorbed through the gut quite readily, by passive transport, and this is the source of the immediacy of its effects upon the central nervous system. The passage of alcohol is dependent upon body weight, and is significantly slowed by the presence of food in the stomach, particularly proteins. Blood alcohol levels (BAL) have essentially vanished in a normal adult within four hours of ingesting a single dose. However, subsequent doses prolong this process additively. The practical consequences of these facts are that social drinking in moderation and low doses can be entirely compatible with normal function, even driving, after a sufficiently long period, and that the accoutrements of the setting in which alcohol is taken are important determinants of the outcome (e.g., "high" versus drunk).

Under ordinary circumstances, the metabolism of alcohol takes place largely in the liver, although kidneys and lungs may become important ultimate disposition routes when there is significant damage to the liver. The oxidation of alcohol is first to acetaldehyde, generally in the presence of the enzyme alcohol dehydrogenase, in the presence of nicotinamide adenine dinucleotide (NAD).

$$NAD^+ + CH_3CH_2OH \rightleftarrows$$
$$NADH + H^+ + CH_3CHO$$

Then, the aldehyde is oxidized to acetate, in the presence of an NAD requiring aldehyde dehydrogenase.

$$NAD^+ + aldehyde \rightarrow$$
$$carboxylic\ acid + NADH + H^+$$

The acetate thus formed is then metabolized further, as for energy production in the heart. The drug disulfuram (Antabuse®) appears to act as a competitive inhibitor, blocking the breakdown of acetaldehyde and allowing either the aldehyde or another resultant toxic product to build up in the body.[10]

Effects of Alcohol Upon the Nervous System

Alcohol belongs to the CNS depressant group of drugs, and there is cross-tolerance between it and minor tranquilizers, such as chlordiazepoxide (Librium®) and meprobamate (Miltown®). Its absorption into the brain is dependent upon its ability to be absorbed by lipids through cell membranes like other depressants.[121]

However, the observed *behavioral* effects of alcoholism on the organism can be quite variable (see below). In general, its effects on the brain are dose-related, and affect the cortex first, releasing inhibitions in many people, and affect lower centers only later, as the quantity of accumulated alcohol grows. The setting, or context, in which drinking is done has much to do with determining the presentation of the induced behavior, as does also the activity level before and during drinking and the *expectations* of the person doing the drinking. For example, it has been shown that the dose-response curve to a number of drugs is related to the previous activity level, and there is a maximum to this effect.[76] It has even been suggested that commonly observed drunken behaviors in our society are *totally* determined by societal expectation, for which suggestion there is some limited cross-cultural evidence.[89]

At present there are a number of promising possibilities for locating the major biochemical effects of alcohol on the CNS. These range from alcohol's effects upon ionic transport across the nerve cell membrane,[69] to their possible role in relation to neuroamine transmitters,[69] to the plausible hypothesis that methanol may be formed in the body and act as a toxin during withdrawal.[90] The congeners present in alcoholic beverages have also been implicated as toxins, although their role in trace amounts is in considerable dispute.

(Etiology

General Considerations

As alcoholism is a multilevel problem, it is not completely correct to speak of a sole causation. Wender, in an excellent discussion, has pointed out the difference between necessary and sufficient explanations in psychiatry.[142]

We will be using the concept of etiology in three different senses in our discussion: (1) Alcoholism may be a condition in which factors operate at more than one system level (for example, biological predisposition and social reinforcement may be necessary for development of the condition). (2) Alcoholism may not be one disease, but rather a mixture of many behaviors, syndromes, and diseases, each of which has its own etiology. (3) Regardless of what the underlying causation is, alcoholism may best be regarded as a final common pathway with underlying causes sometimes unimportant for prognosis and treatment. What is important is an understanding of the factors that are continuing to reinforce and perpetuate the drinking pattern.

Biological Factors

Alcohol is an addicting drug. If a person drinks large amounts of alcohol over a period of time or if alcohol is administered in large doses to laboratory animals, both tolerance and physical dependence will develop.[48,94, 95] Tolerance is a need for increasing levels of a drug to achieve the same behavioral or biochemical results as previously occurred. Physical dependence is the presence of withdrawal symptoms after the drug has been removed. A traditional view in the field is that alcohol is intrinsically addicting, both because of its production of tolerance and physical dependence as well as its actively-sought euphoric effects.

Recent evidence makes the addictive hypothesis more involved. Researchers have been consistently unable to develop experimental animal models of alcoholism.[95] Primates, for example, are remarkably resistant to voluntarily drinking even weak solutions of alcohol, although tolerance and withdrawal have been seen by some when the primates are forced to drink or alcohol is administered parenterally.[41,42,95,101] Evidence from observing alcoholic people in controlled drinking situations has indicated that many alcoholic people, in fact, have dysphoric experiences (or a transient euphoria followed by a longer dysphoria) when drunk, not the euphoric ones that are so widely predicted.[94,100,107,132,133] Other studies have shown that "behavioral tolerance" may be as important as "metabolic tolerance". The alcohol-dependent person consumes up to one quart a day of alcohol without signs of gross inebriation and little impairment of psychomotor functioning, yet little difference can be demonstrated in the metabolism of alcoholics compared to normal subjects.[94,96,98]

Clinical observations are consistent with the research findings. In the United States a relatively small percentage of alcoholic people drink heavily every day (Jellinek's *Delta* alcoholism). A more common pattern is binge drinking or marked day-to-day fluctuations in the amount of alcohol consumed.[24] Thus, while the addicting properties of alcohol as a drug are important, a pattern similar to that of heroin addiction with frequent drug "craving" is not often observed.

Other evidence for biological factors in alcoholism has come from human genetic studies, particularly the work of Donald Goodwin and his colleagues.[57,58,122] In a recent study done in Denmark with adopted children with high-risk potential for alcoholism, they found that children whose biological parents were alcoholic people had a significantly higher chance of developing alcoholism than a controlled group of adopted children whose biological parents were not alcoholic people.[58] However, again the situation is more complicated than at first appears. When "heavy drinkers" were looked at in addition to "alcoholics," the controlled group, in fact, had a higher incidence of heavy drinkers than the

experimental group. The second complication is that there is at present no way of determining whether the alcoholism was inherited as a specific trait or whether a predisposition to psychopathology was inherited which became manifest as alcoholism in a culture where there is a high incidence and encouragement of drinking. Goodwin quotes from Hebb, who, in writing about intelligence, warned against regarding intelligence as due either to heredity *or* to environment; or partly to one, partly to the other. "Each is fully necessary . . . To ask how much heredity contributes to intelligence is like asking how much the width of a field contributes to its area".[66]

Psychological Theories of Etiology

From Freud on, most psychoanalytic writers have emphasized that alcoholic people have severe oral dependency problems.[9,56,83,86,93] Various writers see these oral conflicts as having stemmed either from early childhood deprivation[93] or overindulgence.[83] As a result of the oral fixation, there are associated problems such as poorly-defended-against rage and hostility, sexual immaturity, depression, schizoid object relations, strong dependency wishes, deep mother fixations, and the use of denial as a defense.[146,147] Alcohol then serves as an escape valve for pent-up feelings, allowing the individual to express both dependency and hostility. (For further discussion of these psychodynamic explanations, the reader is referred to the article by Zwerling and Rosenbaum in the first edition of this Handbook).

In addition to oral dependency, another main theme in the psychoanalytic literature emphasizes the issue of latent homosexuality. Because of frustrations in early mothering, boys turn towards the father, establishing homosexual impulses. Fenichel points out that under the influence of alcohol, the homosexual impulses may come to consciousness and may be acted out.[50] This theory has had little empirical verification.

Other psychoanalytic writers have emphasized other aspects. Menninger sees the self-destructive tendency as being more important than oral dependency and suggests that alcoholism may be both a manifestation of the self-destructive trend as well as a way of averting a greater self-destruction.[102] Rado sees all drug cravings as part of a larger disease which he terms "pharmacothymia" in which pharmacological pleasure replaces normal sexual pleasure.[116] Blum, in reviewing various psychoanalytic theories, concludes that there is no pre-alcoholic personality type and supports multiple determination instead of unitary etiology of alcoholism.[14]

McClelland's Work

Recent empirical and theoretical work by McClelland and his colleagues has led to a new hypothesis: that alcoholic men drink out of a heightened personalized power drive. As McClelland states, "men drink primarily to feel stronger. Those for whom personalized power is of particular concern drink more heavily. . . . the experience centers everywhere in men on increased thoughts of power which, as drinking progresses, become more personal and less socialized and responsible. And societies and individuals with accentuated needs for personalized power are most likely to drink more heavily in order to get the feeling of strength they need so much more than others."[92] Wilsnack, as mentioned above, has developed explanations as to why women drink.[145]

Learning Theory Models

As with psychodynamic explanation, there are numerous learning theory models, variously including classical conditioning, operant conditioning, and social learning.[7,76] Miller and Barlow,[103] for example, point out that the reduction of anxiety from drinking is reinforcing. The alcoholic individual is able to exhibit more varied, spontaneous social behavior and gain increased social reinforcement from relatives and friends. Aversive consequences such as hangover, physical problems, loss of family or employment, and arrests may not decrease drinking because of the long delay between the actual drinking behavior and the occurrence of these events.[137] Mendelson and others, however, as previously

mentioned, have demonstrated that alcoholic individuals experience many aversive consequences *while* drinking. He suggests that "black out" phenomena may lead the individual to remember only the transient pleasurable experiences at the beginning of drinking, thus perpetuating the drinking pattern.[100,133] Davis, et al. point out that the observed dysphoria may also be accompanied by adaptive behaviors which are then reinforced, perpetuating both the behaviors and the drinking pattern.[40]

Family Theories of Etiology

Until the late 1950s, alcoholic people were stereotyped as a group of "undersocialized, poorly integrated individuals comprising homeless derelicts, chronic offenders, and the mentally ill".[4] For example, in 1945 Bacon argued that excessive drinking patterns are more incompatible with marriage than with any other social institution because these patterns effectively preclude the close interpersonal relationship necessary for marriage.[3] As more facts about the alcoholic person and his family have emerged, it has become increasingly clear that family factors are important in causing and maintaining alcoholism and that successful therapy may depend upon recognition of these factors.[1]

The first change in perspective consisted in looking at the wife of the alcoholic man. It was recognized that when the alcoholic husband began to improve, many wives began to exhibit psychiatric difficulties. Other clinical patterns were also evinced, such as a woman marrying a man who was just like her alcoholic father, or a woman who was divorced because of her husband's alcoholism only to marry another alcoholic man. Explanations for these patterns resembled the psychoanalytic hypotheses that sought to explain alcoholism itself. Again, there were discussions of unsatisfied oral needs, dependency conflicts, and masochism.[1,4,6,70,143]

The introduction of family therapy and theory and systems theory into psychiatry in the past ten years has led to new perspectives on the role of alcoholism within a family. Alcoholism is now seen not as a result of individual pathology within one of the family members, but as a result of an interaction among all family members or as part of a behavioral program that maintains a family homeostasis. Steinglass and his colleagues, as well as other workers, have discussed in a series of papers how an ongoing alcoholic pattern may serve to stabilize a family system.[40,47,126,127,139] One important dimension of these theories bears emphasis. Family and systems conceptualizations of alcoholism by and large do not look for ultimate causes of behavior. Rather they would hold that drinking is constantly being reinforced because of its systems homeostatic benefits, and that the role of alcohol in maintaining the family system currently must be understood before any therapeutic intervention can be planned.[40]

A clinical illustration may clarify the above points. It is not uncommon to hear family members say that they can best talk to the alcoholic member of their family when he is drunk. In a sense, the situation has evolved in such a family where emotional interaction takes place only when the alcoholic person is drunk. The result is a habitual behavior pattern which is further reinforced. This pattern is perhaps most vividly portrayed in Eugene O'Neill's play *Long Day's Journey Into Night*.

For a provocative and stimulating theory of the development of alcoholism using systems and cybernetic concepts, the reader is referred to the article by Gregory Bateson, who was also the originator of the double-bind hypothesis concerning the etiology of schizophrenia.[8]

Social Forces and the Etiology of Alcoholism

Alcoholism has been viewed as the non-pareil of social diseases as far as sociologists are concerned. A number of major American figures in sociology and anthropology either got their start dealing with questions about alcoholism, or attempted to deal with them at some point in their careers. Many undoubtedly moved into other areas after having burned their fingers on a problem which seemed to defy solution. Once again, the intellectual history of the study of alcoholism is an illustration that: (1) teasing out single, or simple, sets of problems and solutions is extraordinarily difficult, if not impossible in alcoholism, and (2) a systems approach is likely, at this point in time, to prove the most productive methodology.

Possibly the most fruitful studies to date (see above) have been the ongoing longitudinal surveys of attitudes and drinking practices.[21,23,93,129,130] These have yielded a number of interesting results, as well as sharpening our techniques for measuring such elusive variables as "function" and amount of drug ingested over time.[46] One of the earliest, that of Straus and Bacon, demonstrated that there were definite ethnic and religious patterns to drinking behavior, and these suggested some causal relationships to alcoholism. The McCords in the Cambridge-Somerville Project found highly suggestive evidence of consistent family patterns in the later development of alcoholism. For example, the absent or delinquent father, especially if alcoholic himself, was a strong precursor of alcoholism in his sons. This data is also consistent with that of Robins, who traced the subsequent careers of a series of white children treated in a psychiatric clinic.[117] She demonstrated that over a thirty-year period, the psychopathology of fathers tended to be correlated with the development of later problems, including alcoholism, in the children.

Cahalan and co-workers have published a large series of papers, monographs, and books over the past decade in which a large scale door-to-door sampling on American drinking practices has been taken, and repeated.[21,23] As a result, for the first time, a clear picture of numerous issues has been emerging. Sex differences have been sharply delineated for the first time, and it is clear that drinking problems for women have decreased sharply by age 50, whereas for men they are still rising.

Ethnic and religious differences previously described have been borne out, with some added nuances.[112] For instance, Catholics drink more than Protestants and have more alcohol-related problems. To complicate matters, however, *liberal* Protestants are more likely to be heavy drinkers than conservative Protestants, thus suggesting that, on this dimension at least, the more "fundamentalist" Protestant groups, despite their severe, restrictive and ambivalent attitudes towards alcohol, differ little from Catholics. On the other hand, strength of affiliation, as measured by church-going, had a variable relationship to the sect under consideration. In fact, among Catholic men, there was a slightly *higher* tendency to drink heavily if the interviewee was a church attender.

Much can be learned by comparing how drinking customs and alcoholism rates vary among nations and national groups. It is well known that Italians, Jews, Chinese, and Greeks display substantially less public drunkenness and probably have significantly lower rates of alcoholism.[23,26] In Italian families, wine serves a definitely promotive function to mark festive occasions. The rest of the time, however, it is taken for granted. Children begin to try it early in life. Italians generally do not imbibe alcohol between meals, however. Since it seems likely that recollections of early drinking in childhood are inversely correlated with alcoholism later, this cultural patterning may have lifelong implications for outcome.[135] However, it is impossible to separate out the extent to which the family relationships condition the response to tasting alcohol. Correlation does not necessarily imply cause.

By contrast, the French, like Americans, have incorporated a social notion of *machismo* around drinking. A man is measured by his capacity to hold liquor without staggering. The French drink at meals, but unlike the Italians consider the wine an essential part of the atmosphere. Moreover, especially in the working class, wine may serve as a between-meals refresher as well. Aside from showing one of the highest cirrhosis rates in the world, the French have developed a type of alcoholism all their own which corresponds to Jellinek's *Delta* type alcoholic person, one in whom tolerance develops but a steady significant dosage input is necessary to maintain him without evidence of tremors or delirium.[73]

Drinking Versus Drunkenness

Our society often confuses drinking and drunkenness. We once embarked upon a "noble experiment" to eliminate drinking. Yet, during and after Prohibition we have continued to regard drunkenness as a joke and even sometimes as something to be admired. This attitude of condoning irresponsible behavior, of accepting the unacceptable because "I was drunk" or "the poison in the bottle made me do it," will prevent us from making significant progress in the treatment of alcoholism, no matter how much new research is done or how much money is spent.

Styles of drinking behavior, including quantity and frequency of ingestion, are, of course, matters of private decision and likely to remain so. Nevertheless, it is clear that important factors besides conscious decision-making are operative in determining both the process and outcome of drinking alcohol. Those cultures in which alcoholic beverages are of relatively little importance are also the same ones which tend to condemn drunkenness. Chinese and Jews tend to look upon the drunken man not as an object of humor, but of pity or scorn. By contrast, "drunk" jokes are a staple of general American humor.

Alcohol as an Aspect of a Multiple Drug-Taking Culture

Anecdotal reports from numerous centers indicate that cross-addiction to two or more drugs, such as heroin and alcohol, is more common than was previously recognized. It is reasonable to speculate that this is a result of the acceptability of ingesting multiple drugs in our society, whether or not they are physician-prescribed. A series of waves of popularity in the use of particular drugs over the course of the twentieth century has obscured the fact that the availability of a given drug at a given time was the most salient reason for its use. Efforts are being made to coordinate alcohol and drug programs at Federal, State, and local levels in recognition of this fact. However, the success of such joint ventures may depend upon the extent to which drug use is set into the perspective of the social forces at work in our culture.

([Consequences of Alcoholism

Whether drinking alcohol is considered cause or result, there are numerous patterns that develop in the course of dysfunctional drinking behavior. These are described by system level in the sections that follow. None of them should be conceptualized as irreversible. Even in its severe stages, cirrhosis of the liver is known to improve markedly when drinking ceases for months to years. From a practical standpoint, some restoration of function is possible for anyone at any stage of alcoholism.

Biological Consequences

It is a truism rarely observed in practice, that every patient requires a physical examination, whether or not he be labelled a psychiatric or alcoholic case. On the other hand, it is customary in the hospital-based practice of medicine to undertake heroic efforts to correct metabolic imbalances in alcoholic people acutely ill, while passing off the underlying alcoholism problems with a brief psychiatric consultation or a referral to Alcoholics Anonymous. Similarly, it is usual to assess the patient's *dis*ability both medical and psychiatric, whereas his residual *ability*, which is not necessarily measurable in the same ways as his disability, may be much more important in formulating treatment plans and prognosis.

The cardinal measures of "irreversible" tissue damage associated secondarily with alcoholism are brain damage and liver damage. A moderately abnormal EEG, the hallmark of delirium and dementia,[43] which remains abnormal over time, may be quite consistent with recovery from alcoholism, and with the maintenance of relatively stable interpersonal relations, holding a job, and psychological comfort. Although cirrhosis of the liver is generally considered the end stage of persistently

heavy drinking of the drug, the largest number of pathological diagnoses at autopsy, some of which are, of course, alcoholic, are made on previously unsuspected livers.[61] In other words, a substantial number of cirrhotics go undiscovered during life, and are presumably normal people.

Nevertheless, although we deliberately emphasize the constructive uses of alcoholism, we do this as a matter of reapportioning emphasis, not of ignoring possible causal relationships with other diseases. It is known that the greatest single pathological correlate with pancreatitis is alcoholism. The involvement of alcohol ingestion in several forms of cancers is currently being investigated.[65] The role of alcohol in relationship to heart disease has been investigated in various total community surveys and there are preliminary suggestions that in low doses alcohol may actually be protective against myocardial infarction and angina, whereas in high doses it may substantially weaken the myocardium.[82] Similarly, a host of neurological syndromes are well described. Of these, Wernicke-Korsakoff's psychosis, memory loss and confabulation with concomitant internuclear opthalmoplegia, is perhaps the best known, although a relatively unusual entity. More generally, a mild but significant impairment of cognitive function may be present on routine neurological examination when mental status is assessed.

The importance of the crosscurrents between the primary (behavioral) manifestations of alcoholism and the secondary consequences of toxic damage from alcohol is that it is more often than not impossible for any one person to be able to deal with the totality of the patient's medical problems. In much the same way that multiple agencies and persons may be involved in the psychological treatment of the alcoholic person, so, too, in the medical sphere self-reliance by the physician is no virtue.

Alcohol and Other Organ Systems

Alcohol is a food in the sense that it has caloric value. It can, therefore, substitute for other routinely available calories, which are ingested in more nutritious forms (e.g., protein). For this reason, it is quite possible to be "starving amidst plenitude," while ingesting a total daily intake of calories equivalent to an adult minimum. Whether alcohol causes liver damage directly, or only in the presence of relative nutrition deficit, is still a matter of dispute.[39] However, it seems clear that there is some type of interaction between the two, and the result is cirrhosis of the liver. In the end stages of liver damage, hepatic coma may confuse the picture of drunkenness and add to the effects of alcohol ingestion (although no specific product to date has been shown to correlate well with the stages of hepatic coma).

Other fairly frequent physical manifestations of alcohol-induced disease include cutaneous stigmata, cardiomyopathies, skeletal myopathies, peripheral neuritis, and blood dyscrasias (especially anemias).

Psychological Consequences

Many writers have commented on the psychological changes that occur in an alcoholic person once he is trapped in a vicious drinking cycle. Glatt mentions feelings of guilt, inability to discuss problems, grandiose and aggressive behavior, persistent remorse, failure of promises and resolutions, loss of other interest, avoidance of important responsibilities, loss of ordinary willpower, moral deterioration, impaired thinking, indefinable fears, inability to initiate action, and vague spiritual desires as the alcoholic person moves from occasional relief drinking to obsessive drinking in vicious cycles.[54] John Berryman, in his novel *Recovery*, describes what it is like to go through some of these experiences.

We wish to emphasize three aspects of psychological changes, an understanding of which can be helpful for initiating successful treatment. (1) *Concern with alcohol.* The individual who previously drank alcohol only under certain circumstances finds drinking increasing and, perhaps more important, he is often concerned with alcohol when not drinking. It becomes very important for him to know where his next drink is coming from,

and he may start hiding bottles around his house or planning his daily events so that alcohol is always available. It should be emphasized that in some ways knowing where he can get alcohol is more important than the actual drinking. He can increase or decrease his drinking to a considerable degree as long as he knows that he will not be completely cut off from alcohol. (2) *Denial.* As anyone who has a friend or relative who is an alcoholic person knows, the alcoholic individual persistently thinks up rationalizations as to why he does not have a drinking problem. He may talk about the particular type of alcohol he consumes or might insist that he is a heavy drinker and not alcoholic. The denial becomes even more strong when directly challenged, since often an alcoholic person is now defining himself totally by his drinking and a challenge to that identity may represent the challenge to his basic identity. It is important when attempting to challenge the denial of an alcoholic individual that recognition also be given to the beneficial aspects that alcohol is playing in his life as well as recognizing what underlying personality strengths there are that have not been affected by alcohol. (3) *Self-loathing.* Society usually focuses on the harm that the alcoholic individual does to others. A closer look reveals that these manifestations of outward aggression are often in reaction to intense feelings of self-disgust. The alcoholic individual is also caught in a vicious cycle where he acts out one drunk to release those intolerable feelings and winds up loathing himself even more when he sobers up, only to express the anger again during the next drunken episode. It is crucial not to further reinforce the cycle and accept the alcoholic person's low estimate of his self-worth which may be an important precursor of suicide. Working toward an alcoholic individual's better acceptance of himself, again emphasizing his strengths, as well as his weaknesses, can interrupt the vicious cycle.

Family Consequences

The vicious cycle or positive feedback loop that the individual alcoholic person is caught in is usually part of a similar process that exists in the family. The non-alcoholic spouse accuses the alcoholic person of ruining the family life; the alcoholic spouse explains the drinking by saying it is the only way to tolerate the family life that the spouse has created. Mutual recriminations can escalate to separation and divorce, violence, or a situation that everyone considers intolerable but which may persist for years. One very striking aspect of such a situation is the unpredictability of the fluctuation of positions. Promises to stop drinking switch into adamant threats to increase drinking. Threats by the non-alcoholic spouse to leave the impossible situation alternate with decisions to stick out the situation and help the "sick" alcoholic spouse.

Sexual relationships, often not wholly gratifying before the increase in drinking, become a further source of strain. One such pattern in this area is the sexual approach of the alcoholic individual while drunk, the rejection of the approach by the spouse because of drunkenness ("it's disgusting"), and then increased drinking because of hurt pride.

Children in particular are unfortunately affected by such a situation. The rapid fluctuations in the alcoholic spouse, and often, in the non-alcoholic spouse, make consistent parental guidance almost impossible. At times, outright child abuse may occur, but the greater problem is how the child copes with a situation in which he is alternately ignored, smothered with love, and then perhaps blamed for the entire situation.

Some children may attempt to cope with the situation by developing behavioral problems themselves. Others may assume a family role by being over-responsible and in a sense becoming their parents' parent.

Children may also be harmed physically by a mother's heavy drinking. A recent study suggests that there is a greater chance for birth defects in children born to mothers who are heavy drinkers.*

---

* Jones, K. L., Smith, D. W., Ulleland, C. N., Streissguth, A. P. "Pattern of Malformation in Offspring of Chronic Alcoholic Mothers," *Lancet*, 1 (1973) 1267–1271. In a small sample, alcoholism was correlated with fetal malformation.

Some of the long-term sequelae of being raised in a family with alcohol problems are the development of alcoholism, marrying an alcoholic person, or developing other psychiatric disorders. Much future research needs to be done in this area to determine the exact risk to these children, as well as to develop techniques to establish a true primary prevention program.[31,52]

Social Consequences

The reader is referred to M. E. Chafetz and H. W. Demone, Chapter 48, Volume 2 of the *American Handbook of Psychiatry*.

⟮ The Natural History of Alcoholism

In treating any condition it is important to know what its natural history would be if treatment were not offered. The understanding that there is more than one natural history in alcoholism is essential for any formulation of treatment plans. We wish to emphasize that alcoholism is a chronic problem. While we have argued above that the medical model has some usefulness in treating alcoholism, the *acute* medical model so often taught in medical school has very little relevance to most situations. The four categories of natural history patterns offered here are not inclusive and are intended mainly to encourage workers in the field to keep in mind the importance of changes through time in alcoholism.

Downward Spiral

Alcoholism has traditionally been viewed as a progressive disease or condition. The potential alcoholic person starts as a social drinker, becomes increasingly psychologically and physiologically dependent upon alcohol, and eventually reaches the point where alcohol totally dominates his life. According to this viewpoint, there is a corresponding deterioration in the alcoholic's family, work, and social functioning. Eventually, as the downward spiral continues the alcoholic "hits bottom", a point at which he is defeated physically, emotionally, and socially and at which time therapy, particularly the Alcoholics Anonymous approach, can finally be effective to help the alcoholic individual understand the destructive consequences of his drinking. If he does not receive help at this point, the traditional theory would hold that he is likely to wind up a skid-row derelict.

In more recent years, there has been considerable revision of the traditional position. Alcoholics Anonymous now speaks of "high bottom" and "low bottom". A "high bottom" is direct recognition by the alcoholic individual of his powerlessness over his drinking and its consequences without having depleted his social and emotional resources. The alcoholic individual can seek help with his functioning still relatively intact. However, if help is not forthcoming, the traditional view would hold that the downward spiral would continue. More recent observations, however, have indicated that there are a number of alternative courses for alcoholism to take and that the view that all alcoholic persons, if untreated, will show a progressive downhill course is both incorrect and potentially countertherapeutic.

Steady State

The steady state drinker is the one about whom arguments will often develop as to whether he is a social drinker or an alcoholic person. Alcohol plays an extremely important part in his life, but there is no evidence for a downward spiral for many years, if ever. Included in this group is the physiologically addicted individual, classically seen in France, or the Delta alcoholic of Jellinek, who drinks large amounts of alcohol every day, but shows no obvious malfunctioning in his family or work life. Often this person eventually seeks help when physical sequelae of drinking finally appear. Another drinking pattern that might fall in this group is the individual who may only drink one or two drinks a day, but that drinking has an inordinate importance to him. Clearly such an individual is not "sick" by most definitions and such a pattern may

persist unchanged for a lifetime, but care must be paid to the possibility of this pattern's switching into one of the other patterns mentioned here.

Fluctuating State

The most common drinking pattern seen in American society is one that waxes and wanes. There may be a predictable periodicity, such as getting drunk every weekend or going on a binge every six weeks, or drinking episodes may be irregular, often reflecting episodes of psychological, family, or job stress. Frequently in these instances, the use of alcohol and drunken behavior, although clearly having a disruptive effect upon the alcoholic individual and his family, also has a definite adaptive effect, serving as an escape valve for certain tensions that have been building up and are felt to be inexpressible without the assistance of alcohol.

Spontaneous Recovery

Perhaps as many as one-third of people with drinking problems spontaneously recover. Not enough is known at this time as to whether they become social drinkers or become totally abstinent. Similarly it is not known how often they slip back into a pathological drinking pattern. Possible explanations for this pattern include "will-power", a realistic appraisal of the consequences of drinking, and changed family and social circumstances.

(Therapy and Alcoholism

The plethora of theories of causation of alcoholism is matched only by the multiplicity of treatment modalities, some of them quite offbeat and exotic, and perhaps applicable to therapy of other conditions besides alcoholism. The correspondence between theory and therapy is quite low. This should not be surprising from what has been said above. The multifarious threads of causation and participation in the condition of alcoholism are so interwoven that it is unlikely that very many close connections could be made between theory and practice.

In fact, there are essentially as many treatments possible as there are people to receive them. Because a person happens to come through the doors of a clinic or office specializing in a particular brand of treatment does not mean that the client must be molded to fit the Procrustean bed of the available method. What patients want is not necessarily the same as what therapists think they want, unless therapists listen very carefully;[71] what therapists want for patients may not be available in that particular program.[85] Often the client requires an advocate who can help him to navigate the treatment and social systems. Ideally, this should be somebody who is trained for this particular job, such as a counselor into whose job description this is written. However, in the real world, it is likely to be the primary job of the first person who sees him, especially in therapy.

We wish to reemphasize that, whatever the form of therapy, the therapist must keep in mind the positive role alcohol is playing in the patient's life. The negative aspects have been repeatedly emphasized by family, the law, and other "helpers". Recognition of positive behaviors that previously could only be expressed when drunk and the development of a plan to allow expression of them without resorting to alcohol are indispensable for effective treatment.[40]

Some generalizations about therapy are warranted, and a classification scheme is useful for descriptive purposes. We proceed in the following sections from chemobiological therapies, to individual, to family, and to social and other therapies.

Biological Treatment

Biological treatment includes treatment of the sequelae of alcoholism and treatment aimed at preventing and reducing further drinking. In treating the possible sequelae of alcoholism, particular care must be given to prevention and treatment of Wernicke's syndrome and delirium tremens, both of which are relatively rare but potentially quite serious. Any poorly nourished alcoholic person should receive large doses of thiamine and other B-vitamins to prevent Wernicke's syndrome, particularly if he is admitted to the hospital and receiving parenteral glucose. To prevent and treat delirium tremens, it must be recognized that its onset occurs about 72 to 96 hours after withdrawal of alcohol and ends fatally in about 15 percent of untreated cases. The most important aspect of management of delirium tremens is to make sure the patient is well hydrated and to correct any electrolyte imbalances, including magnesium. Use of major or minor tranquilizers may be helpful in decreasing the patient's agitation, but there is, at present, no evidence that they decrease the mortality rate from delirium tremens.[136]

Other withdrawal symptoms from alcohol occur in the first twenty-four to forty-eight hours after cessation of drinking and are not as potentially serious as delirium tremens. Here major and minor tranquilizers are both helpful in decreasing agitation and allowing the patient to sleep. Chlordiazepoxide (Librium®), given either orally or parenterally, is most commonly used although it has not been clearly demonstrated that it has therapeutic advantages over either the major tranquilizers or paraldehyde.[136]

When treating the medical sequelae of alcoholism, it is particularly important to adopt a nonjudgmental, nonmoralistic attitude. Particular care must be given to avoid "scare tactics," since one of the common results of such an approach is to increase subsequent drinking because of the anxiety generated by being confronted with the lurid details of all the possible damage that alcohol can cause. However, neither should a patient's denial of problems be supported. More important than what is said is how it is said. Many medical personnel who work on detoxification units and general medical wards become discouraged with recurrent admissions of alcoholic people for medical problems, but the situation can be changed by both an attitudinal and behavior change on the part of medical personnel, as well as the establishment of a therapy system where the alcoholic person can get meaningful support.

Attempts up to the present to prevent further drinking by biological treatment have had only a limited success. Most commonly used are disulfiram (Antabuse®) and chlordiazepoxide (Librium®). By taking one tablet of Antabuse each morning, the alcoholic person knows that he will be violently ill if he ingests even a small amount of alcohol in any form. Some therapists have found disulfiram very helpful in maintaining an initial sobriety that enables the alcoholic person to become involved in other therapeutic modalities.[10] An occasional patient will prefer to take disulfiram regularly for the rest of his life, helping him to resist any urges to resume drinking. A large number of alcoholic people, however, do not find disulfiram beneficial. If they desire to drink, they merely skip their medicine for one or two days. If they are forced to take medication, by being either institutionalized or forced to report every day for observation to see they take the medication, they often become covertly angry at their treatment and will seize upon the first opportunity to sabotage it.

Chlordiazepoxide and other minor tranquilizers have been widely used in the outpatient treatment of alcoholism by physicians. The rationale is that the medication will decrease the patient's anxiety, thereby lessening the amount of drinking. The results have been quite disappointing. Sometimes the patient may develop an addiction to the medication instead of alcohol or he may even take both the medication and alcohol. Recent studies have indicated that antidepressants and major tranquilizers may be more effective than minor tranquilizers in relieving symptoms of anxiety and depression.[19,20,67,108] It should be emphasized that meaningful interpersonal interaction is more helpful than giving medication for nonspecific reasons. If a psychiatrist finds himself giving medication as a way of getting rid of an alcoholic patient, he would be far better advised to spend a little extra time with the alcoholic person and make an appropriate therapy referral.

Biological treatment toward preventing or diminishing further drinking may be success-ful when there is a concurrent or underlying psychiatric condition that is usually amenable to drug therapy. The manic-depressive patient who drinks, the individual who has an increase in drinking related to becoming severely depressed, or the schizophrenic who drinks as a sort of self-medication may each respond to lithium, significant doses of antidepressants, or phenothiazines. Kline, in addition, has recently found that lithium administered to a group of men who had been hospitalized for detoxification without symptoms of manic-depressive illness significantly reduced the number of future detoxifications although the men continued to drink.[82a] If this study is confirmed, lithium might prove a valuable tool in helping to decrease morbidity associated with alcoholism.

An important area of research at present is an attempt to find the essential blocker of the effects of alcohol similar to cyclazocine or naloxone with opiate addiction as well as to discover a similar or different "sobering-up pill" which an individual could take, for example, when he wished to drive home after a party where he was drinking. Even if such a medication can be developed, it remains to be seen how acceptable it will be both to the general public and to alcoholic people.

Other forms of biological treatment that have been advanced in alcoholism are the use of LSD and megavitamins. Although there were some reports of initial success with LSD, Ludwig's more recent work casts considerable doubt upon the specific value of LSD in the treatment of alcoholism.[88] Megavitamins definitely have a place in treating the sequelae of alcoholism, but there is at present no evidence that they have any other role in treatment.

Individual Therapy

A number of earlier papers have stressed the role of psychodynamics in alcoholism. Oral perversions, based upon deprivations at an early age, have been postulated and utilized in the understanding of the therapeutic process. We now feel that this mode of thinking has only limited usefulness for a limited group of people. Individual therapy can be successful with alcoholic people, but the productivity appears to be lower, both in terms of time input and improvement in function, than with other types of therapies such as group and family therapy. Nevertheless, individual therapy may continue to be a mode of treatment in the field which many will use. Therefore, it is helpful to understand what factors contribute to a happy conclusion for the client.

What therapists whose patients improve seem to have in common is largely their affective characteristics. These include empathy and unconditional warm positive regard.[134] It behooves the therapist of alcoholic people to be an energetic activist. This most emphatically does not mean that he must charge into rescuing the client from each crisis. However, it does mean that he must share of himself as a human being, of what he is feeling at the moment. Alcoholic people in therapy are constantly testing the limits of a therapeutic contract. This creates anger in the therapist. Although inappropriate anger with patients is not useful, sharing with the patient what effect he has on others by his behavior is an important component of helping him to create a new self-awareness.

We have remarked above that the search for an "alcoholic personality" has been largely fruitless. Nonetheless, passive dependency does occur among a significant percentage of alcoholic people who appear for therapy. This is perhaps the most difficult personality trait for most therapists to handle. Again, all therapy is in a sense behavioral in that it requires feedback to the person seeking help about the effects of his behavior. An appropriate goal of therapy for such a person might be to decrease the number of instances of passive resistance *whether or not he understands why this decrease is happening.* Treatment of alcoholism is the paradigm of a therapy in which understanding is not necessarily the ideal end point.

Even when an alcoholic person is engaged with an individual therapist, this rarely turns out to be the only significant person in his treatment. We recommend the provision of a coordinator, who can be of counselor status, to make sure that all the various modalities of help, including social and rehabilitation efforts, are consistent with one another.

Alcoholics Anonymous

Alcoholics Anonymous has historically been the most important modality in treating alcoholism, and it remains very influential.[91] The reader is referred to the chapter by Chafetz and Demone for further discussion of this important modality.

Family Therapy

In the last few years there has been increasing interest in using family therapy to treat alcohol problems. Many alcohol treatment programs now routinely see the spouse of the identified alcoholic and often the children or other extended-family members. If the active drinker refuses to come to sessions, some therapists are now comfortable in holding regular sessions with other family members to examine and change their role in perpetuating the drinking patterns, with the result that these patterns change without the formal participation of the identified alcoholic person.[35]

Techniques used in family therapy of other problems can, with little modification, be used in treating families with alcohol problems. Bowen, for example, has described how he works with alcoholic families in similar ways to other families.[17,18] Alternative methods such as pointing out and actively changing repetitive communicational and behavior patterns and the use of paradoxical instructions can likewise be used.[2,60,119] Therapists and family members have the tactical option of focusing on the role drinking is playing in the relationship or on other family difficulties which the drinking is serving to cover up, or which contribute to the drinking.[15]

An advantage of family therapy is that once destructive drinking has stopped within the family, family therapy can proceed to work on other issues, seeking to establish new relationship patterns that prevent a return of drinking or a future separation of the couple. An opportunity is also presented to work on preventing the transmission of alcoholic drinking patterns to the next generation in the family. If such follow-up therapy is not done, there may occur such phenomena as a spouse becoming depressed, family members consciously or unconsciously manipulating the alcoholic member to resume drinking, separation or divorce, and delinquent behavior or alcoholism in the children.

The importance of treating the entire family has been recognized in the formation of Al-Anon and Al-Ateen as adjuncts to Alcoholics Anonymous. An interesting recent development in Washington, D.C. and perhaps elsewhere is the establishment of a social club for alcoholic people and their spouses, where both can go for social events, as well as for a modified form of couples' group therapy. It seems quite possible that this represents the beginning of a trend to see couples and families together rather than separately, as well as an early recognition that the issue in families is not how a "healthy spouse" deals with a "sick spouse", but how they deal together with a mutual interactional problem in which alcohol plays a very important role.[5,45,47,55]

At the present, there is little more than anecdotal studies that validate the promise of a family therapy approach.[44] In part, this can be explained by the newness of this type of therapy. However, there may also be issues which are qualitatively different in evaluating family therapy compared to individual therapy. For example, is it a success if an alcoholic individual stops drinking, but he or his wife becomes more depressed or gets divorced? Conversely, is it a success if drinking persists at the same level as before, but the family now is able to communicate better with less fighting?

Social Therapy

The concept of the network approach to problems has been elaborated in psychiatry by Ross V. Speck and his co-workers.[124] They attempt to draw as large a community of people together as is necessary to deal with a mental health problem. Their focus is upon those immediately surrounding the family of an identified patient. This approach has been tried on a limited basis in dealing with alco-

holic people. An effort is made to "surround" the drinking person in all major spheres of his life: family, work, personal relations—even the bar where he drinks. A concentrated effort is made to have all the significant people in his life deal with him in fundamentally the same, consistent way.

The notion of networks, however, is worthy of much wider application. First, it is not sufficient to identify a single person in the family as "the problem," nor for that matter, is it usually helpful to isolate a family in a neighborhood by drawing attention to them as the neighborhood black sheep. It can, on the other hand, be quite useful to help communities organize around the issues that are important to them. This implies a two-stage process: at the outset, raising consciousness of the existence of a problem; later, it becomes important to advise on an approach to handling the problem. For example, it is known that alcoholic people have a high rate of suicide within six weeks of a serious loss in their lives. It is possible to institute a community-wide monitoring system of all such losses among the identified alcoholic population, and thereby prevent a significant percentage of suicides.

For a further discussion of social therapy and the establishment of treatment and prevention programs, the reader is referred to Chapter 48 by Chafetz and Demone.

Miscellaneous Therapies

The proliferation of psychiatric treatments has been reflected in alcoholism therapy. Aversion therapy, encounter groups, gestalt therapy, videotape confrontation, transactional analysis, biofeedback, transcendental meditation, psychodrama, have all been used in alcoholism treatment.[25,51,109,125,141] Again, there is no convincing evidence of the utility or lack of utility of these approaches, and we wish to reemphasize the importance of the therapist's recognizing the adaptive and maladaptive consequences of alcohol in his client's life, and using particular techniques in an overall strategy, rather than trying to fit the patient into one particular form of therapy.

Two of the above therapies deserve special

mention. Aversion therapy has received glowing reports by some as a way of eliminating drinking behavior. Patients in whom alcoholism is more of a "bad habit" being currently maintained by forces in his environment and who are freely willing to go through what is an unpleasant experience may indeed benefit from aversion therapy. However, the therapist must be aware that the drinking behavior that is usually extinguished in aversion therapy is only part of the overall picture of alcoholism and that alcoholic people may often behave in a passive, superficially compliant way, while resisting underneath, a pattern that may in fact be reinforced by aversion therapy.

Transactional analysis, which is a particular type of group therapy, has become popular because it is easily understandable by both therapist and patient and because its emphasis on games, roles, and scripts is catchy and often therapeutically useful.[125] Care must be taken to maintain a systems overview of problems encountered by the alcoholic individual rather than saying that everything is a game, also making sure that group therapy does not become an excuse for the venting of the therapist's and group members' aggression upon people who are often not accustomed to protecting themselves.

(Evaluation of Treatment Outcome

As has been emphasized in the previous sections, there are relatively few clear-cut indications for specific treatments in alcoholism. Over the next few years we may become more precise as to what approaches are likely to be successful in specific instances, but we are unlikely ever to reach the point where we can develop standardized protocols for the treatment of alcoholism. For this reason, it is of the utmost necessity for each therapist to establish individualized goals in collaboration with his alcoholic client and his family and then to *evaluate*, again in connection with the alcoholic person and his family, how successfully the goals have been achieved. A useful methodology for establishing goals and evaluating progress is the problem-oriented record as developed by Weed,[140] with the possible addition of Goal Attainment Scaling.[80] Such an approach is widely used at present in medicine, and the field of alcoholism, with its conglomeration of the medical, psychiatric, and social, would seem to be an ideal field in which to expand the use of the problem-oriented record.

(Training and Alcoholism

While many people would probably agree that medicine is the primary discipline for alcohol studies, the need for others to be educated in alcoholism and the specific locus within medicine and the medical school where training should be centered are open to question. Dr. Barry Stimmel of the Mount Sinai School of Medicine in New York has indicated that only 15% of medical students chose elective courses in drugs and alcohol during their first year.[128] Furthermore, despite the listing of more than ten electives for the final year, only four students actually availed themselves of the opportunity to enroll in such courses. One may conjecture the extent to which this reflects the prevailing attitudes of medical faculties despite the major upswing in interest in the subject elsewhere.

The reluctance of medical schools to become involved in developing programs in alcoholism and addiction is reflected in the fact that the National Institute on Alcohol Abuse and Alcoholism and the National Institute on Drug Addiction had been able to make only eighteen awards in the "Career Teachers" program by the end of 1973.[104] This has occurred in spite of the fact that every approved application has been funded. There has been discussion concerning the needs for subspecialties in alcoholism and the addictions. In our view, subspecialties in alcoholism and the addictions would probably lead to a slightly increased supply of specialists without addressing the fundamental question of whether alcoholic people would be better served by specialists or generalists.

We know that in developing our training plans we must think in terms of comprehensiveness. There is a need to focus medical education for alcoholism on primary prevention.

([Toward an Ethos of Responsibility in Drinking

In Chapter 48 of the *Handbook* some concepts of prevention in alcoholism are outlined. To these must be added another dimension: the idea of "responsible drinking." We have indicated that, in our view, whatever the causal relationships in the genesis of alcohol-related problems, alcoholism in its outcome remains primarily a social issue. In essence, and grossly oversimplified, the difficulty lies in our society's ambivalence toward the drunken person (see above for a discussion of Drinking versus Drunkenness). Each member of the society has obligations as part of the social contract, not only to others, but perhaps even more important, to himself. We are accustomed to thinking of self-respect, the dignity of one's self-image, and the sense of well-being as rights. However, they are also duties in several ways, for insofar as we value individual human life we owe it to ourselves to act responsibly. This is exactly what we feel needs to be elaborated and disseminated widely about drinking practices. People who choose to drink alcohol—and most do—need to have knowledge of its effects. In addition, they must have the opportunity to consider the probable consequences of their taking the drug alcohol.

In settings that are reasonable for a given person, with people who will further the individual's responsible use of alcohol, the use of alcohol can and should be healthy. For instance, a number of geriatric programs have come to realize that modest amounts of alcohol are viewed far more positively by participants than tranquilizers to achieve the same

effects with approximately the same risk. There is every reason to expect that such constructive usages can be expanded broadly into other areas.

It is also known that certain drinking practices tend to maximize the desired effects of alcohol and minimize the adverse effects: (1) Drinking small amounts, well-diluted and taken in combination with food; (2) finding congenial and relaxed settings; (3) avoiding drinking to relieve tension; (4) avoiding situations in which drinking is equated with manliness. Although some of these are clearly culture-specific, it involves no value judgment to point out that they can be incorporated to useful effect by other people.

The National Institute on Alcohol Abuse and Alcoholism has recently embarked upon a campaign to promote responsible drinking. The Federal government's only division-level prevention program has been organized, and it will operate with the goal of facilitating a change in the American image of what drinking practices can and should be. One of the first steps will be to draw attention to those subgroups of the culture which do assume a responsible attitude toward drinking alcohol and drug use, and to seek to understand what factors make this possible.

([Bibliography

1. ABLON, J. "Family Structure and Alcoholism," in B. Kissin and H. Begleiter, eds., *Biology of Alcoholism: Social Biology* (Vol. 4). New York: Plenum Press, 1974, in press.

2. ACKERMAN, N. *Treating the Troubled Family.* New York: Basic Books, 1966.

3. BACON, S. D. "Excessive Drinking and the Institution of the Family," in *Quarterly Journal of Studies on Alcohol*, ed., ALCOHOL, SCIENCE, AND SOCIETY. New Haven: Yale Summer School of Alcohol Studies, 1945, 223–238.

4. BAILEY, M. B. "Alcoholism and Marriage: A Review of Research and Professional Literature," *Quarterly Journal of Studies on Alcohol*, 22 (1961), 81 ff.

5. BAILEY, M. B. "Al-Anon Family Groups as an Aid to Wives of Alcoholics," *Social Work*, 10 (1965), 68.

6. BALLARD, R. B. "The Interaction between Marital Conflict and Alcoholism as Seen Through MMPIs of Marriage Partners," *American Journal of Orthopsychiatry*, 29 (1959), 528 ff.

7. BANDURA, A. *Principles of Behavior Modification.* New York: Holt, Rinehart & Winston, 1969.

8. BATESON, G. "The Cybernetics of Self: A Theory of Alcoholism," *Psychiatry*, 34 (1971), 1–18.

9. BERTRAND, S., J. MASLING. "Oral Imagery and Alcoholism," *Journal of Abnormal Psychology*, 74 (1969), 50–53.

10. BILLET, S. L. "Antabuse Therapy," in R. Catanzaro, ed., *Alcoholism: The Total Treatment Approach.* Springfield, Illinois: Charles C. Thomas, 1968.

11. BLANE, H. T. *The Personality of the Alcoholic.* New York: Harper and Row, 1968.

12. BLOCK, M. A. *Alcoholism: Its Facets and Phases.* New York: John Day Co., 1966.

13. BLUM, E. M. "Psychoanalytic Views of Alcoholism: A Review," *Quarterly Journal of Studies on Alcohol*, 27 (1966), 250–290.

14. BLUM, E. M., R. H. BLUM. *Alcoholism: Modern Psychological Approaches to Treatment.* San Francisco: Jossey–Bass, 1967.

15. BOLMAN, W. N. "Abstinence Versus Permissiveness in the Psychotherapy of Alcoholism: A Pilot Study and Review of Some Relevant Literature," *Archives General Psychiatry*, 12 (1965), 456–563.

16. BOURNE, P. G., R. FOX. *Alcoholism: Progress in Research and Treatment.* New York: Academic Press, 1973.

17. BOWEN, M. "Alcoholism as Viewed Through Family Systems Theory and Family Psychotherapy," presentation before Annual Meeting, National Council of Alcoholism, Washington, D.C., April 3, 1973.

18. ———. "Family Therapy and Family Group Therapy" in, Kaplan, H. and Sadock, B., eds., *Comprehensive Group Psychotherapy.* Baltimore: Williams & Wilkins, 1971.

19. BUTTERWORTH, A. T. "Depression Associated with Alcohol Withdrawal: Imipramine Therapy Compared with Placebo," *Quarterly Journal of Studies on Alcohol*, 32 (1971), 343–348.

20. BUTTERWORTH, A. T., R. D. WATTS. "Treatment of Hospitalized Alcoholics with Doxepin and Diazepam: A Controlled Study," *Quarterly Journal of Studies on Alcohol*, 32 (1971), 78–81.

21. CAHALAN, D. *Problem Drinkers.* San Francisco: Jossey–Bass, 1970.

22. CAHALAN, D. and I. H. CISIN. *Report of a Pilot Study of the Attitudes and Behavior of Naval Personnel Concerning Alcohol and Problem Drinking.* BSSR:452. Washington, D.C.: Bureau of Social Science Research, Inc., 1973.

23. CAHALAN, D., I. H. CISIN, H. M. CROSSLEY. *American Drinking Practices.* New Brunswick, New Jersey: Journal of Studies on Alcohol, 1969.

24. CAHALAN, D., I. H. CISIN, G. L. GARDNER and G. C. SMITH. *Drinking Practices and Problems in the U.S. Army 1972.* Report 73–6. Arlington, Virginia: Information Concepts, Inc., 1972.

25. CATANZARO, R. J. *Alcoholism: The Total Treatment Approach.* Springfield, Illinois: Charles C. Thomas, 1968.

26. CHAFETZ, M. E. *Liquor the Servant of Man.* Boston: Little, Brown & Co., 1965.

27. ———. "The Alcoholic Symptom and Its Therapeutic Relevance," *Quarterly Journal of Studies on Alcohol*, 31 (1970), 444–445.

28. ———. "Alcoholism Criteria: An Important Step," *American Journal of Psychiatry*, 129 (1972), 214–215.

29. CHAFETZ, M. E., H. T. BLANE, H. S. ABRAM, J. GOLNER, E. LACY, W. F. McCOURT, E. CLARK and W. MEYERS. "Establishing Treatment Relations with Alcoholics," *Journal of Nervous and Mental Disease*, 134 (1962), 395–409.

30. CHAFETZ, M. E., H. T. BLANE, M. J. HILL, eds. *Frontiers of Alcoholism.* New York: Science House, 1970.

31. CHAFETZ, M. E., H. T. BLANE and M. J. HILL. "Children of Alcoholics," *Quarterly Journal of Studies on Alcohol*, 32 (1971), 687.

32. CHAFETZ, M. E., H. W. DEMONE, JR. *Alcoholism and Society.* New York: Oxford University Press, 1962.

33. CHAFETZ, M. E., H. W. DEMONE. "Alcoholism: Its Cause and Prevention," *New York State Journal of Medicine*, 62 (1962), 1614–1625.

34. CHAFETZ, M. E. and M. J. HILL. "The Alcoholic in Society," in Grunebaum, H., ed., *The Practice of Community Mental*

Health. Boston: Little, Brown and Company, 1970.

35. COHEN, P. C. and M. S. KRAUSE. *Casework with Wives of Alcoholics.* New York: Family Service Association, 1971.

36. THE COMMITTEE ON NOMENCLATURE AND STATISTICS OF THE AMERICAN PSYCHIATRIC ASSOCIATION. *Diagnostic and Statistical Manual of Mental Disorders.* First Edition. Washington, D.C.: American Psychiatric Association, 1952.

37. THE COMMITTEE ON NOMENCLATURE AND STATISTICS OF THE AMERICAN PSYCHIATRIC ASSOCIATION. *Diagnostic and Statistical Manual of Mental Disorders (DSM-II).* Second Edition. Washington, D.C.: American Psychiatric Association, 1968.

38. CRITERIA COMMITTEE, NATIONAL COUNCIL ON ALCOHOLISM. "Criteria for the Diagnosis of Alcoholism," *American Journal of Psychiatry,* 129 (1972), 127–135.

39. DAVIDSON, C. S. "Nutrition, Geography, and Liver Diseases," *American Journal of Clinical Nutrition,* 23 (1970), 427–436.

40. DAVIS, D. I., D. BERENSON, P. STEINGLASS and S. DAVIS. "The Adaptive Consequences of Drinking," *Psychiatry* (in press).

41. DENEAU, G., T. YANAGITA and M. H. SEEVERS. "Self Administration of Psychoactive Substances by the Monkey," *Psychopharmacologia,* 19 (1969), 30–48.

42. ELLIS, F. W. and J. R. PICK. "Ethanol Intoxication and Dependence in Rhesus Monkeys," in, Mello, N. K. and Mendelson, J. H., eds., *Recent Advances in Studies of Alcoholism,* Publication No. (HSM) 71–9045. Washington, D.C.: U.S. Government Printing Office, 1971.

43. ENGEL, G. L. and J. ROMANO. "Delirium, a Syndrome of Cerebral Insufficiency," *Journal of Chronic Disease,* 9 (1959), 260–277.

44. ESSER, P. H. "Evaluation of Family Therapy with Alcoholics," *British Journal of the Addictions,* 66 (1971), 251–255.

45. ———. "Conjoint Family Therapy with Alcoholics—a New Approach," *British Journal of the Addictions,* 64 (1970), 275–286.

46. EWING, J. "Measuring Alcohol Consumption: The Alcohol Quotient," presented before the 30th International Congress on Alcoholism and Drug Dependence, Amsterdam, 1972.

47. EWING, J. A. and R. E. FOX. "Family Therapy of Alcoholism" in, Masserman, J. H., ed., *Current Psychiatric Therapies.* Volume 8. New York: Grune and Stratton, 1968, 86–91.

48. FALK, J. L. "Behavioral Maintenance of High Blood Ethanol and Physical Dependence in the Rat," *Science,* 177 (1972), 811–813.

49. FALLDING, H. *Drinking, Community and Civilization.* New Brunswick, New Jersey: Journal of Studies on Alcohol, in press.

50. FENICHEL, O. *The Psychoanalytic Theory of Neurosis.* New York: W. W. Norton & Company, 1945.

51. FOX, R. *Alcoholism: Behavioral Research, Therapeutic Approaches.* New York: Springer, 1967.

52. ———. "Children in the Alcoholic Family" in, W. C. Bier, ed., *Problems in Addiction: Alcohol and Drug Addiction.* New York: Fordham University Press, 1962, 71–96.

53. GERARD, D. L. and G. SAENGER. *Outpatient Treatment of Alcoholism: A Study of Outcome and Its Determinants.* Toronto: University of Toronto Press, 1966.

54. GLATT, M. M. "Group Therapy in Alcoholism," *British Journal of Addiction,* 54 (1958), 133–147.

55. GLIEDMAN, L. H. "Concurrent and Combined Group Treatment of Chronic Alcoholics and Their Wives," *International Journal of Group Psychotherapy,* 7 (1957), 414–424.

56. GOLDSTEIN, S. G. *The Identification, Description and Multivariate Classification of Alcoholics by Means of the Minnesota Multiphasic Personality Inventory.* Unpublished dissertation, Purdue University, 1968.

57. GOODWIN, D. W. and S. B. GUZE. "Genetic Factors in Alcoholism" in, Kissin, B. and Begleiter, H., eds., *Biology of Alcoholism,* Volume 3, *Clinical Pathology,* 1974, in press.

58. GOODWIN, D. W., F. SCHULSINGER, L. HERMANSEN, S. B. GUZE and G. WINOKUR. "Alcohol Problems in Adoptees Raised Apart From Alcoholic Biological Parents," *Archives of General Psychiatry,* 28 (1973), 238–243.

59. GUSFIELD, J. R. "Status Conflicts and the Changing Ideologies of the American Temperance Movement" in, Pittman, D. J. and Snyder, C. R., eds., *Society, Culture,*

and *Drinking Patterns.* New York: John Wiley and Sons, 1962.

60. HALEY, J. and L. HOFFMAN. *Techniques of Family Therapy.* New York: Basic Books, 1968.

61. HALLEN, J. and J. NORDEN. "Liver Cirrhosis Unsuspected during Life," *Journal of Chronic Disease,* 17 (1964), 951–958.

62. HARFORD, T. Personal Communication.

63. HARRIS L., and ASSOCIATES, INC. Studies of NIAAA Advertising Campaign, prepared on contract, 1972–1973.

64. HARTMANN, H. *Essays on Ego Psychology.* New York: International Universities Press, 1964.

65. HARVEY, A. M., R. J. JOHNS, A. H. OWENS, and R. S. Ross. *The Principles and Practice of Medicine.* New York: Appleton–Century–Crofts, 1972.

66. HEBB, D. O. *A Textbook of Psychology.* Philadelphia: W. B. Saunders, 1968.

67. HERTZMAN, M. and E. A. BENDIT. "Alcoholism and Destructive Behavior" in, A. R. Roberts, ed., *Self-Destructive Behavior.* Charles C. Thomas, forthcoming.

68. HOLLISTER, L. E., et al. "Acetophenazine and Diazepam in Anxious Depressions," *Archives of General Psychiatry,* 24 (1971), 273–278.

69. ISRAEL, Y. and J. MARDONES. *Biological Basis of Alcoholism.* New York: John Wiley & Sons, 1971.

70. JACKSON, J. K. "Alcoholism and the Family" in, Pittman, D. J. and Snyder, C. R., eds., *Society, Culture and Drinking Patterns.* New York: John Wiley & Sons, 1962, 472–492.

71. JACOBSON, A. M., M. W. WILLIAMS, R. J. MIGNONE and S. ZISOOK. "The Walk-In Patient as a 'Customer': A Key Dimension in Evaluation and Treatment," *American Journal of Orthopsychiatry,* 42 (1972), 872–883.

72. JEFFRIES, G. H. "Diseases of the Liver" in, Beeson, P. B. and McDermott, U., eds., *Cecil-Loeb Textbook of Medicine,* Volume II. Philadelphia: W. B. Saunders, 1967.

73. JELLINEK, E. M. *Disease Concept of Alcoholism.* New Haven: Hillhouse Press, 1960.

74. JESSOR, R., T. R. GRAVES, R. C. HANSON and S. L. JESSOR. *Society, Personality, and Deviant Behavior.* New York: Holt, Rinehart & Winston, 1968.

75. KADUSHIN, C. *Why People Go to Psychiatrists.* Chicago: Aldine, 1968.

76. KELLEHER, R. T., W. FRY, J. DEEGAN and L. COOK. "Effects of Meprobamate on Operant Behavior in Rats," *Journal of Pharmacology and Experimental Therapeutics,* 133 (1961), 271–280.

77. KELLER, M. "Alcoholism: Nature and Extent of the Problem," *Annals of the American Academy of Political and Social Sciences,* 315 (1958), 1–11.

78. KELLER, M. and V. EFRON. "The Prevalence of Alcoholism," *Quarterly Journal of Studies on Alcohol,* 16 (1955), 619–644.

79. KENYON, W. H. *About the Illness Alcoholism.* Liverpool, England: Merseyside Council on Alcoholism.

80. KIRESUK, T. and R. E. SHERMAN. "Goal-Attainment Scaling: A General Method for Evaluating Comprehensive Community Mental Health Programs," *Community Mental Health Journal,* 4 (1968), 443–453.

81. KISSIN, B. and H. BEGLEITER, eds., *The Biology of Alcoholism,* Volumes I–IV. New York: Plenum Press, 1971–1974.

82. KLATSKY, A. and G. FRIEDMAN. Presentation before American Heart Association, Atlantic City, New Jersey, 1973.

82-A. KLINE, N. S. "Evaluation of Lithium Therapy In Chronic Alcoholism," Paper Presented before Third Annual Alcoholism Conference, NIAAA, June 21, 1973.

83. KNIGHT, R. P. "The Psychodynamics of Chronic Alcoholism," *Journal of Nervous and Mental Disease,* 86 (1937), 538–548.

84. LEIFER, R. *In the Name of Mental Health.* New York: Science House, 1969.

85. LEVIN, G. "How Well is the Community Mental Health Centers Program Achieving its Goals?" Paper presented before the American Psychological Association. Montreal, Canada: 1973.

86. LISANSKY, E. S. "The Etiology of Alcoholism: The Role of Psychological Predisposition," *Quarterly Journal of Studies on Alcohol,* 21 (1960), 314–343.

87. LUDWIG, A. M. "The Design of Clinical Studies in Treatment Efficacy" in, M. E. Chafetz, ed., *Proceedings of the First Annual Alcoholism Conference NIAAA,* DHEW No. (HSM) 73–9074. Washington, D.C.: U.S. Government Printing Office, 1973.

88. LUDWIG, A. M., J. LEVINE and L. H. STARK.

LSD and Alcoholism. Springfield, Illinois: Charles C. Thomas, 1970.

89. MacAndrew, C. and R. Edgerton. *Drunken Comportment.* Chicago: Aldine, 1969.

90. Majchrowicz, E. and P. Steinglass. "Blood Methanol, Blood Ethanol, and Alcohol Withdrawal Syndrome in Humans," *Federation Proceedings,* 32 (1973), Abstract 2908, p. 728.

91. Maxwell, M. A. "Alcoholics Anonymous: An Interpretation" in, D. J. Pittman and C. R. Snyder, eds., *Society, Culture and Drinking Patterns.* New York: John Wiley & Sons, 1962.

92. McClelland, D. C., W. N. Davis, R. Kalin and E. Wanner. *The Drinking Man: Alcohol and Human Motivation.* New York: Free Press, 1972.

93. McCord, W., J. McCord, and J. Gudeman. *Origins of Alcoholism.* Stanford: Stanford University Press, 1960.

94. Mello, N. K. "Behavioral Studies of Alcoholism" in, B. Kissin and H. Begleiter, eds., *The Biology of Alcoholism: Physiology and Behavior,* Volume II. New York: Plenum Publishing Co., 1972.

95. ————. "A Review of Methods to Induce Alcohol Addiction in Animals," *Pharmacology Biochemistry & Behavior,* 1 (1973), 89–101.

96. ————. "Short-Term Memory Function in Alcohol Addicts During Intoxication" in, M. M. Gross, ed., *Alcohol Intoxication and Withdrawal: Experimental Studies,* Proc. 30th Int. Congress on Alcoholism & Drug Dependency. New York: Plenum Press, 1973.

97. Mello, N. K. and J. H. Mendelson, eds., *Recent Advances in Studies of Alcoholism: An Interdisciplinary Symposium.* National Institute on Alcohol Abuse and Alcoholism, Washington, D.C.: U.S. Government Printing Office, 1971.

98. Mendelson, J. H. "Ethanol-1-C^{14} Metabolism in Alcoholics and Non-Alcoholics," *Science,* 159 (1968), 319–320.

99. ————. "Biological Concomitants of Alcoholism," *New England Journal of Medicine,* 283 (1970), 24–32, 71–81.

100. Mendelson, J. H., J. LaDau and P. Solomon. "Experimentally Induced Intoxication and Withdrawal in Alcoholics, Part 3, Psychiatric Findings," *Quarterly Journal of*

Studies on Alcoholism, Suppl. No. 2 (1969), 40–52.

101. Mendelson, J. H. and N. K. Mello. "Studies of the Development of Alcohol Addiction In Infant Monkeys," *Annals of the New York Academy of Sciences,* 215 (1973), 145–161.

102. Menninger, K. *Man Against Himself.* New York: Harcourt, Brace & Co., 1938.

103. Miller, P. M., D. H. Barlow. "Behavioral Approaches to the Treatment of Alcoholism," *The Journal of Nervous and Mental Disease* 157 (1973), 10–20.

104. Mitnick, L. Personal Communication.

105. Mulford, H. A., D. E. Miller. "Drinking in Iowa, IV. Preoccupation with Alcohol and Definitions of Alcohol, Heavy Drinking and Trouble Due to Drinking," *Quarterly Journal of Studies on Alcohol* 21 (1960), 279–291.

106. Murphy, G. E., E. Robins. "Social Factors in Suicide," *Journal of the American Medical Association* 199 (1967), 81–86.

107. Nathan, P. E., J. S. O'Brien and D. Norton. "Comparative Studies of Interpersonal and Affective Behavior of Alcoholics and Non-alcoholics During Prolonged Experimental Drinking," in, N. K. Mello and J. H. Mendelson, eds., *Recent Advances in Studies of Alcoholism.* Washington, D.C.; U.S. Govt. Print. Office., 1971.

108. Overall, J. E., D. Brown, J. D. Williams and L. T. Neill. "Drug Treatment of Anxiety & Depression in Detoxified Alcoholic Patients," *Archives of General Psychiatry* 29 (1973), 218–221.

109. Paredes, A., et al., "A Clinical Study of Alcoholics Using Audio-visual Self-image Feedback," *Journal of Nervous and Mental Disease* 148 (1969), 449–456.

110. Pattison, E. M. "A Critique of Alcoholism Treatment Concepts; With Special Reference to Abstinence," *Quarterly Journal of Studies on Alcohol* 27 (1966), 49–71.

111. Pattison, E. M., E. B. Headley, G. C. Gleser and L. A. Gottschalk. "Abstinence and Normal Drinking, An Assessment in Changes in Drinking Patterns in Alcoholics After Treatment," *Quarterly Journal of Studies on Alcohol* 29(3) (1968), 610–633.

112. Pittman, D. J., C. R. Snyder, eds., *Society, Culture, and Drinking Patterns.* New York: John Wiley & Sons, 1962.

113. PITTMAN, D. J., C. W. GORDON. *Revolving Door: A Study of the Chronic Police Case Inebriate.* Glencoe, Illinois: The Free Press, 1958.

114. PLAUT, T. F. A., *Alcohol Problems: A Report to the National Cooperative Commission on the Study of Alcoholism.* New York: Oxford University Press, 1967.

115. POPHAM, R. E., ed., *Alcohol and Alcoholism.* Toronto: University of Toronto Press, 1970.

116. RADO, S. "Psychoanalysis of Pharmacothymia," *Psychoanalytic Quarterly*, 2 (1941), 227.

117. ROBINS, L. N., W. M. BATES, P. O'NEAL. *Deviant Children Grown Up: A Sociological and Psychiatric Study of Sociopathic Personality.* Baltimore: Williams & Wilkins, 1966.

118. ROEBUCK, J. B. *The Etiology of Alcoholism: Constitutional, Psychological and Sociological Approaches.* Springfield, Illinois: Charles C Thomas, 1972.

119. SATIR, V. *Conjoint Family Therapy: A Guide.* Palo Alto: Science & Behavior, 1964.

120. SCHEIDLINGER, S. "Identification, the Sense of Belonging and of Identity in Small Groups," *International Journal of Group Psychotherapy*, 14 (1964), 291–306.

121. SCHNEIDER, H. "The Intramembrane Location of Alcohol Anesthetics," *Biochimica Biophysica Acta*, 163 (1968), 451–458.

122. SCHUCKIT, M. A., D. A. GOODWIN and G. WINOKUR. "A Study of Alcoholism in Half Siblings," *American Journal of Psychiatry*, 128(9) (1972), 1132–1136.

123. SOBELL, M. B., L. C. SOBELL. Reported in *The Journal of the Addiction Research Foundation*, 2 (1973), 5.

124. SPECK, R. V., U. RUEVENI. "Network Therapy," in N. W. Ackerman, ed., *Family Process.* New York: Basic Books, 1970.

125. STEINER, C. M. *Games Alcoholics Play.* New York: Grove Press, 1971.

126. STEINGLASS, P., S. WEINER and J. H. MENDELSON. "Interactional Issues as Determinants of Alcoholism," *American Journal of Psychiatry*, 128(3) (1971a), 55.

127. STEINGLASS, P., S. WEINER and J. H. MENDELSON. "A Systems Approach to Alcoholism, A Model and Its Clinical Application," *Archives of General Psychiatry*, 24(5) (1971b), 401.

128. STIMMEL, B. "Integrated Curriculum in Drug Abuse, A Doctor's Perspective," presented before the First Conference on Medical School Curriculum Development in Drug Dependence, State University of New York, Downstate Medical Center, December 3, 1973.

129. STRAUS, R. "Alcohol and Society," *Psychiatric Annals*, 3 (1973), 8–107.

130. STRAUS, R., S. D. BACON. *Drinking in College.* New Haven: Yale University Press, 1953.

131. SZASZ, T. *The Myth of Mental Illness.* New York: Harper & Row, 1961.

132. TAMERIN, J. S. and J. H. MENDELSON. "The Psychodynamics of Chronic Inebriation: Observations of Alcoholics during the Process of Drinking in an Experimental Group Setting," *American Journal of Psychiatry*, 125 (1969), 886–899.

133. TAMERIN, J. A., S. WEINER and J. H. MENDELSON. "Alcoholics' Expectancies and Recall of Experiences During Intoxication," *American Journal of Psychiatry*, 126 (1970), 1697–1704.

134. TRAUX, C. B., R. R. CARKHUFF. *Toward Effective Counseling and Psychotherapy: Training and Practice.* Chicago: Aldine, 1967.

135. ULLMAN, A. D. "First Drinking Experience as Related to Age and Sex," in D. J. Pittman, C. R. Snyder, eds., *Society, Culture, and Drinking Patterns.* New York: John Wiley & Sons, 1962.

136. VICTOR, J. and S. M. WOLFE. "Causation and Treatment of the Alcohol Withdrawal Syndrome," in P. G. Bourne and R. Fox, eds., *Alcoholism: Progress in Research and Treatment* New York: Academic Press, Inc., 1973, 137–169.

137. VOGEL, S. and R. R. BANKS. "The Effect of Delayed Punishment on An Immediately Rewarded Response in Alcoholics and Non-Alcoholics," *Behavior Research & Therapy*, 3 (1965), 69–73.

138. WANBERG, K. W. and J. KNAPP. "Differences in Drinking Symptoms and Behavior of Men and Women Alcoholics," *British Journal of Addiction*, 64 (1970), 347–355.

139. WARD, R. F. and G. A. FAILLACE. "The Alcoholic and His Helpers," *Quarterly Journal of Studies on Alcohol*, 31(3) (1970), 684.

140. WEED, L. L. "Medical Records That Guide

& Teach," *New England Journal of Medicine*, 278 (1968), 593–599 & 652–657.

141. WEINER, H. B. "An Overview of the Use of Psychodrama and Group Psychotherapy in the Treatment of Alcoholism in the U.S. and Abroad," *Group Psychotherapy*, 19 (1966), 159–165.

142. WENDER, P. "On Necessary and Sufficient Conditions in Psychiatric Explanation." *Archives of General Psychiatry*, 16 (1967), 41–47.

143. WHALEN, T. "Wives of Alcoholics: Four Types Observed in a Family Service Agency," *Quarterly Journal of Studies on Alcohol*, 14 (1953), 632.

144. WILKINSON, R. *The Prevention of Drinking Problems*. New York: Oxford University Press, 1970.

145. WILSNACK, S. C. "The Needs of the Female Drinker: Dependency, Power, or What?" Harvard University, June 1972.

146. ZWERLING, I. "Psychiatric Findings In An Interdisciplinary Study of Forty-Six Alcoholic Patients," *Quarterly Journal of Studies on Alcohol*, 20 (1959), 543–554.

147. ZWERLING, I. and M. ROSENBAUM. "Alcoholic Addiction and Personality," in S. Arieti, ed., *American Handbook of Psychiatry*, 1st Edition. New York: Basic Books, 1959.

CHAPTER 19

DRUG ADDICTION

Marie Nyswander

D RUGS WITH A POTENTIAL for addiction may be consdered by the practitioner from several viewpoints: as chemical agents with predictable pharmacological properties; in terms of their psychological effects for the individual concerned; or in terms of the wider sociological implications. Among these, only the pharmacological actions have remained constant with the passage of time and changing environmental conditions.

❪ Addiction Defined

For some years, the term "addiction" has been used chiefly to define a state arising from repeated consumption of a drug capable of inducing *physical* dependence and an overwhelming compulsion to continue its use. The term "habituation" has been reserved more for drugs associated with *psychological* dependence. However, often the terms have been used interchangeably, resulting in confusion as to which drugs actually produce a physical dependence. In recognition, the World Health Organization recently observed that "It has become impossible in practice and is scientifically unsound to maintain a single definition for all forms of drug addiction or habituation."[15] Noting that a feature common to these conditions, as well as to drug abuse in general, is "dependence, psychic or physical, or both, of the individual on a chemical agent," WHO recommended use of the broader term "drug dependence" for "a state arising from the repeated administration of a drug on a periodic or continuous basis." Moreover, since drug dependence may be associated with use of a variety of drugs, the term was qualified further as "drug dependence of the amphetamine type," and so on. This chapter will be devoted chiefly to a discussion of narcotic drug dependence of the morphine type produced by natural derivatives of opium, such as morphine itself, heroin, dilaudid, and codeine, or by synthetic equivalents thereof, for example, meperidine and methadone.

❪ Historical Background

Chemical agents that alter mood and behavior have been known since ancient times. Historical data tell that opium (from the opium poppy, *Papaver somniferum*) was well known to the Egyptians before 1500 B.C.; earlier, at the height of the Sumerian civilization, opium was not only known but given a name it still holds today: "plant of joy." Ancient writings attest to the popularity of opium throughout the rise and fall of the Babylonian, Egyptian, Greek, and Roman empires. Homer referred to the poppy and its properties of "lethal slumber."

Significantly, as opium use increased, presumably for the gratifications it provided, it was acknowledged also as a medically important drug, valuable as a sedative and for its analgesic properties. In the centuries that followed, the use of opium spread throughout Europe and elsewhere in the world. Medical records around the time of the American Revolution attest to the use of opium as an analgesic in various gastrointestinal disorders, to allay the pain of childbirth or of cancer, and in control of fever. It is ironic that despite physicians' familiarity with opium, its addictive properties long remained unsuspected.

With the synthesis of the morphine derivative heroin in 1898, its medical use was encouraged as a nonaddictive substitute for morphine. Rather quickly, heroin became readily obtainable in a number of over-the-counter pharmaceutical preparations. According to records of the time, its availability probably helped to create new addicts in large numbers.

However, an earlier development—invention of the hypodermic needle in 1853—was also encouraging the spread of drug abuse. Introduced to the United States from Europe around 1856, the hypodermic needle was widely used during the Civil War to administer morphine to the wounded and for relieving the symptoms of dysentery. After the war, opium derivatives continued to be taken by any of several routes: orally (in tincture form), rectally (pulverized), or intravenously by hypodermic needle. It was reasoned by many that drug dependence was not possible when administered by a needle—as the drug did not reach the stomach, a "hunger" for it was unlikely to develop. With the advent of heroin at the end of the century, preference for the needle as the means of drug intake was clearly established. Despite its illegality, heroin has been the addict's "drug of choice" since about 1915. Its manufacture or use here has been illegal since the 1920s.

Legal Controls

Early in this century, laws went into effect in virtually all states and many municipalities governing use of opiates. The medical profession, recognizing by then the dangers of drug dependence, had been giving broad publicity to the adverse effects. Lawmakers, as well as the public at large, were increasingly aware that addiction had become a major social problem, although how rapidly incidence was increasing was unknown. (Terry and Pellens[40] estimated the incidence of narcotics addiction in the U. S. Population in 1885 to be between 1 percent and 4 percent.)

Mounting concern over the addiction problem led to the passage of federal legislation (Harrison Narcotic Act of 1914) that could be more vigorously enforced than local or state laws. As is known, the Harrison Narcotic Act sought not to make addiction illegal but to control production and distribution of narcotic drugs so that they would be dispensable only by physicians. One effect was to reduce, temporarily, the number of addicts. Since the passage of the Harrison Narcotic Act, U. S. enforcement policy attempting to regulate the behavior of addicts and the physician-addict relationship has been the most restrictive in the world. (By legal definition, all drugs regulated under the Harrison Narcotic Act and subsequent federal laws are classified as narcotics, although some are non-narcotic in their pharmacological action, for example cocaine and marijuana.)

Unfortunately, in controlling the flow of narcotics from the manufacturer to the physician, the Harrison Narcotic Act and court decisions that followed also limited the physician's role in treating drug dependence. Dispensing of narcotics in diminishing quantities to "break" the drug habit was permissible, but supplying narcotics in a controlled setting for those addicts who were unable to forego drug use was strictly forbidden. It is of interest that prior to these rulings some forty medical clinics throughout the U.S. were dispensing narcotic drugs to addicts as part of a planned treatment program. However, by 1924 all such facilities had been forcibly closed. This action was strongly favored not only by state and local authorities but by the American Medical Association, reflecting the emerging view that drug dependence was a moral evil, in no way to be encouraged. As these policies went into effect, legal difficulties confronted physicians. Referring to this legal harassment of doctors, John Ingersoll,[23] Director of the Bureau of Narcotics and Dangerous Drugs, recently stated:

> Prosecutions and intimidations [during that period] were sufficiently successful to eliminate the interest of the medical profession generally in engaging in the treatment of addicts, other than in the two approved federal hospitals at Lexington (Kentucky) and Fort Worth (Texas). Government policy was broadly supported by existing medical opinion and seems to have achieved the desired end. It was, however, a policy which succeeded in terminating both the sincere and insincere efforts without distinction.

Addiction and Crime

For the addict unable to forego drug use, the only alternative was to turn to illegal sources of supply which prior to that had been a minor factor in the spread of drug abuse. The tragic consequences for the individual addict, and for society at large, have been readily apparent as the incidence of addiction has increased, particularly among the young.[12] In our cities, where drug addiction is most concentrated, the economic decline and deterioration, as well as the increase in crime, have been part of the price paid. Needless to say, the social consequences of addiction vary with the laws governing the use of drugs, as well as the physician-addict relationship. In England, where physicians have long been permitted to prescribe narcotics as part of the management of drug-dependent patients, there has been little association of addiction and crime.[34] Economic background also plays a role. It is well known that in this country the wealthy addict rarely comes to the attention of authorities; in contrast, the poorer addict is too readily forced into a life of crime to meet his increasing need for narcotics.

Failure of Treatment Models

For nearly a thirty-year period ending in 1960, essentially the only treatment facilities for all voluntary patients were at the U.S.P.H.S. hospitals located at Lexington, Kentucky, and Fort Worth, Texas. A major treatment aim was to keep the addict drug-free for a period of time (ranging from four months to five years). It is no secret that the treatment provided proved unsuccessful; the relapse rate following detoxification was in the range of 95 percent. As we now know, this approach was found to fail since the problem of drug abuse is a chronic illness and unlikely to respond to measures involving incarceration or punishment.[28A]

In 1960, New York City pioneered in launching a program for the study and withdrawal treatment of drug dependence. It opened fifty beds in a general hospital, and within a year, to meet the demand, increased the number to some four hundred. After a forty-year absence, physicians were once again participating in the treatment of addiction. In 1965, five years after the return of treatment to the local communities, a new branch of medicine emerged: the medical treatment of narcotic addiction. At the present writing, some 65,000 addicts are receiving medical and rehabilitative services in methadone programs throughout the country, and research is continuing to search for a more effective agent.[14]

Physical Dependence

Physical dependence[26] is in effect a form of physiological adaptation to the presence of a drug. Once such dependence has been established, the body reacts with predictable symptoms if the drug is suddenly withdrawn. The nature and severity of withdrawal symptoms (referred to in their totality as the abstinence syndrome) depend on the drug in question, as well as on the daily dosage level. For example, symptoms of withdrawal from morphine-like narcotics (after as little as eight doses over a two-day period) include neuromuscular twitching, mydriasis, lacrimation, rhinorrhea, shivering, yawning, and sneezing. If allowed to continue, more severe symptoms appear: increased breathing rate and blood pressure, profuse sweating, severe vomiting, and diarrhea. Typically, onset of the abstinence syndrome occurs within eight to twelve hours after the last dose; symptoms peak at thirty-six to seventy-two hours. Death is unlikely, but the intensity of symptoms is such that it is medically negligent to allow them to run their full course. Only administration of a narcotic can bring relief; without doubt, prison suicides of narcotic addicts would occur less often if this were done.

(Tolerance

With the continued use of narcotic drugs, the addict finds he must increase the dose to avoid symptoms of abstinence. This is a consequence of narcotic tolerance. The sedative, analgesic, and respiratory effects may be so greatly diminished that a dose expected to be fatal for a normal individual may be taken without untoward effect. When patients are maintained in a steady state of narcotic tolerance by the regular administration of a long-acting narcotic drug (such as methadone), they are likely to be functioning normally as measured by tests of reaction time,[21] co-ordination, and mental performance.[22] However, high tolerance does not exist in an addict who is not using drugs, and so giving large amounts of a narcotic to such a person is very likely to produce signs of an overdose.

Tolerance can be built up in a pre-exposed addict in a matter of days. Experimentally, it has been demonstrated that a tolerance to 1200 mg. of morphine daily can be established in about four months.[47]

Several theories have been advanced to explain the mechanism of tolerance; thus far, those that have been tested have been pretty well disproven while the others can merely be

speculated upon. Among the possibilities that have been considered are that tolerance is due to changes in enzymatic activity in the liver, to adaptation on a cellular level in the central nervous system, or to altered turnover of a neurotransmitter. It seems certain that metabolic processes are involved both in tolerance and in physical dependence; however, whether they are basic to either or to addiction itself remains to be determined. (A detailed review with bibliography of research in these areas is to be found in the *Annual Review of Biochemistry*.)[3]

Both tolerance and the abstinence syndrome have been well documented with use of experimental animal models;[32,43,33] in most such studies, animals have been repeatedly injected with morphine until the drug is needed to prevent withdrawal symptoms. According to an early experiment by Spragg,[39] animals so treated became "drug-seeking," refusing food, and instead turning to the syringe and narcotics to alleviate their symptoms. In another experiment, animals fitted with an indwelling catheter, to self-administer drugs, became addicted within a few days.[43] Once addicted, they would sustain narcotic dependence by maintaining drug intake at a fairly steady level. Thompson,[41] in an interesting experiment, found that addicted animals given a dose of methodone "self-diminished" the amount of morphine injected in proportion to the dose of methadone given.

In animals as in man, symptoms of abstinence can be curbed only by administration of a narcotic. Tranquilizers and sedatives have proven ineffectual for this purpose.

(Relapse

It has been assumed that once an addict has been withdrawn from physical dependence on a narcotic drug and remains drug-free for a time, he is in effect cured of his drug dependence. On this basis, it is reasoned that if he returns to the use of drugs, it must be for psychological reasons. This tendency to relapse has long been considered due to lack of motivation and/or an inherent weakness in the addict's personality. Hence, according to this theory, the major hope of salvaging the relapsed addict should be through psychotherapy and related techniques. However, psychotherapy has had very limited success. The rate of relapse to drug use following psychotherapy may be as high as 90 percent, which is no better than the result of no treatment.

Research findings[4] suggest an explanation; that relapse may be the result of neurochemical or neurophysiological changes, or perhaps a combination of the two, that persist long after narcotic drugs have been withdrawn.[32] For example, manifestations of the abstinence syndrome—elevated body temperature, mydriasis, increased blood pressure and respiratory rate—may remain for months after withdrawal of a narcotic; this was consistently observed by Himmelsbach in studying detoxified patients at the government facility at Lexington. Confirming these findings, Martin et al.[32] showed that in detoxified addicts abnormalities of metabolism—such as hypothermia and decreased sensitivity of the respiratory center to CO_2—persisted into a later phase of secondary abstinence. Rats withdrawn from high doses of morphine likewise showed lasting metabolic abnormalities. Increased tolerance to the narcotic effects of drugs appears to persist long after drug use has been terminated. According to Cochin and Kornetsky,[2] response to a challenge dose of morphine is significantly different in previously addicted and control rats after as long as a year of abstinence; initially, the former had been given but a single injection of morphine. These findings suggest that the central nervous system of the post-addict remains biochemically and physiologically abnormal after so-called detoxification. The persistence of drug hunger, reflected in relapse after detoxification, may be explainable on this basis.

❮ Clinical Course of Addiction

Despite beliefs to the contrary, narcotics per se do not cause serious impairment to body or mind,[38] as do barbiturates and alcohol. Addicts who have used opiates for as long as fifty years have shown no evidence of mental deterioration. To be sure, addicts neglect themselves physically; the time and money spent in drug-seeking leaves little room for self-care. There is of course the risk of hepatitis from use of contaminated needles, or pulmonary disorders from injected particulate matter, but the pathology seen in addicts does not appear to be due to the opiate.

Typically, the heroin addict is likely to make repeated attempts to be rid of his addiction. Virtually all patients, even recently addicted adolescents, tell of their efforts to find treatment. Most recently, patients applying for treatment have attempted detoxification one to five times a year.

❮ Initial Exposure to Narcotics

Among the misconceptions about drug dependence is the theory that use of marijuana predisposes to heroin addiction;[44] widespread use of both drugs among youths tends to reinforce that belief. Closer analysis reveals that these forms of drug usage tend to involve two different social groups. In the urban ghetto, initial exposure to heroin usually begins without prior experience with other drugs; curiosity and desire to emulate friends or neighbors, plus the availability of heroin, may be sufficient precipitating factors.[44] Economic deprivation, lack of privacy at home, and lack of recreational opportunities outside the home, increase the temptation. Although heroin addiction occurs in privileged middle-class youths, the drugs abused by this group at the present time are more likely to be barbiturates and amphetamines. Apparently, the large majority of college students have tried marijuana without becoming regular users. Drug abuse in this group may be symptomatic of the intense middle-class pressures for achievement, coupled with a sense of alienation. Generally, use of these drugs tends to decrease with time; by the mid-twenties it has usually stopped.

❲ Diagnosis of Addiction

Recognition of the extent of narcotic drug use in various population groups has increased with improved methods of diagnosis. Until quite recently, the diagnosis of active drug addiction was often difficult to establish. The presence of old or new needle marks or "tracks" over the veins of the hands, arms, or legs is certainly good presumptive evidence of heroin addiction,[34] but there may be an absence of other clues. Development of a diagnostic urine test,[5] utilizing thin layer chromatography, has permitted identification of a variety of drugs, including morphine, quinine, barbiturates, amphetamines, cocaine, methadone, and some tranquilizers. Unfortunately, no sooner was the value of the test established than it become subject to misuse, employed for purposes of identifying addicts and refusing them employment or advancement at work. Given the far-reaching consequences when an individual is labeled an addict, a diagnosis should never be made on the basis of a single urine test; moreover, the reliability of the laboratory should be assured. Too often, neither of these requirements is met.

❲ Psychodynamics of Addiction

It is well known that not all individuals exposed to narcotics become addicted. Even with narcotics easily obtainable by city youths "on every street corner," only some people become addicts; others with similar backgrounds of poverty and deprivation do not. This would seem to give support to the thesis that there is a basic personality pattern or character defect that leads to drug dependence or makes a given individual especially vulnerable. The addict is said to be emotionally dependent, unable to form meaningful relationships, driven to seek pleasure through drugs as an escape from reality. Tendencies to opiate addiction and criminality are also closely linked.

These theories implicating psychological or mental abnormality as a cause of addiction have been advanced by a number of investigators over the past thirty years. Once they gained credence, they became part of the dogma concerning addiction; they continue to be cited in textbooks and in teaching. However, the accumulated data from institutions managing large number of addicts have failed to confirm them. No specific personality pattern has emerged.[19] The range of personal characteristics in addicts is as varied as in any other group; comparisons of addicts with other population groups have failed to differentiate between the two. Nor are there psychiatric tests or other measurements that can indicate who is already addicted, or predict who might become addicted with exposure.

Clearly, addiction is the result of the repeated use of an addictive drug. It can and does occur in individuals of all emotional capacities and psychiatric backgrounds. It may occur in psychotics and neurotics, in the mentally retarded, and in persons of high intelligence and productivity. On the other hand, individual differences, as well as the social context in which addiction occurs, do help to explain variations in response to drugs and in drug-seeking behavior. Thus, a physician-addict may contain his addiction to such an extent that he manages to live a productive and useful life; another individual with similar access to drugs may become totally incapacitated.

The view that the tendencies to addiction and criminality are linked, which unfortunately persists, reflects a confusion between consequences and causes of addiction. The reason why one individual becomes an addict after exposure to heroin, and another not, is at present unknown. Whether or not the susceptibility to addiction has a metabolic basis is a question for future research.

❲ Conditioned Reflex Theory

Some investigators think it unlikely that biochemical factors will prove important either in causing addiction or return to use of drugs after detoxification. An alternative explanation of relapse has been offered by Wikler and others.[46,49,20] On the basis of animal experiments in which conditioned associations were established by pairing certain environmental stimuli with drug effects during a cycle of active addiction, it is suggested that relapse may be the result of conditioning.[20] The experiments have involved either classical or operant conditioning in addicted animals (rats or monkeys) subjected to drug withdrawal. In classical conditioning, a neutral stimulus—for example a signal light—becomes associated with the abstinence syndrome by repeated pairing of the signal and the abstinence state; subsequently, the signal is paired with relief of symptoms by provision of the narcotic needed to eliminate them. In operant conditioning, the animal is trained to perform a certain action—pressing a lever, going to a designated area in the cage, moving its head or a limb in a given direction—and rewarded by relief of withdrawal symptoms with a drug injection. There seems an obvious parallel in the behavior of human addicts who resume use of drugs on returning to a familiar neighborhood and meeting old friends. According to histories of addicts, conditioned associations are often involved in relapse after a period of abstinence. However, the observations in animals should not be taken to imply that conditioned associations are likely to be the sole or chief cause of relapse among human addicts. Even if conditioning plays a role, as it undoubtedly does, it may be secondary to narcotic drug hunger having a physiological or biochemical basis.

(Withdrawal Treatment

Methadone has, for twenty years, become the drug of choice for detoxifying heroin addicts.[25] Its use is associated with milder withdrawal symptoms than produced by other narcotics. Adult addicts are initially given 40 mg. of methadone daily in divided doses. The amount of narcotic is slowly reduced over a three-week period; usually, chloral hydrate sleeping medication is given as well. The treatment period may be extended over eight weeks if desired. Detoxification is carried out either within the hospital (on a closed ward) or on an ambulatory basis, in which case the patient reports daily for medication. (The procedure described is that presently used at the Morris J. Bernstein Institute of Beth Israel Hospital in New York City, presently the largest detoxification facility in the country, with which the writer is associated. Other hospitals follow a similar routine.)

Inasmuch as about half of the patients are unable to complete detoxification and virtually all relapse after return to the street, it can no longer be held as an effective therapy of drug abuse. For the "street addict" it offers only brief respite, at least reducing the drug habit. In addition, it brings him into a medical facility, and provides an opportunity for diagnosis and treatment of co-existing medical problems.

(Methadone Maintenance Therapy

The failure of detoxification treatment[1] spurred efforts to find other approaches that might reduce or eliminate the desire for heroin. The experience with the temporary benefits of methadone in detoxification suggested that maintenance therapy with this agent might provide the means. Initial clinical studies begun at Rockefeller University Hospital in New York City in 1964[8] demonstrated that methadone could effectively block the euphoric action of heroin and hence remove drug hunger.[10] Methadone itself produced no euphoric or other narcotic effects when given to patients stabilized on a constant dose. With extension of the program to the Beth Israel Hospital, these observations were confirmed. Methadone tolerance could be maintained without escalation of dosage; moreover, the dosage could be reduced or the drug stopped altogether without creating a desire for methadone itself. The greater duration of action of methadone (twenty-four to thirty-six hours) than of heroin (four to six hours) proved a basic advantage; in addition, it could be taken orally. (There is no indication for dispensing methadone in injectable form, except if a patient is unable to take oral medication for medical or surgical reasons.)

Initially, the patients who were admitted to the methadone research program were addicts with a history of at least four years of "mainline" heroin use and repeated relapses after detoxification. Now, the programs are open to addicts eighteen years or older who have been addicted for two years or more. The diagnosis must be documented by physical signs and urine testing,[5] and the history corroborated by the family and/or medical records. As a measure of the success of these programs, more than 70 percent of patients continuing in one for two years or more have obtained employment or returned to school. Drug-related crime has been reduced to less than 10 percent of the pre-treatment rates.[11]

There appears to be no medical contraindication to use of methadone; in the eight years the program has been operative in New York City, no toxic effects or idiosyncratic reactions have been observed.[42] (More than 10 million doses have been given.)

In initiating maintenance therapy,[8,7,35] the dose must be low at first and increased gradually over a four-to-six-week period. On the first day, 20 to 40 mg. (depending on the amount of heroin being used) can be given in divided doses; increments of 10 mg. daily are added every three or four days, unless the patient complains or appears oversedated.[45] The increase is added to the morning dose so that eventually only one daily dose need be taken. In general, patients feel no drug hunger when maintenance dose is about 50 mg. daily; however, in localities with high narcotic usage, investigators tend to increase the amount to 100 mg. daily; this is to assure a sufficient blocking dose[10,30] should the patient experiment with heroin.

Adjunctive services of methadone maintenance programs should depend on the nature of the population served.[30] In clinics treating chiefly inner city addicts, the services most needed involve housing, jobs, and provision for other essential needs. In programs primarily for the middle class, provision for psychiatric services is usually indicated.

Under some circumstances, physicians can now provide methadone maintenance therapy in their private office.[28] Of course, since methadone is a narcotic, its use anywhere is regulated by federal and state guidelines. In the case of the private physician, specific government provisions must be met.

Despite the success of methadone maintenance therapy, other agents are being tested. [51,50,29] Methadone is dangerous if taken by a nontolerant adult or by a child.[17] (Death of a child after taking a dose intended for a stabilized adult has been described in several reports.) As a narcotic, methadone creates physical dependence; it would be preferable to have an agent equally effective in blocking drug hunger without creating dependence. Ideally, such an agent would be capable of reversing the central nervous system effects of past exposure to heroin or another addictive agent so that treatment would not have to be continued indefinitely.

For the present, whether or not a physician is himself involved in methadone maintenance therapy, he should be aware of the rapid growth of such programs in the past few years.[13] Given the large number of patients being treated, problems of methadone overdose can and do occur.[17] Physicians should be familiar with use of naloxone[6,48] as an antidote (to be given repeatedly over a twenty-four-hour period); hospital emergency rooms should have supplies of the antidote on hand.

❨ Narcotic Antagonists

The possibility that narcotic antagonists might be useful in treatment of heroin addiction was first tested with cyclazocine[31] and more recently with naloxone.[51] When given to detoxified addicts, these agents block the euphoric effect of narcotics; they also have the advantage of being nonaddictive. However, blocking the euphoric effect may not be sufficient to prevent clinical relapse. Experience with cyclazocine in a number of programs over the past six years indicates that only a small minority of patients remain in treatment for more than a year;[36] most return to drug use much sooner. The short blocking action of cyclazocine (less than twenty-hour hours) may be a chief reason why drug hunger remains virtually unaffected. Work with naloxone is proceeding in the hope that it will prove more useful; as yet, there are no definitive results.[29,51]

Therapeutic Communities

Residential facilities managed by former addicts had their start with the founding of Synanon in California in 1958; at present, ex-addicts operate a group of Synanon residences throughout the country; similar programs, modeled after Synanon, include Daytop Village, Phoenix House, Odyssey House, Exodus House, to name but a few.

The theory underlying most such programs is that drug dependence is rooted in specific psychopathology manifested by immaturity and irresponsibility. The aim is to encourage addicts to work toward greater responsibility within the organization. Those who progress are rewarded with more desirable work assignments; those not measuring up are reassigned at a more menial level. Group therapy and "encounter" sessions are an integral part of the program.

Several descriptive accounts of the procedures used have been reported;[30] however, little of the published material provides a detailed analysis of results and, in general, directors of these programs have been reluctant to allow outsiders access for evaluation. From what is known, there seems little question that patients who remain in the therapeutic community fare well, particularly if employed by the program; however, apparently a significant proportion (reportedly about 50 percent) drop out fairly early. Other evidence suggests a high relapse rate among ex-addicts who complete the therapeutic program and return to the community. According to some estimates only 10 percent remain drug-free after two years. Other findings suggest that therapeutic communities may be beneficial to certain addicts, particularly the young middle-

class abuser of amphetamines or barbiturates. The true value of such programs can only be speculated on until more data are available.

Concluding Remarks

Present treatment options in the management of narcotic drug abuse have their basis in either a psychological theory of addiction, or a theory that neurochemical and/or neurophysiological factors[9] may be critical in creating or maintaining drug dependence. The first theory postulates the existence of pre-existing psychiatric problems, plus a need for drugs to escape from reality. According to the second, the initial impulse is likely to reflect a combination of adolescent curiosity and social exposure; and adaptive changes in the central nervous system, induced by physical drug dependence, tend to persist long after the drug is withdrawn.

Naturally, the principles of therapy are dissimilar. Proponents of a psychological basis for drug abuse are apt to ask total abstinence from narcotics; the treatment program may involve confinement in a therapeutic community or another setting providing some form of psychotherapy. Proponents of neurochemical-neurophysiological causation define their successes in terms of behavior, indicated by an addict's ability to pursue a reasonably normal and useful existence despite drug dependence.[11]

To resolve the issue, questions must be answered. Do patients blockaded with methadone exhibit significant residual psychopathology in facing the challenge of giving up heroin and taking on responsibilities of work, school, and family life? According to evaluations from a number of sources,[18] including reports from correctional[27] and social agencies,[16] the large majority of methadone-treated patients are freed of drug hunger and can turn their energies to more productive endeavors. On the other hand, one may ask, are patients treated in a psychologically oriented program with seeming success likely to remain drug-free? It appears, from the evidence, that without continued group reinforcement and perhaps further institutionalization, few are able to do so.

(Bibliography

1. BERLE, B., and M. NYSWANDER. "Ambulatory Withdrawal Treatment of Heroin Addicts," *New York State Journal of Medicine*, 64 (1964), 1846–1848.

2. COCHIN, J., and C. KORNETSKY. "Development and Loss of Tolerance to Morphine in the Rat After Single and Multiple Injections," *Journal of Pharmacology and Experimental Therapeutics*, 145 (1964), 1–10.

3. DOLE, V. P. "Biochemistry of Addiction." *Annual Review of Biochemistry*, 39 (1970), 821–840.

4. ———. "Narcotic Addiction, Physical Dependence and Relapse," *New England Journal of Medicine*, 286 (1972), 988–992.

5. DOLE, V. P., A. CROWTHER, J. JOHNSON, M. MONSALVATAGE, B. BILLER, and S. NELSON. "Detection of Narcotic, Sedative and Amphetamine Drugs in Urine," *New York State Journal of Medicine*, 72 (1972), 471–476.

6. DOLE, V. P., F. F. FOLDER, H. TRIGG, J. W. ROBINSON, and S. BLATMAN. "Methadone Poisoning," *New York State Journal of Medicine*, 71 (1971), 541–543.

7. DOLE, V. P., and M. NYSWANDER. "Rehabilitation of the Street Addict," *Archives of Environmental Health*, 14 (1967), 477–480.

8. ———. "A Medical Treatment for Diacetylmorphine Addiction," *Journal of the AMA*, 193 (1965), 646–650.

9. ———. "Methodone Maintenance and Its Implication for Theories of Narcotic Addiction," in *The Addictive States*, pp. 359–366. Baltimore: Williams and Wilkens, 1968.

10. DOLE, V. P., M. NYSWANDER, and M. J. KREEK. "Narcotic Blockade," *Archives of Internal Medicine*, 118 (1966), 304–309.

11. DOLE, V. P., M. NYSWANDER, and A. WARNER. "Successful Treatment of 750 Criminal Addicts," *Journal of the AMA*, 206 (1968), 2708–2711.

12. DUPONT, R. L. "Profile of a Heroin Addiction Epidemic," *New England Journal of Medicine*, 285 (1971), 320–324.

13. DUPONT, R. L., and R. N. KATON. "A Heroin-Addiction Treatment Program," *Journal of the AMA*, 216 (1971), 1320–1324.

14. EDDY, N. B. "The Search for a Potent Nonaddicting Analgesic," in E. L. Way, ed., *New Concepts in Pain and Its Clinical Management*, pp. 65–84. Philadelphia: Davis, 1967.

15. EDDY, N. B., H. HALBACH, H. ISBELL, and M. H. SEEVERS. "Drug Dependence: Its Significance and Characteristics," World Health Organization, 32 (1965), 721–733.

16. GEARING, F. "A Road Back from Heroin Addiction." *Proceedings of the Fourth National Conference on Methadone Treatment*, San Francisco, Cal., Jan. 1972, pp. 157–158.

17. ———. "Death Before, During and After Methadone Maintenance Treatment in New York City." *Proceedings of the Fourth National Conference on Methadone Treatment*, San Francisco, Cal., Jan. 1972, pp. 493–494.

18. ———. "Evaluation of Methadone Maintenance Treatment Program," *International Journal of Addictions*, 5 (1970), 517–543.

19. GENDREAU, P., and L. P. GENDREAU. "The 'Addiction Prone' Personality: A Study of Canadian Heroin Addicts," *Canadian Journal of Behavioral Science*, 2 (1970), 18–25.

20. GOLDSTEIN, A. "Heroin Addiction and the Role of Methadone in Its Treatment," *Archives of General Psychiatry*, 26 (1972), 291–297.

21. GORDON, N. B. "Reaction Times of Methadone Treated Ex-heroin Addicts," *Psychopharmacologia*, 16 (1970), 337–344.

22. GORDON, N. B., A. WARNER, and A. HENDERSON. "Psychomotor and Intellectual Performance Under Methadone Maintenance." Presented to the Committee on Problems of Drug Dependence, National Academy of Sciences, National Research Council, 1967.

23. INGERSOLL, J. Testimony before Subcommittee on Public Health and Environment, U.S. Senate, 1971.

24. ISBELL, H. "Addiction to Barbiturates and the Barbiturate Abstinence Syndrome," *Annals of Internal Medicine*, 33 (1950), 108–121.

25. ISBELL, H., and V. VOGEL. "The Addiction Liability of Methadone and Its Use in the Treatment of Morphine Abstinence Syn-

drome," *The American Journal of Psychiatry*, 105 (1949), 909–914.

26. JAFFE, J. "Drug Addiction and Drug Abuse," in Goodman and Gilman, eds., *The Pharmacological Basis of Therapeutics*, pp. 285–311. New York: Macmillan, 1965.

27. JOSEPH, H., and V. P. DOLE. "Methadone Patients on Probation and Parole," *Federal Probation*, (1970), 91–93.

28. KARKUS, H. "Methadone Failures: Patient or Program?" *Proceedings of the Fourth National Conference on Methadone Treatment*, San Francisco, Cal., Jan. 1972, pp. 401–403.

28A. KRAMER, J. C. "The State versus the Addict: Uncivil Commitment," *Boston University Law Review*, 50 (1970).

29. LEVINE, R., A. ZAKS, M. FINK, and A. FREEDMAN. "Naloxone Pamoate: A Long Acting Opiate Antagonist," (to be published).

30. LOWINSON, J., and I. ZWERLING. "Group Therapy with Narcotic Addicts," in J. Kaplan, and J. Sadock, eds., *Comprehensive Group Psychotherapy*, pp. 602–622. Baltimore: Williams and Wilkens, 1971.

31. MARTIN, W. R. "Opioid Antagonists," *Pharmacological Review*, 19 (1967), 463–521.

32. MARTIN, W. R., A. WIKLER, C. G. EADES, and F. T. PESCOR. "Tolerance to and Physical Dependence on Morphine in Rats," *Psychopharmacologia*, 4 (1963), 247–260.

33. NICHOLS, J. R. "How Opiates Change Behavior," *Scientific American*, 212 (1965), 80–88.

34. NYSWANDER, M. *The Drug Addict as a Patient*. New York: Grune & Stratton, 1956.

35. ———. "The Methadone Treatment of Heroin Addiction," *Hospital Practice*, 2 (1967), 27–33.

36. RESNICK, R., M. FINK, and A. FREEDMAN. "Cyclazocine Treatment of Opiate Dependence, a Progress Report," *Comprehensive Psychiatry* (in press).

37. SEEVERS, M. H., and G. A. DENEAU. W. S. Root, and F. G. Hofmann, eds., in *Physiological Pharmacology*, pp. 565–640. New York: Academic Press, 1963.

38. SOLITAIRE, G. B. "Neuropathologic Aspects of Drug Dependence, (Narcotic Addiction)," *Human Pathology*, 3 (1972), 85–89.

39. SPRAGG, S. D. S. "Morphine Addiction in Chimpanzees," *Comparative Psychology Monographs*, 15 (1940), 1.

40. TERRY, C. E., and M. PELLENS. *The Opium Problems*. New York: Bureau of Social Hygiene, 1928. (Reprinted by Patterson Smith Co., Montclair, N.J., 1970.)

41. THOMPSON, T. "Drugs as Reinforcers: Experimental Addiction," *International Journal of Addictions*, 3 (1968), 199–206.

42. WALLACH, R. C., E. JEREZ, and G. BLINICK. "Pregnancy and Menstrual Function in Narcotics Addicts Treated with Methadone," *American Journal of Obstetrics and Gynecology*, 105 (1969), 1226–1229.

43. WEEKS, J. R. "Experimental Narcotic Addiction," *Scientific American*, 210 (1964), 46–52.

44. WEPPNER, R. S., and M. H. AGAR. "Immediate Precursors of Heroin Addiction," *Journal of Health and Social Behavior*, 12 (1971), 10–18.

45. WIELAND, W., and C. CHARLES. "Methadone Maintenance: A Comparison of Two Stabilization Techniques," *Journal of Addictions*, 5 (1970).

46. WIKLER, A. "Some Implications of Conditioning Theory for Problems of Drug Abuse," *Behavioral Science*, 16 (1971), 92–97.

47. ———. "A psychodynamic study of a patient during experimental self-regulated re-addiction to morphine." *Psychiatry Quarterly*, 26:270–293, 1952.

48. ———, H. F. FRASER, and H. ISBELL. "N-allylnor-morphine: Effects of Single Doses and Precipitation of Acute 'Abstinence Syndromes' During Addiction to Morphine, Methadone on Man (Postaddicts)," *Journal of Pharmacology and Experimental Therapeutics*, 109 (1953), 92–101.

49. ——— and F. T. PESCOR. "Classical Conditioning of a Morphine Abstinence Phenomenon, Reinforcement of Opioid-drinking Behavior and 'Relapse' in Morphine-addicted Rats," *Psychopharmacologia*, 10 (1967), 255–284.

50. ZAKS, A., M. FINK, and A. M. FREEDMAN. "Levomethadyl in Opiate Dependence," *Journal of the AMA*, 220 (1972), 811–813.

51. ZAKS, A., T. JONES, A. M. FREEDMAN, and M. FINK. "Naloxone Treatment of Opiate Dependence," *Journal of the AMA*, 215 (1971), 2108–2110.

CHAPTER 20

THE USE OF PSYCHOTOMIMETIC AND RELATED CONSCIOUSNESS-ALTERING DRUGS

George U. Balis

THE TERM "PSYCHOTOMIMETIC" DESIGNATES a large class of psychoactive compounds, variously known as hallucinogenic, psychedelic, psycholytic, psychotogenic, psychodysleptic, mysticomimetic, and phantastica. The decision as to which drugs should be included under these names is to some extent arbitrary, since there is no precise definition of the pharmacological category of these compounds. They are generally described as substances that produce primarily alterations in perception, thought, and mood in the absence of changes in conscious awareness.[129] This definition excludes drugs that induce delirious states (deliriants), generally characterized by an altered state of consciousness accompanied by clouding of awareness,

and also drugs that are variously classified as sedative-anesthetic, narcotic, inebriant, euphoriant, or stimulant. Nevertheless, there is considerable overlapping in the pharmacological profile of these drugs, since, one way or the other, they alter some aspect of the conscious experience, a psychotropic effect that greatly depends on dosage, route of administration, and combination with other drugs, as well as on the idiosyncrasy, personality, and mental set of the user, and the setting in which the drug is taken. In general, this chapter deals with those drugs which alter the state of consciousness with regard to the quality and intensity of the various parameters of the conscious experience, especially perception, cognition, and affectivity.

When drug-induced changes in these experiential parameters occur in a clear sensorium, the effect is described in its typical form as "psychedelic" or "hallucinogenic." On the other hand, when these changes occur in a clouded sensorium, that is, in a state of confusion, disorientation, diminished awareness, and impaired subsequent recall of the drug experience, the drug response is described as "delirium." However, this distinction is to some extent arbitrary, because overlapping intermediate states may be induced by both categories of drugs. Furthermore, the two psychotomimetic syndromes reach "psychotic" proportions only when the mental functioning of the subject is sufficiently impaired to result in profound alterations of mood or in serious deficits in the areas of reality testing, perception, and cognition. Actually, the usual reaction to most of these drugs can hardly be described as "psychotic." Since the most important characteristic of the effect of these drugs is alteration of consciousness, it is pertinent to consider in some detail the concept of consciousness and its vicissitudes under the influence of psychotomimetic drugs.

(Drugs and the Vicissitudes of Consciousness

Attempting to define consciousness is fraught with as many difficulties as trying to define the "ghost in the machine." The class of phenomena denoted by the term "consciousness" represents not only a conceptual construct but also an empirical datum, the *sui generis* nature of which transcends any measure of objectivity. As a conceptual construct, the term has various meanings when used in a philosophical or metaphysical context, but has very little heuristic value in scientific research. As an empirical datum, consciousness was defined by Jaspers[154] as a phenomenon of psychic life understandable in terms of our own introspection or of our patient's reported introspection, and constituting an immediate experience of the total psyche—analogous to a stage—within which the phenomena of perception,

cognition, memory, and affect occur. Jaspers further distinguished three aspects of consciousness, namely, (i) the actual inner awareness that accompanies consciousness, (ii) the awareness that defines the boundaries of the self (the subject-object dichotomy), and (iii) the knowledge of the conscious self, or self-awareness. Another important aspect of consciousness is its "anticipatory" nature in the context of hindsight and foresight. The subjective experience of awareness, although a "private datum," represents the most substantive aspect of consciousness, the phenomenology of which can only be understood through introspection. On the other hand, the inspective study of observable behavioral and neurophysiological variables associated with the phenomena of consciousness is primarily concerned with the subject's responsiveness to his environment, but yields no information about the introspected or experienced aspect of this state. The reticular activating system seems to play an important role in the activation as well as the integration of the processes that subserve consciousness.

The state of consciousness may undergo alterations in many clinical conditions including epilepsy (twilight states), dissociative forms of hysteria (fugue states, somnambulism), psychoses, delirium, stupor, and coma, as well as in hypnotic states, dreaming, religious "conversion" experiences, and transcendental or mystical experiences. These conditions may involve changes in the content, intensity, and/or quality of the conscious experience. For instance, the content of consciousness—thoughts, memories, percepts—may become pathologic in nature, as in psychoses (delusions, hallucinations), or it may be quantitatively reduced, as in dementias. Disturbances related to the intensity gradient of consciousness—viewed as a continuum ranging from hypervigilance to coma—are seen in acute panic states or drug-induced stimulation on the one hand, and in the various stages of coma and anesthesia on the other. In describing the latter states, reference is made to levels or depths of coma or anesthesia. In delirious states, there is primarily an interference with integrative processes, which results in the dissolution of the "Gestalt" of consciousness that is referred to as awareness. In the psychedelic experience induced by hallucinogens, there is primarily an alteration in the quality of the introspected correlate of consciousness associated with heightened awareness.[25]

The "Psychedelic" (LSD) Experience

This drug response is induced by LSD-25, mescaline, psilocybin, and other hallucinogens. The experiential content of the reaction is greatly influenced by the "set" (the subject's expectations of what the drug will do to him in relation to his personality) and the "setting" (the total milieu) in which the drug is taken. A description of the LSD-induced psychedelic experience will be presented as a prototype. The sequence of occurrences following the ingestion of effective doses of LSD—popularly known as the "trip"—usually begins half an hour after taking the drug, reaches a peak in about two to three hours, and terminates after a total duration of six to twelve hours. The reaction[64,86,104,128,129] begins with a prodromal phase of autonomic effects, lasting about one hour, and including pupillary dilation, nausea and occasional vomiting, pallor or flushing, tremor, dizziness, and restlessness associated with dysphoria. The vegetative phase is followed by a period of perceptual changes involving distortions of body image characterized by sensations of changed body size and shape, and altered perceptions of the subject's relationship to his body and its parts. Body boundaries may become fluid, or fused with the surroundings, or may acquire a pulsating quality. As the reaction progresses, the subject increasingly experiences feelings of derealization and depersonalization characterized by a peculiar awareness of "apartness" or a feeling of "double consciousness," in which there is a splitting of the self into a passive, detached, and observing monitor—the "spectator ego"—and an experiencing self. Other perceptual changes include vivid illusions which are mostly visual, distortions in the three-dimensional space, and, rarely, hallucinations. Freedman[104] asserts that "illusions

can be imaginatively or regressively elaborated in hallucinations," and "memories can emerge as clear images competing for the status of current reality." Subjects report a phantasmagoria of kaleidoscopically perceived visual experiences variously described as space full of geometric patterns and weird objects, brilliant colors, lights, objects which appear to fluctuate, to change in size and shape or fuse with the background, faces of people distorted in a caricaturistic or frightening way, fluid boundaries, perseveration of images, synesthesias, such as "color-hearing" and "sound-seeing," and, in general, an endless description of perceptual alterations, the nature of which is greatly influenced by set and setting. Subjects may show the whole spectrum of affective responses ranging from exhilaration, ecstasy, and euphoria (accompanied by uncontrollable giggling and laughing) to depression, despair, or panic. Investigators have emphasized the subject's fear of loss of control in the area of intellect, emotion, and bodily function, which may result in panic reactions. While some subjects show euphoria and "ego expansiveness," others react with apathy, psychomotor retardation, and "ego constriction." Most cognitive functions have been reported to suffer significant impairment, even under moderate doses, especially immediate memory,[21] attention, concentration, recognition and recall, problem-solving and spatial discrimination,[266] judgment and comprehension, and learning.[21] Reported disturbances of thought processes include blocking, flight of ideas, and incoherence.[128] Rorschach responses reveal a tendency towards concrete thinking, decreased productivity of responses, and an exaggeration of basic personality characteristics.[85] Perceptual tests have shown impairment in discrimination in color perception,[125] alterations in perception of size, direction, and distance,[262] and distortions in the sense of time.[20] The telescoping of past and future and the overvaluation of "nowness" during the LSD-experience may be the result of the alterations in time perception, probably related to the impairment of immediate memory, a phenomenon also reported with marijuana smoking.[200,201] The compelling immediacy of the psychedelic experience may also contribute to this "here-and-now" orientation.[104] Other effects of the drug, which are greatly dependent on the expectations of the user, include the experience of a self-revealing transcendental state, the attainment of stunning "insights," and the enhancement of creativity, either during the experience or thereafter.[142,177] These controversial effects have been attributed to subjective convictions resulting from the peculiar experiential state of the subject. Under the influence of the drug, objects that are void of any aesthetic, emotional, or intellectual connotation become overwhelmingly beautiful, or are invested with new and profound significance. According to Freedman,[104] "qualities become intense and gain a life of their own; redness is more interesting than the object which is red, meaningfulness more important than what is specifically meant. Connotations balloon into cosmic allusiveness. This can be experienced religiously, aesthetically, sensually." Also, in this state, the familiar acquires the characteristics of a *jamais vu* quality, and becomes novel and "portentous." It is "the capacity of the mind to see more than it can tell, to experience more than it can explicate, to believe in and be impressed with more than it can rationally justify, to experience boundlessness and 'boundaryless' events, from the banal to the profound," that Freedman calls "portentousness." The claim that the drug experience enhances creativity has been challenged by several writers.[104,109,188,254,272] Mamlet[188] has called attention to the "consciousness-limiting" side effects of these so-called consciousness-expanding drugs. Others believe that these potential forms of consciousness may open up avenues of creativity but are not creative themselves,[227] or, as William James asserts, they "may determine attitudes though they cannot furnish formulas and open a region though they fail to give a map."[152]

The "Euphoric" (Marijuana) Experience

The term "euphoria" is loosely used in the literature to describe a variety of affective states including a heightened sense of well-being, or a pleasurable (hedonic) feeling of variable quality. Euphoria does not seem to represent a distinct affect or to be associated with a specific stimulus or a specific psychological state. It is an overinclusive term that encompasses such qualitatively different feelings as those induced by narcotics (opiates), inebriants and intoxicants (ethanol, ether), stimulants (amphetamines), or moods experienced by manic patients. The euphoric experience or "high" induced by marijuana and its products is a complex psychological response characteristic of this drug. Although with small doses the marijuana effect is primarily euphoric and comparable to that of alcohol, with larger doses it is mainly "psychedelic" comparable to that of LSD. There is wide variation of response to marijuana, depending not only on the type and quality of the cannabis product (tetrahydrocannabinol content), but also on the user (his personality, motivation, expectations, and previous experience with the drug), and the environment in which it is taken. There are also variations in the effect, depending on whether marijuana is smoked or ingested. With marijuana smoking the effects occur rapidly (within ten to thirty minutes) and last for two to four hours; also, the level of intoxication can be easily titrated. With oral administration, the onset is slower (thirty minutes to one hour) and the effects last longer (five to twelve hours).[121,238] The initial effects of marijuana on the naïve user have been described as unpleasant or ambiguous.[31,32,44,264] It has been suggested that "before the smoker can derive agreeable sensations from cannabis, he must first go through the discomforts of habituation,"[44] a phenomenon that has been attributed to a learning process involving not only the learning of the correct technique of inhaling but also learning to appreciate and define the effects of the drug as pleasurable.[31,32] The alternative hypothesis, however, "that getting high on marijuana occurs only after some sort of pharmacological sensitization takes place"[264] has received recent support from metabolic studies on tetrahydrocannabinol which indicate that active metabolites are formed in the liver by inducible enzymes activated by repeated exposures to the drug.[178,198] A characteristic aspect of marijuana effect is its wave-like quality, a waxing and waning phenomenon which has also been reported to characterize the psychedelic experience produced by hallucinogens, like LSD.[66] The predominant psychological effect is euphoria.[14,15,44,49,62,112,195] Other affective changes may include elation and sense of well-being, confidence, and adequacy, hilarity and uncontrollable laughter.[44,112] Anxiety has been frequently reported, especially in the inexperienced user, and when the drug is taken in nonsupportive settings.[15,48,49,62,163] Somnolence is invariably present. Perceptual changes include heightened sensitivity to external stimuli, shifting attention with focusing on details that would ordinarily be overlooked, micropsias and occasionally macropsias, disturbances of body image, depersonalization and the phenomenon of "double consciousness," distortions in the perception of time and space, and enhancement in the aesthetic appreciation or insightful understanding of what is perceived or experienced.[15,44,49,121,238,250] Other, less frequently reported perceptual changes include synesthesias,[48,49,195,250] illusions, and hallucinatory-like experiences.[15,44,48,49,66,164,195] In a recent questionnaire study of forty-two marijuana users, Keeler et al.[104] found that about 40 percent of the subjects had experienced hallucinations. In another questionnaire study by Tart,[250] marijuana users reported the following perceptual changes experienced under the influence of the drug:

"When looking at pictures, they may acquire an element of visual depth, a third dimensional aspect . . . contours stand out more sharply against the background." When listening to music, the subjects felt that "spatial separation between various instruments sounds greater, as if they were physically apart," and with eyes closed, they felt that the space "becomes an auditory space, a space where things are arranged according to their sound characteristics instead of visual geometric characteristics." There were also distortions from other sensory modalities: "My sense of touch is more exciting, more sensual . . .

Smells become richer and more unique . . . Taste sensations take on new qualities," "distances seem to get greater," "time passes very slowly . . . certain experiences seem outside of time, are timeless."

The exaggeration of the sense of time is considered as one of the most conspicuous effects of marijuana and has been attributed to a characteristic congnitive impairment involving primarily immediate memory.[65,66,90,200,201] The interrelationship between changes in time perception and impairment of immediate memory was ingeniously demonstrated by Melges and associates,[200] who found that subjects given marijuana-extracted tetrahydrocannabinol show a definite impairment on a complex test for immediate memory. The impairment was labeled "temporal disintegration," which they defined as "difficulty in retaining, coordinating, and serially indexing those memories, perceptions, and expectations that are relevant to the goal . . . (an individual) is pursuing." Temporal disintegration was also found to be associated with the loosening of verbal associations and the lack of goal-directedness in speech.

In another study, using a test in which the subjects judged for themselves how well they were able to co-ordinate the past, present, and future, as well as how well goal-directed they felt, Melges and associates[201] concluded that the distorted time perception induced by marijuana was also associated with the subject's tendency to focus on the present to the exclusion of the past and future. This telescoping of time, also reported with LSD, was closely related to the degree of depersonalization experienced by the subject. There is considerable controversy as to whether marijuana smoking produces any significant impairment in cognitive functions and task performance. In general, marijuana users feel that they can "turn off" the "high" at will, and that they have a degree of self-control that allows them to pursue any goal-directed activity.[250] This ability to "compensate" when performing on a task has been reported by several investigators,[42,52,67,83,159,264] who have found that the administration of marijuana does not produce any significant impairment in various simple motor and mental performance tests. Weil and associates[264] reported that although marijuana-naïve persons demonstrate impaired performance on simple intellectual and psychomotor tests, experienced marijuana users show very little impairment. Similarly, Crancer and associates,[83] using experienced marijuana smokers to compare the effect of alcohol and marijuana on performance in a driving simulator apparatus, found that there were no significant differences in terms of total scores, except for speedometer errors, when the subjects were under the influence of marijuana, whereas there was marked impairment in all measures of the test, with the exception of steering errors, when the subjects were under the influence of alcohol. It has been suggested that Crancer's enthusiastic marijuana smokers were probably eager to prove that marijuana is safe and alcohol dangerous.[240]

More recently, Meyer and associates[202] compared the effect of marijuana on heavy and casual marijuana users by using a placebo, a fixed dose of marijuana, and a self-selected ad lib dose. Their subjects showed a modest decrease in perception and psychomotor task performance with both types of marijuana dose, though casual users demonstrated a greater degree of impairment than did heavy users. Other investigators have similarly reported that the administration of increased doses of marijuana does not produce increased performance decrements.[52,66,83,264] The question of dose-response relationship in perceptual and cognitive functions was recently studied by Dornbush and associates,[90] who found that memory and retention time were significantly affected by the higher doses, whereas time estimation was not differentially affected by either lower or higher doses. Studies using more complex tests have shown that marijuana produces considerable impairment in performance.[66,189] Thus, Clark and associates,[66] using tests which involved a prolonged and intricate task, concluded that "marijuana intoxication has significant effects on complex reaction time (largely through sporadic im-

pairment of vigilance), recent memory, recall and comprehension of written information, and accuracy of time estimation," and also that "the processes involved in selective perception (and, conversely, habituation to irrelevant stimuli), immediate recall of preceding thoughts in order to keep on track, and capacity for goal-directed systematic thinking are particularly sensitive to relatively low doses of marijuana." In spite of this cognitive impairment, many marijuana users claim that the drug makes them think insightfully and creatively.[250] Using objective measures of perceptiveness, Jones and Stones[159] found that subjects under the influence of marijuana were less perceptive than when sober, and retrospectively regarded many of their marijuana-produced "insights" as nonsense. It is likely that the marijuana-induced feeling that things look novel and original, a phenomenon comparable to the clinically occurring experiences of *jamais vu*, might account for the subjective reports of originality, insightfulness, and creativity. Others have attributed it to heightened suggestibility and faulty perception, impaired judgment, and enhanced awareness.[121,238]

The effects of tetrahydrocannabinol (THC) —the major psychoactive substance contained in cannabis—were first studied by Isbell and associates.[146] These investigators administered progressively increasing doses of THC by smoking (50 to 200 mcg./kg) and oral ingestion (120 to 480 mcg./kg). The psychological changes induced by the drug were dose-dependent. Lower doses produced euphoria, alterations in sense of time, and heightened visual and auditory perception. Higher doses produced marked perceptual distortions, derealization, depersonalization, and hallucinations, both auditory and visual. Studies comparing the subjective experience produced by THC and LSD have shown that the effect of the two drugs is very similar.[137,147] The only significant difference is that with LSD the subjects are extremely alert, whereas with THC they become sedated and fall asleep. Also, THC tends to produce prominent and persistent euphoria; on the other hand, the prominent effect in LSD experience is awe and fear. Subjects generally describe the THC experience as more pleasant than that of LSD.

The "Delirious" (Toxic) Experience

This is a primitive "high" characterized by gross disturbances of consciousness and cognitive functions, frequently associated with perceptual distortions and affective changes ranging from euphoria to panic or rage. It represents a crude assault to conscious experience and is sought primarily for the initial inebriating effect that precedes the confusional excitement. Deliriant drugs commonly used to obtain this type of "high" include ether, nitrous oxide, and various industrial solvents containing hydrocarbons (e.g., glue-sniffing).[216,217] In general, the drug response is the result of an acute brain syndrome characteristic of a "toxic psychosis." In delirium, there is characteristic reduction of the level of awareness, ranging from mild sluggishness of grasp to stupor or unconsciousness. In a typical case, the patient is disoriented, confused, bewildered, and incoherent. In more severe cases, thinking is disjoined, irrelevant, and frequently delusional. Delusional ideas are poorly organized, shifting in content, dream-like, and often persecutory in nature. They usually occur in the context of perceptual distortions, illusory misinterpretations (usually misinterpreting the unfamiliar for the familiar), and hallucinatory experiences, mainly visual. The mood of the delirious patient is often characterized by perplexity, apprehension, and fear, which often reaches panicky proportions. In his panic, the patient may become highly impulsive, destructive, and suicidal. Motor activity may vary from marked retardation to severe excitement with uncontrollable hyperactivity. The electroencephalographic (EEG) findings in delirium consist of generalized slow frequencies in the delta-theta range. The degree of synchronization of the EEG seems to correlate with the severity of the disturbances of consciousness. Upon recovery from the episode, the patient shows spotty amnesia of his experiences during the delirium; the amnesia is proportional to the degree of the impairment of consciousness.[25]

❡ Pharmacology of Psychotomimetic Drugs

Classification

The psychotomimetic drugs may be classified into two major categories: (1) Those producing heightened awareness, properly labeled as "psychedelic;" and (2) those producing clouded awareness, known as "deliriant."

1. *The Psychedelic Group* includes a number of drugs of synthetic or plant origin which can be subdivided, from a chemical point of view, into the following three subgroups:

  a. *The Indole (Tryptamine) Compounds*, which include LSD-25 (d-lysergic acid diethylamide), psilocybin (4-phosphoryloxy-N,N-dimethoxytryptamine), psilocin (dephosphorylated derivative of psilocybin), and the dimethyl homolog of psilocin, DMT (N,N-dimethyltryptamine), DET (N,N-diethyltryptamine), DPT (N,N-dipropyltryptamine), Alpha-MT (dl-alpha-methyltryptamine), harmine and its tetrahydrogenated derivative, tetrahydroharmine, and ibogaine. The psychotomimetic action of two other indole derivatives, bufotenine and serotonin, is not definitely established. A number of plants shown to possess psychotomimetic properties associated with naturally occurring indole compounds are also included in this group. The snuff called "cohoba" prepared by Haitian natives from the seeds of *Piptadenia peregrina* contains bufotenine, DMT, and several other indoles. The Mexican "hallucinogenic" mushrooms ("teonanactyl") which belong to the *Psilocybe* species contain psilocybin. The fly-agaric mushrooms (*Amanita muscaria*) contain bufotenine, muscarine, and piltzatropine. The African shrub "iboga" (*Tabernanthe iboga*), used by some inhabitants of West Africa and Congo to increase endurance and as an aphrodisiac, contains ibogaine. The psychotomimetic substances contained in the plants *Banisteropsis caapi* and *Prestonia amazonicum*, which are used by the Indians of Peru, Ecuador, Colombia, and Brazil for their hallucinogenc properties, include harmine and tetrahydroharmine. Finally, the morning glory plants (*Ololiuqui*), which belong to the *Convolvulaceae* species (*Rivea corybosa*), contain several ergot alkaloids, including lysergic acid amide and isolysergic acid amide.

b. *The Catecholamine (Adrenaline) Compounds* include the *phenylethylamine derivatives*, the most important member of which is mescaline (3,4,5-trimethoxyphenyethylamine), and the *amphetamine derivatives*, which include TMA (trimethoxyamphetamine), MDA (methylenedioxyamphetamine), DMA (2,5-dimethoxyamphetamine), DOM (2,5-dimethoxy-4-methylamphetamine), known in the hippie vernacular as "STP," DOET (2,5-dimethoxy-4-ethylamphetamine), MMDA (3-methoxy-4,5-methylenedioxyamphetamine), and DMMDA (2,5-dimethoxy-3,4-methylenedioxyamphetamine).

In this category belong the following psychotomimctic plants containing adrenaline-type derivatives: The cactus plant peyote, which contains mescaline; nutmeg, a household spice derived from the tree *Myristica fragrans* grown in the Molucca Islands, and which contains the psychoactive substance myristicin, a methylenedioxy-substituted compound resembling mescaline and ephedrine; khat, derived from the plant *Catha edulis*, is a mild stimulant and euphoriant widely used in many parts of Africa and Arabia, which contains the ephedrine-like compounds cathine, cathidine, and cathinine; kava-kava, derived from the plant *Piper methysticum*, is another mild social euphoriant containing the active substance methysticin, used by the inhabitants of the Pacific islands in the form of a beverage.

Finally, we will add to this category the various *sympathomimetic amines*, which include amphetamine, methamphetamine (Methedrine), methylphenidate (Ritalin), and phenmetrazine (Preludin). These central stimulants, although not psychotomimetic in the usual clinical doses, do produce psychotomimetic reactions when given in toxic doses.

c. *Tetrahydrocannabinols*, of which Delta-9-tetrahydrocannabinol (TCH) is considered to be the active substance contained in marijuana (*Cannabis sativa*) and other hemp products (hashish).

2. *The Deliriant Group* is the second large category of psychotomimetic drugs. The deliriants may further be classified into the following three subgroups:

a. *Anticholinergic Compounds*, which include the belladonna alkaloids (atropine), the piperydil-benzilates (Ditran), the diphenylmethane compounds (diethazine), and a number of other anticholinergic compounds (antiparkinsonian drugs).

b. *Anesthetic Compounds*, including Sernyl, alpha chloralose, and other anesthetic drugs which are characterized by a prolonged Stage II anesthesia (chloroform, ether, nitrous oxide).

c. *Various Volatile Hydrocarbons*, used primarily as industrial solvents (benzine, toluene, carbon tetrachloride), the sniffing of which reprcsents an increasing aberrant behavior among young adolescents.

LSD-25

LSD is a semisynthetic derivative of the fungus ergot of rye and belongs to the ergobasine group. Its psychotomimetic effect was discovered accidentally by Hofmann in 1943.[130] In the past twenty-five years there has been published a voluminous literature on the actions of this drug, stimulated primarily by the interest in producing a "model psychosis" for the understanding of schizophrenia, and by the controversial use of the drug as a psychotherapeutic tool. The widespread abuse of the drug by the young during the 1960s, and the possible dangers associated with it, gave a new impetus to LSD research and added new controversies. The "serotonin hypothesis" concerning the biochemical site of action of LSD is based on the notion that the drug may produce its effect by interfering with the action of serotonin in the brain. Although most of the data tend to support the view that LSD alters synaptic transmission by antagonizing serotonin, the hypothesis still remains unproven. The literature on this subject has been reviewed elsewhere.[9,129] The neurophysiological actions of LSD, and its effects on animal behavior have also been reviewed elsewhere.[17,120,178] The minimal effective (threshold) dose of LSD in humans is 25 mcg. However, the usual effective dose for eliciting a typical psychedelic experience ranges from 100 to 250 mcg, although much higher doses have been used by various investigators.[129] The duration of the reaction to LSD (eight to twelve hours), and the variations of its intensity correlate with the biological half-life of the drug in the plasma.[106] Chronic administration of LSD does not result in physical dependence or withdrawal reaction. There is, however, a dose-contingent tolerance, which develops rapidly after repeated doses, requiring a free period of four to six days before a complete experience can recur.[5,105,106,148] Cross-tolerance among various hallucinogens (LSD, mescaline, psilocybin) has been demonstrated in both animals[18,19,105] and man.[6,145,148] There is no cross-tolerance, however, between LSD and amphetamine[149] or tetrahydrocannabinol.[147] Drugs which tend to enhance and prolong the subjective experience to LSD include reserpine, sympathomimetic amines, and anticholinergic drugs;[129] on the other hand, chlorpromazine and other phenothiazines are very effective in attenuating the LSD effect.[18,128] LSD has a mild desynchronizing effect on the electroencephalogram characterized by a reduction in alpha frequency and an increase in beta activity.[100] Monroe and associates,[206] using depth electrodes, reported that LSD and mescaline produce subcortical paroxysmal activity in the hippocampal, amygdaloid, and septal regions, and that this activity correlated with an increase of psychotic behavior in schizophrenic subjects; these changes were blocked by chlorpromazine but not by reserpine. Many investigators have studied the effect of LSD on schizophrenic patients and have reported controversial findings as to whether these patients react in the same way as normals, whether they are more resistant in terms of dose, and whether they develop tolerance more quickly.[61,128,129,133] The physiological changes induced by LSD in human subjects consist primarily of pupillary dilatation and increase in deep tendon reflexes, an increase in pulse rate, and a rather inconsistent rise in systolic blood pressure; LSD has also been reported to produce slight ataxia, analgesia, increased salivation, and antidiuretic effect.[103,129,133] The only significant biochemical changes induced by LSD consist of an increase in free fatty acid levels, and a decrease in inorganic phosphorus excretion.[133,138]

Other Indole (Tryptamine) Derivatives

Psilocybin. The psychotomimetic compound contained in the mushrooms of the *Psilocybe* species, which have been used by Mexican Indians for centuries in religious and ceremonial practices. The psychotomimetic effect of psilocybin is very similar to that induced by LSD, though shorter in duration. The clinical changes after parenteral injection start within five minutes and terminate after five hours;

the intensity of the experience is dose-dependent.[132] Threshold doses up to 4 mg. of psilocybin produce a pleasant sensation of relaxation associated with feelings of mild detachment, and floating sensations. With higher doses (5 to 12 mg.) a typical psychotomimetic experience is elicited, characterized by perceptual alterations, depersonalization, heightened awareness, and mood changes. As with other hallucinogens, the reaction is preceded by vegetative symptoms. The phenomena of tolerance and cross-tolerance with other hallucinogens have been reported in repeated uses of psilocybin.[129,132,148]

DMT (N,N-dimethyltryptamine). An idole derivative which occurs naturally in various plants (*Piptadena peregrina, Prestonia amazonicum*), used by South American Indians as a snuff (cohoba) for ceremonial and religious purposes. In doses of 20 to 75 mg., DMT produces a short but intense psychotomimetic reaction, which develops rapidly and is characterized by a greater variety of visual experiences; strong feelings of loss of control may lead to panic states. With 75 mg. of DMT, given intramuscularly, Szara[245] reported strong autonomic changes consisting of nausea, mydriasis, increased blood pressure and pulse rate, trembling and choreoathetoid movements, as well as euphoria and vivid illusory-hallucinatory experiences; the symptoms disappeared after three-quarters to one hour.

DET (N,N-diethyltryptamine). Also a potent hallucinogen whose action has been compared to that of DMT.[247] With intramuscular doses ranging from 0.70 to 0.80 mg./kg. of weight, DET has been reported to produce vegetative symptoms, paresthesias, and psychic changes characteristic of other psychotomimetic drugs; however, the majority of cases experience some clouding of consciousness characteristic of delirious states. Other indole derivatives which have been demonstrated to possess psychotomimetic activity include DPT, alpha-MT, ibogaine, and harmine.

Mescaline

Mescaline is the principal psychoactive substance contained in the peyote, a cactus plant (*Lophophora williamsii*) found in the southwestern part of the United States and the northern part of Mexico. Peyote has been used for centuries by Mexican Indians in the context of religious ceremonies, and in the past one hundred years by the members of the native American Church of North America, a Christian-derived religion followed by North American Indians. The members of this religious group eat liberal amounts of peyote during collective all-night "meetings" held in the home of one of the participating families, a sacramental practice that enables the faithful to commune with God for curative and other beneficial purposes. Weir Mitchell, Havelock Ellis, and more recently, Aldous Huxley,[142] have written fascinating descriptions of the mescaline effects in self-experimentation. Louis Lewin, in his classic 1924 monograph, "Phantastica, Narcotic and Stimulating Drugs,"[182] presented a thorough discussion of the mescaline-induced psychological changes. In the early 1900s, there was considerable research interest in investigating the pharmacological properties of the drug, and this early work represents the first scientific attempts to study the phenomena associated with the use of psychotomimetic drugs. Peyote contains numerous alkaloids which are biogenetically interrelated, including two major classes: (a) the phenylethylamines, among which the most important is mescaline, and (b) the tetrahydroisoquinolines. Most of the phenylethylamines present in the cactus have sympathomimetic properties and produce experimental catatonia in animals.[129] The reported pharmacological, physiological, and behavioral effects of mescaline are very similar to those of LSD.[17,129,173] The active psychotomimetic dose of mescaline is in the range of 300 to 500 mg. The clinical effects of this drug are also similar to those of LSD, with minor differences: The duration of the action of mescaline is longer than that of LSD and is characterized by stronger autonomic effects; it is also thought that mescaline produces a more "sensual" experience than does LSD. Tolerance develops after repeated doses of mescaline, although more slowly than with LSD.[125,128] [129,138]

Mescaline Analogs (Amphetamine Derivatives)

The psychotomimetic effects of these drugs are much less known, but appear to be similar to those produced by LSD and other hallucinogens, with some differences in the nuances of the subjective effects, and variations in onset and duration of action.

DOM (2,5-dimethoxy-4-methylamphetamine). Known in the "hippie" subculture as "STP," DOM has been shown to produce in doses greater than 5 mg. pronounced hallucinogenic effects, which begin about one hour after administration of the drug, reach a peak between three and five hours, and subside after seven to eight hours.[81,239,240] The somatic, perceptual, and psychic changes are similar to those of LSD. In lower doses, it produces mild euphoria; the minimal perceptible dose is 2 mg. Although DOM was rumored to be more potent than LSD ("megahallucinogen"), recent findings[240] indicate that it is only about one-thirtieth as potent as LSD. The illicit product STP has been reported to produce severe and prolonged psychotic-like reactions which may persist for seventy-two hours,[242] and that administration of chlorpromazine may precipitate cardiovascular shock, with fatal consequences in some cases, attributed to an alleged atropine-like effect of the drug. However, Synder and associates[81,239,240] have demonstrated that there is no accentuation of any DOM effects by chlorpromazine; this finding suggests that street STP might contain atropine-like substances, which might also account for the reported prolonged reactions.

DOET (2,5-dimethoxy-4-ethylamphetamine). The ethyl homologue of DOM, the action of which appears to differ in its spectrum of psychological effects from other psychotomimetic drugs.[240] Over a five-fold range of dosage (0.75 to 4 mg.), DOET was shown to produce mild euphoria and enhanced self-awareness in the absence of hallucinogenic or other psychotomimetic effects. The drug produced no changes in blood pressure and pulse rate; there was slight pupil dilation with effects most marked at four hours.

TMA (3,4,5-trimethoxyamphetamine). The amphetamine analogue of mescaline, TMA is an active psychotomimetic agent, twice as potent as mescaline. Doses of 50 to 100 mg. of TMA produce giddiness and excitement characterized by hyperactivity, talkativeness, and decreased inhibitions, while at higher doses (200 mg.) it induces marked psychological changes (hostility, grandiosity, euphoria, and visual imagery) preceded by prodromal autonomic symptoms.[234]

A large number of isomeres of amphetamine derivatives (trimethoxyamphetamines, methylenedioxyamphetamines, methoxymethylenedioxyamphetamines, dimethoxymethylenedioxyamphetamines) have been synthesized; the relative activities of several of these compounds have been confirmed in animal behavioral tests. MDA and MMDA have been reported to produce psychotomimetic effects in man in the same dose range as mescaline.[233]

Amphetamines and Other Sympathomimetic Amines

These compounds, although not psychotomimetic by definition, are included here because they produce psychotomimetic-like syndromes when given in large doses, and especially through the intravenous route.[120,] [174,185] They include amphetamine, dextroamphetamine (Dexedrine), methamphetamine (Methedrine), phenmetrazine (Preludin), methylphenidate (Ritalin), and diethylpropion hydrochloride (Tenuate). It appears that the central stimulatory action of amphetamine and its peripheral sympathomimetic effects are mediated through the release of catecholimines. Numerous studies have demonstrated that amphetamine has facilitating effects on learning and goal-directed or operant behavior. The central adrenergic effects of amphetamines include arousal and heightened awareness, wakefulness, euphoria, mild antidepressant effect, and hyperactivity. These drugs produce desynchronized electro-encephalographic patterns characterized by a decrease in the abundance of alpha activity and an increase in beta frequencies.[150] With therapeutic doses, amphetamines commonly produce anorexia, dryness of the mouth, tachycardia, restlessness, and insomnia; with larger doses, subjects show marked euphoria, pressure of speech, restlessness, and irritability. Other effects include mydriasis, elevation of blood pressure, brisk reflexes, fine tremor of the limbs, cardiac arrhythmias, palpitation, dizziness, vasomotor disturbances, as well as dysphoria, apprehension, and agitation.[81] Chlorpromazine has been reported to be effective in the symptomatic treatment of acute amphetamine poisoning.[96] There is recently accumulating evidence which suggests that the intravenous use of large doses of amphetamines and related compounds may produce predictable psychotomimetic reactions, characterized primarily by paranoid ideation.[120,175] Louria[185] reports that in Sweden the major drug problem is the intravenous administration of amphetamine-type drugs, especially phenmetrazine (Preludin). These drugs are believed to have a substantial aphrodisiac effect when taken intravenously. During a "central-stimulant binge," popularly known as "speeding," there is a cyclic pattern in the intravenous use of these drugs, characterized by repeated injections ("runs") of increasing amounts of the drug every few hours around the clock for a period of three to six days.[175,185] After each injection, the user experiences a sudden overwhelming, pleasurable feeling called a "flash" or a "rush." With increasing doses in each "run" (as tolerance to the drug develops), the subject shows "recurrent affective lability," hyperacousia, compulsive patterns of behavior (a stereotyped mechanical-like hyperactivity), and finally he may develop paranoid ideas and illusory experiences.[185] After the cycle is terminated—often by the administration of a barbiturate—

the subject goes into profound and prolonged sleep, and upon awakening he feels lethargic, apathetic, and depressed ("crushed"), and experiences marked hunger for food. When the drug use becomes an established pattern, the dosage ranges from 100 to 300 mg. of methamphetamine, although much higher doses have been reported. Although chronic use of amphetamines leads to the development of tolerance and psychological dependence, there is no convincing evidence of physiological dependence. The lethargy and depression that invariably follow the discontinuation of the drug after prolonged use has been described as representing an abstinence syndrome by some writers,[175,271] but this has been disputed by others.[120]

Marijuana and Tetrahydrocannabinol

Cannabis sativa (or *C. indica*, or *C. americana*), commonly known as hemp or marijuana, has been used for its psychoactive properties since ancient times. Until about 1000 A.D., cannabis was mainly used in India and to much lesser extent in China. In the following centuries, its use spread to the Middle East and Near East, and in the nineteenth century, during the Napoleonic era, it was introduced from Egypt to Europe. It was during this period that the first literary and medical descriptions of marijuana effects were published in the Western world. Theophile Gautier, Charles Baudelaire, and Alexander Dumas wrote colorful and perceptive accounts of their hashish experiences. Cannabis extracts became a popular medication, prescribed for a variety of conditions, and especially used as sedative, analgesic, muscle relaxant, and anticonvulsant. The use of cannabis in medical practice gradually declined, mainly because of the variable potency of its preparations and its replacement by more effective anodynes and sedatives. The use of marijuana as a euphoriant drug was first introduced to the United States during the first quarter of this century, via Mexico to New Orleans, where it was reported to have reached epidemic proportions in the 1920s and 1930s. It was during this period that marijuana received its publicity as the "marijuana menace" and the "killer drug," and the public upheaval created by the news media finally culminated with the passing of the Marijuana Tax Act in 1936.[121,238]

Cannabis sativa is a ubiquitous annual plant, varying in botanical characteristics and properties according to the geographic and climatic conditions in which it is grown.[14,41,62,89,112] Strains grown in warmer climates (Mexico, India) are reported to produce more of the resin that contains the psychoactive material than strains from colder climates. Other factors that determine the psychoactive potency of cannabis include conditions of cultivation, and conditions of harvesting, preparation, and storage.[89] There are three rough grades of intoxicating material that are usually prepared from cannabis: (a) Low potency forms, prepared chiefly from the leaves of the entire plant, and variously known as marijuana (United States), bhang (India), dagga (S. Africa), or kif (N. Africa); (b) medium potency forms, ganjia (India), prepared from the leaves of the flowering tops; and (c) high potency forms, containing pure resin scraped from the leaves near the flowering tops, and known as hashish or charas (India). The variable content of these products in psychoactive material is the most significant factor that accounts for the reported great differences in their pharmacological effects.

CANNABIS CHEMISTRY AND METABOLISM

Although the major active components of cannabis, the cannabinoids, had been known for several decades, a number of them were subsequently proven to be psychotomimetically inactive (cannabinol, cannabidiol, cannabichromene, cannabinoid acids). With the isolation and synthesis of tetrahydrocannabinol (THC),[111,199] a number of derivatives have been synthesized, characterized by variable potency and properties.[198] Research during the last few years has shown that the major psychoactive THC contained in cannabis is Delta 9-THC (or Delta 1-THC). However, the active Delta 8-THC (or Delta 1(6)-THC) isomer may also be present in varying amounts. Delta 9-THC is a labile resi-

nous substance that is easily isomerized by acids to the more stable Delta 8-THC, and is slowly oxidized by air to cannabinol.[198] On the other hand, there is evidence indicating that during smoking of marijuana the inactive cannabidiol may be partially converted into Delta 9-THC through the pyrolytic process. This finding may partly explain the observation that cannabis is more active when smoked than when taken orally. Although the THC content of marijuana varies greatly, it is estimated that marijuana generally available in the United States averages about 1 percent THC. In view that approximately 50 percent of the THC originally contained in a marijuana cigarette is destroyed by the combustion process, it is estimated that a cigarette (1 gram) can deliver a maximum of 5 mg. THC.

Several *in vitro* studies have shown that the metabolism of Delta 9- and Delta 8-THC by the post-mitochondrial fraction obtained from the liver homogenates of various species proceeds by allylic hydroxylation to 11-hydroxy metabolites.[50,102,196,211] Although the potency of these compounds varies depending on structure and route of administration, they produce similar behavior effects in animals.[63,230] The 11-hydroxy-Delta 9-THC has been shown in mice to be fifteen to twenty times more active than the parent compound, and it is postulated that it may represent the active form of Delta 9-THC on the molecular level.[63,196] It has been suggested that these hydroxylated metabolites of THC are formed in the liver, possibly by inducible microsomal enzymes.[198] Induction of these enzymes is implied by the observation of shortened barbiturate sleeping time in animals pretreated with THC. These findings may partly explain the phenomenon of "inverse tolerance" reported in experienced marijuana users,[269] who may have a ready supply of the microsomal oxidase for a rapid conversion of THC to the 11-hydroxy metabolite. Recent studies show that THC and its metabolites can be found in body tissues for a considerable length of time after administration.[11,178] In man, THC metabolites continue to circulate for at least eight days after administration. The plasma half-life of injected radioactive THC was found to be fifty-six hours in marijuana naïve subjects, but much shorter in the experienced user.[178]

PHARMACOLOGICAL EFFECTS OF
MARIJUANA AND THC

As Grinspoon points out,[121] "In evaluating the various reports of the effects of marijuana, the problem of relative potency, stability, dosage level, and means of administration of marijuana or synthetic analogues rates second to bias or prejudice." The most consistent physiological changes during marijuana or THC intoxication, regardless of route of administration, include injection of conjuctivae[14,15,41,62,146] and increased pulse rate.[14,62,90,146] Both these signs tend to parallel clinical effects. Increased appetite, especially for sweets, is commonly reported, although less consistently.[13,62,134] Several studies have shown that the marijuana-induced hunger is not related to changes in blood glucose levels.[90,137,264] Although several writers have reported pupillary dilatation,[14,41,44,62] recent evidence[146,264] has failed to corroborate this finding. Also, contrary to earlier reports,[14,62] marijuana, as well as THC, do not appear to affect respiratory rate, systolic and diastolic blood pressure, or tendon reflexes.[90,134,264] Other less frequently reported symptoms include inco-ordination, tremors, ataxia, and muscle weakness, as well as thirst, dryness of the mouth and throat, nausea, vomiting, diarrhea, headache, vertigo, perspiration, palpitations, urinary urgency, and paresthesias.[14,15,34,41,44,49,62,112] There are inconsistent reports about the electroencephalographic (EEG) effects of marijuana.[15,59,90,203] Dornbush and associates[90] recently reported EEG changes consisting of transient increase in percent time alpha and decrease in percent time theta and beta activities. Contrary to the reported "inverse tolerance" in experienced users, recent evidence indicates that tolerance does develop to the effects of marijuana and THC in animals and in man. Tolerance to THC is marked and rapid and extends across species;[196] it is also prolonged. There is cross-tolerance among tetrahydrocannabinols, but not to LSD and mescaline.[147] No withdrawal syndrome develops following abrupt discontinuation of marijuana or THC. With regard to psychological changes, marijuana has a biphasic action, with an initial period of stimulation (anxiety, heightened perception, euphoria) followed by a period of sedation and somnolence.[139] Higher doses produce definite psychotomimetic effects.[146]

Deliriant Psychotomimetic Compounds

ANTICHOLINERGIC DRUGS

This group includes the belladonna alkaloids (atropine, l-hyoscyamine, and l-scopolamine), the synthetic piperydil-benzilates (Ditran), diphenylmethane compounds (benactyzine), and other anticholinergic drugs (diethazine, procyclidine, benzotropine, methane sulfate, trihexyphenidyl, and others). The solanacea (belladonna alkaloids) have been known for inducing psychosis since ancient times. The clinical picture of atropine psychosis is characterized by confusion, drowsiness, ataxia, dysarthria, restlessness, overactivity, visual hallucinations, and excitement; the reaction may last several days.[23] Scopolamine has a strong narcotic effect and, for this reason, it was used to produce a "twilight sleep" during labor. The EEG changes induced by atropine and scopolamine consist of a disappearance of alpha activity and a decrease in amplitudes with a concurrent increase in theta and beta activities.[100] The piperydil-benzilates (glycolate esters) include a large series of anticholinergic compounds, many of which have been shown to possess psychotomimetic activity.[1,2] Among them, Ditran, when given in doses of 10 to 20 mg., produces excitement, hallucinations, confusion, disorientation, confabulation, and considerable amnesia for the delirious episode.[129,150]

ANESTHETIC DRUGS

A number of anesthetic drugs, including phenylcyclidine (Sernyl), alpha chloralose and, in general, anesthetics whose action is characterized by a prolonged Stage II anesthesia (e.g., chloroform, nitrous oxide, ether), produce psychotomimetic effects of the delirious type.[129] Phenylcyclidine administered intravenously (0.1 mg./kg.) induces feelings of depersonalization and derealization, hallucinations, delusions, loss of sense of time, hostile attitudes, and panic.[24,27] Alpha chloralose, used as an EEG activating agent, may induce psychotic-like reactions.[26] Also, nitrous oxide (laughing gas) is a well-known deliriant with a considerable potential for abuse.

VOLATILE HYDROCARBONS (SOLVENT SNIFFING)

In the past ten years, there has been a marked increase in the use by inhalation of a wide variety of volatile organic solvents for the purpose of inducing states of intoxication.[58,216,217] This form of drug abuse is most common among juveniles between the ages of ten to fifteen. The industrial products involved in solvent sniffing (plastic cements, model cements, and household cements or glues, fingernail polish remover, lacquer thinners, lighter fluid, cleaning fluid, gasoline) contain various volatile hydrocarbons, including toluene, acetone, aliphatic acetates, benzine, petroleum naphtha, perchlorethylene, tricholorethane, carbon tetrachloride, and others. In general, the acute effects of inhaling the vapors of these compounds are similar to those produced by the inhalation of anesthetic drugs (ether, nitrous oxide). The initial state of intoxication is characterized by mild euphoria, feelings of drunkenness, dizziness, and impaired control and judgment. During this phase, the user may experience "feelings of reckless abandon, grandiosity and omnipotence,"[216] which may presumably account for the impulsive and antisocial behavior that has often been reported to occur in these individuals during a "high." Depending upon the intensity of the exposure, this phase may progress into a transient overt psychotic behavior of a delirious nature characterized by excitation, perceptual distortions of space, delusions, and sometimes hallucinations occurring in a state of variable clouding of consciousness, and with subsequent spotty amnesia of the events surrounding the intoxication. Hallucinogenic activity has been reported to be associated with the sniffing of gasoline,[254]

toluene,[59,217,232] and lighter fluid.[7] With increasing concentrations, the narcotic effect of these substances may result in loss of consciousness. The duration of the acute effects is variable, depending on the intensity of the exposure, and may range from fifteen minutes to a few hours.[217] Tolerance has been reported to develop with most of these substances in chronic sniffers.[7,93,116,226,244] There is no clear evidence that the chronic use of these substances produces physical dependence.[28,217] Also, there is no sufficient evidence at the present to support the claims that solvent sniffing produces transient or permanent brain damage, although this possibility has not been ruled out. However, a number of fatalities related to solvent sniffing have been reported, most of them attributed to suffocation by the plastic bag used in the method of inhalation.[30,217]

❰ Adverse Effects of Psychotomimetic Drugs

LSD and Other Hallucinogens

The widespread illicit use of LSD and other psychotomimetic drugs in the recent years has resulted in an alarming number of reports of acute and long-term adverse drug effects. These adverse effects may be classified into (a) psychological and (b) mutogenic (teratogenic).

ADVERSE PSYCHOLOGICAL REACTIONS

Since the first reports were published,[73,76,77] there has been considerable literature accumulated which has unequivocally established the dangerous psychological consequences associated with the misuse or abuse of LSD and related drugs.[40,73,74,76,77,99,109,115,139,192,194,220,242,256,257,258,270] It is estimated that approximately 10 percent of LSD "trips" can be potentially upsetting. On the other hand, with skilled therapists using LSD, 1 percent or less of drug experiences may be traumatic.[104] These reactions may be classified into the following categories:

a. *Acute panic reactions* ("bad trips" or "freak-outs") occur while the subject is under the influence of the drug. This is the most common adverse effect, and it usually consists of a transient panic reaction which subsides within twenty-four hours. These reactions are greatly dependent on the affective and anticipatory state of the individual and on the setting in which the drug is taken, and are usually associated with a fear of loss of control or fear of "losing one's mind" in the absence of outside support and reality orientation. Confused motives and unstable nonsupportive environments are likely to precipitate them.[104] The majority of the cases do not require hospitalization and are effectively managed with proper support and reassurance. More severe cases failing to respond to this approach may require the use of sedatives (e.g., pentobarbital), minor tranquilizers (e.g., chloridazepoxide), or phenothiazines (e.g., chlorpromazine). It is generally advisable, however, to avoid the administration of drugs because of the potential risk of precipitating serious complications in an individual who has taken an unknown drug, not infrequently available in the illicit market in combination with other drugs, such as atropine (i.e., "STP"), strychnine, opiates, or animal tranquilizers.

b. *Acute psychotic episodes* represent more serious psychiatric complications which may or may not be dependent on the occurrence of a panic reaction. In the state of hypervigilance, impaired control of critical and discriminatory functions, dissolution of "body ego" organization, impaired autonomy and labile affect of the psychodelic experience, there is a tenuous contact with reality which may easily lead to misinterpretations, ideas of reference, delusions, or catatonic-like postures, to impulsive, aggressive, or self-destructive behavior, and to marked disorganization of personality. These reactions are usually diagnosed as acute schizophrenic episodes, dissociative states, or acute brain syndromes (toxic psychosis),[256] may last several days, and generally require hospitalization. Treatment is primarily supportive and may necessitate the administration of phenothiazines or other antipsychotic agents for the control of symptoms.

c. *Prolonged psychotic reactions*, such as schizophrenia or schizophreniform psychosis, may develop in certain "predisposed" individuals following the use of these drugs. They are believed to be of a functional origin, making the significance of the drug incidental rather than causative. The premorbid personality of these individuals has been described as unstable, schizoid, paranoid, hysterical, borderline, or psychopathic.[258] It is of interest, however, that several investigators have failed to find any significant premorbid psychopathology in many of these patients.[115,258] It is not clear, therefore, whether some of these protracted psychotic reactions associated with repeated use of LSD might represent a type of psychosis in which LSD is more than a precipitating factor. The therapeutic management of these cases is similar to that of the spontaneously occurring psychoses. Some of these patients require prolonged treatment or show a refractory response to it.[115]

d. *Intermittent recurrence of LSD-related symptoms*, commonly called "flashbacks," involve the recurrence of various symptoms experienced during a previous LSD exposure, and may include anxiety, paranoid feelings, or hallucinations, described as a type of "echo phenomenon." They may occur days, weeks, or even months after the drug was taken, and are characteristically elicited during some stressful situation, or following the ingestion of other drugs, such as marijuana or amphetamine. Although the experience may be a pleasant one, most frequently it is dysphoric and is usually associated with the fear of losing one's mind. Their occurrence while driving may become a hazard.[270]

e. *Chronic personality changes*, attributed to the effects of continued and frequent use of LSD and related drugs among the so-called "acid-heads," represent a controversial issue. Reports are often presumptive or based on retrospective evaluations. The common pattern of multiple drug use among the chronic users renders the identification of LSD effects even more difficult. The so-called "amotivational syndrome," which is thought to occur in chronic marijuana smokers, has also been associated with the chronic use of LSD.[123,125,268] There is no evidence that repeated use of LSD might result in demonstrable brain damage.[40,192] The rate of serious emotional disturbances among peyote- (mescaline) using American Indians has been reported to be very low.[37]

MUTOGENIC AND TERATOGENIC EFFECTS OF LSD

Since 1967, there has been considerable research activity centered around the possible genetic damage resulting from LSD. This research was stimulated by the initial report of Cohen and associates[68] which indicated a higher chromosomal aberration rate in cultures of white blood cells (WBC) to which LSD was added (6.7 to 36.8 percent) than in untreated control cultures (3.7 percent). This *in vitro* study was followed by a series of *in vivo* studies on LSD users, which resulted in both positive[28,69,71,95,144,210,273] and negative correlations.[35,82,141,160,184,243,252,261] Subsequent studies have focused on investigating the effect of LSD on the chromosomes of germ cells—reporting both positive[72] and negative findings—[151] and on the drug's ultimate effect on the offspring of animals (teratogenicity). Positive results on the teratogenic effect of LSD administered to pregnant animals[12,22,98,113] have not been corroborated by others.[87,225,260] Several studies concerning the effect of LSD on the human fetus, in women who had taken the drug during pregnancy, have reported high incidence of abortion, few cases of congenital malformations of the extremities,[55,273] and persisting chromosomal defects that tended to repair incompletely.[38] It has been suggested that future sterility and reproduction of congenital defects in next-generation offsprings may result from such unrepaired chromosomal defects.[46] There is considerable skepticism regarding studies on alleged human LSD users because the purity of the illicitly obtained drug cannot be accurately determined. Furthermore, these subjects frequently experiment simultaneously with other psychotomimetic drugs. Factors

underlying the reported contradictory findings in animals may include strain differences, individual threshold differences, genetic susceptibility, coexisting subclinical viral infections, purity of the drug, and other factors.[225] In conclusion, the evidence that the drug produces embryonic malformations and chromosomal damage in human users and animals is inconsistent and continues to remain equivocal.

Adverse Effects of Marijuana

In the past decade there has been an unprecedented increase in the use of marijuana in this country, especially among high school and college students, a phenomenon that has raised highly controversial issues centering primarily on evaluating the dangers associated with the use of this drug. Among the alleged dangers that have been used as reasons to justify strict legal control of marijuana are that its use is criminogenic, addicting, leading to sexual promiscuity and to the use of narcotics ("stepping stone" theory). Since it is beyond the scope of this chapter to discuss all these issues at any length, the reader is referred to the available literature.[121,185,238] We will limit our discussion to the adverse psychological effects of the drug. There is no doubt that the use of cannabis may result in one of several types of adverse psychological effects, variously described by different authors as "panic reactions," "toxic psychosis," "psychotomimetic reactions," "flashbacks," "depressive reactions," and "functional psychoses." The development of these reactions appears to be overdetermined, that is, multiple factors contribute to their occurrence, although in varying degrees, depending on the nature of the reaction. Thus, some of these effects are primarily dose-dependent (psychotomimetic reactions), while others are greatly influenced by the set and setting (panic reactions), others by "idiosyncratic" factors (toxic psychosis), and others by factors related to the underlying basic personality structure of the individual (functional psychosis).

PANIC REACTIONS

These are acute anxiety reactions of variable intensity which may reach panic proportions and constitute by far the majority of the adverse reactions to marijuana in this country. These reactions can be best understood in terms of the subject's psychological response to the experience of the marijuana effect, within the context of his anticipatory attitudes towards it and its consequences, and in relation to his conscious and unconscious intepretive distortions of the drug effect, as perceived by him in terms of the significant experiences of his past life, and as reflected in his immediate relationships with others. During this reaction, the subject may feel that he is dying or "losing his mind" and, in general, he perceives the drug effects (depersonalization, derealization) and their consequences as catastrophic. Sometimes, this state of anticipatory hypervigilance may result in the emergence of paranoid ideas which are commonly associated with the subject's apprehensive expectation of retaliatory retributions for using the drug, an act considered illicit in this country and, largely, culturally deviant. This adverse effect is mostly commonly seen among novice users of marijuana, and especially those who are ambivalently motivated in using it. The significant role that the set and setting play in the occurrence of these reactions is exemplified by Weil's[263] observation that their frequency varies greatly in different communities. They may be extremely rare (e.g., 1 percent of all reactions to marijuana) in communities where marijuana is well accepted as a "recreational intoxicant," or, on the other hand, very common (25 percent of the persons trying it for the first time) in places where use of the drug represents a greater degree of social deviance. These reactions are generally self-limited and show a marked response to simple reassurance. It is possible, however, that the occurrence of panic reaction in subjects with an unstable or precariously compensated personality may produce a much more serious ego disorganization, characteristic of a psychotic state, the outcome of which may crucially depend on a number of factors related not only to the individual's capacity for reintegration but also to the support he receives from others, and most importantly, to the way he is handled by the physician.[263]

PSYCHOTIC REACTIONS

One of the most controversial issues about marijuana is its alleged role in precipitating a "true" psychosis, such as schizophrenia, or producing a psychosis specific for the drug, referred to as "cannabis psychosis." The literature is replete with polarized categorical views, as well as "objective" analyses of the problem, in which the subtlety of creeping biases becomes the main virtue of objectivity. There are few, if any, reliable data, a fact that makes obvious the need for more and better studies. In reviewing the world literature, there is a definite dichotomy on this subject.[121] Authors from Eastern countries (India, Egypt, Morocco) are largely in agreement that there is direct relationship of cannabis (charas, hashish) to the development of psychosis. On the other hand, Western literature (especially American) generally presents a contrary view. This controversy is not by any means recent. A voluminous literature on "cannabis insanity" had already been accumulated during the latter part of the nineteenth century. These reports have been criticized on the grounds that they were largely based on inadequate and circumstantial evidence. The *Report of the Indian Hemp Commission*[190]—appointed in 1893 by the British government to investigate all facts about hemp drugs in India—concluded that "Moderate use of these drugs produced no injurious effect except in persons with a marked neurotic diathesis. Excessive use indicates and intensifies mental instability. Moderate use produces no moral injury whatsoever." Two major studies conducted in India[62] and Morocco[34] have reported a high incidence of psychosis secondary to the chronic use of the more potent cannabis preparations, charas and hashish. Both studies, however, have been criticized on several accounts, including inadequate methodology, and a tenuous cause and effect relationship. In the United States, there have been few studies, and they consist primarily of sporadic clinical case reports.[14,15,48,49] The findings of the *LaGuardia Report*,[191] conducted by a committee charged with the task of assessing the marijuana problem in New York City, were largely similar to those reported by the Indian Hemp Commission. Several earlier survey studies involving chronic marijuana users in this country revealed no cases of psychosis.[60,107,112] Also, recent survey studies of drug abusers, seen in hospitals or clinics, report no cases of marijuana psychosis.[126,236,237] It appears, therefore, that the current pattern of marijuana use in this country does not constitute a significant danger with regard to the development of prolonged psychotic reactions.

ACUTE TOXIC PSYCHOSIS

Cannabis may induce clinical syndromes characteristic of a toxic psychosis and consisting of confusion, disorientation, and cognitive impairment of various degrees. These symptoms may be associated with vivid illusory and hallucinatory experiences, suspiciousness and paranoid thinking, excitement and marked affective changes, characterized predominantly by anxiety or panic. Patients recover invariably within a few days, as is the case with delirious reactions. It has been suggested that confusional psychosis is dose-dependent, and more common when marijuana is taken orally.[121,263] Nevertheless, high doses of THC, administered orally or by smoking, have been shown to produce typical psychotomimetic reactions of the LSD-type, without clouding of consciousness.[146] Idiosyncratic factors might be important; it is also likely that other substances contained in cannabis might have toxic effects responsible for the development of the delirium.

DEPRESSIVE REACTIONS

Sporadic cases of transient depressive reactions, most commonly of the reactive type, have been reported.[14,48,53,122,162,263] Clinical material is too limited to warrant any further discussion.

RECURRENCE OF PSYCHOTOMIMETIC SYMPTOMS

The phenomenon of recurrences (flashbacks) has also been reported to occur after the use of marijuana.[165] They mainly consist of a recurrence of feelings of unreality and altered perception experienced during a marijuana "high." Marijuana may also elicit a "flashback" to a previous LSD experience.[263]

LONG-TERM PERSONALITY CHANGES

Habitual use of marijuana has been reported to lead to serious personality changes, described in the earlier literature as "deterioration,"[62] and more recently as the "amotivational syndrome."[13,161,195,268] Although a highly controversial issue, it appears that a potential long-term effect of marijuana (and especially hashish) on personality deserves the most compelling consideration. The reports presented by the Indian Hemp Commission,[190] the LaGuardia Committee,[191] and the British Advisory Committee on Drug Dependence,[54] and several other studies,[48,107] have asserted that there are no reliable observations to support the alleged syndrome of mental deterioration from the habitual use of cannabis. It appears that the term "deterioration," which reflects the prevailing biases about marijuana, has been used to imply not only gross intellectual and psychological impairment but also social, cultural, and even moral deficit. Nevertheless, one common observation that emerges from many Eastern studies is the description of the chronic cannabis user as passive and nonproductive. In a recent study conducted in Greece, Miras[203] described marked personality changes in a group of chronic heavy hashish smokers, including loss of drive and ambition, apathy, and social disengagement.

Similar personality changes have been described in chronic marijuana users ("potheads") in this country, constituting what is referred to as the "amotivational syndrome," and including apathy, loss of effectiveness, inward turning and passivity, loss of drive for achievement, tendency toward magical thinking, and other amotivational personality characteristics leading to a state of relaxed and careless drifting.[13,161,195,268] These subjects were also described as being "less able to carry out long-term plans, endure frustration, concentrate for extended periods, follow routines, or successfully master new material (learning) with the same ease as before."[13] However, the causal relationship between chronic marijuana use and the development of the "amotivational syndrome" reported in these retrospective studies has been challenged on the grounds that these alleged personality characteristics have probably existed prior to the use of marijuana. Grinspoon[121] argues that "assuming this is a clinical entity . . . there is the question whether or not this syndrome is truly a manifestation of personality deterioration or even change" rather than "manifestations of a purposeful and extensive change in life style, one involving ideology, values, attitudes, dress, social norms, and many aspects of behavior." It appears that there are some striking similarities when one attempts to compare the alleged personality characteristics attributed to the "amotivational syndrome" of the "potheads" with the ideology and life style of the emergent hippie subculture of the 1960s. The intimate relationship that exists between this youth subculture and the use of marijuana and LSD does not seem to represent a simple cause-effect relationship but rather a complex and multilevel interrelationship in which drug use is only one aspect of a pluralistic and overdetermined phenomenon. The habitual marijuana and LSD users or "heads," as described by Carey,[56] have minimal attachments to customary institutions of society, and show signs of estrangement in their appearance, which are also sources of commitment to their style of life. Their ethos includes the rejection of societal values, the dropping out of conventional social affiliations, and the dissociation from conventional roles. Their distinctive attitude towards time, characterized by a focus of interest in the present, is intimately connected with the disavowal of ambition, and the life style of "hanging out." Several other studies have em-

phasized in these subjects such personality and cultural characteristics as humanistic and social orientation, passivity and unaggressiveness, nonconformism, introspectiveness, pleasure-seeking, and rejection of societal values and norms, especially those regarding competitiveness and achievement.[70,104,118,131,204,231,274] The reported "cultogenic"[204] and "sociogenic"[118] effects of LSD and marijuana are thought to contribute to the formation of the tribal affiliations of fringe groups and the development of the characteristic drug subculture of the "heads," who generally view the use of these drugs as the central and most significant aspect of their life-patterns.[56,268,274] In a study of chronic LSD users, Blacker and associates[40] noted that the group shared a set of mystical-magical beliefs and profound nonaggressive attitudes, which were attributed to learned consequences of frequent, intense LSD experiences in susceptible individuals. A study by McGlothlin and associates[194] on the effect of one LSD experience on the personality of normal subjects revealed some evidence of a more introspective and passive orientation in the experimental group in the postdrug period. On the other hand, the findings relating personality variables to attitude toward and response to the taking of LSD confirmed the commonly reported observation that persons who place strong emphasis on structure and control generally have no interest in the experience, and tend to respond minimally if exposed. Those who respond intensely tend to prefer a more unstructured, spontaneous, inward-turning life, and to be less aggressive, less competitive, and less conforming. One might hypothesize that individuals possessing the latter personality characteristics to a marked degree, when repeatedly exposed to the effects of hallucinogenic drugs or marijuana, are more likely to continue taking these drugs and to adopt the values, attitudes, and life styles of a suitable ideology. Those aspects of LSD and marijuana experience that might be most significant in enhancing these personality characteristics may include the blurring of spatial and temporal boundaries, as experienced in the feelings of depersonalization and derealization, as well as the experience of compelling immediacy in the LSD effects,[104] and the phenomenon of "temporal disintegration" described in the marijuana effects,[200,201] both of which diminish the importance of past and future and result in the overvaluation of "nowness" and loss of goal-directedness. It is likely that the process of "temporal disintegration" in the marijuana user and its consequent telescoping effect on the subject's ability to project himself into past and future, when experienced repeatedly by certain predisposed individuals, may result in the enhancement of some of the alleged long-term personality changes associated with the "amotivational syndrome." Furthermore, this pathogenetic mechanism may involve an operant reinforcement of these personality changes, which are consciously rationalized and further reinforced by the adoption of a suitable ideological framework provided by the hippie subculture.

Adverse Effects of Amphetamines

The recent increase of amphetamine abuse in this country, as well as in Sweden, England, and other countries,[80,81,92,119,175,179,185,207] has raised great concern about the possible dangers associated with the use of these drugs, especially with regard to the development of the so-called amphetamine psychosis.[16,33,59,79,127,179,251,265] The clinical picture of this psychosis is characterized by ideas of reference, delusions of persecution, and auditory and visual hallucinations in a setting of clear consciousness, and is described as being indistinguishable from that of paranoid schizophrenia. These reactions are usually short-lived, although prolonged psychotic states, some of them refractory to treatment, may also occur.[179,251] They are thought to develop in certain susceptible individuals. However, in a recent study by Griffith and associates,[120] it was demonstrated that repeated and progressively increasing intravenous doses of d-amphetamine can precipitate a brief paranoid psychotic reaction resembling a schizophrenic psychosis, without causing appreciable alterations in sensorium or orientation, and it was

concluded that a personality defect is not an essential factor for its occurrence. It was also noted that the sequence of symptoms preceding the onset of psychosis and the type of psychosis elicited were remarkably similar in all subjects. In the prodromal phase, once the cumulative dose exceeded 50 mg., the initial mild euphoria observed with smaller doses was followed by depressive-like symptoms, some loss of interest, and hypochondriasis. Several hours before the onset of the psychotic episode, the subjects became withdrawn and taciturn. The psychotic reaction developed quite abruptly and was characterized by ideas of reference and paranoid ideas of a persecutory nature; there were no visual or auditory hallucinations. There is no evidence to support the claim that amphetamine psychosis is a withdrawal phenomenon.[271] Also, the reported chronic brain damage in chronic amphetamine users requres further substantiation.[175,179] The observed syndrome of apathy, lethargy, and depression, which invariably follows the discontinuation of a prolonged use of excessive doses of amphetamines, does not seem to represent a withdrawal reaction, for it has primarily the features of a depletion state rather than of a release phenomenon.

⦗ Therapeutic Uses of Psychotomimetic Drugs (LSD)

The dramatic psychic changes experienced under the influence of psychotomimetic drugs, and especially LSD, have led many investigators to formulate hypotheses about their potential therapeutic use in psychiatry, and therefore, to apply them in the treatment of various psychiatric conditions, including alcoholism, drug addiction, psychoneuroses, homosexuality, psychopathy, chronic schizophrenia, as well as in autistic children and dying patients. Although chemical abreactive aids to psychotherapy (e.g., sodium amytal, methedrine) have been used since World War II,[224] it was Busch and Johnson[51] who first introduced in 1950 the use of LSD as a means of facilitating recall and bringing about a cathartic release of emotions during psycho-therapy. The use of LSD as an adjunct to psychotherapy received considerable popular-ity in the subsequent years,[3,4,64,222,227,229] especially with regard to the treatment of chronic alcoholism, and has resulted in the publication of many enthusiastic reports that have become the focus of a continuing con-troversy. The techniques employed in LSD therapy vary greatly, according to the theoret-ical framework that is used to conceptualize the mechanism or the process by which the desired therapeutic effect is achieved. Thus, LSD has been used for emotional abreac-tions,[51] for facilitating insight psychotherapy as in psychoanalysis [3,4,227] (removing resis-tances, increasing tolerance to anxiety, inten-sifying transference phenomena), for enhanc-ing the patient's emotional tone, or for induc-ing regression to an earlier period of his life and the relieving of emotionally charged memories,[222] or for producing a profound psychedelic experience of a spiritual, mystical, or transcendental nature.[64,176,228] These tech-niques are generally classified into psyche-delic, psycholytic and hypnodelic.

a. *Psychedelic therapy.* This technique was originally developed for the treatment of al-coholics, and was based on the assumption that alcoholic patients view the occurrence of delirium tremens as a "turning point" in their struggle for sobriety, a change in orientation thought to be associated with the realization of "hitting bottom." It was hypothesized that the LSD-induced psychotomimetic effect might serve as a model experience of "hitting bottom" and thus become the springboard for establishing sobriety.[64,129] The recognition of the occurrence of mystical or transcendental ("psychedelic") experiences under LSD led later to an emphasis on the manipulation of the setting as a means of facilitating and en-hancing the occurrence of the psychedelic experience. Typically, the procedure involves a single session with a large dose of LSD (300 to 600 mcg.). As modified by Savage and as-sociates,[176,227] the procedure consists of sev-eral weeks of intensive psychotherapy, incor-porating one high-dose LSD session.

b. *Psycholytic therapy.* This technique con-

sists of a series of drug sessions in which small doses of LSD (100 to 200 mcg.), are given to a number of patients in an outpatient setting. These sessions are associated with individual or group therapy and involve an interpretive handling of the material experienced under LSD within the psychoanalytic frame of refer-ence. The method was developed by Leu-ner[180] and is the most popular LSD therapy in Europe.

c. *Hypnodelic therapy.* This utilizes the combined use of hypnosis and LSD.[181,187]

The reported therapeutic efficacy of the psychedelic drugs in the treatment of alco-holism and other conditions has been the sub-ject of several reviews[84,129] and has been challenged in heated controversies. Criticism has primarily centered on methodological grounds: lack of objective criteria for measur-ing change, insufficient follow-up, insufficient control groups, inadequate statistical analysis of data, and uncritical or even biased report-ing. Others have found it difficult to accept the apparent absurdity of producing a transi-ent "psychosis" for therapeutic purposes, or to condone a practice that allegedly takes unwar-ranted risks with a drug that is reputed to be dangerous. With regard to the treatment of chronic alcoholism, the reported high rates of improvement in the earlier studies[64,155,213,235] were subsequently shown to disappear when controlled and longer follow-up studies were used.[88,137,156,157,186] Although several other studies have shown variable success,[176,213] it appears that improvement occurs with both LSD and control treatments and that in the majority of cases it is not maintained beyond the initial post-treatment period.[137,186]

(Use and Abuse of Psychotomimetic Drugs

Defining a pattern of drug use as "abuse" is a controversial matter. The term "abuse" is vari-ously employed to describe a certain type of behavior which may be viewed as socially deviant, pathological, or criminal, depending on one's biases and perspectives. The politics of semantics in this area reflect the prevailing radicalization of views on a complex and poorly understood phenomenon, whose definition as a "problem" has various social, political, medical, and legal implications. For instance, Szasz[248] regards freedom of self-medication as a fundamental human right and feels that the term "drug abuse" places this behavior in the category of ethics, "for it is ethics that deals with the right and wrong uses of man's power and possessions." However, many view this issue within the context of restrictive practices that have emerged from "the interaction between the rights and responsibilities of the individual and of his society,"[75] a position which, although universally accepted, has always been the focus of controversy as to how one defines the collective rights and obligations of the state and those of the individual. Criteria for defining a certain pattern of drug use as dangerous to the individual or to his society vary greatly, depending not only on the amount of scientific knowledge of the drug's action that is available, but also on the prevailing cultural values and social norms that characterize a particular period of man's history. The recent widespread use of drugs among the young represents an unprecedented phenomenon with regard to its magnitude, epidemiological characteristics, and social implications. It has raised questions that go far beyond mere medical or public health considerations; it has been associated with such issues as ideology, social change, and the quality of man's life.

Prevalence and Patterns of Drug Use

For epidemiological purposes, drug users are usually classified in terms of frequency of and motivation for drug use, as well as in terms of single or multiple drug use. There are four major categories with regard to frequency: (i) the "experimenting" user (maximum of few drug trials); (ii) the "casual" user, who uses drugs occasionally and sporadically, and generally when offered the opportunity; (iii) the "social" or "recreational" user, who takes drugs regularly but infrequently; and (iv) the "habitual" user or "head," whose drug-dependent behavior is an established pattern characterized by a regular and frequent use of drugs. This last group is characterized by considerable psychopathology, which seems to play a part in the motivation to use drugs. The great majority of drug users fall into the first three categories. Geller and Boas[114] divided marijuana users into five categories: (i) urban minority groups (Negroes, Puerto Ricans); (ii) rural minority groups (Mexican Americans and Negroes); (iii) white middle-class students; (iv) hippies; and (v) over-thirty artists, intellectuals, and writers.

Any meaningful discussion of prevalence of drug use must take into consideration the rapid changes that the "drug scene" is constantly undergoing. As Scher[231] pointed out, "So varied, complex and changing is drug use, depending on shifting styles of use or abuse, altering availability, the introduction of new agents, changing group structure, membership, or mores in one location or different sections of the country, as well as police or legislative intensifications, that the picture is one of kaleidoscopic twists, and turns at any particular moment." Consequently, little is known about incidence and prevalence of current drug use. Most of the available evidence is concerned with drug use by college students.[29,43,94,101,143,169,171,183,193,205,215] Estimates vary greatly. Studies conducted at various campuses before or during 1967 showed rates of marijuana use ranging from 12 to 20 percent, and LSD use from 2 to 9 percent.[171,193,215] Blum's[43] survey of five campuses, which ended in 1967, reported an incidence of marijuana use from 10 to 33 percent, and LSD from 2 to 9 percent. One campus which was resurveyed one-and-a-half years later showed an increase in marijuana use from 21 to 57 percent, and in LSD use from 6 to 17 percent. In a large survey of college student drug use in the Denver-Boulder metropolitan area, conducted in the fall of 1968, Mizner and associates[205] found that 26 percent of the students had used marijuana, 5 percent had used LSD, and 26 percent amphetamines without a doctor's prescription. Almost half of the users reported that they had used only marijuana, and 14 percent had used only amphetamines; almost all LSD users had also tried marijuana and most had also used amphetamines. Of the single drug users, 76 percent fell into the experimental (maximum of two trials) and casual (maximum of nine trials) use category. Of the polydrug users, 75 percent were in the moderate to heavy category (ten trials or more). On the other hand, current drug use for the total sample was estimated to be 2.8 percent for LSD, 7.4 percent for amphetamines, and 16.4 percent for marijuana. Their data also supported Blum's observation that the drug use rate in college populations tends to be higher in private schools with a predominance of students of upper socioeconomic status, and among students majoring in the humanities and social sciences. Engineering and physical science students are less likely to experiment with drugs. Drug use is also reported to be higher in the East and West Coast states. Keniston[169] draws a close correlation between the "intellectual climate" of a college and the incidence of drug use on its campus. The highest rates are found at small, progressive liberal arts colleges which place higher value on academic independence and intellectual interest for students. The lowest rates occur in colleges noted for their practical orientation, and an emphasis on fraternity life and sports. In a recent survey[183] of medical students at four medical schools in different geographic regions, it was found that 50 percent of the students had tried marijuana at least once, and 30 percent identified themselves as current users. Nearly 10 percent of the total sample had used marijuana over one hundred times, and of them, 93 percent said that they were using it currently. There were significant differences in the rates among the four schools, ranging from 17 to 70 percent. On the basis of the students' responses, it was also suggested that marijuana use could be expected to increase with a favorable change in its legal status.

Data concerning the rates of drug use among adults are very limited. In a sequence of studies[65] conducted in the San Francisco Bay area in 1969, it was found that 14 percent of adults in San Francisco and 12 percent in the Contra Costa suburbs had used marijuana at least once. In spite of differences in population composition, there were no striking differences between city and suburb in major correlates of marijuana use. In both locales, about half of the young men aged eighteen to twenty-four and about one-third of the women in the same age range reported having used marijuana at some time. In both locales, the use rate among persons aged eighteen to thirty-four was 29 percent. Those who were more likely to have used marijuana were tobacco smokers, heavier alcohol drinkers, single persons, childless married persons, individuals who were prone to take drugs without prescription, and persons who had sought help from a psychiatrist. Data regarding drug use among Negroes are also sparse. Marijuana appears to be the most widely available and extensively used drug among both Negro teenagers and adult Negro men.[218] Several studies have surveyed the incidence of drug use among enlisted men in the army.[39,57,78,223] In a sample of 5,482 enlisted men on active duty, Black and associates[39] found that 27 percent of the subjects reported having used marijuana, amphetamines, LSD, or heroin. Of those admitting drug use, 83 percent had used marijuana, 26 percent had used LSD, and 37 percent had used amphetamines. Also, 61 percent of the marijuana users had used the drug more than ten times and 30 percent had used it over one-hundred times. A recent review of the literature on the use of marijuana by GI's in Vietnam[78] concluded that there has been an increasing rate of use of the drug among lower-grade enlisted men. The two most recent studies showed that 25 to 31 percent of the users are beyond the experimentation stage.

Profiles of Drug Users

The fluidity of the ideology, ethos, and lifestyle that characterizes the drug subculture makes any description of the profiles of drug users obsolete. In general, the most important groups are the "social" users and the "habitual" users.

"Social" or "Recreational" Users

According to Carey,[56] these users represent a cross-section of student population, and constitute the majority of those who use drugs. They use mainly marijuana in a fairly regular way, especially during leisure time. Many of them have tried other drugs, particularly LSD, but few use them with any regularity. Their views of drugs are essentially an extension of attitudes about alcohol. Keniston,[169] however, believes that they use marijuana to explore new domains of awareness in their search for "truth and meaningful experience." They are more likely to be found in liberal colleges of higher "intellectual climate," or majoring in one of the social sciences or humanities. They consider themselves as liberals or radicals politically, as well as critical, open-minded, sensitive, and intellectually oriented. Their lives are very much patterned by their student status. Although disillusioned with society and quite critical of its values, they are closely tied to the conventional world in terms of friendships and career aspirations[56] and, in general, they are not in any systematic way "alienated" from American society.[169]

"Habitual" Users or "Heads"

They are popularly known as "potheads" (marijuana users), "acidheads" (LSD users), and "pillheads" (multiple drug users), and are found among those who use drugs with considerable frequency. They generally live in a distinct subculture, with its own values, life style, and particular rituals, and jargon. Drugs are a focal point in their lives and are used with great casualness and regularity, particularly marijuana, which is smoked every day or several times a day.[56] The use of LSD is not likely to occur more than once a week. The amphetamines are used by some of them. Many of them use LSD as a means of expanding self-awareness and cosmic consciousness, as an avenue for mystical or religious experience, and as a way of finding solutions to personal problems. Marijuana is an important aspect of this culture and is thought by some to provide a "social ritual," "a focus of guiltless lawbreaking," and a means to "relieve unde-

sired feelings of anger and aggression."[268] The "heads," according to Carey,[56] are "status disclaimers," reject the traditional values and roles of society, and place a great deal of emphasis on "choice that gives one the unlimited freedom to change." "The major choice is to drop out of conventional society and opt for independence in personal relationships." Keniston[169] described them along the same lines, as "genuinely alienated from American society," and rejecting the prevalent social values which they criticize largely on cultural and humanistic grounds. They rarely stay involved for long in the pursuit of political or social causes, because for them the "basic societal problem is not so much political as aesthetic." "What matters is the interior world and, in the exploration of that world, drugs play a major role." In classifying marijuana users, Bloomquist[41] refers to an "upper-caste" and "lower-caste." The lower-caste user has a hedonistic orientation and is merely interested in experiencing "the bizarre effect of the drug for the effect alone." Until recently, most marijuana users belonged to the lower-caste; however, with "the entrance of the intellectual into the cannabis drug community," according to Bloomquist, there is a growing group of users, constituting the upper-caste, the members of which "take the drug to 'maintain' and to explore themselves and the infinite. To 'maintain' . . . is to defer the enjoyment to better understand one's inner self and rid oneself of his hangups." As Grinspoon[121] points out, Bloomquist's dichotomy assumes an evaluative-judgmental stance closely related to the Puritan ethic.

❪ Determinants of Drug Use

Drug use is an extraordinarily complex phenomenon that can only be understood in a multidimensional frame of reference. As Keniston[166] points out, ". . . like any broad social phenomenon, [it] must be viewed simultaneously in two contexts: in the context of each individual life in which it occurs, and in the context of the social, political and historical situation of the generation in which it occurs."

Historical-Ideological Perspective

Man's "chemophilic" interest in the use of drugs as a means of altering his conscious experience dates probably back to the primordial era of his emergence as an introspective being capable of manipulating his unique ability for self-awareness. By accident or serendipity, he learned to appreciate and respect their effects, to seek the euphoria, blissfulness, awe, or fear produced by them, and look upon them, not only as a source of pleasure, but also as a means for mystical and religious experiences. Whether it was alcohol, opium, cannabis, peyote, or hallucinogenic mushrooms, man has always associated the use of psychoactive drugs with both hedonistic-convivial or mystical-ceremonial practices. This dichotomy, reflecting man's eternal philosophical vacillation between a "Dionysian" and an "Apollonian" view of himself, is exemplified by such drug practices as the orgiastic excitement of the Dionysian festivals or the Pythian oracles of the Delphic mysteries in ancient Greece; the use of cannabis for escapism and pleasure by the poor outcast, or for mystical revelation by the ascetic in India; the use of the fly-agaric mushrooms by the "berserkers" among the Vikings and the Siberian Koryaks, or the use of peyote for religious purposes by the Mexican Indians; and in our contemporary society, the use of marijuana by a hedonistic lower-caste and a revelation-seeking upper-caste.[41]

The current "drug scene" in this country is intimately connected with the ideological currents and the sociocultural changes that occurred during the 1960s, a period characterized by such historical events as the civil-rights movement, the black ghetto uprisings, the campus revolts, the assassination of political leaders, the hippie movement, and the war in Indochina. Seen from a vantage point that is still too close for proper perspective, this decade's mood, style, and reverberating themes have been described in terms of a "counterculture," a "social revolution" or a "protest movement" associated with a "greening" change in national "consciousness" that

brought out a chasmal "generation gap." This has been the epoch of confrontation by an iconoclastic youth that challenged traditional values and symbols, tampered with old taboos, rejected parental authority, as well as established institutional order and structure, and sought to bring about a pervasive change in every aspect of life style and social conduct. Although one can easily understand the concurrent "black movement" within traditional historical precedents, the counterculture of the 1960s represents a historical paradox, a middle-class phenomenon, which sprang explosively in the midst of economic affluence as an expression of protest by a "privileged" youth that felt oppressed. The major characteristics of this youth movement include freedom from binding and constrictive social rituals, and freedom to experiment and to seek the novel, a preoccupation with nonconformism, a need for commitment and involvement coupled with a demand for participation in the institutionalized decision-making process, a quest for relevancy and meaning, and a hedonistic focusing on the "here-and-now" that emphasizes the supremacy of the immediate experience over the contemplation of the future and the reverence of the past. The extreme fringes of this movement represent radical departures from most established norms of current social behavior, characterized by a radical activism or anarchism on the one hand, and the hippie subculture on the other hand; they espouse an escape from technological society and bring a message of a psychedelically-induced transcendental union among all mankind within the ideology of a quasi-religious mysticism, sloganeering love, peace, and brotherhood. The glorification of deviance in both behavior and ideology in this latter group, couched in a new and ever-changing language, became intimately connected with the use of psychedelic drugs.

Those outside the counterculture interpreted it as an expression of defiance of parental authority, a rebellion against societal restrictions, or a reaction to the Indochina war, the threat of an atomic holocaust, environmental pollution, urban decay, racial injustice, or rapid social change. Others viewed it as the primitization of man's experience, or the vulgarization of culture, or as a flight into Utopia. Some saw in the new ethos the messianic salvation of man from himself, the ascendancy of the "psychological man" whose ecstatic venture into the mystical and visionary experience of the occult—instantly gained through the use of drugs—would lead to his blissful union with the universe and to the redemption of his lost soul. Others saw in it the alienated man's escape from his anomic loneliness and powerlessness imposed upon him by a technocratic society, or his quest to recapture the experience of intimacy, compassion, and togetherness, as well as his long-cherished ideals of free choice, self-determination and self-actualization, by seeking the emotional exchange of an "encounter" and the revelations of confrontation. Commenting on the "insurgent mood" of the 1960s, Hughes[140] emphasized "its peculiar blend of political puritanism and personal license, its cult of 'confrontation' as a quasi-religious act of witness," "a basically unpolitical aspiration to see through, to unmask, to strip," the goal of which was psychological or spiritual. Various attempts to understand the preceding "silent generation" of the 1950s have been based on the machine ideal that emerged from the postwar triumph of technology and the system of free enterprise. The young collegians of that era were described as earnest, ambitious, pragmatic, and reality-oriented conformists, pursuing conventional roles that promised maximum engagement into the established social system. Their value system emphasized success, comfort, security, status-striving, competition, power, and role-playing.[97,140,168,269] They were described as having a "hyperactive and rigid ego,"[168] leading to a state of "ego restriction."[97] The younger generation of the 1960s, on the other hand, is thought to represent the postindustrial man[269] whose values include the establishment of personal identity, cooperation, mutuality, and the pursuit of "authentic" relations with others. The emphasis, as Evans[97] points out, is on what might be called "ego relaxation," referring to the demand for immediacy, sensuality, and regressive experiences, as well as receptivity to new experiences, confrontation, and action.

The prevailing ideologies of the counterculture are drawn primarily from the writings of the existentialists (J.-P. Sartre, Simone de Beauvoir, A. Camus), the "beats" (A. Ginsberg, J.C. Holmes), and the mystical writings of the East, especially Zen Buddhism, popularized by Alan Watts and others.[56] Roszak[221] points out that one can discern "a continuum of thought and experience among the young which links together the New Left sociology of Mills, the Freudian Marxism of Herbert Marcuse, the Gestalt-therapy anarchism of Paul Goodman, the apocalyptic body mysticism of Norman Brown, the Zen-based psychotherapy of Alan Watts, and finally Timothy Leary's impenetrably occult narcissism." The renaissance of the mystical-religious interest and the widespread preoccupation with the occult (Zen, Hinduism, primitive shamanism, theosophy, astrology, numerology) are seen by Roszak as the youthful opposition to the skeptical intellectuality and positivism of a severely secularized technocratic society that has no place for mystery, myth, and ritual, the cultural elements that "weave together the collective fabric of society" and which "are meant to be shared in for the purpose of enriching life by experience of awe and splendor." Roszak views the "disaffected" youth's effort to capture the "counterfeit infinity" through the use of psychedelic drugs as essentially "an exploration of the politics of consciousness" and as representing youth's most radical rejection of the parental society. He further asserts that the psychedelic preoccupation at the level of the alienated youth is a symptom of cultural impoverishment, diminishing consciousness by way of fixation, and reducing culture to an esoteric collection of peer-group symbols and slogans. He points out that ". . . instead of culture, we get collage: a miscellaneous heaping together, as if one had simply ransacked the Encyclopedia of Religion and Ethics and the *Celestia Arcana* for exotic tidbits." According to Brody,[47] "Values are part of the cultural symbolic-meaningful matrix in which all behavior occurs" and are regarded "as key elements of the shared symbolic experience that constitutes the cultural mainstream holding the members of any society together." He further views values as "the organizing factors in all ideologies and hence in most sustained collective behaviors." They develop "through social interaction as signs become invested with meaning through shared cumulative experience and move away from the status of representing particular external-world entities. This movement in the direction of abstraction and generalization results ultimately in the development of relative autonomy for the symbol as a method of transmitting information, motivating behavior, or categorizing individual experience." With regard to the subculture of the disaffiliated youth, there is a continuous shifting of values and symbols, which fail to become integrated into a "cultural symbolic-meaningful matrix," emerging and submerging as transient phenomena characterizing a developmentally transient adolescent population. Such fluid cultural systems fail to become institutionalized and traditionalized, with the result of having a tenuous impact on the individual and little sustaining effect on the collective behaviors of the group. They represent abortive imitations and caricatures of the cultogenic process, a sort of "instant culture" which is not internalized but acted out.

Social Determinants of Drug Use

The sociological approach to the understanding of the motivation for drug use takes into consideration such variables as social disorganization, alienation, anomie, rapid culture change, role conflict or value conflict, peer pressure, and others. Drug use, viewed in the context of deviant behavior, is thus conceptualized as being the result of a dysfunctional social structure, regardless of the personality characteristics of the individual. This dysfunctional social structure has been viewed as creating a dissociation between culturally defined aspirations and socially structured means to achieve these aspirations, resulting in the inaccessibility of legitimate avenues for attain-

ment and self-fulfillment, thus forcing the individual to adopt deviant patterns of behavior.[56] This process, as well as the syndrome produced by it, has been described as "alienation." The concept of alienation has been widely used to understand a number of contemporary problems, including youth rebellion and drug use. It was Durkheim,[91] in his study of suicide, who first focused on alienation by his concern with modern man's isolation from traditional society, and resultant state of "anomie." He identified industrialism, secularism, and mass democracy as the alienating factors. To Fromm,[108] alienated is the person who has become estranged from himself and from others as a result of his loss of control over a complicated social machine which was created to administer an ever-expanding technological world. Alienation has been traditionally associated with poverty, old age, minority groups, social exclusion, oppression, and lack of choice and opportunity. With the urbanization of the industrial man, the disappearance of close relationships between people, and the dissolution of the extended family—especially in the large metropolitan areas where life has become anonymous and impersonal, and work mechanized and bureaucratic—have resulted in cultural disaffection and social isolation. According to Keniston,[167] what is new about alienation in our modern society is a sense of estrangement secondary to affluence, increasing rates of social change, lack of creativity in work, and a decline in utopian ideas. Also, automation together with increased longevity has resulted in dramatic changes in work practices and has given modern man a large measure of free time and leisure, for which he is emotionally unprepared, leading him to alienation from self.[56,167] Among the most important conditions for the development of the drug subculture, Carey[56] asserts, "is the unavailability of means to express protest or grievances among a population suffering from some kind of strain." One factor that contributes to this strain is the "deprivation of participation," and the sense of powerlessness that leads to disaffection and disillusionment. He further postulates that this social strain was produced by "internal migration" that led to the concentration of population in large cities after World War II, and a shift in the composition of the population secondary to increased birth rate. The "baby boom" of the preceding decades that has resulted in the contemporary adolescent population explosion has not only disturbed the balance of intergenerational dynamics, but it has also taxed the available community resources, social systems, and institutions that are responsive to the needs of youth.

Carey emphasizes the sense of "disillusionment" and consequent alienation that leads to questioning the legitimacy of society's norms as the initial stage in the sequence of events in the involvement in the drug scene. Furthermore, the potential user must be in a setting where drugs are available and also he must be introduced to drugs by someone he holds in esteem. With regard to marijuana, Becker[31,32] believes that the whole sequence, from curious experimentation to habitual use of the drug, comprises a definite learning process in which there are three distinct consecutive phases: The first step is learning the proper technique of its use through participation in a marijuana-using group; second, the naïve user must learn to perceive the effects of being "high"; and finally, he must learn to enjoy the effect that he has previously learned to perceive. His further use of the drug depends not only on his ability to continue to answer "Yes" to the question, "Is it fun?" but also on his response to awareness that society disapproves of his smoking of marijuana. Becker focuses on the sequence of events which allegedly constitute the causal process of drug-taking behavior; in his framework, the motives do not precede this behavior but are generated in the process of its development. He also places major emphasis on the role that the group plays in influencing this process. Marijuana, LSD, and other hallucinogens have been described as exerting a "sociogenic"[118] or "cultogenic"[104] effect. Drug taking is a communal affair. Goode[118] asserts that "being 'turned on' for the first time is a group experience" and that "marijuana use, even in its very inception, is *simultaneously*

participation in a specific social group." He further states that "Marijuana is not merely smoked in groups, but is also smoked in *intimate* groups. The others with whom one is smoking are overwhelmingly *significant* others." The continuous use of the drug serves as "a catalyst in generating and reaffirming commitment to a drug using subculture," and is richly invested with the elements of a "tribal ritual," including its symbolic reaffirmation of membership in the subcommunity of users, the strong feelings of brotherhood, belonging, and loyalty, the sharing of something of value and of special meaning, and the development of a distinct mythology. According to Freedman,[104] "For this group, magical transformation of reality, omniscient union rather than painful confrontation of separateness and effort is a lure." It has been shown that LSD is a mutual component with heavy marijuana use and that the more one uses marijuana, the greater is the likelihood that the user will take at least one of the psychedelic drugs.[118] Peer or group pressure associated with curiosity has been cited as a major motivation for experimentation with drugs.[104,121,185] Taking the drug does not only satisfy the urgent adolescent need for belonging, but also provides the user with the opportunity for a challenging deed that evokes interest among friends and can offer the basis for a loose group cohesion.[104] Several commentators have attributed the spread of the "psychedelic mystique" to the "irresponsible, alluring and provocative advertising" of the mass communication media,[104] to the "glorification of the hippie culture by the establishment, and the exploration of the psychedelic movement by business,"[185] and to the proselytizing ideology of the "apologists" of the psychedelic use.[142,177] Other factors that have been mentioned to be related to the development of the "drug epidemic" include inadequate leadership, parental hypocrisy, excessive permissiveness in both family and society, disorganization of the family unit, poverty with its compelling need to escape from a boring and frustrating reality, and economic affluence.[185] For some, affluence results in a "sensate society, the ascendancy of hedonism, the cult of experience,"[185] and for others, in an immense prolongation of adolescence through prolongation of education, a new stage of life in which "individuals are in an experimental age, a stage of seeking for meaning and significance, often sought through drugs."[166]

Psychological Determinants of Drug Use

The psychological approach to the understanding of the motives for habitual drug use is based on two major theoretical assumptions: (i) the concept of "psychological dependence," and (ii) the concept of "susceptibility" or "predisposition" to drug use as determined by pre-exising personality factors and the inherent vulnerabilities associated with the developmental vicissitudes of adolescence.

PSYCHOLOGICAL DEPENDENCE

The concept of psychological dependence refers to a pattern of repetitive use of drugs assumed to be maintained by irresistible psychological factors. It is postulated that these factors reach certain autonomy in the psychic organization of the so-called habitual user, and operate as an acquired drive system that is motivating drug-dependent behavior. It is further assumed that there is a prerequisite state of individual predisposition or susceptibility ("psychological readiness") which requires the presence of certain environmental contingencies (social milieu, availability of drugs, culture values, ideology) for the pattern to develop. The affective component of this predispositional state has been variously described as tension, anxiety, depression, boredom, feelings of alienation, or "tense depression," thus implying a psychopathological origin of this state. Frustration is the most commonly mentioned underlying determinant of the affective component of this state. In this context, the alloplastic pattern of drug use serves as a means of relieving the dysphoria produced by frustrating experiences, and subsequently, this tension-reducing mechanism further reinforces the drug-dependent behavior as a conditioned response of the operant

paradigm. The hedonistic variant of this hypothesis conceptualizes the predispositional state as being characterized by an ascendancy of pleasure-seeking behavior, described in terms of experiencing euphoria ("getting high"), or as an intellectually rewarding pursuit rationalized as gaining insights or expanding conscious experience.

Drug-dependent behavior, maintained by factors related to psychological dependence, can be viewed within the framework of the drive theory as representing a substitutive behavior response pattern for "frustrated" drives (e.g., sexual, aggressive, achievement, self-fulfillment) whose original responses or goals have been thwarted or have failed to occur. These responses generally have the characteristics of short-term goals, that is, urgency and immediacy of action, and upon repetition are highly learnable. In this situation, the "excitatory" component of the frustrated drive continues to energize the behavior of the individual, while the "directional" component of the same drive undergoes changes and becomes redirected, resulting in the substitutive response of drug-taking, further maintained through the reinforcing effect of frustration reduction (discharge of tension) produced by the drug. It is generally assumed that the motivational state of the individual who is prone to develop psychological dependence on a drug is characterized primarily by ascendant drives for immediate goals, which tend to pre-empt drives for long-term goals. Habitual drug users, as well as alcoholics, are described as "narcissistic" individuals who are motivated by "immature" drives for immediate goals, and who demand immediate gratification of their exaggerated needs. Furthermore, these individuals are described as being continuously frustrated, due to excessive needs which they are unable to satisfy.

DEVELOPMENTAL-PSYCHODYNAMIC APPROACH

Drug-taking behavior among the young does not appear to represent an obligatory component of any particular syndrome or personality pattern. It is generally viewed as a maturational phenomenon associated with the nature of adolescent process, which in our culture has further extended into early adulthood. In our modern society, the adolescent's difficult developmental task of reaching integration of individual maturation that leads to the formation of a stable identity and to the acceptance of adult roles has been further burdened by a number of emergent factors that are primarily related to rapid social change. Evans[97] describes three "drive-defense constellations" representing adaptational modes characteristic of the contemporary adolescent's effort to deal with stage-specific maturational tasks: (i) Protective regression of ego function, as manifested in the adolescent's tenuous, idealized, and narcissistic way of relating to external objects; (ii) rebellion, which is interpreted as the externalization of the adolescent's ambivalent emancipatory strivings; and (iii) dislocation, a clinical term for alienation.

The transition through adolescence is fraught with a "sense of crisis," according to King,[172] which is more likely to occur at times of rapid social change when transition points and the rites of passage of the adolescent receive less attention and less social endorsement, and the lines of demarcation between the child and the adult roles are less clear. King further asserts that in an affluent society, as in a family setting which overindulges the child's wishes, this crisis may lead to the fantasy of omnipotence served by what Murray[208] has described as "narcissistic entitlement," the feeling that things are owed a person without his doing anything to earn them. Narcissism, however, may take another form in crisis, ". . . that of destructive rebellion, or the form of withdrawal, or regression to the real or fantasied gratifications of earlier phases of development, including the belief in magical solutions to problems. Drugs provide one avenue to withdrawal, and represent one way of responding to crisis. The danger lies in abrogating the task of maturing in a rapidly changing society for which there is no blueprint providing safe guidelines into the future."[172] Other sources of difficulties for the adolescent brought about by rapid social change include, according to Settlage,[241] "the sparsity of suitable models for identification in

bridging the gap from childhood to adulthood," and the "lack of consensus and conviction regarding values on the part of the society that tends to deprive parents of convictions and support in their child-rearing practices and also tends to deprive children of the benefit of relatively clear-cut limits and guidelines for their impulses and behavior."

Considerable interest has been focused on the syndrome of adolescent "alienation" as a major factor associated with both the phenomena of youth unrest and drug-taking behavior. Halleck[123] describes alienation from a psychiatric viewpoint as a "syndrome which represents a psychological arrest in growth and maturity," reflecting Blos's[241] view of the alienated older adolescent as one who "has settled down in a transitory stage of adolescence." For Halleck, alienation constitutes a distinct personality pattern disturbance and a specific clinical syndrome which results from the adolescent's failure to resolve childhood conflicts and prepare himself for the complexities and frustrations of the student role. Halleck describes the alienated student's family setting as being characterized by an "image of loving permissiveness" in which love "was more talked out than provided," by an "identification of the parents with their child in an attempt to impose role responsibilities upon him which more appropriately belonged to them," and by paratactical communication or "double binds." In this family setting, the adolescent learns to adopt a pseudomature pose in which he is just rebellious enough and just conforming enough to please his parents. When he leaves home and begins life at the university, where there are no restraints to serve his need for structure and guidance, he reacts to his new freedom with strong guilt feelings which eventually lead to a peculiar kind of apathy and withdrawal. Referring to the "middle-class, white, alienated, generation-gap-minded, drug-taking, uncommitted older adolescent," Blos[241] emphasizes the "enormous dependency on a caretaking tension-reducing environment, which represents a displacement from the family." Blos describes the alienated adolescent's tribal affiliations as "sham independence" in a "self-built ghetto."

He further asserts that "Adolescent phase-specific regression, finding no adequate societal support or rescue, leads to the formation of adolescent groups, which contain flagrant ego inadequacies or put them to self-protective and adaptive use." The adaptive element of this activity is further supported by the reparative nature of self-medication in drug-taking behavior, which may be viewed as the alienated youth's attempt to "treat himself" in order to relieve his symptoms of depression and anxiety.

Several authors have emphasized the presence of depression in the alienated drug user.[123,126,209,242,257,267] Unwin[259] has pointed out the striking clinical similarities between the "alienated syndrome" and the "amotivational syndrome"[195] described in heavy marijuana users, both of which, in his view, appear to be characterized by a "masked nuclear depression." The dynamics of this depression, according to Unwin, are "a function of the ego-ideal and a feeling of shame, rather than a function of superego and a feeling of guilt with which depressive reactions are traditionally associated." Nicholi[209] has also described this depression as being "related not to object loss but to the disparity between the ideal self as a uniquely gifted intellectual achiever and the real self as one of thousands of students struggling in a competitive and threatening environment." Similarly, Settlage,[241] in his discussion of alienated youth, notes "a rather grim and unrelenting attempt to measure up to the excessive high standards of one's ego ideal in order to maintain self-esteem," and feels that "if the gap between personal standards and performance is too great . . . the results can be a depressive picture of varying degrees of severity," which may eventually lead to experimentation with drugs and to "an increasing disengagement from truly meaningful relationships with people, with an accompanying rationalization of the activity as a means of discovering the self and the true meaning of life." Goodman[241] also associates the use of drugs with "the urgent wish for an escape from conflict and anxiety into a sense of omnipotence and omniscience by way of a magic potion."

Adler[8] views the contemporary hippie subculture as representing a "crisis of values" which has resulted in the emergence of a specific personality configuration: the "antinomian personality" of the hippie. According to Adler, the "antinomian" fears diffusion and depersonalization, seeks out "haptic irritations" to overcome boredom and insensibility, and plays at throwing away what is lost to maintain the illusion of self-determination and freedom. His life style, including his introspective LSD "trips," represent his attempts to demonstrate a capacity to control self and objects and to reinstate both self- and object-constancy. Boredom has been mentioned by others as playing an important role in drug use,[121,185] especially in the late adolescent. Grinspoon[121] assumes that boredom may reflect a maladaptive control of unacceptable sexual and aggressive impulses, which are unsuccessfully sublimated. However, this special ennui may also be related to an increased need for self-stimulation, a low motivational level, or masked depression.

Other writers[45,117] have attempted to relate the use of drugs to needs for interpersonal closeness, a wish for fusion with others, and fantasied introjection of strength, or to an "ambivalent loneliness"[185] in which drugs fulfill the need for an episodic establishment of intimacy. To Grinspoon,[121] drug use may also represent "identification with, or modeling after, a generation that has legitimized the taking of drugs," a viewpoint that has been elaborated by many others. Grinspoon further asserts that "to some extent, at least, young people are acting out some of the repressed unconscious wishes of their parents" for antisocial behavior and sexual promiscuity, symbolized or fantasized in the taking of marijuana.

In concluding the discussion of the determinants of drug use, it is important to emphasize the following points: (1) The ubiquitous phenomenon of drug use among adolescents, although symptomatic of the strains associated with the vicissitudes of the developmental process, is not specific of these strains. (2) The preferential use of the so-called psychotomimetic or mind-altering drugs by the contemporary youth may be viewed as an age-contingent phenomenon only within the presently existing sociocultural and ideological contexts. Future preferential patterns of drug use for any age group should be expected to undergo changes dependent upon the evolving culture and ideology of a society. (3) The pervasive use of drugs in our modern society represents one example of the emergence of phenomena of a new order, the increasing magnitude of which is not merely the result of increased population. These phenomena constitute the expression of the complex interaction and reverberation of processes characteristic of large-scale systems. Among them, the processes of rapid and wide dissemination ("megaprocesses"), developed by recent technological advances—telecommunication, mass information media, and mass transportation—not only facilitate the massive and distal spreading of localized, episodic, or sporadic phenomena that were previously controlled by small-scale systems, but also account for the information overload that is continuously and instantly impinging upon large masses of people, with far-reaching consequences on man's personality, behavior, culture, and society. Any serious consideration of the social control of drug use must take into account these points.

❲ Bibliography

1. ABOOD, L. G. "The Psychotomimetic Glycolate Esters," in A. Burger, ed., *Medicinal Research Series, II: Drugs Affecting the Central Nervous System.* New York: Marcel Dekker, 1968.

2. ABOOD, L. G., and J. H. BIEL. "Anticholinergic Psychotomimetic Agents," *International Review of Neurobiology,* 4 (1962), 217–273.

3. ABRAMSON, H. A. "LSD-25: III. As an Adjunct to Psychotherapy with Elimination of Fear of Homosexuality," *Journal of Psychology,* 39 (1955), 127–155.

4. ———, ed., *The Use of LSD in Psychotherapy and Alcoholism.* Indianapolis: Bobbs-Merrill, 1967.

5. ABRAMSON, H. A., M. E. JARVIK, M. H. GORIN, and M. W. HIRSCH. "Lysergic Acid Diethylamide (LSD-25): XVII. Tolerance Development and Its Relationship to a Theory of Psychosis," *Journal of Psychology,* 41 (1956), 81–105.

6. ABRAMSON, H. A., B. SKLAROFSKY, and M. D. BARON. "Lysergic Acid Diethylamide (LSD-25) Antagonists. II: Development of Tolerance in Man to LSD-25 by Prior Administration of MLD-41 (1-methyl-d-lysergic acid diethylamide)," *Archives of Neurology and Psychiatry,* 79 (1958), 201–207.

7. ACKERLY, W. C., and G. GIBSON. "Lighter Fluid 'Sniffing,'" *The American Journal of Psychiatry,* 120 (1964), 1056–1061.

8. ADLER, N. "The Antinomian Personality: the Hippie Character Type," *Psychiatry,* 31 (1968), 325–338.

9. AGHAJANIAN, G. K., and D. X. FREEDMAN. "Biochemical and Morphological Aspects of LSD Pharmacology," in D. E. Efron, ed., *Psychopharmacology—A Review of Progress 1957–1967.* Public Health Service Publication No. 1836, 1968.

10. AGHAJANIAN, G. K., and O. H. L. BING. "Persistence of Lysergic Acid Diethylamide in the Plasma of Human Subjects," *Clinical Pharmacology and Therapeutics,* 5 (1964), 611–614.

11. AGURELL, S., I. M. NILSSON, A. OHLSSON, and F. SANDBERG. "Elimination of Tritium-Labelled Cannabinols in the Rat with Special Reference to the Development of Tests for the Identification of Cannabis Users," *Biochemical Pharmacology,* 18 (1969), 1195–1201.

12. ALEXANDER, G. J., B. E. MILES, G. M. GOLD, and B. E. ALEXANDER. "LSD: Injection Early in Pregnancy Produces Abnormalities in Offspring of Rats," *Science,* 157 (1967), 459–460.

13. ALLEN, J. R., and L. J. WEST. "Flight from Violence: Hippies and the Green Rebellion," *The American Journal of Psychiatry,* 125 (1968), 364–370.

14. ALLENTUCK, S., and K. M. BOWMAN. "The Psychiatric Aspects of Marihuana Intoxication," *The American Journal of Psychiatry,* 99 (1942), 248–251.

15. AMES, F. "A Clinical and Metabolic Study of Acute Intoxication with Cannabis Sativa and Its Role in the Model Psycho-

ses," *Journal of Mental Science*, 104 (1958), 972–999.

16. ANGRIST, B. M., J. W. SCHWEITZER, S. GERSHON, and A. J. FRIEDHOFF. "Mephentermine Psychosis: Misuse of the Wyamine Inhaler," *The American Journal of Psychiatry*, 126 (1970), 1315–1317.

17. APPEL, J. B. "The Effects of 'Psychotomimetic' Drugs on Animal Behavior," in D. E. Efron, ed., *Psychopharmacology—A Review of Progress 1957–1967*. Public Health Service Publication No. 1836, 1968.

18. APPEL, J. B. and D. X. FREEDMAN. "Chemically-Induced Alterations in the Behavioral Effects of LSD-25," *Biochemical Pharmacology*, 13 (1964), 861–869.

19. ———. "Tolerance and Cross-Tolerance among Psychotomimetic Drugs," *Psychopharmacologia*, 13 (1968), 267–274.

20. ARONSON, H., A. B. SILVERSTEIN, and G. D. KLEE. "Influence of Lysergic Acid Diethylamide (LSD-25) on Subjective Time," *Archives of General Psychiatry*, 1 (1959), 469.

21. ARONSON, H., C. E. WATERMANN, and G. D. KLEE. "The Effect of D-Lysergic Acid Diethylamide (LSD-25) on Learning and Retention," *Journal of Clinical and Experimental Psychopathology*, 23 (1962), 17–23.

22. AUERBACH, R., and J. A. RUDOWSKI. "Lysergic Acid Diethylamide: Effect on Embryos," *Science*, 157 (1967), 1325–1326.

23. BAKER, J. P., and J. D. FARLEY. "Toxic Psychosis Following Atropine Eye-Drops," *British Medical Journal*, II (1958), 1390–1392.

24. BAKKER, C. B., and F. B. AMINI, "Observations on the Psychotomimetic Effects of Sernyl," *Comprehensive Psychiatry*, 2 (1961), 269–280.

25. BALIS, G. U. "Delirium and Other States of Altered Consciousness," in Tice's *Practice of Medicine*, 10 (1970), Chapter 39, 17–29.

26. BALIS, G. U., and R. R. MONROE. "The Pharmacology of Chloralose: A Review," *Psychopharmacologia*, 6 (1964), 1–30.

27. BAN, T. A., J. J. LOHRENZ, and H. E. LEHMAN. "Observations on the Action of Sernyl—A New Psychotropic Drug," *Canadian Psychiatric Association Journal*, 6 (1961), 150–157.

28. BARKER, G. H., and W. T. ADAMS. "Glue Sniffers," *Sociology and Social Research*, 47 (1963), 299.

29. BASS, D. "The Pot-Smoking UC Law Students," *San Francisco Chronicle*, (Oct. 27, 1969), 1.

30. BASS, M. "Sudden Sniffing Death," *Journal of the AMA*, 212 (1970), 2075–2079.

31. BECKER, H. S. "Marihuana Use and Social Control," *Social Problems*, 3 (1955), 35–44.

32. ———. "Becoming a Marijuana Smoker," in *The Outsiders*. New York: Macmillan, 1963.

33. BELL, D. S. "Comparison of Amphetamine Psychosis and Schizophrenia," *British Journal of Psychiatry*, 111 (1965), 701–707.

34. BENABUD, A. "Psycho-pathological Aspects of the Cannabis Situation in Morocco: Statistical Data for 1956," *United Nations Bulletin on Narcotics*, 9 (No. 4) (1957), 1–16.

35. BENDER, L., and D. V. S. SANKAR. "Chromosomal Damage Not Found in Leukocytes of Children Treated With LSD-25," *Science*, 159 (1968), 749.

36. BERGEN, J. R., D. M. KRUS, and G. G. PINCUS. "Suppression of LSD-25 Effects in Rats by Steroids," *Proc. Soc. Exp. Biol.*, 105 (1960), 254.

37. BERGMAN, R. "Navajo Peyote Use: Its Apparent Safety," *The American Journal of Psychiatry*, 128 (1971), 695–699.

38. BERLIN, C. M. "Effects of LSD Taken by Pregnant Women on Chromosomal Abnormalities of Offspring," *Pediatric Herald*, (Jan. and Feb. 1969), 1.

39. BLACK, S., K. L. OWENS, and R. P. WOLFF. "Patterns of Drug Use: A Study of 5,482 Subjects," *The American Journal of Psychiatry*, 127 (1970), 420–423.

40. BLACKER, U. H., R. T. JONES, G. C. STONE, and D. PFEFFERBAUM. "Chronic Users of LSD: The 'Acid Heads'," *The American Journal of Psychiatry*, 125 (1968), 341–351.

41. BLOOMQUIST, E. R. *Marijuana*. Beverly Hills: Glencoe Press, 1968.

42. ———. "Marijuana: Social Benefit or Social Detriment?," *California Medicine*, 106 (1967), 346–353.

43. BLUM, R. F. *Students and Drugs*. San Francisco: Jassey-Bass, Inc., 1970.

44. BOUQUET, R. J. "Cannabis," *Bulletin of Narcotics*, 2 (1950), Part I, 14–30; and 3 (1951), Part II, 22–45.

45. BOWERS, M., A. CHIPMAN, A. SCHWARTZ, and O. T. DANN. "Dynamics of Psychodelic Drug Abuse: A Clinical Study," *Archives of General Psychiatry*, 16 (1967), 560–566.

46. BRAZELTON, T. B. "Effect of Prenatal Drugs on the Behavior of the Neonate," *The American Journal of Psychiatry*, 126 (1970), 1261–1266.

47. BRODY, E. B. "Culture, Symbol and Value in the Social Etiology of Behavioral Deviance," in *Social Psychiatry*. New York: Grune & Stratton, 1968.

48. BROMBERG, W. "Marihuana, a Psychiatric Study," *Journal of the AMA*, 113 (1939), 4–12.

49. ———. "Marihuana Intoxication: A Clinical Study of Cannabis Sativa Intoxication," *The American Journal of Psychiatry*, 91 (1934), 303–330.

50. BURSTEIN, S. H., F. MENEZES, E. WILLIAMSON, and R. MECHOULAM. "Metabolism of Delta 1(6)-Tetrahydrocannabinol, an Active Marihuana Constituent," *Nature*, 225 (1970), 87–88.

51. BUSCH, A. K., and W. C. JOHNSON. "LSD-25 as an Aid in Psychotherapy," *Diseases of the Nervous System*, 11 (1950), 241–243.

52. CALDWELL, D. F., S. A. MYERS, E. F. DOMINO, et al. "Auditory and Visual Threshold Effects of Marihuana in Man," *Perceptive Motor Skills*, 29 (1969), 755–759.

53. CAMPBELL, D. R. "The Electroencephalogram in Cannabis Associated Psychosis," *Canadian Psychiatric Association Journal*, 16 (1971), 161–165.

54. CANNABIS: REPORT BY THE ADVISORY COMMITTEE ON DRUG DEPENDENCE. London: Her Majesty's Stationery Office, 1968.

55. CARAKUSHANSKY, G., R. L. NEU, and L. I. GARDNER. "Lysergide and Cannabis as Possible Teratogens in Man," *Lancet*, 1 (1969), 150–151.

56. CAREY, J. T. *The College Drug Scene*. Englewood Cliffs: Prentice-Hall, 1968.

57. CASPER, E., J. JANECEK, and H. MARTINELLI, JR. "Marihuana in Vietnam," *USARV Medical Bulletin*, 11 (1968), 60–72.

58. CHALOUT, L. "*Revue de la litterature: Les Solvants Organiques*," *Canadian Psychiat-*

ric Association Journal, 16 (1971), 157–160.

59. CHAPEL, J. L., and D. W. TAYLOR. "Glue Sniffing," *Missouri Medicine*, 65 (1968), 288–292.

60. CHAREN, S., and L. PERELMAN. "Personality Studies of Marihuana Addicts," *The American Journal of Psychiatry*, 102 (1946), 674–682.

61. CHOLDEN, L. W., A. KURLAND, and C. SAVAGE. "Clinical Reactions and Tolerance to LSD in Chronic Schizophrenia," *Journal of Nervous and Mental Disease*, 122 (1955), 211–221.

62. CHOPRA, I. C., and R. N. CHOPRA. "The Use of Cannabis Drugs in India," *Bulletin of Narcotics*, 9 (1957), 4–29.

63. CHRISTENSEN, H. D., et al. "Activity of Delta 8- and Delta 9-Tetrahydrocannabinol and Related Compounds in the Mouse," *Science*, 172 (1971), 165–167.

64. CHWELOS, N., D. B. BLEWETT, C. M. SMITH, and A. HOFFER. "Use of LSD-25 in the Treatment of Alcoholism," *Quarterly Journal of Studies on Alcohol*, 20 (1959), 577–590.

65. CISIN, I. H., and D. I. MANHEIMER. "Marijuana Use Among Adults in a Large City and Suburb," in A. J. Singer, ed., *Marijuana: Chemistry, Pharmacology, and Pattern of Social Use*. Annals of New York Academy of Science, 1971.

66. CLARK, L. D., R. HUGHES, and E. N. NAKASHIMA. "Behavioral Effects of Marihuana: Experimental Studies," *Archives of General Psychiatry*, 23 (1970), 193–198.

67. CLARK, L. D., and E. N. NAKASHIMA. "Experimental Studies of Marihuana," *The American Journal of Psychiatry*, 125 (1968), 379–384.

68. COHEN, M. M., K. HIRSCHHORN, and W. A. FROSH. "In Vivo and in Vitro Chromosomal Damage Induced by LSD-25," *New England Journal of Medicine*, 277 (1967), 1043–1049.

69. COHEN, M. M., et al. "The Effect of LSD-25 on the Chromosomes of Children Exposed in Utero," *Pediatric Research*, 2 (1968), 486–492.

70. COHEN, M. M., and D. F. KLEIN. "Drug Abuse in a Young Psychiatric Population," *American Journal of Orthopsychiatry*, 40 (1970), 448–455.

71. COHEN, M. M., M. J. MARINELLO, and N. BACK. "Chromosomal Damage in Hu-

man Leukocytes Induced by Lysergic Acid Diethylamide," *Science*, 155 (1967), 1417–1419.

72. COHEN, M. M., and A. B. MUKHERJEE. "Meiotic Chromosome Damage Induced by LSD-25," *Nature*, 219 (1968), 1072–1074.

73. COHEN, S. "LSD Side Effects and Complications," *Journal of Nervous and Mental Disease*, 130 (1960), 30–40.

74. ———. "A Classification of LSD Complications," *Psychosomatics*, 7 (1966), 182–186.

75. ———. "A Commentary on 'The Ethics of Addiction,'" *The American Journal of Psychiatry*, 128 (1971), 547–550.

76. COHEN, S., and K. S. DITMAN. "Complications Associated with Lysergic Acid Diethylamide (LSD-25)," *Journal of the AMA*, 181 (1962), 161–162.

77. ———. "Prolonged Adverse Reactions to Lysergic Acid Diethylamide," *Archives of General Psychiatry*, 8 (1963), 475–480.

78. COLBACH, E. "Marihuana Use by GIs in Viet Nam," *The American Journal of Psychiatry*, 128 (1971), 204–206.

79. CONNELL, P. H. *Amphetamine Psychosis*. Maudsley Monograph No. 5. London: Maudsley, 1958.

80. ———. "Clinical Manifestations and Treatment of Amphetamine Type of Dependence," *Journal of the AMA*, 196 (1966), 718–723.

81. ———. "The Use and Abuse of Amphetamines," *Practitioner*, 200 (1968), 234–243.

82. COREY, W. J., et al. "Chromosome Studies on Patients (In Vivo) and Cells (In Vitro) Treated with Lysergic Acid Diethylamide," *New England Journal of Medicine*, 282 (1970), 939–943.

83. CRANCER, A., J. M. DILLE, J. C. DELAY, et al. "Comparison of the Effects of Marihuana and Alcohol on Simulated Driving Performance," *Science*, 164 (1969), 851–854.

84. CROCKETT, R., R. A. SANDISON, and A. WALK, eds. *Hallucinogenic Drugs and Their Therapeutic Use*. London: Lewis, 1963.

85. DELAY, J., P. PICHOT, B. LAINE, and J. PERSE. "Changes in Personality Produced by LSD: A Study Using the Rorschach Test," *Annales de Medico-Psychologi*, 112 (1954), 1.

86. DESHON, H. J., M. RINKEL, and H. C. SOLOMON. "Mental Changes Experimentally Produced by LSD," *Psychiatric Quarterly*, 26 (1952), 33–53.

87. DIPAOLO, J. A., H. M. GIVELBER, and H. ERWIN. "Evaluation of Teratogenicity of Lysergic Acid Diethylamide," *Nature*, 220 (1968), 490–491.

88. DITMAN, K. S., M. HAYMAN, and J. WHITTLESEY. "Nature and Frequency of Claims Following LSD," *Journal of Nervous and Mental Disease*, 134 (1962), 346–352.

89. DOORENBOS, N. J., M. X. QUINTBY, and N. J. TURNER. "Cultivation, Extraction, and Analysis of Cannabis Sativa," I., in A. J. Singer, ed., *Marijuana: Chemistry, Pharmacology, and Pattern of Social Use*. Annals of New York Academy of Science, 1971.

90. DORNBUSH, R. L., M. FINK, and A. FREEDMAN. "Marijuana, Memory, and Perception," *The American Journal of Psychiatry*, 128 (1971), 194–197.

91. DURKHEIM, E. *Suicide: A Study in Sociology*. J. A. Spaulding and G. Simpson, eds. Glencoe: Free Press, 1951. (Original work, 1897.)

92. DURRANT, B. W. "Amphetamine Addiction," *Practitioner*, 194 (1965), 649–651.

93. EASSON, W. M. "Gasoline Addiction in Children," *Pediatrics*, 29 (1962), 250–254.

94. EELS, K. "A Survey of Student Practices and Attitudes with Respect to Marijuana and LSD," *Journal of Consulting Psychology*, 15 (1968), 459–467.

95. EGOZCUE, J., S. IRWIN, and C. A. MARUFFO. "Chromosomal Damage in LSD Users," *Journal of the AMA*, 204 (1968), 214–218.

96. ESPELIN, D. E., and A. K. DONE. "Amphetamine Poisoning: Effectiveness of Chlorpromazine," *New England Journal of Medicine*, 278 (1968), 1361–1365.

97. EVANS, J. L. "The College Student in the Psychiatric Clinic: Syndromes and Subcultural Sanctions," *The American Journal of Psychiatry*, 126 (1970), 1736–1742.

98. FABRO, S., and S. M. SIEBER. "Is Lysergide a Teratogen?," *Lancet*, 1 (1968), 639.

99. FINK, M., J. SIMEON, W. HAQUE, and T. M. ITIL. "Prolonged Adverse Reactions in LSD in Psychotic Subjects," *Archives of General Psychiatry*, 15 (1966), 450–454.

100. FINK, M., and T. M. ITIL. "Neurophysiology of Phantastica: EEG and Behavioral Relations in Man," in D. E. Efron, ed.,

Psychopharmacology—A Review of Progress 1957–1967. Public Health Service Publication No. 1836, 1968.

101. FISHER, D. D. "Frequency of Hallucinogenic Drug Use and Its Implications," *Journal of American College Health Association*, 16 (1967), 20–22.

102. FOLTZ, R. L., A. F. FENTIMAN, JR., E. G. LEIGHTY, et al. "Metabolite of (−)-Trans-Delta 8-Tetrahydrocannabinol: Identification and Synthesis," *Science*, 168 (1970), 844–845.

103. FORRER, G. R., and R. D. GOLDNER. "Experimental Physiological Studies with Lysergic Acid Diethylamide (LSD-25)," *Archives of Neurology and Psychiatry*, 65 (1951), 581–588.

104. FREEDMAN, D. X. "On the Use and Abuse of LSD," *Archives of General Psychiatry*, 18 (1968), 330–347.

105. FREEDMAN, D. X., and G. K. AGHAJANIAN. "Time Parameters in Acute Tolerance, Cross Tolerance, and Antagonism to Psychotogens," *Federation Proceedings*, 18 (1959), 390.

106. FREEDMAN, D. X., J. B. APPEL, F. R. HARTMAN, and M. D. MOLLIVER. "Tolerance to the Behavioral Effects of LSD-25 in Rat," *Journal of Pharmacology and Experimental Therapeutics*, 143 (1964), 309–313.

107. FREEDMAN, H. L., and M. J. ROCKMORE. "Marihuana: A Factor in Personality Evaluation and Army Maladjustment," *Journal of Clinical Psychopathology*, 7 (1946), 765–782 (Part I), and 8 (1946), 221–236 (Part II).

108. FROMM, E. *The Sane Society.* New York: Holt, Rinehart and Winston, 1955.

109. FROSCH, W. A., E. ROBBINS, L. ROBBINS, and M. STERN. "Motivation for Self-Administration of LSD," *Psychiatric Quarterly*, 41 (1967), 56–61.

110. FROSCH, W., E. ROBBINS, and M. STERN. "Untoward Reactions to LSD Requiring Hospitalization," *New England Journal of Medicine*, 273 (1965), 1235–1239.

111. GAONI, Y., and R. MECHOULAM. "Isolation, Structure and Partial Synthesis of an Active Constituent of Hashish," *Journal of American Chemical Society*, 86 (1964), 1646–1648.

112. GASKILL, H. S. "Marihuana, an Intoxicant," *The American Journal of Psychiatry*, 102 (1945), 202–204.

113. GEBER, W. F. "Congenital Malformations Induced by Mescaline, Lysergic Acid Diethylamide and Bromlysergic Acid in the Hamster," *Science*, 158 (1967), 265–266.

114. GELLER, A., and M. BOAS. *The Drug Beat.* New York: Cowles Book Co., 1969.

115. GLASS, G. S., and M. B. BOWERS, JR. "Chronic Psychosis Associated with Long-Term Psychotomimetic Drug Abuse," *Archives of General Psychiatry*, 23 (1970), 97–103.

116. GLASSER, H. H., and O. N. MASSENGALE. "Glue-Sniffing in Children: Deliberate Inhalation of Vaporized Plastic Cements," *Journal of the AMA*, 181 (1962), 300–303.

117. GLICKMAN, L., and M. BLUMFIELD. "Psychological Determinants of 'LSD Reactions'," *Journal of Nervous and Mental Disease*, 145 (1967), 79–83.

118. GOODE, E. "Multiple Drug Use Among Marijuana Smokers," *Social Problems*, 17(1) (1969), 48–64.

119. GRIFFITH, J. "A Study of Illicit Amphetamine Drug Traffic in Oklahoma City," *The American Journal of Psychiatry*, 123 (1966), 560–569.

120. GRIFFITH, J. D., J. H. CAVANAUGH, and J. A. OATES. "Psychosis Induced by the Administration of D-Amphetamine to Human Volunteers," in D. E. Efron, ed., *Psychotomimetic Drugs.* New York: Raven Press, 1970.

121. GRINSPOON, L. *Marihuana Reconsidered.* Cambridge: Harvard University Press, 1971.

122. GROSSMAN, W. "Adverse Reactions Associated With Cannabis Products in India," *Annals of Internal Medicine*, 70 (1969), 529–533.

123. HALLECK, S. L. "Psychiatric Treatment for the Alienated College Student," *The American Journal of Psychiatry*, 124 (1967), 642–650.

124. HANAWAY, J. K. "Lysergic Acid Diethylamide: Effects on the Developing Mouse Lens," *Science*, 164 (1969), 574–575.

125. HARTMAN, A. M., and L. E. HOLLISTER. "Effect of Mescaline, Lysergic Acid Diethylamide and Psilocybin on Color Perception," *Psychopharmacologia*, 4 (1963), 441–451.

126. HEKIMIAN, L. J., and S. GERSHON, "Characteristics of Drug Abusers Admitted to a Psychiatric Hospital," *Journal of the AMA*, 205 (1968), 125–130.

127. HERMAN, M., and S. H. NAGLER. "Psychoses Due to Amphetamine," *Journal of Nervous and Mental Disease*, 120 (1954), 268–272.

128. HOCH, P. H. "Pharmacologically Induced Psychoses," in S. Arieti, ed., *American Handbook of Psychiatry*, Vol. 2. New York: Basic Books, 1959.

129. HOFFER, A., and H. OSMOND. *The Hallucinogens*. New York: Academic Press, 1967.

130. HOFMANN, A. "Psychotomimetic Drugs: Chemical and Pharmacological Aspects," *Acta Physiologica et Pharmacologica Nederlandica*, 8 (1959), 240–258.

131. HOGAN, R., et al. "Personality Correlates of Undergraduate Marijuana Use," *Journal of Consulting Clinical Psychology*, 35 (1970), 58–63.

132. HOLLISTER, L. E. "Clinical, Biochemical and Psychologic Effects of Psilocybin," *Archives of International Pharmacodynamics*, 130 (1961), 42–52.

133. ———. "Human Pharmacology of Lysergic Acid Diethylamide (LSD)," in D. E. Efron, ed., *Psychopharmacology—A Review of Progress 1957–1967*. Public Health Service Publication No. 1836, 1968.

134. ———. "Status Report on Clinical Pharmacology of Marijuana," in A. J. Singer, ed., *Marijuana: Chemistry, Pharmacology, and Pattern of Social Use*. Annals of New York Academy of Science, 1971.

135. HOLLISTER, L. E., J. J. PRUSMACK, J. A. PAULSEN, and N. ROSENQUIST. "Comparison of Three Psychotropic Drugs (Psilocybin, JB-329 and IT-190)," *Journal of Nervous and Mental Disease*, 131 (1960), 428–434.

136. HOLLISTER, L. E., R. K. RICHARDS, and H. K. GILLESPIE. "Comparison of Tetrahydrocannabinol and Synhexyl in Man," *Clinical and Pharmacological Therapeutics*, 9 (1968), 783–791.

137. HOLLISTER, L. E., J. SHELTON, and G. KRIEGER. "A Controlled Comparison of LSD and Dextroamphetamine in Alcoholics," *The American Journal of Psychiatry*, 125 (1969), 1352–1357.

138. HOLLISTER, L. E., and B. J. SJOBERG. "Clinical Syndromes and Biochemical Alterations Following Mescaline, Lysergic Acid Diethylamide, Psilocybin and a Combination of the Three Psychotomimetic Drugs," *Comprehensive Psychiatry*, 5(3) (1964), 170–178.

139. HOROWITZ, M. J. "Flashbacks: Recurrent Intrusive Images After the Use of LSD," *The American Journal of Psychiatry*, 126 (1969), 565–569.

140. HUGHES, H. S. "Emotional Disturbance and American Social Change, 1944–1969," *The American Journal of Psychiatry*, 126 (1969), 21–28.

141. HUNGERFORD, D. A., K. M. TAYLOR, C. SHAGAS, et al. "Cytogenetic Effects of LSD 25 Therapy in Man," *Journal of the AMA*, 206 (1968), 2287–2291.

142. HUXLEY, A. *The Doors of Perception*. New York: Harper Colophon, 1963.

143. IMPERI, L. L., H. D. KLEBER, and J. C. DAVIE. "Use of Hallucinogenic Drugs on Campus," *Journal of the AMA*, 204 (1968), 87–90.

144. IRWIN, S., and T. EGOZCUE. "Chromosomal Damage," *Science*, 159 (1968), 749.

145. ISBELL, H., R. E. BELLEVILLE, H. F. FRASER, et al. "Studies on Lysergic Acid Diethylamide (LSD-25)," *Archives of Neurology and Psychiatry*, 76 (1956), 468–478.

146. ISBELL, H., C. W. GORODETZSKY, C. W. JASINSKI, et al. "Effects of Delta 9-Trans-Tetrahydrocannabinol in Man," *Psychopharmacologia*, 11 (1967), 184–188.

147. ISBELL, H., and D. R. JASINSKI. "A Comparison of LSD-25 with (−) Delta 9-Trans-Tetrahydrocannabinol (THC) and Attempted Cross-Tolerance Between LSD and THC," *Psychopharmacologia*, 14 (1969), 115–123.

148. ISBELL, H., A. B. WOLBACH, A. WIKLER, and E. J. MINER. "Cross Tolerance Between LSD and Psilocybin," *Psychopharmacologia*, 2 (1961), 147–159.

149. ISBELL, H., A. WOLBACH, and D. ROSENBERG. "Observations on Direct and Cross Tolerance with LSD and Dextroamphetamine in Man," *Federation Proceedings*, 2 (1962), 416.

150. ITIL, T., and M. FINK. "Anticholinergic Hallucinogens and Their Interaction with Centrally Active Drugs," in P. Bradley and M. Fink, eds., *Anticholinergic Hallucinogens: Progress in Brain Research*. Amsterdam: Elsevier, 1968.

151. JAGIELLO, G., and P. E. POLANI. "Mouse Germ Cells and LSD-25," *Cytogenetics*, 8 (1969), 136–147.

152. JAMES, W. *Varieties of Religious Experience*. New York: Longmans, Green & Co., 1916.

153. JASINSKI, D. R., C. A. HAERTZEN, and H. ISBELL. "Review of the Effects in Man of Marijuana and Tetrahydrocannabinols on Subjective State and Physiological Functioning," in A. J. Singer, ed., *Marihuana: Chemistry, Pharmacology, and Pattern of Social Use*. Annals of New York Academy of Science, 1971.

154. JASPERS, K. *General Psychopathology*. Chicago: University of Chicago Press, 1963.

155. JENSEN, S. E., and R. RAMSEY. "Treatment of Chronic Alcoholism with Lysergic Acid Diethylamide," *Canadian Psychiatric Association Journal*, 8 (1963), 182–188.

156. JOHNSON, F. G. "LSD in the Treatment of Alcoholism," *The American Journal of Psychiatry*, 126 (1969), 481–487.

157. ———. "A Comparison of Short-Term Treatment Effects of Intravenous Sodium Amytal-Methedrine and LSD in the Alcoholic," *Canadian Psychiatric Association Journal*, 15 (1970), 493–497.

158. JONES, R. T. "Tetrahydrocannabinol and the Marijuana-Induced Social 'High' or the Effects of the Mind on Marijuana," in A. J. Singer, ed., *Marijuana: Chemistry, Pharmacology, and Pattern of Social Use*. Annals of New York Academy of Science, 1971.

159. JONES, R. T., and G. C. STONE. "Psychological Studies of Marijuana and Alcohol in Man," *Psychopharmacologia*, 18 (1970), 108–117.

160. JUDD, L. L., W. W. BRANDKAMP, and W. H. McGLOTHLIN. "Comparison of the Chromosomal Patterns Obtained from Groups of Continued Users, Former Users, and Nonusers of LSD-25," *The American Journal of Psychiatry*, 126 (1969), 626–635.

161. KAUFMAN, J., J. R. ALLEN, and L. J. WEST. "Runaways, Hippies, and Marihuana," *The American Journal of Psychiatry*, 126 (1969), 717–720.

162. KEELER, M. H. "Adverse Reaction to Marihuana," *The American Journal of Psychiatry*, 124 (1967), 674–677.

163. ———. "Motivation for Marihuana Use: A Correlate of Adverse Reaction," *The American Journal of Psychiatry*, 125 (1968), 386–390.

164. KEELER, M. H., J. A. EWING, and B. A. ROUSE. "Hallucinogenic Effects of Marijuana as Currently Used," *The American*

Journal of Psychiatry, 128 (1971), 213–216.

165. KEELER, M. H., C. B. REIFLER, and M. D. LIPZIN. "Spontaneous Recurrence of the Marijuana Effect," *The American Journal of Psychiatry*, 125 (1968), 384–386.

166. KENISTON, K. "Search and Rebellion Among the Advantaged," in *Drug Dependence*. Chicago: Committee on Alcoholism and Drug Dependence, Council on Mental Health, AMA, 1970.

167. ———. *The Uncommitted: Alienated Youth in American Society*. New York: Harcourt, Brace and World, Inc., 1965.

168. ———. "The Sources of Student Dissent," *Journal of Social Issues*, 23(3) (1967), 108–137.

169. ———. "Heads and Seekers: Drugs on Campus, Counter-Cultures and American Society," *The American Scholar*, 38 (1968–69), 97–112.

170. KEUP, W. "Psychotic Symptoms Due to Cannabis Abuse," *Diseases of the Nervous System*, 30 (1970), 119–126.

171. KING, F. W. "Marijuana and LSD Usage Among Male College Students: Prevalence Rate, Frequency, and Self-Estimates of Future Use," *Psychiatry*, 32 (1969), 265–276.

172. KING, S. H. "Youth in Rebellion: An Historical Perspective," in *Drug Dependence*. Chicago: Committee on Alcoholism and Drug Dependence, Council on Mental Health, AMA, 1970.

173. KOELLA, W. P. "Invited Discussion of Dr. J. Appel's Paper: 'Neurophysiological Effects of Psychotomimetic Substances' (A Supplemental Review)." in D. E. Efron, ed., *Psychopharmacology—A Review of Progress 1957–1967*. Public Health Service Publication No. 1836, 1968.

174. KRAMER, J. C. "Introduction to Amphetamine Abuse," *Journal of Psychedelic Drugs*, 2 (1970), 1–15.

175. ———, V. S. FISCHMAN, and D. C. LITTLEFIELD. "Amphetamine Abuse: Pattern and Effects of High Doses Taken Intravenously," *Journal of the AMA*, 201(5) (1967), 305–309.

176. KURLAND, A. A., S. UNGER, J. W. SHAFFER, and C. SAVAGE. "Psychodelic Therapy Utilizing LSD in the Treatment of the Alcoholic Patient: A Preliminary Report,"

The American Journal of Psychiatry, 123 (1967), 1202–1209.

177. LEARY, T., and R. ALPERT. "The Politics of Consciousness Expansion," *Harvard Review,* 1 (1963), 33–37.

178. LEMBERGER, L., S. D. SILBERSTEIN, J. AXELROD, and I. J. KOPIN. "Marihuana: Studies on the Disposition and Metabolism of Delta-9-Tetrahydrocannabinol in Man," *Science,* 170 (1970), 1320–1322.

179. LEMERE, F. "The Danger of Amphetamine Dependency," *The American Journal of Psychiatry,* 123 (1966), 569–572.

180. LEUNER, H. "Present State of Psycholytic Therapy and Its Possibilities," in H. A. Abramson, ed., *The Use of LSD in Psychotherapy and Alcoholism.* Indianapolis: Bobbs-Merrill Co., Inc., 1967.

181. LEVINE, J., and A. M. LUDWIG. "Alterations in Consciousness Produced by Combinations of LSD, Hypnosis and Psychotherapy," *Psychopharmacologia,* 7 (1965), 123–137.

182. LEWIN, L. *Phantastica, Narcotic and Stimulating Drugs, Their Use and Abuse.* London: Routledge & Kegan Paul, 1931.

183. LIPP, M. R., S. G. BENSON, and Z. TAINTOR. "Marijuana Use by Medical Students," *The American Journal of Psychiatry,* 128 (1971), 207–212.

184. LOUGHMAN, W. D., T. W. SARGENT, and D. M. ISRAELSTAM. "Leukocytes of Humans Exposed to Lysergic Acid Diethylamide: Lack of Chromosomal Damage," *Science,* 158 (1967), 508–510.

185. LOURIA, D. B. *Overcoming Drugs.* New York: McGraw-Hill, 1971.

186. LUDWIG, A. M., and J. LEVINE. "A Controlled Comparison of Five Brief Treatment Techniques Employing LSD, Hypnosis and Psychotherapy," *American Journal of Psychotherapy,* 19 (1965), 417–435.

187. ———. "Hypnodelic Therapy," in J. Masserman, ed., *Current Psychiatric Therapies,* Vol. 7. New York: Grune and Stratton, 1967.

188. MAMLET, L. N. " 'Consciousness-Limiting' Side Effects of 'Consciousness-Expanding' Drugs," *American Journal of Orthopsychiatry,* 37 (1967), 296–297.

189. MANNO, J. E., G. F. KIPLINGER, N. SCHOLTZ, and R. B. FORNEY. "The Influence of Alcohol and Marihauna on Motor and Mental Performance," *Clinical and Pharma-*

cological Therapeutics, 12 (1971), 202–211.

190. *Marijuana: Report of the Indian Hemp Drugs Commission 1893–1894.* Silver Spring: Thomas Jefferson Publishing Co., 1969.

191. MAYOR LAGUARDIA'S COMMITTEE ON MARIHUANA. *The Marihuana Problem in the City of New York.* Lancaster: Jacques Cattell Press, 1944.

192. MCGLOTHLIN, W. H., D. O. ARNOLD, and D. X. FREEDMAN. "Organicity Measures Following Repeated LSD Ingestion," *Archives of General Psychiatry,* 21 (1969), 704–709.

193. MCGLOTHLIN, W. H., and S. I. COHEN. "The Use of Hallucinogenic Drugs Among College Students," *The American Journal of Psychiatry,* 122 (1965), 572–574.

194. MCGLOTHLIN, W., S. COHEN, and M. S. MCGLOTHLIN. "Long Lasting Effects of LSD on Normals," *Archives of General Psychiatry,* 17 (1967), 521–532.

195. MCGLOTHLIN, W. H., and L. J. WEST. "The Marihuana Problem: An Overview," *The American Journal of Psychiatry,* 125 (1968), 370–378.

196. MCMILLAN, D. E., and W. L. EEWEY. "Characteristics of Tetrahydrocannabinol Tolerance," in A. J. Singer, ed., *Marijuana: Chemistry, Pharmacology, and Pattern of Social Use.* Annals of New York Academy of Science, 1971.

197. MCMILLAN, D. E., L. S. HARRIS, J. M. FRANKENHEIM, and J. S. KENNEDY. "1-Delta 9-Trans-Tetrahydrocannabinol in Pigeons: Tolerance to the Behavioral Effects," *Science,* 169 (1970), 501–503.

198. MECHOULAM, R. "Marihuana Chemistry," *Science,* 168 (1970), 1159–1166.

199. MECHOULAM, R., and Y. GAONI. "A Total Synthesis of dl-Delta 1-Tetrahydrocannabinol, the Active Constituent of Hashish," *Journal of American Chemical Society,* 87 (1965), 3273–3275.

200. MELGES, F. T., J. R. TINKLENBERG, L. E. HOLLISTER, and H. K. GILLESPIE. "Marihuana and Temporal Disintegration," *Science,* 168 (1970), 1118–1120.

201. ———. "Temporal Disintegration and Depersonalization During Marihuana Intoxication," *Archives of General Psychiatry,* 23 (1970), 204–210.

202. MEYER, R. E., R. C. PILLARD, L. M.

SHAPIRO, and S. M. MIRIN. "Administration of Marijuana to Heavy and Casual Marijuana Users," *The American Journal of Psychiatry*, 128 (1971), 198–203.

203. MIRAS, C. J. "Experience with Chronic Hashish Smokers," in *Drugs and Youth*. Springfield: Charles C. Thomas, 1969.

204. MIRIN, S. M., et al. "Casual Versus Heavy Use of Marijuana: A Redefinition of the Marijuana Problem," *The American Journal of Psychiatry*, 127 (1971), 54–60.

205. MIZNER, G. L., J. T. BARTER, and P. H. WERME. "Patterns of Drug Use Among College Students: A Preliminary Report," *The American Journal of Psychiatry*, 127 (1970), 15–24.

206. MONROE, R. R., R. G. HEATH, W. A. MICKLE, and R. C. LLEWELLYN. "Correlation of Rhinencephalic Electrograms with Behavior: A Study on Humans Under the Influence of LSD and Mescaline," *Electroencephalography and Clinical Neurophysiology*, 9 (1957), 623–642.

207. MORIMOTO, K. "The Problem of the Abuse of Amphetamines in Japan," *Bulletin of Narcotics*, 9 (1957), 8–12.

208. MURRAY, J. M. "Narcissism and the Ego Ideal," *Journal of American Psychoanalytic Association*, 12 (1964), 477–511.

209. NICHOLI, A. M. "Harvard Dropouts: Some Psychiatric Findings," *The American Journal of Psychiatry*, 124 (1967), 651–658.

210. NIELSEN, J., U. FRIEDRICH, and T. TSUBOI. "Chromosome Abnormalities and Psychotropic Drugs," *Nature*, 218 (1968), 488–489.

211. NILSSON, I. M., S. AGURELL, T. L. C. NILSSON, et al. "Delta 1-Tetrahydrocannabinol: Structure of a Major Metabolite," *Science*, 168 (1970), 1228–1229.

212. NORTON, W. A. "The Marihuana Habit: Some Observations of a Small Group of Users," *Canadian Psychiatric Association Journal*, 13 (1968), 163–173.

213. O'REILLY, P. O., and A. FUNK. "LSD in Chronic Alcoholism," *Canadian Psychiatric Association Journal*, 9 (1964), 258–260.

214. PACE, H. B., W. M. DAVIS, and L. A. BORGEN. "Teratogenesis and Marijuana," in A. J. Singer, ed., *Marijuana: Chemistry, Pharmacology, and Pattern of Social Use*. Annals of New York Academy of Science, 1971.

215. PEARLMAN, S. "Drug Use and Experience in an Urban College Population," *American Journal of Orthopsychiatry*, 38 (1968), 503–514.

216. PRESS, E., and A. K. DONE. "Solvent Sniffing: Physiologic Effects and Community Control Measures for Intoxication from the Intentional Inhalation of Organic Solvents, I," *Pediatrics*, 39 (1967), 451–461.

217. ———. "Physiologic Effects and Community Control Measures for Intoxication from the Intentional Inhalation of Organic Solvents, II," *Pediatrics*, 39 (1967), 611–622.

218. ROBINS, L. N., and G. E. MURPHY. "Drug Use in a Normal Population of Young Negro Men," *American Journal of Public Health*, 57 (1967), 1580–1596.

219. ROSENBERG, D. E., H. ISBELL, and E. J. MINER. "Comparison of a Placebo, N-Dimethyltryptamine, and 6-Hydroxy-N-Dimethyltryptamine in Man," *Psychopharmacologia*, 4 (1963), 39–42.

220. ROSENTHAL, S. H. "Persistent Hallucinosis Following Repeated Administration of Hallucinogenic Drugs," *The American Journal of Psychiatry*, 121 (1964), 238–244.

221. ROSZAK, T. *The Making of a Counter Culture*. Garden City: Doubleday & Co., Inc., 1969.

222. SANDISON, R. A., A. M. SPENCER, and J. D. A. WHITELAW. "The Therapeutic Value of LSD in Mental Illness," *Journal of Mental Science*, 100 (1954), 491–507.

223. SAPOL, E., and R. A. ROFFMAN. "Marihuana in Vietnam," *International Journal of Addictions*, 5 (1970), 1–42.

224. SARGANT, W., and H. J. SHOVRON. "Acute War Neuroses," *Archives of Neurology and Psychiatry*, 54 (1945), 231–240.

225. SATO, H., E. PERGAMENT, and V. NAIR. "LSD in Pregnancy: Chromosomal Effects," *Life Sciences*, 10 (1971), 773–779.

226. SATRAN, R., and V. N. DODSON. "Toluene Habituation," *New England Journal of Medicine*, 95 (1968), 304–305.

227. SAVAGE, C. "The Resolution and Subsequent Remobilization of Resistance by LSD in Psychotherapy," *Journal of Nervous and Mental Disease*, 125 (1962), 434–437.

228. SAVAGE, C., A. A. KURLAND, S. UNGER, and

J. Shaffer. "Therapeutic Application of LSD," in P. Black, ed., *Drugs and the Brain*. Baltimore: The Johns Hopkins Press, 1969.

229. Savage, C., M. Stolaroff, W. Harman, and J. Fadiman. "The Psychodelic Experience," *Journal of Neuropsychiatry*, 5 (1963), 4–5.

230. Scheckel, C. L., E. Boff, P. Dahlen, and T. Smart. "Behavioral Effects in Monkeys of Racemates of Two Biologically Active Marijuana Constituents," *Science*, 160 (1968), 1467–1469.

231. Scher, J ."Patterns and Profiles of Addiction and Drug Abuse," *Archives of General Psychiatry*, 15 (1966), 539–551.

232. Shanholtz, M. I. "Glue Sniffing: A New Symptom of an Old Disease," *Virginia Medical Monthly*, 95 (1968), 304–305.

233. Shulgin, A. T. "3-Methoxy-4, 5-Methylenedioxy Amphetamine, A New Psychotomimetic Agent," *Nature*, 201 (1964), 1120–1121.

234. Shulgin, A. T., S. Bunnell, and T. Sargent. "The Psychotomimetic Properties of 3, 4, 5-Trimethoxyamphetamine," *Nature*, 189 (1961), 1011–1012.

235. Smith, C. M. "A New Adjunct to the Treatment of Alcoholism: The Hallucinogenic Drugs," *Quarterly Journal of Studies on Alcohol*, 19 (1958), 406.

236. Smith, D. E. "Acute and Chronic Toxicity of Marijuana," *Journal of Psychedelic Drugs*, 2 (1968), 37–47.

237. ———. "Health Problems in a "Hippie" Subculture: Observations by the Haight-Ashbury Medical Clinic," *Clinical Pediatrics*, 8 (1969), 313–316.

238. Snyder, S. H. *Uses of Marijuana*. New York: Oxford University Press, 1971.

239. ———, L. Faillace, and L. Hollister. "2, 5-Dimethoxy-4-Methyl-Amphetamine (STP): A New Hallucinogenic Drug," *Science*, 158 (1967), 669–670.

240. Snyder, S. H., H. Weingartner, and L. A. Faillace. "DOET (2, 5-Dimethoxy-4-Ethylamphetamine) and DOM (STP) (2, 5-Dimethoxy-4-Methylamphetamine), New Psychotropic Agents: Their Effects in Man," in D. H. Efron, ed., *Psychotomimetic Drugs*. New York: Raven Press, 1970.

241. Solnit, A. J., C. F. Settlage, S. Goodman, and P. Blos. "Youth Unrest: A Symposium," *The American Journal of Psychiatry*, 125 (1969), 1145–1159.

242. Solursh, L. P., and W. R. Clement. "Hallucinogenic Drug Abuse: Manifestations and Management," *Canadian Medical Association Journal*, 98 (1968), 407–410.

243. Sparkes, R. S., J. Melnyk, and L. P. Bozzetti. "Chromosomal Effect in Vivo of Exposure to Lysergic Acid Diethylamide," *Science*, 160 (1968), 1343–1344.

244. Sterling, J. W. "A Comparative Examination of Two Modes of Intoxication—An Exploratory Study of Glue Sniffing," *Journal of Criminal Law, Criminology and Police Science*, 55 (1964), 94.

245. Szara, S. "The Comparison of the Psychotic Effect of Tryptamine Derivatives with the Effects of Mescaline and LSD-25 in Self-Experiments," in S. Garattini and V. Ghetti, eds., *Psychotropic Drugs*. Amsterdam: Elsevier, 1957.

246. ———. "Dimethytryptamine: Its Metabolism in Man; The Relation of Its Psychotic Effect to the Serotonin Metabolism," *Experientia*, 12 (1956), 441–442.

247. Szara, S., L. H. Rockland, D. Rosenthal, and J. H. Handlon. "Psychological Effects and Metabolism of N, N-Diethyltryptamine in Man," *Archives of General Psychiatry*, 15 (1966), 320–329.

248. Szasz, T. S. "The Ethics of Addiction," *The American Journal of Psychiatry*, 128 (1971), 541–546.

249. Talbott, J. A., and J. W. Teague. "Marihuana Psychosis," *Journal of the AMA*, 210 (1969), 299–302.

250. Tart, C. T. "Marijuana Intoxication: Common Experiences," *Nature*, 226 (1970), 701–704.

251. Tatetsu, S. "Methamphetamine Psychosis," *Folia Psychiatrica et Neurologica Japonica*, 7 (Suppl.) (1963), 377–380.

252. Tinklenberg, J. R., et al. "Marijuana and Immediate Memory," *Nature*, 226 (1970), 1171–1172.

253. Tjio, J., W. N. Pahnke, and A. A. Kurland. "LSD and Chromosomes: A Controlled Experiment," *Journal of the AMA*, 210 (1969), 849–856.

254. Tolan, E. J., and F. A. Lingl. "Model Psychosis Produced by Inhalation of Gasoline Fumes," *The American Journal of Psychiatry*, 120 (1964), 757–761.

255. TONINI, G., and C. MONTANARI. "Effects of Experimentally Induced Psychoses on Artistic Expression," *Confinia Neurologica*, 15 (1955), 225–239.

256. UNGERLEIDER, J. T., D. D. FISHER, and M. FULLER. "The Dangers of LSD: Analysis of Seven Months' Experience in a University Hospital's Psychiatric Service," *Journal of the AMA*, 197 (1966), 389–392.

257. UNGERLEIDER, J. T., and D. D. FISHER. "The Problems of LSD and Emotional Disorders," *California Medicine*, 106 (1967), 49–55.

258. UNGERLEIDER, J. T., D. D. FISHER, M. FULLER, and A. CALDWELL. "The 'Bad Trip'— The Etiology of the Adverse LSD Reaction," *The American Journal of Psychiatry*, 124 (1968), 1483–1490.

259. UNWIN, J. R. "Depression in Alienated Youth," *Canadian Psychiatric Association Journal*, 15 (1970), 83–86.

260. WARKANY, J. "Lysergic Acid Diethylamide (LSD): No Teratogenicity in Rats," *Science*, 159 (1968), 731–732.

261. WARREN, R. J., D. L. RIMOIN, and W. S. SLY. "LSD Exposure in Utero," *Pediatrics*, 45 (1970), 466–469.

262. WECKOWICZ, T. E. "The Effect of Lysergic Acid Diethylamide (LSD) on Size Constancy," *Canadian Psychiatric Association Journal*, 4 (1959), 255–259.

263. WEIL, A. T. "Adverse Reactions to Marihuana: Classification and Suggested Treatment," *New England Journal of Medicine*, 282 (1970), 997–1000.

264. WEIL, A. T., N. E. ZINBERG, and J. M. NELSEN. "Clinical and Psychological Effects of Marihuana in Man," *Science*, 162 (1968), 1234–1242.

265. WEINER, I. B. "Differential Diagnosis in Amphetamine Poisoning," *Psychiatric Quarterly*, 38 (1964), 707–716.

266. WEINTRAUB, W., A. B. SILVERSTEIN, and G. D. KLEE. "The Effect of LSD on the Associative Process," *Journal of Nervous and Mental Disease*, 128 (1959), 409–414.

267. WELPTON, D. F. "Psychodynamics of Chronic Lysergic Acid Diethylamide Use," *Journal of Nervous and Mental Disease*, 147 (1968), 377–385.

268. WEST, L. J., and J. R. ALLEN. "Three Rebellions: Red, Black, and Green," in J. H. Masserman, ed., *The Dynamics of Dissent: Scientific Proceedings of the American Academy of Psychoanalysis*. New York: Grune and Stratton, 1968.

269. WINTHROP, H. "The Alienation of Post-Industrial Man," *Midwest Quarterly*, 9 (1968), 121–138.

270. WOODY, G. E. "Visual Disturbances Experienced by Hallucinogenic Drug Abusers While Driving," *The American Journal of Psychiatry*, 127 (1970), 683–686.

271. YOUNG, G. Y., C. B. SIMSON, and C. E. FROHMAN. "Clinical and Biochemical Studies of an Amphetamine Withdrawal Psychosis," *Journal of Nervous and Mental Disease*, 132 (1961), 234–238.

272. ZEGANS, L. S., J. C. POLLARD, and D. BROWN. "The Effects of LSD-25 on Creativity and Tolerance to Regression," *Archives of General Psychiatry*, 16 (1967), 740–749.

273. ZELLWEGER, H., J. S. McDONALD, and G. ABBO. "Is Lysergic Acid Diethylamide a Teratogen?," *Lancet*, 2 (1967), 1066–1068.

274. ZINBERG, N. E., and A. T. WEIL. "A Comparison of Marijuana Users and Non-Users," *Nature*, 226 (1970), 119–123.

PART SIX

Functional Psychoses and Related Conditions

CHAPTER 21

AFFECTIVE DISORDERS: MANIC-DEPRESSIVE PSYCHOSIS AND PSYCHOTIC DEPRESSION[*]

Manifest Symptomatology, Psychodynamics, Sociological Factors, and Psychotherapy

Silvano Arieti

A s VARIABLE AS THEIR clinical pictures are, as controversial as their etiology continues to be, as unconfirmed as their dynamic interpretation remains in our time, affective disorders nevertheless strike the student of psychiatry for the facility with which their clinical concepts are grasped even by the beginner.

It is therefore appropriate to start the section on functional psychoses with the study of these conditions, for it can serve, in part, as an introduction to the study of other psychotic disorders that even at a manifest clinical level appear more complicated.

Needless to say, every psychotic disorder is multidimensional and any aspect of simplicity that we can see in it is only apparent or relative.

[*] In this chapter is included the study of the disorders which, according to the official nomenclature of the American Psychiatric Association, are called:
296 Major affective disorders: 1 Manic-depressive illness, manic; 2 depressed; 3 circular; 8 other.
298.0 Psychotic depressive reaction.
Involutional Melancholia will be discussed in Chapter 30.

❰ Introductory Remarks

Already, at this point, several questions may have occurred to the reader, on account of the fact that we have labeled these disorders "functional psychoses." Why psychoses, and why functional? Since many cases of affective psychoses are mild, and the percentage of these mild cases seems to increase in relation to the total incidence of the disorders, it would seem logical at first to call the conditions psychoneuroses rather than functional psychoses. The term "psychosis," however, does not indicate only an actual or potential severity of the disorders (a severity which may be reached even by some psychoneuroses), but also connotes the fact that the psychopathological way of living was, in a certain way, accepted by the patient. No matter what transformation the psychotic patient has undergone (either a predominantly symbolic transformation as in schizophrenia, or a predominantly emotional transformation as in affective psychoses, or a predominantly cognitive defect as in organic conditions), that transformation becomes his way of relating to himself and others and of interpreting the world.

The patient suffering from an affective psychosis does not fight his disorder, as does the psychoneurotic, but lives in it. In this respect he resembles persons who are affected by character neuroses and who do not even know of the pathological nature of their difficulties. The distortions of the character neuroses, however, are susceptible of at least partial adaptation to the demands of society, whereas in psychoses such adaptation is not possible.

Several psychiatric authorities sharply oppose the use of the word "functional" on the grounds that each condition is at the same time organic and functional, since an organ must always be there to mediate a function. Cobb,[21] for example, states that "every symptom is both functional and organic."

In the neuropsychiatric frame of reference, this statement is perfectly valid: Every symptom is functional inasmuch as it consists of a physiological function of the organ, and organic inasmuch as it requires the organ that mediates it, either in its anatomical integrity or in its pathological alterations. The statement carries the implicit admission that such states as the functional and the organic do exist. Neither state, however, can exist without the other; we may conceive them separately as abstract concepts, but in the physical world they are always together.

How is it then that the term "functional" has been retained in American psychiatry and is so widely used? According to the present writer, its use is not maintained merely through semantic inertia. Like many other words in every language, it has enlarged some of its meanings and lost some others, and has come to convey a group of concepts which, at the present stage of our knowledge, may still be useful.

A functional point of view about a psychiatric disorder does not exclude the possibility of a hereditary or constitutional predisposition that makes the functional transformation possible. It does not exclude recognition that any function is accompanied by a physical, molecular substratum. It does not even refer to the fact that functions are generally transitory and reversible, whereas organic alterations are not, because this is not true in every case. A memory trace may be permanent, and an anatomical alteration may reverse completely. The functional point of view focuses on the fact that no matter what the complex causality of the disorder may be, it is the particular form of functioning with its content that constitutes the predominant and primary (although not exclusive) essence of the disorder and leads to secondary sequels, both organic and functional.

It also implies that the dysfunction is predominantly determined by, or connected with, an emotional maladaptation, which, in its turn, is at least partially provoked by a human environment. For instance, it is obvious that functional cases differ from psychoses occurring with tumors of the cerebral hemispheres. Here, the normal functionality is made impossible by the anatomical alteration.

It is certain that the last word has not been

said on this imporatnt subject; for the time being, however, the concept of functional disorder is found useful by many, and therefore retained in the classification adopted in this handbook. In the European literature, functional psychoses are generally called endogenous. This classification implies that these psychoses are based primarily on heredito-constitutional factors or causes within the nervous system, in contrast to the disorders that are exogenous—that is, originating from causes outside of the nervous system. This classification is not accepted by the majority of American psychiatrists.

The following definitions of affective psychoses are based on the fundamental Kraepelinian concepts, and we shall use them only as elementary clinical notions, without any etiological or dynamic implication:

By *manic-depressive psychoses* is meant a group of mental disorders characterized by periodic attacks of melancholia or elation of marked proportions, accompanied by retardation or hyperactivity.

By *psychotic depression* is meant a mental disorder characterized by a single attack or periodic attacks of severe melancholia, in the absence of marked mood swings.

In this chapter, we shall give most attention to manic-depressive psychosis, which offers the most diversified or complete picture of the affective disorders. We shall describe psychotic depression separately only in those aspects in which it differs from manic-depressive psychosis. Involutional depression will be described and discussed in Chapter 30 of this volume by Rosenthal.[68]

(Historical Notes

The reader who is particularly interested in the historical perspective of the concept of manic-depressive psychosis is referred to the excellent article by Jelliffe[39] and to the monograph by Zilboorg[81] for the prepsychoanalytical literature; for a historical survey of the analytical literature, the reader is referred to Lewin's monograph.[51] In this volume, we shall restrict our discussion to a brief exposition.

Ancient Times

As Zilboorg wrote, manic-depressive is a condition which has been known since antiquity. According to Jelliffe, the disorder is "the only form [of psychosis] whose chief features may be unequivocally recognized down through the ages." According to Koerner,[44] the earliest record in Indo-Germanic cultures is that of the melancholia of Bellerophon in the Homeric epics. In the writings of Hippocrates, we find many references to mania and melancholia. He considered manic and melancholic states to be chronic conditions, although he admitted the possibility of recovery in some cases. He distinguished various forms of melancholia and swings of mood, although it seems certain that he did not make any connection between the elation of the manic and the melancholia of the depressed patient.

Not until several centuries later, when Aretaeus appeared on the scene, was any additional contribution made to this subject. According to several authors, Aretaeus lived in the second century of the Christian era, but other authors, such as Cumston and Zilboorg, think that he lived toward the end of the first century. Aretaeus was born in Cappadocia, a kingdom in a region of Asia Minor. The kingdom of Cappadocia was part of the Roman Empire, and it is possible that Aretaeus practiced most of his life in Imperial Rome. He was particularly interested in the condition that we call manic-depressive psychosis. His observations are so exact and deep as to be comparable to the modern views on this disorder. He not only described the symptomatology of manias and melancholias but also saw a connection between the two states. He observed that young people are more susceptible to mania and older people to melancholia, and that, although the two states are related, mania is not always an outcome of melancholia. He seems thus to have anticipated by at least seventeen centuries the contributions of Kraepelin. In certain ways, he went even further than Kraepelin, for he felt that spontaneous remissions were not reliable. The intermittent character of the illness was clear to him. He also described very well the religious, guilt-ridden, and self-sacrificing attitudes of the melancholic, and the gay and overactive behavior of the manic. He reported how a severe case of melancholia, about whom many physicians were pessimistic, recovered fully after the patient had fallen in love.

Classical Period of Psychiatry

The teachings of Aretaeus were soon forgotten or ignored, and not until 1851 did a French psychiatrist, Falret,[27] again describe the condition and grasp its intermittent and circular character.* Kahlbaum's attempts in 1863 to consider mania and melancholia as two simple states of *vesania typica* (the general form in which he included all functional psychoses, with the exception of paranoia) were not successful.

Kraepelin,[47] who was obviously influenced by the works of Falret and Baillarger (another French psychiatrist who made important studies of this condition, at approximately the time of Falret), studied many patients and conceived the concept of manic-depressive psychosis as one syndrome which, in its many varieties, included simple mania, most cases of melancholia, and the periodic and circular insanity. It included also "some cases of amentia" and some affective moods, which, although not of such severe proportions as the previously mentioned disorders, were regarded by him as "rudiments" of the latter. Kraepelin's reason for including all these syndromes in a large nosologic entity was based on the fact that these syndromes, in spite of many external differences, (1) have common fundamental features, (2) not only cannot be easily differentiated but may replace each other in the same patient, and (3) have a uniform benign prognosis. The outcome was thus,

* According to Cameron,[19] earlier authors grasped the intermittently manic and depressed character of the psychosis: Bonet in 1684, Schacht in 1747, and Herschel in 1768 (all quoted by Cameron).

for Kraepelin, as important a nosologic characteristic for manic-depressive psychosis as it was for dementia praecox. Kraepelin worked in the field of manic-depressive psychosis for many years, but it was only in the sixth edition of his *Lehrbuch der Psychiatrie*, published in 1899, that he used the term "manic-depressive insanity," and only in the eighth edition (1913) that he fully expanded this nosologic concept.

At first, Kraepelin's concepts were not unanimously or universally accepted.[74] Later, however, his concepts were generally accepted, although many psychiatrists continued to separate the single or recurring depressions from the complete manic-depressive circular syndrome.

Psychoanalytic Approaches

We must turn to the psychoanalytic school to find an attempt to go beyond descriptive and nosological concepts. Exceptionally, it is not Freud himself who introduced manic-depressive psychosis into the field of psychoanalysis, but his pupil Abraham.[1] In 1912, Abraham had the original idea of comparing melancholic depression with normal grief. Both conditions are due to a loss that the person has suffered, but, whereas the normal mourner is interested in the lost person, the depressed patient is tormented by guilt feelings. The unconscious hostility that he had for the lost object he now directs toward himself. Abraham also assumed that there was a regression to an ambivalent pregenital stage of object-relationships, that is, a return to an anal-sadistic stage.

Freud,[29] in the paper titled "Mourning and Melancholia," accepted Abraham's ideas that there is a relation between mourning and melancholia and pointed out that, whereas in mourning the object is lost because of death, in melancholia there was an internal loss because the lost person had been incorporated. The sadism present in the ambivalent relationship is then directed against the incorporated love-object. This concept of introjection helped Freud to develop the concepts of ego ideals and, later, of superego. In a subsequent work published in 1921 (*Group Psychology and the Analysis of the Ego*), Freud advanced the idea that in mania there is a fusion between the ego and the superego. Thus, the energy previously used in the conflict between the two parts of the psyche is now available for enjoyment. Freud also pointed out that this fusion between ego and superego may be based on biologically determined cycles (something similar to the cyclic fusion of the ego and id, which periodically occurs every night during the state of sleep).

In later works, Abraham confirmed Freud's findings and clearly postulated the factors that are prerequisites for manic-depressive psychosis: (1) a constitutional and inherited over-accentuation of oral eroticism; (2) a special fixation of the libido on the oral level; (3) a severe injury to infantile narcissism, brought about by disappointments in love; (4) the occurrence of this disappointment before the Oedipus complex was resolved; and (5) the repetition of the primary disappointment in later life.

After Abraham and Freud, Rado and Melanie Klein have, perhaps, made the most important psychoanalytic contributions to this subject. For Rado,[62,63] "melancholia is a despairing cry for love." The ego tries to punish itself in order to prevent the parental punishment. The patient attempts to repeat the sequence—guilt, atonement, forgiveness—which, according to Rado, is connected with a previous sequence occurring in the infant—wakening rage, hunger, appearance of the mother's breast, and ensuing satisfaction. The excitement of being nursed by the mother is compared to a sexual orgastic experience, and mania is compared to an oral fusion, an equivalent of the breast situation.

Freud's and Abraham's theories about the incorporation of the object received further elaboration by Rado. He believed that there is a splitting of the incorporated object: The good part of it, by which the child wants to be accepted and loved, remains in the superego, whereas the bad part of it, which the child despises and even wants to kill, becomes part of the ego.

Melanie Klein[43] saw in the infant baby the mechanism which may develop later into full psychosis. She described the paranoid position and the depressive position. Whereas the first consists of mechanisms by which the child "spits out" or eliminates or projects to others what is unpleasant, the second or depressive position occurs at the time of weaning, that is, around the sixth month of life. The child has an innate fear of death, and the "positions" are defenses to guarantee the survival. Thus, for Melanie Klein, this depressive position is a normal event in the life of every child.* It is the inability to solve this position adequately that presumably leads, later, to the disorder. The mother who before was seen as two persons (one good and one bad), according to Klein is seen as one person; she continues, however, to be internalized as a good or bad object. The child is afraid that his instinctual aggressive impulses will destroy the good object, and interprets the loss of mother's breast and milk at the time of weaning as the result of the destructive impulses.

Bibring[14] considered depression a conflict within the ego, rather than between ego and superego. Predisposition to depression is not always caused by "oral fixation" but is often the result of "the infant's or little child's shock-like experience of and fixation to the feeling of helplessness." A loss of self-esteem is the main factor in depression. According to Bibring, "The emotional expression of a state of helplessness and powerlessness of the ego, irrespective of what may have caused the breakdown of the mechanisms which establish the self-esteem, contributes the essence of the condition." Cohen et al.[22] studied twelve manic-depressive patients and tried to differentiate some psychodynamic patterns. Their patients depended on approval from others, were conventional, and adhered to the expec-

---

* This point of view has been sharply criticized by Spitz,[72] who has found infantile depressions (which he calls anaclitic) only in pathological conditions and determined by the fact that the mother was removed from the child between the sixth and eighth months for an approximate period of three months.

Several of Klein's conceptions seem only adult personifications of the infantile psyche. Although these conceptions are thought-provoking, there is nothing to indicate that they relate to the processes or activities of the infant's cerebrum.

tations or mores of the group to which they belonged, and to status consciousness.

Among the contributions of the neo-Freudian schools are to be mentioned those of Beck,[10] Bemporad,[12] and Arieti.[2,5,6,7,8,9] According to Beck, depression is predominantly a cognitive disorder. The mood of depression is caused by three major cognitive patterns that force the individual to view himself, the world, and his future, in an idiosyncratic way. Beck believes that early in life the individual develops a wide variety of concepts and attitudes about himself and the world. The vulnerability of the depression-prone person is attributable to the constellation of enduring negative attitudes about himself, about the world, and about the future. A special feedback mechanism is often established: The more negatively the patient thinks, the worse he feels; the worse he feels, the more negatively he thinks.

Bemporad[12] considers depression:

as an affective reaction elicited by the individual's realization that an important source of self-esteem and meaning is lost. The sense of loss is intensified by the awareness that the deprivation is final; it cannot be repaired. What is lost is not simply a love object, but the source of meaning and satisfaction in one's life. . . . What seems to be characteristic about the depressive is that he seems to depend almost exclusively on some external agency for his self-esteem.

Psychoanalytic and predominantly psychodynamic views of affective disorders have been criticized by various authors, not only by authors who follow an exclusively biological approach, like Kraines,[48] but even by such scholarly students of psychoanalysis as Grinker[35] and Mendelson.[59]

Grinker et al. wrote:

From these theoretical psychoanalytic discussions, there has developed a stereotype of the psychodynamics of depression which is unrelated to the variations in the clinical picture. It is this stereotype which has influenced psychiatrists today to assume that, once given a symptomatology of depression, the formation of the psychodynamics can be reeled off with facile fluency. These basic formulations, stereotyped though they may be and agreed upon as they are by so many, have

never been validated and despite their universal acceptance by many authors, they are far from applicable to individual cases or groups of cases.

In concluding his book on psychoanalytic concepts of depression, Mendelson wrote:

It would have been pleasing to be able to report that this body of literature represented, in essence, a progress through the years of a Great Investigation. It does so in part. But perhaps even more does it represent a Great Debate with the rhetorical rather than scientific implications of this word. Indeed at times it bears the stigmata not of an exchange of ideas but of a Monologue—a Not-So-Great Monologue.

Mendelson later adds that his book represents the summary of an era:

This era was chiefly characterized by boldly speculative theoretical formulations and by insightful clinical studies. It was a richly productive era in which sensitive and intuitive observers mapped out whole continents of the mind that had previously been unexplored. It was an era of large scale conceptualizations and generalizations. This era is drawing to a close.

I dare say that Mendelson's prediction is premature, and I hope to demonstrate this point of view in the rest of this chapter.

The Existentialist School*

It is difficult, within the limits of the assigned space, to give an adequate account of the contributions of the existentialist approach to manic-depressive psychosis. Any account presupposes a familiarity with existentialist philosophy, and especially with the works of Heidegger, which most psychiatrists do not have. Moreover, the interpretation of these writings is not an easy task for those who are not well acquainted with the intricacies of German philosophical language. A brief résumé will, however, be attempted here.

In the existentialist school, manic-depressive psychosis is not, as a rule, studied as a unit; mania and melancholia are the objects of separate studies. Contrary to what we find in the

* See Chapter 41, Volume One, for a succinct, comprehensive presentation of the existentialist approach. See also Kahn.[40]

other schools (particularly in the psychoanalytic schools, where melancholia receives the main consideration), it is mania which has attracted the interest of the existentialists. Binswanger[15,16] has devoted six long articles to mania. He asks himself the usual existentialist question: What, for the manic, is the way of being in the world? It is a world of festivity, of the victory of the instinct over restraint and inhibitions. It is a world that tends to abolish logic and real difficulties; it is a direct and immediate world, the world of optimism itself. Optimism is a special style of thinking and living. In this way of living the patient becomes big and the world small.

In the flight of ideas, we have three factors —the regression, the play on words, and the logorrhea. Because of the regression, language ceases to be a means of communication and ends by becoming an end in itself, a kind of play at the service of the existential joy (*Daseinfreude*). Playing has invaded the whole human structure of the manic, and play on words is part of it. The logorrhea manifests a *grossmauling* way of existence.

The ambivalence of the manic-depressive is different from that of the schizophrenic. Whereas the latter may hate and love at the same time, the manic-depressive, at certain periods of time, may only love or hate, although alternately he does both.

Binswanger attributes to the flight of ideas the following characteristics: (1) an affective tone of optimism, (2) a particular way of experiencing space and time, (3) a volatile and confused character of thought and meanings, and (4) the prevalence of projections.

Existentialist studies of depressions have been made by LeMappian (quoted by Roi[67]) and by Ey.[26] For these authors, as well as for other existentialists, the depressed state is constituted by an arrest or insufficiency of all the vital activities. It is a "pathetic immobility, a suspension of existence, a syncope of time" according to Ey. As a consequence, the patient experiences a feeling of incompleteness, of unreality, and of impotence; a special, inhibitory way of living then ensues. Most authors emphasize the particular attitude of the patient toward time. Only the past counts; it

extends into the present to torture the patient and to remind him of his guilt, his unworthiness, and his inability to accomplish. "Time was lost," the future is not even contemplated. Sommer[69] points out how the patient, although self-accusatory, does not want to repair; he wants to be punished.

The studies of the existentialist authors give us a more accurate account of the uniqueness of the subjective experiences of the patient, permitting us to become more aware of their particular ways of living, and offering an enrichment of the understanding obtained by the dynamic, sociocultural, and formal approaches.

❡ The Manifest Symptomatology of Manic-Depressive Psychosis

In 1944, Zilboorg[81] wrote that manic-depressive psychosis seems to have changed comparatively little in its symptomatology since antiquity—much less than other mental disorders. This statement, correct in 1944, is no longer so today. Changes such as the less frequent occurrence of the disorder, the relative mildness of many attacks, the relative rarity of the manic episodes, and others to be described, are now noticed and may have appeared at other times in history.

What seems to have remained unchanged from the time of Hippocrates to the early 1960s was the picture of an intense state of depression in which one could almost always recognize a profound and overwhelming theme of self-blame, hopelessness, and self-depreciation. Although cases with this classic picture are still common, others, with a picture which this writer calls claiming depression, occur with increasing frequency.

Manic-depressive psychosis manifests itself with recurring attacks of depression and of manic elation in various forms and cycles. We shall take into consideration (1) the classical or self-blaming type of depression, (2) the claiming type of depression, (3) other varieties of depression, (4) the manic attack, (5) the course of the disorder, (6) the specific characteristics of pure psychotic depression, as an entity separate from manic-depressive psychosis, (7) diagnostic criteria.

Classical Depression

Depression is characterized by the following triad of psychological symptoms: (1) a pervading feeling of melancholia; (2) a disorder of thought processes, characterized by retardation and unusual content, and (3) psychomotor retardation. In addition, there are accessory somatic dysfunctions.

The pervading mood of depression at times has its onset quite acutely and dramatically, at other times slowly and insidiously. The patient generally had previous attacks of depression which, because they were mild in intensity, passed unnoticed or were considered by the patient and his family as normal variations of mood. Even the psychotic attack is misunderstood at first. An unpleasant event, such as the death of a close relative or a grief of any kind, has occurred, and a certain amount of depression is justified. When, however, a certain period of time has elapsed and the depressed mood should have subsided, it seems instead to become more intense. The patient complains that he cannot think freely, feels unable to work, cannot eat, and sleeps only a few hours a night.

As the symptoms increase in intensity, the patient himself may request to be taken to a physician; often, however, the illness is advanced to such a degree that the patient is no longer able to make such a decision and he has to consult a physician at the initiative of the members of the family. When the patient is seen by the physician, the latter is impressed by his unhappy, sad appearance. He looks older than his age, his forehead is wrinkled, and his face, although undergoing very little mimic play, reveals a despondent mood. In some cases, the main fold of the upper lip at the edges of its inner third is contracted upward and a little backward (sign of Veraguth).

In most cases, the examiner is often taken astray by the complaints of the patient, which consist of physical pain, a feeling of discomfort, digestive difficulties, lack of appetite, and

insomnia. The physician may interpret these complaints as simple psychosomatic dysfunctions; in the majority of cases, however, the mood of melancholia is prominent and leads to an easy diagnosis.

The patient is often at a loss in describing the experience of melancholia. He says that his chest is heavy, his body is numb; he would like to sleep but he cannot; he would like to immerse himself in activities, but he cannot; he would even like to cry, but he cannot. "The eyes have consumed all the tears." "Life is a torment." There is at the same time a desire to punish oneself by destroying oneself, and at the same time to end one's suffering. Suicidal ideas occur in about 75 percent of patients, and actual suicide attempts are made by at least 10 to 15 percent. Often, the suicide attempt occurs when it is not expected, because the patient seems to have made some improvement, as the depression is less pronounced. In a minority of suicide attempts, the suicidal idea was carefully concealed from the members of the family. The desire to end life applies only to the life of the patient himself, with one important exception, to be kept in mind always: Young mothers who undergo psychotic depressions often plan to destroy not only themselves but their children, who are presumably considered by the patient as extensions of herself. Newspaper reports about mothers who have killed themselves and their little children in most cases refer to patients suffering from unrecognized attacks of manic-depressive psychosis or psychotic depression.

The second important symptom of depression concerns the content and type of thinking. As far as the content is concerned, the thoughts of the patient are characterized by gloomy, morbid ideas. In some cases, at the beginning of the attack, ideas occur which cannot be recognized as part of the ensuing picture of psychotic depression. They seem to be neurotic obsessions, phobias, what the patient calls "unclean thoughts." They are followed by discouraging ideas which acquire more and more prominence. The patient feels that he will not be able to work, he will lose his money, something bad will happen to his family, somebody is going to get hurt, or the family is in extreme poverty. There is no great variety in the patient's thoughts. It is almost as if the patient purposely selected the thoughts which have an unpleasant content. *They are not thoughts as thoughts; they are chiefly carriers of mental pain.* The distortion caused by the unpleasantness of the mood at times transforms these melancholic thoughts into almost delusional ideas or definite delusions. They often represent distortions of the body image and hypochondriasis. The patient thinks he has cancer, tuberculosis, syphilis, etc. His brain is melting, his bowels have been lost, the heart does not beat, etc. Delusions of poverty are also common. Ideas of guilt, sin, and self-condemnation are very pronounced, especially in serious cases. At times, these self-accusatory ideas are so unrealistic that the name "delusion" seems appropriate for them. "It is all my fault," "It is all my responsibility." In some cases, the tendency to blame oneself reaches the absurd; the patient blames himself for being sick or for "succumbing to the illness." In some cases, he feels that he is not really sick but acts as if he would be sick. This impression is almost the opposite of that which we find in some schizophrenics. In the latter, there is the idea that what happens in the world is an act, a play, the world is a big stage. The depressed patient, on the contrary, feels that he is acting the part of the sick person. This idea, incidentally, occurs generally when the patient starts to recover from the depressed attack.

These delusional ideas cannot always be traced back to an exaggeration or distortion of mood. In cases that have a mixed paranoid and melancholic symptomatology, the delusions are more inappropriate and bizarre and are in no way distinguishable from those of paranoid patients.

In this classical or traditional type of psychotic depression the main theme remains a self-blaming attitude. In severe cases, the patient seems to transmit the following message to the observer: "Do not help me. I do not deserve to be helped. I deserve to die."

Together with this peculiar content of thought, there is retardation of thinking processes. The patient complains that he cannot concentrate, he cannot focus his attention. At first, he can read but cannot retain what he reads. Writing is more difficult for him because composing a letter requires tremendous effort. If the patient was a student, he cannot study any longer. Thoughts seem to follow each other at a very slow pace. Talk is also slow. In a severe state of stupor, the patient cannot talk at all.

Hallucinations are described by many authors in manic-depressive psychosis, especially in the old textbooks. According to the experience of many psychiatrists, however, they are much less common in manic-depressive psychosis than they used to be. This difference is not apparent, in the sense that patients who hallucinate are now diagnosed as schizophrenics. According to the present author, hallucinations do occur, although rarely, in some severely depressed patients. They have the following characteristics:

1. They are very rare in comparison to their occurrences in schizophrenia.
2. They do not have the distinct perceptual and auditory quality that they have in schizophrenia. The patients often cannot repeat what the voices say; they sound indistinct. The patients describe them as "as if rocks would fall," or as "bells which ring," etc. Often, they seem more illusions than hallucinations, or as transformations of actual perceptions.
3. Much more easily than in schizophrenia, they can be related to the prevailing mood of the patient. Their secondary character, that is, secondary to the overall mood, is obvious. They are generally depressive in content, and denigratory, often commanding self-destruction or injury.
4. More frequently than in schizophrenic patients, they seem to occur at night, seldom during the day. The manic-depressive, who is more in contact with external reality than the schizophrenic, possibly needs the removal of diurnal stimuli in order to become aware of these inner phenomena.

The third important sign of the classic type of depression is psychomotor retardation. The actions of the patient decrease in number, and even those which are carried out are very slow. Even the perceptions are retarded. Talking is reduced to a minimum, although a minority of patients retain the tendency to be loquacious. Solving of the usual small daily tasks of life is postponed or retarded. The patient avoids doing many things but continues to do what is essential. Women neglect their housework and their appearance, discontinue the use of make-up, and always wear the same dress. Every change seems a tremendous effort. Interpersonal relations are cut off. In some mild cases, however, the opposite seems to occur at first. The patient, who is prone to accuse himself and extoll others, becomes more affectionate toward the members of the family and willing to do many things for them in an unselfish manner. Later, however, when the disorder increases in intensity, he becomes indifferent to everybody.

The accessory physical symptoms that accompany classic depressive attacks are reduction in sleep, decrease in appetite, and considerable loss in weight. These symptoms do not seem to be due to a specific or direct physiological mechanism, but rather are related to, or a consequence of, the depression. Many patients complain of dryness of the mouth, which is to be attributed to decreased secretion of the parotid glands.[73]

Other frequent symptoms are backache and amenorrhea. There is a definite decrease in sexual desire, often to the point of complete impotence or frigidity. In many patients, sugar is found in the urine during the attack. The basal metabolism tends to be slightly lower than normal. Kennedy[42] believes that in many patients the symptomatology consists almost exclusively of these somatic dysfunctions. He calls these syndromes "manic-depressive equivalents."

The Claiming Type of Depression

As we have already mentioned, since the late 1950s there has been a decline in the number of cases showing the classic type of depression, as part of manic-depressive psychosis or as pure depression. Moreover, the cases that we see seldom reach those severe degrees which used to be very common. Another type of depression is frequently observed now, whose symptomatology has the appearance of an appeal, a cry for help. The patient is anguished, but wants people near him to become very aware of his condition. All the symptoms seem to imply the message, "Help me; pity me. It is in your power to relieve me. If I suffer, it is because you don't give me what I need." Even the suicidal attempt or prospect is an appeal of "Do not abandon me," or "You have the power to prevent my death. I want you to know it." In other words, the symptomatology, although colored by an atmosphere of depression, is a gigantic claim. Now, it is the Gestalt of depression that looms in the foreground with the claim lurking behind; now, it is the claim that looms with the depression apparently receding. Badly hidden are also feelings of hostility for people close to the patient, like members of the family who do not give the patient as much as he would like. If anger is expressed, feelings of guilt and depression follow. Whereas the patient with the self-blaming type of depression generally wants to be left alone, the claiming type of patient is clinging, dependent, and demanding. Self-accusation and guilt feelings play a secondary role or no role at all in this type of depression.

Whereas in the self-blaming type of depression there is a decrease of appetite and insomnia, in the claiming type the appetite is not necessarily diminished and quite often there is a need and ability to sleep longer than usual. In several cases, the patient does not want to get up from bed and wishes to return to it several times during the day.

Clinical Varieties of Depression

Some authors distinguish several varieties of depression: the simple, the acute, the paranoid, and the depressive stupor.

Simple depression is characterized by a relative mildness of the symptoms and may make the diagnosis of psychosis difficult. Delusions and hallucinations are absent. Although retarded, the patient is able to take care of the basic vital needs. Suicidal ideas and attempts, however, occur in this type, too. In recent years, cases of simple depression seem to have increased in number, relative to the total incidence of manic-depressive psychosis.

In *acute depression*, the symptoms are much more pronounced. Self-accusation and ideas of sin and poverty are prominent. Some depressive ideas, bordering on delusions, are present. The loss of weight is very marked.

In *paranoid depression*, although the prominent feature remains the depressed mood, delusional ideas play an important role. The patient feels that he is watched, spied on, or threatened. Somebody wants to hurt him. Hypochondriacal delusions with pronounced distortion of the body image may occur. As in the case of hallucinations, these delusions are secondary to the prevailing mood of the patient. They disappear easily when the mood changes. Hallucinations may also occur, although rarely.

Depressive stupor is the most pronounced form of depression. Here there is more than retardation: The movements are definitely inhibited or suppressed. The patients are so absorbed in their own pervading feeling of depression that they cannot focus their attention on their surroundings. They do not seem to hear; they do not respond. They are mute, with the exception of some occasional utterances. Since they cannot focus on anything, they give the impression of being apathetic, whereas they are actually the prey of a deep, disturbing emotion. These patients cannot take care of themselves. Generally, they lie in bed mute, and have to be spoon-fed.

Unless they are successfully treated during the attack, physical health may suffer severely. They lose up to a hundred pounds in certain cases; they are constipated, and their circulation is enfeebled.

The Manic Attack

In the manic attack, as in depression, the symptomatology is characterized by (1) a change in mood, which is one of elation; (2) a disorder of thought processes, characterized by flight of ideas and happy content; and (3) an increased mobility. Accessory bodily changes also occur.

It is difficult in many instances to determine the beginning of an attack. The patient is often in a lively mood. His personality is described as that of an extrovert, active individual who likes to talk a lot and do many things. At the time of the attack, however, the overjoyousness of the patient seems somewhat out of proportion, occasionally even inappropriate, as, for instance, when he easily dismisses things which should make him sad and continues to be in his happy mood. The patient seems exuberant, very sociable, and, at times, even succeeds in transmitting his happiness to the surrounding persons. This mood, however, although pronounced, is not a constant or solid one. We are not referring here to the alternations with depression but to the fact that this euphoric mood may easily change into one of irritation, or even rage and anger, especially when the patient sees that the environment does not respond to his enthusiasm, or does not react in accordance with the exalted opinion that he has of himself.

The thinking disorder is prominent and reveals itself in the verbal productions of the patient. The patient talks very fast, and cannot concentrate on any subject for more than a few seconds. Any marginal idea is expressed; any secondary, distracting stimulus is allowed to affect the patient. The thoughts expressed are not disconnected but maintain some apparent ties. We can always determine that the individual ideas are connected by the elementary laws of association, but the talk as a whole is verbose, circumstantial, not directed toward any goal, or toward the logical demonstration of any point which is discussed. The ensemble of these thought and language alterations is called "flight of ideas."

Actually, this type of verbal behavior has a goal—that of maintaining this superficial effervescent euphoria, and of escaping from intruding thoughts which may bring about depression. In not too-pronounced cases, the patient realizes that he unduly allows details to interfere with the original goal of his conversation and tries to go back to it, but again he is lost in many details.

In this incessant logorrhea, the patient makes jokes. The propensity toward associations leads to repeated clang associations, which the patient uses to make jokes, puns, etc.[4] In some rare cases, the lack of thought inhibition facilitates a certain artistic propensity, which does not, however, lead to achievement because of the lack of concentration.

Lorenz and Cobb[53] and Lorenz,[52] who made an accurate study of speech in manic patients, reported that in manic speech there is a quantitative change in the use of certain speech elements, namely: (1) a relative increase in the use of pronouns and verbs; (2) a relative decrease in the use of adjectives and prepositions; and (3) a high verb-adjective quotient (that is, the proportion of adjectives is decreased). These authors found no gross disorganization at the level of structural elements and postulated that the defect in manic speech occurs at higher integrative levels of language formulation. They concluded that "If the assumption of a correlation between emotional states and verb-adjective quotient is correct, the manic patient's speech gives objective evidence of a heightened degree of anxiety."

The rapid association ability that the manic possesses enables him to grasp immediately some aspects of the environment which otherwise would pass unnoticed. The patient is in the paradoxical situation in which his ability to observe and grasp environmental stimuli has increased, but he cannot make use of it because of his distractibility.

The content of thought often reveals an exalted opinion of himself. The patient may boast that he is very rich, a great lover, a famous actor, a prominent businessman, etc. These statements receive flimsy support. When asked to prove them, the patient attempts to do so but is soon lost in a web of unnecessary details. If he is reminded of the goal of the conversation, he may become excitable. Disturbances of the sensorium are generally of minimal intensity and are caused by the exalted mood or distractibility rather than by intellectual impairment.

The motor activity is increased. The patients are always on the go. They are in a state that ranges from mild motor excitement to incessant and wild activity. They talk, they sing, they dance, they tease, destroy, move objects, etc. In severe states, these actions or movements remain unfinished, purposeless. In spite of this constant activity, the patients do not feel tired and have tremendous endurance.

Accessory somatic symptoms consist in loss of weight, generally not as pronounced as in depression, decrease in appetite, and constipation. Insomnia is marked. The blood pressure is generally lowered. Menstruations are irregular. Sexual functions, although frequently increased in hypomanic states, are eventually decreased or disturbed in various ways.

As in the states of depression, many forms of manic states have been described by the early authors. Following is a brief description of them:

MANIC VARIETIES

In *hypomania*, the symptoms are not of a marked intensity. As mentioned before, it is difficult at times to say whether what the patient shows is his usual "extrovert" personality or the beginning of the illness. He seems full of pep and in a good humor. He wants to do many things. His verbal abilities are accentuated. Although he always had a talent for foreign languages, now he speaks many of them without hesitation, unconcerned with the mistakes he may make. Some of these patients increase their activities to such an exaggerated degree as to show very poor judgment. Actually, they do so compelled by their inner excitability and by their exalted mood. They may walk for miles and miles. Generally, they have a goal (for instance, to reach the next village), but not a necessary one. They may send out hundreds of unnecessary letters or greeting cards and make a large number of lengthy telephone calls. They often go on spending sprees, with disastrous economic consequences. The sexual activity is increased, and lack of control may bring about unpleasant results. Illegitimate pregnancies in hypomanic women and venereal diseases in hypomanic men and women are relatively common.

The excitability, richness of movements, and euphoric mood, give a bizarre flavor to the behavior. A female patient, in order to show a sore to a physician, completely undressed in front of him. Occasionally, even thefts and fraudulent acts are committed. The patient retains the ability to rationalize his actions, at times to such an extent that the layman is confused and believes in the patient's sanity.

In *acute mania*, the symptoms are much more pronounced. They may have become marked gradually from a previously hypomanic state, or rapidly from a normal condition. The patient is in a state of such extreme restlessness that his behavior may be very disturbing and difficult to control. He may disrupt theatrical audiences, sing or scream in the street, or ring bells. If an attempt is made to control him, he may become belligerent. The mood is one of such exaltation that spontaneous thoughts of self-aggrandizement are immediately accepted.

A subtype, which Kraepelin differentiated from acute mania, is delusional mania, characterized by an abundance of grandiose delusional ideas reminiscent of those found in the expansive type of general paresis.

Delirious mania represents an extreme stage of excitement. The patient is incoherent, disoriented, restless, and agitated. He may easily injure himself and others in his aimless activity. Restraint, chemical or physical, is an absolute necessity to avoid exhaustion which may lead to death. Hallucinations and delusions frequently occur.

In addition to the above-mentioned types, Kraepelin has described *mixed states* which are characterized by a combination of manic and depressive symptoms. He distinguished the following six principal types: (1) manic stupor; (2) agitated depression; (3) unproductive mania; (4) depressive mania; (5) depression, with flight of ideas; and (6) akinetic mania.

The names given to these types indicate the combinations of the chief symptoms. Of the six types the most common is, perhaps, agitated depression. In this condition, a motor restlessness, more typical of a manic excitement, is superimposed on a markedly depressive symptomatology.

Course

Although the various types of manic-depressive psychoses have been described as if they were separate entities, all the types are related, as Kraepelin saw when he formulated the large nosological concept of manic-depressive psychosis.

The melancholic attack and the manic, which at first sight seem so different, have an intrinsic similarity. In fact, the same mental functions are altered, although the alterations are, in a certain way, opposite. Whereas in depression the mood is one of melancholia, in the manic attack it is one of elation; whereas in depression the thought processes and motor activity are retarded, in the manic attack one finds a flight of ideas and increased motility.

One of the main characteristics of manic-depressive psychosis is the recurrence of the attacks, which has conferred on the disorder the designation, often used in Europe, "intermittent psychosis."

The attack may occur in different successions, which old textbooks of psychiatry described at great length and with many illustrations (which represented the manic attack as a positive wave and the depression as a negative wave). If we have a sequence of a manic and a depressed attack (or an attack of depression followed by a manic one), we have the typical circular psychosis. We may observe, however, that the attacks of depression far outnumber those of mania. Some patients may undergo a conspicuous number of depressions without ever having a manic attack.

There seems to be no relation between the duration of the attack and the normal intervals. At times, short attacks recur several times in short succession, but frequently the series is interrupted by a long interval. I have seen several cases in which an attack of depression in the patient's early twenties was not followed by a second one until he had reached his middle sixties or even seventies. Many attacks of depression which occur later in life and which by many authors are considered as a subtype of senile psychosis, must be considered instead as late occurrences or relapses of manic-depressive psychosis, as Kraepelin illustrated. This fact has been confirmed by the recovery that these patients make as a result of convulsive electric treatment; the genuine senile patients do not improve.

According to Pollock et al.,[61] 58.1 percent of patients have only one attack; 26.1 percent have two attacks; 9.3 percent have three attacks; and 6.5 percent more than three. Occasionally, one finds a patient who has had twenty-five or more attacks.

The age at which the first attack occurs varies. It may happen in childhood, in rare cases. By far the largest number of first attacks occurs between the ages of twenty and thirty-five. Manic attacks are slightly more frequent between ages twenty and forty. After forty, their ratio to depressive attacks decreases further. Women are more susceptible to this psychosis than men. (About 70 percent of patients are women.)

The illness generally results in recovery, as far as the individual attack is concerned. Repeated attacks usually cause very little intellectual impairment. Death, however, may occur in two instances: suicide in depression, and exhaustion or cardiac insufficiency in cases of delirious mania. Another situation, which we shall discuss later, is the change of the manic-depressive symptomatology into a schizophrenic one, either shortly after the onset of the illness or even after many years of hospitalization.*

Prognostic criteria as to the future course of the condition are very difficult when the patient is examined only from the point of view of the manifest symptomatology. Much more rarely than in schizophrenia, the manifest symptomatology of manic-depressive psychosis will permit prediction as to whether the patient will have only the present attack, a few, or many, in his lifetime. The prognosis is almost always good as to the individual attack but is uncertain as to the possibility of recurrence. Rennie,[64] in an accurate statistical study, found that the prognosis is worse when attacks occur after the age of forty. He found that 70 percent of all patients have a second attack; 63.5 percent a third; and 45 percent a fourth. The more frequent the attacks, the worse the prognosis.

Psychotic Depression

Psychotic depression, or as it is called by some authors, "psychotic depressive reaction," is a psychosis which is distinguishable from the depression occurring in manic-depressive psychosis by virtue of the following characteristics: (1) absence of manic attacks or even cyclothymic mood swings; (2) obvious importance of environmental precipitating factors. Among these precipitating factors, the following are frequent: death of husband or wife, death of a parent, death of a child, death of a sister or brother, disappointment in love, loss of position, business failure, etc. It is really debatable whether the presence of a definite precipitating factor is enough to establish the differential diagnosis from manic-depressive psychosis. As a matter of fact, the present author is convinced that the same precipitating factors may unchain specific attacks of manic-depressive psychosis. A recurrence of depressive episodes is also not enough to exclude the diagnosis of psychotic depression. In my experience, psychotic depressions tend to recur unless adequately treated with psychotherapy. It seems to this writer that the only differential diagnosis consists in the absence of manic at-

---

* There are many psychiatrists who would deny such a statement. They feel that if a manic-depressive seems later to become schizophrenic it is because the right diagnosis (schizophrenia) was not made. At the present time, the prevalent opinion of people who have worked for many years in the same hospital is that some patients who once presented what appeared to be a typical manic-depressive symptomatology later disclose a typical schizophrenic symptomatology. This point of view, of course, does not exclude the possibility of wrong diagnoses being made in some cases, especially during the first psychotic attack.

tack or of marked mood swings which indicate a cyclothymic personality.

Diagnostic Criteria

Typical cases of manic-depressive psychosis are generally easy to diagnose, even if the examination is limited to the study of the manifest symptoms, although the beginner may have some difficulties in some cases.

An elderly man, who has lost a lot of weight, is depressed, and complains that he may have cancer, may be mistaken for a manic-depressive or for a person suffering from psychotic depression when actually he really has some sort of malignancy with reactive depression. An accurate physical examination will determine the condition. In psychiatric practice, however, the opposite occurrence is more common: An elderly patient has lost weight, has many hypochondriacal complaints, fear of cancer, and is depressed; negative physical findings, retardation, and insomnia, as well as the past history, will generally determine that he is suffering from a depression.

Some patients, who are very retarded, have lost accessory movements, and present a mask-like expression on their faces, are occasionally confused with postencephalitics.

According to the *Diagnostic and Statistical Manual of Mental Disorders* of the American Psychiatric Association (DSM-II), the differentiation between psychotic depression and depressive neurosis "depends on whether the reaction impairs reality testing or functional adequacy enough to be considered a psychosis." The reality testing in this case concerns the mood of depression. Does the patient consider his depression justified? Does he want to maintain it? Does it transform drastically his appreciation of his life? If the answers are yes, the diagnosis is bound to be one of affective psychosis.

Whether a different biological constitution is prerequisite for having psychotic depression instead of manic-depressive psychosis is a question which will not be discussed in this chapter. A differentiation in the psychodynamics is again impossible to make, except that in typical manic-depressive psychosis the early events of life seem more important than in psychotic depression. The reverse is true for the later life events.

For the differential diagnosis between psychotic depression and involutional melancholia, the reader is referred to Chapter 30 of this volume.

Manic states may be confused with the following conditions:

1. *Psychomotor epilepsy.* Epileptic exaltation is impulsive but is deprived of elation. Furthermore, the electroencephalogram will lead to an easy diagnosis.
2. *Toxic deliriums* (or amential states). The wealth of disconnected hallucinations and the poverty of external perceptions (or of reactivity to the environment) will lead to recognition of the delirium.
3. *General paresis.* The physical symptoms of general paresis, and the serological findings, will lead to a diagnosis. Moreover, in the paretic, the sensorium is more defective and the actions and thoughts are more incongruous than the degree of exaltation would permit, and superficial delusions more numerous.
4. *Catatonic excitement.* The excitement precedes or follows the catatonic state. The actions are more aimless, absurd, and deprived of any conscious feeling of guilt, the mood is more incongruous and inappropriate, and hostility toward others is more pronounced.
5. *Attack of exaltation* occurring in any mental diseases, including mental deficiency. The subsequent course will reveal the correct diagnosis.

(Psychodynamic Mechanisms

The characteristics that we have described in the previous section constitute the manifest aspects of processes of a much more subtle nature that were unfolding for a long time. Because psychotherapy of manic-depressive patients or patients suffering from psychotic depression presents great difficulties in a large number of cases (even greater than those presented by schizophrenic patients), our knowledge of the psychodynamics of these cases is still fragmentary. Some fundamental factors, however, stand out sufficiently to permit us to explain grossly some of the most common mechanisms.

The Childhood of the Manic-Depressive Patient

It seems to be a fairly well-established clinical fact that the early childhood (at least the first year of life) of the future manic-depressive patient was not so traumatic as that of people who tend to become schizophrenics or even seriously neurotic.

The future manic-depressive is generally born in a home which is willing to accept him and care for him. The word "accept" has a special meaning here: The mother is duty-bound and willing to administer to the baby as much care as he requires; she is willing to provide for him everything that he needs. This willingness of the mother is, in turn, accepted by the child, who is willing to accept everything he is offered; that is, early in life the child appears very receptive to the influence (or giving) of the significant adult (parent). There are no manifestations of resistance toward accepting this influence, as, for instance, the autistic manifestations or attempts to prevent or retard socialization, as one finds in schizophrenia.[3] If we use Buber's terminology,[18] we may say that the "Thou," that is, the other, is immediately accepted and introjected. The "Thou" is at first the mother, but this receptivity to the mother enhances a receptivity for both parents and all the important surrounding adults, and promotes a willingness to accept them with their symbols and their values. It promotes also a certain readiness to accept their food (either the milk of the mother or regular food) and thus predisposes some people (but by no means all) to overeating, obesity, and the seeking of compensation in food when other satisfactions are not available.

This receptiveness to the others and willingness to introject the others determine at this early age some aspects of the personality of the patient. He tends to become an "extrovert"; at the same time, he tends to be a conformist, willing to accept what he is given by his surroundings (not only in material things but also in terms of habits and values), and to rely less than the average person on his own resources or on his own world. This readiness to accept, this psychological receptivity, will predispose him also to pathological (or exaggerated) introjection.

In the second year of life (earlier, according to some authors), a new attitude on the part of the mother drastically changes the environment in which the child was growing, and exposes him to a severe trauma. The mother will continue to take care of the child, but considerably less than before, and now she makes many demands on him. The child will receive care and affection provided he accepts the expectations that the parents have for him and tries to live up to them.

This brusque change in the parents' attitude is generally the result of many things; predominantly, their attitude toward life in general tends to evoke in the child an early sense of duty and responsibility—what is to be obtained is to be deserved. The parents are generally dissatisfied with their own life and harbor resentment, at times, toward the children, who represent increased work and responsibility. This hostility, however, is seldom manifested openly; generally, it is manifested by the fact that the parents increase their expectations too much.

Thus, the child finds himself changed from an environment which predisposes to great receptivity to one of great expectation. These dissimilar environments are actually determined by a common factor: the strong sense of duty that compelled the mother to do so much for the baby is now transmitted at an early age to the child. Generally, the families of manic-depressive patients have many children, and often, when the future manic-depressive patient is in his second year of life, a sibling is already born and the mother is now lavishing her care on the newborn with the same duty-bound generosity that she previously had for the patient. This, of course, makes the change in the environment more marked for the patient.

This displacement by a younger sibling seems to be important in the dynamics of many cases of manic-depressive psychosis and of psychotic depression, although, again, no statistical proof of it can be given.* Statistical studies have so far concerned themselves more with birth order.†

In many cases, the brusque change had to occur because of unexpected events, such as the child had to be abandoned by the mother because of illness, economic setback, forced emigration, political persecution, etc. The child was then left in custody of an aunt, grandmother, cousin, stranger, or orphan asylum, and was subjected to a violent and unmitigated experience of loss.

For several patients, the abrupt change that we have described has already taken place at the time of weaning. Future affective patients are generally breast-fed in their infancy and then suddenly deprived of mother's milk. No bottles, no rubber nipples, and no pacifiers are used. There is a sharp transition from the breast to the glass. In a minority of patients, this loss of the breast plays an important role.

In many other patients, the abrupt change occurs later, but generally still in the preschool years.

How does the child try to adjust to the new threatening situation? The child who is likely later to develop an affective psychosis tends to adopt special mechanisms. A common one, although decreasing in frequency, is that of

finding security by accepting parental expectations, no matter how onerous they are. The child does not reject the parents emotionally, or avoid them (as the schizoid often does), but consciously accepts them. He must live up to their expectations no matter how heavy the burden. It is only by complying, obeying, and working hard, that he will recapture the love or state of bliss which he used to have as a baby, or at least maintain that moderate love which he is receiving now. Love is still available, but not as a steady flow. The flow is intermittent, conditioned, and therefore does not confer security. The child feels that if he does not do what he is supposed to, he will be punished—mother may withdraw her love totally. At the same time that the anxiety of losing mother's love sets in, hope is given to the child that he will be able to retain this love, or to recapture it, if and when it is lost. The child thus feels he has choice, the freedom of retaining the parental love or not. No matter what he chooses, however, he has a hard price to pay: submission or rejection. He also feels that mother is not bad, in spite of her appearance, but, on the contrary, that she is good. She is good even in punishing him, because by punishing him she wants to redeem him, make him again worthy of her love. Thus, the mechanism is different from that occurring in many preschizophrenics; although the preaffective patient has an image of himself as bad, he does not feel that he is beyond the possibility of redemption, as the preschizophrenic often feels. The anxiety about being unable to fulfill parental expectations changes into guilt feelings. If affection or forgiveness is not forthcoming, the child feels that it is his own fault; he has not lived up to what was expected of him, and he feels guilty. When he feels guilty, he again expects punishment. He wants to be punished, because punishment is the lesser of the evils. He would rather be punished than lose mother's love. If he is not punished, he often works harder in order to punish himself.

A little later, but still at a very early age, many of these children assume responsibilities such as the support of the family. If they engage in a career, it is often in order to bring

---

* I have observed this displacement by a sibling to be an important factor also in the psychodynamics of milder depressions, which cannot be classified as cases of manic-depressive psychosis.

† Some statistical works seem to indicate that the first-born child is more liable to manic-depressive psychosis. Of course, the first-born is more liable to be displaced. Berman,[13] in a study of 100 manic-depressives, found that forty-eight were first-born, fifteen second, ten each third and fourth, and seventeen fifth or later. Pollock and coworkers[61] found that 39.7 percent were first-born and 29.7 percent were second-born. Malzberg[54] and Katz[41] could not find any relationship between birth order and manic-depressive psychosis.

honor and prestige to the family. In a relatively large number of cases, the family belongs to a "marginal" group of society because of religious or ethnic minority status, and the child feels that it is his duty to rescue the family with his own achievement.

In addition, in several patients, incestuous wishes toward parents and, as frequently, toward siblings of opposite sex elicit strong guilt feelings which the patient feels must be atoned.

Other facts make the picture more complicated and difficult to understand, for instance, the impression often received that the parents of several patients are not strict but overindulgent. This is due to the fact that, in this second stage of childhood, the parents do not need to enforce any rules with their actions. The rules, the principles, have already been incorporated by the patient. As a matter of fact, some of the parents now regret that the children take rules with such seriousness.

The parents of the patient generally give a picture of cohesiveness and stability. There is no serious talk of divorce; the family seems on stable ground, reinforced by the conventions of society. Those family conflicts or schisms described in schizophrenia are not seen as frequently in the family of patients suffering from affective psychoses.

The second important mechanism by which the child tries to cope with the sudden change in environmental circumstances is an attempt to make himself more babyish, more dependent. If the child makes himself aggressively dependent, the mother or other important adults will be forced to re-establish an atmosphere of babyhood and of early bliss. The child, and later the adult, will develop a very demanding and at the same time clinging, dependent type of personality.

Since the 1950s, this second type of mechanism has become much more common, at least in the United States.

Secondary mechanisms also occur concomitantly with the two main ones. The child harbors a strong resentment against the parental figure who, in the first type of mechanism, has made so many impositions, or who, in the second type, has not given enough. Such resentment mainfests itself in attacks of rage, anger, rebellion, or even violence. When such anger becomes manifest, it often is enough to dispel an oncoming feeling of depression. For this reason, some therapists believe that any depression hides an underlying anger. This is true only to a limited extent. The anger is consequent to a situation that already existed and was unacceptable to the child. Anger alone is not a solution to the conflictful situation, although it may be a temporary defense against future depression.

In many cases feelings of anger are promptly checked and repressed, not only in childhood but throughout the life of the patient. Sadistic thoughts and impulses are, at times, very pronounced but seldom acted out. Together with the consequent guilt feelings brought about by these impulses are feelings of unworthiness and depression. The patient soon learns that rebellion does not pay; on the contrary, it increases the atonement he must undergo later. The stronger his sadistic impulses, the stronger become the masochistic tendencies. He soon desires peace at any cost; any compromise is worthy of peace. The mechanisms which will permit him to maintain a certain equilibrium is the repression of this resentment. The resentment is, however, retained unconsciously, as it appears from dreams and occasional outbursts which reach consciousness.

An additional dynamic mechanism which is found in some cases of manic-depressive psychosis is the following:

The child senses that the acceptance or introjection of parents is too much of a burden and, without realizing it, shifts the directions of his incorporations; other adults in the environment (much older siblings, uncles, aunts, grandparents, friends, etc.) tend then to be internalized instead of parents. Not only is the common tendency of children to introject adults exaggerated here, but peripheral adults become parentlike figures. The child unconsciously resorts to this mechanism in order to decrease the burden of the parental introjection, but in many cases this defense does not prove useful. As Fromm-Reichmann[32] noted, there will be no single significant adult to whom the patient will be able to relate in a meaningful way. The relationship with these other grown-ups again is determined by a utilitarian purpose, duty, or role. The introjection of such adults eventually fails to provide what is needed and may end by confusing the child (How can he satisfy all the adults?) and increasing his burden and feeling of guilt.

(Prepsychotic Personality

The prepsychotic personality of the patient who will develop an affective psychosis is colored by one or the other of the main psychodynamic mechanisms which we have mentioned in the previous section and by some reactions to these mechanisms.

We shall describe first the personality of patients who have tried to overcome the initial trauma by living up to ideal parental expectations. The strong tendency of these patients to introject parental figures will also produce strong feelings of patriotism, religiosity, and loyalty to a political party. They often wish to have a military or ecclesiastic career. These organizations are not parent substitutes but additional parents. Group loyalty and *esprit de corps* play an important part in the psychological constellation of these people. Actually, under the pretense of belonging to a group, to a close-knit family, or to an organization, the individual hides his loneliness.

In many cases, we find a self-conscious individual, always motivated by duty, of the type of personality Riesman[66] has called "inner-directed." Unless he overcomes some of his difficulties, the individual cannot become a creative person, but remains an imitator. However, what he tries to do, he does well. He has deep convictions, and his life is motivated by principles. He must be a dedicated person. He is generally efficient, and people who do not know him too well have the impression that he is a well-adjusted, untroubled individual. On the contrary, he is not a happy person. He selects a mate not because he loves her but because she "needs" him. Later, he will never divorce the mate because she is in terrible

need of him. At the same time, he blames himself for being so egotistic as to think that he is indispensable. The necessity to please others and to act in accordance with the expectations of others, or in accordance with the principles that he has accepted, makes him unable to get really in touch with himself. He does not listen to his own wishes; he does not know what it means to be himself. He works incessantly and yet has feelings of futility and emptiness. At times, he conceals his unhappiness by considering what he has accomplished, just as he conceals his loneliness by thinking of the group to which he belongs. But when he allows himself to experience these feelings of unhappiness, futility, and unfulfillment, he misinterprets them again. He tends to believe that he is to be blamed for them. If he is unhappy, if he finds no purpose in life, it must be his fault, or he must not be worthy of anything else. A vicious circle is thus established which repeats itself and increases in intensity, often throughout the life of the patient, unless fortunate circumstances or psychotherapy intervene.

The patient often has partial insight into his own mechanisms but does not know how to solve them. For instance, he is willing to accept the role in the family and in society which has been assigned to him, and yet later he scolds himself for playing this role, for not being spontaneous. But if he tries to refuse the role, he has guilt feelings. The conclusion is that no matter how he tries to solve his problems, he will feel he has made the wrong choice. A female patient told me that she "felt like a little girl who pretends to be grown up but is not. I am acting." But she must live in that way; that's her duty. It is her fault that she "acts" and does not accept social behavior as spontaneous or real life.

The patient also tends to put his superiors or teachers in a parental authoritarian role. Again, and quite often, he feels angry at them as they seem to expect too much, or they themselves have been found at fault. The patient does not know how to act: Should he continue to accept the authority of these people and the burden that this acceptance implies, or should he remove them from the pedestal? But if he removes them, a void will be left. His authorities are part of him, of his values, and of the symbolic world upon which he sustains himself, and to do without them is impossible. Furthermore, he would feel very guilty. The patient often realizes (as Cohen and co-workers have illustrated[22]) that he tends to understimate himself. It is his "duty" to "undersell" himself. On the other hand, he tends to blame himself for underestimating himself and giving himself no chance to develop his own talents and potential abilities.

In spite of the fact that this type of patient may at times give the impression of living independently or of being involved in his work, the equilibrium he has been able to maintain, even if precarious, is sustained mainly or exclusively in relation to one person in his immediate environment. I have called this person the *dominant other*.[5] The dominant other provides the patient with the evidence, real or illusory, or at least the hope, that acceptance, love, respect, and recognition of his human worth and meaning of his life are acknowledged by at least another person. The dominant other is represented most often by the spouse. Far less often, in order of frequency, follow the mother, a person to whom the patient is romantically attached, an adult child, a sister, the father. Also, frequently, the dominant other is represented, through anthropomorphization, by the firm where the patient works, or a social institution to which he belongs, like the church, the political party, the army, the club, and so forth. All these dominant others are symbolic of the depriving mother, or to be more accurate, of the once giving and later depriving mother. If the real mother is still living and is the dominant other, she will act in two ways—as her present role is actual in the present and also symbolic of her old one. If the dominant other dies, he becomes even more powerful through the meanings attached to his death. A relationship of subtle dependency exists between the patient and the dominant other.

The relationship of dependency is not so subtle in the other type of prepsychotic personality, which has adopted the mechanism of obvious leaning on mother and maternal substitutes after the initial trauma. Contrary to the persons described above, this type includes people who, even at a superficial examination, appear maladjusted. These patients have never forgotten the bliss of the first year of life and still expect or demand a continuation of it. They demand and expect from others, feel deprived and sad when they do not get what they expect. They are demanding but not aggressive in the usual sense of the word, because they do not try to get what they want through their own efforts: they *expect* it from others. They have not developed that complex of duty and hard work typical of the accepting, introjecting patient.

These patients alternate between feeling guilty and having the desire to make other people feel guilty. They generally find one person on whom to depend, and they make this other person feel guilty if he does not do what the patient wants. The sustaining person (generally the spouse) is empowered with the capacity to make the patient happy or unhappy and is supposed to be responsible for the despair and helplessness of the patient. Relatively often, we find in this group women who depend entirely on their husbands, who are generally much older. In these cases, the dominant other is not only the person who is supposed to accept, love, respect, but also the person who protects and gives material things. At times, the request is immense; the patient seems almost to request, metaphorically speaking, milk or blood.

In some cases, there is an apparent variation in the picture inasmuch as the patient tries desperately to submerge himself into work and activities, hoping that eventually he will find something to do which will make him worthy of recognition from other people. Whereas the first type of prepsychotic personality looked inwardly for a solution to his conflicts, the second type looks externally.

A third type of prepsychotic personality is observed in some cases either as the prevailing type or as a temporary characterological structure which replaces from time to time one of the two structures previously described. This third type, the forerunner of the manic, is lively, active, hearty, and friendly. On closer scrutiny, the apparent health and liveliness are found to be superficial. In a certain way, the patient actually escapes into actions or into reality but remains shallow and dissatisfied. If he happens to be engaged in work in which not concentration but action is required, he may do well and maintain a satisfactory level of adjustment; otherwise, he may sooner or later get into trouble. He claims that he has many friends, but, although the interpersonal relations seem warm and sincere, they are superficial and lack real kinship. One patient said, "I joke, I laugh, I pretend; I appear radiant and alive, but deep down I am lonely and empty." This type of person is, only in certain respects, the opposite of the duty-bound individual. He tries to escape from his inner directions, but he does not correspond to what Riesman has called the "other-directed" person. Imitating Riesman's terminology, we could call this hypomanic-like person "outer-directed," but not "other-directed." He does not escape into others, he escapes *from* his inner self (because the inner self has incorporated the burdening others). As we shall see later, he does make an attempt to contact others, but not to integrate with them. He escapes into the world of superficial reality where meditations, reflections, or deep emotions are unnecessary. Such an individual may, at times, seem so free as to be considered psychopathic. Actually, his deep concern with conventional morality often necessitates this pseudopsychopathic escape. Some of the pseudopsychopathic hypomanics have shown asocial behavior since childhood, when, for example, in order to escape from inner and external restrictions, they run away from home or school.

The above-described affective prepsychotic personality types are seldom seen in pure culture. When the patient changes or alternates from one of the first two types of personality to the third, he presents the so-called cyclothymic personality.

Precipitating Factors

The three types of personality that we have described lead not to a stable equilibrium but to an almost constant state of dissatisfaction and mild depression (or hypomanic denial of depression). In this unstable background, we generally find precipitating factors that bring about the full-fledged psychosis.

These precipitating situations may be classified into three categories: (1) the death of a person important to the patient; (2) the realization on the part of the patient of the failure of an important relationship (generally with the spouse); and (3) a severe disappointment in a relationship to an institution or work activity to which the patient had devoted his whole life, or the most important part of his time. This disappointment threatened the self-image which the patient cherishes. It may force a re-evaluation of the self which is hard for the patient to accept.

It is obvious that these situations are considered separately for didactic reasons, but actually may be reduced to a single cause: the loss of something very valuable. This "something," even if represented by a tangible object or concrete situation, is in reality something with a profound and vast psychological and spiritual meaning. At times, although the loss has not yet occurred, the fact that it is impending seems so certain that the patient experiences depression rather than anxiety. Anxiety is the emotion associated with the expectancy of danger; depression is the emotion associated with the experience of loss—the dangerous event has already come and has produced its havoc.*

All the precipitating situations are interpreted by the patient as the proof of abandonment, of having lost the battle and consequently the purpose of life—the love of mother. The present situation reactivates the childhood threat of fear of loss of the mother's love and assumes the emotional form of the old feeling—with much greater intensity, however, because the threatened loss has already and finally occurred. All the efforts of the patient to prevent such loss (either by

---

* It is not implied here that the feeling of depression removes the feeling of anxiety. Some anxiety, at times even to a pronounced degree, is retained by every melancholic patient, in connection with additional possible losses, but depression is the general feeling.

respect of duties and work, or by excessive, demanding dependency, or by hypomanic-like fervor) have failed.

The death of a person dear to the patient is a symbolic reproduction of parental abandonment. The patient feels depressed not only because he feels he has been finally abandoned—that is, deprived of the sources of love—but also because he feels responsible and guilty. The guilt feelings arise from two different levels. On one level, the patient feels that he has "killed" the dead person; his bad behavior has made the person unhappy and sick and more likely to die, or has made this person want to leave the patient. On another level, the patient feels guilty because he recognizes that, in those moments of re-emerging resentment, he wished the death of the lost person. The wish has now become reality; to the wish is attributed the primitive power of producing the reality; consequently, the patient feels guilty for having entertained the murderous desire.

On the other hand, if the patient, in his prepsychotic period, had the dependent, demanding type of personality that we have described, he becomes aware that he cannot depend any more on the dominant other for his self-esteem. As Bemporad[12] noted, it becomes obvious that he is incapable of autonomous gratification.

The second precipitative situation is the full realization of the failure of an important interpersonal relationship. The symbolic parent, generally the marital partner, is recognized, or half-consciously recognized, as a tyrant who took advantage of the compliant, submissive attitude of the patient, rather than as a person to be loved and cherished. The patient has tolerated everything, wanted peace at any cost, but it is impossible for him to continue to do so. He feels that he has wasted his life in devoting himself intensely to the spouse, in loving her or forcing himself to love her at any cost. The realization that the spouse deserves not devotion but hate (actually, in many cases what she got was only devotion, not love) is something the patient cannot accept because it would undermine the foundation of his whole life, would prove the futility of all his efforts. Thus, he tries to repress this hate; he will deny to his friends that he hates the spouse; on the contrary, he will blame himself, for if he does not love the spouse he will be found to be unworthy and will be finally abandoned. Again if the patient used to be a very demanding and dependent person, he now realizes that he cannot depend any more on this interpersonal relationship.

In the third instance, the loss is less personal. A sudden event, such as a dismissal or a failure to obtain a promotion, makes the patient realize that his whole life has been a failure. The institution to which he has devoted so much of himself has badly disappointed him, and again the patient blames himself. In this third instance, too, the patient might have depended on this external agency for self-esteem. He may experience deprivation and lack of autonomous gratification.

Loss of employment is a relatively common precipitating factor. Malzberg[55] found that during the economic depression of 1929 to 1937 the effect of loss of employment or of financial loss was statistically evident in manic-depressive patients. For instance, in the year 1933, 26.2 percent of first-admission patients in New York State hospitals diagnosed as manic-depressive psychotics presented as the precipitating factor loss of employment or financial loss, whereas in the same year only 9.6 percent of first-admission patients with the diagnosis of dementia praecox presented the financial loss as a precipitating factor.

In some patients, an attack is apparently precipitated not by a loss but by what even seems a pleasant event. For instance, women in their forties or fifties, who may have undergone previous subliminal attacks of depression, can develop a severe attack shortly after the marriage of an only son or daughter. Here, the event is experienced by the patient not as a pleasant happening but as a loss. The child whom the mother needed so much, and who was her only purpose and satisfaction in life, is now abandoning her. These cases belong to the second category.

In other cases, an attack occurs after a

promotion, which is interpreted by the patient as a new imposition. The patient is tired of new duties; furthermore, the new position with added responsibility removes the security the patient had established with painstaking effort. In other cases, the individual, faced with promotion, dreads the expected envy and rage of previous associates to whom he is closely bound. The expectation of such emotions in others separates him from them and thus leads to the depressive reaction.

Often, depressions are precipitated in a young parent by the birth of a child whom he had ostensibly wanted. Here, again, several mechanisms are put into operation by the birth. One is the desperation at the expectation of the increase in duty that the child will require, and a brooding again about the futility of life. In some young fathers, the birth of a child reactivates the trauma of replacement by a new sibling. In these cases, one finds unconscious fantasies about the lost breast (for now the baby will have the breast of the mother-wife). It is interesting that whereas the birth of the child precipitates a schizophrenic psychosis only in the mother, it may precipitate an attack of depression in fathers, too. As a whole, however, postpartum depressions are much less frequent than they used to be, and much less frequent than schizophrenic reactions. Zilboorg,[79] who has made a detailed study of postpartum depressions, explained them as the result of a psychosexual conflict. Nevertheless, postpartum psychotic depressions do occur and may reach very severe proportions. This author has seen several severe postpartum depressions, at first unrecognized or just dismissed as postpartum "blues."

The patient, who has just given birth, identifies with her own mother, who once deprived her of love; therefore, she feels sorry for the newborn who also will be deprived of love. She also identifies with the child, deprived of love. The mother of the patient, during pregnancy, labor, and puerperium, retains the status of dominant other, but the patient believes that the mother will no longer supply her with approval and love, because she will discover that the patient is not able to be a good mother. In these cases, generally, the husband has never become a dominant other.

Postpartum manic states are less common.

In many other cases, psychotic attacks do not seem to be precipitated by any definite happening or loss. Here, the precipitating factor is not a specific happening but a total reappraisal of life. The patient becomes more and more discontented; he claims that everything is all right, but an inner dissatisfaction, an inability to experience *la joie de vivre*, possesses him, and he finally becomes openly depressed. *It is the denial of the dissatisfaction that has led many psychiatrists to believe that attacks of affective psychosis often occur without any psychogenic cause.* At other times, the precipitating event seems to be so small as to make the psychiatrist disregard the significance of it. Kraepelin,[47] to show the relative unimportance of psychogenic factors, reported a woman who had had three attacks of depression, the first after the death of her husband, the second after the death of her dog, and the third after the death of her dove. Now, from what we have so far discussed, it is apparent that each of these deaths in itself was not the cause of the psychosis. One may guess that the death of the dove reactivated the sorrow the patient had experienced at the previous deaths, and was also symbolic of a much greater loss, perhaps that of the meaning or purpose of life.

Manic attacks are often precipitated by seeming successes. The patient wants to keep up the fervor that the success has produced, lest he find himself later in a state of depression. A girl, who later in life had several attacks, both manic and depressive, had her first manic attack, of a few days' duration, at the age of nineteen, after winning a local radio debating contest. She was supposed to participate again in a subsequent national contest, but she became so excited, hyperactive, and euphoric that this was impossible. The opponent whom she had defeated on the local contest won. Here, again, it is difficult to ascertain whether it was the success or the fear of not retaining it that precipitated the attack.

Often, however, manic attacks occur as a sudden reaction to creeping depression.

The Psychotic Attack

When the precipitating event or the precipitating situation reveals to the patient that he has "lost," the attack ensues either in the form of depression or in the form of mania.

What is the meaning of the psychotic attack? Does the patient really mourn his loss? Does he punish himself? Does he want to punish others? He probably does all these things in an intense degree.

As we have mentioned in describing the manifest symptomatology, the patient now assumes a prevailing self-blaming or claiming attitude. If he blames himself, he seems to send a message: "I do not deserve any pity, any help. I deserve to die; I should do to myself what you should do to me, but you are too good to do it." On the other hand, although he mourns his loss and feels guilty for the loss, he may want to make a desperate effort to redeem himself by punishing himself. The mechanism described earlier is again in effect, but in a more pronounced form. As Rado[62] says, "Melancholia is a despairing cry for love." Probably, the patient feels: "Punish yourself as parents would do to you and you will be accepted again. You are acceptable but not accepted. Forgiveness is eventually available. The intermittent love will be given again."

At this point, we must try to understand the meaning of the suicide attempt. Three possibilities must be considered: The patient (1) wants relief from suffering; (2) wants to punish himself; or (3) attempts to kill the introjected person (parent or spouse).

The first two possibilities are self-contradictory or self-exclusive until seen from the standpoint of the emotional state of the patient. The feeling that it is better to die than to suffer so much is certainly experienced. The patient would not carry out the suicidal ideas, however, if these ideas were not reinforced or sustained by the other idea that he deserves to die and that he must inflict on himself the supreme punishment. Thus, these two motiva-

tions, logically self-contradictory, coexist, and reinforce each other.

The more orthodox Freudian interpretation holds that suicide represents the attempt to kill the detested incorporated person.

According to our original interpretation of the psychological growth of the child in accordance with Buber's concepts of I and Thou, it appears that the manic-depressive patient, much more than the normal person, has accepted the Thou since his early infancy. At times, he let the Thou suffocate or smother the I. In this light, the suicidal attempt is the culmination of this process: It is the Thou who finally kills the I, not the I who kills the Thou. If the I would kill the Thou, there would be a complete and sudden reversal of the previous and constant trend of denial of the self. Rado[63] has ingeniously tried to solve the problem by assuming that the superego (the Thou) is divided into two parts, one which the patient wants to love, and one which the patient wants to kill. I am convinced, however, that, at least in my personal clinical experience, the patient really wanted to kill himself. By killing himself, he achieved a complete acceptance or a complete introjection of a distorted image of the Thou.

There are several other factors that support this point of view. First of all, many cases of suicide seem to occur not when the state of melancholia is at its peak but at an early stage of remission, when the worst is over. This characteristic may, of course, be interpreted in various ways. The first explanation is a simple and mechanical one. When the patient is very depressed, in, or almost in, stupor, he cannot act, is extremely slow or immobile, cannot move or think co-ordinatedly, and therefore cannot carry out his intentions. When he becomes less retarded, more capable of co-ordinating his thoughts, he goes ahead with his destructive intention. There is the alternative possibility that the patient, who has gone through terrible experiences at the acme of the depression, is afraid that these experiences may recur and, rather than face them again, he prefers to die (this, of course, corresponds to the first possibility mentioned).

Yet, neither of these interpretations seems

adequate in my opinion. It seems more likely that the patient feels that even the depth of depression has not been enough, has not succeeded in relieving him entirely of his guilt feeling, and that only by killing himself will he entirely redeem himself.

This interpretation is supported by other factors. Significantly, there is almost complete relief after the suicide attempt, whereas the Freudian interpretation would lead one to expect an increase in guilt feeling (for having attempted to, but not actually succeeded in, killing the superego) and a consequent increase in depression. As Weiss[76] and others have emphasized, in the attempt itself, that is, in the gambling with death, the patient feels that he has been punished adequately. He has done what the Thou wanted and now he can live peacefully. Often, of course, there is no need for the suicide attempt; after having gone through the acme of the depression, the patient feels suddenly relieved, and a marked improvement occurs.*

According to Kolb,[45] "The suicidal maneuver is often determined by family indicated permission for acting out." In his clinical experience, the psychodynamic explanation for acting out which has been given for other antisocial acts is valid also for suicide. "In families where suicide has occurred the likelihood of suicide for the manic-depressive patient is much higher than otherwise. Where suicide has not occurred, one usually finds threats of suicide or intimidating actions suggesting suicide on the part of parents."

The relief experienced by the patient after the acute depression is remarkable. The patient feels guilt-free and accepted, and wants to settle down in his own life. Even reality seems pleasant now; he does not want to be alone; he feels that he wants to be close to his mate. This attempt, however, will not work out unless psychotherapy intervenes. Other attacks of depression are not acute and tend to assume a chronic course, unless successful therapy intervenes or the circumstances of life change radically.

As we have mentioned earlier, in the claim-

ing type of depression the suicidal attempt seems to convey the message, "Do not abandon me. You have the power to prevent my death. You will feel guilty if you don't give me what I need and let me die." If we remember the involved psychodynamic mechanisms, it will be easy to recognize that in claiming depression the patient is still claiming the lost paradise or the state of bliss of the early life, when he was completely dependent on the duty-bound mother. The patient makes himself dependent on the dominant other and becomes more and more demanding the more deprived he feels. Any unfulfilled demand is experienced as a wound, a loss, and brings about depression.

The attack of psychotic depression, like every other psychotic defense, offers not a solution but a pseudosolution. When the patient cannot find relief with the end of the depression, he may, in order to avert the danger of recurrence, develop hypomanic traits which may eventually explode into a complete manic attack. We then have the typical circular psychosis. The manic attack thus must also be considered a defense against the depression. But in the manic attack the Thou is not eliminated or projected to the external world; it is only disregarded. The patient must continue to force himself into a distracted and frenzied mood, which shuts out introspection. In the manic state, there is no elimination of the Freudian superego, as perhaps there is in some psychopathics. The superego remains, and the manic frenzy is a method of dealing with it.

But neither the depression nor the manic state actually brings about a solution to the deeply rooted conflicts. Even after having paid the penalty of the psychotic attack, the patient, after a more or less free interval, will tend to be affected again with the same difficulties, which will be channeled in the same patterns, and the cycle will repeat itself.

Until the late 1950s, psychiatrists treated patients who, after having experienced one or more attacks of affective psychosis, developed a typical schizophrenic symptomatology. These cases still occur, but since the early 1960s they have become less common. In these

---

* For further discussion of suicide, see Chapter 33 of this volume.

cases, psychodynamic analyses indicate that there were always some projective tendencies present along with strong introjective tendencies. Once the manic-depressive mechanism has failed, the individual resorts to the projective mechanisms, which until then had occupied only a secondary role. In some cases, these schizophrenic symptoms consist only of delusional, persecutory trends, and they are not in themselves of grave prognostic meaning, but if a typical hebephrenic picture ensues, the prognosis is serious.

As is mentioned in Chapter 24, the opposite sequence prevails today. An increasing number of cases, which had presented a typical schizophrenic symptomatology at the onset of the disorder, develop later a syndrome of depression.

(Depression as a Feeling and as a Mechanism

We have so far attempted to retrace the psychodynamic developments that lead to depression (or more seldom elation), but we have not yet studied the question why depression is the outcome of these developments. In other words, what is the phenomenon of depression itself and why does the psyche experience it after the sequence of the events that we have described? Books of psychiatry generally fail to explain what depression is or they take for granted that the student, having experienced at times depression in his own life, has a certain knowledge of it. Of course, we all experience depression at times. Depression may be a normal emotion, a symptom, or a clinical entity. Some authors refer only to depression or melancholia when the emotion is considered abnormal. They use the terms "sadness," "dejection," "low spirits," and "anguish" when the depression is normal or supposed to be normal. It is obvious that all these emotional states are related, even if they vary in degree, and even if some are considered normal and others abnormal. It is obvious that it will be difficult to understand abnormal depression (or melancholia) if we do not

know what normal depression (or sadness) is.

Although practically all human beings have at some time experienced depression, this emotional state is among the most difficult to describe and to analyze.[7] It is a pervading feeling of unpleasantness accompanied by such somatic conditions as numbness, paresthesias of the skin, alterations of muscle tone, and decreases in respiration, pulsation, and perspiration. The head of the depressed person has the tendency to bend; the legs flex; the trunk tilts forward. The face assumes a special expression because of increased wrinkles and decreased mimic play. There is also retardation of movements, rigidity in thinking, and a general feeling of weakness. These characteristics vary in intensity, of course, from very mild to very pronounced, in accordance with the degree of the depression.

It is, however, at the mental rather than the somatic level that depression has more specific characteristics. Whereas anxiety is characterized by an expectancy of danger, depression is accompanied by a feeling that the dangerous event has already occurred, that the loss has already been sustained. For instance, a cherished love or a deep friendship has been destroyed, a loved person has died, a good position has been taken away, a business venture has failed, an acceptable image of the self can no longer be maintained, an ideal has been dismissed. If the feeling is one of pure and profound depression and is not mixed with anxiety, there is also a more or less marked sense of despair, of unpleasant finality, as if the loss could not be remedied. The loss is deemed to have repercussions on the present as well as the future.

From these examples it is evident that, at least in conditions considered normal, depression follows other psychological processes, such as evaluations and appraisals. Cognitive processes, generally some ideas or clusters of ideas, have preceded depression.

Such considerations would make depression a uniquely human emotion, different from more primitive emotions, such as fear, rage, and some forms of anxiety that occur also in much lower animals. This point, of course, is debatable. Inasmuch as animals cannot verbalize their feelings, it is an open question whether or not the belief that animals become depressed is an anthropomorphization. A dog, for instance, may appear depressed when his master is away, but it is doubtful that this is either a feeling involving the future or a sense of loss that transcends the immediate discomfort. A feeling of deprivation rather than despair seems to be involved here. On the other hand, these uncomfortable feelings of deprivation, which even animals are capable of experiencing, may be the precursors of human depression.[7] Depression must have a significance and possibly a special function in the fabric of the psychological organism. If depression had only or predominantly negative survival value, species capable of experiencing it probably would not have procreated themselves in the course of evolution. Other emotions have survival value.[6] Anxiety, for instance, is a warning of forthcoming danger.

What is the biological meaning of depression? Depression or anguish is mental pain, an experience to which the name pain is often given because of the similarity to physical pain. It is not implied here that depression is the only form of mental pain, but that it is the most typical, and that it is the evolutionary outcome at a human symbolic-interpersonal level of the biologic nociceptive pain.

Physical pain is a sensation which informs the conscious organism that a loss to the continuity of the proper functioning of the body has taken place. By being unpleasant, pain becomes a warning that something is wrong. It becomes a signal that a discontinuity of the integrity of the organism has occurred and may increase unless the animal removes the source of pain. Pain is thus a translation of an abnormal state of the organism into a subjective experience. In lower species, an attempt at removal of pain is made by withdrawal from the source of pain. In higher species, especially in man, a voluntary action generally attempts to remove the source of pain, so that the regenerative potentialities of the organism will permit healing. We may see something similar in that form of mental pain, depression. The depression follows the appreciation of a loss of what we consider a normal and generally important ingredient of our psychological life.

For example, an individual hears the news of the unexpected death of a person he loved. After he has understood and almost instantaneously evaluated what that death means to him, he experiences shock, then sadness. For a few days, all thoughts connected with the deceased person will bring about a painful, almost unbearable feeling. Any group of thoughts even remotely connected with the dead person will elicit depression. The individual cannot adjust to the idea that the loved person does not live any more. And, since that person was so important to him, many of his thoughts or actions will be directly or indirectly connected with the dead person and therefore will elicit sad reactions.

Nevertheless, after a certain period of time, that individual adjusts to the idea that the person is dead. By being unpleasant, the depression seems to have a function—its own elimination. It will be removed only if the individual is forced to reorganize his thinking, to search for new ideas so that he can rearrange his life. He must rearrange especially those ideas that are connected with the departed, so that the departed will no longer be considered indispensable. Like pain, depression thus stimulates a change in order to be removed, but it is a psychological change, an ideational change, a rearrangement of thoughts, and clusters of thoughts. Eventually, the actions of the individual, too, will alter as a consequence of this cognitive rearrangement.

Depression, however, is not always a normal emotion. Its importance in the field of psychiatry is probably second only to another emotion, anxiety. Depression is deemed abnormal when it is excessive relative to the antecedent event or events that have elicited it; when it is inappropriate in relation to its known cause or precipitating factor; when it is a substitution for a more appropriate emotion, for instance, when it takes the place of hostility or anxiety; or when it does not seem to have been caused by any antecedent factor of which the person is aware.

In abnormal depression, the process of cognitive change and reorganization, mentioned in relation to normal depression, fails. Another process occurs which brings about several degrees of pathology. The depression, rather than forcing a reorganization of ideas, slows down the thought processes. In this case, the psychological mechanism seems to have the purpose of decreasing the quantity of thoughts in order to decrease the quantity of suffering. At times, the slowing down of thought processes is so pronounced (as in the state of stupor) that only a few thoughts of a general or atmospheric quality are left; these are accompanied by an overpowering feeling of melancholy. Thus, the slowing down of thought processes is a self-defeating mechanism. A vicious circle is produced which aggravates the condition. The decrease in motility, formed in the psychotic depressed, is secondary to the slowing down of thought processes, so that even the ideomotor activity, preceding movements and actions, is decreased.

When the depression becomes overwhelming, it seems to possess the whole psyche, to leave no room for ideas or thinking. The patient reduces his thinking to a minimum. He becomes aware only of the overpowering feeling of depression. As a matter of fact, if we ask the patient why he is depressed, he may say that he does not know. In patients who have recurring depressions, severe or even moderate in intensity, often the ideas or thoughts that have triggered off the depression become almost immediately submerged by the depression. They become unconscious, and the patient is not able to say why he is depressed. Some patients say things like the following: "I woke up this morning, and I was immediately overpowered by an intense feeling of depression." In these cases, the depression has, among others, the function that repression has in other psychiatric conditions. Perhaps, it is a special type of repression; the cognitive part is repressed, but the painful feeling is very intensely experienced at the level of consciousness.

Another type of defense that the individual may resort to in the presence of depressive thoughts is the escape into action and fugitive thoughts. This defense is available in typical manic-depressive patients, who, although they do not have clear-cut manic episodes, go through periods of hyperactivity. This defense, which is not as frequent as the deep depression just described, is the formal counterpart of the outer-directed, hypomanic-like, or merely cyclothymic personality. This defense may be so effective as to prevent the occurrence of the psychosis throughout the life of the patient. Thoughts must be very fugitive, must be changed very rapidly, because any constellation of organized thoughts about practically any topic sooner or later brings about the depression. Pleasant thoughts are searched for; actions that may replace ideas are sought.

The patient resorts to this defense either in order to prevent the depression or in order to escape from the depression (as when he slips from the melancholic into the manic state).

At times, he succeeds in using this defense in an acceptable, or at least tolerable way, retaining, or even increasing, normal abilities. The ability to recall masses of detail, shown by some hypomanic patients when reporting their experiences, may be useful if channeled into activities that require accurate descriptions. Often, however, the wealth of details is useless and irritating. The escape into words, into social symbolism, and into observation of reality almost to a photographic level is obvious.

The following are some excerpts from a woman's conversation during a hypomanic interval: (She has had three previous psychotic depressions.)

"The telephone rang; it was the doctor who treated my husband, Dr. B. He told me that I should go to see him right away. I put on my spring coat. It must have been spring, as I remember, because I wore the spring coat. The doctor lived a few blocks away in an apartment in the Hotel Plaza. I went there, took the elevator. They lived at the fourth floor, fourth or fifth. I don't think it makes much difference. I rang the bell. The wife came to open the door. She is such a short woman, and her husband, the doctor, is so tall. . . ."

These details were, of course, useless and irrelevant to the goal of the conversation. Logicalness, however, was retained. Similar behavior may be tolerated. Often, however, when the looming depression is very intense, the patient must resort to more pronounced manic mechanisms.

The foregoing exposition may create the impression that the manic pleasure consists only in the escape from depression, in the removal of the negative. Not every pleasure, however, is the removal of the negative, or a decrease in the tension that produced pain; it is my impression that the manic does not try only to escape from the pain of depression but to gain by extending or enlarging his contacts with the world. Such contacts must remain superficial, however, if depressing connections are to be avoided. A further consideration is the fact that pain elicits in the organism a reaction of *moving away* from the source. At the level of human depression, no movement or moving away is visible, because the moving away is only from depressive thoughts (unless, as we have seen before, the depression is very intense). In pleasure, there is not only a moving away from the source of pain but also a *moving toward* the object which will confer pleasure. And the increased motility of the manic must be considered as an attempt to *move toward* the source of pleasure.

The manic mechanisms, however, fail on account of their pathologic proportions. In order to avoid unpleasant constellations, thoughts must be so rapid that they cannot be organized or, therefore, capable of achieving rewarding actions. The pleasant ideas cannot be sustained and eventually leave the patient with the realization that they are futile. When the manic fervor is exhausted or cannot be sustained any longer, depression ensues or returns.

It is still not clear why some patients are able to avail themselves of the manic defenses and others are not. Perhaps constitutional, cultural, and dynamic factors play roles that cannot yet be ascertained. Studying the literature, however, one gets the impression that in so-called primitive cultures the manic attacks are much more numerous than the depressions.

The incidence of manic attacks is much lower than that of depressions, and many writers today feel that one cannot classify as manic-depressive the many patients who undergo depressions but never have a manic attack.

More conservative psychiatrists, however, tend to retain the manic-depressive syndrome as a unit, a position that can be justified on the grounds that our understanding of its partial manifestations is increased by our acceptance of its unitary concept.

([The Study of Affective Psychoses from the Point of View of Sociocultural Psychiatry

Affective psychoses offer a special field of inquiry for social and cultural psychiatry because of two clinical variations that seem correlated to changes in the sociocultural environment.

The first variation consists of a marked decrease in recent times in the incidence of typical manic-depressive psychosis. The second variation is represented by the increasing frequence of the claiming type of depression, and the relative decrease of the traditional self-blaming type. We shall consider these two phenomena separately.

The decline in frequency of typical manic-depressive psychosis is reflected also by a decline of interest among psychiatrists in the condition. Whereas at the time of Kraepelin this psychosis received an amount of consideration equal, or almost equal, to that of dementia praecox, a relative but progressive disinterest has gradually been evident in the last few decades. Books and articles continue to be written,[10,11,20,34,35,36,48,56,58,59] but schizophrenia appears much more often in the literature, particularly in the United States.

Practicing psychiatrists justify their decrease of interest with the statement that they encounter this disorder much less frequently. The statistics seem to support this observation, made at a clinical level. In 1928, in New York, there were ten first hospital admissions of manic-depressive patients per 100,000 inhabitants; in 1947, this incidence decreased to 3.7 per 100,000. The percentage of first admissions of manic-depressive psychosis in 1928 was 13.5 percent of all admissions; in 1947, the percentage was reduced to 3.8. Similar statistical trends are obtained in most of the other states. The statistics point out a definite decrease of this psychosis, but their interpretation is difficult because, as in all cases of psychiatric vital statistics, there are many variables involved. Bellak[11] offers three possible explanations: (1) an actual lessening of the relative frequency of this disease; (2) greater toleration by the healthy population of milder cases of manic-depressive psychosis; and (3) changing diagnostic trends.

To these three hypotheses a fourth can be added. New therapeutic methods administered at the beginning of the illness produce such improvement or recovery that the patients do not need to be hospitalized. One thinks here in particular of electric shock treatment, which is capable of rapidly ending a manic-depressive attack. But this hypothesis will not withstand close examination. The first reports on electric shock by Cerletti and Bini appeared in 1938. Electric shock was introduced into the United States in 1939 but did not receive wide application, especially in private offices with nonhospitalized patients, until 1942–1943. The statistics indicate, on the other hand, that the decline in first admissions of manic-depressive psychoses started in 1928. What I have said in reference to electric shock treatment could be reported with even more emphasis about antidepressant drug therapy or lithium therapy in manic cases, which were introduced long after a marked decrease in affective psychosis had taken place.

There are some factors that tend to weaken Bellak's third hypothesis, that changing diagnostic trends are completely responsible for this decrease. It is correct that many patients with a mixed symptomatology today are classified not as manic-depressives but as cases of reactive depression, senile depression, schizophrenia, obsessive-compulsive psychoneurosis, etc. The pertinent question here is, Why are we reluctant to make the diagnosis of manic-depressive psychosis?

It can be argued justifiably that this reluctance is not merely caprice but is determined by the fact that in many cases today the manic-depressive features play only a secondary role, whereas in the past they played the predominant one. We have already mentioned that an increase has recently been noticed of cases in which depression follows a typical initial schizophrenic symptomatology. In these cases, obviously, preference is given to the initial, and much more marked, symptomatology. Moreover, often schizophrenic residues are detectable in these cases even when the depressive features prevail.

Relevant information has been gathered in other parts of the world. Gold[33] found a relatively larger incidence of manic-depressive than schizophrenic psychoses in the lands of the Mediterranean basin, as well as in Ireland. He reported that in Oriental countries, especially where Hinduism and Buddhism prevail, manic-depresive psychosis again becomes much less common, but in the Fiji Islands manic-depressive patients are numerous. He wrote further that, whereas in India the incidence of manic-depressive psychosis is low and that of schizophrenia higher, the reverse is true for the Indians who have emigrated to Fiji. While I was visiting mental hospitals in Italy immediately after World War II, I had the impression that classical or pure manic-depressive patients were more numerous there than in the United States. The official statistics in Italy corroborated this clinical impression. In 1949, in the United States, the rate of admissions was 4.7 for manic-depressive psychosis and 16.1 for schizophrenia; in Italy, it was 10.0 for manic-depressive psychosis and 8.2 for schizophrenia.* Italian psychiatrists, however, state that since the late 1940s, in

* Italian statistics were kindly provided by Professor Francesco Bonfiglio of Rome. To be exact, first admissions of schizophrenics in Italy totaled 3,541 in the year 1947, 3,780 in the year 1948, and 3,854 in 1949. First admissions of manic-depressive totaled 4,298 in 1947, 4,562 in 1948, and 4,791 in 1949. The rate of admission per 100,000 represents the annual average of the triennial period 1947–1949.

Italy, too, manic-depressive psychosis has decreased in number, especially the manic type, approximately by now as much as in the United States.

Another important point to consider concerning diagnostic trends is whether the differentiation of such categories as "involutional paranoid state" and "involutional melancholia" is responsible for the statistical differences. In other words, patients previously diagnosed as manic-depressive may now be diagnosed as suffering from the involutional syndromes. Here, again, it is difficult to evaluate all the factors. Previously, involutional patients might have been diagnosed as paranoid conditions, paraphrenia, etc. It is only in the case of pure involutional melancholia that competition with the diagnosis of manic-depressive psychosis exists. It is doubtful whether the cases of pure involutional melancholia, if added to the official figures of manic-depressive psychosis, would reverse the apparent decline or explain the great difference existing today, between the rate of first admissions of schizophrenia and that of manic-depressive psychosis. Again, the trend is demonstrated sharply by the statistics. Bellak reports that, of first admissions to New York State hospitals for the year ending March 1947, 27.7 percent were diagnosed as dementia praecox, 7.0 percent as involutional psychosis, and 3.8 percent as manic-depressive psychosis. (Involutional and manic-depressive combined were 10.8 percent.)

The second hypothesis of Bellak, that the healthy population has more tolerance for milder cases, is difficult to accept. Bellak states that the "full-of-pep-and-energy" salesman type of person is now an accepted type. He is correct, but, in spite of some similarities, this person corresponds not to the cyclothymic hypomanic who is liable to become manic-depressive, but rather to the "marketing personality" of Fromm[31] and the "other-directed" person of Riesman.[66]

These observations and considerations seem to lead to the conclusion offered by Bellak's first hypothesis that the decline in the number of manic-depressive patients is real rather than apparent. Statistics further indicate that if the same trends continue in the United States, manic-depressive psychosis may disappear entirely or reappear later in a near or distant future. Although this decline is not universal, it seems to affect many countries, especially Western countries, but not with the same speed.

It seems apparent that a clear understanding of the reasons for this decline can lead to conclusions relevant to the fields of mental hygiene in particular, and of psychiatry in general. In order to understand this, we must resort to social psychiatry, that discipline which, as Rennie[65] has defined it, "is concerned not only with facts of prevalence and incidence . . . [but] searches more deeply into the possible significance of social and cultural factors in the etiology and dynamics of mental disorder."

There may be a relation between what Riesman calls the "inner-directed" personality and culture, and manic-depressive psychosis. When this type of personality and culture tend to disappear, this psychosis tends also to disappear.

Riesman explains the establishment of the inner-directed society as the result of demographic and political changes. At certain times in history, a rapid growth of population determines a diminution of material goods and a psychology of scarcity. Although this type of society has existed several times in history, we are particularly concerned with the recurrence which had its beginning at the time of the Renaissance and the Reformation. As Fromm[30] noted, at that time the security that the individual enjoyed in the Middle Ages by virtue of membership in his closed-class system was lost, and he was left alone on his own effort. The religious doctrines of Luther and, indirectly, Calvin, gave the individual the feeling that everything depended on his own efforts. Deeply felt concepts of responsibility, duty, guilt, and punishment, which, up to that time had been confined to a few religious men, acquired general acceptance and tremendous significance and came to color every manifestation of life. This type of culture, which originated during the Renaissance and developed during the Reformation, sooner or later permeated all Western countries; only recently has it faced replacement by another type of culture, the "other-directed." In some countries, such as the United States, this replacement is taking place at a rapid rate; in others, it is taking place more slowly.

In the "inner-directed" society, the parent is duty-bound and much concerned with the care of the newborn child. It is this duty-bound care and the ensuing burdening of the child with responsibilities and the sense of duty and guilt that may permit the child to develop the strong introjective tendencies that play such a prominent role in the development of manic-depressive psychoses.

The similarities between the pattern of life of the manic-depressive patient and the typical "inner-directed" person are apparent.

1. Very early in the life of the child, the parent is duty-bound and gives such tremendous care to the child as to determine in the latter strong introjective tendencies.

2. A drastic change will occur later when the child is burdened with responsibility. This change will produce the trauma of the paradise lost.

3. The individual feels responsible for any possible loss. He reacts by becoming compliant, working hard, and harboring strong feelings of guilt. Life becomes a purgatory. (At this point many manic-depressive patients deviate from the "inner-directed" personality, as they develop instead an excessively dependent or a hypomanic-like outer-directed personality.)

4. This tremendously burdened life leads to depressive trends, or to inactivity which leads to guilt feelings, or as a reaction, to activity which appears futile. These negative states and feelings are misinterpreted as proof of one's unworthiness, and reactivate the expectancy of losing the paradise again, this time forever. A vicious circle is thus formed.

Other social studies point out a relation which is more than coincidental between manic-depressive psychosis and "inner-directed" society. The research by Eaton and Weil[23],[24] on the Hutterites may throw additional weight behind this hypothesis, although these authors do not speak of "inner-directed" society. The Hutterites are a group of people of German ancestry who settled in the Dakotas, Montana, and the prairie provinces of Canada. Their life is very much concerned with religion, and their birth rate is very high, the average family having ten children. This type of society seems to be a typically "inner-directed" one. In a population of 8,542 people, Eaton and Weil found only nine persons who some time in their life had been suffering from schizophrenia and thirty–nine who had been suffering from manic-depressive psychosis. In other words, among the Hutterites, manic-depressive psychosis was 4.33 times more frequent than schizophrenia, whereas in the general population of the United States the incidence of schizophrenia by far exceeded that of manic-depressive psychosis.

The "inner-directed" society actually offers a high degree of security to the individual, for it leaves his fate in his own hands rather than in the control of mysterious, omnipotent, and unpredictable forces. Thus, obviously, I do not mean to suggest that the "inner-directed" culture is "the cause of" manic-depressive psychosis; rather, I speculate that this type of culture tends, in certain cases, to elicit family configurations and interpersonal conflicts that are generally those that lead to manic-depressive psychosis. What is supported here is a psychosocial or biosocial position similar to that expounded by Opler[60] and by Lemkau and his collaborators.[50]

Additional cultural factors either add to or detract from the importance of the structure of the society in the formation of various disease entities. Immigration to a foreign country, with consequent problems of maladjustment, seems to elicit a propensity toward this as well as other psychiatric disorders. Some additional explanation for the various incidences of manic-depressive psychosis may be found in epidemiologic studies.

In 1939, Faris and Dunham[28] published a study, *Mental Disorders in Urban Areas*, in which they found that while schizophrenia is prevalent in the central areas of the cities of Chicago and Providence—that is, in areas of social disorganization (where delinquency, crime, prostitution, and drug addiction are also frequent)—and gradually declines in number toward the outskirts of the city, no definite pattern of distribution was found for the cases of manic-depressive psychosis.

The contrast between the ecological distribution of manic-depressive psychosis and schizophrenia was so marked that Faris and Dunham saw in it another proof of the distinct nature of the two disorders. Faris and Dunham believed that precipitating factors probably have a more important causal relation to manic-depressive psychosis than to other disorders. We have seen that precipitating factors are undoubtedly important in manic-depressive psychosis. On the other hand, it is my impression that manic-depressive psychosis is not necessarily connected with a milieu that offers "extremely intimate and intense social contacts," but rather with a structural, well-organized "inner-directed" milieu, removed from the disorganization or relative looseness of organization that we find either in some "other-directed" societies or, for entirely different reasons, in low economic or socially unstable elements of the population.

A difference in the occurrence of the two major psychoses is also illustrated by the size of the communities involved. The highest proportion of manic-depressives comes from cities of 100,000 to 200,000 population and from rural areas, whereas the largest proportion of schizophrenic cases comes from metropolitan or urban areas.[58]

Other studies seen to point out that the economic level of the manic-depressive tends to be higher than that of the schizophrenic. It is debatable, however, whether the low economic condition of the latter is related to the effect of, rather than to the etiology of, the disorder. Manic-depressives are affected by their condition later in life and less seriously.

In sum, there is much presumptive evidence that ecological, cultural, and social factors are important in either engendering or at least predisposing to manic-depressive psychosis.

We have observed in relation to affective psychoses the increase of the claiming type depression and the decrease of the self-blaming type. Of course, what we have discussed in reference to the decline of manic-depressive psychosis applies in particular to the self-blaming type. It cannot be necessarily repeated for the claiming type. A person who tends to rely on others for autonomous gratification is also a person who may be "other-directed," a person who since early childhood has resorted to the external environment for most kinds of stimulation and has been less prone to internalize or conceive distant values and goals. In my book, *The Will To Be Human*,[9] I describe how the most pronounced forms of this type of personality are not just "other-directed." They are immediacy-directed. Inasmuch as they cannot be in touch with any sustaining inner life, I consider them as suffering from a special type of alienation not previously described. They search excessive external stimulation; they do not even conform, they respond. They are at the mercy of the environment. When they feel deprived, they become depressed, especially if early in life they had undergone traumas that had sensitized them to losses.

⟮ Choice of Therapy

The treatment of affective psychoses should be considered under four headings: (1) psychotherapy; (2) hospitalization; (3) drug therapy; (4) shock therapy. A discussion of the last three will be confined to a few general remarks, since they are discussed extensively in Volume 5 of this Handbook. Here we will consider primarily the psychotherapeutic approach.

Hospitalization must be considered especially when there is danger of suicide. However, we must realize that a suicidal risk exists in practically every patient suffering from a psychotic form of depression. It is up to the psychiatrist to determine whether the risk is great, moderate, or minimal, and there are no infallible methods to make such distinction. If the danger is deemed great and the patient cannot be under proper surveillance at home, hospitalization becomes necessary. Often it is more difficult to convince the relatives than the patient that he should be hospitalized. The depressed patient, perhaps in a masochistic spirit, at times is ready to enter the hospital, whereas the relatives would prefer to send him on vacation. It is more difficult to hospitalize a manic, as he himself prefers to take trips and to escape into actions. When the risk is moderate or minimal, the decision is more difficult. At times the risk is worth taking in view of the fact that long psychotherapy is not possible in the hospital (with some exceptions), and that the possibility of suicide is not completely eliminated even in a hospital setting. Moreover, in some cases a certain amount of risk remains for an indefinite but prolonged period of time, because the patient does not benefit from any type of therapy; he would thus have to be hospitalized for an indefinite period of time with great damage to his self-image and increased feeling of hopelessness. All these possibilities, of course, should be discussed openly with the members of the family. The responsibility for the decision must be made in a spirit of collaboration and possible unanimity among patient, family, and therapist.

Drug therapy at times diminishes the risk of suicide, but in my experience is not sufficient in most cases to cure affective psychoses even from the manifest symptomatology. Lithium therapy, however, often produces good results in manic attacks.

Electric shock therapy is very efficient in terminating many (but not all) acute and subacute attacks of severe depression. At times, merely a few electric shock treatments are sufficient to produce a temporary recovery from a depression. A manic attack may require a longer course, and the result is more uncertain than the one obtained with lithium.

In my opinion, these physical therapies do not change the basic personality of the patient. The fundamental problems remain unsolved, although they may be forgotten or poorly integrated because of the effects of electric shock treatment. Drug therapy makes the patient less sensitive to his depression or elation; but the potentiality for affective disorders remains, once the therapy is discontinued.

Psychotherapy, if successful, will prove to be the best type of treatment, because it will change the psychological prerequisites for the disorder. On the other hand, psychotherapy, too, has many disadvantages: (1) in extremely severe cases, where the patient is in stupor or near stupor, it may be difficult to establish contact or to elicit an atmosphere of participation necessary for the treatment; (2) the risk of suicide is often great and the patient cannot be allowed to go to the therapist (unless, of course, psychotherapy is given in a hospital setting or the patient is accompanied by a reliable person).

Psychotherapy should be instituted also in (1) patients whose acute attacks have ended spontaneously; (2) patients who have received convulsive treatment, as soon as the organic effects of the treatment, such as forgetfulness, mild confusion, etc., have decreased in intensity.

Psychotherapy

Psychotherapy of affective psychoses is still in the pioneer stage. It is true that depression has been treated with psychotherapy for a long time, but generally in cases which had not reached the psychotic level. It is also true that unlike schizophrenia, psychotic depression has been treated psychoanalytically relatively early in the history of psychoanalysis. However, these cases have been very few and have as a rule been treated in the intervals during the attacks of depression. Manic attacks have been treated with uncertain results by psychoanalytic and existentialist therapists.

The intensity of the depression should not deter the therapist from making psychotherapeutic attempts. Certainly, it is difficult to make contact with a depressed person but not impossible.

Contrary to what happens in schizophrenia, where the psychosis is a consequence to a failure of cosmic magnitude, involving as a rule the relation with the whole interpersonal world, the failure of the depressed patient is experienced mainly or exclusively in relation to what we have previously designated as the dominant other.[6] It is one of the first tasks of the therapist to detect and study the failure of this relation.

We have seen that the dominant other is generally a person, most often the spouse, less often the mother, a person to whom the patient is romantically attached, an adult child, a sister, the father. We have also seen that the dominant other at times is not a person but a group of persons, like the family as a whole, the firm where he works, or an organization to which he belongs. This changed relation with the dominant other produces or precipitates a sense of loss, which triggers off the depression. The dominant other, who used to nourish the patient with approval, love, guidance, or hope, is no longer there, either because he has died, dissolved, or is seen by the patient in a different light.

When the therapist enters the life of a very depressed person and proves his genuine desire to help, to reach, to nourish, to offer certainty or at least hope, he will often be accepted, but only as a *dominant third*. Immediate relief may be obtained, because the patient sees in the therapist a new and reliable love-object. Although the establishment of this type of relatedness may be helpful to the subsequent therapy, it cannot be considered a real cure; as a matter of fact, it may be followed by another attack of depression when the patient realizes the limitation of this type of therapeutic situation.

The therapist must be not a *dominant third*, but a *significant third*—a third person, in addition to the patient and the dominant other, a third person with a forceful, sincere, and unambiguous type of personality, who wants to help the patient without making threatening demands.

In the case of a predominantly self-blaming type of depression, the relation with the dominant other has to be studied, especially in some aspects described in previous sections of this chapter. The dominant other quite often, because of repressed hostility or because of perfectionistic, ultramoralistic, or obsessive-compulsive attitudes, unwittingly increases the patient's feeling of guilt, duty, and denial of himself. Such sentences as "You are too sick to do the housework now," or, "For many years you took care of me; now I take care of you" increase the guilt feeling of the patient. With the permission of the patient, in some cases it is important to discuss with the dominant other several environmental changes and the climate of the relationship, in order to relieve as much as possible the patient's feeling of unbearable yoke, guilt, responsibility, unaccomplishment, loss.

On the other hand, we must clarify to the patient that he did not know how to live for himself. He never listened to himself, he was never able to assert himself, but cared only about obtaining the approval, affection, love, admiration, or care of the dominant other.

As we have already mentioned, the dominant other is not necessarily a person, but in some cases may be the whole family or a special group or organization. The patient must be guided by the significant third on how to live for whatever meaning he wants to give to his life, and not just in order to obtain the gratifying psychological supply from the dominant other.

If the therapist succeeds in making some indentations in the patient's psyche, several developments may occur. The patient may become less depressed, but angry either at the dominant other or the therapist, whom he would like to transform into a dominant third. The anger and hostility toward the dominant other (most frequently the spouse), is at times out of proportion. Once repressed or unconscious ideations come to the surface, the dominant other may be seen as a tyrant, a domineering person who has subjugated the patient. At this point, the therapist has a difficult task in clarifying the issues involved. At times, the dominant other has been really overdemanding and even domineering, taking advantage of the placating, compliant qualities of the patient. Often, however, it is the patient himself who, by being unable to assert himself and by complying excessively, has allowed certain patterns of life to develop and persist. Now, when he wants to change these patterns, he attributes the responsibility for them to the dominant other. No real recovery is possible unless the patient understands the role that he himself has played in creating the climate and pattern of submissiveness.

We have so far referred to the patient as "he" and we shall continue to do so. However, we must remind the reader that almost two-thirds of these patients are women, and if the language required referring to the most common sex involved, we would use the pronoun "she." Perhaps, society will change and the so-called woman's liberation movement will alter the cultural climate or at least the frequency of certain developments. At the present time, the prevailing patriarchal character of our society makes it easier for a woman to assume the attitude of dependency on a male dominant other, or even on a female dominant other. By tradition, many more women than men have overtly or in subtle ways been trained to depend on others for support, approval, appreciation. Some of them actually live a vicarious life.

The fact that society and culture have facilitated these developments does not exonerate the female patient from recognizing the role she has played. By omission or commission, the patient has, so to say, allowed the dominant other to assume that specific position in her life. Many husbands, certainly helped by the prevailing patriarchal character of society, are not even aware of having played the role of dominant other. When they come to such realization, they may try to deny certain facts, are busy in defending themselves as if they had been accused, and may require psychotherapy (or family therapy together with the patient). The same remarks can be made, although less frequently, for dominant others, other than husbands.

The realization of these factors on the part of the patient does not yet relieve the depression, although in most cases it diminishes it. Generally, the patient continues to be depressed because he broods (1) over what he did not have; (2) has a feeling of self-betrayal (by accommodating to the dominant other, he

has not been true to himself); (3) has some sort of realization that many gratifications he desired in life had to be given up; (4) has a feeling of hopelessness about remedying or retrieving what he has lost, the opportunities he did not grasp.

As mentioned earlier, ideas of this type are not kept in consciousness for a long time. The ensuing depression covers up these cognitive components. The therapist must train the patient to catch himself in the act of having these ideas, or in an attitude in which he expects to be or to become depressed. If he becomes aware of these ideas and of expecting to be consequently depressed, he may stop the depression from occurring, or at least from reaching the previous intensity. Then, he must, of course, discuss with the therapist these depression-prone cognitive components. If the patient understands that he had a role in this dynamic complex, he will abandon a state of helplessness and hopelessness. In the present and in the future, he may act differently and learn to assert himself and to obtain what is really meaningful to him and gratifying. Any feeling of loss or disappointment is no longer translated into self-accusation and/or guilt.

Obviously, he must, with the help of the therapist, change his ways of living and interrelating with the dominant other. The patient cannot devote his life to the dominant other or live vicariously through him. On the other hand, the patient may be afraid of going overboard, of being too hostile and angry at the dominant other. However, this stage will be also outgrown when the dominant other will be recognized to be not as the patient consciously or unconsciously used to see him in recent years, but as the early childhood situation has made the patient envision him. In other words, the trauma over the alleged or real loss of love, sustained in childhood, and the mechanisms adopted in the attempt to re-obtain this love or its equivalents (admiration, approval, affection, care), have led to a series of events where the patient had to create or to choose as a mate a person who would fit the role of dominant other. The patient has also misperceived some attributes of the dominant other, in order to see him in that role. When the patient will no longer be concerned with the dominant other, in his recent role, and will concentrate on his childhood's situation, treatment will be at an advanced stage. However, even then, the patient may become easily depressed since depression has become his fundamental mode of living. Depressive thoughts should not be allowed to expand into a general mood of depression, but must retain their discrete quality and content, which have to be analyzed. The patient must learn that because of this pattern of depression even innocent thoughts at times have the power of eliciting a depression. Little disappointments or losses that lead the patient to self-accusation, guilt, or severe depression are actually symbolic of an earlier, greater disappointment, or of lifelong disappointment. But, now, the early losses or the recurring losses are no longer likely to be repeated, because the patient is learning to assert and fulfill himself.

It is not possible to eliminate historically the original trauma of childhood, but it is possible to change the pattern by which the patient tried to remedy or undo the original trauma. Finally, the original traumas and these patterns will lose their significance and the compulsive qualities that caused their persistence or recurrence.

The handling of irrational guilt feeling is still important in the self-blaming cases of depression, even at advanced stages of treatment. The pattern that the patient has learned, throughout many years of life, is the following: guilt feeling → atoning → attempted redemption. Guilt about what? Originally, of course, the child attributed to himself the responsibility for the traumatic loss. He was naughty, terrible, evil. By atoning (that is, by placating, obeying, working hard, doing his duty, denying himself, by wanting peace at any cost), he felt he could obtain the love, approval, or admiration that he desired. But if he did not get it, he felt guilt again for not having done enough, for not having atoned enough. The cycle thus repeated itself. Since this pattern has become so ingrained in him, the patient will often change other psychological mechanisms into this guilt complex, for

instance, anxiety into guilt feeling. For example, the patient does not go to church on Sunday or does not accompany her child to grammar school. Now, the patient has something to feel guilty about. As painful as the guilt feeling is, the patient is aware that the possibility of suffering and thus of redeeming himself is in his power, whereas with anxiety he is at a loss; he does not know what to do about it.

The obsessive-compulsive symptoms that complicate a minority of cases of severe depression are attempts to channel guilt feelings and find measures to relieve them, so that the lost love or approval will be re-acquired. Actually, they aggravate the situation instead of solving it. For instance, the patient may have the obsession of thinking about something profane or sacrilegious, or about the coming death of a relative, and he feels guilty about having such thoughts. Similarly, compulsions may obligate the patient to perform actions condemned by the ritual of his religion, and again he feels guilty.

During therapy, it will be possible to show the patient how he tends to translate anxiety into guilt and depression. Finally, he will learn to face anxiety rather than to reproduce the sequence that will lead to the depression. He will also recognize the cognitive components that lead to anxiety. If the therapeutic climate established with the therapist is a sound one, the patient will realize that he can manifest and consequently share his anxiety with the therapist. His anxiety, that is, his negative attitude toward what is uncertain or what is about to come, will progressively change into hope, that is, into a positive attitude toward what is uncertain or what is about to come.

The therapist will eventually learn to handle little relapses, to understand and explain little psychological vicious circles that are formed or stumbling blocks that are encountered and tend to re-establish a mood of depression. For instance, the patient may become depressed over the fact that he may so easily become depressed; any little disappointment triggers off the state of sadness or guilt. Again, he has to be reminded that the little disappointment is symbolic of a bigger one. Another difficulty consists of the fact that some clusters of thought seem harmless to the therapist and are allowed to recur; actually, they lead to depression because of the particular connections that they have only in the patient's frame of reference. Eventually, however, the emotional pitch of the therapist will become more and more attuned to that of the patient.

At times, we encounter patients who do not seem to have had the relation with a dominant other that we have described. It is true that the patient has experienced mild disappointments, like broken friendships, but they hardly seem traumatic loss situations. If we analyze these patients carefully, we discover that once in their life a dominant other existed, and that these little disappointments are symbolic. In a few cases, however, the dominant other has not been a person, not even a group of persons or an organization, but an ideology, an ideal, a grandiose aspiration about oneself and the world. The patient has lived for this ideological dominant other, which eventually has proved to be false, unworthy of a lifetime sacrifice, or unrealizable. Whereas the stable person, the artist, or the philosophically inclined individual may accept the impossibility of realizing certain goals, and understand it in terms of the human limitations, the severely depressed person may interpret it again as proof of his defeat, guilt, unworthiness of himself, or of life in general. Again, a great deal of explanation and sharing of anxiety is necessary on the part of the significant third.

The treatment of the claiming type of depression is also difficult. Before starting treatment, the patient has become more and more demanding on the dominant other, the more deprived he felt. Any unfulfilled demand was experienced as a wound, a loss, and increased the depression. When treatment starts, the patient wants to find in the therapist a substitute for the dominant other who has failed. To the extent that the patient's demands are plausible or realistic, the therapist should try to go along with these requests and satisfy some of the needs for affection, consideration, companionship. Even clinging and nagging have to be accepted.

Kolb,[45,46] English,[25] and Cohen et al.[22] emphasized this excessive clinging as one of the main problems encountered in intensive psychotherapy with manic-depressives. Some patients do not want to leave at the end of the hour; they claim to suddenly remember many things they must say, plead for help, and attempt to make the therapist feel guilty if they are not improving. As Kolb[46] described, these patients have learned proper or apparently suitable social manners, and, with pleading and tenacity, they are often capable of eliciting in the therapist the reaction they want.

Occasionally, we have to prolong the session for a few minutes, as at the last minute the patient feels the urge to make new demands or to ask "one more question." The recommended attitude may seem a too indulgent one, but, especially at the beginning of treatment, we cannot expect the patient to give up mechanisms he has used for a long time.

Many patients, especially at the beginning of the session, are not able to verbalize freely, and should not be requested to explain their feelings in detail or to go into a long series of associations. On the contrary, the therapist should take the initiative and speak freely to them, even about unrelated subjects. As a patient of Thompson's[75] said, the words of the analyst are often experienced as gifts of love by the depressed person. Following the suggestions made in Spiegel's studies,[70,71] the therapist will soon learn to communicate with the depressed, at times even in spite of his lack of imagery and the poverty of his verbalizations. It is in the feeling itself, rather than in verbal symbols, that he often expresses himself.

When this immediate craving for being given acceptance is somewhat satisfied, the claiming depression will considerably diminish, but not disappear. However, now the depression will no longer be in the form of a sustained mood, but will appear in isolated, discrete fits. At this stage, it will be relatively easy to guide the patient to recognize that the fit of depression comes as a result of the following conscious or unconscious sequence of thoughts or of their symbolic equivalents: "I am not getting what I should → I am deprived → I am in a miserable state." The patient is guided to stop at the first stage of this sequence, because these words mean, "I would like to go back to the bliss of babyhood. I do not want to be a person in my own right, with self-determination." Can the person substitute this recurring idea and aim for another one, for instance, "What ways, other than aggressive expectation and dependency, are at my disposal in order to get what I want?" In other words, the patient is guided to reorganize his ways of thinking, so that the usual clusters of thoughts will not recur and will not reproduce the old sequence. The psychological horizon will enlarge and new patterns of living will be sought. However, the patient will be able to do so only if the new relationship with the therapist has decreased his feeling of deprivation and his suffering, so that the old pathogenic sequence will not reproduce itself automatically and with such tenacity. Excursions into paths of self-reliance will be made more and more frequently by the patient. At the same time, gradual limitations are imposed on the demands made on the therapist. Once the fits of depression have disappeared, the treatment will continue along traditional lines. The patient will learn to recognize his basic patterns of living that had led him to the depression, and the special characteristics of his early interpersonal relationships that led to the organization of such patterns. Such characteristics as superficiality, insensitivity, marked extroversion covered by depression, recurrence of clichés, infantile attitudes, such as "love me like a baby," will be recognized as defense mechanisms and disappear.

At an advanced stage of treatment with any type of depression, therapy should consist in going over again and again the life patterns the patient has adopted and in explaining how his present dealings with current life situations are often in accordance with the old psychogenetic patterns. Sooner or later, the patient, who has understood by now the psychodynamics of his life history, learns to avoid the old mechanisms, as he recognizes in them pseudosolutions and vicious circles. In some patients, the old mechanisms will tend to recur even after they have been completely understood. As a matter of fact, even discussion of them will evoke strong emotional reactions that are not congruous with the gained insight but are the usual affective components of the original symptoms. For, even after the patient has understood the meanings of his symptoms and behavior patterns, he has more familiarity with the old patterns.

It must, for example, be pointed out constantly to the patient that he should learn to ask himself what he wants, what he really wishes. Quite often, his attempted answer will be only a pseudoanswer. He may say, "I wish first of all for peace; I wish for the happiness of my children." He must learn—and relearn —that peace at any cost implies satisfying others before oneself, and that even the happiness of children, although a natural wish of every parent, is not a wish predominantly related to the individual himself.

In other words, the patient must learn to listen to himself and to reduce the overpowering role of the Thou. At the same time, he must make a voluntary effort to develop inner resources. In the attempt to imitate others, or even to surpass others in proficiency and technique, the patient has never relied on himself. He cannot be alone (unless he is depressed), and alone he cannot do anything that gives him satisfaction; he must work for the benefit of others or take flight into common actions. He must learn that he, too, may have artistic talent, and if he has the capacity to search for it, he may find it. Creative upsurges in apparently uncreative conventional manic-depressive personalities are a good prognostic sign. Transient and short feelings of depression will be tolerated at this point, indicating, as Zetzel[78] puts it, a measure of the ego strength.

As we have already mentioned, the therapist must be alert to spot early signs of depressions, at times precipitated even by trivial disappointments or even by chance associations of ideas. As Jacobson[37] and Kolb[46] emphasize, the recurring depression must immediately be related by the therapist to its precipitating cause. Dream interpretations are very useful.

What is advocated here is in a certain way a psychotherapeutic approach that will attempt to reproduce the healthy formal mechanisms which constitute a normal reaction to depression and loss—reconstructions of thought constellations, rather than the self-perpetuating depression or the manic flight.

Orthodox psychoanalytic procedure, with the use of the couch and free associations, is not indicated in manic-depressive psychosis even during the interval periods. Many failures in treatment of these patients were due to the adoption of the classical psychoanalytic technique. Many therapists feel today that the retarded or hyperactive patients generally should be treated with less frequent sessions— from one to three a week. Many patients, especially elderly ones, seem to do well with one session a week. The therapist must play a relatively active role, not one that conveys to the patient the feeling that he is being pushed or under pressure, nor one in which the passivity of the therapist is too much in contrast with the natural extroversion of the patient. Whenever the therapist feels that he has succeeded in reaching some conclusions or in understanding the feelings of the patient, he should verbalize them freely. Often, the patient prefers to keep quiet, not because he is unable to put things together, as in the case of the neurotic or the schizophrenic, but because he feels guilty or ashamed to express his feelings of rage, hostility, and, paradoxically, even of guilt and depression.

The treatment of hypomanic patients is far more difficult, as the flight of ideas prevents any significant contact. Here, an opposite procedure is to be followed. The patient is asked to cut out details, so that irritation and rage are purposely engendered, or he is reminded that he must talk about certain subjects (the subjects that are liable to induce depression). A conversion to a mild depression is therapeutically desirable. In many cases, however, it will not be possible to induce mild depression exclusively with active intervention of the therapist, and chlorpromazine (Thorazine) must be resorted to. This drug, either by decreasing the intensity of the manic or hypomanic state or by eliciting a mild depression, can be a valuable adjunct to psychotherapy.

Needless to say, not every therapist is suit-

able to treat manic-depressive patients. Some therapists who have been quite competent in treating psychoneurotic or schizophrenic patients have been utterly unsuccessful with manic-depressive patients, especially of the manic-hypomanic type. The verbose, circumstantial talk, or the photographic reproductions of past experiences with no signs of originality, the lack of any fantasy or of symbolic material, may tire the therapist. The immediate recognition of these characteristics as defense measures, and of their variation in accordance with the transference situation, can help the therapist in his trying efforts.

(Bibliography

1. ABRAHAM, K. "Notes on the Psycho-Analytical Investigation and Treatment of Manic-Depressive Insanity and Allied Conditions," in *Selected Papers on Psychoanalysis*. New York: Basic Books, 1953.
2. ARIETI, S. "The Decline of Manic-Depressive Psychosis: Its Significance in the Light of Dynamic and Social Psychiatry," in *American Handbook of Psychiatry*, 1st ed., Vol. 1. New York: Basic Books, 1959.
3. ———. *Interpretation of Schizophrenia*. New York: Brunner, 1955.
4. ———. "New Views on the Psychology and Psychopathology of Wit and of the Comic," *Psychiatry*, 13 (1950), 43.
5. ———. "The Psychotherapeutic Approach to Depression," *American Journal of Psychotherapy*, 16 (1962), 397–406.
6. ———. *The Intrapsychic Self: Feeling, Cognition and Creativity in Health and Mental Illness*. New York: Basic Books, 1967.
7. ———. "Depressive Disorders," in *International Encyclopedia of the Social Sciences*. New York: Free Press, 1968.
8. ———. "The Intrapsychic and the Interpersonal in Severe Psychopathology," in E. Witenberg, ed., *Interpersonal Explorations in Psychoanalysis*. New York: Basic Books, 1973.
9. ———. *The Will To Be Human*. New York: Quadrangle Books, 1972.
10. BECK, A. T. *Depression: Clinical, Experimental, and Theoretical Aspects*. New York: Hoeber, 1967.
11. BELLAK, L. *Manic-Depressive Psychosis and*

Allied Conditions. New York: Grune and Stratton, 1952.

12. BEMPORAD, J. R. "New Views on the Psychodynamics of the Depressive Character," in S. Arieti, ed., *The World Biennial of Psychiatry and Psychotherapy*, Vol. 1. New York: Basic Books, 1970.

13. BERMAN, H. H. "Order of Birth in Manic-Depressive Reactions," *Psychiatric Quarterly*, 12 (1933), 43.

14. BIBRING, E. "The Mechanisms of Depression," in P. Greenacre, ed., *Affective Disorders.* New York: International Universities Press, 1953.

15. BINSWANGER, L. *"Die Ideenflucht," Schweizer Archiven für Neurologie und Psychiatrie*, Vols. 28, 29, and 30, 1931–1932.

16. ———. *Über Ideenflucht.* Zurich: Orrell-Fussli, 1933.

17. BONFIGLIO, F. Personal communication.

18. BUBER, M. *I and Thou.* Translated by R. E. Smith. Edinburgh: Clark, 1953.

19. CAMERON, N. "The Functional Psychoses," in J. McV. Hunt, ed., *Personality and Behavior Disorders*, Vol. 2. New York: Ronald Press, 1944.

20. CAMPBELL, J. D. *Manic-Depressive Disease.* Philadelphia: Lippincott, 1953.

21. COBB, S. *Borderland of Psychiatry.* Cambridge: Harvard University Press, 1943.

22. COHEN, M. B., G. BAKER, R. A. COHEN, F. FROMM-REICHMANN, and E. V. WEIGERT. "An Intensive Study of Twelve Cases of Manic-Depressive Psychosis," *Psychiatry*, 17 (1954), 103.

23. EATON, J. W., and R. J. WEIL. *Culture and Mental Disorders.* Glencoe: Free Press, 1955.

24. ———. "The Mental Health of the Hutterites," in A. M. Rose, ed., *Mental Health and Mental Disorder.* New York: Norton, 1955.

25. ENGLISH, O. S. "Observations of Trends in Manic-Depressive Psychosis," *Psychiatry*, 12 (1949), 125.

26. EY, H. *Études Psychiatriques*, Vol. 3. Paris: Desclée de Brouwer, 1954.

27. FALRET, J. P., SR. *"Leçons."* Quoted by Koerner, Ref. 44.

28. FARIS, R. E. L., and H. W. DUNHAM. *Mental Disorders in Urban Areas.* Chicago: University of Chicago Press, 1939.

29. FREUD, S. "Mourning and Melancholia," in *Collected Papers*, Vol. 4. New York: Basic Books, 1959.

30. FROMM, E. *Escape from Freedom.* New York: Rinehart, 1941.

31. ———. *Man for Himself.* New York: Rinehart, 1947.

32. FROMM-REICHMANN, F. "Discussion of a Paper by O. S. English," *Psychiatry*, 12 (1949), 133.

33. GOLD, H. R. "Observations on Cultural Psychiatry During a World Tour of Mental Hospitals," *The American Journal of Psychiatry*, 108 (1951), 462.

34. GREENACRE, P. *Affective Disorders.* New York: International Universities Press, 1953.

35. GRINKER, R. R., J. MILLER, M. SABSHIN, R. NUN, and J. C. NUNNALLY. *The Phenomena of Depressions.* New York: Hoeber, 1961.

36. HOCH, P. H., and J. ZUBIN. *Depression.* New York: Grune and Stratton, 1954.

37. JACOBSON, E. "Transference Problems in the Psychoanalytic Treatment of Severly Depressed Patients," *The American Journal of Psychiatry*, 2 (1954), 395.

38. ———. *Depression: Comparative Studies of Normal, Neurotic, and Psychotic Conditions.* New York: International Universities Press, 1971.

39. JELLIFFE, S. E. "Some Historical Phases of the Manic-Depressive Synthesis," in *Manic-Depressive Psychosis*, Vol. 11. Baltimore: Williams & Wilkins, 1931.

40. KAHN, E. "An Appraisal of Existential Analysis," *Psychiatric Quarterly*, 31 (1957), 203.

41. KATZ, S. E. "The Family Constellation as a Predisposing Factor in Psychosis," *Psychiatric Quarterly*, 8 (1934), 121.

42. KENNEDY, F. "Neuroses Related to Manic-Depressive Constitutions," *M. Clin. North America*, 28 (1944), 452.

43. KLEIN, M. *Contributions to Psycho-Analysis.* London: Hogarth Press, 1950.

44. KOERNER, O. *Die Ärztliche Kenntnisse in Ilias und Odysse*, 1929.

45. KOLB, L. C. Personal Communication.

46. ———. "Psychotherapeutic Evolution and Its Implications," *Psychiatric Quarterly*, 30 (1956), 579.

47. KRAEPELIN, E. *Manic-Depressive Insanity and Paranoia.* Edinburgh: Livingstone, 1921.

48. KRAINES, S. H. *Mental Depressions and Their Treatment.* New York: Macmillan, 1957.

49. LANDIS, C., and J. D. PAGE. *Society and Men-*

tal Disease. New York: Rinehart, 1938.

50. LEMKAU, P., B. PASAMANIK, and M. COOPER. "The Implications of the Psycho-genetic Hypothesis for Mental Hygiene," *The American Journal of Psychiatry,* 110 (1953), 436.

51. LEWIN, B. *The Psychoanalysis of Elation.* New York: Norton, 1950.

52. LORENZ, M. "Language Behavior in Manic Patients. An Equalitative Study," *Archives of Neurology and Psychiatry,* 69 (1953), 14.

53. LORENZ, M., and L. COBB. "Language Behavior in Manic Patients," *Archives of Neurology and Psychiatry,* 67 (1952), 763.

54. MALZBERG, B. "Is Birth Order Related to Incidence of Mental Disease?" *American Journal of Physical Anthropology,* 24 (1937), 91.

55. ———. *Social and Biological Aspects of Mental Disease.* Utica: State Hospital Press, 1940.

56. MASSERMAN, J. H., ed. *Depressions: Theories and Therapies.* New York: Grune and Stratton, 1970.

57. MATZ, P. B., and O. C. WILLHITE. "A Study of Manic-Depressive Psychosis Among Ex-Service Men," in *Manic-Depressive Psychosis,* Vol. 11. Baltimore: Williams & Wilkins, 1931.

58. MENDELS, J. *Concepts of Depression.* New York: Wiley, 1970.

59. MENDELSON, M. *Psychoanalytic Concepts of Depression.* Springfield: Charles C Thomas, 1960.

60. OPLER, M. K. *Culture Psychiatry and Human Values.* Springfield: Charles C Thomas, 1956.

61. POLLOCK, H. M., B. MALZBERG, and R. G. FULLER. *Hereditary and Environmental Factors in the Causation of Manic-Depressive Psychosis and Dementia Praecox.* Utica: State Hospital Press, 1939.

62. RADO, S. "The Problem of Melancholia," *International Journal of Psycho-Analysis,* 9 (1928), 420.

63. ———. "Psychodynamics of Depression from the Etiologic Point of View," *Psychosomatic Medicine,* 13 (1951), 51.

64. RENNIE, T. A. L. "Prognosis in Manic-Depressive Psychosis," *The American Journal of Psychiatry,* 98 (1942), 801.

65. ———. "Social Psychiatry—A Definition," *International Journal of Social Psychiatry,* 1 (1955), 5.

66. RIESMAN, D., with N. GLAZER and R. DENNEY. *The Lonely Crowd.* New Haven: Yale University Press, 1950.

67. ROI, G. "*Stati depressivi e Psicoterapia,*" *Riv. sperim-di freniatria,* 81 (1957), 392.

68. ROSENTHAL, S. H. "Involutional Depression," in S. Arieti, ed., *American Handbook of Psychiatry,* Second Edition, Vol. 3. New York: Basic Books, 1974.

69. SOMMER, A. "*Analogies et Differences des États Maniaques et Mélancoliques.*" *Evol. Psychiat.,* (1949).

70. SPIEGEL, R. "Specific Problems of Communication in Psychiatric Conditions," in S. Arieti, ed., *American Handbook of Psychiatry,* 1st ed., Vol. 1 New York: Basic Books, 1959.

71. ———. "Communication in the Psychoanalysis of Depression," in J. Masserman, ed., *Psychoanalysis and Human Values.* New York: Grune and Stratton, 1960.

72. SPITZ, R. A. "Anaclitic Depression," in *The Psychoanalytic Study of the Child,* Vol. 2. New York: International Universities Press, 1946.

73. STRONGIN, E. I., and L. E. HINSIE. "Parotid Gland Secretions in Manic-Depressive Patients," *The American Journal of Psychiatry,* 94 (1938), 1459.

74. TANZI, E. *A Text-Book of Mental Diseases.* New York: Rebruan, 1909.

75. THOMPSON, C. M. "Analytic Observations During the Course of a Manic-Depressive Psychosis, *Psychoanalytic Review,* 17 (1930), 240.

76. WEISS, J. M. A. "The Gamble with Death in Attempted Suicide," *Psychiatry,* 20 (1957), 17.

77. ———. "Suicide," in S. Arieti, ed., *American Handbook of Psychiatry,* Second Edition, Vol. 3. New York: Basic Books, 1974.

78. ZETZEL, E. R. "Depression and the Incapacity to Bear It," in M. Schur, ed., *Drives, Affects, Behavior,* Vol. 2. New York: International Universities Press, 1965.

79. ZILBOORG, G. "Depressive Reactions Related to Parenthood," in *Manic-Depressive Psychosis,* Vol. 11. Baltimore: Williams & Wilkins, 1931.

80. ———. *A History of Medical Psychology.* New York: Norton, 1941.

81. ———. "Manic-Depressive Psychoses," in S. Lorand, ed., *Psycho-Analysis Today.* New York: International Universities Press, 1944.

CHAPTER 22

BIOLOGICAL ASPECTS OF AFFECTIVE ILLNESS[*]

J. Mendels

DURING THE PAST DECADE, there has been a major upsurge of investigation into biological correlates of mood disturbance. The development of pharmacological agents that alleviate the symptoms of depression and mania or induce symptoms resembling clinical depression has encouraged efforts to explore and define the biological changes associated with affective illness.

At this time, there is no final resolution to the question of whether affective illness results from a psychological or biological disturbance or from alterations in one system interacting with some pre-existing vulnerability in the other. It is, however, clear that there are alterations in the central nervous system, autonomic nervous system, and endocrine system, in association with changes in mood, regardless of whether the psychopathological symptoms are primary or secondary.

In this chapter, we are concerned with the biological changes associated with depressive illness. It must be remembered that the syndrome of depression (and perhaps mania) probably represents a heterogeneous group of conditions in terms of etiology, pathology, and symptomatology. These issues have been discussed in detail elsewhere,[166,193,217,218,220,225,289] and need not be repeated here. However, the fact that we are probably dealing with several distinct conditions suggests that the biological correlates will not be necessarily the same for all. A major difficulty in current investigations of the psychobiology of depression has been the frequent failure to distinguish between specific groups of depressed patients.

There are many analogies in general medicine. For example, the recognition that pernicious anemia constitutes a separate condition with a unique pathology, etiology, and treatment, separate from other forms of anemia, required the recognition of the relationship

[*] I wish to thank Bernard J. Carroll, Elizabeth Dorus, Alan Frazer, and Steven K. Secunda, for their comments and suggestions in the preparation of this chapter. Portions of this chapter represent work done in collaboration with them. The work was supported in part by research funds from the Veterans Administration and by USPHS Grant No. 1 R10 MH21, 411, awarded by the National Institute of Mental Health.

between this syndrome and vitamin B_{12} deficiency. Treating 100 consecutive patients with anemia (i.e., a significant reduction in hemoglobin concentration) with vitamin B_{12} alone would be of no significant value. Similarly, the separation of phenylketonuria from the broad syndrome of mental deficiency required the recognition of the unique features of this condition. It is possible that similar problems are relevant to the study of clinical depression. Thus, the failure to define consistent and specific biological alterations in depression may be at least in part a function of the fact that investigators have studied mixed groups of patients. For example, there are now reports of possibly important differences between groups of depressed patients with and without a previous history of mania.

Much of the information which underlies the psychobiological hypotheses of the affective illnesses derives from pharmacological rather than from clinical studies. While this information is of importance, we remain without a real understanding of the biological changes in our patients. To a large extent, this is the result of the limitation on the type of experiments which can be conducted in patients. We do not have the techniques to study the details of brain function or the relationship between brain function and mood and behavior in man. Therefore, much of the research has been indirect, concerned with changes in peripheral systems or in electrical measurements of brain function.

It must also be remembered that the demonstration of a biological alteration in patients with a particular psychiatric syndrome (albeit a consistent abnormality) does not necessarily mean that this is the cause of the condition. The change may be a result of another and perhaps undetectable biological change or may result from psychological events. Further, the complex interrelationships between multiple biological systems in man have yet to be clearly understood and defined, let alone explored systematically in clinical depression.

In spite of these problems, there has been progress in developing models of the psychobiology of depression, together with the in-

vestigation of these in patients. Alterations in a number of different systems have been observed or postulated. These include a genetic predisposition; alterations in biogenic amine function (norepinephrine, dopamine, serotonin), and perhaps in other neurotransmitters; changes in electrolyte metabolism (sodium, potassium, magnesium, and calcium); neuroendocrine changes including hypothalamic-pituitary activity, adrenocortical function, growth hormone release, and thyroid function; studies of electrophysiological activity, such as cortical evoked potential, electromyography, and sleep electroencephalography; and, more recently, suggestions of alterations in receptor sensitivity, cell membrane function and in adenyl cyclase-cyclic AMP activity.

For purposes of convenience, these will be reviewed separately, but it should be remembered that the interrelationships between these systems are very important. It is essential to recognize and define these interrelationships and to begin to incorporate them into a meaningful hypothesis.

(Genetics

There is considerable evidence that genetic factors play an important role in the etiology of affective illness. There is a significant difference between concordance rates for manic-depressive illness in monozygotic and dizygotic twin pairs. A review of six twin studies[370] indicated a concordance rate for monozygotic twins of 74 percent, whereas the concordance rate for dizygotic twins was only 19 percent. A comparable concordance rate was found in a review of case reports of twelve monozygotic twins reared apart.[281] Although these findings suggest a substantial genetic component, twin studies do have important methodological limitations.[149]

The prevalence of affective illness in the first-degree relatives of manic-depressive patients is approximately 20 percent, while in uniphasic patients it is estimated to be 13 percent.[7,8,9,270] This contrasts with an estimated incidence in the general population of only 1 percent.[370] It is of interest to note that while most studies have shown depression in general to be more common in females than in males (a mean of male-female ratios of 0.69 has been reported,[332] this difference may not occur among manic-depressives.[270] Here the incidence is the same in both sexes, whereas among uniphasic depressives it is higher among women.

Twin studies and family history studies have provided evidence of a genetic factor but have not provided unequivocal support for the specific mode of genetic transmission. The hypothesized modes of transmission include a single dominant autosomal gene with incomplete penetrance, polygenic transmission, and an X-linked dominant gene with incomplete penetrance.

The hypothesis of a single dominant autosomal gene has been supported by similar prevalences of affective illness in parents, siblings, and children of patients.[295] A prevalence rate of less than 50 percent in the siblings and children of patients, the fact that not all patients have an affected parent, and that not all monozygotic twins are concordant, suggest incomplete penetrance of the gene.

The hypothesis of polygenic mode of transmission is also supported by similar prevalences in parents, siblings, and children of probands, as well as by the continuum of manic and depressive characteristics, ranging from mild to severe, in the general population. A single dominant autosomal gene transmission and polygenic transmission would both have prevalence rates among relatives which decrease toward the population prevalence at different rates, as more and more remote relatives are examined. One test to discriminate between a single dominant autosomal gene and polygenic transmission in a disorder with a population incidence of approximately 1.0 percent would be the relative prevalence of the disorder in second- and first-degree relatives, respectively. The single dominant autosomal gene hypothesis suggests that the ratio should be approximately 1:2, while the polygenic hypothesis suggests approximately 1:4.

The available data are equivocal,[332] and more data are needed on second-degree and more remote relatives. It is also of interest to note that polygenic models of transmission assume random mating with regard to the trait or disorder in question. This assumption has been challenged by a report indicating a significantly higher prevalence of affective illness in wives (and in their family history) of male patients with affective illness than would be expected with random mating.[150]

A dominant X-chromosome with incomplete penetrance has also been proposed as the mode of transmission.[364,366,367] This would be consistent with a higher prevalence of affected females than males and with the report of an absence of father-son pairs in a sample of bipolar patients.[366] However, other investigators[271,332] have documented cases of similarly affected father-son pairs, and thus, if one assumes that these cases do not represent undetected transmission by the mother, an additional genetic factor (or factors) must be postulated.

The suggestion of X-linkage in manic-depressive illness led to investigation of the possibility of linkage between manic-depressive illness and X-linked marker traits. Linkage can be demonstrated when two genes, each affecting a different trait, are in close enough proximity on a chromosome that they do not assort independently. Thus, greater than chance association between two such traits would support the X-linkage hypothesis. Reports of linkage between manic-depressive illness and both Xg blood system[367] and deutan and protan color blindness[284,366] have been made. They provide more compelling evidence of X-linked transmission than family psychiatric history data in general.

([Biogenic Amines

Following the discovery by Walter Cannon in 1915 that animals exposed to rage- or fear-inducing situations secrete increased amounts of epinephrine (adrenalin), there has been an increasing interest in the association between emotional behavior, epinephrine, and the other biogenic amines. The subsequent description of the behavioral syndrome induced by reserpine administration to rats,[33] and the recognition that this was associated with a depletion of brain catecholamines (dopamine and norepinephrine) and serotonin,[75] have led to an extensive series of investigations designed to explore the relationship between brain amine function and behavior. The widespread use of reserpine for the treatment of hypertension, and the development of a syndrome thought by some to be a model for clinical depression,[2,122,146,249,334] spurred investigation of the association between depression and brain biogenic amine metabolism. These investigations and the observations that most antidepressant drugs have pharmacological actions that presumably increase the amount of the amine available at receptor sites led to the formulation of the biogenic amine hypothesis of affective disorders. This states that clinical depression is associated with a functional deficiency of norepinephrine or serotonin at significant receptor sites in the brain, whereas mania is associated with an excess of the amine. These hypotheses are based mainly on indirect pharmacological observations with limited evidence from clinical studies. Much of this material has been reviewed elsewhere,[59,61,63,94,241,275,315,319] and will only be summarized here. Likewise, the reader is referred to several reviews for a detailed discussion of the metabolism and pharmacology of the biogenic amines.[21,29,144,177,245,328,347,354]

Recently, several investigators have questioned the view that the syndrome induced by reserpine is a model for depression.[36,159,228] It may rather be the result of sedation and psychomotor retardation in certain susceptible individuals, particularly those with a history of previous depressive episodes. Furthermore, recent evidence indicates that the gross behavioral syndrome produced by reserpine is likely to result from dopamine depletion, as a consequence of reserpine's inhibition of the uptake of dopamine into storage granules and its storage within such granules,[3,4,76] rather

than from reserpine's effect on norepinephrine or serotonin, as was originally emphasized in the development of the biogenic amine theories.

Catecholamines: Antidepressant Drugs

A major impetus for the catecholamine hypothesis derived from the study of the pharmacological action of the antidepressant and antimanic drugs. While these drugs are probably of value,[114,115,192] they are not uniformly effective.

The monoamine oxidase inhibitors (MAOI), such as tranylcypromine, nialimide, increase the intraneuronal concentration of norepinephrine, dopamine, and serotonin, by inhibiting the action of the enzyme monoamine-oxidase, which is responsible for the oxidative deamination of those compounds.[115,192] They may also decrease the re-uptake of amines into the neurons from which they were released. This re-uptake process is normally the main mechanism for terminating catecholamine activity.[22]

While the MAOIs do increase tissue concentration of amines in man,[181] there is as yet no conclusive evidence that they produce increased functional activity at central aminergic receptor sites. Indeed, patients receiving MAOI do not have symptoms indicative of an increase in sympathetic nervous system activity. In fact, the hypotensive effect of MAOIs may result from *decreased* sympathetic activity,[254] as a consequence of feedback inhibition of tyrosine hydroxylase[354] or false transmitter formation.[201]

The tricyclic antidepressants, such as amitryptyline and imipramine, potentiate the actions of endogenously released norepinephrine by blocking its re-uptake into the nerve terminal.[158,175] Iprindol is an antidepressant drug,[131] chemically related to the tricyclic compounds and yet it does not block norepinephrine or serotonin uptake as do the other tricyclic drugs, raising the question of whether the blockage of amine re-uptake is the critically important variable in determining the clinical efficacy of the drugs.[158]

Catecholamines: Urinary Metabolites

There are a number of reports dealing with the concentration of amines and their metabolites in the urine of depressed and manic patients. This strategy must be interpreted with caution in that it probably provides little, if any, information about central nervous system amine metabolism. Almost all of the urinary compounds are derived from peripheral metabolism and we do not know whether or not there is an association between changes in peripheral and in brain amine metabolism.

Robins and Hartmann[290] have summarized the findings from nine studies which included both depressed and manic patients and in which norepinephrine, epinephrine, dopamine, metanephrine, normetanephrine, and 3-methoxy-4-hydroxy mandellic acid (VMA) were measured.

The studies involved 281 determinations of these compounds. They concluded that twenty-one observations from the depressed patients were consistent with the catecholamine hypothesis of depression, whereas seventy-one were inconsistent. The manic patients provided twenty-two determinations that were consistent, and six that were inconsistent with the hypothesis. The remaining 161 determinations were equivocal. Thus, studies of urinary metabolites of catecholamines in depressed patients have not contributed to confirmation of the hypothesis. Observations in manic patients are more consistent with the hypothesis, but may be the result of increased activity in these patients.

A more recent strategy has involved the measurement of the urinary concentration of 3-methoxy-4-hydroxyphenylglycol (MHPG). Some observers have suggested that it may be the major metabolite of brain norepinephrine and that the percentage of urinary MHPG coming from the brain may be higher than the percentage of the other metabolites.[212,312,313] While this conclusion has been questioned,[88,102] several investigators have measured urinary MHPG in groups of psychiatric patients and found it to be reduced in some depressed

patients.[164,210] However, this finding has not been confirmed.[278] It is possible that abnormalities in urinary MHPG (and perhaps in other amine metabolites) in depressed and manic patients may simply be the result of the differences in the level of physical activity in these patients.[124] There is a preliminary suggestion that depressed patients with low urinary MHPG concentrations are more likely to respond favorably to imipramine than are patients with normal MHPG concentration,[211] while a few patients with normal urinary MHPG concentration seemed to have a superior response to amitriptyline.[316] Much more investigation is needed to clarify the exact relationship between urinary MHPG and brain norepinephrine and changes in this compound in depression.

Catecholamines: Brain and CSF Studies

Bourne et al.[45] found no difference in hypothalamic and hindbrain norepinephrine concentrations or in caudate dopamine concentration after death by suicide as compared with nonsuicide death.

Cerebrospinal fluid (CSF) concentration of homovanillic acid (HVA), the primary metabolite of dopamine and of MHPG, has been measured in depressed and manic patients. There are inconsistent reports of a reduction in HVA concentration while depressed, with increases to normal values after clinical improvement.[47,230] There is also an increase in CSF HVA concentration after the oral administration of L-DOPA to depressed patients.[161] However, there is no accompanying clinical improvement,[80,242] suggesting the possibility that the CSF HVA level may not be directly associated with the clinical state of the patient but may reflect changes in motor activity.[353] Others have not found an association between CSF HVA concentration and psychomotor activity.[230,361] Further, lumbar fluid HVA may not originate from brain dopamine solely, but may derive from spinal cord capillaries.[31]

There are several studies of CSF MHPG concentration in depressed and manic patients.[163,327,361] In the main, CSF MHPG has been found to be normal in depressives.[327,361] One study has reported low values,[163] but some of the control subjects had values as low or lower than some depressives, indicating that there is no clear-cut relationship between mood and CSF MHPG concentration. An elevation in CSF MHPG was noted in a few manic patients.[361] However, some manics had normal values[361] and a group of schizophrenics also had a raised concentration.[327] In view of these findings and the demonstration that MHPG concentration in urine may be in part a reflection of physical activity,[124] it is possible that the reports of low values in a few depressed patients and elevated values in a few manics are the result of the fact that these patients had psychomotor retardation (or hyperactivity) rather than due to the depressed (or manic) mood per se. One study [273] has not found this to apply to CSF MHPG concentration in spite of changes in CSF HVA and HIAA concentrations. There is still uncertainty over the precision of the method used to assay CSF MHPG, which may account for some of the confusion.

Catecholamines: Enzyme Studies

An alternative strategy for investigation involves the measurement of some of the enzymes involved in catecholamine metabolism. Catechol-o-methyltransferase (COMT) is the main enzyme involved in the extraneuronal deactivation of norepinephrine.[21] Most of the norepinephrine which is released into the synapse is deactivated by re-uptake into the neuron; the remainder is acted on by COMT. Erythrocyte COMT activity has been measured in several groups of psychiatric patients, recognizing that it is unknown whether it is an index of brain COMT activity or not. A large reduction in COMT activity in women with unipolar depression and some reduction in women with bipolar depression has been found.[91,120] It is possible that estrogens interact with other hormones to influence COMT activity.[90] COMT activity did not change when these patients improved clinically or when four of them became manic.

This persistence in the reduction of COMT activity suggests that it may reflect an underlying genetic abnormality. It has been proposed that COMT activity is an index of adrenergic receptor activity,[17] and the reduction in activity in these patients is compatible with the hypothesis that there is a reduction in adrenergic receptor function in some depressed patients (infravide).[121,278] However, it could equally well be argued that the reduced COMT activity would allow more circulating norepinephrine to reach the receptors. Alternatively, it is possible that norepinephrine metabolism is only abnormal in the manic phase of manic depressive illness and not in the depressed phase.[67] Roberts and Broadly[288] had originally speculated that there might be an abnormality in COMT activity in some depressives, resulting in the formation of an abnormal norepinephrine metabolite, noradnamine.

Monoamine Oxidase (MAO) activity in platelets has been found to be significantly reduced in bipolar depressed patients as compared with control subjects and unipolar depressives.[250] Others have reported normal[135] and elevated[190,256] MAO activity in mixed groups of depressed patients. MAO activity is higher in women and in the elderly,[291] which may be relevant to the higher incidence of depression in these groups. However, it has been shown that several different forms of MAO exist in the brain,[169,310] and it is unclear what the relevance of these findings might be for brain activity.

Very preliminary studies of plasma *dopamine beta hydroxylase (DBH) activity* indicate no difference between patients with affective illness and control subjects.[19] An elevation in *histamine-n-methyltransferase activity* has been noted in depressed women.[90]

Indoleamines

There have been extensive investigations into serotonin metabolism in parallel with the studies of changes in catecholamines.[157,176, 206,241] For example, the antidepressant drugs have pharmacological effects on serotonin metabolism which are similar to their effects on norepinephrine.[168]

Studies of the CSF concentration of 5-hydroxyindoles or 5-hydroxy-indoleacetic acid (5HIAA), the principal metabolite of serotonin, of depressed patients have more often than not found its concentration to be reduced.[13,48,96,117,230,352] Not all investigators have confirmed this.[263] Further, the rate of accumulation of 5HIAA in lumbar fluid after the administration of probenecid* (which blocks the egress of 5HIAA from CSF) is less in depressed patients than control subjects.[294,344,351,352] This has been interpreted as reflecting a reduction in central serotonin turnover in depressed patients. Two related findings are of interest. A number of patients have been found to have a continued reduction in CSF 5HIAA concentrations after clinical recovery,[14,96,230] and a similar reduction in 5HIAA has been found in some manic patients.[48,96,230] Not all investigators have confirmed these observations,[258,263,294] and there are also reports that some schizophrenic patients may also have low CSF 5HIAA concentration.[13,48] There is disagreement as to whether the concentration of metabolites in lumbar fluid is a measure of brain serotonin activity or whether it derives primarily from the spinal cord.[62]

While a number of investigators have reported CSF 5HIAA concentration to be low in depressives, there is disagreement which may in part be due to age,[47] diagnosis (e.g., may be lower in unipolar than bipolar depressives),[13] psychosis,[230] or physical activity.[141]

It has been hypothesized that the postulated reduction in brain serotonin in depression may be the result of an increase in hepatic tryptophan pyrrolase activity.[109,206] There is an increase in plasma corticosteroids in some depressed patients, which could stimulate pyrrolase activity,[196] resulting in an increased conversion of tryptophan to kynurenine and a reduction in the amount of tryptophan available for conversion into serotonin. However, the amount of corticosteroids required to achieve this effect in animal studies is much higher than the increase found in depressed patients and it is questionable whether this mechanism is applicable.

An alternative strategy has been to study the metabolism of tryptophan, the precursor of serotonin, in depressed patients. Tryptophan is normally converted into kynurenine and its metabolites, and into tryptamine and serotonin. In the tryptophan load test an oral dose of tryptophan is followed by the measurement of kynurenine metabolites together with tryptamine.[92,281] Several investigators[85,110] have reported findings which they have interpreted as supporting the pyrrolase hypothesis. Cazzullo et al.[85] reported an increase in basal urinary xanthurenic acid excretion. This did not increase abnormally after oral tryptophan administration. While these findings have been advanced as evidence for the enhanced metabolism of tryptophan along the kynurenine pathway in depression,[110,299] they do not really support this conclusion. The dose of tryptophan used in this study was very high, and the patients received large amounts of pyridoxine prior to and during the study which render the findings difficult to interpret.

Curzon and Bridges[110] reported that female patients with endogenous depression excreted increased amounts of kynurenine and 3-hydroxy-kynurenine but not of their subsequent metabolite, 3-hydroxy-anthranillic acid, after an oral dose of 30 mg./kg. of tryptophan, as compared with nine psychiatric patients without endogenous depression. The increase in kynurenine and hydroxykynurenine was presumed to be caused by an increase in hepatic tryptophan pyrrolase activity. However, some control subjects had a similar response, some depressed patients did not have this response, and several of the patients had an even greater excretion of these metabolites after recovery, as compared to when they were ill. In neither of these two studies[85,110] were there controls for dietary, drug, or hormonal factors which may have influenced tryptophan metabolism. In a more carefully controlled study, Frazer et al.[143] were unable to replicate these findings in a group of male

---

* Recently, there have been reports that probenecid may itself influence brain tryptophan-serotonin metabolism, thus complicating interpretations of these findings.[8] Also, the varying rates of absorption and blood levels of probenecid could distort the results with big variations in its effects from subject to subject.

depressed patients. There was no significant difference between tryptophan metabolism in these patients and a group of psychiatric control subjects. There are reports of a reduction in urinary tryptamine in depressed patients,[98,278] while others have found normal values.[143]

Careful consideration of all of the available data leads to the conclusion that there is no significant evidence to support the hypothesis of an enhanced metabolism of tryptophan along the kynurenine pathway (at least in male depressed patients), and no evidence of enhanced tryptophan pyrrolase activity in these patients.

CSF tryptophan concentration has been reported to be low in depressed patients (and also in three manic patients).[95] Total plasma tryptophan concentration was normal, but it is probable that free tryptophan (as opposed to the protein-bound fraction) would be a more critical measure.[195] It is known that increasing plasma tryptophan concentration will result in an increase in brain tryptophan concentration and may alter the rate of serotonin synthesis.[125,137] A low CSF tryptophan *may* reflect a reduced brain tryptophan concentration producing a reduction in brain serotonin. There are also reports of a reduction in hindbrain serotonin concentration of people who died from suicide, as compared with control subjects,[264,326] as well as a relatively low concentration of 5HIAA.[45,326] These findings are difficult to interpret because of the large number of factors which may have influenced the results, including ingestion of drugs, age differences, and post-mortem effects.

Amine Depletion Studies

As discussed above, considerable attention has been directed to the behavioral syndrome found in animals and some people after reserpine administration.

The development of this syndrome is in part related to dose, but more significantly, to a previous history of depression.[159,228] There is doubt whether this syndrome is an appropriate model for clinical depression.[36,159,228] It is possible that sedation and/or psychomotor retardation may be more important complications, with depression occasionally developing as a secondary complication in vulnerable individuals. When treatment with reserpine is associated with prospective evaluation of the patient's clinical state, no significant depression occurs.[36]

One major disadvantage of the use of reserpine is that it not only affects biogenic amine metabolism but also involves other systems, such as acetylcholine, making interpretation of results more difficult. A more selective approach to depletion of individual brain amines has been attempted under both experimental and clinical conditions, with results that do not support the hypothesis that a general depletion of brain amines in itself necessarily leads to a clinical depression.

Several strategies have been adopted. The intraventricular injection of 6-hydroxydopamine (6OHDA) results in a significant and permanent decrease in brain norepinephrine and depending on dose, of dopamine,[69,349] with probably little significant effect on serotonin.[38,50,174] There is also a long-lasting interference with tyrosine hydroxylase activity, resulting in a reduction in the synthesis of new catecholamines.[253] In spite of these profound and persistent effects, there are few significant persistent behavioral changes. While there is an increased irritability and an enhancement of aggressive behavior, there are no changes suggestive of clinical depression, when brain norepinephrine is reduced by 60–70 percent.[38,50,174,207] It is probable that some form of "supersensitivity" of the postsynaptic cell may develop,[262,348] countering the effects of its reduction in concentration and turnover.

Likewise, the administration of alpha-methyl-paratyrosine (AMPT), which inhibits tyrosine hydroxylase, the rate limiting enzyme in catecholamine synthesis,[252] with a decrease in the production and tissue stores of dopamine and norepinephrine,[336] is not associated in animal or man with behavioral changes suggestive of clinical depression.[86,129,151,329] There is some sedation and decreased spontaneous motor activity.

The chronic administration of AMPT to *Maccaca speciosa* is reported to produce behavioral changes analogous to human depression.[282,283] These included a decrease in total social interactions and initiatives, postural and facial changes suggestive of withdrawal, diminished motor activity, together with a continued willingness to remain close to other monkeys in the colony and to respond appropriately to their social initiatives. It is difficult to determine whether this is an appropriate model for clinical depression. These animals apparently were willing to remain within the group and had normal social responses, which is often not the case in depressed individuals who are withdrawn and "nonreactive" in spite of social initiatives. Further, these animals did not have the loss of appetite, weight, and libido, and the insomnia often seen in depressives. The administration of relatively large doses of AMPT to medical[129,329] and to schizophrenic[86,149] patients was not associated with the development of clinical depression, in spite of a significant reduction in catecholamines.[129,329] One possible exception to these findings is the report of an aggravation of clinical state in three depressed patients given AMPT.[55] However, these patients had significant psychomotor retardation prior to the administration of AMPT, and in view of AMPT's sedative effects, it is possible that the apparent aggravation in depression may have been the result of further sedation of patients who were already "slowed down."

The administration of para-chlorophenylalanine (PCPA) which, by inhibiting tryptophan hydroxylase, produces a depletion of serotonin,[198] as well as a moderate reduction in norepinephrine,[355,356] is also not associated with behavioral changes suggestive of clinical depression. This casts doubt on the suggestion that depression results from a simple reduction in brain serotonin. The effects of PCPA administration vary considerably with species, dose, and duration of administration, but there are frequent reports of increases in sexuality, aggressiveness, and insomnia,[200,338] which, if anything, are compatible with manic behavior.[3,247]

These approaches to depleting brain biogenic amines have not provided evidence to confirm the hypothesis that clinical depression is associated with a reduction in these amines. However, they do not necessarily disprove the hypothesis. For example, it has been suggested that there is a "functional" intraneuronal pool from which norepinephrine is utilized at a rapid rate, and a "storage" pool which serves as a reserve depot.[328,341,354] Thus, depletion of brain norepinephrine may have its major effect on the "storage" pool, but leave the "functional" pool sufficiently intact (with newly synthesized norepinephrine) to prevent development of a depression. A similar mechanism may apply to serotonin.

Alteration in Receptor Sensitivity

A functional deficiency of biogenic amine activity could arise in the presence of normal or even increased amounts of the amine if there was an abnormality of the receptor site on which the amine exerts its action. For example, depressives have been reported to have a reduced blood pressure response to norepinephrine infusion,[276] which could be the result of a decreased receptor sensitivity. Prange et al.[278] have suggested that their finding that small amounts of tri-iodothyronine will enhance the antidepressant effect of imipramine in depressed females may be due to the ability of thyroid hormone to increase the sensitivity of adrenergic receptors.[277] As discussed above, the finding of a reduction in erythrocyte COMT activity[91] may also be compatible with this view. A reported increase in plasma norepinephrine levels in depressed patients[368] may reflect an effort to compensate for a decreased receptor sensitivity. However, the increase in plasma norepinephrine may have been more closely related to the anxiety component of the syndrome than to the depression per se.

Adenyl Cyclase-Cyclic AMP

Adenosine 3', 5'-monophosphate (cyclic AMP), the product of enzymatic degradation of adenosine triphosphate by adenyl cyclase, has a critical role in regulating the effects of many hormones and neurotransmitters.[101,171,292,342] Adenyl cyclase's ubiquitous location in most cell membranes makes it readily accessible to stimulation by the many hormones that act upon it. The hormones initiate an increase in adenyl cyclase activity and are often referred to as the "first messenger," while cyclic AMP is known as the "second messenger." The "first messenger" carries the information to the cell, where the "second messenger" transfers the information to the cell's internal mechanisms. Thus, adenyl cyclase plays an integral part in hormonal (including catecholamine) activity.[292]

Consequently, it is reasonable to consider the possibility that there may be some abnormality in cyclic AMP function in affective illness. There are reports of a decrease in urinary cyclic AMP excretion in depression with an elevation in mania.[1,267] Further, a marked elevation in the urinary excretion of cyclic AMP was observed on the day of an acute change from a depressed state into a manic state in six manic-depressed patients.[265,266]

The relationship of these changes in urinary cyclic AMP concentration to the disease process is unclear in that a high percentage of urinary cyclic AMP is derived from the kidney,[184] and its concentration may be influenced by physical activity[126] and endocrine changes.[87,184] Thus, reports of levels of cyclic AMP in the urine of depressed and manic patients must be interpreted with caution.

A study of CSF cyclic AMP levels in twelve depressed, six manic, and fifteen neurological subjects showed that the depressives had higher basal levels than the other two groups.[106] Physical activity did not seem to affect these values. However, the study of the rate of accumulation of cyclic AMP after probenecid administration led to the tentative conclusion that this was relatively low in the depressives and relatively high in two manics, suggesting a possible deficit in cyclic AMP function in the depressed patients.

Acetylcholine

It has been suggested that acetylcholine may serve as a synaptic transmitter in the brain, but there is little conclusive evidence as to its real role.[134,199,274] Relatively little attention

has been paid to a possible disturbance of cholinergic function in depression. However, drugs which, *inter alia*, increase brain acetylcholine activity will produce central nervous system depression (reserpine, morphine, barbiturates, general anesthetics, etc.),[10,346] while drugs which are associated with decreased brain acetylcholine activity cause excitation and convulsions.[134,333]

The tricyclic antidepressants have definite anticholinergic effects[34,340] and Fink[138] has suggested that electroconvulsive therapy acts through the cholinergic nervous system.

Janowsky et al.[180] have reported that the intravenous administration of physostigmine, an acetyl-cholinesterase inhibitor, will significantly reverse symptoms of mania, and under some conditions induce symptoms of depression, including feelings of hopelessness and uselessness, lethargy, psychomotor retardation, social withdrawal, and irritability. They suggest that increasing acetylcholine activity will reduce mania and may induce depression. In an effort to integrate this view with the biogenic amine theories of affective illness, they have postulated the need for a critical balance between the cholinergic and the aminergic systems, with a relative preponderance of amines over acetylcholine in mania, and a relative preponderance of cholinergic activity in depression.

While there is no direct evidence to incriminate the cholinergic system in the genesis of affective illness, there is sufficient circumstantial evidence and preliminary experimental observations to indicate that this system does warrant further investigation.[10,138,180,340]

(Neuroendocrine Studies

Hypothalamic-Pituitary-Adrenal Function

The hypothalamus is a vital integrating and regulating center whose functioning may be disturbed in depression. Kraines[203] has reviewed much of the evidence in favor of an abnormal hypothalamic functioning in affective illness. This includes the findings that cer tain hypothalamic lesions are associated with mood disturbance; that an intense affective state can be induced by hypothalamic stimulation; that the hypothalamus is involved in the regulation of appetite, sexual activity, menstruation, and aggression, which are frequently abnormal in depressives; and that it is part of the link between the cerebral cortex and the neuroendocrine system. He suggested that depression results from a persistent, gradually intensifying inhibition of hypothalamic function. While it is probable that aspects of hypothalamic function are altered in depression, there is at this time insufficient evidence to support the hypothesis that this is the primary disturbance.

Patients with hyperadrenalism (Cushing's Syndrome) may be either euphoric or depressed,[44,128,293,337] while patients with hypoadrenalism (Addison's Disease) have many symptoms suggestive of clinical depression.[89,128] The administration of adrenocortical hormones for therapeutic reasons may be associated with symptoms of both depression or mania. Butler and Besser[71] found that tests of adrenal and pituitary function did not distinguish between patients with Cushing's syndrome and patients with severe depression. Antidepressant treatment and clinical improvement reversed the abnormal endocrine function in the depressed patients.

It is known that adrenocortical hormones do directly influence brain function. Cortisol is present in brain tissue and the concentration of cortisol in the brain is responsive to alterations in plasma cortisol levels.[127]

Depressed patients do have a number of changes in adrenocortical function, which point to alterations in glucocorticoid production.[78,81,133,298] These changes include an elevation in plasma 17-hydroxycorticosteroids, 11-hydroxycorticosteroids and cortisol, and in urinary corticosteroids and free cortisol.[6,39,40,52,57,65,68,108,152–155,209,301,302] There is also an increase in the cortisol secretion rate.[154,155] There is a report of an abnormal response to the metapyrone test involving an increased excretion of 11-deoxycorticoids, suggesting an increase in ACTH secretion.[179] Some, but not all, investigators have found alterations in the

normal circadian rhythm of plasma cortisol.[52,57,71,119,133,216,308]

Some, but not all, investigators have found a resistance to the normal suppression of plasma cortisol following dexamethasone administration.[71,81,83,133,155,339] Dexamethasone is a synthetic glucocorticoid which normally reduces endogenous ACTH release, with a subsequent lowering of plasma cortisol. Finally, it has been shown that the plasma cortisol response to an insulin hypoglycemia is impaired in depressed patients and returns to normal with recovery.[79,305]

There is disagreement over whether these changes in adrenocortical function are simply a reflection of the "stress" of the illness or result from a more fundamental disturbance. It is known that a variety of stress experiences will cause an increase in adrenocortical activity, and it has been suggested that either the stress of hospitalization, the nonspecific stress of the illness, or perhaps fluctuations in emotional distress and turmoil in individual patients, are sufficient to account for the changes. An example of this might be the increase in urinary 17-hydroxycorticoids found in some depressed patients prior to suicide attempts.[133]

Sachar[303] has reported that apathetic depressed patients with little emotional arousal have no significant change in cortisol production, while anxious depressed patients have a moderate increase in cortisol, and psychotic depressed patients with severe anxiety have marked increases. He suggests that the elevation in glucocorticoid output may reflect individual distress and pain with disruption of ego defenses, and that cortisol production returns to normal when the disruption passes, even though there may be no real alleviation of the depression.

Other investigators[81,339] have argued that changes, such as the abnormal response to dexamethasone, indicate a disturbance of the normal hypothalamic control over adrenal function which *may* contribute to the genesis of the illness. This dysfunction may involve the limbic system which exerts a regulatory effect on the hypothalamus.

Alterations in *ketosteroid* metabolism,[204,205]

including a reduction in urinary ketogenic steroids,[136] in 11-deoxy-17-ketosteroids (especially dehydro-epiondrosterene),[136] and in the urinary C19 compound, androstenol (with normal 17 ketosteroids),[56] have also been reported. Morning plasmatestosterone concentration was found to be normal in a preliminary study of male depressives.[303] There is a report of an elevation in 11-oxy-17-ketosteroids, as compared with the 11-deoxy-17-ketosteroids, in a group of eight male depressed patients.[219] Values returned to normal with clinical improvement.[218] These preliminary findings suggest the possibility of a disturbance in androgen metabolism in depression.[219]

Epidemiological studies of depression have drawn attention to its association with endocrine state and change. Depression is more common in females than in males (a male:female ratio of 0.69);[332] this may only apply to recurrent depressive illness, rather than to manic-depressive illness, and is more likely to occur at times of life associated with endocrine changes: premenstrually,[*111,214] postpartum, and during the involutional period.[257] There are also conflicting reports of depression occurring in women receiving oral contraceptives.[185]

In addition to the possibility that these endocrine changes may in themselves contribute to the development of mood changes, there are important functional links between them, biogenic amines, and electrolytes. For example, progesterones increase monoamine oxidase activity, while estrogens may decrease it.[191,190,197] Further, biogenic amines play a critical role in hypothalamic control of endocrine function.

Thyroid

There is some circumstantial evidence pointing to a possible association between thyroid function and affective illness. Hypothyroid patients often have features of clinical depression,[360] together with symptoms of an organic confusional state. Measures of thyroid function, such as protein-bound iodine and ankle reflex time, have not produced any conclusive findings in depressives.

L-tri-iodothyronine (T3) and thyroid-stimulating hormone (TSH) have been reported to accelerate the antidepressant effects of imipramine[278,279] and of amitriptyline[358] in female patients, an effect which has been attributed to the action of thyroid hormone in increasing the sensitivity of adrenergic receptors.[276,277]

There are also reports[187] that the intravenous injection of thyrotropin-releasing factor (TRF) will produce a temporary symptomatic relief in some depressed patients. TRF is the hypothalamic polypeptide which, inter alia, stimulates the release of TSH from the pituitary. There was also less of an increase in plasma TSH levels in the depressed patients than in normal control subjects in response to TRF. It has been suggested that the antidepressant effect of TRF may be due to a central action rather than its effect on the thyroid gland.

Growth Hormone

The release of growth hormone from the pituitary gland is also under hypothalamic regulation[285] and is believed to involve dopamine[186] and possibly other biogenic amines.[58] The capacity of the pituitary to release growth hormone into the bloodstream after such stimuli as L-DOPA,[49,186,248] or apomorphine administration, insulin hypoglycemia,[297] or soon after sleep onset,[343] provides another measure of the hypothalamic-pituitary functional state. There are initial reports of deficiency in the release of growth hormone after L-DOPA administration, during sleep, and in response to insulin hypoglycemia in depressed patients.[79,244,304] These findings must await confirmation in larger studies involving age-matched control subjects.

❲ Electrolyte Metabolism

Electrolytes play a crucial role in the maintenance of the resting potential across the cell membrane, in the transmission of electrical

---

* The premenstrual mood changes may be associated with changes in electrolyte and water distribution.

impulses within the nervous system, and in the changes associated with synaptic excitation and inhibition. In addition, they have a critical role in the metabolism of the biogenic amines and are involved in the mechanisms that govern the release, re-uptake, and storage of amines from the neurone. Thus, alterations in the concentration or distribution of certain cations can profoundly affect neuronal functioning through either a direct action on cell membrane activity and electrochemical potential or by altering biogenic amine metabolism. Changes in the ratio of one cation to another are probably very important. For example, the passage of norepinephrine across the membrane is believed to involve a carrier with a high affinity for the amine at the outer neuronal membrane surface (where sodium concentration is high and potassium concentration is low), and a low affinity for the amine at the inner surface (where potassium concentration is high and sodium concentration is low).[41,42] Alterations in sodium-potassium concentrations and of their ratio to each can thus alter norepinephrine metabolism. The maintenance of the normal ionic gradient is an active process governed in part by (Na + K) Mg adenosinetriphosphatase (ATPase).[330] Further, the transport of norepinephrine into the storage granule involves a carrier system with an affinity for sodium at the low concentration found intraneuronally.

Further, the effectiveness of the cation lithium in the treatment and prophylaxis of various phases of manic-depressive and depressive illness[23,123,222,239,240] has stimulated additional interest in ionic metabolism in depression. The interested reader is referred to several recent reviews describing the physiology of electrolyte metabolism and their role in brain function.[24,188]

SODIUM

Depressed patients are reported to have an increase in sodium retention, followed by an increased excretion of sodium on recovery.[26,25,152] The correlation between exchangeable body sodium and clinical improvement has been shown to be close. For example, Gibbons[152] found that sixteen depressed patients who were successfully treated with electroconvulsive therapy had a mean decrease in exchangeable body sodium of 209 mEq, which represented an almost 10 percent reduction in their total exchangeable body sodium. In contrast, eight similar patients also treated with electroconvulsive therapy who did not improve had no significant alteration in exchangeable body sodium.

Similar changes have been found in association with relatively minor mood changes in normal subjects. For example, there is a report of an association between transient periods of depression of mood and a decrease in urinary sodium excretion in a group of normal subjects.[320]

Coppen and Shaw[97] suggested that the extra sodium was mainly being retained in the "residual sodium" compartment (comprised of intracellular sodium and exchangeable bone sodium). They also found an increase in residual sodium in manic patients.[98] However, the method they used for the calculation of residual sodium is relatively imprecise, and their results remain unconfirmed.

It is possible that the sodium retention may result from an increase in cortisol production, and a significant correlation between sodium and water retention and elevated urinary 17-hydroxycorticosteroids has been found.[25]

A logical consequence of these findings has been the effort to directly measure intracellular sodium in depressed patients.

Mendels et al.[229] found erythrocyte sodium concentration to be relatively normal in hospitalized male depressives. Further, the depressed patients who improved with lithium treatment tended to have an increase in erythrocyte sodium concentration over time (in association with lithium administration), whereas the patients who did not respond to lithium tended to have little change (or even a decrease) in erythrocyte sodium concentration.[229,227]

There is also a report that patients who responded to lithium had a significantly greater increase in twenty-four-hour exchangeable sodium that did nonresponders.[25] These findings have led to the suggestion that depressed patients who show an increase in intracellular (or exchangeable) sodium during lithium therapy are more likely to improve than patients who do not show these changes.[229] These findings indicate that there is a difference in the cell membrane function governing electrolyte transport between the lithium responders and nonresponders. This requires further investigation.

An alternative strategy has involved the measurement of the rate of entry of sodium from plasma into the cerebrospinal fluid. This measure may provide an indication of the retention and rate of turnover of sodium by the central nervous system. While there are conflicting reports, the consensus of several investigators[27,81,84,93,141] is that there is a decrease in the rate of entry of sodium into lumbar fluid for depressed and manic patients, in comparison with either control subjects or recovered depressed or manic patients. There was no significant difference between manic and depressed patients.[81]

POTASSIUM

No consistent significant changes in potassium have been found in depression or mania. Studies of exchangeable potassium,[152] potassium balance,[300] and of plasma and erythrocyte potassium concentrations,[232] have produced essentially normal findings. There is an unconfirmed report of a decrease in intracellular potassium in depression, which persisted after clinical recovery.[325]

MAGNESIUM

Magnesium is important for nervous system activity,[74] serving *inter alia* as a necessary cofactor in the ATPase system which regulates ion and perhaps biogenic amine flux across the neuronal membrane.[323,330] There are reports that depressed patients have elevated[72,139] or reduced[147] plasma magnesium concentrations, and of increased plasma and erythrocyte magnesium concentrations in both depressed and manic patients.[72,139,255] Nielson[255] found no significant differences in erythrocyte magnesium concentrations between depressed and manic patients. Some of these findings are difficult to interpret and additional carefully controlled studies, as well as measures of ionized

(unbound) magnesium, will be important in clarifying whether or not there is an important alteration in magnesium metabolism in depression.

CALCIUM

Calcium plays an important role in several aspects of neuronal function. Thus, studies of calcium metabolism are potentially important. Methodological problems have impeded work in this area in that the measurement of total plasma calcium does not provide a reliable index of the functional or ionized portion. At the time of writing, no reliable studies of ionized plasma calcium have been conducted in depressed patients. There are reports of an increased calcium retention with a reduction in urinary calcium excretion in depressed patients in association with clinical improvement.[132,140] These investigators suggested that there might be some alteration in calcitonin activity in depression.

⟪ Psychophysiological Studies

A variety of psychophysiological measures have been studied in depressed patients on the assumption that they provide a measure of brain function or nerve conduction. Studies of the *resting encephalographic pattern* in depressed patients have not produced any significant findings, except for the suggestion of a nonspecific "electrophysiologic instability."[116]

Studies of the *sleep electroencephalogram* have attracted the most attention. In general, most depressed patients have a reduction in actual sleep time, an increased frequency of wakening through the night (especially in the last third of the night) and a reduction in delta-wave sleep (Stages 3 and 4). In addition, the depressed patient takes longer to fall asleep, wakes significantly earlier in the morning, and has an increase in Stage 1 sleep and in drowsiness.[170,172,173,233,234,235,236,237,238,335,372] In most respects, sleep appears to be lighter and more susceptible to disruption by external stimuli.

Reports of changes in Stage 1 Rapid Eye Movement (REM) sleep or dreaming sleep are not as consistent. There were a number of initial reports of a reduction in Stage 1 REM sleep during depression.[172,233] However, more recent careful longitudinal studies show an increase in the amount of Stage 1 REM sleep in some depressives.[170,224,237,238,259] There is also evidence of an increased pressure to achieve REM sleep, which is reflected by a reduced latency to the first REM period of the night in some patients.[224]

There is considerable variation in the sleep pattern from night to night and from patient to patient, which may be the result of differences in diagnostic category, severity of the illness, or fluctuations in clinical state from day to day.

There is evidence that some of the abnormal sleep features revert to normal, prior to complete clinical improvement. A notable exception to this is delta-wave sleep, which may continue below normal values after clinical improvement,[234] although it does eventually reach control values.[224] Several patients whose sleep was studied on an intermittent basis for one or two years after clinical recovery developed abnormal changes in their sleep pattern while asymptomatic. Several weeks later, these patients relapsed.[224] If this finding were confirmed, it would indicate that there are important alterations in brain physiology *prior* to clinical manifestation of the illness.

It is known that the biogenic amines, and perhaps acetylcholine, histamine, and other possible central neurotransmitters, play an important role in the mediation of sleep.[182,362] Attempts are being made to relate the postulated role of these substances in the control of sleep with their hypothesized involvement in the affective disorders.[235]

Alpha suppression in response to stimuli is reported to be more persistent in depressed patients than controls. A prolongation of the recovery phase of the *cortical evoked potential* beyond the normal 20 milliseconds has been noted in psychotically depressed patients.[321,][322] These two findings suggest the possibility of an increased activity of the reticular activating system.

Two patterns of abnormality in the *auditory evoked cortical response* in depressed patients have been reported: hyperrecovery and hyporecovery.[311] The former patients may have increased CNS excitability whereas the latter may have decreased excitability. There is some preliminary evidence that these two patterns of recovery are associated with the presence or absence of a positive family history of affective disorder, as well as with a different response to chemotherapy.

Perez-Reyes[268,269] used intravenous sodium pentothal to determine the inhibition threshold for the galvanic skin response (GSR), and the sleep threshold. He found significant differences between neurotic depressives, psychotic depressives, and control subjects, suggestive of a "basic difference" in CNS activity among the three groups. He suggested that the neurotic depressives have an increased central excitatory state, a decreased central inhibitory state, or a combination of both. In contrast, the psychotically depressed patients may have a decreased central inhibitory state or a combination of both.

Most of the findings from these studies of psychophysiological function (with the exception of the sleep studies) must be regarded as preliminary. Further, it is difficult to come to any clear conclusion as to their significance, in view of our limited understanding of the multiple mechanisms involved in their mediation.

(General

Investigators have studied a number of the biological parameters in depressed patients, and in a few instances also proposed specific theories. These remain very limited findings, which are still to be confirmed and whose significance is uncertain. As such, they will only be noted in summary form here.

(a) Alterations in glucose utilization.[5,350]
(b) An increase in blood acetaldehyde levels.[16]
(c) An increase in plasma triglycerides and cholesterol.[30]

(d) An elevation of residual motor activity (muscle tension) termed "hyperponesis."[357]

(e) A reduction in salivation.[70,261]

(f) Proposal to divide monoamines into excitant and depressant types with abnormalities in balance between two types.[118]

(g) A defect in the normal rhythmic homeostatic mechanism which may underline at least some forms of manic-depressive illness and which may involve some abnormal "switch mechanism."[67]

Manic-Depressive and Recurrent Depressive Illness

Among the many efforts that have been made to divide depressed patients into meaningful subgroups,[166,193,217,218,220,225,289] one of the more promising involves the distinction between manic-depressive illness and recurrent depressive illness. This distinction is made on the basis of whether or not the patient has a previous history of mania, or has only a history of recurrent depressive episodes. The terms "bipolar" or "biphasic" illness and "unipolar" and "uniphasic" illness have been applied.[270]

When depressed patients are divided according to this classification, a number of potentially important differences have been found. Biphasic depressed patients (in contrast with uniphasic depressed patients) have, in addition to a previous history of manic episode(s), the following distinctive features: A different genetic history with a high incidence of biphasic illness in first-degree relatives;[7,54,208,270,365] a more equal frequency of the illness in males and females;[270] an alteration in erythrocyte catechol-o-methyl-transferase levels (in female patients);[91,120] an increased frequency of pacing, physical complaints, and anger;[32] an increased likelihood of responding to lithium carbonate;[123,160,223] an increased likelihood of developing symptoms of psychomotor activity after the administration of L-DOPA[251] or of developing a manic response to tricyclic antidepressants;[69]

lower urinary 17-hydroxycorticosteroids;[121] more frequent augmentation with increased stimulus intensity on cortical evoked potential;[60] reduced platelet monoamine oxidase activity;[250] an earlier age of onset;[54,73,270] a more frequent history of postpartum depression;[28] and a lower sedation threshold.[270]

Thus, it is reasonable to proceed on the assumption at this time that these may be separate conditions.

Relationship Between Depression and Mania

Many investigators regard mania and depression as representing opposite ends of the affective spectrum—the bipolar concept of manic-depressive illness. This is implied in the catecholamine hypothesis of affective illness, which postulates a relative deficiency of norepinephrine in depression and a relative excess in mania. However, there are a number of observations which suggest the possibility that depression and mania share a number of important features and that their relationship may not be bipolar. These observations include: Symptoms of depression are frequent in manic patients; steroid therapy may precipitate either depression or elation; depression and mania both occur in Cushing's Syndrome; total body water and intracellular water concentration are altered in both manic and depressed patients; CSF 5HIAA are low in both manic and depressed patients; CSF tryptophan concentration is low in depressed and manic patients; sleep changes in hypomanic and depressed patients have many features in common; erythrocyte COMT activity is reduced in both mania and depression; sodium transfer into the CSF is reduced in both depressed and manic patients; plasma and RBC magnesium concentrations are reported to be elevated in both mania and depression; electroconvulsive therapy is an effective treatment for both manic and selected depressed patients; lithium carbonate is effective in the treatment of manic and some depressed patients; phenothiazines are useful in the treatment of manic and of some selected depressed patients.

These observations, of course, do not prove that mania and depression are the same. Clearly, they have many important features that distinguish between them. However, it is also apparent that it may not be correct to regard them as bipolar states, and that the eventual unraveling of the biological features of these two conditions may reveal a certain important communality. This concept has been discussed in more detail elsewhere.[103,104,221,223,359]

(Conclusion

Complex interrelationships exist between the metabolic systems discussed here. It seems likely that a meaningful hypothesis of the biology of depression must eventually account for this.[231] Such interrelationships include the critical effect of the electrolytes in the synthesis release, re-uptake, and storage of biogenic amines;[41,42] the effect of changes in hypothalamic function on pituitary adrenal activity, which in turn can alter electrolyte distribution and metabolism (and thus affect amine metabolism); alterations in catecholamine metabolism affecting hypothalamic function; changes in the (Na+K) ATPase system as a result of alterations in cortisol metabolism, with a consequent effect on both electrolyte and amine activity, and the central role of cyclic AMP in so many neuroendocrine and amine activities, amongst others. Research is only beginning to explore the implications of these and other interactions for an understanding of the biology of affective illness.

(Bibliography

1. ABDULLA, Y. H., and K. HAMADAH. "3',5' Cyclic Adenosine Monophosphate in Depression and Mania," *Lancet*, 1 (1970), 378–381.
2. ACHOR, R. W. P., N. O. HANSON, and R. W. GIFFORD. "Hypertension Treated with Rauwolfia Serpentina (Whole Root) and with Reserpine," *Journal of the AMA*, 159 (1955), 841–845.
3. AHLENIUS, S., H. ERIKSSON, K. LARSSON, K. MODIGH, and I. SODERSTEN. "Mating Behavior in the Male Rat Treated with P-Chlorophenylalanine Methyl Ester Alone and in Combination with Pargyline," *Psychopharmacologia*, 20 (1971), 383–388.
4. ANDEN, N.-E. "Effects of Amphetamine and Some Other Drugs on Central Catecholamine Mechanisms," in E. Costa, and S. Garattini, eds., *Amphetamines and Related Compounds*, pp. 447–462. New York: Raven Press, 1970.
5. ANDERSON, W. McC., and J. DAWSON. "The Clinical Manifestations of Depressive Illness with Abnormal Acetyl Methyl Carbinol Metabolism," *Journal of Mental Science*, 108 (1962), 80–87.
6. ———. "Variability of Plasma 17-Hydroxycorticosteroid Levels in Affective Illness and Schizophrenia," *Journal of Psychosomatic Research*, 9 (1965), 237–248.
7. ANGST, J. "Zur Aetiologie und Nosologie Endogener Depressiver Psychosen," *Monographien aus dem Gesamtgebiete der Neurologie und Psychiatrie*, 112 (1966), 1–118.
8. ANGST, J., and C. PERRIS. "Zur Nosologie Endogener Depressionen. Vergleich der Ergebnisse Zweier Untersuchungen," *Archiv für Psychiatrie und Nervenkrankheiten*, 210 (1968), 373–386.
9. ———. "The Nosology of Endogenous Depression: Comparison of the Results of Two Studies," *International Journal of Mental Health*, 1 (1972), 145–158.
10. APRISON, M. H., T. KARIYA, J. N. HINGTGEN, and M. TORU. "Neurochemical Correlates of Behaviour. Changes in Acetylcholine, Norepinephrine and 5-Hydroxytryptamine Concentrations in Several Discrete Brain Areas of the Rat During Behavioural Excitation," *Journal of Neurochemistry*, 15 (1968), 1131–1139.
11. ARONOFF, M. S., R. G. EVENS, and J. DURELL. "Effect of Lithium Salts on Electrolyte Metabolism," *Journal of Psychiatric Research*, 8 (1971), 139–159.
12. ASHCROFT, G. W., and D. F. SHARMAN. "5-Hydroxyindoles in Human Cerebrospinal Fluids," *Nature*, 186 (1960), 1050–1051.
13. ASHCROFT, G. W., P. W. BROOKS, R. L. CUNDALL, D. ECCLESTON, L. G. MURRAY, and I. A. PULLAR. "Changes in the Glycol Metabolites of Noradrenaline in Affective

Illness." Presented at the Fifth World Congress of Psychiatry, Mexico City, Mexico, 1971.

14. ASHCROFT, G. W., T. B. B. CRAWFORD, D. ECCLESTON, D. F. SHARMAN, E. J. MacDOUGALL, J. B. STANTON, and J. K. BINNS. "5-Hydroxyindole Compounds in the Cerebrospinal Fluid of Patients with Psychiatric or Neurological Disease," Lancet, 2 (1966), 1049–1052.

15. ASHCROFT, G. W., D. ECCLESTON, L. G. MURRAY, A. I. M. GLEN, T. B. B. CRAW-FORD, I. A. PULLAR, P. J. SHIELDS, D. S. WALTER, I. M. BLACKBURN, J. CONNEC-HAN, and M. LONERGAN. "Modified Amine Hypothesis for the Aetiology of Affective Illness," Lancet, 2 (1972), 573–577.

16. ASSAEL, M., and M. THEIN. "Blood Acetaldehyde Levels in Affective Disorders," The Israel Annals of Psychiatry and Related Disciplines, 2 (1964), 228–234.

17. AXELROD, J. "Methylation Reactions in the Formation and Metabolism of Catecholamines and Other Biogenic Amines," Pharmacological Reviews, 18 (1966), 95–113.

18. ———. "Noradrenaline: Fate and Control of Its Biosynthesis," Science, 173 (1971), 598–606.

19. ———. "Dopamine-β-Hydroxylase: Regulation of Its Synthesis and Release From Nerve Terminals," Pharmacological Reviews, 24 (1972), 233–243.

20. AXELROD, J., R. A. MUELLER, J. P. HENRY, and P. M. STEPHENS. "Changes in Enzymes Involved in the Biosynthesis and Metabolism of Noradrenaline and Adrenaline After Psychosocial Stimulation," Nature, 225 (1970), 1059–1060.

21. AXELROD, J., and R. TOMCHICK. "Enzymatic O-methylation of Epinephrine and Other Catechols," Journal of Biological Chemistry, 233 (1958), 702–705.

22. AXELROD, J., H. WEIL-MALHERBE, and R. TOMCHICK. "The Physiological Disposition of H³-epinephrine and Its Metabolite Metanephrine," Journal of Pharmacology and Experimental Therapeutics, 127 (1969), 251–256.

23. BAASTRUP, P. C., J. C. POULSEN, M. SCHOU, K. THOMSEN, and A. AMDISEN. "Prophylactic Lithium: Double Blind Discontinuation in Manic Depressive and Recurrent-Depressive Disorders," Lancet, 2 (1970), 326–330.

24. BAER, L. "Electrolyte Metabolism in Psychiatric Disorders," in J. Mendels, ed., Textbook of Biological Psychiatry, pp. 199–234. New York: John Wiley & Sons, 1973.

25. BAER, L., J. DURELL, W. E. BUNNEY, JR., B. S. LEVY, and P. V. CARDON. "Sodium-22 Retention and 17-hydroxy corticosteroid Excretion in Affective Disorders," Journal of Psychiatric Research, 6 (1969), 289–297.

26. BAER, L., J. DURELL, W. E. BUNNEY, JR., D. MURPHY, B. S. LEVY, K. GREENSPAN, and P. V. CARDON. "Sodium Balance and Distribution in Lithium Carbonate Therapy," Archives of General Psychiatry, 22 (1969), 40–44.

27. BAKER, E. F. W. "Sodium Transfer to Cerebrospinal Fluid in Functional Psychiatric Illness," Canadian Psychiatric Association Journal, 16 (1971), 167–170.

28. BAKER, M., J. DORZAB, G. WINOKUR, and R. CADORET. "Depressive Disease: The Effect of the Postpartum State," Biological Psychiatry, 3 (1971), 357–365.

29. BALDESSARINI, R. J. "Biogenic Amines and Behavior," Annual Review of Medicine, 23 (1972), 343–354.

30. BANDRUP, E., and A. BANDRUP. "A Controlled Investigation of Plasma Lipids in Manic Depressives," British Journal of Psychiatry, 113 (1967), 987–992.

31. BARTHOLINI, G., R. TISSOT, and A. PLET-SCHER. "Brain Capillaries as a Source of Homovanillic Acid in Cerebrospinal Fluid," Brain Research, 27 (1971), 163–168.

32. BEIGEL, A., and D. L. MURPHY. "Differences in Clinical Characteristics Accompanying Depression in Unipolar and Bipolar Affective Illness," Archives of General Psychiatry, 24 (1971), 215–220.

33. BEIN, H. J. "Zur Pharmakologie des Reserpin, eines Neven Alkaloids, aus Rauwolfia Serpentina Benth," Experientia, 9 (1953), 107–110.

34. BENESOVA, O. "The Relation of Imipramine-like Drugs to the Cholinergic System," in S. Garattini, and M. N. G. Dukes, eds., Antidepressant Drugs, pp. 247–254. Amsterdam: Excerpta Medica, 1969.

35. BERGSMAN, A. "Urinary Excretion of Adrenalin and Noradrenalin in Some Mental Diseases: Clinical and Experimental Study," Acta Psychiatrica and Neurologica Scandinavica, 34 (Suppl. 133) (1959), 5–107.

36. BERNSTEIN, S., and M. R. KAUFMAN. "A Psychological Analysis of Apparent Depression Following Rauwolfia Therapy," *Journal of Mt. Sinai Hospital*, 27 (1960), 525–530.

37. BERTILSSON, L., and L. PALMER. "Indole-3-acetic Acid in Human Cerebrospinal Fluid: Identification and Quantification by Mass Fragmentography," *Science*, 177 (1972), 74–76.

38. BLOOM, F. E., S. ALGERI, A. GROPPETTE, A. REVUELTA, and E. COSTA. "Lesions of Central Norepinephrine Terminals with 6-OH-dopamine: Biochemistry and Fine Structure," *Science*, 166 (1969), 1284–1286.

39. BOARD, F., H. PERSKY, and D. A. HAMBURG. "Psychological Stress and Endocrine Functions: Blood Levels of Adrenocortical and Thyroid Hormones in Acutely Disturbed Patients," *Psychosomatic Medicine*, 18 (1956), 324–333.

40. BOARD, F., R. WADESON, and H. PERSKY. "Depressive Affect and Endocrine Functions. Blood Levels of Adrenal Cortex and Thyroid Hormones in Patients Suffering From Depressive Reactions," *AMA Archives of Neurology and Psychiatry*, 78 (1957), 612–620.

41. BOGDANSKI, D. F., and B. B. BRODIE. "Role of Sodium and Potassium Ions in Storage of Norepinephrine by Sympathetic Nerve Endings," *Life Sciences*, 5 (1966), 1563–1569.

42. BOGDANSKI, D. F., A. TISSARI, and B. B. BRODIE. "Role of Sodium, Potassium, Ouabain and Reserpine in Uptake, Storage and Metabolism of Biogenic Amines in Synaptosomes," *Life Sciences*, 7 (Part 1) (1968), 419–428.

43. BOND, P. A., F. A. JENNER, and G. A. SAMPSON. "Daily Variations of the Urine Content of 3-Methoxy-4-Hydroxyphenylglycol in Two Manic-Depressive Patients," *Psychological Medicine*, 2 (1972), 81–85.

44. BORMAN, M. C., and H. C. SCHMALLENBERG. "Suicide Following Cortisone Treatment," *Journal of AMA*, 146 (1951), 337–338.

45. BOURNE, H. R., W. E. BUNNEY, JR., R. W. COLBURN, J. M. DAVIS, J. N. DAVIS, D. M. SHAW, and A. J. COPPEN. "Noradrenaline, 5-Hydroxytryptamine, and 5-Hydroxyindoleacetic Acid in Hindbrains of Suicidal Patients," *Lancet*, 2 (1968), 805–808.

46. BOWERS, M. B. "Clinical Measurements of Central Dopamine and 5-Hydroxytryptamine Metabolism: Reliability and Interpretation of Cerebrospinal Fluid Acid Monoamine Metabolite Measures," *Neuropharmacology*, 2 (1972), 101–111.

47. BOWERS, M. B., and F. A. GERBODE. "Relationship of Monoamine Metabolites in Human Cerebrospinal Fluid to Age," *Nature*, 219 (1968), 1256–1257.

48. BOWERS, M. B., G. R. HENINGER, and F. GERBODE. "Cerebrospinal Fluid 5-Hydroxyindoleacetic Acid and Homovanillic Acid in Psychiatric Patients," *International Journal of Neuropharmacology*, 8 (1969), 255–262.

49. BOYD, A. E., III, H. E. LEBOVITZ, and J. B. PFEIFFER. "Stimulation of Human Growth Hormone Secretion by L-DOPA," *New England Journal of Medicine*, 283 (1970), 1425–1429.

50. BREESE, G. R., and T. D. TRAYLOR. "Effect of 6-Hydroxydopamine on Brain Norepinephrine and Dopamine Evidence for Selective Degeneration of Catecholamine Neurons," *Journal of Pharmacology and Experimental Therapeutics*, 174 (1970), 413–420.

51. ———. "Depletion of Brain Noradrenaline and Dopamine by 6-Hydroxydopamine," *British Journal of Pharmacology*, 42 (1971), 88–99.

52. BRIDGES, P. K., and M. T. JONES. "Personality, Physique and the Adrenocortical Response to a Psychological Stress," *British Journal of Psychiatry*, 112 (1966), 1257–1261.

53. BRODIE, B. B., and W. D. REID. "Serotonin in Brain: Functional Considerations," *Advances in Pharmacology*, 6b (1968), 97–113.

54. BRODIE, II. K. H., and M. J. LEFF. "Bipolar Depression—A Comparative Study of Patient Characteristics," *The American Journal of Psychiatry*, 127 (1971), 1086–1090.

55. BRODIE, H. K. H., D. L. MURPHY, F. K. GOODWIN, and W. E. BUNNEY, JR. "Catecholamines and Mania: The Effect of Alpha-Methyl-Para-Tyrosine on Manic Behavior and Catecholamine Metabolism," *Clinical Pharmacology and Therapeutics*, 12 (1971), 219–224.

56. BROOKSBANK, B. W. L. "Urinary Steroids

and Mental Illness," *Lancet*, 2 (1962), 150–151.

57. BROOKSBANK, B. W. L., and A. COPPEN. "Plasma 11-Hydroxycorticosteroids in Affective Disorders," *British Journal of Psychiatry*, 113 (1967), 395–404.

58. BROWN, G. M., and S. REICHLIN. "Psychologic and Neural Regulation of Growth Hormone Secretion," *Psychosomatic Medicine*, 34 (1972), 45–61.

59. BRYSON, G. "Biogenic Amines in Normal and Abnormal Behavioral States," *Clinical Chemistry*, 17 (1971), 5–26.

60. BUCHSBAUM, M., F. GOODWIN, D. L. MURPHY, and G. BORGE. "AER in Affective Disorders." *The American Journal of Psychiatry*, 128 (1971), 19–25.

61. BUENA, J. R., and H. E. HIMWICH. "A Dualistic Approach to Some Biochemical Problems in Endogenous Depressions," *Psychosomatics*, 8 (1967), 82–94.

62. BULAT, M., and B. ZIVKOVIC. "Origin of 5-Hydroxyindoleacetic Acid in the Spinal Fluid," *Science*, 173 (1971), 738–740.

63. BUNNEY, W. E., JR., and J. M. DAVIS. "Norepinephrine in Depressive Reactions. A Review," *Archives of General Psychiatry*, 13 (1965), 483–494.

64. BUNNEY, W. E., JR., and J. A. FAWCETT. "Possibility of a Biochemical Test for Suicide Potential: An Analysis of Endocrine Findings Prior to Three Suicides," *Archives of General Psychiatry*, 13 (1965), 232–239.

65. BUNNEY, W. E., JR., J. W. MASON, and D. A. HAMBURG. "Correlations Between Behavioral Variables and Urinary 17-Hydroxycorticosteroids in Depressed Patients," *Psychosomatic Medicine*, 27 (1965), 299–308.

66. BUNNEY, W. E., JR., J. W. MASON, J. F. ROATCH, and D. A. HAMBURG. "A Psychoendocrine Study of Severe Psychotic Depressive Crises," *The American Journal of Psychiatry*, 122 (1965), 72–80.

67. BUNNEY, W. E., JR., D. L. MURPHY, F. K. GOODWIN, and G. F. BORGE. "The Switch Process From Depression to Mania: Relationship to Drugs Which Alter Brain Amines," *Lancet*, 1 (1970), 1022–1027.

68. BUNNEY, W. E., JR., and D. L. MURPHY. "The Behavioral Switch Process and Psychopathology," in J. Mendels, ed. *Biological Psychiatry*, pp. 345–367. New York: John Wiley & Sons, 1973.

69. BURKARD, W. P., M. JALFRE, and J. BLUM. "Effect of 6-Hydroxydopamine on Behaviour and Cerebral Amine Content in Rats," *Experientia*, 125 (1969), 1295–1296.

70. BUSFIELD, B. L., H. WECHSLER, and W. J. BARNUM. "Studies of Salivation in Depression," *Archives of General Psychiatry*, 51 (1961), 472–477.

71. BUTLER, P. W. P., and G. M. BESSER. "Pituitary-Adrenal Function in a Severe Depressive Illness," *Lancet*, 2 (1968), 1234–1236.

72. CADE, J. F. J. "A Significant Elevation of Plasma Magnesium Levels in Schizophrenia and Depressive States," *Medical Journal of Australia*, 1 (1964), 195–196.

73. CADORET, R., G. WINOKUR, and P. CLAYTON. "Family History Studies. VII. Manic Depressive Disease Versus Depressive Disease," *British Journal of Psychiatry*, 116 (1970), 625–635.

74. CALDWELL, P. C. "Factors Governing Movement and Distribution of Inorganic Ions in Nerve and Muscle," *Physiological Reviews*, 48 (1968), 1–64.

75. CARLSSON, A., and M. LINDQVIST. "Metatyrosine as a Tool for Selective Protection of Catecholamine Stores Against Reserpine," *European Journal of Pharmacology*, 2 (1967), 192–197.

76. CARLSSON, A., E. ROSENGREN, A. BERTLER, and J. NILSSON. "Effect of Reserpine on the Metabolism of Catecholamines," in S. Garattini, and V. Ghetti, eds., *Psychotropic Drugs*, pp. 363–372. Amsterdam: Elsevier, 1957.

77. CARPENTER, W. T. "Serotonin Now: Clinical Implications of Inhibiting Its Synthesis with Para-Chlorophenylalanine," *Annals of Internal Medicine*, 23 (1970), 607–629.

78. CARPENTER, W. T., and W. E. BUNNEY, JR. "Adrenal Cortical Activity in Depressive Illness," *The American Journal of Psychiatry*, 128 (1970), 31–40.

79. CARROLL, B. J. "Hypothalamic-Pituitary Function in Depressive Illness: Insensitivity to Hypoglycaemia," *British Medical Journal*, 3 (1969), 27–28.

80. ———. "Monoamine Precursors in the Treatment of Depression," *Clinical Pharmacology and Therapeutics*, 12 (1971), 743–761.

81. ———. In B. Davies, B. Carroll, and R. M. Mowbray, eds., *Depressive Illness: Some*

Research Studies. Springfield: Thomas, 1972.

82. CARROLL, B. J., and B. M. DAVIES. "Clinical Associations of 11-Hydroxycorticosteroid Suppression and Non-Suppression in Severe Depressive Illnesses," *British Medical Journal*, 1 (1970), 789–791.

83. CARROLL, B. J., F. I. R. MARTIN, and B. M. DAVIES. "Resistance to Suppression by Dexamethasone of Plasma 11-OHCS Levels in Severe Depressive Illnesses," *British Medical Journal*, 3 (1968), 285–287.

84. CARROLL, B. J., L. STEVEN, R. A. POPE, and B. M. DAVIES. "Sodium Transfer From Plasma to CSF in Severe Depressive Illness," *Archives of General Psychiatry*, 21 (1969), 77–81.

85. CAZZULLO, C. L., A. MANGONI, and G. MASCHERPA. "Tryptophan Metabolism in Affective Psychoses," *British Journal of Psychiatry*, 112 (1966), 157–162.

86. CHARALAMPOUS, K. D., and S. BROWN. "A Clinical Trial of Alpha-Methyl-Paratyrosine in Mentally Ill Patients," *Psychopharmacologia*, 11 (1967), 422–429.

87. CHASE, L. R., and G. D. AURBACH. "Renal Adenyl Cyclase: Anatomically Separate Sites for Parathyroid Hormone and Vasopressin," *Science*, 159 (1968), 545–547.

88. CHASE, T. N., G. R. BREESE, E. K. GORDON, and I. J. KOPIN. "Catecholamine Metabolism in the Dog: Comparison of Intravenously and Intraventricularly Administered (^{14}C) Dopamine and (^{3}H) Norepinephrine," *Journal of Neurochemistry*, 18 (1971), 135–140.

89. CLEGHORN, R. A. "Adrenal Cortical Insufficiency: Psychological and Neurological Observations," *Canadian Medical Association Journal*, 65 (1951), 449–454.

90. COHN, C. K., and J. AXELROD. "The Effect of Estradiol on Catechol-O-Methyltransferase Activity in Rat Liver," *Life Sciences*, 10 (1971), 1351–1354.

91. COHN, C. K., D. L. DUNNER, and J. AXELROD. "Reduced Catechol-O-Methyl-Transferase Activity in Red Blood Cells of Women With Primary Affective Disorder," *Science*, 170 (1970), 1323–1324.

92. COON, W. W., and E. NAGLER. "The Tryptophan Load as a Test For Pyridoxine Deficiency in Hospitalized Patients," *Annals of the New York Academy of Science*, 166 (1969), 30–43.

93. COPPEN, A. J. "Abnormality of the Blood-Cerebrospinal Fluid Barrier of Patients Suffering From a Depressive Illness," *Journal of Neurology, Neurosurgery and Psychiatry*, 23 (1960), 156–161.

94. ———. "The Biochemistry of Affective Disorders," *British Journal of Psychiatry*, 113 (1967), 1237–1264.

95. COPPEN, A. J., B. W. L. BROOKSBANK, and M. PEET. "Tryptophan Concentration in the Cerebrospinal Fluid of Depressive Patients," *Lancet*, 1 (1972), 1393.

96. COPPEN, A. J., A. J. PRANGE, JR., P. C. WHYBROW, and R. NOGUERA. "Abnormalities of Indoleamines in Affective Disorders," *Archives of General Psychiatry*, 26 (1972), 474–478.

97. COPPEN, A. J., and D. M. SHAW. "Mineral Metabolism in Melancholia," *British Journal of Medicine*, 2 (1963), 1439–1444.

98. COPPEN, A. J., D. M. SHAW, J. P. FARRELL, and R. COSTAIN. "Mineral Metabolism in Mania," *British Medical Journal*, 1 (1966), 71–75.

99. COPPEN, A. J., D. M. SHAW, and A. MANGONI. "Total Exchangeable Sodium in Depressive Illness," *British Medical Journal*, 5300 (1962), 295–298.

100. COPPEN, A. J., D .M. SHAW, A. MALLESON, E. ECCLESTON, and G. GUNDY. "Tryptamine Metabolism in Depression," *British Journal of Psychiatry*, 3 (1965), 993–998.

101. COSTA, E., and N. H. NEFF. "Importance of Turnover Rate Measurements to Elucidate the Functions of Neuronal Monoamines," in I. Rabinowitz, and R. Meyerson, eds., *Topics in Medicinal Chemistry*, 3 (1968), 65–95.

102. ———. "Estimation of Turnover Rates to Study the Metabolic Regulation of the Steady-State Level of Neuronal Monoamines," in A. Lajtha, ed., *Handbook of Neurochemistry*. New York: Plenum Press, 1970.

103. COURT, J. H. "Manic-Depressive Psychosis: An Alternative Conceptual Model," *British Journal of Psychiatry*, 114 (1968), 1523–1530.

104. ———. "The Continuum Model as a Resolution of Paradoxes in Manic-Depressive Psychosis," *British Journal of Psychiatry*, 120 (1972), 133–141.

105. COX, B., and D. POTKONJAK. "The Effect of Ambient Temperature on the Actions of Tremorine on Body Temperature and on

the Concentration of Noradrenaline, Dopamine, 5-Hydroxytryptamine and Acetylcholine in Rat Brain," *British Journal of Pharmacology and Chemotherapy*, 31 (1967), 356–366.

106. CRAMER, H., F. K. GOODWIN, R. M. POST, and W. E. BUNNEY, JR. "Effects of Probenecid and Exercise on Cerebrospinal Fluid Cyclic A.M.P. in Affective Illness," *Lancet*, 1 (1972), 1346–1347.

107. CREMATA, V. Y., JR., and B. K. KOE. "Clinical-Pharmacological Evaluation of p-Chlorophenylalanine: A new Serotonin-Depleting Agent," *Clinical Pharmacology and Therapeutics* 7 (1966), 768–776.

108. CURTIS, B. C., R. A. CLEGHORN, and T. L. SOURKES. "The Relationship Between Affect and the Excretion of Adrenaline, Noradrenaline, and 17-Hydroxycorticosteriods," *Journal of Psychosomatic Research*, 4 (1960), 176–184.

109. CURZON, G. "Tryptophan Pyrrolase—A Biochemical Factor in Depressive Illness?" *British Journal of Psychiatry*, 115 (1969), 1367–1374.

110. CURZON, G., and P. K. BRIDGES. "Tryptophan Metabolism in Depression," *Journal of Neurology, Neurosurgery and Psychiatry*, 33 (1970), 698–704.

111. DALTON, K. "Menstruation and Acute Psychiatric Illnesses," *British Medical Journal*, 1 (1959), 148–149.

112. DAVIES, B. M., B. J. CARROLL, and R. M. MOWBRAY. *Depressive Illness*. Springfield: Thomas, 1972.

113. DAVIS, J. M. "Theories of Biological Etiology of Affective Disorders," in C. C. Pfeiffer, and J. R. Smythies, eds., *International Review of Neurobiology*, Vol. 12, pp. 145–175. New York: Academic Press, 1970.

114. DAVIS, J. M., and W. E. FANN. "Lithium," *Annual Review of Pharmacology*, 11 (1971), 285–303.

115. DAVIS, J. M., G. L. KLERMAN, and J. J. SCHILDKRAUT. "Drugs Used in the Treatment of Depression," in D. H. Efron, ed., *Psychopharmacology: A Review of Progress, 1957–1967*, pp. 719–738. Washington: U.S. Government Printing Office, 1968.

116. DENBER, N. C. B. "Electroencephalographic Findings During Chlorpromazine-Diethazine Treatment," *Journal of Nervous and Mental Disease*, 126 (1958), 392–398.

117. DENCKER, S. J., U. MALM, R. E. ROOS, and B. WERDINIUS. "Acid Monoamine Metabolites of Cerebrospinal Fluid in Mental Depression and Mania," *Journal of Neurochemistry*, 13 (1966), 1545–1548.

118. DEWHURST, W. G. "Cerebral Amine Functions in Health and Disease," in M. Shephard, and D. L. Davies, eds., *Studies in Psychiatry*, pp. 289–317. London: Oxford University Press, 1968.

119. DOIG, R. J., R. V. MUMMERY, M. R. WILLS, and A. ELKES. "Plasma Cortisol Levels in Depression," *British Journal of Psychiatry*, 112 (1966), 1263–1267.

120. DUNNER, D. L., C. K. COHN, E. S. GERSHON, and F. K. GOODWIN. "Differential Catechol-O-Methyl-Transferase Activity in Unipolar and Bipolar Affective Illness," *Archives of General Psychiatry*, 25 (1971), 348–353.

121. DUNNER, D. L., F. K. GOODWIN, E. S. GERSHON, D. L. MURPHY, and W. E. BUNNEY, JR. "Excretion of 17-Hydroxycorticosteroids in Unipolar and Bipolar Depressed Patients," *Archives of General Psychiatry*, 26 (1972), 360–363.

122. DUSTAN, H. P., R. D. TAYLOR, A. C. CORCORAN, and I. H. PAGE. "Clinical Experience With Reserpine (Serpasil): A Controlled Study," *Annals of the New York Academy of Science*, 59 (1954), 136–140.

123. DYSON, W. L., and J. MENDELS. "Lithium and Depression," *Current Therapeutic Research*, 10 (1968), 601–608.

124. EBERT, M. H., R. M. POST, and F. K. GOODWIN. "Effect of Physical Activity on Urinary M.H.P.G. Excretion in Depressed Patients," *Lancet*, 2 (1972), 766.

125. ECCLESTON, D., G. W. ASHCROFT, T. B. B. CRAWFORD, J. B. STANTON, D. WOOD, and P. H. McTURK. "Effect of Tryptophan Administration on 5HIAA in Cerebrospinal Fluid in Man," *Journal of Neurology, Neurosurgery and Psychiatry*, 33 (1970), 269–272.

126. ECCLESTON, D., R. LOOSE, I. A. PULLAR, and R. F. SUGDEN. "Exercise and Urinary Excretion of Cyclic A.M.P.," *Lancet*, 2 (1970), 612–613.

127. EIK-NES, K. B., and K. R. BRIZZEE. "Concentration of Tritium in Brain Tissue of Dogs Given $(1,2-{}^3H_2)$ Cortisol Intravenously," *Biochimica et Biophysica Acta*, 97 (1965), 320–333.

128. ENGEL, G. L., and S. G. MARGOLIN. "Neuro-

psychiatric Disturbances in Addison's Disease and the Role of Impaired Carbohydrate Metabolism in Production of Abnormal Cerebral Function," *AMA Archives of Neurology and Psychiatry*, 45 (1941), 881–884.

129. ENGELMAN, K., D. HORWITZ, E. JEQUIER, and A. SJOERDSMA. "Biochemical and Pharmacologic Effects of Alpha-Methyltyrosine in Man," *Journal of Clinical Investigation*, 47 (1968), 577–594.

130. EVERETT, G. M., and R. G. WIEGAND. "Central Amines and Behavioral States. A Critique and New Data," in B. Uvnas, ed., *Mode of Action of Drugs*, Vol. 8, pp. 85–92. New York: Pergamon Press, 1962.

131. FANN, W. E., J. M. DAVIS, D. S. JANOWSKY, J. S. KAUFMANN, J. D. GRIFFITH, and J. A. OATES. "Effect of Iprindole on Amine Uptake in Man," *Archives of General Psychiatry*, 26 (1972), 158–162.

132. FARAGALLA, F. F., and F. F. FLACH. "Studies of Mineral Metabolism in Mental Depression. I. The Effects of Imipramine and Electric Convulsive Therapy on Calcium Balance and Kinetics," *Journal of Nervous and Mental Disease*, 151 (1970), 120–129.

133. FAWCETT, J. A., and W. E. BUNNEY, JR. "Pituitary Adrenal Function and Depression. An Outline for Research," *Archives of General Psychiatry*, 16 (1967), 517–535.

134. FELDBERG, W. "Present Views on Mode of Action of Acetylcholine in Central Nervous System," *Physiological Review*, 25 (1945), 596–642.

135. FELDSTEIN, A., H. HOAGLAND, K. K. WONG, M. R. OKTEM, and H. FREEMAN. "MAO Activity in Relation to Depression," *The American Journal of Psychiatry*, 120 (1966), 1192–1194.

136. FERGUSON, H. C., A. C. G. BARTRAM, H. C. FOWLIE, D. M. CATHRO, K. BIRCHELL, and F. L. MITCHELL. "A Preliminary Investigation of Steroid Excretion in Depressed Patients Before and After Electroconvulsive Therapy," *Acta Endocrinologica*, 47 (1964), 58–68.

137. FERNSTROM, J. D., and R. J. WURTMAN. "Brain Serotonin Content: Physiological Dependence on Plasma Tryptophan Levels," *Science*, 173 (1971), 149–152.

138. FINK, M. "CNS Effects of Convulsive Therapy: Significance for a Theory of Depressive Psychosis", in J. Zubin, and F. A.

Freyhan, eds., *Disorders of Mood*, pp. 93–112. Baltimore: Johns Hopkins Press, 1972.

139. FITZGERALD, R., A. FRAZER, S. SECUNDA, and J. MENDELS. "Magnesium and Affective Disorders: Plasma and Red Blood Cell Concentrations and Effect of Lithium." In preparation.

140. FLACH, F. F. "Calcium Metabolism in States of Depression," *British Journal of Psychiatry*, 110 (1964), 588–593.

141. FOTHERBY, K., G. W. ASHCROFT, J. W. AFFLECK, and A D. FORREST. "Studies on Sodium Transfer and 5-Hydroxyindoles in Depressive Illness," *Journal of Neurology, Neurosurgery and Psychiatry*, 26 (1963), 71–73.

142. FRAZER, A., J. MENDELS, S. SECUNDA, C. M. COCKRANE, C. P. BIANCHI. "The Prediction of Brain Lithium Concentrations From Plasma or Erythrocyte Measures," *Journal of Psychiatric Research*, 10 (1973), 1–7.

143. FRAZER, A., G. N. PANDY, and J. MENDELS. "Metabolism of Tryptophan in Depressive Disease," *Archives of General Psychiatry*, 29 (1973), 528–535.

144. FRAZER, A., and J. L. STINNETT. "Distribution and Metabolism of Norepinephrine and Serotonin in the Central Nervous System," in J. Mendels, ed., *Biological Psychology*, pp. 35–64. New York: John Wiley & Sons, 1973.

145. FREEMAN, J. J., K. W. MILLER, J. V. DINGELL, and F. SULSER. "On the Mechanism of Amphetamine Potentiation by Iprindole," *Experientia*, 26 (1970), 863–864.

146. FREIS, E. D. "Mental Depression in Hypertensive Patients Treated for Long Periods With Large Doses of Reserpine," *New England Journal of Medicine*, 251 (1954), 1006–1008.

147. FRIZEL, D., A. COPPEN, and V. MARKS. "Plasma Magnesium and Calcium in Depression," *British Journal of Psychiatry*, 115 (1969), 1375–1377.

148. FULLERTON, D. T., F. J. WENZEL, F. N. LOHRENZ, and H. FAHS. "Circadian Rhythm of Adrenal Cortical Activity in Depression. A Comparison of Depressed Patients with Normal Subjects," *Archives of General Psychiatry*, 19 (1968), 674–681.

149. GERSHON, E. S., D. L. DUNNER, and F. K. GOODWIN. "Toward a Biology of Affective Disorders: Genetic Contributions," *Ar-*

chives of General Psychiatry, 25 (1971), 1–15.

150. GERSHON, E. S., D. L. DUNNER, L. STURT, and F. K. GOODWIN. "Assortative Mating in the Affective Disorders." Presented at the Annual Meeting of the American Psychiatric Association, Washington, D.C., May 1971.

151. GERSHON, S., L. J. HEKIMIAN, A. FLOYD, JR., and L. E. HOLLISTER. "Alpha-Methyl-p-Tyrosine (AMT) in Schizophrenia," *Psychopharmacologia*, 11 (1967), 189–194.

152. GIBBONS, J. L. "Total Body Sodium and Potassium in Depressive Patients," *Clinical Science*, 19 (1960), 133–138.

153. ———. "Electrolytes and Depressive Illness," *Postgraduate Medical Journal*, 39 (1963), 19–25.

154. ———. "Cortisol Secretion Rate in Depressive Illness," *Archives of General Psychiatry*, 10 (1964), 572–575.

155. GIBBONS, J. L., and T. J. FAHY. "Effect of Dexamethasone on Plasma Corticosteroids in Depressive Illness," *Neuroendocrinology*, 1 (1966), 358–363.

156. GIBBONS, J. L., and P. R. McHUGH. "Plasma Cortisol in Depressive Illness," *Journal of Psychiatric Research*, 1 (1962), 162–171.

157. GLASSMAN, A. H. "Indoleamines and Affective Disorders," *Psychosomatic Medicine*, 2 (1969), 107–114.

158. GLOWINSKI, J., and J. AXELROD. "Inhibition of Uptake of Tritiated-Noradrenaline in the Intact Rat Brain by Imipramine and Structurally Related Compounds," *Nature*, 204 (1964), 1318–1319.

159. GOODWIN, F. K., and W. E. BUNNEY, JR. "Depressions Following Reserpine: A Re-evaluation," *Seminars in Psychiatry*, 3 (1971), 435–448.

160. GOODWIN, F. K., D. L. MURPHY, and W. E. BUNNEY, JR. "Lithium Carbonate Treatment in Depression and Mania. A Longitudinal Double-Blind Study," *Archives of General Psychiatry*, 21 (1969), 486–496.

161. GOODWIN, F. K., D. L. MURPHY, H. K. H. BRODIE, and W. E. BUNNEY, JR. "L-DOPA, Catecholamines and Behavior: A Clinical and Biochemical Study in Depressed Patients," *Biological Psychiatry*, 2 (1970), 341–366.

162. GOODWIN, F. K., D. L. MURPHY, D. L. DUNNER, and W. E. BUNNEY, JR. "Lithium Response in Unipolar Versus Bipolar De-

pression," *The American Journal of Psychiatry*, 129 (1972), 44–47.

163. GORDON, E. K., and J. OLIVER. "3-Methoxy-4-Hydroxyphenylethylene Glycol in Human Cerebrospinal Fluid," *Clinica Chimica Acta*, 35 (1971), 145–150.

164. GREENSPAN, K., J. J. SCHILDKRAUT, E. K. GORDON, L. BAER, M. S. ARANOFF, and J. DURELL. "Catecholamine Metabolism in Affective Disorders. III. MHPG and Other Catecholamine Metabolities in Patients Treated with Lithium Carbonate," *Journal of Psychiatric Research*, 7 (1970), 171–183.

165. GREENSPAN, K., J. J. SCHILDKRAUT, E. K. GORDON, B. LEVY, and J. DURELL. "Catecholamine Metabolism in Affective Disorders. II. Norepinephrine, Normetanephrine, Epinephrine, Metanephrine, and VMA Excretion in Hypomanic Patients," *Archives of General Psychiatry*, 21 (1969), 710–716.

166. GRINKER, R. R., SR., J. MILLER, M. SABSHIN, R. NANN, and J. C. NUNNALLY. *The Phenomena of Depressions*. New York: Hoeber, 1961.

167. GYERMEK, L. "Effects of Imipramine-Like Antidepressant Agents on the Autonomic Nervous System," in D. H. Efron, and S. S. Kety, eds., *Antidepressant Drugs of Non-MAO Inhibitor Type*, pp. 41–62. Washington: U.S. Government Printing Office, 1966.

168. ———. "The Pharmacology of Imipramine and Related Antidepressants," *International Review of Neurobiology*, 9 (1966), 95–143.

169. HARTMAN, B. K. "The Discovery and Isolation of a New Monoamine Oxidase from Brain," *Biological Psychiatry*, 4 (1972), 147–156.

170. HARTMANN, E. "Longitudinal Studies of Sleep and Dream Patterns in Manic-Depressive Patients," *Archives of General Psychiatry*, 19 (1968), 312–329.

171. HAUGAARD, N., and M. E. HESS. "Actions of Autonomic Drugs on Phosphorylase Activity and Function," *Pharmacological Review*, 17 (1965), 27–69.

172. HAWKINS, D. R., and J. MENDELS. "Sleep Disturbance in Depressive Syndrome," *The American Journal of Psychiatry*, 123 (1966), 682–690.

173. ———. "The Psychopathology and Psycho-

physiology of Sleep," in J. Mendels, ed., *Biological Psychiatry*, pp. 297–330. New York: John Wiley & Sons, 1973.

174. HERMAN, Z. S., K. KMIECIAK-KOLADA, and R. BRUS. "Behaviour of Rats and Biogenic Amine Level in Brain After 6-Hydroxydopamine," *Psychopharmacologia*, 24 (1972), 407–416.

175. HERTTING, G., J. AXELROD, and L. G. WHITBY. "Effect of Drugs on the Uptake and Metabolism of H³-Norepinephrine," *Journal of Pharmacology and Experimental Therapeutics*, 134 (1961), 146–153.

176. HIMWICH, H. E., and H. S. ALPERS. "Psychopharmacology," *Annual Review of Pharmacology*, 10 (1970), 313–324.

177. HOOPER, G., ed. *Metabolism of Amines in the Brain*. London: Macmillan, Ltd., 1968.

178. HORDERN, A. *Depressive States, a Pharmacotherapeutic Study*. Springfield: Thomas, 1965.

179. JAKOBSON, T., A. STENBÄCK, L. STRANDSTRÖM, and P. RIMON. "The Excretion of Urinary 11-Deoxy- and 11-Oxy-17-Hydroxy-Corticosteroids in Depressive Patients During Basal Conditions and During the Administration of Methopyrapone," *Journal of Psychosomatic Research*, 9 (1966), 363–374.

180. JANOWSKY, D. S., M. K. EL-YOUSEF, J. M. DAVIS, and H. J. SEKERKE. "A Cholinergic-Adrenergic Hypothesis of Mania and Depression," *Lancet*, 2 (1972), 632–635.

181. JONES, A. B. B., C. M. B. PARE, W. J. NICHOLSON, K. PRICE, and R. S. STACEY. "Brain Amine Concentrations After Monoamine Oxidase Inhibitor Administration," *British Medical Journal*, 1 (1972), 17–19.

182. JOUVET, M. "The Role of Monoamines and Acetylcholine in the Regulation of the Sleep-Waking Cycle," in R. H. Adrain, E. Helmreich, H. Holzer, et al., eds., *Reviews of Physiology*, pp. 166–307. Berlin: Springer-Verlag, 1972.

183. KALLMAN, F. "Genetic Aspects of Psychoses," in *Biology of Mental Health and Disease*, 27th Annual Conference of the Milbank Memorial Fund, pp. 283–302. New York: Hoeber, 1952.

184. KAMINSKY, N. I., A. E. BROADUS, J. G. HARDMAN, D. J. JONES, J. H. BALL, E. W. SUTHERLAND, and G. W. LIDDLE. "Effects of Parathyroid Hormone on Plasma and Urinary Adenosine 3′,5′-Monophosphate in

Man," *Journal of Clinical Investigation*, 49 (1970), 2387–2395.

185. KANE, F. J. "Clinical Psychiatric Symptoms Accompanying Oral Contraceptive Use," *Comments on Contemporary Psychiatry*, 1 (1971), 7–16.

186. KANSAL, P. C., J. BUSE, O. R. TALBERT, and M. G. BUSE. "The Effect of L-DOPA on Plasma Growth Hormone, Insulin, and Thyroxine," *Journal of Clinical Endocrinology and Metabolism*, 34 (1972), 99–105.

187. KASTIN, A. J., D. S. SCHALCH, R. H. EHRENSING, and M. S. ANDERSON. "Improvement in Mental Depression with Decreased Thyrotropin Response After Administration of Thyrotropin-Releasing Hormone," *Lancet*, 2 (1972), 740–742.

188. KATZ, B. *Nerve Muscle and Synapse*. New York: McGraw-Hill, 1966.

189. KERRY, R. J., and G. OWEN. "Lithium Carbonate as a Mood and Total Body Water Stabilizer," *Archives of General Psychiatry*, 22 (1970), 301–303.

190. KLAIBER, E. L., D. M. BROVERMAN, W. VOGEL, Y. KOBAYASHI, and D. MORIARTY. "Effects of Estrogen Therapy on Plasma MAO Activity and EEG Driving Responses of Depressed Women," *The American Journal of Psychiatry*, 128 (1972), 1492–1498.

191. KLAIBER, E. L., Y. KOBAYASHI, D. M. BROVERMAN, and F. HALL. "Plasma Monoamine Oxidase Activity in Regularly Menstruating Women and in Amenorrheic Women Receiving Cyclic Treatment with Estrogens and a Progestin," *Journal of Clinical Endocrinology and Metabolism*, 33 (1971), 630–638.

192. KLEIN, D. F., and J. M. DAVIS. *Diagnosis and Drug Treatment of Psychiatric Disorders*. Baltimore: Williams and Wilkins, 1969.

193. KLERMAN, G. L. "Clinical Research in Depression," *Archives of General Psychiatry*, 24 (1971), 305–319.

194. KLERMAN, G. L., and J. O. COLE. "Clinical Pharmacology of Imipramine and Related Antidepressant Compounds," *Pharmacological Reviews*, 17 (1965), 101–141.

195. KNOTT, P. J., and G. CURZON. "Free Tryptophan in Plasma and Brain Tryptophan Metabolism," *Nature*, 239 (1972), 452–453.

196. KNOX, W. E., and V. H. AUERBACH. "The

Hormonal Control of Tryptophan Peroxidase in the Rat," *Journal of Biological Chemistry*, 214 (1955), 307–313.

197. KOBAYASHI, T., T. KOBAYASHI, J. KATO, and H. MINAGUCHI. "Cholinergic and Adrenergic Mechanisms in the Female Rat of Hypothalamus with Special Reference to Feedback of Ovarian Steroid Hormones," in G. Pincus, et al., eds., *Steroid Dynamics. Symposium on the Dynamics of Steroid Hormones, Tokyo, 1965*, pp. 303–339. New York: Academic Press, 1966.

198. KOE, B. K., and A. WEISSMAN. "P-Chlorophenylalanine: A Specific Depletion of Brain Serotonin," *Journal of Pharmacology and Experimental Therapeutics*, 154 (1966), 499–516.

199. KOELLE, G. B. "Acetylcholine—Current Status in Physiology, Pharmacology and Medicine," *New England Journal of Medicine*, 286 (1972), 1086–1090.

200. KOELLA, W. P., A. FELDSTEIN, and J. S. CZICMAN. "The Effect of Para-Chlorophenylalanine on the Sleep of Cats," *Electroencephalography and Clinical Neurophysiology*, 25 (1968), 481–490.

201. KOPIN, I. J., G. R. BREESE, K. R. KRAUSS, and V. K. WEISE. "Selective Release of Newly Synthesized Norepinephrine from the Cat Spleen During Sympathetic Nerve Stimulation," *Journal of Pharmacology and Experimental Therapeutics*, 161 (1968), 271–278.

202. KOPIN, I. J., J. E. FISCHER, J. M. MUSACCHIO, W. D. HORST, and V. K. WEISE. "False Neurochemical Transmitters and the Mechanism of Sympathetic Blockade by Monoamine Oxidase Inhibitors," *Journal of Pharmacology and Experimental Therapeutics*, 147 (1965), 186–193.

203. KRAINES, S. H. "Manic-Depressive Syndrome: A Physiologic Disease," *Diseases of the Nervous System*, 27 (1966), 3–19.

204. KURLAND, H. D. "Steroid Excretion in Depressive Disorders," *Archives of General Psychiatry*, 10 (1964), 554–560.

205. ———. "Physiologic Treatment of Depressive Reactions: A Pilot Study," *The American Journal of Psychiatry*, 122 (1965), 457–458.

206. LAPIN, I. P., and G. F. OXENKRUG. "Intensification of the Central Serotoninergic Processes as a Possible Determinant of the Thymoleptic Effect," *Lancet*, 1 (1969), 132–136.

207. LAVERTY, R., and K. M. TAYLOR. "Effects of Intraventricular 2,4,5-Trihydroxyphenylethylamine (6-Hydroxydopamine) on Rat Behaviour and Brain Catecholamine Metabolism," *British Journal of Pharmacology*, 40 (1970), 836–846.

208. LEONHARD, K. *Aufteilung der Endogen Psychosen*. Berlin: Akademik Verlag, 1959.

209. LINGIAERDE, P. S. "Plasma Hydrocortisone in Mental Diseases," *British Journal of Psychiatry*, 110 (1964), 423–432.

210. MAAS, J. W., J. FAWCETT, and H. DEKIRMENJIAN. "3-Methoxy-4-Hydroxyphenylglycol (MHPG) Excretion in Depressive States," *Archives of General Psychiatry*, 19 (1968), 129–134.

211. ———. "Catecholamine Metabolism, Depressive Illness, and Drug Response," *Archives of General Psychiatry*, 26 (1972), 252–262.

212. ———, and D. H. LANDIS. "*In Vivo* Studies of the Rates of Appearance in Urine of Metabolites of Brain Norepinephrine," *Federation Proceedings*, 26 (Abstract 1156) (1967), 463.

213. MALLESON, A., D. FRIZEL, and V. MARKS. "Ionized and Total Plasma Calcium and Magnesium Before and After Modified ECT," *British Journal of Psychiatry*, 114 (1968), 631–633.

214. MANDELL, A., and M. P. MANDELL. "Suicide and the Menstrual Cycle," *Journal of the AMA*, 200 (1967), 792–793.

215. MASON, J. W. "A Review of Psychoendocrine Research on the Pituitary-Adrenal Cortical System," *Psychosomatic Medicine*, 30 (1968), 576–607.

216. McCLURE, D. J. "The Diurnal Variation of Plasma Cortisol Levels in Depression," *Journal of Psychosomatic Research*, 10 (1966), 189–195.

217. MENDELS, J. "The Prediction of Response to Electroconvulsive Therapy," *The American Journal of Psychiatry*, 124 (1967), 153–159.

218. ———. "Depression: The Distinction Between Symptom and Syndrome," *British Journal of Psychiatry*, 114 (1968), 1549–1554.

219. ———. "Urinary 17-Ketosteroid Fractionation in Depression: A Preliminary Report," *British Journal of Psychiatry*, 115 (1969), 581–585.

220. ———. *Concepts of Depression*. John Wiley & Sons, New York: 1970.

221. ———. "Relationship Between Depression and Mania," *Lancet*, 1 (1971), 342.
222. ———. *Textbook of Biological Psychiatry.* New York: John Wiley & Sons, 1973.
223. ———. "Lithium and Depression," in S. Gershon, et al., eds., *The Lithium Ion.* New York: Raven Press (1937), 253–267.
224. MENDELS, J., and D. CHERNIK. "REM Sleep and Depression," in M. H. Chase, W. C. Stern and P. L. Walter, eds. *Sleep Research*, Vol. 1, Los Angeles: Brain Information Service—Brain Research Institute, 1972.   1
225. MENDELS, J., and C. COCHRANE. "The Nosology of Depression: The Endogenous-Reactive Concept," *The American Journal of Psychiatry*, 124 (Supplement) (1968), 1–11.
226. MENDELS, J., and C. COCHRANE. "Syndromes of Depression and the Response to E.C.T.," in preparation.
227. MENDELS, J., and A. FRAZER. "Intracellular Lithium Concentration and Clinical Response: Towards a Membrane Theory of Depression," *Journal of Psychiatric Research*, 10 (1973), 9–18.
228. ———. "Brain Biogenic Amine Depletion and Mood." *Archives of General Psychiatry*, in press.
229. MENDELS, J., A. FRAZER, C. COCHRANE, and P. BIANCHI. "Sodium and Lithium Erythrocyte Concentration in Affective Disorders" (Abstract), Psychiatric Research Society, Washington, D.C., 1972.
230. MENDELS, J., A. FRAZER, R. FITZGERALD, T. A. RAMSEY, and J. STOKES. "Biogenic Amine Metabolites in the Cerebral-Spinal Fluid of Depressed and Manic Patients," *Science*, 175 (1972), 1380–1382.
231. MENDELS, J., A. FRAZER, S. SECUNDA, and J. STOKES. "Biochemical Changes in Depression," *Lancet*, 1 (1971), 448–449.
232. MENDELS, J., A. FRAZER, and S. K. SECUNDA. "Intraerythrocyte Sodium and Potassium in Manic-Depressive Illness," *Biological Psychiatry*, 5 (1972), 165–171.
233. MENDELS, J., and D. R. HAWKINS. "Sleep and Depression: A Controlled EEG Study," *Archives of General Psychiatry*, 16 (1967), 344–354.
234. ———. "Sleep and Depression: A Follow-up Study," *Archives of General Psychiatry*, 16 (1967), 536–542.
235. ———. "Sleep and Depression: Further

Considerations," *Archives of General Psychiatry*, 19 (1968), 445–452.
236. ———. "Longitudinal Sleep Study in Hypomania," *Archives of General Psychiatry*, 25 (1971), 274–277.
237. ———. "Sleep and Depression: IV. Longitudinal Studies," *Journal of Nervous and Mental Disease*, 153 (1972), 251–272.
238. ———. "Sleep Studies in Depression," in T. Williams, M. Katz, and J. Shields, eds., *Recent Advances in the Psychobiology of the Depressive Illnesses.* Washington: U.S. Government Printing Office, 1972.
239. MENDELS, J., and S. SECUNDA. *Lithium: Clinical and Research Aspects.* New York: Gordon and Breech, 1972.
240. MENDELS, J., S. K. SECUNDA, and W. L. DYSON. "A Controlled Study of the Antidepressant Effects of Lithium," *Archives of General Psychiatry*, 26 (1972), 154–157.
241. MENDELS, J., and J. STINNETT. "Biogenic Amine Metabolism, Depression and Mania," in J. Mendels, ed., *Biological Psychiatry*, pp. 99–131. New York: John Wiley & Sons, Inc., 1973.
242. MENDELS, J., J. L. STINNETT, D. BURNS, and A. FRAZER. "A Controlled Trial of L-DOPA and L-Tryptophan in Depression," in preparation.
243. MESSIHA, F. S., D. AGALLIANOS, and C. CLOWER. "Dopamine Excretion in Affective States and Following Li_2CO_3 Therapy," *Nature*, 225 (1970), 868–869.
244. MEULLER, P., G. HENNINGER, and R. MAC-DONALD. "Insulin Tolerance Test in Depression," *Archives of General Psychiatry*, 21 (1969), 587–594.
245. MOLINOFF, P., and J. AXELROD. "Biochemistry of Catecholamines," *Annual Review of Biochemistry*, 40 (1971), 465–500.
246. MONGONI, A., V. ANDRIOLI, F. CABIBBE, and V. MANDELLI. "Body Fluid Distribution in Manic and Depressed Patients Treated with Lithium Carbonate," *Acta Psychiatrica Scandinavica*, 46 (1970), 244–257.
247. MOURET, J., P. BOBILLIER, and M. JOUVET. "Insomnia Following Para-Chlorophenylalanine in the Rat," *European Journal of Pharmacology*, 5 (1968), 17–22.
248. MULLER, E. E., P. D. PRA, and A. PECILE. "Influence of Brain Neurohumours Injected Into the Lateral Ventricle of the Rat on Growth Hormone Release," *Endocrinology*, 83 (1968), 893–896.
249. MULLER, J. C., W. W. PRYOR, J. E. GIB-

bons, and E. S. Orgain. "Depression and Anxiety Occurring During Rauwolfia Therapy," *Journal of the AMA*, 159 (1955), 836–839.

250. Murphy, D. L., and R. Weiss. "Reduced Monoamine Oxidase Activity in Blood Platelets from Bipolar Depressed Patients," *The American Journal of Psychiatry*, 128 (1972), 1351–1357.

251. Murphy, D. L., H. K. H. Brodie, F. K. Goodwin, and W. E. Bunney, Jr. "L-DOPA: Regular Induction of Hypomania in Bipolar Manic-Depressive Patients," *Nature*, 229 (1971), 135–136.

252. Nagatsu, T., M. Levitt, and S. Udenfriend. "Tyrosine Hydroxylase, the Initial Step in Norepinephrine Biosynthesis," *Journal of Biological Chemistry*, 239 (1964), 2910–2917.

253. Nakamura, K., and H. Thoenen. "Increased Irritability: A Permanent Behavior Change Induced in the Rat by Intraventricular Administration of 6-Hydroxydopamine," *Psychopharmacologia*, 24 (1972), 359–372.

254. Nickerson, M. "Antihypertensive Agents and the Drug Therapy of Hypertension," in L. S. Goodman, and A. Gilman, eds., *The Pharmacological Basis of Therapeutics*, pp. 728–744. New York: Macmillan, 1970.

255. Nielson, J. "Magnesium-Lithium Studies. I. Serum and Erythrocyte Magnesium in Patients with Manic States During Lithium Treatment," *Acta Psychiatrica Scandinavica*, 40 (1964), 190–196.

256. Nies, A., D. S. Robinson, C. L. Ravaris, and J. M. Davis. "Amines and Monoamine Oxidase in Relation to Aging and Depression in Man," *Psychosomatic Medicine*, 33 (1971), 470.

257. Nikula-Baumann, L. "Endocrinological Studies on Subjects With Involutional Melancholia," *Acta Psychiatrica Scandinavica* (Suppl.) 226 (1971).

258. Nordin, G., J.-O. Ottosson, and B.-E. Roos. "Influence of Convulsive Therapy on 5-Hydroxyindoleacetic Acid and Homovanillic Acid in Cerebrospinal Fluid in Endogenous Depression," *Psychopharmacologia*, 20 (1971), 315–320.

259. Oswald, I., R. J. Berger, R. A. Jarmillo, K. M. G. Keddie, P. C. Olley, and H. G. B. Plunke. "Melancholia and Barbiturates: Controlled EEG, Body and Eye Movement Study of Sleep," *British Journal of Psychiatry*, 109 (1963), 66–78.

260. Overall, J. E., L. E. Hollester, F. Meyer, I. Kimbell, Jr., and J. Shelton. "Imipramine and Thioridazine in Depressed and Schizophrenic Patients. Are There Specific Antidepressant Drugs?" *Journal of the AMA*, 189 (1964), 605–608.

261. Palmai, G., B. Blackwell, A. E. Maxwell, and F. Morgenstern. Patterns of Salivary Flow in Depressive Illness and During Treatment," *British Journal of Psychiatry*, 113 (1967), 1297–1308.

262. Palmer, G. C. "Increased Cyclic AMP Response to Norepinephrine in the Rat Brain Following 6-Hydroxydopamine," *Neuropharmacology*, 11 (1972), 145–149.

263. Papeschi, R., and D. J. McClure. "Homovanillic and 5-Hydroxyindoleacetic Acid in Cerebrospinal Fluid of Depressed Patients," *Archives of General Psychiatry*, 25 (1971), 354–358.

264. Pare, C. M. B., D. P. H. Yeung, K. Price, and R. S. Stacey. "5-Hydroxytryptamine in Brainstem, Hypothalamus and Caudate Nucleus of Controls and of Patients Committing Suicide by Coal-Gas Poisoning," *Lancet*, 2 (1969), 133–135.

265. Paul, M. I., H. Cramer, and W. E. Bunney, Jr. "Urinary Adenosine 3′,5′-Monophosphate in the Switch Process from Depression to Mania," *Science*, 171 (1971), 300–303.

266. Paul, M. I., H. Cramer, and F. K. Goodwin. "Urinary Cyclic AMP Excretion in Depression and Mania," *Archives of General Psychiatry*, 24 (1971), 327–333.

267. Paul, M. I., B .R. Ditzion, G. L. Pauk, and D. S. Janowsky. "Urinary Adenosine 3′,5′-Monophosphate Excretion in Affective Disorders," *The American Journal of Psychiatry*, 126 (1970), 1493–1497.

268. Perez-Reyes, M. "Differences in Sedative Susceptibility Between Types of Depression: Clinical and Neurophysiological Significance," in T. A. Williams, M. M. Katz, and J. A. Shield, eds., *Recent Advances in the Psychobiology of the Depressive Illnesses*, pp. 119–130. Washington: U.S. Government Printing Office, 1972.

269. ———. "Differences in the Capacity of the Sympathetic and Endocrine Systems of Depressed Patients to React to a Physiological Stress," in T. A. Williams, M. M. Katz, and J. A. Shield, eds., *Recent Advances in*

the Psychobiology of the Depressive Illnesses, pp. 131–135. Washington: U.S. Government Printing Office, 1972.

270. PERRIS, C. "A Study of Bipolar (Manic-Depressive) and Unipolar Recurrent Depressive Psychoses," *Acta Psychiatrica Scandinavica*, 42 (Suppl. 194) (1966).

271. ———. "The Genetics of Affective Disorders," in J. Mendels, ed., *Biological Psychiatry*, pp. 385–415. New York: John Wiley & Sons, 1973.

272. PLETSCHER, A. "Monoamine Oxidase Inhibitors: Effects Related to Psychostimulation," in D. H. Efron, ed., *Psychopharmacology Review of Progress, 1957–1967*, pp. 649–654. Washington: U.S. Government Printing Office, 1968.

273. POST, R. M., J. KOTIN, and F. K. GOODWIN. "Psychomotor Activity and Cerebrospinal Fluid Amine Metabolites in Affective Illness." Presented at the Annual Meeting of American Psychiatric Association, Dallas, Texas, 1972.

274. PRADHAN, S. N., and S. N. DUTTA. "Central Cholinergic Mechanism and Behavior," in C. C. Pfeiffer, and J. R. Smythies, eds., *International Review of Neurobiology*, 13 (1971), 173–231.

275. PRANGE, A. J., JR. "The Pharmacology and Biochemistry of Depression," *Diseases of the Nervous System*, 25 (1964), 217–221.

276. PRANGE, A. J., JR., R. L. McCURDY, and C. M. COCHRANE. "The Systolic Blood Pressure Response of Depressed Patients to Infused Norepinephrine," *Journal of Psychiatric Research*, 5 (1967), 1–13.

277. PRANGE, A. J., JR., J. L. MEEK, and M. A. LIPTON. "Catecholamines: Diminished Rate of Synthesis in Rat Brain and Heart After Thyroxine Pretreatment," *Life Sciences*, 9 (1970), 901–907.

278. PRANGE, A. J., JR., I. C. WILSON, A. E. KNOX, T. K. McCLANE, B. R. MARTIN, L. B. ALLTOP, and M. A. LIPTON. "Thyroid-Imipramine Clinical and Chemical Interaction: Evidence for a Receptor Deficit in Depression," *Journal of Psychiatric Research*, in press.

279. PRANGE, A. J., JR., I. C. WILSON, A. M. RABON, and M. A. LIPTON. "Enhancement of Imipramine Antidepressant Activity by Thyroid Hormone," *The American Journal of Psychiatry*, 126 (1969), 457–469.

280. PRICE, J. "The Genetics of Depressive Behavior," in A. Coppen, and A. Walk, eds.,

Recent Developments in Affective Disorders. British Journal of Psychiatry, Special Publication #2, pp. 37–54, 1968.

281. PRICE, J. M., R. R. BROWN, and N. YESS. "Testing the Functional Capacity of the Tryptophan-Niacin Pathway in Man by Analyses of Urinary Metabolites," *Advances in Metabolic Disorders*, 2 (1965), 159–225.

282. REDMOND, D. E., J. W. MAAS, A. KLING, and H. DEKIRMENJIAN. "Changes in Primate Social Behavior After Treatment With Alpha-Methyl-Para-Tyrosine," *Psychosomatic Medicine*, 33 (1971), 97–113.

283. REDMOND, D. E., J. W. MASS, A. KLING, C. W. GRAHAM, and H. DEKIRMENJIAN. "Social Behavior of Monkeys Selectively Depleted of Monoamines," *Science*, 174 (1971), 428–431.

284. REICH, T., P. CLAYTON, and G. WINOKUR. "Family History Studies: V. The Genetics of Mania," *The American Journal of Psychiatry*, 125 (1969), 1358–1369.

285. REICHLIN, S. "Hypothalamic Control of Growth Hormone Secretion and the Response to Stress," in R. D. Michael, ed., *Endocrinology and Human Behaviour*, pp. 256–283. New York: Oxford Avenue Press, 1968.

286. RICKLES, K., C. H. WARD, and L. SCHUT. "Different Populations, Different Drug Responses. A Comparative Study of Two Anti-Depressants, Each Used in Two Different Patient Groups," *American Journal of the Medical Sciences*, 247 (1964), 328–335.

287. RIMON, R., A. STEINBACK, and E. HUHMAR. "Electromyographic Findings in Depressive Patients," *Journal of Psychosomatic Research*, 10 (1966), 159–170.

288. ROBERTS, D. J., and K. J. BROADLEY. "Treatment of Depression," *Lancet*, 1 (1965), 1219–1220.

289. ROBINS, E., and S. GUZE. "Classification of Affective Disorders: The Primary-Secondary, the Endogenous-Reactive, and the Neurotic-Psychotic Concepts," in T. A. Williams, M. M. Katz, and J. A. Shield, eds., *Recent Advances in the Psychobiology of the Depressive Illnesses*, pp. 283–293. Washington: U.S. Government Printing Office, 1972.

290. ROBINS, E., and B. K. HARTMAN. "Some Chemical Theories of Mental Disorders," in R. W. Albers, G. J. Siegel, R. Katzman,

and B. W. Agranoff, eds., *Basic Neurochemistry*, pp. 607–644. Boston: Little, Brown, 1972.

291. ROBINSON, D. S., J. M. DAVIS, A. NIES, C. L. RAVARIS, and D. SYLWESTER. "Relation of Sex and Aging to Monamine Oxidase Activity of Human Brain, Plasma and Platelets, *Archives of General Psychiatry*, 24 (1971), 536–539.

292. ROBISON, G. A., R. W. BUTCHER, and E. W. SUTHERLAND. *Cyclic AMP.* New York: Press, 1971.

293. ROME, H. P., and F. J. BRACELAND. "Psychological Response to Corticotropin, Cortisone, and Related Steroid Substances, Psychotic Reaction Types," *Journal of the AMA*, 148 (1952), 27–30.

294. ROOS, B.-E., and R. SJÖSTRÖM. "5-Hydroxyindoleacetic Acid and Homovanillic Acid Levels in the Cerebrospinal Fluid After Probenecid Application in Patients With Manic-Depressive Psychosis," *Pharmacologia Clinica*, 1 (1969), 153–155.

295. ROSENTHAL, D. *Genetic Theory and Abnormal Behavior.* New York: McGraw-Hill, 1970.

296. ROSS, S. B., A. L. RENJI, and S.-O. OGREN. "A Comparison of the Inhibitory Activities of Iprindole and Imipramine on the Uptake of 5-Hydroxytryptamine and Nonadrenaline in Brain Slices," *Life Sciences*, 10 (1971), 1267–1277.

297. ROTH, J., S. M. GLICK, R. S. YALOW, and S. A. BERSON. "Hypoglycemia: A Patent Stimulus to Secretion of Growth Hormone," *Science*, 140 (1963), 987–988.

298. RUBIN, R. T., and A. J. MANDELL. "Adrenal Cortical Activity in Pathological Emotional States: A Review," *The American Journal of Psychiatry*, 123 (1966), 387–400.

299. RUBIN, R. T. "Adrenal Cortical Activity Changes in Manic Depressive Illness. Influence on Intermediatry Metabolism of Tryptophan," *Archives of General Psychiatry*, 17 (1967), 671–679.

300. RUSSEL, G. F. M. "Body Weight and Balance of Water, Sodium and Potassium in Depressed Patients Given Electroconvulsive Therapy," *Clinical Science*, 19 (1960), 327–336.

301. SACHAR, E. J. "Corticosteroids in Depressive Illness. A Re-Evaluation of Control Issues and the Literature," *Archives of General Psychiatry*, 17 (1967), 544–553.

302. ———. "Corticosteroids in Depressive Illness. A Longitudinal Psychoendocrine Study," *Archives of General Psychiatry*, 17 (1967), 554–567.

303. ———. "Endocrine Factors in Psychopathological States," in J. Mendels, ed., *Biological Psychiatry*, pp. 175–197. New York: John Wiley & Sons, 1973.

304. SACHAR, E. J., J. FINKELSTEIN, and L. HELLMAN. "Growth Hormone Responses in Depressive Illness. I. Response to Insulin Tolerance Test," *Archives of General Psychiatry*, 25 (1971), 263–269.

305. SACHAR, E. J., L. HELLMAN, D. K. FUKUSHIMA, and T. F. GALLAGHER. "Cortisol Production in Depressive Illness. A Clinical and Biochemical Clarification," *Archives of General Psychiatry*, 23 (1971), 289–298.

306. SACHAR, E. J., S. S. KANTER, D. BUIE, R. ENGLE, and R. MEHLMAN. "Psychoendocrinology of Ego Disintegration," *The American Journal of Psychiatry*, 126 (1970), 1067–1078.

307. SACHAR, E. J., J. M. MACKENZIE, W. A. BINSTOCK, and J. E. MACK. "Corticosteroid Responses to Psychotherapy of Depressions," *Archives of General Psychiatry*, 16 (1967), 461–470.

308. SAKAI, M. "Diurnal Rhythm of 17-Ketosteroid and Diurnal Fluctuation of Depressive Affect," *Yokohama Medical Bulletin*, 11 (1960), 352–367.

309. ———. "Corticosteroid Responses to Psychotherapy of Reactive Depressions. II. Further Clinical and Physiological Implications," *Psychosomatic Medicine*, 30 (1968), 23–44.

310. SANDLER, M., and M. B. H. YOUDIM. "Multiple Forms of Monoamine Oxidase: Functional Significance," *Pharmacological Reviews*, 24 (1972), 331–348.

311. SATTERFIELD, J. H. "Auditory Evoked Cortical Response Studies in Depressed Patients and Normal Control Subjects," in T. A. Williams, M. M. Katz, and J. A. Shield, eds., *Recent Advances in the Psychobiology of the Depressive Illnesses*, pp. 87–98. Washington: U.S. Government Printing Office, 1972.

312. SCHANBERG, S. M., G. R. BREESE, J. J. SCHILDKRAUT, E. K. GORDON, and I. J. KOPIN. "3-Methoxy-4-Hydroxyphenylglycol Sulfate in Brain and Cerebrospinal Fluid," *Biochemical Pharmacology*, 17 (1968), 2006–2008.

313. SCHANBERG, S. M., J. J. SCHILDKRAUT, G. R. BREESE, and I. J. KOPIN. "Metabolism of Normetanephrine-H3 in Rat Brain Identification of Conjugated 3-Methoxy-4-Hydroxyphenylglycol as the Major Metabolite," *Biochemical Pharmacology*, 17 (1968), 247–254.

314. SCHANBERG, S. M., J. J. SCHILDKRAUT, and I. J. KOPIN. "The Effects of Psychoactive Drugs on Norepinephrine-³H Metabolism in Brain," *Biochemical Pharmacology*, 16 (1967), 393–399.

315. SCHILDKRAUT, J. J. "The Catecholamine Hypothesis of Affective Disorders: A Review of Supporting Evidence," *The American Journal of Psychiatry*, 122 (1965), 509–522.

316. SCHILDKRAUT, J. J., P. R. DRASKOCZY, E. S. GERSHON, P. REICH, and E. L. GRAB. "Effects of Tricyclic Antidepressants on Norepinephrine Metabolism: Basic and Clinical Studies," in B. T. Ho, and W. M. McIsaac, eds., *Brain Chemistry and Mental Disease*, pp. 215–236. New York: Plenum Press, 1971.

317. SCHILDKRAUT, J. J., E. K. GORDON, and J. DURELL. "Catecholamine Metabolism in Affective Disorders. I. Normetanephrine and VMA Excretion in Depressed Patients Treated with Imipramine," *Journal of Psychiatric Research*, 3 (1965), 213–228.

318. SCHILDKRAUT, J. J., R. GREEN, E. K. GORDON, and J. DURELL. "Normetanephrine Excretion and Affective State in Depressed Patients Treated with Imipramine," *The American Journal of Psychiatry*, 123 (1966), 690–700.

319. SCHILDKRAUT, J. J., and S. S. KETY. "Biogenic Amines and Emotion," *Science*, 156 (1967), 21–30.

320. SCHOTTSTAEDT, W. W., W. J. GRACE, and H. G. WOLFF. "Life Situations, Behaviour, Attitudes, Emotions and Renal Excretion of Fluid and Electrolytes. IV. Situations Associated with Retention of Water, Sodium and Potassium," *Journal of Psychosomatic Research*, 1 (1956), 287–291.

321. SHAGASS, C. *Evoked Brain Potentials in Psychiatry*. New York: Plenum Press, 1972.

322. SHAGASS, C., and M. SCHWARTZ. "Cerebral Cortical Reactivity in Psychotic Depressions," *Archives of General Psychiatry*, 6 (1962), 235–242.

323. SHANES, A. M. "Electrochemical Aspects of Physiological and Pharmacological Action in Excitable Cells. I. The Resting Cell and its Alteration by Extrinsic Factors," *Pharmacological Reviews*, 10 (1958), 59–164.

324. SHAW, D. M. "Mineral Metabolism, Mania, and Melancholia," *British Medical Journal*, 2 (1966), 262–267.

325. SHAW, D. M., and A. COPPEN. "Potassium and Sodium Distribution in Depression," *British Journal of Psychiatry*, 112 (1966), 269–276.

326. SHAW, D. M., F. E. CAMPS, and E. G. ECCLESTON. "5-Hydroxytryptamine in the Hindbrain of Depressive Suicides," *British Journal of Psychiatry*, 113 (1967), 1407–1411.

327. SHOPSIN, B., S. WILK, S. GERSHON, K. DAVIS, and M. SUHL. "Cerebrospinal Fluid MHPG: An Assessment of Norepinephrine Metabolism in Affective Disorders," in press.

328. SHORE, P. A. "Transport and Storage of Biogenic Amines," *Annual Review of Pharmacology*, 12 (1972), 209–226.

329. SJOERDSMA, A., K. ENGELMAN, and S. SPECTOR. "Inhibition of Catecholamine Synthesis in Man with Alpha Methyl Tyrosine, an Inhibitor of Tyrosine Hydroxylase," *Lancet*, 2 (1965), 1092–1094.

330. SKOU, J. C. "Further Investigations on a Mg Ion- and Na Ion-Activated Adenosintriphosphatase, Possibly Related to the Active, Linked Transport of Na Ion and K Ion Across the Nerve Membrane," *Biochimica Biophysica Acta*, 42 (1960), 6–23.

331. SLATER, E. "Psychiatric and Neurotic Illness in Twins," in *Medical Research Council Special Report Series*, No. 278. London: Her Majesty's Stationery Office, 1953.

332. SLATER, E., and V. COWIE. *The Genetics of Mental Disorders*. London: Oxford University Press, 1971.

333. SLATER, P., and J. ROGERS. "The Effects of Triethylcholine and Hemicholinium-3 on Tremore and Brain Acetylcholine," *European Journal of Pharmacology*, 4 (1968), 390–394.

334. SMIRK, F. H., and E. G. McQUEEN. "Comparison of Rescinnamine and Reserpine as Hypotensive Agents," *Lancet*, 269 (1955), 115–116.

335. SNYDER, F. "NIH Studies of EEG Sleep in Affective Illness," in T. A. Williams, M. M. Katz, and J. A. Shield, eds., *Recent Advances in the Psychobiology of the Depressive*

Illnesses, pp. 171–192. Washington: U.S. Government Printing Office, 1972.

336. SPECTOR, S., A. SJOERDSMA, and S. UDEN-FRIEND. "Blockade of Endogenous Nor-epinephrine Synthesis by a-Methyl Tyrosine, an Inhibitor of Tyrosine Hydroxylase," *Journal of Pharmacology and Experimental Therapeutics*, 147 (1965), 86–95.

337. STEFANINI, M., C. A. ROY, L. ZANNUS, and W. DAMESHEK. "Therapeutic Effect of Pituitary Adrenocorticotropic Hormone (ACTH) in Case of Henoch-Schönlein Vascular (Anaphylactoid) Purpura," *Journal of the AMA*, 144 (1950), 1372–1374.

338. STEVENS, D. A., O. RESNICK, and D. M. KRUS. "The Effects of P-Chlorophenylalanine, a Depletor of Brain Serotonin, on Behavior. I. Facilitation of Discrimination Learning," *Life Sciences*, 6 (1967), 2215–2220.

339. STOKES, P. E. "Studies on the Control of Adrenocortical Function in Depression," in T. A. Williams, M. M. Katz, and J. A. Shield, eds., *Recent Advances in the Psychobiology of the Depressive Illnesses*, pp. 199–220. Washington: U.S. Government Printing Office, 1972.

340. SULSER, F., M. H. BICKEL, and B. B. BRODIE. "The Action of Desmethylimipramine in Counteracting Sedation and Cholinergic Effects of Reserpine-Like Drugs," *Journal of Pharmacology and Experimental Therapeutics*, 144 (1964), 321–330.

341. SULSER, F., and E. SANDERS-BUSH. "Effect of Drugs on Amines in the CNS," *Annual Review of Pharmacology*, 11 (1971), 209–230.

342. SUTHERLAND, E. W., I. ØYE, and R. W. BUTCHER. "The Action of Epinephrine and the Role of the Adenyl Cyclase System in Hormone Action," *Recent Progress in Hormone Research*, 21 (1965), 623–646.

343. TAKAHASHI, Y., D. KIPNIS, and W. DAUGHADAY. "Growth Hormone Secretion During Sleep," *Journal of Clinical Investigation*, 47 (1968), 2079–2090.

344. TAMARKIN, N. R., F. K. GOODWIN, and J. AXELROD. "Rapid Elevation of Biogenic Amine Metabolites in Human CSF Following Probenecid," *Life Sciences*, 9 (1970), 1397–1408.

345. TISSARI, A. H., P. S. SCHONHOFER, D. F. BOGDANSKI, and B. B. BRODIE. "Mechanism

of Biogenic Amine Transport," *Molecular Pharmacology*, 5 (1969), 593–604.

346. TORU, M., J. N. HINGTEN, and M. H. APRISON. "Acetylcholine Concentrations in Brain Areas of Rats During Three States of Avoidance Behavior: Normal, Depression, and Excitation," *Life Sciences*, 5 (1966), 181–189.

347. UDENFRIEND, S., and W. DAIRMAN. "Regulation of Norepinephrine Synthesis," in G. Weber, ed., *Advances in Enzyme Regulations*, Vol. 9, pp. 145–165. New York: Pergamon Press, 1971.

348. UNGERSTEDT, U. "Postsynaptic Supersensitivity After 6-Hydroxydopamine Induced Degeneration of the Nigro-Striatal Dopamine System," *Acta Physiologica Scandinavica* (Suppl.), 367 (1971), 69–93.

349. URETSKY, N. J., and L. L. IVERSEN. "Effects of 6-hydroxydopamine on Noradrenaline-Containing Neurones in the Rat Brain," *Nature*, 221 (1969), 557–559.

350. VAN PRAAG, H. M., and B. LEISNSE. "Depression, Glucose Tolerance, Peripheral Glucose Uptake and Their Alterations Under the Influence of Antidepressive Drugs of the Hydrazine Type," *Psychopharmacologia*, 8 (1965), 67–78.

351. VAN PRAAG, H. M., J. KORF, and J. PUITE. "5-Hydroxyindoleacetic Acid Levels in the Cerebro-Spinal Fluid of Depressive Patients Treated with Probenecid," *Nature*, 225 (1970), 1259–1260.

352. VAN PRAAG, H. M., and J. KORF. "Endogenous Depressions With and Without Disturbances in the 5-Hydroxytryptamine Metabolism: A Biochemical Classification?" *Psychopharmacologia*, 19 (1971), 148–152.

353. ————. "A Pilot Study of Some Kinetic Aspects of the Metabolism of 5-Hydroxytryptamine in Depressed Patients," *Biological Psychiatry*, 3 (1972), 105–112.

354. WEINER, N. "Regulation of Norepinephrine Biosynthesis," *Annual Review of Pharmacology*, 10 (1970), 273–290.

355. WELCH, A. S., and B. L. WELCH. "Effect of Stress and Parachlorophenylalanine Upon Brain Serotonin, 5-Hydroxyindoleacetic Acid and Catecholamines in Grouped and Isolated Mice," *Biochemical Pharmacology*, 17 (1968), 699–708.

356. ————. "Failure of Natural Stimuli to Accelerate Brain Catecholamine Depletion After Biosynthesis Inhibition With Alpha-

Methyltyrosine," *Brain Research*, 9 (1968), 402–405.

357. WHATMORE, G. B., and R. M. ELLIS, JR. "Further Neurophysiologic Aspects of Depressed States: An electromyographic Study," *Archives of General Psychiatry*, 6 (1962), 243–253.

358. WHEATLEY, D. "Potentiation of Amitriptyline by Thyroid Hormone," *Archives of General Psychiatry*, 26 (1972), 229–233.

359. WHYBROW, P. C., and J. MENDELS. "Toward a Biology of Depression: Some Suggestions from Neurophysiology," *The American Journal of Psychiatry*, 125 (1969), 1491–1500.

360. WHYBROW, P. C., A. PRANGE, and C. TREADWAY. "Mental Changes Accompanying Thyroid Gland Dysfunction," *Archives of General Psychiatry*, 20 (1969), 48–63.

361. WILK, S., B. SHOPSIN, S. GERSHON, and M. SUHL. "Cerebrospinal Fluid Levels of MHPG in Affective Disorders," *Nature*, 235 (1972), 440–441.

362. WILLIAMS, H. L., "The New Biology of Sleep," *Journal of Psychiatric Research*, 8 (1971), 445–478.

363. WILLIAMS, T. A., M. M. KATZ, and J. A. SHIELD, eds. *Recent Advances in the Psychobiology of the Depressive Illnesses.* Washington: U.S. Government Printing Office, 1972.

364. WINOKUR, G. "Genetic Principles in the Clarification of Clinical Issues in Affective Disorders," in A. J. Mandell, and M. P. Mandell, eds., *Psychochemical Research*

in Man. New York: Academic Press, 1969.

365. WINOKUR, G., and P. J. CLAYTON. "Family History Studies, I. Two Types of Affective Disorders Separated According to Genetic and Clinical Factors," *Recent Advances in Biological Psychiatry*, 9 (1967), 35–50.

366. WINOKUR, G., P. J. CLAYTON, and T. REICH. *Manic Depressive Illness.* St. Louis: Mosby, 1969.

367. WINOKUR, G., and V. TANNA. "Possible Role of X-Linked Dominant Factor in Manic Depressive Disease," *Diseases of the Nervous System*, 30 (1969), 89–94.

368. WYATT, R. J., B. PORTNOY, D. J. KUPFER, F. SNYDER, and K. ENGELMAN. "Resting Plasma Catecholamine Concentrations in Patients With Depression and Anxiety," *Archives of General Psychiatry*, 24 (1971), 65–70.

369. YUWILER, A., L. WETTERBERG, and E. GELLER. "Relationship Between Alternate Routes of Tryptophan Metabolism Following Administration of Tryptophan Peroxidase Inducers or Stressors," *Journal of Neurochemistry*, 18 (1971), 593–599.

370. ZERBIN-RÜDIN, E. "*Endogene Psychosen,*" in P. E. Becker, ed., *Humangenetic, ein Kurzes Handbuch*, Volume 5. Stuttgart, Georg Thieme Verlag, 1967.

371. ZUBIN, J., and F. A. FREYHAN. *Disorders of Mood.* Baltimore: Johns Hopkins Press, 1972.

372. ZUNG, W. W. K., W. P. WILSON, and W. E. DODSON. "Effect of Depressive Disorders on Sleep EEG Responses," *Archives of General Psychiatry*, 10 (1964), 439–445.

CHAPTER 23

SCHIZOPHRENIA: THE MANIFEST SYMPTOMATOLOGY

Jules R. Bemporad and Henry Pinsker

SINCE ITS INITIAL DESCRIPTION in 1896, there has been continuous debate about whether schizophrenia is a disease of organic etiology, a group of separate entities, not delineated, but with enough common features to be characterized as a syndrome, a reaction to severe stress, latent in all individuals, or an accumulation of maladaptive behavior patterns. Despite these controversies, the setting apart of schizophrenia as a nosological entity has stood the test of time. It is usually described as an entity with unknown etiology and variable course. Commonly, psychiatrists speak of schizophrenia in the singular, while agreeing that there is a group of schizophrenias. In this chapter, we will be concerned with the signs and symptoms, the clinical manifestations which make possible diagnosis of schizophrenia, and which set it apart from other psychiatric disorders.

While in certain cases it is not difficult to make the diagnosis of schizophrenia, at other times it may be exceedingly difficult. The difficulty may reflect the psychiatrist's bias against an ominous-sounding diagnosis, his concept of psychiatric nosology, or diagnostic habits to which he was educated. For example, schizophrenia is diagnosed more frequently in the United States than in any other country— thirteen times more frequently per unit of population, for example, than in the Netherlands.[64] Even within the United States, statistics vary from hospital to hospital. Despite these differences, there is general agreement that schizophrenia is a disorder that affects the total personality in all aspects of its functioning: emotion, volition, outward behavior, and most particularly, the thinking process. While not all patients show the same range or magnitude of disturbances, and even the same patient's symptoms will vary in time, the hallmark of this disorder is that it permeates every aspect of the individual's functioning.

(Historical Review

The Classical Period

Kraepelin,[54] in 1896, was the first psychiatrist to delineate schizophrenia as a separate diagnostic entity. He termed the new disease entity *dementia praecox*,* meaning mental deterioration occurring early in life. As he wrote two decades later:

I got the starting point of the line of thought which in 1896 led to dementia praecox being regarded as a distinct disease, on the one hand from the overpowering impression of the states of dementia quite similar to each other which developed from the most varied clinical symptoms, on the other hand from experienced connected with the observation of Hecker that these peculiar dementias seemed to stand in relation to the period of youth.

Kraepelin separated two major groups of patients: those who despite the severity of their acute symptoms achieve recovery in a short time, and those who showed a chronic and steady deterioration. The former were delineated as having manic-depressive psychosis, which Kraepelin eventually believed to be a constitutional or genetic illness, and the latter were classified as dementia praecox, which he believed to be an acquired, organic condition.

Within this newly established entity, Kraepelin unified a number of separately described syndromes, demonstrating that although the disorder could begin from a variety of clinical forms, ultimately a similar type of dementia ensued. These syndromes included catatonia,

---

* The term *dementia praecocée* had been used previously by Morel, a Belgian psychiatrist, in his description of a fourteen-year-old boy who after a history of excellent scholastic achievement became melancholic and withdrawn, expressed homicidal wishes toward his father, and eventually lapsed into a seclusiveness and lethargy.

previously described by Kahlbaum in 1874, hebephrenia, fully reported by Hecker in 1871, and dementia paranoides. Ultimately, Kraepelin added other subtypes so that in his final works he listed nine types of dementia praecox.[14] While Kraepelin made an exhaustive descriptive study of dementia praecox, he particularly stressed specific symptoms. Among these was hallucination, especially of the auditory type. He believed that hearing of voices was specifically characteristic of the disorder, ranging from the milder illusory belief that real noises have been transformed into messages to the extreme hallucinatory verbigeration, during which the patient's thoughts are constantly interrupted by a stream of meaningless phrases. Other pertinent symptoms were the delusion that one's thoughts were being influenced by external forces or that one's thoughts were known by others, and conversely that one could read the thoughts of others. Delusions of almost any type formed a prominent part of the symptom picture.

The faculty of judgment was also severely impaired. Kraepelin writes:

What surprises the observer anew is the quiet complacency with which the most nonsensical ideas can be uttered by them and the most incomprehensible actions carried out. One has the impression that the patients are not in a position to accomplish that mental grouping of ideas which is requisite for their survey and comparison, their subordination among one another and for the discovery of contradiction.

Other prominent symptoms were disturbances of emotional expression, bizarre and stereotyped behavior, and, often, negativism. What differentiated this disorder from the commonly seen toxic psychoses was the absence of delirium or gross defect of the intellectual faculties, at least prior to the terminal phase. Memory, orientation, and comprehension remained intact despite gross incapacitation in other areas of functioning.

Kraepelin's great contribution lay in recognizing that a number of clinical syndromes could be seen as forms of one disease, and in differentiating this new entity from other psychoses (manic-depressive illness and paraphrenia). However, he triggered a controversy which is still with us by making prognosis as well as symptoms criteria for diagnosis. Dementia praecox was expected to end eventually in deterioration. Other psychiatrists, while applauding his genius for observation and classification, were critical of his fatalistic outlook. Kraepelin eventually conceded that about 13 percent of such patients did achieve some form of recovery, that, in a sense, dementia praecox did not always lead to dementia, and if it did, it did not always develop precociously. Finally, the idea that correct diagnosis could be made only when the course of the illness was known is incompatible with the usual medical approach, which requires that diagnosis be made on the basis of available information and recognizes that all diagnoses are tentative and may be corrected in the light of subsequent data, including the course of the illness.

In the United States, Adolph Meyer[61,62] extensively criticized Kraepelin's pessimistic view of dementia praecox, as well as his view of the disorder as analogous to an organic illness. Meyer argued that each patient be studied longitudinally and that premorbid life events be carefully investigated. If this were done, Meyer proposed, then dementia praecox could be seen as the culmination of accrued "faulty habits" and maladaptive reactions to environmental demands. Schizophrenic symptoms were extreme "substitutive reactions" which replaced effective action in the real world. Innocuous behavior such as daydreaming or such mild traits as a tendency to be uncomfortable in social situations gradually developed into autistic retreat with compensatory delusions or hallucinations. Meyer's contributions are extremely important in demonstrating that illness does not arise *de novo* but is an extension of and continuous with the past life of each patient. On the other hand, Meyer has been criticized for being vague in defining where "faulty habits" end and true psychosis begins, that is, in not appreciating that in psychosis there is extensive alteration of the total personality.

Bleuler,[12] a Swiss psychiatrist, accepted most of Kraepelin's observations but attempted to go beyond a purely descriptive approach. In his classic monograph, *Dementia Praecox, or the Group of Schizophrenias*, published in 1911, Bleuler made many fundamental and lasting contributions to the study of schizophrenia. To the three previous subtypes he added the simple type, previously described by Diem. He recognized that the majority of schizophrenic patients were not so severely ill as to require hospitalization, and that deterioration to dementia was not inevitable.

Perhaps of greater importance was Bleuler's attempt to define the basic disorder of schizophrenia. He believed the fundamental defect was a splitting of the functions of the personality, so that the mind lost its natural harmonious integration. The will was no longer co-ordinated with cognitive processes which in turn were split off from emotions. Therefore, he proposed the term "schizophrenia" (from the Greek *schizein*, to divide, and *phren*, mind) to replace Kraepelin's dementia praecox.

Bleuler separated the symptoms of schizophrenia into two major categories: the *primary symptoms*, which were basic manifestations of the disorder, and the *secondary symptoms*, which were psychological adaptations to the primary difficulty. The primary symptoms, which Bleuler ultimately believed to be due to an organic disease, consisted of (1) a *loosening of associative linkages* in the flow of thought, so that one thought no longer logically followed another and the associative flow of cognition became fragmented; (2) *autism*, which consisted of a paritcular type of thinking and acting that are not bound by external reality but follow the inner fantasy world of the individual; (3) *ambivalence*, meaning the simultaneous occurrence of contradictory feelings, wishes, or thoughts (his descriptions making clear that he considered only incongruous or paralyzing ambivalence pathological, and that the mixed emotions of everyday life were not intended to be diagnostic of schizophrenia); and (4) *disorders of affect*, such as indifference and lack of emotional expression, persistence of a basic mood unaffected by external events, or inconsistency between affective expression and the expressed thought or circumstances.

Bleuler believed that these primary symptoms were pathognomonic of schizophrenia, because they were manifestations of the disharmony or splitting of the personality. However, they were rarely seen in pure form, because the more florid secondary symptoms dominated the clinical picture. Secondary symptoms included delusions, hallucinations, gestures, disturbances of speech and writing, and catatonic symptoms (impulsiveness, automatisms, negativism, sterotypy). All these symptoms were elaborated differently in individual patients and formed the clinical basis for the classical subtypes of schizophrenia— paranoid, hebephrenic, catatonic, and simple. These symptoms were the result of the individual's attempt to cope with the primary disorder and could be understood in the context of his past experience. Bleuler, who was familiar with Freud's early work, undertook to demonstrate that the meaning of hallucinations and delusions was not random, but related to the patient's life and susceptible to being understood by study of the patient's life.

In addition, Bleuler also differentiated between fundamental and accessory symptoms. The fundamental symptoms were only found in schizophrenia and thus pathognomonic of the disorder, while the accessory symptoms could also be found in other psychiatric conditions. It appears that the distinction between fundamental and accessory symptoms was made on a phenomenological basis, while the difference between primary and secondary symptoms aimed at an etiological concept of schizophrenia.

In summary, Bleuler's monumental contributions include the demonstration that schizophrenia does not inevitably end in deterioration, a broadening of the subtypes included in the category, an attempt to show that symptoms have meaning, and an effort to grasp the fundamental defect of schizophrenia as the splitting of the functions of the personality. His specific emphasis on the defect of the associative process has persisted, so that even today schizophrenia is often referred to as primarily a disorder of thinking.

Jung,[47] while a student of Bleuler, made significant contributions to the meaning of schizophrenic symptoms; he was also one of the first psychiatrists to perform psychological tests on schizophrenic patients. In *The Psychology of Dementia Praecox*, published in 1903, Jung postulated the existence of autonomous unconscious "complexes," or groups of ideas and feelings, which had been repressed but during psychosis involuntarily intrude into conscious thought, accounting for the schizophrenic's discontinuity of themes in speech. Furthermore, through the use of word association tests, Jung found that similar or related ideas would recur to a variety of stimulus words. Jung proposed a psychosomatic theory of schizophrenia in which excess affect and trauma cause the release of a hypothetical toxin, which in turn destroys the hierarchical arrangement of the ego, so that archaic, repressed material emerges in a dramatic and overwhelming manner. Jung thus related psychosis to dreams and the schizophrenic to an awake dreamer, in that unconscious themes break into consciousness due to a weakening of the ego.

Although they were later to break with Freud, both Bleuler and Jung relied heavily on the then newly formulated principles of psychoanalysis in their interpretation of symptoms. Much of what Freud had written about distortion in dreams was found to be applicable to schizophrenic symptoms in terms of repressed themes and their symbolic representation in conscious life in the form of symptoms. They appear to be equally indebted to the studies of Janet on hysteria, in which he suggested an organic "weakening" of the mind allowing for the emergence of "fixed ideas" and pathologic behavior.

The Psychoanalytic Approach

While Freud's revolutionary theories have found their greatest application to an understanding and therapy of the neuroses, they are no less relevant to the study of schizophrenia.

His work on dreams describes the elaboration of symbolism, the regression to perceptual rather than conceptual modes of experience, the simultaneous expression of incompatible ideas, and mental mechanisms such as condensation and displacement, which are useful in describing schizophrenic symptoms. Freud's formulation of two major classes of cognition into primary and secondary processes has influenced much of psychiatric thought regarding psychoses. The primary process was postulated as being solely concerned with the attainment of pleasure and a release of tension. It does not follow logical rules and utilizes any means to attain expression. The primary process is essentially the mode of the unconscious and the id; it becomes manifest in dreams, slips of the tongue, various symptoms, and most blatantly, in psychosis. On the other hand, the secondary process is concerned with the individual's relationship to his environment, rather than with release of instinctual energy. It is characterized by logical, coherent cognitive forms and typifies most of our everyday conscious experience. In schizophrenia, there occurs a massive regression, with the overwhelming of the ego by primary-process mentation, accounting for the peculiarities of thought and behavior. Concomitant with regression, Freud postulated a withdrawal of libido or interest from the external world and its redirection onto the self, so that wishes are satisfied thrugh hallucinations or delusions, rather than through actual behavior.[36]

The libidinal decathexis of external reality accounts for the "end of the world" and other cataclysmic fantasies found in schizophrenia. In the analysis of Schreber's diary of his own psychotic episode, Freud[35] hypothesized that the megalomaniacal, hypochondriacal, and egocentric preoccupations result from an attempt to deal with the loss of external reality, and delusions and hallucinations are re-creations of a personal, fantasied reality to compensate for the loss of actual relationships. For Freud, then, schizophrenia represented a massive regression to a self-contained or narcissistic state, in which a fantasy world is substituted for the lost reality and in which the id and primary-process cognition overwhelm the

ego's hold on reality, leading to a condition where unconscious wishes and drives are freely expressed and the environment distorted to fit these needs. Freud often compared the schizophrenic state to the dream process, showing that in schizophrenia behavior and language are subjected to the same mechanisms that create dream images out of latent and repressed instinctual desires.

Arlow and Brenner[5] have explained how Freud's concepts of decathexis and recathexis do not fit clinical experience with most psychotic patients, for Freud selected only certain symptoms of schizophrenia, attributing to them unjustified primacy. Many schizophrenic patients do not show the extensive withdrawal from reality described by Freud, many do not have restitutive delusions or hallucinations, and delusions of world destruction, although not uncommon, are by no means characteristic of schizophrenia. Psychosis may be understood, within the context of evolving psychoanalytic theory, as a widespread disturbance of ego and superego function, a regression employed as a defense against anxiety related to intrapsychic conflict.

Since the schizophrenic, according to Freud, has given up relating to his environment, such a patient would be unable to form a transferential relationship to a therapist and would thus be untreatable by psychotherapeutic means. Sullivan,[82] and later Fromm-Reichmann, argued against this therapeutic pessimism and engaged in the psychoanalytic treatment of schizophrenic patients; as a result, they altered much of the psychoanalytic theory of psychoses. Sullivan dismissed the idea that instinctual and biological processes were predominant in psychopathology and instead stressed the importance of early interpersonal relationships. He believed that schizophrenia was a result of extremely destructive experiences with significant adults which prevent the individual from forming a satisfactory self-image and from developing adequate modes of dealing with anxiety, so that throughout life he must distort perceptions of himself and others in order to escape being overwhelmed by anxiety. During life crises, the individual can no longer defend himself from early fears and the repressed experiences of early childhood re-emerge in a symbolic and often terrifying manner. Sullivan thus saw the symptoms of schizophrenia as signifying modes of previous relationships which were played out again in adult life with substituted protagonists. Sullivan's work is extremely relevant in showing the interpersonal nature of symptoms, as well as in opening the way to family studies of schizophrenia, but his greatest contributions are perhaps in the sphere of treatment.

Whether or not the psychoanalytic study of schizophrenia has succeeded in explaining the causes of the illness, it has contributed much to the understanding of the behavior and suffering of the schizophrenic patient, and has shown how similar mental processes can be found in healthy individuals.

The Existential Approach

While receiving limited attention in the United States, the existential approach to schizophrenia has attracted a number of adherents in Europe. Binswanger[11] and Minkowski[63] have attempted "existential" analyses of schizophrenic patients, utilizing basic categories of experience, rather than relying on extra-experiential constructs, such as libido or defenses. They attempt to reconstruct the mode of being of the patient, his subjective view of his world, what he feels, rather than how he behaves. According to Binswanger, for example, the world of the schizophrenic becomes flattened and constricted, dominated by a few recurrent themes. He is described as losing his freedom and existing as a passive object, subject to external forces instead of being motivated by internal desires. Minkowski emphasizes distortions in the perception of time and space, relating these alterations to manifest symptomatology. Jaspers has also used a phenomenological approach to schizophrenia, stressing the ability of the examiner to empathize with the patient. If the patient appears as an enigma to the examiner and the latter cannot make contact with or understand the patient, then a diagnosis of "true" schizophrenia is indicated, rather than that of a re-

active psychosis. This somewhat subjective approach to a diagnosis has been furthered by Rumke[73] in differentiating types of schizophrenias. The point is that true schizophrenia is an organic condition that defies empathic understanding.

Cognitive Approach

Study of the cognitive defects of schizophrenia has never been formalized into a "school" or doctrine, but attempts to elucidate the nature of the basic disturbances in thought or conceptual processes have occupied the attention of workers in the field from the start. Kraepelin, in his initial description of dementia praecox, noted that "the most different ideas follow one another with the most bewildering want of connection." Bleuler, influenced by the association psychology prevalent at the time, stressed a loosening of the associations as a primary and fundamental symptom of schizophrenia. Since that time, thousands of studies have appeared, yet Kreitman et al.[55] found thought disorder to be one of the symptoms least likely to be agreed upon by clinicians. Reed,[71] in a recent review of the literature on thought disorder concludes:

> . . . much of what is found in schizophrenic thought, speech and writing also occurs in normal people and what is observed as schizophrenic thought disorder is not due to a qualitatively abnormal mechanism, but rather to the use of normal ones in a quantitatively abnormal way.

STUDIES OF CONCRETENESS OF THOUGHT

In the 1920s the Russian psychologist Vigotsky[87] began to experiment with categories of thought in schizophrenic patients. He was influenced by his own work on the development of language and thought in childhood, as well as by the studies of Piaget. Vigotsky and Luria devised a test employing blocks of different shapes, sizes, and colors. The test tasks required, for success, classifying the blocks in a way more complex than simple sorting by color or size. They found that the schizophrenic patients were unable to go beyond a concrete appreciation of the test material and concluded that they were unable to make higher order generalizations. Kasanin[49] duplicated Vigotsky's work, and further concluded that schizophrenics had lost their former ability to generate abstract hypotheses and that their thinking was limited to concrete, realistic, matter-of-fact terms, in which things have personal rather than symbolic values. Goldstein,[38] utilizing a sorting test which he had developed for the study of brain-damaged patients, found that schizophrenic patients as well as brain-damaged ones lost the "abstract attitude" and centered on the concrete aspects of their environment. Goldstein added that schizophrenics could concentrate on only one aspect of a problem at a time and that they were unable to see common properties of different objects, so that each object was judged as unique. This inability to generalize was seen as part of the over-all loss of abstraction ability. Benjamin[9] found that schizophrenics interpreted proverbs literally, being unable to realize the existence of underlying abstract or figurative meaning.

While many workers have asserted that schizophrenics can be expected to give concrete responses, others, including Harrow, et al.,[42] have reported that strange, idiosyncratic thinking is a more important characteristic, both in acute and chronic schizophrenia. Similarly, McGaughran[59] found that the difficulty in schizophrenia is not an over-all inability to go beyond literal, concrete meanings, but rather a tendency to give personalized and unusual meanings to test material. Rapaport et al.,[70] too, using an object-sorting test, could find no evidence for marked concreteness. Whitbeck and Tucker[89] have suggested that what has often been called "concreteness" is actually a defect in metaphorical thinking. The schizophrenic is described as unable to understand one object on the model of another. Reed[71] has pointed out that in the early studies any atypical response was considered concrete, which magnified the prevalence of this finding. Low intelligence and the low energy output associated with chronic illness and prolonged hospitalization also increase the incidence of concrete responses.

At present, concreteness of thought is viewed as one of the many possible symptoms found in schizophrenia, rather than as a basic or universal defect. Some have claimed that overabstract thinking is also found in schizophrenia; however, what is described as "overabstract," is usually a pattern of speech dominated by words and phrases which, when used by most people, would be used to express abstract ideas, but which are used as inexact substitutes for specific terms, and which convey private symbolism rather than abstraction. Thus, a patient asked to explain how he would repair the cord of an electric clock described the clock as a "span of time" and talked about eliminating the cord and having the clock operated by solar rays or by light.

STUDIES OF OVERINCLUSION

In a series of studies dating back to the 1930s, Cameron[17,18,19] has reported his own investigation into cognitive disturbances in schizophrenia. On the basis of sentence completion tests and the Vigotsky sorting test, Cameron described a number of cognitive abnormalities. Schizophrenics displayed "asyndetic thinking," which Cameron described as the juxtaposition of cognitive elements without adequate linkages, similar to the loosening of associations previously noted by Kraepelin and Bleuler. Also noted were "metonymic distortions," described as the characteristic displacement of a precise term by an approximation. Related rather than exact terms were used in the context of speech. For example, Cameron quoted a patient saying he had three "menus," rather than three meals a day. Another finding was "interpenetration of themes," in which preoccupations of the patient intrude into his appraisal of the environment. On the basis of these findings, Cameron developed the concept of "overinclusive thinking" as a basic disorder in schizophrenia. By this term, Cameron meant that the boundaries of concepts become blurred, so that irrelevant ideas become incorporated into the formation of concepts. As a result, thinking is imprecise and vague, replete with unessential details and highly personal material. For example, a patient included in one category of a sorting test the blotter, the desk, and the examiner. Such overinclusion was seen as responsible for the interpenetration of themes, since categories are no longer logically firm but may include all sorts of unrelated objects or events.

Payne[67] has continued the study of overinclusive thinking, and found that it occurs not only in schizophrenia, but in manic states and, to a milder degree, in neurosis. He found it in schizophrenics only when thought disorder was clinically obvious, and it disappeared in them when the acute illness subsided. Harrow et al.,[41] on the other hand, subdividing the phenomenon into behavioral and conceptual overinclusion, reported that while chronic patients, as described by Payne, showed less overinclusive behavior, they continued to show overinclusive thinking.

COGNITIVE STYLE

A distinction between thought disorder and "cognitive style" was made by Wynne and Singer.[90] Cognitive style was described as a continuum that had analytic thinking at one end, global thinking at the other. Analytic thinking was described as orderly, systematic, discriminating. Global thinking was described as loose, diffuse, erratic, field-dependent, with problems approached as a whole, with random rather than systematic efforts made toward solution. They found that when thought disorder occurred in an analytic thinker, it was of a type they designated "fragmented." It was loose, characterized by intrusions that could not be harmoniously integrated into experiences or speech, and illogical leaps between ideas as the individual attempted to explain. Discontinuity between life compartments made for intact thinking in some areas, disordered in others. When the global thinker manifested thought disorder, it was of an "amorphous" type. By this they meant woolly or fuzzy percepts, improverished thought, vague, perseverative, lacking in purpose or goal, unable to elaborate ideas into more complex concepts, rambling, interpenetrating themes, blocking, and drifting off.

STUDIES OF MENTAL SET AND STIMULUS FILTRATION

Related to theories of overinclusive thinking have been hypotheses stressing the schizophrenic's inability to filter out irrelevant stimuli or to maintain a prolonged state of attention. Payne, in fact, seems to have shifted his interest from overinclusion to problems in selective attention. The major researcher in this area, however, has been Shakow[76,77] who has spent half a century studying the psychological aspects of schizophrenia. Shakow asserts that schizophrenics lose the ability to maintain a major set that would allow for sustained concentration in completing a task or following a complex sequence of thought. Instead, the schizophrenic's behavior is a result of momentary, shifting, "segmental" sets, so that attention is constantly diverted toward immediate stimuli that are irrelevant to the attempted task. The schizophrenic becomes bombarded by details and distractions, so that his actions appear erratic and disconnected. Shakow compares this state to that of a centipede who was so concerned with how each of his feet moved that he lost sight of where he was going. Some support for Shakow's hypothesis has come from the studies of Freeman et al.,[33] who reported schizophrenics as describing themselves as "flooded" with unwanted stimuli.

In a study of associative structure, O'Brian and Weingartner[65] observed that schizophrenic subjects gave more deviant responses on a word association test than did normals. But when asked to select from a list the words most related to the stimulus words, the schizophrenic subjects performed well, suggesting that they were able to recognize normal associations, but were unable to filter out idiosyncratic associations on an unstructured test.

On the basis of clinical reports of recovered schizophrenics, Arieti[3] has found that perceptions become fragmented, so that whole constructs are no longer appreciated. This observation was confirmed in a study[8] in which schizophrenics were presented with ambiguous cards that could be perceived as whole or disconnected partial percepts. While normal controls immediately perceived the whole percept, schizophrenic subjects perseverated on partial and fragmented percepts. Chapman and McGhie[21] found an intensification of schizophrenic symptoms when patients were transferred to a busy, noisy ward, presumably representing an increase of stimulation. On the basis of various tests, Orzack and Kornetsky[66] have reported evidence of overarousal in schizophrenics.

Despite these reports, reviews of the literature compiled by Shakow[77] and by McGhie[60] reveal that overarousal or segmental set is an inconsistent finding. Here, again, the type of patient can greatly bias the results: Hebephrenic schizophrenics showed difficulties in maintaining a given mental set, but paranoid schizophrenics proved to be more attentive than controls. With this avenue of research, the same conclusions seemed to have been reached as with the studies of concreteness or overinclusive thinking, namely, that some patients show the disability while others do not, and that the specific defect characterizes only some of the schizophrenic population, rather than being a pathognomonic sign.

Studies of Logical Processes

Another attempt to define the psychological deficit in schizophrenia has been the elucidation of the logical properties of thought disorder. Von Domarus,[24] who first attempted a logical analysis, described the thought of schizophrenics as "paralogical," defining its formal aspects as follows: "Whereas the logician accepts identity only upon the basis of identical subjects, the paralogician accepts identity on the basis of identical predicates." As an example, Von Domarus describes a schizophrenic patient who believed that Jesus, cigar boxes, and sex were identical. Investigation revealed that the link connecting these disparate items was the concept of being encircled: Jesus' head is encircled by a halo, cigar boxes by a tax band, and women by the sex glance of a man. Thus, the slightest similarity between items or events becomes a connecting link that makes them identical.

Stimulated by the work of Von Domarus, Arieti[3] has formulated a detailed analysis of

the formal mechanisms of schizophrenia. According to Arieti, the symptoms of schizophrenia are part of a "progressive teleologic regression." By "regression," Arieti intends a return to older phylogenetic modes of cognition and expression; by "teleologic" is meant that the regression is purposeful in defending against anxiety and re-establishing some sort of psychic equilibrium; and by "progressive" is meant that this regressive attempt fails to protect the individual and elicits more symptoms or a clinical disintegration. The schizophrenic cannot integrate at this lower level of cognition and so is doomed to a downward spiral of conceptual disorganization. The use of "predicate thinking," which equates as identical any items or events that have even the slightest similarity, is used to give the schizophrenic some semblance of meaning and to protect him from the anguish that a realistic appraisal of his environment would engender. Arieti's often-quoted patient who believed she was the Virgin Mary because she also was a virgin, demonstrates how this "paleological" identification serves to bolster a shriveling sense of self and defend against feelings of worthlessness.

Arieti has attempted a synthesis of the psychodynamic and cognitive points of view in his approach to schizophrenia.[4] He has delineated four stages of the disorder, showing how defense from anxiety at each stage is expressed by specific cognitive aberrations. He views schizophrenic symptoms as not only purposeful in the psychodynamic sense but utilizing particular mental mechanisms, such as concretization of concepts, desymbolization, and desocialization.

Other psychiatrists have also approached schizophrenic symptoms from the standpoint of logical analysis, the most pertinent being the symptom of "context shifting," which consists of shifting from one frame of reference to another in order to protect against anxiety-laden ideas. Burnham[16] gives several examples of such maneuvers as follows:

Interviewer: You seem to want to avoid all possible pain.

Patient: I remember reading about Thomas Paine in a history course.

I: You seem to fear that if you develop any close friends, they will desert you.

P: I wonder what's for dessert today.

It is obvious in this example that with the play on words the patient shifts the context of a meaningful word to one that is less likely to lead to painful realizations. Possibly, once the habit of shifting contexts is established, it is applied to nonsignificant as well as significant ideas. Also, any word or phrase might, to a schizophrenic patient, have a meaning unsuspected by others. Much of what has been described as the irrelevant, loose, or even delusional thoughts of some patients stems from this shifting, which frequently cannot be grasped readily by examiners.

Schizophrenia, more than any other psychiatric disorder, is characterized by aberrations in conceptual process. These aberrations have been described in terms of overinclusion, paleologic thought, shifting contexts, decreased filtration, or concreteness. Schizophrenia, it must be remembered, probably consists of several entities. Extensive study tends to dilute the magnitude of any single finding that appears important in schizophrenia. A characteristic that persists is variability. Whatever aspect of schizophrenia is being studied, there is a tendency for the pluses and the minuses to cancel each other out, leaving averages that call attention away from the aberrations characteristic of schizophrenics as a group, but not of each individual.

(Sign and Symptoms of Schizophrenia

Onset of Schizophrenia

While truly sudden onset can occur, especially in catatonic forms of schizophrenia, what often appears as sudden to the bystander, even to close family, is usually the culmination of a period of weeks or months of mounting inner turmoil and sense of ill-being. There is no single pathognomonic sign of early schizophrenia, and no valid predictors of potential for schizophrenia. Polatin and Hoch[68] reported that those who eventually become schizophrenic were apt to have been shy, seclusive, timid, with marked mood fluctuations and free-floating anxiety of overwhelming proportions, but this does not mean that those diagnosed schizoid personality are all potentially schizophrenic. The patient becomes increasingly restless, loses his appetite, becomes unable to sleep, often because of disturbing dreams, which may deal with calamitous destruction, humiliation, or unaccustomed primary-process material.

There may be inability to think, often explained as consequence of having too many thoughts at one time. This experience, seen briefly in normal individuals as an aspect of happy excitement, is, when prolonged, usually associated with a feeling of pressure or pain in the head. The patient begins to fear that he is becoming insane or losing his mind, that he will lose control, will never be able to think again, or, simply, that he will explode.

Here, as in most descriptions of the experience of mental illness, it is the verbal, introspective people who have provided the information. Those who are habitually nonverbal, however, appear to have the same suffering. If questioned about the presence of feelings or experiences known to be characteristic of the illness, they recognize, with relief, the description of what they have been experiencing. In the development of illness, the choice of symptoms, the manner in which they are elaborated, the attempts to deal with them, are all related to the patient's underlying personality, his sophistication, his current family relationships, and culturally determined patterns of illness and help-seeking.

Insidiously developing schizophrenias may appear to lack the painful mental experiences described above. The young person may become excessively shy, feel embarrassed with others, but become more withdrawn than other self-conscious adolescents, possibly develop ideas of reference. Instead of anxiety, there is avoidance, which may be so rationalized that it appears to be a neurotic defense. A young man with many symptoms of schizophrenia dropped out of college, explaining that he became too anxious to sit in class, fearing that he would have to urinate and not be able to get out in time. He was unable to speak with girls, but simply attributed this to shyness.

Compulsive behavior may appear, or, if already present, become intense. Occurrence of multiple or disabling compulsive symptoms in a young person suggests the possibility of schizophrenia. An eighteen-year-old, struggling with continuous sexual fantasies and uncontrollable feelings of inexplicable misery, each day emptied his drawers and closets, washed them, then carefully rearranged all his possessions. His parents offered little objection until he began to require a tube of toothpaste each day in his frantic efforts to become clean. The person who is trying to defend against overwhelming anxiety, or to deny the painfulness of being unable to maintain contact with other people may apply himself with considerable competence to a single intellectual pursuit, such as mathematics, chess, or religion, with room for little else. Friends are, in such cases, limited to one or two people with whom the activity and little else is shared. Far more common is a dwelling on abstractions, such as time, the nature of life, solutions to political and social problems. The individual may appear deep or intellectual to his neighbors, but if he records his thoughts in notebooks, as is often done, it can be seen that the ideas are usually lacking in depth or systematic approach, tend to be expressed in dramatic or cryptic but inconsistent phrases, fraught with significance only for the writer. Mark Twain described a youth who memorized thousands of verses of Scripture, received a gold medal, then went mad. Today, a young person with similar problems, instead of memorizing Scripture, might contemplate for months his own inner experiences and relationships.

The development of illness may often be recognized by a change in behavior. The new behavior may not be inherently pathological— the sociable person may become withdrawn, or the retiring person may become expansive. Behavioral changes that develop as defense against emerging psychosis may be mistakenly identified as healthy efforts to improve adaptation. In early stages of illness, a person may quit his job, leave his spouse, marry unwisely, or make other major life changes, in futile attempt to solve problems that, although related to his environment, arise from within. A feeling of depression, sadness, hopelessness is often present coincident with early schizophrenia. Suicide is not uncommon.

Subtle alterations of perception, as described by Chapman,[20] may occur during the premonitory period. Objects may appear larger or smaller, brighter or duller, take on unusual characteristics, fluctuate in size, appear to have outlines, or dance about. The patient may be unable to distinguish between object and background. Movement or change in perspective may create a sense of puzzlement and the visual scene may become incomprehensible. Extraneous stimuli may prove so distracting that organized activity becomes impossible.*

"Things just don't make sense," is a description often offered by patients in the early stages of a schizophrenic episode. People's speech becomes too fast to be understood. It becomes impossible to shift from one idea to another with the usual facility. The signs on buses or streets suddenly seem divorced from meaning, although ability to read is unimpaired. When this happens, an individual may become lost while traveling routes he has traveled before. There is a loss of mental efficiency and an impairment of ability to organize and synthesize perceptions into meaningful patterns. Many complain that they feel doped, or dazed, or robot-like.

Psychiatric examination at this point may reveal loosened associations, increased incidence of idiosyncratic use of words or concepts, blending of one concept into another, with ideas following one another in profusion. There may be circumstantiality, a constant elaboration of detail. The affect is likely to be anxiety or perplexity. Frequently, there is a disruption of the boundaries that normally separate inner experience from perceptions,

---

* Tucker et al.[83] have shown that existence of perceptual disturbance may be related to high anxiety, and is not pathognomonic of schizophrenia.

self from others, thoughts from actions. The patient who, upon first meeting a new physician, speaks as if a relationship already existed is subtly blurring the distinction between his inner need for a relationship and the environmental facts. The patient who "adjusts" to the hospital with ease and rapidity inconsistent with the outward disturbance illustrates a sensitivity to the surroundings which overrides the inner disturbance. In the course of an early interview, florid psychosexual material may be presented, material that most people would repress or conceal until a therapeutic relationship existed.[44]

If the illness continues, disturbances of perception and testing of reality may occur. Trivial stimuli, such as subway signs, television commercials, overheard bits of conversation, the facial expressions of strangers, may begin to have special meaning. Illusions and hallucinations may become intense and frightening. While voices (phonemes) are the most common hallucinations in schizophrenia, hallucinations of all sensory modalities can be readily discovered by careful questioning.[39] Olfactory hallucinations are usually foul odors, often related to sexual or excretory products. Tactile hallucinations may take the form of embarrassing sexual sensations.

People may be misidentified, or their actions misinterpreted. A patient admitted to a hospital in which staff wore street clothes rather than uniforms was too distracted to notice the name badges that distinguished staff from patients. He assumed that someone must be a doctor there to observe him, and selected the patient who seemed most intelligent and declared him to be the psychiatrist. He accepted medication, but soon became quite disturbed, having concluded that the medication was LSD, given him to make him crazy in order to justify his being held in a psychiatric hospital.

Delusions are common when an early schizophrenic illness has fully developed. Usually, these are fragmentary explanations for things not otherwise understood. They are not systematized or believed with conviction. The patient may experience "psychotic insight." Suddenly, everything becomes clear. He understands what has been happening to him, he understands the significance of hitherto unexplained perceptions, sensations, or thoughts. The usual rules of causality or evidence are ignored. This acceptance of private (autistic) thoughts and explanations is what is commonly but imprecisely termed a "break with reality." Body processes, ordinarily not noticed, may be suddenly detected and thought of as symptoms of illness. Various sensations in the chest, for example, may be perceived as manifestations of grave heart disease.

Recurrences of Schizophrenia

The course of schizophrenic illness most commonly seen is a series of recurrences and remissions, occurring against a background of chronic disability. Some of the classical manifestations of chronic schizophrenia, such as clang associations, neologisms, mutism, grossly bizarre behavior, are now seen often in acute episodes, but tend to fade away. It is thought by many that prolonged hospitalization in an environment dominated by other chronic patients encouraged continuance of such extreme symptoms. It had been hoped that elimination of prolonged hospital care would eliminate the chronic illness, but this has not been the case. Despite the enthusiasm of many workers, most studies have shown recurrences to occur, no matter what treatment has been employed. Several studies[29,31] have shown that patients who take prescribed medication are less likely to be rehospitalized. Careful follow-up studies by Davis et al.[22] of patients who had initially done well with intensive home care instead of hospitalization showed that they were, when the intensive care ceased, as likely to experience recurrences.

When symptoms recur, each episode of illness may develop as described in the section on onset of schizophrenia. Many patients, having learned from experience which mental phenomena are signs of illness, recognize what is happening and seek help. Hallucinations are readily recognized as such by many patients, delusions less often. Repeated episodes tend to be characterized by less affective response, but there is often a complaint of unpleasant affect, often described by the patient, for want of better vocabulary, as either "anxiety" or "depression."

Types of Schizophrenia

Hebephrenia, catatonia, and dementia paranoides, once known as separate entities, were united as forms of one disease by Kraepelin, described as types of schizophrenias by Bleuler. The International Classification of Diseases continues to recognize these subtypes, although their clinical utility is debatable. Patients who manifest the classical symptoms of each type continue to appear, but in time different manifestations appear, or, as the illness becomes chronic, lose the differentiating features. What once appeared to be entities, and later subtypes, are best viewed now as pathological behavior patterns.

Simple schizophrenia is said to be characterized by insidious reduction of external attachments and interests, apathy, impoverishment of interpersonal relations, poverty of thought, and an absence of florid schizophrenic symptoms. The repetition of almost identical descriptions in many texts suggests that clinical experience has contributed little to the descriptions. In concluding a review of the literature on simple schizophrenia, Stone et al.[81] state, "It is a vague and inherently unreliable diagnosis without foundation in psychological theory or psychiatric practice." They found that the diagnosis was seldom made, but when it was, just as in cases reported in the literature, hallucinations and delusions were often present, despite the fact that the condition is defined as a form of schizophrenia without these accessory symptoms. Apathy, indifference, and absence of anxiety, although described as characteristic of patients in this and other diagnostic entities, are often defenses that have proven impenetrable to the examiner, rather than intrinsic aspects of the illness. Uncommunicative patients often have anxiety, hallucinations, delusions, desires, and opinions, which they do not share with their families or psychiatrists. Since diagnostic terms are operationally defined, simple schizophrenia can be diagnosed when there is some tangible evidence of schizophrenia in a patient whose behavior is characterized by apparent emptiness, apathy, poverty of thought, and for whom no other diagnosis is appropriate.

Doubt has also been expressed about the validity of *hebephrenic schizophrenia* as a subtype. Markedly differing criteria for use of this diagnostic term have been provided by different authorities. In Bleuler's time, almost any schizophrenic patient who was not catatonic and not paranoid was likely to be called hebephrenic. Slater and Roth[79] describe as hebephrenic all cases of schizophrenia in which thought disorder is the leading symptom. Leonhard, as cited in Fish,[30] has proposed an independent classification of chronic schizophrenias. Disturbance of affect is the outstanding disorder of the four types of hebephrenia he describes, and the range of disturbance includes marked silliness, depressive flat effect, apathy, and autism.

In current American usage, characteristics are disorganized thinking, shallow and inappropriate affect, unpredictable giggling, silly behavior, and mannerisms. Hallucinations or delusions may be bizarre, disorganzed, and transient.

Illustration: A woman of thirty, who had been hospitalized several times before with different manifestations of schizophrenia, was a constant source of irritation to staff and patients alike because of her child-like attention-seeking behavior. She lay on the floor in the corridor, turned the radio loud, jumped and stamped, shouted at her psychiatrist from the far end of the ward. When milk was spilled on the table, she licked it. She initiated conversation with a man by apologizing for having ugly, dirty thoughts about men, and said that she wanted to cut off her hair because it was a symbol of power. When she was reprimanded for walking nude from the shower, she responded by throwing eggs in all directions. She would suddenly throw her arms around people. Thought process disturbance was illustrated in a response to discussion of her unkempt appearance: "You are saying that I am filthy and dirty . . . the hands are mostly used for masturbation—that's what you mean by talking about my dirty fingernails." A few weeks later, she had returned to her usual sad, discouraged state, and was able to discuss her inability to maintain relationships, to control her intrusive fantasies, or to be free of anxiety.

Hebephrenic behavior is seen, acutely, as a form of clowning, acting-crazy behavior, defensively similar to mania, in chronic schizophrenic individuals. Classically, hebephrenic schizophrenia is one of the forms which begins in adolescence, and when this does occur, the prognosis is poor. Brill and Glass[15] studied a group of hospitalized hebephrenic patients and concluded that the syndrome represented an end-stage of illness, indicative of greater severity of schizophrenic illness, rather than being a special subtype.

Catatonic behavior may occur in any form of schizophrenia and is also seen at times with organic brain disease.[6] Catatonic schizophrenia is diagnosed when volitional disturbance is the predominant characteristic of illness. Catatonic schizophrenia may occur as an acute illness, one of the reactive schizophrenias, or as a form of chronic illness. The acute catatonic episode is usually characterized by rather sudden onset of mutism, often accompanied by marked reduction in motor activity. The patient looks blank, but the pulse is rapid, suggestive of fear, and the eyes may dart about. Usually, he passively allows himself to be directed, admitted to a hospital. Placed in a bed, the catatonic patient may attract no attention. A suble turning away, a resistance to being moved, discloses the characteristic negativism. The patient may be rigid when examined, may hold his head above the bed if the pillow is removed, but relax when alone. The most classical sign of catatonia is wax-like flexibility—if a limb is placed in an unnatural position, the patient retains the position for a short while, then, like melting wax, the limb gradually returns to natural position. This sign is not often seen; it may occur when a patient, having an arm placed above his head, for example, tries to co-operate by holding it there, until he fatigues. This behavior illustrates a suspension of volition, also expressed by echolalia or echopraxia. In the early stages of a catatonic episode, the patient may refuse food, but, if liquids are available, drink surreptitiously, so signs of dehydration are of greater management significance than recorded intake. Prolonged inanition presents considerable danger. Usually, one or two feedings through a nasogastric tube are followed by resumption of less unpleasant methods of food intake. Most catatonic patients understand fully what is going on around them, and may integrate what they hear with fantastic illusions and delusions, often on themes of destruction. Some later report that they have been blank, or unaware of the passage of time. Rapid recovery is often seen, but if this does not happen, electrotherapy can be expected to produce dramatic improvement, and should be recognized as a potentially life-saving treatment. A patient whose immobility was so extreme that he developed large decubiti and severe dehydration recovered after a few shock treatments and explained that he had been convinced that if he moved a muscle, even an eye muscle, he would instantly die. Another, who would function for weeks, then spend an entire day standing immobile or lying in bed explained that only by doing so could she be sure she would not kill herself.

Chronic catatonic schizophrenia has a poor prognosis. In the past, every large mental hospital had some patients who stood in one spot day after day, developing stasis edema of the legs eventually, or patients who had to be tube-fed for years. Unusual repeated movements of the entire body, posturing, or of lesser extent, stereotypy, were common. The stereotyped behavior, or repeated utterances, usually have some symbolic significance, not readily recognized because the separate parts of the miniature pantomime become condensed, abbreviated, and distorted.

Illustration: A chronic catatonic man, who had not spoken more than a few words at a time for over a year, regularly attended a day hospital, spending most of his time standing in the corridor, posturing, grimacing, and laughing to himself. He usually made some fragment of a comment when a staff member was absent, and he stood near meetings or group therapy without participating. As part of a research project on attitudes toward work, he was asked to write sentence completions. His response revealed some of his previously unexpressed, bizarre thoughts, and demonstrated the severe thought process disturbance that justifies inclusion of this condition among the schizophrenias.* His responses included: When my co-workers are around, I: "feel like hair sprouting out all over." The more responsibility a worker is given: "the less important he takes himself." If I were working: "omnisciently empowered. If only I was working omnisciently empowered." Sometimes I feel that my supervisor: "uses medieval techniques." I feel that my co-workers: "plot." What I want most from a job is: "friendly people." If the boss criticized me, I would: "spit in his face." Taking orders at work: "mutely."

Catatonic excitement, characterized by ceaseless activity, can be one of the few dangerous conditions in psychiatric practice. Whereas the paranoid patient who becomes dangerous is usually defending himself against what he perceives as an attack or an attacker, the excited catatonic patient may thrash out wildly, possibly continuously, without apparent reason or target. Fortunately, this condition is not common. Potential for catatonic excitement can be detected when a typically slowed patient seems to be struggling to maintain control or when he communicates, nonverbally, a disturbing feeling of tension.

Of all clinical types of schizophrenia, the *paranoid* type is the most homogeneous and the least variable.[78] Whether recurrent or continuous, the symptoms may be relatively unchanged over the years. Disturbances of verbal process or affect may be absent or very subtle. This is the most frequent form of schizophrenia developing in middle life, often in individuals who have been capable of forming relationships and performing well at work. Paranoid schizophrenia is characterized by prominent delusional thinking.

* Mute patients will often speak under sodium amobarbital, narcohypnosis, disclosing both current fears and underlying thought disorder.

A primary delusion, also known as autochthonous or apophanous, as described originally by Gruhle (according to Slater and Roth[79]), is a fundamental disturbance. A perception is suddenly understood as having a unique meaning, such as the description by a patient, "I saw the neon sign flashing on the building across the street and suddenly I knew it was being done to tell me that I was a failure in life." The primary delusion springs to mind fully formed, without precursor or explanation, and it carries a sense of conviction. It is not a product of disturbed thought process, mistaken information, or altered perception.

Secondary delusions, also known as delusional elaborations or delusional interpretations, are efforts to apply reason to explain what is happening. They are characterized by arbitrary or idiosyncratic connections, and inability to even consider the possibility of alternative explanations. A patient who constantly complained that she was given injections of medication while she slept during the night was explaining, in an arbitrary fashion, why she felt dull and uneasy each morning. All efforts to suggest alternative explanations for these common symptoms were rejected as being inconsistent with the "obvious" facts. Then, having accepted the idea that someone was entering her apartment during the night, it seemed plausible to her that strangers were being brought in to look at her. Dynamically, this implied that she was of interest to many people. In answer to her own question of how this could go on, she explained that such crimes could go on only if people in high places were involved, which then made her feel more helpless, but also more important.

Delusional individuals often say that they do not know why they are persecuted, that it must be a result of mistaken identity, but usually there is a deep-seated conviction that they are the target of animosity from someone who is threatened by their power or righteousness. The patient whose delusions are frankly grandiose may identify himself as a member of the FBI, usually on a secret mission, a friend of the President, and a veteran of many important but secret triumphs. If hospitalized, he is there to observe the staff.

Somatic delusions may occur in all forms of schizophrenia and in depressions, but they are especially common in paranoid schizophrenia. The patient may believe that part of his body is missing, rotting, shrunken, or malfunctioning. The hypochondriac seeks treatment to restore him to health, but the delusional individual is un-reassurable. The somatic delusions in schizophrenia may be bizarre, as the belief that the heart has stopped, or, as one man described his problem, "I have a gas-oil leak inside." It is difficult to distinguish between somatic delusion, somatic hallucination, and the strange descriptions given by some patients of sensations arising from the brain or other organs not associated with perceived sensation.

Paranoid schizophrenia is associated with far less disruption of personality and less disturbance of function than any other schizophrenia. The patient may relate well to others, may have maintained relationships in the past, may have normal affective responses, and, often, no gross evidence of thought process disturbance. Careful examination or use of projective tests may elucidate subtle thought disorder. In all patients, thought disorder is most likely to be manifest when the patient is speaking about a topic that is emotionally significant to him. The paranoid schizophrenic patient may demonstrate thought process disorder only when explaining his delusional beliefs.

A delusion is described as "systematized" when the patient attempts to explain everything as a consequence of one cause. If this is accomplished, there is reduction of anxiety and greater acceptance of pathological view of things by the patient, thus systematization of delusions is prognostically unfavorable. Most of the time, delusions are but tentative explanations, doubly useful in that they spare the patient the need to think about his personal troubles. The diagnosis of paranoia, a rare entity, can be made only in the presence of an isolated, fixed, systematized delusion, without evidence of other psychopathologic process.

Not all false beliefs are delusions. False beliefs may have been learned, or they may be products of distortion, selective attention, disturbance of identity, or faulty reasoning. The diagnosis of delusion should always be based upon demonstration of arbitrary or idiosyncratic thinking and denial of the possibility that alternatives could exist.

Hallucinations are found in all types of schizophrenia, and may be prominent in the paranoid type. Voices (phonemes) are the most abundant form. They may be accusatory, derogatory, condemning, commanding, or they may offer a continuous commentary or description of actions and thoughts. Voices may be a primary experience, with delusional elaboration to account for them. Distinction between hallucinations which are recognized as such, designated as "pseudohallucinations" by Sedman,[75] and hallucinations believed to be the voice of a real person, is of doubtful clinical significance.

Kasanin[50] coined the term *schizoaffective psychosis* to characterize individuals who appeared to have a schizophrenic episode, but whose course was similar to those with affective disorders, i.e., they recovered or had remissions. In subsequent years, the definition of schizoaffective was changed, and it is now applied to patients who are clearly schizophrenic but who have significant disturbances of affect. Included in this group are some patients who present with symptoms of recurrent or continual depression, but who are discovered by careful study to be predominantly self-absorbed and to have magical, irrational, and idiosyncratic thinking. Impetus for acceptance of this compromise term, straddling affective disorder and schizophrenia, came from the studies[58] which revealed that many patients, initially diagnosed manic-depressive, were subsequently found to be hospitalized as chronic schizophrenics.

The subtype of schizophrenia most often diagnosed in North America is *chronic undifferentiated* type, which was introduced to the nomenclature in 1952. It had been recognized that as time passed, patients whose early illness could be readily characterized as hebephrenic or catatonic, or at times paranoid, developed signs or symptoms of other types, and that the manifestations of chronic illness were similar for all patients. Also, there were always patients whose symptoms seemed to fit neither in one category nor in another. This diagnostic entity seemed appropriate for large numbers of patients, and, since it was so useful, interest in differentiating the other entities declined.

Chronic Schizophrenia

Most descriptions of chronic schizophrenic patients, based upon observations of the chronically hospitalized, have emphasized that they are bizarre, inexplicable, stereotyped, uncommunicative. Return of many seriously impaired patients to the community may provide opportunities for discovering which manifestations are caused by the illness and which by institutional care. The manifestations of illness within hospitals have changed, reflecting in part the influence of learned patterns and social forces in shaping the symptoms, or in creating conditions that allow a patient to be excused as sick or to get assistance. A century ago, religious preoccupations, mutism, and grossly impaired behavior, were far more common.[53]

The chronic manifestations of schizophrenia are similar in patients who began as catatonic or as paranoid, in those who became ill at forty, and those whose illness began in childhood. Thought process disturbance may be severe and global, or it may be detectable only in certain areas of thought. Conversation may be vague, stilted, superficial, repetitious, marked by cliches and explanations that fail to explain. Those who are extremely autistic may dwell on their own thoughts and not attempt to respond to others. Past events and present ideas may be intermixed. Referents may be omitted, so that the patient's statements lack context and appear incoherent.

Delusions and hallucinations may persist; reality-testing may be adequate, or may be very poor. Inexplicable physical symptoms are common, and may include total body pain, diffuse weakness, unsteadiness of gait, vomiting, choking. Any symptom is possible, but often the patient just cannot find words to describe the over-all bad feeling. Affective response may be dull, incongruous, or there may be a sustained mood, perhaps cheerfulness, but more often stubborn irritability.

Anergy, or disturbances of volition, have at times been incorrectly described as apathy. The patient who, without knowing why, is unable to act, may defensively say that he does not care. During recovery from a schizophrenic episode, patients may be abnormally tired, fatigue easily, and experience clinical depression.[80] The chronic schizophrenic may sit blankly for long periods, unaware of the passage of time, even giving the impression that he has organic brain disease. He may remain in bed when he intended to look for a job, avoid or put off without reason any activity that is new, unfamiliar, or outside of his routine. A patient referred to a clinic may fail to attend because he dreads going to a new place, or he may stop attending if personnel change, rather than meet someone new. Life is routine, constricted, empty. He may sleep most of the day, be awake during the night. The chronic schizophrenic in the community may fear contact with strangers, be unable to maintain a flexible approach to buying food, and consequently live on a monotonous, deficient diet. He may be unable to cope with externally caused changes in environment or to meet the complex depends of welfare departments. Years of interpersonal isolation may make him appear to lack common sense. He cannot anticipate other people's reactions or understand what impression he makes upon others.

Personal hygiene and habits may be neglected; there may be reluctance to change clothes, for the body image and the garments may be intertwined. Thus, he may apply for a job looking disheveled, and if employed, may insist on doing the job his way, not the employer's way. He may be unable to handle common social skills of any sort, such as breaking off conversation if he does not want to talk to the person, or refusing if asked to do something he does not want to do, or asking someone to go to a movie with him. There may be a constant fear of hurting others, or a remarkable lack of concern or even awareness of the feelings of others.

Many chronic schizophrenic individuals are unable to handle excessive external stimuli or multiple simultaneous stimuli. They think slowly, have difficulty concentrating, become unable to function by disorganization of behavior or protective withdrawal if too much happens at one time, if the system becomes overloaded. External events, thoughts, bodily sensations, all may compete for attention and lead to overload. Some patients appear to be unable to differentiate self from environment, and to experience internal and external sensations as a continuum. Freeman et al.[34] consider this loss of "ego feeling" to be the basic disturbance in chronic schizophrenia.

Early studies suggested deterioration of intellectual skills and capacities in chronic schizophrenia. There does seem to be slowing of learning and quick loss of what has been learned. To a large extent, the defects once thought to be deterioration appear to be related to attention and motivation. Test results can be improved when the outwardly apathetic patient can be motivated.

Arieti[4] has differentiated states of schizophrenia which summarize the changes that take place as schizophrenia progresses, without implying that this is the inevitable course for all patients.

The first stage extends from the beginning of impairment of perception of sensory reality to the formation of the characteristic symptoms of schizophrenia. It is characterized by the presence of anxiety in the patient, and a tendency to fight the external world in an attempt to vindicate his illness. Three substages have been recognized: (1) substage of panic, when the patient begins to perceive things in a different way, is frightened, and does not know how to explain the strange things that are happening; (2) substage of psychotic insight—he puts things together in a pathological way; (3) substage of multiplication of symptoms—symptoms become more and more numerous as the patient vainly attempts to solve his conflicts and remove his anxiety with them.

The second, or advanced, stage is characterized by an apparent acceptance of the illness. All the classic symptoms are present and they do not seem to bother the patient as much as before. Life has become more and more restricted and lacking spontaneity. Routine and stereotyped behavior are outstanding.

In the third, or preterminal, stage,[2] which may occur five to fifteen years after onset, many symptoms seem to have burned out and the types of schizophrenia resemble each other. At this stage, primitive habits, such as that of hoarding useless objects and decorating oneself in a bizarre manner are conspicuous.

In the fourth, or terminal, stage,[1] the behavior of the patient is even more impulsive and reflex-like. Hoarding of objects is replaced by food-grabbing and later by ingestion of small objects, edible or not. Later in the fourth stage, although occasionally in the third stage, many patients present what appears to be perceptual deficiency. They seem insensitive to pain, temperature, and taste, although they still react to olfactory stimuli. Incontinence of urine and feces may be constant or occasional. The most organic-appearing behavior may, in some instances, prove reversible if the patient's withdrawal and negativism are overcome.

Residual type is the official diagnostic term to be applied to the patient who no longer shows psychotic evidences of schizophrenia, but does have other evidences. This term, although plausible, has never become widely used, probably because the appearance and disappearance of psychotic symptoms is recognized as a fluid matter. Chronic schizophrenic patients may be more or less psychotic, more or less incapacitated.

Late schizophrenia is not an officially accepted term, and many deny the existence of such an entity. Kay and Roth[51] described carefully the schizophrenias that appear in later life. There has been a tendency to diagnose involutional psychosis too glibly among those in the 1950s or 1960s, and to assume that any older patient must have a senile or arteriosclerotic problem. Illnesses recognizable as schizophrenia of late onset are usually dominated by delusional thinking. There are no major evidences of organic brain dysfunction. When the patients are admitted to hospitals, they do not show the rapid deterioration of physical and mental condition characteristic of those with arteriosclerotic brain disease. The prognosis for recovery from the delusional illness is poor. The individual who develops late schizophrenia has usually been seclusive, eccentric, or very tense throughout adult life.

Borderline Syndromes

Whether this group should be included among the schizophrenias is a source of much controversy. Rarely are such patients thought of as schizophrenic in Europe, where they are diagnosed as neurotic or having a character disorder. Terms that have been applied to at least some portion of the patients in this group include "borderline schizophrenia," "borderline personality," "borderline syndrome," "ambulatory schizophrenia," "larval schizophrenia." In ICD-8 and DSM-II, these conditions are included among schizophrenia, latent type. This is an unfortunate term, but at least it allows patients who are clinically similar to be classified together. In DSM-I, patients in this so-called borderline group were classified among the chronic undifferentiated, which then created the odd situation of the sickest and most chronic patients sharing a category with patients thought by many not to be schizophrenic at all.

In 1949, Hoch and Polatin[45] coined the term "pseudoneurotic schizophrenia" to describe patients who had multiple, shifting neurotic symptoms (pan-neurosis), continual, pervasive anxiety (pan-anxiety), and chaotic sexuality. Careful examination revealed Bleulerian signs to a mild degree, and on follow-up many developed clear-cut schizophrenia. Zilboorg[91,92] described mild schizophrenias, making the point that tuberculosis could be diagnosed before cavitation developed, and appendicitis before peritonitis. His original use of the term "ambulatory schizophrenia" referred to the patients' tendency to wander about, but subsequently he accepted the popular usage that equates ambulatory and non-hospitalized. Dunlaif and Hoch[25] described

pseudopsychopathic schizophrenias, characterized by antisocial behavior as a consequence of an irrational view of reality, inappropriate responses in human relationships, disturbance of affect, and profusion of neurotic and hypochondriacal complaints. Patients may become psychotic when their antisocial behavior is prevented by incarceration.

The term *latent schizophrenia* has a long history of use analogous to the use of "latent" in most medical conditions, as Bleuler's[13] explanation that he would diagnose schizophrenia only in disturbances unquestionably psychotic in terms of social adjustment; if the schizophrenia was assumed to be present but has not advanced to the level of psychosis, he called it "latent." In ICD-8 and DSM-II, the conditions described above, plus others termed "larval" or "incipient schizophrenia" are classified as schizophrenia, latent type.

"Borderline state," "borderline schizophrenia," "borderline personality," "borderline syndrome," are terms applied to a condition that resembles personality disorders in that it is stable and not especially likely to develop into psychosis or overt schizophrenia,[88] but that resembles schizophrenia when diagnosis is based on disturbance of ego function. Grinker et al.,[40] studying hospitalized patients, delineated four subtypes within this group. In these conditions, there is diffuse impairment of most ego functions, moderate in severity. "Micropsychotic" episodes may occur under stress. Such patients are never considered schizophrenic in England,[52] and even in the U.S. many are troubled by the existence within the schizophrenias of a diagnostic entity defined as nonpsychotic. Psychotherapeutically, the approach to these patients is more like the approach to severe schizophrenia than to neurosis.

(Approaches to Diagnosis

In much of the world, the diagnosis of schizophrenia is made only when the patient is clearly psychotic. British psychiatrists are likely to make a diagnosis of affective disorder if there is significant disturbance of mood, or if delusions or hallucinations are explainable as products of altered mood.[26,52] The diagnosis of affective disorders almost died out in the United States after follow-up studies of patients initially diagnosed manic-depressive showed that many subsequently became unmistakably schizophrenic. The situation was epitomized by Lewis and Piotrowski:[58]

Even a trace of schizophrenia is schizophrenia and has a very important prognostic as well as diagnostic significance. Many patients with few and mild schizophrenic signs and with a strong affective element fail to improve. ... ... schizophrenics are qualitatively different from all other people.

After schizophrenia is diagnosed, it becomes apparent that prognosis is quite variable. The attempts to dichotomize the schizophrenias have been reviewed by several authors.[37,43,48] Of the many pairs of terms proposed, "process" and "reactive" have gained the widest usage. *Process schizophrenia* is characterized by gradual or insidious onset, without precipitants, isolation, impoverishment of thought, poor premorbid adjustment. This form of schizophrenia most often reaches the level of psychosis in late adolescence or early adult years. Prognosis is poor. Patients in this group are considered schizophrenic in every diagnostic school.

Reactive schizophrenias appear to develop in response to some psychological stress in individuals whose adjustment has been adequate. Onset is rapid, with gross disturbance, such as catatonic or paranoid symptoms. There may be severe disturbances of reality perception and testing. This form of schizophrenia may appear at any age, often in the late thirties or forties. Prognosis is good for recovery from each episode.

When schizophrenia is defined narrowly, the course of illness is apt to be one of progressive impairment, corresponding to Kraepelin's original concept. When this approach to diagnosis is followed, the patient who has what some would call a schizophrenic illness with recovery, is given another diagnosis.

Langfeldt[56] introduced the term "schizophreniform psychoses" to describe patients who did not manifest "splitting phenomena with clear consciousness." By "splitting phenomena" he meant "clear ideas and feelings of passivity (resulting, among other things, in thought-reading, thought-stealing, etc.), derealization and depersonalization, which are accepted by the patient without comment." The schizophreniform psychoses were more likely to have symptoms that were psychologically intelligible and to have an acute onset related to some precipitating emotional event. Schizophreniform psychoses were thought to be psychogenic, and schizophrenia organic. In many long follow-up studies,[27,57] 77 percent of the patients diagnosed schizophreniform when hospitalized have done relatively well, half of them were free of symptoms or working. Of those diagnosed schizophrenic, fewer than 20 percent were able to live outside the hospital, and most of those not hospitalized were not self-sufficient.

More recently, Robins and Guze[72] reviewed selected literature on prognosis and concluded that schizophrenia with good prognosis is not a mild form of schizophrenia, but a different illness, probably related to affective disorders.

One of the clearest presentations of the narrow delineation of schizophrenia is that of Schneider.[74]

Schneider's Diagnostic Criteria

Schneider designates a group of phenomena as being of first-rank importance, not because they are thought to be basic disturbances, or related to any theory of schizophrenia, but because they have special value in making the diagnosis of schizophrenia. He describes the following as being of first-rank importance, cautioning that they might at times be found in other psychotic states.

1. Hallucinations:
    (a) Audible thoughts: hearing one's own thoughts as an auditory experience;

(b) Voices conversing with one another;

(c) Voices that keep up a running
commentary on the patient's behavior.

2. Somatic Passivity Experiences: experiences (not delusions) of physical interference, which may include somatic
hallucinations, attributed to various
devices, rays, hypnotic influence, frequently of a sexual nature.

3. Thought Process:

(a) Thought-withdrawal or interruption of thought attributed to some
outside person or force. Also,
thoughts ascribed to others who
intrude their thoughts upon the
patient.

(b) Diffusion or broadcasting of
thoughts: private thoughts are
known to others. This is a change
in the experience of thinking, not
a deluson or a hallucination.

4. Delusional Perception: abnormal significance, usually with self-reference, is
attached to a genuine preception without any comprehensible, rational, or
emotional justification. The significance
is almost always urgent, personal, and of
great import.

5. Will: actions, feelings and impulses felt
as the products of others, as well as
influenced or directed by them.

According to Schneider, signs and symptoms which, although seen often in schizophrenia, are also seen often in other conditions, or in normals, are not useful in establishing diagnosis. His list of inconclusive symptoms includes some that have been associated
with schizophrenia since Kraepelin and Bleuler. Thought withdrawal is seen in severe depression, he says; disconnected thought is seen
in normal individuals, especially when upset;
the opinion of an examiner that the patient's
affective response is inadequate, is undepend-
able; rapport with the examiner cannot be
accurately determined; lack of drive or impulsive conduct are seen in other conditions.

Ego Function

The concept of schizophrenias as conditions
characterized by disturbances of the ego has
received increasing attention. Several authors
have attempted to define the ego in terms of
its specific characteristics. Beres[10] presented a
list of seven functions of the ego, explaining
that the development of the ego can be understood only in terms of its several functions.
Bellak[7] has for many years been developing
scales for measuring ego functions. He has
formulated twelve functions. The description
of ego function disturbances below does not
correspond precisely to either Beres or Bellak.
While psychoanalysis may explain the disturbance of ego and superego in schizophrenia as
regression employed as a defense against anxiety arising from intrapsychic conflicts, it is not
necessary to accept the validity of analytic
concepts in order to employ the descriptive
terms related to ego dysfunction.

1. Thought process: defects of association,
concreteness, inability to use figurative language, excessive use of overabstract language,
impaired logic, autistic or idiosyncratic use of
words, blocking.

2. Reality:

(a) Perception of reality: hallucinations, illusions, perceptual distortion, ideas of reference, delusions.

(b) Testing of reality: inability to
recognize that perception does not
correspond to the external world or
that thinking is arbitrary and does
not follow socially shared methods
of establishing proof or correctness.

(c) Sense of reality: depersonalization,
derealization, loss of ego boundaries, feelings of dissolution, oceanic
feelings, disturbances of sense of
identity.

3. Object Relations (interpersonal relations): withdrawal, social isolation, extreme
self-absorption or egocentricity; inability to
maintain relationships of mutuality.

4. Regulation and Control of Drives, Affects, and Impulses: inability to delay, to tolerate frustration; direct expression of basic aggressive and sexual drives.

5. Defensive Functioning: inability to maintain repression, emergence of primary-process thinking, inability to develop or maintain stable defenses.

6. Autonomous Functioning: disturbances of language, memory, will, inability to work, disturbance of motor skills.

7. Snythetic-Integrative Functioning: feeling of confusion, splitting, disorganized behavior, inability to maintain goal-direction or sense of causality.

8. Stimulus Barrier: overawareness of internal or external stimuli, overresponse to stimuli; tendency to become disorganized in presence of excess stimuli.

This approach to diagnosis allows all the schizophrenias, from the nonpsychotic "latent" to the most disabled, to be ordered on one continuum of operationally defined terms. It does not imply that all the schizophrenias thus diagnosed are forms of a single disease entity.

(Prognosis in Schizophrenia

Prognosis for recovery from an acute episode is good, but it is not possible to predict the future course at the time of a first episode. The ICD-8 terms, "reactive confusion," "reactive excitation," and "reactive psychosis, unspecified," employed in some countries, but not in the U.S., allow a neutral diagnosis of a psychotic episode which may or may not mark the onset of a chronic illness. If a second episode occurs and is again followed by recovery, it may be argued that the correct diagnosis should be manic-depressive illness. In terms of the North American practice of diagnosing schizophrenia in rather broad terms, it can be said that the course may be (1) a single psychotic episode followed by remission, (2) psychotic episodes with no impairment between them, (3) recurrent episodes with pro-

gressive impairment of ability to function, (4) continuous psychosis, and (5) continuous psychosis with progressive apparent impairment of intellectual capacity. Changes in approach to treatment render obsolete many of the earlier studies that were done when prolonged hospitalization was a frequent form of treatment. At this time, it can be said that if the diagnosis of schizophrenia is firmly established (excluding latent types) in a hospitalized patient, the patient is likely to be hospitalized again and is likely to experience impaired ability to be self-sufficient.

Studies of prognostic criteria and outcome have led to the conclusion that the standard subtypes of schizophrenia (catatonic, paranoid, etc.) lack prognostic value. Indicators of good prognosis, according to Vaillant's[85,86] review, are rapid onset, recognizable psychological stresses, presence of confusion, presence of depression, good premorbid adjustment (i.e., nonschizoid), and family history of affective disorder.

(Differential Diagnosis

Perhaps the most important rule in diagnosing schizophrenia is that *no one symptom is pathognomonic*, but that a constellation of specific symptoms is necessary. Schizophrenia is a complex disorder characterized by a withdrawal into a private fantasy world, which is maintained through the use of personal beliefs, idiosyncratic thought patterns, and precepts that are not culturally shared.

Schizophrenia can at times be confused with both functional and organic conditions. Among functional disorders, the emotional excesses of the hysterical personality sometimes present a diagnostic problem. However, while bizarre behavior and extreme mood swings can be seen in hysteria, there is no withdrawal from others and the hysteric is extremely susceptible to environmental influences. Gross stress reactions, such as the "three-day psychosis" seen in military settings, are often indistinguishable from acute schizophrenic episodes. The patient is typically agitated and anxious, has hypochondriacal complaints and some paranoid ideation. However, as in hysteria, there is no withdrawal from others, but rather a fear of being left alone, and extreme compliance. There is a history of prolonged fatigue and psychological stress. Similarly, in manic states, there is a constant effort to be involved with others. Finally, none of these conditions demonstrates the disturbance of thinking or the excessive reliance on internal interpretation of events, as found in schizophrenia.

Psychiatric disorders of adolescence present specific difficulties in diagnosis, since this is so often the age of onset for schizophrenia. Nonschizophrenic adolescents frequently show eccentric behavior, extreme mood swings, hypochondriacal concerns, social withdrawal, and preoccupation with overly abstract ideas. Careful observation reveals that the intellectualization or romanticized view of things does not represent thought disorders or delusional thinking. Of diagnostic importance is the ability of the adolescent to experience pleasure. Prolonged feelings of hopelessness or despair—the anhedonia described by Rado[69] —is an ominous sign in this age group.

The occurrence of a schizophrenia-like illness in patients who have had temporal lobe epilepsy for a mean duration of 14.1 years was described by Slater et al.[78] Davison and Bagley[23] have reviewed the literature and reported a more than chance incidence of schizophrenia-like psychosis associated with the following: epilepsy, cerebral trauma, cerebral tumor, encephalitis, basal ganglia diseases (including paralysis agitans, Wilson's disease, Huntington's chorea), presenile degeneration, Friedreich's ataxia, motor neurone disease, multiple sclerosis, narcolepsy, cerebrovascular disorders, carbon monoxide poisoning, cerebral anoxia, hypoglycemia, thallium poisoning, phenylketonuria, vitamin B_{12} and folic acid deficiency. Any of these may at times be mistakenly diagnosed schizophrenia.

In the past, toxic disorders did not present a diagnostic problem in that disorientation, memory difficulties and altered intellectual functions absent in schizophrenia were prominent symptoms. With the current usage of psychedelic compounds, such as LSD, mescaline, and psilocybin, toxic psychoses similar to schizophrenia are more frequently seen.

Freedman[32] reports that almost all of the symptoms of acute schizophrenic episodes can be produced by LSD, and that in the early phases of an LSD psychosis it may be impossible to differentiate the two. In a few hours, however, the individual's ability to structure his world despite the toxic effect of the drug is different than the misinterpretation seen in schizophrenia. In general, these hallucinogens produce fragmented visual hallucinations (vivid colors, patches of flowers), rather than the conceptual auditory hallucinations of schizophrenia. Also, in many cases, part of the self is unaffected by the drug and remains rational while observing the drug-induced distortions, so there is not the total panic and anxiety that correspond to the gross involvement of the personality in schizophrenia. Diagnosis may be difficult when a schizophrenic youth using hallucinogens in his efforts to eliminate anxieties about identity finds the toxic psychosis a trigger for functional psychosis.

In contrast to the hallucinogens, chronic use (or even a few doses in susceptible individuals) of amphetamines can produce a syndrome undistinguishable from paranoid schizophrenia.[84] Ideas of reference, distortions of the body image, delusions of persecution, and auditory hallucinations in the presence of clear consciousness have been reported.[28] These patients usually recover within a week of withdrawal from amphetamines, during which they exhibit prolonged sleep, extreme hunger, and severe mental depression. Without a history of amphetamine ingestion, diagnosis may be impossible, unless high urinary amphetamine levels are discovered.

The Clinical Concept of Schizophrenia

From the disparity and great variety of symptom pictures described above, it must be questioned whether an entity such as schizophrenia exists, and if the concept of it as a unitary psychiatric disorder is valid. In view of our present state of knowledge, schizophrenia may be best conceptualized as a clinical syndrome, rather than a classic disease with a single etiology, symptom picture, and course. Schizophrenia represents the singularly human ability to substitute an internal world for external reality through an alteration of thought and perception, and the creation of an idiosyncratic set of symbolic criteria through which to interpret experience. The attempt to identify and define the mechanisms of these distorting processes may ultimately shed light on the higher reaches of the human mind, as well as on its disintegration.

As Jung[46] wrote over half a century ago, "We healthy people who stand with both feet in reality, see only the ruin of the patient in this world, but not the richness of the psyche that is turned away from us." An appreciation for this hidden richness should be the task of every student of psychiatry.

(Bibliography

1. ARIETI, S. "Primitive Habits and Perceptual Alterations in the Terminal Stage of Schizophrenia," *Archives of Neurology and Psychiatry*, 53 (1945), 378–384.

2. ———. "Primitive Habits in the Preterminal Stage of Schizophrenia," *Journal of Nervous Mental Disease*, 102 (1945), 367–375.

3. ———. *Interpretation of Schizophrenia.* New York: Brunner, 1955.

4. ———. "Schizophrenia" in S. Arieti, ed., *American Handbook of Psychiatry*, 1st ed., Vol. 1. New York: Basic Books, 1959.

5. ARLOW, J. A., and C. BRENNER. "Psychoanalytic Concepts and the Structural Theory," *Journal of the American Psychoanalytic Association Monograph*, Series #3. New York: International Universities Press, 1964.

6. BELFER, M. I., and C. C. D'AUTREMONT. "Catatonia-like Symptomatology," *Archives of General Psychiatry*, 24 (1971), 119–120.

7. BELLAK, L., and M. HURVICH. "A Systematic Study of Ego Functions," *Journal of Nervous and Mental Disease*, 148 (1969), 569–585.

8. BEMPORAD, J. "Perceptual Disorders in Schizophrenia," *The American Journal of Psychiatry*, 123 (1967), 971–976.

9. BENJAMIN, J. "A Method of Distinguishing and Evaluating Formal Thinking Disorders in Schizophrenia," in J. S. Kasanin, ed., *Language and Thought in Schizophrenia.* New York: W. W. Norton, 1964.

10. BERES, D. "Ego Deviation and the Concept of Schizophrenia," in *The Psychoanalytic Study of the Child*, Vol. 11. New York: International Universities Press, 1956.

11. BINSWANGER, L. *Being-in-the-World*, J. Needleman, transl. New York: Basic Books, 1963.

12. BLEULER, E. *Dementia Praecox, or the Group of Schizophrenias*, J. Zinkin, transl. New York: International Universities Press, Press, 1952.

13. BLEULER, M. "The Concept of Schizophrenia," *The American Journal of Psychiatry*, 111 (1954), 382–3.

14. BRACELAND, F. J. "Kraepelin, His System and His Influence," *The American Journal of Psychiatry*, 114 (1957), 871–876.

15. BRILL, N. Q., and J. F. GLASS. "Hebephrenic Schizophrenic Reactions," *Archives of General Psychiatry*, 12 (1965), 545–551.

16. BURNHAM, D. L. "Varieties of Reality Restructuring in Schizophrenia," in R. Cancro, ed., *The Schizophrenic Reactions.* New York: Bruner/Mazel, 1970.

17. CAMERON, N. "Reasoning, Regression and Communications in Schizophrenics," *Psychological Monographs*, 50 (1938), 1–33.

18. ———. "Schizophrenic Thinking in a Problem-Solving Situation," *Journal of Mental Science*, 85 (1939), 1012–1035.

19. ———. "Experimental Analysis of Schizophrenic Thinking," in J. S. Kasanin, ed., *Language and Thought in Schizophrenia.* Univ. of Calif. Press, Berkeley, 1946.

20. CHAPMAN, J. "The Early Symptoms of Schizophrenia," *British Journal of Psychiatry*, 112 (1966), 255–261.

21. CHAPMAN, L. J., and A. McGHIE. "An Approach to the Psychotherapy of Cognitive Dysfunction in Schizophrenia," *British Journal of Medical Psychology*, 36 (1963), 253–260.

22. DAVIS, A. E., S. DINITZ, and B. PASSAMANICK. "The Prevention of Hospitalization in Schizophrenia: Five Years After an Experi-

mental Program," *American Journal of Orthopsychiatry*, 42 (1972), 375–388.

23. Davison, K., and C. S. Bagley. "Schizophrenia-like Psychoses Associated with Organic Disorders of the Central Nervous System: A Review of the Literature," in R. N. Herrington, ed., *Current Problems in Neuropsychiatry. British Journal of Psychiatry* Special Publication #4, 1969.

24. Domarus, E. von. "The Specific Laws of Logic in Schizophrenia," in J. S. Kasanin, ed., *Language and Thought in Schizophrenia*. New York: W. W. Norton, 1964.

25. Dunlaif, S. L., and P. Hoch. "Pseudopsychopathic Schizophrenia," in P. Hoch, and J. Zubin, eds., *Psychiatry and the Law*. New York: Grune and Stratton, 1955.

26. Edwards, G. "Diagnosis of Schizophrenia: An Anglo-American Comparison," *British Journal of Psychiatry*, 120 (1972), 385–390.

27. Eitinger, L., et al. "The Prognostic Value of the Clinical Picture and the Therapeutic Value of Physical Treatment in Schizophrenia and the Schizophreniform States," *Acta Psychiatrica et Neurologica Scandinavica*, 33 (1957), 33–53.

28. Ellinwood, E. H. "Amphetamine Psychosis: I. Description of the Individuals and Process," *Journal of Nervous and Mental Disease*, 144 (1967), 273–283.

29. Englehardt, D. M., et al. "Phenothiazines in Prevention of Psychiatric Hospitalization, IV. Delay or Prevention of Hospitalization —A Reevaluation," *Archives of General Psychiatry*, 16 (1967), 98–101.

30. Fish, F. *Schizophrenia*. Bristol: John Wright and Sons, Ltd., 1962.

31. Forest, F. M., et al. "Drug Maintenance Problems of Rehabilitated Mental Patients: The Current Drug Dosage 'Merry-Go-Round'," *The American Journal of Psychiatry*, 12 (1964), 33–40.

32. Freedman, D. X. "On the Use and Abuse of LSD," in S. C. Feinstein, P. L. Giovachini, and A. A. Miller, eds., *Adolescent Psychiatry*. New York: Basic Books, 1971.

33. Freeman, T., et al. *Studies on Psychoses*. London: Tavistock Publications, 1966.

34. Freeman, T., J. L. Cameron, and A. McGhie. *Chronic Schizophrenia*. New York: International Universities Press, 1958.

35. Freud, S. "Psychoanalytic Notes on an Auto-biographical Account of a Case of Paranoia," in Standard Edition, Vol. 14. London: Hogarth Press, 1958.

36. ———. "On Narcissism: An Introduction," in Standard Edition, Vol. 14. London: Hogarth Press, 1958.

37. Garmezy, N. "Process and Reactive Schizophrenia: Some Conceptions and Issues," *Schizophrenia Bulletin*, 2 (1970), 20–74.

38. Goldstein, K. "Methodological Approach to the Study of Schizophrenic Thought Disorder," in J. S. Kasanin, ed., *Language and Thought in Schizophrenia*. New York: W. W. Norton, 1964.

39. Goodwin, D. W., P. Alderson, and R. Rosenthal. "Clinical Significance of Hallucinations in Psychiatric Disorders," *Archives of General Psychiatry*, 24 (1971), 76–80.

40. Grinker, R. R., B. Werble, and R. C. Drye. *The Borderline Syndrome*. New York: Basic Books, 1968.

41. Harrow, M., et al. "Schizophrenic Thought Disorders After the Acute Phase," *The American Journal of Psychiatry*, 128 (1972), 824–829.

42. Harrow, M., G. J. Tucker, and D. Adler. "Concrete and Idiosyncratic Thinking in Acute Schizophrenic Patients," *Archives of General Psychiatry*, 26 (1972), 433–439.

43. Higgins, J. "Process-Reactive Schizophrenia: Recent Developments," *Journal of Nervous and Mental Disease*, 149 (1969), 450–472.

44. Hill, L. B. "The Nature of Extramural Schizophrenia," in A. H. Rifkin, ed., *Schizophrenia in Psychiatric Office Practice*. New York: Grune and Stratton, 1957.

45. Hoch, P., and P. Polatin. "Pseudoneurotic Forms of Schizophrenia," *Psychiatric Quarterly*, 23 (1949), 248–276.

46. Jung, C. G. "The Content of the Psychoses," in *Collected Works*, Vol. 3, R. F. C. Hull, Transl. New York: Pantheon Books, 1960.

47. ———. *The Psychology of Dementia Praecox*. New York: Nervous and Mental Disease Pub. Co., 1936.

48. Kantor, R. E., and W. G. Herron. *Reactive and Process Schizophrenia*. Palo Alto: Science and Behavior Books, Inc., 1966.

49. Kasanin, J. "The Acute Schizoaffective Psychoses," *The American Journal of Psychiatry*, 90 (1933), 97–126.

50. Kasanin, J. S. "The Disturbance of Concep-

tual Thinking in Schizophrenia," in J. S. Kasanin, ed., *Language and Thought in Schizophrenia*. New York: W. W. Norton, 1964.

51. KAY, D. W. K., and M. ROTH. "Environmental and Hereditary Factors in the Schizophrenias of Old Age ('Late Paraphrenia') and Their Bearing on the General Problem of Causation in Schizophrenia," *Journal of Mental Science*, 107 (1961), 649–686.

52. KENDELL, R. E. "Diagnostic Criteria of American and British Psychiatrists," *Archives of General Psychiatry*, 25 (1971), 123–130.

53. KLAF, F. F., and J. G. HAMILTON. "Schizophrenia—A Hundred Years Ago and Today," *Journal of Mental Science*, 107 (1961), 819–827.

54. KRAEPELIN, E. *Dementia Praecox and Paraphrenia*. 8th German edition translated by R. M. Barclay, and G. M. Robertson. Edinburgh: Livingstone, 1919.

55. KREITMAN, N., et al. "The Reliability of Psychiatric Assessment in Analysis," *Journal of Mental Science*, 107 (1961), 887–908.

56. LANGFELDT, G. *The Schizophreniform States*. London: Oxford University Press, 1939.

57. ———. "The Prognosis in Schizophrenia and the Factors Influencing the Course of the Disease," *Acta Psychiatrica et Neurologica Scandinavica*, Suppl. 13, 1937.

58. LEWIS, N. D. C., and Z. S. PIOTROWSKI. "Clinical Diagnosis of Manic Depressive Psychosis," in P. H. HOCH, and I. ZUBIN, eds., *Depression*. New York: Grune and Stratton, 1937.

59. McGAUGHRAN, L. S. "Differences Between Schizophrenia and Brain-Damaged Groups in Conceptual Aspects of Object Sorting," *Journal of Abnormal and Social Psychology*, 54 (1957), 44–49.

60. McGHIE, A. *Pathology of Attention*. Baltimore: Penguin Books, 1969.

61. MEYER, A. "Fundamental Conceptions of Dementia Praecox," *British Medical Journal*, 2 (1906), 757–760.

62. ———. "The Dynamic Interpretation of Dementia Praecox," *American Journal of Psychology*, 21 (1910), 385–403.

63. MINKOWSKI, E. "Findings in a Case of Schizophrenic Depression," in R. May, E. Anzel, and H. F. Ellenberger, eds.,

Existence. New York: Basic Books, 1958.

64. MOSHER, L. R., and D. FEINSILVER. *Special Report on Schizophrenia*. Washington: U. S. Dept. of Health, Education and Welfare, 1970.

65. O'BRIAN, J. P., and H. WEINGARTNER. "Associative Structure in Chronic Schizophrenia," *Archives of General Psychiatry*, 22 (1970), 136–142.

66. ORZACK, M. H., and C. KORNETSKY. "Attention Dysfunction in Schizophrenia," *Archives of General Psychiatry*, 14 (1966), 323–326.

67. PAYNE, R. W. "Cognitive Defects in Schizophrenia: Over-Inclusive Thinking," in J. Hellmuth, ed., *Cognitive Studies*, Vol. 2. New York: Bruner/Mazel, 1971.

68. POLATIN, P., and P. HOCH. "Diagnostic Evaluation of Early Schizophrenia," *Journal of Nervous and Mental Disease*, 105 (1947), 221–230.

69. RADO, S. "Schizotypal Organization, Preliminary Report on a Clinical Study of Schizophrenia," in S. Rado, ed., *Psychoanalysis of Behavior*, Vol. 2. New York: Grune and Stratton, 1962.

70. RAPAPORT, D., et al. *Diagnostic Psychological Testing*. Chicago: Year Book Publishers, 1945.

71. REED, J. L. "Schizophrenic Thought Disorder: A Review and Hypothesis," *Comprehensive Psychiatry*, 11 (1970), 403–431.

72. ROBINS, E., and S. B. GUZE. "Establishment of Diagnostic Validity in Psychiatric Illness: Its Application to Schizophrenia," *The American Journal of Psychiatry*, 126 (1970), 938–987.

73. RUMKE, H. C. "The Clinical Differentiation within the Group of Schizophrenias," *Proceedings of the Second International Congress of Psychiatry*, Vol. 1, 1957.

74. SCHNEIDER, K. *Clinical Psychopathology*, M. W. HAMILTON, transl. New York: Grune and Stratton, 1959.

75. SEDMAN, G. "A Phenomenological Study of Pseudohallucinations and Related Experiences," *Acta Psychiatrica Scandinavica*, 42 (1966), 35–70.

76. SHAKOW, D. "Segmental Set: A Theory of the Formal Psychological Deficit in Schizophrenia," *Archives of General Psychiatry*, 6 (1962), 1–17.

77. ———. "Psychological Deficit in Schizo-

phrenia," *Behavioral Science*, 8 (1963), 275–305.

78. SLATER, E., A. W. BEARD, and E. GLITHERO. "The Schizophrenia-like Psychoses of Epilepsy," *British Journal of Psychiatry*, 109 (1963), 95–150.

79. SLATER, E., and M. ROTH. *Mayer-Gross Slater and Roth Clinical Psychiatry*, 3rd Ed. Baltimore: Williams and Wilkins Co., 1969.

80. STEINBERG, H. R., R. GREEN, and J. DURELL. "Depression Occurring During the Course of Recovery from Schizophrenic Symptoms," *The American Journal of Psychiatry*, 124 (1967), 699–702.

81. STONE, A. A., et al. "Simple Schizophrenia—Syndrome or Shibboleth," *The American Journal of Psychiatry*, 125 (1968), 305–312.

82. SULLIVAN, H. S. *The Interpersonal Theory of Psychiatry*. New York: Norton, 1953.

83. TUCKER, G., et al. "Perceptual Experiences in Schizophrenic and Non-Schizophrenic Patients," *Archives of General Psychiatry*, 20 (1969), 159–166.

84. UNWIN, J. R. "The Contemporary Misuse of Psychoactive Drugs by Youth," in S. Arieti, ed., *World Biennial of Psychiatry and Psy-*

chotherapy. New York: Basic Books, 1971.

85. VAILLANT, G. E. "The Prediction of Recovery in Schizophrenia," *Journal of Nervous and Mental Disease*, 135 (1962), 534–543.

86. ———. "Prospective Prediction of Schizophrenic Remission," *Archives of General Psychiatry*, 11 (1964), 509–518.

87. VIGOTSKY, L. S. "Thought in Schizophrenia," *Archives of Neurology and Psychiatry*, 31 (1934), 1063–1077.

88. WERBLE, B. "Second Follow-up Study of Borderline Patients," *Archives of General Psychiatry*, 23 (1970), 3–7.

89. WHITBECK, C., and G. J. TUCKER. "Thought Disorder: Implications of a New Paradigm." Presented at the 125th Annual Meeting of the American Psychiatric Association, Dallas, Tex., May, 1972.

90. WYNNE, L., and M. T. SINGER. "Thought Disorder and Family Relations of Schizophrenics, II. A Classification of Forms of Thinking," *Archives of General Psychiatry*, 9 (1962), 199–206.

91. ZILBOORG, G. "Ambulatory Schizophrenias," *Psychiatry*, 4 (1941), 149–155.

92. ———. "The Problem of Ambulatory Schizophrenias," *The American Journal of Psychiatry*, 113 (1952), 519–525.

CHAPTER 24

SCHIZOPHRENIA: THE PSYCHODYNAMIC MECHANISMS AND THE PSYCHOSTRUCTURAL FORMS

Silvano Arieti

OR THE PSYCHODYNAMICALLY ORIENTED psychiatrist the onset of the manifest symptomatology of schizophrenia is a beginning as well as an end—the end of a special nonpsychotic personal history which in its adverse characteristics started much earlier in life, in some cases at the time of birth.

A psychodynamic approach retraces in reverse this long history and correlates it with the present psychosis in order to understand its development, meanings, effects, and potentialities.

Inherent in the manifest symptomatology of schizophrenia (described in Chapter 23) are also unusual psychological structures and forms which must be studied beyond their immediate clinical appearance.

The first part of this chapter will deal with the psychodynamics, the second with the formal psychological structure of the disorder. The knowledge of these two aspects of schizophrenia is of the greatest help to the psychotherapist (see Chapter 27).

(Psychodynamics of Schizophrenia

We have already mentioned that the road leading to adult schizophrenia has its beginning in the remote past of the patient, in some cases at the time of his birth or shortly afterwards. Some authors (for instance, Fodor[35]) push the beginning further back, to the intrauterine life. Others feel that the parental attitudes which are so important in determining the conflicts of the patient have their roots in sociological, historical, political, and geographical conditions. It is generally agreed that the psychodynamic studies should include only the psychological life experiences of the patient and the interaction with his close interpersonal environment, leaving the connections with the larger environment to epidemiological, sociological, or community psychiatry studies. Such division is purely conventional and arbitrary, because, as I expressed elsewhere,[17] the sociological factors affect the patient psychodynamically by direct, or, most of the time, indirect routes. Other experiences, such as physical illnesses, unless studied in reference to their psychological impact, cannot be included among the psychodynamic factors.

Although these psychodynamic aspects have so far revealed nothing that can be considered absolutely specific of the life of schizophrenics, certain constellations of circumstances, and their consequences, cluster more frequently in the life of these patients than in that of the average individual.

A psychodynamic understanding of any human being and, in our particular case, of a person who will eventually suffer from schizophrenia, requires that we take into consideration (1) the world which the child meets; (2) the child's way of experiencing that world, especially in its interpersonal aspects; (3) the way the child internalizes that world; (4) the ways by which the sequence of later experiences weaken, reinforce, distort, neutralize, expand, or restrict the effects of the early experiences.

The world the child meets consists overwhelmingly of his family, and it is this family's world which we shall study in the following section. In this author's frame of reference, the life pattern of the schizophrenic is divided into four periods, of which only the last one can be considered psychotic.* We shall examine them separately.

* In previous publications I used the terms, "first, second, third, and fourth stages" to designate the different parts of the patient's life history. Inasmuch as these parts do not represent actual stages of an illness, but portions of time, characterized by certain events and processes, the term "period" seems to me more

⟨ The Family of the Schizophrenic

The reader must be aware that all the studies of the family of schizophrenics were made after the patient became obviously sick and in most cases had grown to be an adult. The assumption is made that the study of how the family is at the time of the illness and the eliciting of past history give an adequate picture of the family environment during the time preceding the psychosis. Moreover, often the appraisal of the family was in many studies strongly influenced by the personal account of it given by the patient himself. Nevertheless, there is no doubt that one of the first vivid impressions that we get in dealing with patients and their relatives is that the family of the patient is not a happy one, or at least was not so in the formative years of the patient. The unhappiness, although aggravated at times by realistic situations such as poverty and physical illness, was as a rule determined by psychological factors, predominantly by the unhappy marriage of the parents. The marriage was unhappy not only because of the character incompatibility and personality difficulties of the parents but also because such difficulties, instead of being compensated for or countered by less destructive defenses, were enormously aggravated by the process of living together. This atmosphere of unhappiness and tension, although all-pervading and pronounced, in many cases is not apparent to the casual observer, as an attempt is made by all concerned to conceal it not only from the external world but also from themselves. At times, it is almost totally repressed and replaced by psychological insensitivity.

Mostly because of the pioneer work of Ackerman,[1,2] the family has been studied as a unity, or a constellation, having an impact on the future patient, which is greater than the sum of the effects of the individual members. For instance, it is not just the attitude of the mother toward the child that has to be taken

appropriate. Moreover, in this way we avoid confusion with the different stages of the disorder, once the illness has started its manifest course.

into consideration, but also how the attitude of the mother affects the whole family, and how the result of this attitude toward the whole family indirectly affects the child.

Many authors have described special family constellations in schizophrenics. In the first edition of *Interpretation of Schizophrenia*,[4] I described one which I have encountered frequently. A domineering, nagging, and hostile mother, who gives the child no chance to assert himself, is married to a dependent, weak man, too weak to help the child. The father does not dare to protect the child because of fear of losing his wife's sexual favors, or simply because he is not able to oppose her strong personality. By default more than by his direct doing he becomes as crippling to the child as mother is.

Occurring less frequently in the United States, but still frequently enough, is the opposite combination: a tyrannical or extremely narcissistic father is married to a weak mother who tries to solve her problems by unconditionally accepting her husband's rules. These rules do not allow her to give enough love to the child and to be considerate enough of his affective requirements. In these families, the weak parent, whether mother or father, becomes antagonistic and hostile toward at least one child, because she or he (the parent) displaces her or his anger from the spouse, who is too strong to be a suitable target, to the child. In 1957, Lidz et al.[59] described the same type of family constellation, to which they gave the name of "marital skew."

Lidz and his associates[58-64] found that the role of each spouse in the family cannot be well established and that no attempt is made by them to complement or to help each other. There is no possibility of getting together, of reciprocal understanding and co-operation, no mutual trust, no confidence, but rivalry, undercutting of worth, threat of separation, and enrollment of the children's support against the other. Each partner is disillusioned in the other: the husband sees the wife as a defiant and disregarding person who also fails as a mother. The wife is disappointed because she does not find in her husband the father figure she expected. In this background, the family is often split into two factions by the overt *marital schism* of the parents. Generally, the children belong to one side of the schism or to the other and have to contend with problems of guilt because of their divided loyalty.

I have found other frequent constellations in the family of schizophrenics. One of them consists of a family in which each member is intensely involved with the others. Each member experiences not just a feeling of competition with the others, but an extreme sense of participation, reactivity, and sensitivity to the actions of the others, often interpreted in a negative way. In these cases, the members of the family want to help each other, but because of their neurotic entanglement, anxiety, distrust, and misinterpretation, they end up by hurting one another.

I have observed also a different type of family, which is almost the opposite, or perhaps a reaction formation of the one described. The family can be compared to an archipelago. Each member lives in emotional isolation and communicates very little with the others in spite of physical proximity.

In evaluating the families of schizophrenics in a general way, Lidz and Fleck[62] wrote of the possibilities of something being fundamentally wrong with the capacity of the "parents to establish families capable of providing the integrative development of their offspring." They spoke more specifically of three categories of deficiency: (1) parental nurturance; (2) the failure of the family as a social institution; (3) defect in transmitting the communicative and other basic instrumental techniques of the culture. Lidz and collaborators feel also that the irrationality of the parents is transmitted directly to the patient.

An important problem that has interested some authors[70] is the persistence of abnormal interaction patterns. An outsider could at first be inclined to believe that if a pattern of living leading to undesirable results has been formed in a family, the pattern would be corrected and equilibrium restored. The opposite, however, occurs in the family of schizophrenics. The same unhealthy "homeostasis" at times lasts decades.

Don Jackson[44] made the pertinent observation that families of schizophrenics are not disturbed in the sense of being disorganized. On the contrary, the family of the schizophrenic is highly more organized than the normal family, in the sense that "such family utilizes relatively few of the behavioral possibilities available to it." According to Jackson, the bizarre, maladaptive behavior of the family is indication of the restriction of the behavioral repertory, which does not allow variations, or other roles to be followed. Some authors see the family of the schizophrenic as conferring on the patient the role of scapegoat or as a responsible ally of one parent. This role would maintain the pathogenetic interaction patterns of the whole family. Searles[78] and Wolman[91] believe that the child maintains the morbid role because he loves mother and wants to give to her. He believes that without him she would be in a disastrous situation.

Even before the family of the patient was studied as a unity, the various members, and especially the parents, were studied individually, although, as already mentioned, often by relying greatly on how the patient experienced them. Some authors have followed Fromm-Reichmann in referring to the mother as "schizophrenogenic." They have described her as overprotective, hostile, overtly or subtly rejecting, overanxious, cold, distant, etc. Because of these characteristics, she was unable to give herself to the child and was unfit for motherhood. Rosen[76] referred to her perverse sense of motherhood. In the writings of a large number of authors, she was described as a malevolent creature, and portrayed in an intensely negative, judgmental way (Sullivan,[82,83] Rosen,[75,76] Hill,[41] Limentani,[65] Bateson et al.,[19] Lu,[66] Lidz and Fleck[63]).

The father of the schizophrenic has also been studied by Lidz and his associates.[53,64] Whereas previous authors had emphasized the weakness, aloofness, and ineffectiveness of the father in the paternal role, Lidz and associates described him as insecure in his masculinity, in need of great admiration for the sake of bolstering his shaky self-esteem, occasionally paranoid or given to paranoid-like irrational behavior.

I shall present my own conclusions, based on over thirty years of personal clinical experience and on the study of the literature.

1. Practically all the authors, including this writer, agree that serious tension, anxiety, hostility, or detachment and turbulent conflicts existed in the family of the patient, especially during his formative years. However, these findings could never be submitted to accurate statistical analysis. Some authors[87] have found family disturbances less frequently among schizophrenics than in control studies.

2. It is common knowledge that family disturbances, similar to those reported by most of the quoted authors, exist also in families in which there has not been a single case of schizophrenia in the two or three generations which could be investigated.

3. It is not possible to prove that adult schizophrenics, studied in family research, were potentially normal children whose lives were warped only by environmental circumstances.

4. The only point of agreement of all the authors is that *in every case of schizophrenia studied psychodynamically, serious family disturbance was found.* Unless we think that biases have grossly distorted the judgment of the investigators, we must believe that serious disturbance existed.

5. This conclusion indicates that although serious family disturbance is not *sufficient* to explain schizophrenia etiologically, it is presumably a *necessary* condition. To have differentiated a necessary, though not sufficient causative factor, is important enough to make this factor the object of full consideration.

6. The concept of the so-called schizophrenogenic mother needs revision. We have seen that the mother of the schizophrenic has been described as a malevolent creature, deprived of maternal feeling or having a perverse sense of motherhood. She has been called a monstrous human being. At times, it is indeed difficult not to make these negative appraisals because some of these mothers, who to us seem typical, fit that image. Quite often, however, an unwarranted generalization is made. The mother of the patient is not a monster or an evil-doer, but a person who has been overcome by the difficulties of living.

These difficulties have become enormous because of her unhappy marriage, but most of all because of her neurosis and the neurotic defenses that she built up in interacting with her children. Moreover, we must take into account the fact that the studies of these mothers were made at a time which preceded by a decade or two the "women's liberation" era. It was a period during which the woman had to contend fully but most of the time tacitly with her newly emerged need to assert equality. She could not accept submission any longer, and yet she strove to fulfill her traditional role. These are not just social changes; they are factors that enter into the intimacy of family life and complicate the parental roles of both mothers and fathers.

Since the early sixties, I have made some private studies and compiled statistics that differ from what other authors have reported, and from what I myself have described in the first edition of *Interpretation of Schizophrenia*.[4] Although personal biases cannot be excluded and the over-all figures are too small to be definitive, I have reached the tentative conclusion that only 25 percent of the mothers of schizophrenics fit the image of the schizophrenogenic mother. Why then have so many different authors generalized to all cases what is found in a minority of cases?

Of course, there is the possibility that I have not recognized what was not apparent. However, it is hard for me to believe that I have grown insensitive in my psychiatric work or less aware of the intangible and subtle family dynamics. Repeated observations have led me to different tentative conclusions. As we shall see in greater detail in Chapter 27 of this volume, schizophrenics who are at a relatively advanced stage of psychodynamically oriented psychotherapy, often describe their parents, especially the mother, in negative terms. Therapists, including the present writer, have believed what the patients told us. Inasmuch as a considerable percentage of mothers have proved to be that way, we have considered this percentage as typical and we have made an unwarranted generalization, which includes all the mothers of schizophrenics. The

psychotherapists of schizophrenics have made a mistake reminiscent of the one made by Freud when he came to believe that neurotic patients had been assaulted sexually by their parents. Later, Freud realized that what he had believed as true was, in by far the majority of cases, only the product of the fantasy of the patient. The comparison is not exactly similar, because in possibly 25 percent of the cases, the mothers of schizophrenic patients have really been nonmaternal, and we do not know what percentage of mothers of non-schizophrenics has been nonmaternal.

If this conclusion is correct, we must inquire why many patients have transformed the image of the mother or of both parents into one which is much worse than the real one. The answer to this problem will be provided by the intrapsychic study of the patient, especially in his early childhood.

❨ First Period: Early Childhood

A characteristic unique to the human race—prolonged childhood with consequent extended dependency on adults—is the most important factor in the psychodynamics of schizophrenia. What occurs at any subsequent age is also relevant and may bring about the decisive turns of events which trigger off the psychosis. The childhood situation, however, provides the preparatory factors which have a fundamental role, inasmuch as they narrow the range of choices of life directions, thwart the possibility of compensation, determine basic orientations, and facilitate abnormal sequence of events.

The first period of the psychodynamic pattern leading to schizophrenia extends from birth to approximately the time when the child enters grade school. We shall summarize here some salient aspects of normal development during this period in order to understand the deviations occurring in individuals likely to develop schizophrenia later in life.

The newborn human being needs other members of his own species in order to survive and to grow physically and psychologically.

This growth will proceed in accordance with its potentialities if the child, with the help of others, obtains a state of *satisfaction* and a state of *security*.[82] A state of satisfaction of the physical needs, such as food, sleep, rest, warmth, and contact with the body of the mother, is enough for the growth of lower species, and for the growth of the human being in the first months of life. But, in order to continue to grow normally after the first nine-twelve months, the human being needs, in addition to a state of satisfaction, a state of security. Before the others acquire "a significant" or symbolic importance, the life of the child is almost entirely governed by simple psychological mechanisms, like reflexes, conditioned and unconditioned, autonomous functions, nonsymbolic learning, imitation, and empathic processes.

Things are soon taken for granted by the child; they are expected to occur, as they have occurred before. After a certain stimulus, hunger, for instance, a subsequent act—the appearance of the mother's breast—is expected. Later, the child comes to feel that all things in life are due to others or depend on others. It is up to mother to give him the breast, to keep him on her lap, to fondle him. The child learns to see everything in a teleologic way—everything depends on the will or actions of others. But, together with the feeling that everything depends on others, there is also the feeling that people will do these wonderful things. In other words, the child expects these wonderful things to happen; he trusts adults. At first, of course, these feelings of the child are vague, indefinite. Since the child is deprived of the use of abstract words to describe these phenomena, his expression of these feelings remains at a primitive level. We may describe them as diffuse feelings, postural attitudes, physiological preparation for what is expected, nonverbal symbolism, and so forth.

Later, the child also expects approval from others. That is, the child expects the significant adults to expect something of him; the child *trusts* that the adults will *trust* him. In other words, there is a reciprocal trust that things are going to be well, that the child will be capable of growing up to be a healthy and mature man. The child perceives this faith of the mother and accepts it, just as he used to accept the primitive responses to the usual stimuli. He finally assimilates the trust of the significant adults, and he *trusts* himself.[5] Thus, things will no longer depend exclusively on others, but also on himself.

This feeling of trust in oneself and this favorable expectancy, which at first is limited to the immediate future, becomes extended to the immediate contingencies of life and then expands into a feeling of favorable anticipation as far as a more or less distant future is concerned. A basic optimism, founded on basic trust, is thus originated. Security consists of these feelings. If we consider this feeling of security or basic trust in its more social or interpersonal aspect, we may state that its interpersonal counterpart is what can be called a state of *communion*.

This atmosphere, first of satisfaction, then of security and communion (at least with the mother), facilitates the introjection in the child of the symbolic world of the others. It is this introjection that actually permits the emergence and the growth of the self, especially the introjection of the attitudes, feelings, verbal symbolisms, etc., emanating from the mother.

Using Buber's useful terminology and concepts, we may say that an "I-Thou" relationship exists.[23] Psychologically, this means that without others and trust in them there would be no I, no development of the self.*

The development of the self, emerging by the incorporation of the Thou while a state of satisfaction and security exists, permits the child to attain a stable self-image. The self-image consists of (1) body-image, (2) self-identity, and (3) self-esteem. As to the body-image, the child will have a realistic appraisal of himself and will be able to identify with his own sex. As to self-identity, the child will become aware of his role in the family and in society. As to self-esteem, he will trust himself and will have a sense of confidence and optimism.

It is toward the end of the first year of life,

* Buber's "I-Thou" expression corresponds approximately to Sullivan's "me-you" expression.

generally from the ninth month, that the child starts to build an inner life, or psychic reality, which is a counterpart to the external reality in which he is involved. Internalization occurs first through cognitive mechanisms belonging predominantly to what Freud called the primary process, and later more and more to what Freud called the secondary process.

The child continues to participate in the world through nonsymbolic ways, like simple or direct learning derived from perceptions, conditioned reflexes, etc. Now, however, he develops symbolic mechanisms, the most primitive of which constitute primary-process cognition. They are images, endocepts, and paleologic thinking.* Except in pathological conditions, these primitive mechanisms are replaced and overpowered by more mature secondary processes. Although examples of primitive mechanisms occur also in normal adult life, it is difficult to find pure forms of these even in children, if they are normal. By "pure" we mean forms that are not affected by concomitant secondary-process mechanisms.

The image is a memory trace which assumes the form of a representation. It is almost an internal reproduction of a perception which does not require the corresponding external stimulus in order to be evoked. The image is indeed one of the earliest and most important foundations of symbolism, if by symbolism we mean something that stands for something else which is not present. Whereas previous forms of cognition and learning permitted an understanding that was based on what was directly experienced and perceived, from now on cognition will rely also on what is absent and inferred. For instance, the child closes his eyes and visualizes his mother. She may not be present, but her image is with him; it stands for her. The image is obviously based on the memory traces of previous perceptions of the mother. The mother then acquires a psychic reality which is not tied to her physical presence.

Image formation introduces the child into that inner world which I have called "phan-

tasmic."[16] The image becomes a substitute for the external object; it is a primitive inner object.

The endocept is a mental construct representative of a level intermediary between the phantasmic and the verbal. It derives from memory traces, images, and motor engrams. Its organization results in a construct that does not tend to reproduce reality, and that remains at a nonrepresentational, preverbal, and preaction level. It is just a disposition to feel, to act, to think, and is accompanied by a vague awareness and at times undefinable, diffuse emotions.

Paleologic thinking occurs for a short period of time early in childhood, from the age of one to three. It is a way of thinking that seems illogical by adult standards or normal logic, and it is based on a confusion between similarities and identities. A salient part or characteristic which two persons or objects have in common is enough to make them appear identical, or belonging to the same category or class (formation of primary classes).[14] All men are "daddies" because they look like daddy.

Normal maturation controls the inhibition of these primitive forms and enhances the replacement by mature or secondary forms of cognition. That young children have greater difficulty in dealing with objects similar to those already known to them than with objects completely unknown has been recently confirmed by Kagan,[46] which formulated the discrepancy principle. As a result of the infant's encounters with the environment, he acquires mental representations of events, called schemata. Events that are moderately different from an infant's schema (or discrepant events) elicit longer spans of attention than either totally familiar events or totally novel events. For instance, in one experiment the child was shown a two-inch orange cube on six separate occasions. The infant was shown either a smaller orange cube (a discrepant event) or a yellow rippled cylinder (a novel event). Kagan reports that infants between seven and twelve months became excited by the discrepant small cube, whereas they remained calm by the appearance of the novel rippled cylinder. Discrepant objects or

---

* For a more elaborate analysis of images, endocepts, and paleologic thinking, see Volume 1, Chapter 40, Section C. Also, see *The Intrapsychic Self.*[16]

events are similar. A tendency exists in children to overcome the problem of how to deal with similar events by reacting to them as if they were identical. Normal maturation controls the inhibition of all these primitive forms of cognition as well as their replacement by mature or secondary forms.

In the families of schizophrenics, maturation and psychological development do not have the normal course that we have described. We find, instead of a state of satisfaction and security, an atmosphere of anxiety. Anxiety occurs in the absence of a state of satisfaction or security, or both. The anxiety due to lack of satisfaction would not alone lead to schizophrenia, because it is based on mechanisms more primitive than those involved in the pathogenesis of this disorder. Some schizophrenics were not deprived of satisfaction during the first year of life, but of security later, for many parents are capable of functioning as such when the child is a baby who has not yet developed a will of his own and is completely dependent. In many other cases, however, the patient was deprived of both his early need for satisfaction and his later need for security. A state of communion was never reached. Immature cognitive mechanisms persist and mature forms are delayed. As we have already mentioned, similarity is confused with identity. Often, the salient parts of stimuli are perceived and the background is ignored. The difficulty spreads backward from cognition to perception, and part-perception tends to replace whole perception. Generalizations follow primary class formation. For instance, certain characteristics of the mother are generalized to all women. Verbal thinking is underdeveloped. Most cognitive processes are mediated by images, predominantly visual. The child who has been raised in an adverse environment tends to participate as little as possible in the unpleasant external reality. He tends to be by himself, and this aloofness favors an overdevelopment of fantasy life or life images. If a few images have pleasant connotations, they urge the child to search for the corresponding external objects which are gratifying. Thus, pleasant images tend to be substituted by overt behavior and mostly unpleasant images and paleosymbols remain as durable inner objects. The result is that inner life in these children is mainly disagreeable at this level of development. Images become associated with others and spread an unpleasant affective tonality to all inner objects. Parents are experienced as clusters of disagreeable images, later paleologically transformed into terrifying fantasy figures.

To summarize what has been said so far, there is an unbalance in these children between external and internal forces. The child escapes from the external life, but the inner life in which he takes refuge is not pleasant either.

The cognitive immaturity of the child brings about other difficulties. These difficulties exist also in normal children, but to a minimal degree only. Psychological life in which images prevail predisposes to adualism: that is, to an inability to distinguish inner reality from external reality. Inasmuch as life of images is in these children predominantly unpleasant, the result is a negative appraisal of the world. Another difficulty consists in the uncertain appreciation of causality. The child cannot very well ask himself why certain things occur. At first, he expects things to happen in a sort of naïve acausality; but past experiences have predisposed him to a state of ominous expectancy, in contrast to the feeling of basic trust of the normal child. Later, he will be more and more under the impression that whatever occurs is brought about by the will of those unpleasant clusters of images that represent the parents, especially the mother.

Some of these experiences tend later to be transformed into endocepts (or imageless thoughts). All these primary-process mechanisms are slowly substituted by others that are verbal and conceptual.

It is obvious from the foregoing that we are not studying only intrapsychic processes in the child, or only interpersonal processes between the child and the family, but both types and their interconnections.

In the families of schizophrenics, there is at first no emotional detachment. All are involved with each other without helping each other, but the little child cannot entirely accept the others, or the Thou, because the Thou is too threatening, is a carrier of too much anxiety. *This is the beginning of the schizophrenic cleavage, this never-complete acceptance of the Thou, or the social self, of that part of the self that originates from others.* This Thou tends to remain unintegrated or to become dissociated like a foreign body, which later in life can be more readily externalized in forms of projection and hallucination.

These difficulties in accepting the Thou are manifested by the reluctance of these children to acquire the language and ways of the surrounding adults and by the emergence of such autistic ways and expressions as neologisms. Autistic tendencies exist even in normal children to a minimum degree, but they are more pronounced in pathological conditions—that is, when the child is afraid of the first interpersonal relations. In some cases, autistic manifestations become so pronounced as to offer the picture of childhood schizophrenia or of "early infantile autism," as originally described by Kanner.[47-50] In most cases, however, even of preschizophrenics, these autistic tendencies are repressed and the individual acquires the symbols of the others, but a propensity to lose them and to return to one's private autistic ways will persist.

Why is it so difficult for the child to accept the Thou, or its most significant component and representative, the mother? We must return to the basic question: Why does the future patient transform the image of his mother or of both parents into one which is much worse than the real one? In my opinion, what happens in the majority of cases is the following: The mother has definite negative characteristics—excessive anxiety, hostility, or detachment—and the future patient becomes particularly sensitized to these characteristics. He becomes aware only of them, because they are the parts of mother which hurt and to which he responds deeply. He ignores the others. His use of primary-process cognition makes possible and perpetuates this partial awareness, this original part-object relationship, if one wants to use Melanie Klein's terminology. The patient who responds mainly to the negative parts of mother will try to make a whole out of these negative parts, and the resulting whole will be a monstrous transformation of mother. In later stages, this negative image may attract other negative aspects of the other members of the family or of the family constellation, so that her image will be intensified in her negative aspect. This vision of mother is somewhat understood by the mother who responds to the child with more anxiety and hostility. A vicious circle is thus organized, which produces progressive and intense distortions and maladaptations. Mother becomes the malevolent Thou, the malevolent mother of a part of the psychiatric literature, and her image becomes the malevolent image of mother. What I have said in relation to the mother could, in a smaller number of patients, be more appropriately said in reference to the father. Moreover, this feeling of expected malevolence is extended to any adult who may become experienced as a malevolent other. Communion is now perhaps lost forever, any interpersonal relation is experienced with a sense of being ill-at-ease, or even of suspiciousness, possible danger.

Two tendencies may develop: one, to repress from consciousness the reality of the mother-child relationship, but this is not a task which can be easily achieved; the other, to displace or project to some parts of the external world this state of affairs. But, this tendency is also not possible unless a psychosis occurs, and for the time being it remains only a potentiality.

The self-image of the future patient deserves to be studied already during this first period or early childhood. Sullivan conceived the self and self-esteem as constituted of reflected appraisals. Although Sullivan[82,83] stressed the point that the patient "selectively inattends" certain parts of these appraisals and is mostly aware of that part called "the bad me," this concept, as it is generally used, represents an approximation of the truth.

The young child does not respond equally to all appraisals and roles attributed to him. Those elements that hurt him more stand out and are integrated disproportionally. Thus, the self of the future patient, although related to the external appraisals, is not a reproduction but a grotesque representation of them. Moreover, the self is constituted of all the defenses that are built to cope with these appraisals and their distortions. The more disturbed the environment, the more prominent the role and lingering of primary cognition. Others factors undoubtedly play a role in making the self-image so different from reflected appraisals. These factors are connected with environmental conditions and with biological individual characteristics which are difficult to ascertain. This grotesque self-image, the image of the "bad me," is very painful, and would become even more painful if the future patient continued to be aware of it and continued to connect it with an increasing number of ramifications and implications. Fortunately, to a large extent this image is repressed from awareness. The individual would not be able to bear it.

One of the relatively common characteristics of the self-image of children who later in life become schizophrenic is their uncertain gender and/or sex identification. Feeling rejected by both parents, they may have difficulty in identifying with either sex and gender. Later, they may not be able to find a complete heterosexual or homosexual identification, and may maintain even through their whole life some unconscious sexual uncertainty.

Another frequent characteristic in the childhood of preschizophrenics, found from the second to the fifth year of life, is a certain inconsistency in what is repressed from consciousness. The image of the malevolent mother and of the "bad me" threaten to come back to awareness, as the normal mechanism of removing unpleasant constructs from consciousness is less efficient in these children. Often, the repressed images tend to become conscious again, or to be transformed into symbolic forms later on in life, or to be projected to other people. In a minority of cases, the malevolent image of the mother is totally repressed and replaced by the image of the good, omnipotent mother, corresponding to the image the child had built during babyhood, when his needs for satisfaction were well taken care of. This image of the mother,

however, predisposes to regression and total dependency. If the child should become a baby again, mother will love and protect him. In spite of the anomalies, dreariness, and intense difficulties of this period, relatively few children succumb to child psychosis. The psyche of the individual has many resources, and even in the situation of the children so far described, permits them to enter without obvious or gross pathology the second part of childhood, which covers generally the grammar-school period.

❲ Second Period: Late Childhood

Mechanisms of repression, suppression, or denial are already in full swing. The malevolent mother and malevolent other are now only "distressing others" who make life difficult but possible. The image of the "bad me" has been transformed into the image of the "weak me." The child will see himself as weak, in a world of strong and distressing adults. Although in the children that we are describing primary-process mechanisms continue to function for a period of time longer than in normal circumstances, the primary process is eventually overcome and to a large extent replaced by secondary-process mechanisms. The latter are easily accepted as they seem to offer solutions to many of the patient's problems. The child learns the language of the community, as well as the prevailing ways of thinking, ideas, and mores. The prevailing of secondary-process mechanisms, which are similar to those of the surrounding adults, does not imply, however, that normal relatedness is established between the future patient and the members of his family. There is an abnormal dialogue between the patient and his parents and siblings. No language of basic trust, no taken-for-granted acceptance, no easiness of communication exist, but lack of clarity of meaning, excessive contradictions, unexpressed or distorted emotions, suspiciousness, or, at best, very pronounced cautiousness. Many authors have done much research to elucidate the disturbed communications in the family.

For instance, Bateson and associates[19] have advanced the so-called double bind theory, by which to a large extent they explained schizophrenia etiologically. According to Bateson and associates, the future patient receives, predominantly from his mother, a message with two or more logical meanings so related to each other as to induce painful conflict. In the words of Don Jackson,[44] "It's a sort of game, or gambit, set up by mother so that the child is damned if he does and damned if he doesn't"; he does not know to which of the messages to respond. Bateson gives the following example as an illustration: The child cries and the mother goes to him; her impulse is to get rid of the child, perhaps to kill him, but her feelings about this impulse compel her to feign acceptance or love; the child perceives the original impulse and the simulated love (the double bind) and becomes confused and anxious.

Such situations undoubtedly occur more often in the childhood of schizophrenics than in the childhood of other people and may be considered to be among the factors responsible for the general state of anxiety that eventually leads to the disorder. However, it would be unjustified to attribute to the double-bind mechanism too much importance.[9,18] Double-bind situations are a characteristic of life, not just of schizophrenia. They represent not necessarily pathology, but the complexity of human existence. If we were called upon to deal not with double binds but only with single messages, in a sort of reflex or conditioned reflex manner, life undoubtedly would be much simpler and offer much less anxiety, but it would not deserve to be called human; it would be a unidimensional life. Culture itself exposes the individual to many double-bind situations, that is, to conflictful situations. The healthy child learns to deal with them more or less adequately. But for the child who is to become schizophrenic, the double bind is one of the many carriers of parental difficulty in communication, and also of hostility and anxiety. The child is ill equipped to handle the many aspects of the communication at the same time. In conclusion, it is not the double-bind mechanism per se which is pathogenetic,

but either the use of it in a pathogenetic situation, or the fact that the child is unable to tolerate any ambivalence, any plurality of dimensions.

During the second period of childhood, the child has to repress to a large extent the unpleasantness of the first period. Although he will have difficulties in identifying with the significant adults in his life, he will be able now to build up some kind of less undesirable self-image, including identification with one sex rather than the other. Sexual confusion or homosexual tendencies are repressed and the child's identification with his own sex is achieved. This patched-up self-image and these identifications are not deeply rooted in the core of his being. They are more superficial reflections of how he feels people deal with him than a well-integrated vision of the self. Obviously, this child does not live in a state of communion with others, but in one of uneasiness. He still has to learn ways of relating to people. The basic patterns of relating will constitute his personality. They are defensive types of personality. The two most common types of prepsychotic personality in the future schizophrenic are the *schizoid* and the *stormy*. Although they may be found during the whole life of the patient and some of the most pronounced characteristics will appear at a later age, we shall describe them here. In fact, it is in late childhood that they acquire sufficient characteristics to be recognized.

The schizoid personality is found not only in people who are liable to become schizophrenic but also in neurotics, in people with character disorders, and in a mild form even in people who are considered normal. In the potential schizophrenic, however, it is particularly pronounced and has additional characteristics.

The person who has a schizoid personality appears aloof, detached, less emotional than the average person, and less involved. This emotional detachment originated as a defense against those intense interpersonal relations which occurred in early childhood and which proved destructive. Neurotic children may find defenses in other ways against similar family situations—that is, they may become compliant and submit to the parents unconditionally or become aggressive and fight the parents, and/or develop several neurotic symptoms, such as phobias, compulsions, etc. The person who is becoming schizoid selects instead a pattern similar to the one Horney[42] described as "moving away from people." Emotional detachment will permit the child to be less concerned or to suffer less on account of the bad images he has formed of his parents, and on account of his self-image and the general difficulties in life.

In addition to this emotional detachment, or rather as a consequence of it, the schizoid person limits his life experiences—his social contacts, his activities, his usual functions. The "object-relationships" are decreased in number.

It is important to remember that the schizoid personality is only a character armor, a defense the patient has evolved in order to fight the anxiety in living. Actually, the schizoid person is very sensitive; it is because of his oversensitivity that he has to defend himself with this character armor. By decreasing his contacts with society, he shows paradoxically how involved he is with society, and how afraid he is of people.

Although this defense may protect the patient so that he can remain schizoid for the rest of his life, it may also become more destructive than constructive unless treatment or other circumstances change his basic attitudes. When the patient had to contend only, or predominantly, with his family, this character armor may have been an adequate defense, but at about the time of puberty the patient discovers that not only his family but the world at large makes demands on him. He feels "pushed around" when environmental forces compel him to do things in spite of his detachment. On the one hand, reduction of his experiences in living has made him unprepared, hesitant, awkward, fearful; on the other, the early unhealthy experiences, which he may have forgotten, continue to alter or to give a particular flavor to his present experiences. Symbolically, and unconsciously, every interpersonal situation is experienced as a reproduction of the old parent-child relationship. As a matter of fact, a compulsive attitude often compels the patient to make this reproduction more like the original situation than it actually is.

At times, the patient himself is not satisfied with his withdrawal and harbors strong desires to make excursions into life, but every time he tries, he is burdened with anxiety, is awkward and ineffective, and meets defeat. Defeat in its turn reinforces his inferiority feelings, and a vicious circle is thus perpetuated. According to Guntrip,[40] the schizoid wants to escape from life and return to the womb, for safety, not for pleasure. The schizoid pattern of living is a compromise, since the return to the womb is impossible. It is a half-way house position, according to Guntrip, neither in life nor out.

I would say that the schizoid pattern is *a way of dealing with the distressing other*. The distressing other may be realistically distressing, just as the malevolent other may have been really malevolent. However, in most cases, the patient behaves almost automatically toward every "other" as if he were a distressing other. The patient is predisposed to see any other according to the introject or image which he has formed of the distressing other. His awkward, suspicious, or remote ways may actually elicit in other people unpleasant behavior toward him. In his turn, he may interpret this unpleasant behavior as a proof of the validity of the image of the distressing other. Thus, his schizoidism is reinforced.

In addition to the schizoid personality, which is well known in the psychiatric literature, the present author has described another type of personality frequently found in persons who are apt to become schizophrenic. This is the *stormy* personality. It must be added that since the early 1960s, schizophrenics with a prepsychotic stormy personality have increased in number, especially in large urban centers, whereas there has been a gradual but steady decrease of schizophrenics with a prepsychotic schizoid personality. Sociocultural factors, which I have analyzed elsewhere, are partially responsible for the change in frequency of the two types by acting on the family structure.[8,18] Whereas the schizoid presents a classic type of alienation (remoteness from one's feelings and from others), the stormy may present either psychological instability or a new type of alienation.[18] In this new form of alienation, the person is not capable or prone to listening to his inner self, but is busy in contacting others, adjusting to others, and responding to external stimulation.

People with a stormy personality did not find a defense in emotional detachment or withdrawal. They tried many possible ways; at times, submersion in external perpetual stimulation; at other times, extreme submissiveness; at other times, aggressiveness; at other times, even schizoid detachment. This variety of dealing with people was often determined by the inconsistency of the parents. The distressing you they contend with is not only distressing but also unpredictable and inconsistent. The distressing you does not become only an unpredictable distressing other, but, unless detachment is present, remains a *you*; that is, the members of the family (and at times even other adults) are still experienced as close, perhaps manifesting that pseudomutuality that Wynne et al. have described.[92] People with a stormy personality have developed an even less workable enduring pattern of living than have the schizoids. Their self-images and self-indentifications are even more indistinct than those of the schizoid. They keep trying to reach people, but each attempt leads to hurt. In a certain way, they are like schizoid persons who have been deprived of the character armor of indifference and therefore experience a tremendous amount of conscious anxiety. They are very vulnerable; every minor event can unchain a crisis. Life is generally a series of crises, frequently precipitated by little happenings, which are magnified by the patients who unconsciously see in them symbolic reproductions of original anxiety-producing situations. At other times, the patients seem actively to precipitate crises. They search actively for a meaningful way of living, but the inappropri-

ateness of their actions (bizarre marriages, love affairs, absurd jobs, etc.) leads them to repeated crises. They actually live a stormy life; often, they resort to excessive use of drugs and alcohol in order to abate the storms.

Returning specifically to the second period of childhood of our future patients, we can state that the defenses are generally built as reaction to chronic, undramatic danger, not to immediate fear, and as tepid responses to poorly expressed states of anxiety.

With relatively few exceptions, the psychological picture seems much improved toward the last period of childhood. The family has learned to live less inadequately with the patient, who is now less immature, less dependent, and less demanding. Although the child's earlier basic impressions and feelings about the world will linger, he is to a considerable extent able to alter them through the use of secondary-process mechanisms. These modifications are generally useful, even when at first they would seem to have an adverse effect. For instance, if the mother seemed to the child a terrible parent during the first period of childhood, the emotional detachment may have repressed the feeling associated with the maternal image. Moreover, the child might have also assumed, at an unverbalized level, that mothers are all this way; that's how the world is. In other words, in this case, he still makes a primary-process generalization. Later, he discovers that culture and society, as a whole, represent or take for granted an image of mother which is much better than that of his own mother. At first impression, one would think that the child will suffer when he discovers this discrepancy. Certainly, it would be better if such discrepancy did not exist, and to a certain extent he does suffer. However, he acquires some hope in life. He becomes more and more aware that the family does not constitute the whole world. He thinks that he will discover the world at large in the future. More and more, he appreciates the importance of the future in one's life and he builds hopes for his own.

Fortunately, in the majority of cases, there is no subsequent evolution toward schizophrenia. The individual succeeds in building up adequate defenses, in adjusting more or less to life, and the psychosis never occurs. When these defenses do not prove adequate, the patient enters the third period.

(Third Period: Adolescence, Youth, Adulthood

Since the early experiences have made the future patient awkward socially, clumsy in his activities, and somewhat inadequate in coping with life in general, his defeats become more evident in adolescence and youth, since he has to deal with a greater range of situations.

The schizoid or stormy personalities become more marked. Many of the schizoid youngsters appear markedly detached, as if something unnatural and strange divided them from the world. In spite of this apathy and aloofness, little signs can be detected in them which indicate how their original sensitivity is ready to erupt. They lack a sense of humor, cannot stand jokes or teasing, and are poor losers in games. In some cases, they find acceptable ways, like entering a monastery, in order to withdraw from life. In some cases, the schizoid person becomes a member of a marginal or fringe group: a beatnik, a bohemian, a hippie, or a marginally asocial person. A common defense among schizoid people is that of decreasing their needs to an almost unbelievable extent. Many of them live alone in furnished rooms, cut relations with their families, have no social contacts of any kind, except those which are absolutely necessary.

Young people with a stormy personality do not establish an adequate sense of self-identity. The series of crises they go through decreases their self-esteem and their hope.

Although the third period of the course toward schizophrenia may extend to or become manifest as late as the fourth or fifth decade of life, it generally starts around the time of puberty. These wide variations are related to the particular climate of the historical era and of the culture, and to individual occurrences in the patient's life.

The third period starts when the defenses begin to be less effective. We have to examine in detail how the process of ineffectiveness and inability to cope with events starts.

In order to understand this period, we have to unlearn or modify early psychiatric concepts. Repression from awareness does not pertain only to early childhood memories. Sexual maturity does not constitute the only problem of the adolescent; and, as a matter of fact, in many cases it is not the most important per se; it becomes important because of its implications. What may prove most pathogenetic is not instinctual impulses or instinctual deprivations, but *ideas*—the cognitive part of man, which has been so neglected in psychoanalysis, as well as in general psychiatry. The secondary-process mechanisms, which during the so-called latency period (our second stage) had protected him from the unpleasant generalizations and the paleologic terror of the first stage, now increase the discomfort of the preschizophrenic adolescent.

The patient finally comes to believe that not only his family, but the world at large is unwilling to accept his inadequacy. He has tried to adjust to a difficult world by resorting to heroic defenses, but he has not succeeded. The family drama or the social drama, involving the patient and his milieu, becomes more intense. Let us remember, however, that as long as this drama remains social or intrafamilial, we are still not dealing with schizophrenia. The work of all those authors who, following the lucid and penetrating example of Lidz, have illustrated the importance of the family in the pathogenesis of schizophrenia, has to be complemented by the study of the intrapsychic. The same could be repeated for the work of those authors who have studied the disorder as a social process. As a matter of fact, we may even state that as long as the drama remains an interpersonal one and is not internalized in abnormal ways, we do not have schizophrenia. In order to lead to schizophrenia, the drama must injure the self very much and become a drama of the self, by virtue of high symbolic processes.

As Vygotsky[86] has illustrated, conceptual thinking starts early in life, but it is in adolescence that it acquires prominence. Conceptual life is a necessary and very important part of mature life. Some people, however, make an exaggerated use of concepts, tend to put things into categories, and forget individual characteristics. Some adolescents, who later become schizophrenics, tend to select the formation of concepts and categories that have a gloomy emotional load, and these categories are given an absolute, exceptionless finality.

Individual memories that have escaped repression continue to bother the patient, no longer as individual facts, but as concepts. Their emotional tonality is extended to whole categories and clusters of concepts which become complexes. Old concepts change connotation. Let us take again, as an example, the concept of mother. We have seen how in the prepubertal period the earlier concept of mother, derived from individual experiences, undergoes improvement, because of the acquisition of the image of mother provided by the culture. The child was thus actually able to overcome the formation of a primary-process generalization and was no longer including all mothers in one category. But now, because of his unsuccessful dealings with the world, he has come to the conclusion that all adults, and consequently mothers, are not loving creatures. They are also fakers, like his own mother.

From a psychiatric point of view, perhaps the most important aspect of this expansion of conceptual life is the fact that the image of the self from then on will consist mostly of concepts. The image of the self varies through the ages. At first, it consists of a bulk of feelings, sensations, kinesthetic perceptions, and bodily movements; later, of the image of one's own body. After several other transformations in adolescence, it consists of remnants of previous images, but predominantly of concepts.

The concept-feelings of personal significance, of self-identity, of one's role in life, of self-esteem, now constitute a great part of the self. The self will consist of concepts which have adverse emotional components. This devastating self-image compels one to change concepts about other matters, and these changes, in their turn, will do further damage

to the concept of the self. Let us examine again the example of the concept of mother. We have seen how at the beginning of the third period the patient generalizes and sees all mothers as bad and insincere. Later, he develops another concept of mothers which, even if it remains unverbalized, has a more ominous effect than the previous one. He comes to believe that no matter what woman would be his mother, even the best, she would be a bad mother for him, because he himself is so undeserving and so bad that he elicits badness in others who try to be close to him.

Sexual life does not appear as desirable to many troubled adolescents and young adults but as something that has to be controlled and yet is very difficult to control. In the preschizophrenic, however, the problem does not lie simply in lack of gratification or difficulty of control, but predominantly in the image of the self that he will acquire as a consequence of sexual life. Either because he sees himself in the image of a sexually inadequate person or a homosexual, or an undesirable sexual partner, or lacking sexual control, or having no definite sexual identity, much more than other disturbed adolescents the patient will develop a concept of himself which may become very pathogenetic.

We have seen that in the second period the future acquires importance, and this could be repeated for adolescence and young adulthood, too. In order to feed his present self-esteem and maintain an adequate self-image, the young individual has, so to say, to borrow from his expectations and hopes for the future. "One day it will happen," he secretly says to himself. It is when he believes that the future has no hope, the promise of life will not be fulfilled, and the future may be even more desolate than the present, that the psychological decline, characteristic of this third stage, reaches its culmination. He feels threatened from all sides, as if he were in a jungle. It is not a jungle where lions, tigers, snakes, and spiders are to be found, but a jungle of concepts, where the threat is not to survival, but to the self-image. The dangers are concept-feelings, such as those of being unwanted, unloved, unlovable, inadequate, unacceptable, inferior, awkward, clumsy, not belonging, peculiar, different, rejected, humiliated, guilty, unable to find his own way among the different paths of life, disgraced, discriminated, kept at a distance, suspected, etc. Is this a man-made jungle created by civilization in place of the jungle to which primitive tribes are exposed? The answer is in the understanding of a circular process. To a large extent, the collectivity of man, in its historical heritage and present conditions, has made this jungle; but, to a large extent the patient, too, has created it. Sensitized as he is, because of his past experiences and crippling defenses, he distorts the environment. At this point, his distortion is not yet a paranoid projection or a delusion in a technical sense. It is predominantly experienced as anguish, increased vulnerability, fear, anxiety, mental pain. Now, the patient not only feels that the segment of the world which is important to him finds him unacceptable, he also believes that as long as he lives, he will be unacceptable to others. He is excluded from the busy, relentless ways of the world. He does not fit; he is alone. He experiences ultimate loneliness; and inasmuch as he becomes unacceptable to himself, too, he becomes somewhat alienated from himself. It is at this point that the *prepsychotic panic* occurs.

This panic is at first experienced as a sort of strange emotional *resonance* between something which is very clear (as the devastating self-image brought about by the expansion of the secondary process and of the conceptual world), and something which is unclear, yet gloomy, horrifying. These obscure forces, generally silent but now re-emerging with destructive clamor, are the repressed early experiences of the first period and their transformations in accordance with the laws of the primary process. In other words, the ineluctable conceptual conclusions reached through secondary-process mechanisms and their emotional accompaniment reactivate primary-process mechanisms and contents, not only because of their strength but also because of their fundamental similarity. These resurging mechanisms reinforce those of the secondary

process, as they are in agreement with them, and the result is of dire proportions and consequences.

It is this concordance or unification of the primary and secondary processes that first reawakens the primary process, and secondly completes and magnifies in terrifying ways the horrendous vision of the self. In the totality of his human existence, and through the depth of all his feelings, the individual now sees himself as totally defeated, without any worth and possibility of redemption. Although in the past he has undergone similar experiences, they were faint, whereas now these experiences are vivid. They are vivid, even though they are not verbalized and occur in a nonrepresentational, almost abstract, form. They include experiences that cannot be analyzed or pinned down into pieces of information, yet are accompanied by increasingly lugubrious feelings. The patient does not dare to express these feelings in words. He would not be able to do so.* Nevertheless, in some circumstances, he tries to appeal for help. This occurs at times in youngsters who are away in camps or colleges. These appeals are often misunderstood. Occasionally, an almost "magic encounter" occurs with a person who is able to reach a patient, change his secondary-process vision of the world, and arrest the psychosis.

⟨ Fourth Period: The Psychosis

In most cases only one solution, one defense, is still available to the psyche: to dissolve the secondary process, the process that has brought about conceptual disaster and has acquired ominous resonance with the archaic primary process. It is at this point that the fourth, psychotic period begins. The psychotic period covers the whole psychosis from its onset to termination. In Chapter 23 of this volume, Bemporad and Pinsker reported how I divide the psychosis, which proceeds to a full course, into four stages: initial, advanced, preterminal, and terminal. Elsewhere, I present a detailed description and interpretation

---

* His understanding is to some extent endoceptual again, as it was during the first period.

of the four stages.[4,18] In this chapter, I shall limit the discussion to the initial stage, which is the most important one from a psychodynamic point of view. Furthermore, cases that advance beyond the first stage are now fortunately sharply declining in number.

When the secondary process starts to disintegrate, it loses control of the primary process, which now starts to prevail. The patient acquires not-learned, not-imitated habits, which will constitute his schizophrenic ways of dealing with the world and himself. They are archaic and to a large extent unpredictable ways. They have the flavor of myth and primitivity. They finally do change the unbearable concepts into hallucinated lions and tigers, and mother and father into persecutors or kings and fairies. In other words, the individual now evaluates some aspects of the external world and reassesses some of his past experiences in accordance with the modes of the primary process.

Here, we shall discuss from a general point of view the psychodynamic significance of the psychotic episode. For didactic purposes, we shall describe only the acute variety of the paranoid type, which is the most common and the easiest to interpret. I must refer the reader to other publications[4,18] for the study of other types. We must keep in mind that in many cases the psychosis assumes a non-acute course. Also, at times the prepsychotic panic and the psychosis blend or progress gradually by almost imperceptible steps. At times, the gradual changes are so minimal that neither the patient nor his relatives are aware of them. An acquaintance, however, who has not seen the patient for a long time generally recognizes the change at once.

During the prepsychotic panic, the patient has, so to say, protected the world from blame, and to a large extent considered himself responsible for his own defeat. Now, again, he externalizes this feeling. He senses a vague feeling of hostility. The world is terrible. A sensation of threat surrounds him. He cannot escape from it.

The psychosis starts not only when these feeling-concepts are projected to the external world, but also when they become specific and concrete. The indefinite feelings become finite, the imperceptible becomes perceptible, the vague menace is transformed into a specific threat. It is no longer the whole horrible world that is against the patient, "they" are against him. No longer has he a feeling of being under scrutiny, under the eyes of the world, no longer a mild sense of suspiciousness toward his unfriendly neighbors. The sense of suspiciousness becomes the conviction that "they" are following him. The conceptual and abstract are reduced to the concrete, the specific. The "they" is a concretization of external threats; later, "they" are more definitely recognized as FBI agents, neighbors, or other particular persecutors. Whereas during the third period the patient often felt that millions of authorities were justified in having the lowest opinion of him, now he feels that a few malevolent, powerful people are unfair toward him and cause him troubles. There is thus a return to a situation similar to the one he experienced in his childhood, when he felt that a few powerful people were responsible for his difficulties, but now there is a displacement in his attributing the responsibility. In the majority of cases with definite psychotic features, not the parents but other people are considered the wrongdoers. This displacement permits, even during the psychosis, a partial repression of the bad image of the parent. In many cases, the displacement is later extended to a whole category of persons who are identified with the original wrongdoers. But, whether a whole category of people, or a few persons, or only an individual, are seen as the persecutor or persecutors, such people are experienced as persons, as "malevolent Thou" or malevolent you. The malevolent you, who had been transformed, introjected, tamed, and transformed into a distressing other, is now extrojected, projected, appears strong, and often in the most unusual fantasied forms. At times, the patient refers not to a person as the persecutor, but to a machine, rays, electricity, with the tacit or manifest understanding that these means are used by some malevolent human beings.

The patient often experiences some phenomena that convince him that something is done or ordained against him. He is the victim of a plot. He is accused of being a spy, a murderer, a traitor, a homosexual. He hears hallucinatory voices which repeat these accusations. He is unhappy, fearful, often indignant.

At first impression, one would think that the development of these symptoms is not a defensive maneuver at all. The patient is indeed suffering. It is not difficult to recognize, however, that the externalization (or projection) and the reduction (or concretization) of some of the psychodynamic conflicts into these psychotic symptoms, prove to be advantageous to him. As unpleasant as it is to be accused by others, it is not as unpleasant as to accuse oneself. It is true that because of the cognitive transformation the accusation assumes a specific form. For instance, the projected feeling of being a failure does not become a belief of being accused of being a failure, but of being a spy or a murderer. These accusations seem worse than the original self-accusations, but are more easily projected to others. The patient who believes he is accused, feels falsely accused. Thus, although the projected accusation is painful, it is not injurious to the self-esteem. On the contrary, in comparison with his prepsychotic state, the patient experiences a rise in self-esteem, often accompanied by a feeling of martyrdom. The really accused person now is not the patient, but the persecutor who is accused of persecuting the patient. What was an intrapsychic evaluation of the self now becomes an evaluation or an attitude of others who reside in the external world. No longer does the patient consider himself "bad"; the others unfairly think he is bad. The danger which used to be an internal one is now transformed by the psychosis into an external one. *In this transformation lies the psychodynamic significance of the paranoid psychosis.*

An incomplete form of the transformation mechanism is found in some neurotic, borderline, prepsychotic, and even psychotic patients. In these cases, the patient continues to accuse, hate, and disparage himself at the same time that he thinks that other people have the same feelings toward him. Thus, there is a partial projection to other people of the feelings which the patient nourishes toward himself, but there is no repudiation of this self-accusatory or self-effacing component of his psyche.

Some external events often precipitate a psychotic attack and seem at first to contradict the opinion expressed that what hurts the patient mostly is a sense of inner, not external, danger. Although many cases of psychosis are not preceded by any particular significant external event, others occur after such circumstances as marriage, childbirth, loss of a position, accident at work, automobile accident, traveling, being away from home, flunking examinations, romantic disappointments, striking up a new friendship, quarreling with one's boss or co-workers, etc.

An observation made quickly and repeatedly—and generally valid as a rule of thumb—is that the more important the precipitating event, the better the prognosis. This situation is easy to understand. The precipitating event is singular and recent, and therefore its effects can be removed or remedied more easily than those durable alterations that are the result of the life history of the patient.

As a matter of fact, we may parenthetically state that it is this relatively good prognosis of cases triggered off by a precipitating event that has made many authors (for instance, Kantor and Herron[51]) postulate two kinds of schizophrenia: reactive schizophrenia and process schizophrenia. Process schizophrenia would be a full-fledged psychosis with an insidious, chronic course, and based on organic pathology. The reactive form would be a schizophrenic-like reaction to the stress of external events.

The present writer cannot subscribe to this view. First of all, all gradations are seen in clinical practice between the apparent reactive acute type and the apparent chronic process type. The more accurately we study cases of the so-called process type, the more evident will be the presence of serious psychological factors. They did not affect the patient with obvious acute impact, but were slow, hidden, difficult to uncover, interpret, understand, and more destructive in their relentless, insidious course.

If we analyze the precipitating events, we recognize in them the capacity to increase anxiety to a marked degree and to inflict additional and serious blows to the self-image of the patient. Some events, like marriage, new position, may be experienced by the patient as challenges he cannot cope with. Other events, like accidents, disappointments in love, occupational failures, etc., may be interpreted as the final and irrevocable proof of the patient's inadequacy.

At times, a sudden friendship with a person of the same sex may rekindle or bring to the level of consciousness homosexual desires that the patient had tried to repress. Latent homosexuality, however, does not seem to be such a frequent precipitating event as it was once assumed by the Freudian school. The importance of homosexuality seems to lie in the fact that it causes anxiety to the patient who knows that this form of sexuality is not accepted in most segments of his environment. Childbirth is a frequent precipitating factor of schizophrenia (in what is commonly called postpartum psychosis). Many authors attribute the onset of postpartum psychosis to the stress of labor or to hormonal or other metabolic changes. Although these physical factors may play some role, the main factors may be psychogenetic in nature. Schizophrenic psychosis is not the only condition that may develop after childbirth; all psychiatric conditions may occur, including manic-depressive psychosis, reactive depressions, and exacerbations of previous neuroses. The symptoms may occur acutely after the birth or even gradually, and at times may be recognizable only a few months after the delivery.

If the condition remains at a neurotic level, we generally have one of these two pictures: Either the mother feels that she is not able to take care of the baby and is very distressed about it, or she is afraid that she may harm the child, and even kill him. These obsessive ideas and phobias are very distressing. In other cases, a pre-existing character disorder becomes much more pronounced.

In cases where schizophrenic panic occurs, the confusion is more acute. The patient presents a sudden inability to face facts. She states that she cannot take care of the baby. She wants to run away, leave her home, her husband, her baby. At other times, she alternates between these feelings and the feelings that she is guilty, worthless, not even capable of being a mother. She identifies with her own mother, who was a bad mother, and with her child, who is the victim of a bad mother. Any human contact increases her feeling of inadequacy and her anxiety. The family is unable to help at all. The family generally consists of three people in addition to the patient, and these three people are perceived by the patient as strangers. The first stranger is the baby, who is seen not as a source of love but as a source of anxiety, because it will disclose her failure as a mother, her ungiving qualities, her inadequacy. The second stranger is the mother of the patient who, as in the past, is incapable of reassuring the patient. As a matter of fact, she seems to scold the patient for her failure to be a mother and, paradoxically, she herself seems to the patient to be the prototype of bad motherhood. In many but not all cases, there is a third stranger: the husband who is also caught in a situation he does not know how to cope with. Although he tries to control himself, he cannot comfort or express sympathy for the wife who is not able even to be a real woman, a mother for his child. Instead of sympathizing with her, he bemoans his destiny for having married such a woman.

Although the mother and husband try most of the time to conceal these feelings, the real feelings are conveyed to the patient. Her anxiety and confusion increase, the fear reaches the proportion of panic, perceptual reality becomes more and more distorted, and finally a full-fledged psychotic episode, often hebephrenic or catatonic in type, ensues. In some cases, what follows is an acute or more or less chronic paranoid state. I have also seen lasting postpartum quasi-delusional states where the distortion never reached psychotic dimensions.

Space limitations do not permit me to discuss the psychodynamics of all the types of schizophrenia or all varieties even of the para-noid type. The reader is referred to my more complete works for my personal approach to this topic.[4,18] Important works of other authors are those by Fromm-Reichmann,[37] Hill,[41] Rosen,[75,76] Searles,[78] and Will.[90]

Other authors have given a different psychodynamic interpretation to the schizophrenic psychotic episode. For some authors (especially Lidz,[63] Wynne,[93] and Jackson[44]), the psychosis is the outcome of irrationality directly transmitted from the parents or the family to the patient. For instance, a female patient hears a hallucinatory voice calling her a prostitute. But we know from the history of the patient that the mother used to call her a "whore," just because she was wearing lipstick. The present writer cannot subscribe to this point of view, as he strongly feels that we cannot equate psychodynamics with the whole psychopathology. The irrationality of schizophrenia is not transmitted from generation to generation with such simple mechanisms as are language, manners, or mores. Direct transmission is not a mechanism that can explain the characteristics of schizophrenic thinking, delusional ideas, hallucinations, etc. If the parents of the schizophrenic presented the same irrationality and used the same forms of cognition as the patient, they themselves would be recognized as schizophrenics, but they are not, except in a relatively small percentage of cases. They may be peculiar, odd, eccentric. Certainly, their children may adopt their peculiarities, but they are not to be diagnosed schizophrenic because they learned them. Eccentricity in itself is not schizophrenia. Schizophrenia is not learned, although it may be acquired by virtue of certain relations with parents and family. The family affects the patient psychodynamically, so that eventually under the stress of conflicts the secondary-process mechanisms weaken or disintegrate, primary-process mechanisms acquire predominance, and the psychosis occurs. Psychotic symptoms do reflect or echo the family conflicts, just as a dream may reflect family conflicts. Family conflicts, however, could never explain the characteristics of dreams, such as reduction of ideas to visual images, special

ways of thinking, confusion of reality with imagination, etc.

Other authors interpret the illness as a result of unfavorable social factors. Siirala[79,80] sees a prophetic value in many apparent delusions of schizophrenics. He sees the patient as a victim and as a prophet to whom nobody listens. These prophecies consist of insights into our collective sickness, into the murders that we have committed for many generations and which we have buried, so that they will not be noticed. For Laing,[55,56] schizophrenia is not a disease but a broken-down relationship. The environment of the patient is so bad that he has to invent special strategies in order "to live in this unlivable situation." Not only the family but society at large with its hypocrisies and masks make the situation unlivable. In some ways echoing Szasz,[84] Laing goes to the extent of saying that the diagnosis of schizophrenia is a political one.

There is no doubt that society at large enters into the psychodynamics of mental illness, but these authors have not described accurately how society puts into action unhealthy mechanisms that may favor the psychosis. The statements made by these authors seem to indicate a direct and simple cause-and-effect relation. The disorder would be a normal reaction to an abnormal social situation. In my opinion, the disorder is an *abnormal way of coping with an abnormal situation*. The way the schizophrenic deals with the adverse environmental factors is not a normal one. This topic is too complex to be treated here;[8,17,18] on the other hand, we must stress that the numerous social or epidemiological studies of schizophrenia published so far have not been well integrated with their psychological significance. For instance, it is not enough to find out that the incidence of schizophrenia is increased among minorities, or people living in slums or poverty. We must be able to translate these statistical data in terms of human suffering. For instance, we must investigate whether these social factors become pathogenetic or not by decreasing in a certain group of people the possibility of either becoming good parents or of providing good parenthood.

I wish to stress again that the psychodynamic development of schizophrenia, which I have for didactic purposes divided into four periods, should not be considered an ineluctable course of events once the first period has taken place. Perhaps we can reformulate part of what I have said in the frame of reference of von Bertalanffy's general system theory.[20,21,22] Prior to becoming schizophrenic, the patient can be seen as an open system in a steady state. His final state, or any state, is not unequivocally determined by the initial conditions. Thus, psychiatrists who stress only early childhood and overlook the fact that the individual is always open to new possibilities that may alter the cycle of life, ignore the principle of equifinality. Any individual may increase negative entropy, and develop toward states of increased order and organization, even if he has to cope with a great deal of psychodynamic pathology, inside and outside himself. But when he becomes schizophrenic, that is, when his way of living accords with the prevalence of the primary process, he tends to become a closed system, to follow the second principle of thermodynamics, and to move toward progressive simplification and homogeneity. The aim of therapy is to reopen the system. By re-establishing relatedness with the patient, we shall feed him negative entropy again. By understanding his psychodynamics and by learning special techniques, the patient will become able to choose to be less homogeneous, less passive, and more complex, and to accept more and more his autonomous meeting with the world. (See Chapter 27 of this volume.)

We must now take into specific consideration the passage from a predominantly psychodynamic frame of reference to one that is predominantly psychostructural or formal. In other words, we must see how the psychodynamic conflicts become mediated during the fourth period by schizophrenic cognition.

(Schizophrenic Cognition

Schizophrenic cognition in some aspects corresponds to the primary process of the Freudian school. Freud originally described the primary process in Chapter 7 of *The Interpretation of Dreams*,[36] and he took into particular consideration the mechanism of displacement and condensation. The primary process is represented as an immature functioning of the psyche, which appears ontogenetically prior to the more mature secondary process. After this important contribution, Freud did not make other significant discoveries about the structure of the primary process. He became particularly interested in the primary process as a carrier of unconscious motivation.

It has been one of my main focuses of interest to study the primary process, predominantly as a kind of cognitive organization. It was always difficult for me to understand how the followers of the orthodox Freudian school could conceive the id and the primary process, respectively, as an amorphous reservoir of energy and as a way of dealing with energy. Very recently, however, some classical psychoanalysts, for instance Schur[77] and Holt, have started to study the primary process from a cognitive point of view.

In my studies on cognition, I have adopted a comparative developmental approach which is a derivation of the one proposed by Werner.[88,89] I see primary-process cognition as a less differentiated, premature, microgenetic, or intermediary process in the complicated hierarchy of mechanisms, which eventually leads to the secondary process. Although it is true that primary-process cognition is not as elaborate as that of the secondary process, it is by no means a random conglomeration of psychic functions. The primary process presents immature forms that occur also in the three types of development, phylogeny, ontogeny, and microgeny. The concept of microgeny, as formulated by Werner,[89] is less known and requires some explanations.

As I expressed elsewhere,[13,15,16] microgeny is the immediate unfolding of a phenomenon, that is, the sequence of the necessary steps inherent in the occurrence of a psychological process. For instance, to the question, "Who is the author of *Hamlet*?" a person answers "Shakespeare." He is aware only of the question (stimulus) and of his answer (conscious response), but not of the numerous steps that led him in a remarkable short time to give the correct answer. Why did he not reply "Sophocles" or "George Bernard Shaw"? How did he reach the correct answer? There are numerous proofs that the answer was not necessarily an established and purely physical or neuronic association between *Hamlet* and Shakespeare, but that an actual unconscious search went on. In fact, if the same question is asked of a mental patient or a person who is very sleepy or drunk or paying little attention, he may reply "Sophocles" or "George Bernard Shaw." These are wrong but not haphazard answers, inasmuch as they refer to playwrights. The mental search required by the answer had at least reached the category of playwrights. The numerous steps that a mental process goes through constitute its microgenetic development.

These three developments, phylogeny, ontogeny, and microgeny, unfold in time, although with great variation in the quantity of time: from periods as long as geological eras in phylogeny to periods as short as fractions of a second in microgeny. What is of fundamental importance is that the three types of development tend to use the same structural plans. I do not mean that microgeny recapitulates phylogeny, but that *there are certain formal similarities in the three fields of development and that we are able to individualize schemes of highest forms of generality that involve all levels of the psyche in its three types of development.* Here, we may find a beginning of a general system theory of cognition.

When the primary process takes over, the whole psychological picture undergoes a transformation. The relation to the external world changes. Not only does inner reality become much more important than external reality, but it is confused with external reality. The patient becomes adualistic, that is, unable to distinguish the two worlds, that of his own mind and the external. Consensual validation as well as intrapsychic feedback mechanisms become defective. The patient is less and less in contact with the external world and, like people during sensory deprivation experiments, becomes more and more dependent on the primary process. In other words, whereas

secondary process mechanisms need contact with reality or feedback mechanisms to maintain such contact with reality, primary-process mechanisms feed more and more on themselves.[71]

In my research, I have studied some mechanisms of the primary process not fully studied by Freud from the point of view of cognition. I have illustrated such phenomena as the mechanisms of active concretization, the principle of von Domarus, the imbalance between the connotative, denotative, and verbal values of language, altered causality, perceptualization of the concepts, and related processes. I have also tried to trace back the biological origin of primary-process cognition.[10,14,16] These studies do not purport to reveal what goes on in the interplay of neurons, but they may be viewed as heuristic psychological formulations that help us to understand how primary-process cognition works, at least in schizophrenia.

The Process of Active Concretization

The process of active concretization may be best illustrated in the paranoid type of schizophrenia. We have seen that prior to the outbreak of the psychosis, the patient experiences feelings of despair and inadequacy and an impression that the whole world is hostile toward him. Some of these feelings are vague, all-pervasive, indefinite, and imperceptible. They represent the culmination of his disastrous life history, particularly in the presence of a new challenge with which he cannot cope. After the onset of the psychosis, these feelings become definite and concrete. Now, the patient believes that "someone" or "they" are against him. Another patient who prior to the onset of the psychosis had the feeling that he had a "rotten personality" channels this concept into a concrete olfactory hallucination; he smells a bad odor emanating from his body. From now on, the patient is concerned with his body, which stinks, and forgets his personality. In this aspect, the schizophrenic is similar to the dreamer, the fine artist, and the poet, who transform abstract concepts into perceptual images. The higher level impinges itself upon a lower form. Contrary to what happens in artistic production, however, in schizophrenic cognition the abstract level disappears within the concrete form and the patient is no longer aware of it.

Goldstein[38,39] was one of the first to see the schizophrenic process as an expression of the concrete attitude. According to him, the schizophrenic abandons the realm of the abstract and withdraws into the concrete. There is no doubt that Goldstein has opened a path of fruitful inquiry. Nevertheless, we must recognize that his formulations are incomplete and at times even inaccurate, suffering from the fact that originally Goldstein worked predominantly with patients with organic dysfunctions. Life, experienced only or predominantly at a concrete level, is a reduced life, but not necessarily a psychotic one. A brain-injured patient may not be able to solve problems of higher mathematics, but may remain in the realm of a limited reality. Goldstein himself stated that the concrete attitude may be a realistic one. The subhuman animal, which does not possess the ability to conceive categories or platonic universals, lives in a limited but nevertheless realistic world. Goldstein also realized that the concreteness of the schizophrenic is not the same as that of the organically diseased patient, but he interpreted the difference simply as the result of different levels of concreteness.

This explanation is not satisfactory. We find different degrees of concreteness in various organic defects and also in mental deficiencies, but these conditions are not necessarily accompanied by psychosis. To this writer, schizophrenic cognition seems to result not from a reduction to a concrete level but from a process of *active concretization*. It is not just a question here of different semantics. The process is viewed differently. By active concretization is meant that the psyche is still capable of conceiving the abstract but not of sustaining it, because it is too anxiety-provoking and disintegrating. It has to transform it immediately into a concrete representation.

The most advanced form of active concretization is the perceptualization of the concept, as found in hallucinations. For instance, the patient who smelled an awful odor emanating from his body changed his feeling toward himself into an olfactory hallucination.

In the intermediary stages between the abstract level and the perceptualization of the concept, the patient undergoes peculiar experiences. At times, but especially at the beginning of the first psychotic attack, these subjective experiences are felt as a struggle, "a fight against a tendency to give in." The patient tries to resist the temptation of accepting this limited, perceptual world and is afraid that sooner or later he will succumb. Succumbing would somewhat relieve a state of confusion and panic.

At other times, the opposite process occurs: The patient searches actively for corroborative perceptual evidence.

In patients who have auditory hallucinations and, through psychotherapy, have acquired some understanding of their symptoms, three states could be recognized in the hallucinatory experience: First, the patient is in a state of anxiety. (A situation that would not arouse too much anxiety in an ordinary person has acquired a particular meaning for the patient and provokes great turmoil—for instance, returning to a lonely home from a party, after having vainly hoped for a date.) Second, the patient puts himself in the *listening attitude*. He expects to hear something derogatory. (This would be the evidence he searches for.) For instance, he must try to listen to what the neighbors say. Third, the patient actually hears; he *hallucinates*.

Most patients are aware only of the third stage. As a rule, only during intense psychotherapy do they acquire awareness of the first two stages.

Let us now examine hallucinations in their three important characteristics: (1) perceptualization of the concept; (2) projection to the external world of the inner experience; and (3) the extremely difficult corrigibility of the experience.

The perceptualization of the concept is an extreme degree of concretization. It is not the only type of perceptualization of concept, dreaming being another important one. In dreams, thoughts acquire the form of visual perceptions. In hallucinations, they acquire the forms of many types, but predominantly of the auditory. Thoughts, which ordinarily consist of images (verbal, visual, auditory, etc.) use a lower mechanism—the mechanism of perception.

The second important characteristic of hallucination, projection to the external world of the inner subjective experience, also exists in dreams. The dreamer believes that the action of the dream actually takes place in the external world. This characteristic of hallucinations may be easily understood if we remember that it is also present in every normal perception. If I see an object in front of me, the perception of that object occurs inside me, around my calcarine fissure, but my organism projects this perception again into the external world. Thus, in hallucination, the most important fact is not that the subjective experience is externalized, because this externalization or projection occurs in every perception, but that an abstract thought has been perceptualized and follows the law of perception instead of those of thinking.

In a previous publication, I called the third characteristic the "incorrigibility of the experience." I think now that the term "difficult corrigibility" is more appropriate, because patients in psychotherapy learn to recognize and correct the hallucinatory experiences, although with great difficulty. (See Chapter 27.) In the majority of not-treated patients, however, hallucinations are not corrected. The patient not only has the dynamic wish to believe the content of the hallucination but also the need to interpret experiences in accordance with the levels of mentality to which he regresses.

The concretization and perceptualization of the concept (for instance, in the case of the patient who smells an awful odor emanating from his body) may seem metaphorical and symbolic. Let us remember, however, that these experiences are metaphorical and symbolic only for us, who retain our usual way of thinking or at least the possibility of shifting from one to another of different ways of think-

ing. But these experiences are not metaphorical for the patient. They are intensely lived; they are his reality.

⟨ Paleologic Thought

The patient struggling in his attempts to resist the "fascination" of the lower levels is in a very unpleasant state of mental confusion. Often, in this state, he suddenly experiences what has been called "psychotic insight."[4,18] For instance, given a sequence of events such as noticing, during the course of a few days, that several people glance at him and then hearing his doorbell ring twice in an evening, the patient will suddenly think that these are not coincidences—there is a relation between the events; agents of the FBI are watching him in order to prove that he is a spy.

If the patient were resorting only to the process of concretization of the concept, he would not begin to use this method of interpretation. But here he regresses to a lower level of rationality; he no longer operates with Aristotelian logic but rather uses a logic *sui generis*, which has been called paleologic. Paleologic is, to a great extent, based on a principle enunciated by von Domarus.[33,34] This author, as a result of his studies on schizophrenia, formulated a principle which, in slightly modified form, is as follows: *Whereas the normal person accepts identity only upon the basis of identical subjects, the paleologician accepts identity based upon identical predicates.*

For instance, if a schizophrenic happens to think: "The President of the United States is a person who was born in the United States; John Doe is a person who was born in the United States," in certain circumstances he may conclude, "John Doe is the President of the United States." This conclusion, which to a normal person appears delusional, is reached because the identity of the predicate of the two premises, "a person who was born in the United States," makes the schizophrenic accept the identity of the subjects, "the President of the United States" and "John Doe." Of course, two additional factors permit him to reach such a conclusion: first, the over-all state of anxiety makes the use of the highest levels of mentation less efficient; second, he has an emotional need to believe that John Doe is the President of the United States, a need which will arouse additional anxiety if it is not satisfied. It is not difficult, then, to see how, in a teleologic way, the patient grasps the re-emerging paleologic level in order to reach the conclusion that he desires. A patient thought that she was the Virgin Mary. Her thought process was the following: "The Virgin Mary was a virgin; I am a virgin; therefore, I am the Virgin Mary." The delusional conclusion was reached because the identity of the predicates of the premises (the state of being virgin) made the patient accept the identity of the two subjects (the Virgin Mary and the patient). She needed to identify herself with the Virgin Mary because of the extreme closeness and spiritual kinship she felt for the Virgin Mary.

A patient, quoted by Bleuler, thought that he was Switzerland. How can we explain such a bizarre thought? Switzerland was one of the few free countries in the world, and the patient had selected the name of this country for the concept of freedom with which he had the impelling need to identify.

It must be emphasized that the schizophrenic does not necessarily adopt paleologic thought for all or even most of his thinking processes. Especially in the early stages of the illness, paleologic thought is found only when it involves the complexes of the patient. Later, however, it tends to extend to other areas. In this early selectivity for the emotionally determined complexes, paleologic thinking differs from organically determined mechanisms which apply indiscriminately to any content. In the light of von Domarus' principle, even bizarre and complex schizophrenic delusions can be interpreted.[3,4,6,7,18]

Occasionally, the schizophrenic has insight into his mode of thinking and makes his deductions consciously. Usually, however, this process is as automatic as the normal person's application of Aristotelian logic.

The application of von Domarus' principle

extends far beyond schizophrenia. The whole phenomenon of Freudian symbolism may be interpreted from a formal point of view as an application of this type of logic. The symbol is not only something that stands for something else but also something that has at least a common characteristic (predicate) with the thing it symbolizes. Freud demonstrated that a person or object A, having certain characteristics of B (that is, a common predicate with B), may appear in dreams as B or a composite of A and B. The wife of a dreamer may appear in a dream as having the physical appearance of the dreamer's boss. The two persons are identified in the dream because the dreamer is concerned with a characteristic common to them (domineering attitude).

Of course, we do not attribute to the word "predicate" only the meaning usually given to it in logic or grammar. The term, as used here, refers to an attribute of the subject, in the broadest sense. It may also be a tangible part of the subject. Thus, in this type of thinking there is a tendency to identify a part with the whole—e.g., a room with the house to which the room belongs. Expressed differently, $a=a+b+c$ because the two terms of the equation have a in common. The predicate, furthermore, may refer not only to a quality inherent in the objects but also to spatial and temporal contiguity. The predicate that leads to the identification is called the *identifying link*.

Often, what should be only an *associative link* becomes, for the schizophrenic, an *identifying link*. According to my own studies,[4] this mechanism underlies the disturbances of association in schizophrenia. It is beyond the purpose of this chapter to describe and interpret all alterations of association that may occur in schizophrenia. It will be enough to mention that regressed schizophrenics substitute associative words for those actually appropriate. For instance, if a regressed schizophrenic is asked the name of the President of the United States, he may reply, "White House." The idea of "White House" is a normal association to the idea of President of the United States, but in the regressed schizophrenic, associated ideas are identified and substituted for one another. The understanding of this transformation of associative links into identifying links will lead to the interpretation of word-salad, which otherwise appears an incomprehensible phenomenon.

Paleologic thinking can be interpreted with formulations which seem to differ from von Domarus' principle, but actually refer to the same phenomena. We may, for instance, state that the cognitive faculty of the schizophrenic organizes classes or categories which differ from those of normal thinking. For normal persons *a class is a collection of objects to which a concept applies.* For instance, Washington, Jefferson, Lincoln, Roosevelt, Truman, etc., form a class of objects to which the concept "President of the United States" applies. In paleologic thinking (or thinking which follows the primary process), *a class is a collection of objects that have a predicate or part in common, and which, by virtue of having such predicate or part in common, become identified or equivalent.* Whereas the members of a secondary (or normal) class are recognized as being similar (and it is actually on their similarity that their classification is based), the members of a primary class become equivalent, that is, they are freely interchanged (for instance, the patient becomes the Virgin Mary). Not only do they all become equivalent, but one of them may become equivalent to the whole class. It is easy to understand why it is so. In primary classification, it is only the common element that counts; all the rest is not important, or not noticed or responded to by the psyche.

Other authors have given different interpretations of schizophrenic thinking. Cameron,[24,25] an author who has made important contributions, considers schizophrenic thinking: (a) *asyndetic*, that is, having few causal links; (b) *metonymic*, or lacking precise terms and using words with approximate or related meaning (like "menu" for "meal"); (c) having interpenetrations, or intrusions with unrelated themes; (d) overinclusive, including material that has only peripheral connection; (e) requesting changing the conditions with which problems are solved; (f) presenting incongruity between acts and words; (g) ineffec-

tive in changing generalizations and hypotheses; (h) disorganized.

Of all the characteristics described by Cameron, *overinclusion* is the one that has received the greatest consideration. Some authors believe that if the patient's thinking is overinclusive, it comprehends more than it should, and therefore cannot be considered restricted or concrete. According to Payne,[72,73] the schizophrenic thought disorder could be due to inability to develop and maintain a normal set. Normal mechanisms of inhibition would be broken down. Ideas distantly related are thus included in thoughts. Similarly, the patient is unable to disregard perceptual stimuli, ignored by most people, and their perception, too, becomes overinclusive.

In my opinion there is no contradiction between "overinclusion" in the sense used by Cameron and Payne and the concepts of concreteness and paleologic thinking. "Overinclusive" means inability to exclude the non-essential and to abstract the essential. The nonessential, related to the essential only by a whimsical or peripheral similarity, is retained in the new categories formed by the schizophrenic. In other words, overinclusion implies a defect in the formation of Aristotelian or secondary classes. This inability of the schizophrenic is related to stimulus generalization, as Mednick and Freedman[69] think, or to increased equivalence of stimuli,[53,54] or to what I have called primary generalization.[16] In other words, schizophrenic generalization tends to be at the level of non-differentiation. It is not the type of generalization that follows the Pavlovian technique of discrimination. Thus, contrary to what Payne and Mednick and Freedman believe, overinclusion is not the converse of concreteness or paleologic way of thinking, but an expression of it. This point of view has also been reaffirmed by Sturm.[81]

Piro[74] believes that there is a semantic dissociation in schizophrenia. This dissociation is linguistic and does not refer to thinking per se. For him, dissociation means loosening the connection between the verbal sign and its meaning, cognitive and emotional. The word is no longer applied to the original semantic structure. According to Piro, in normal persons every word has a *semantic halo,* or a personal extension of meaning, which allows a certain ambiguity and indetermination in its use. In schizophrenia, the semantic halo is either increased or decreased. I agree with Piro that words have different meanings for the schizophrenic, but I have related this phenomenon to the difficulty in forming Aristotelian categories.

Loren J. Chapman, alone,[28] and with collaborators,[29,30,31] wrote a series of important papers on schizophrenic cognition. McGhie and J. Chapman[67] attribute great importance to disorders of attention in schizophrenic thinking. There is no doubt that attention is very much impaired in many schizophrenics and that this defect may lead to conceptual impairment. However, it is not always present, nor can it explain most delusional thinking. For instance, how can impaired attention lead the patient to believe he is Jesus Christ?

A large number of authors have directly studied schizophrenic thinking from the point of view of family or social interaction and transaction. Wynne[93] has written many of these works in collaboration with several authors, but there is no doubt that he is the architect of this large and interesting area of work. I have already expressed the opinion earlier in this chapter that this work is very important in elucidating some aspects of the psychodynamics of schizophrenia, but not in explaining the specific formal characteristics of the thought disorder.

(Desymbolization and Desocialization

The individual during his childhood introjects symbols and roles from the surrounding adults. During the schizophrenic psychosis, he tends to lose these introjected symbols and roles. Desocialization or withdrawal in the schizophrenic means much more than being at a physical distance from the interpersonal environment and living in an ivory tower (as the schizoid does). For the schizophrenic patient,

desocialization implies a change in the process of symbolizing, change that will permit the loss of the introjected symbols which originate from others, and the replacement with more primitive ones.

In order to understand this process, a brief discussion of the process of symbolization in the human mind is necessary.*

The symbolic property of the mind permits the human being *to go beyond* what is given by the perceptual apparatus. Sense perceptions give information about what is here and now, that is, present in the spatiotemporal world in which the subject lives and by which he is stimulated, but symbols and the symbolic apparatus will permit him to become aware even of what is not given.

We may recognize a hierarchy of symbols. The simplest is the sign, which we have in common with infrahuman animals. The smell of a mouse, which is not seen, is, for the cat, the sign that the mouse is around. The physician sees a rash on the skin of the child and he realizes that that rash is the sign of measles. Signs are parts or cues of objects or situations and stand for the whole objects or situations that are *present or about to be present.* We may even say that the *sign* is that predicate of the subject, which makes the observer become aware of the presence or imminent presence of the subject. *Symbols* must be considered as belonging to higher levels than signs because they stand for something which is not present.

As we have seen in a previous section of this chapter, the image is the most primitive form of symbol. The external object is no longer present, but the individual retains an internal image which tends to reproduce the past perception of the object. Thus, the image of the mother may be with the child even when the mother is not present.

The image, however, tends to be private and cannot be externalized. We have seen that the same characteristics are found in the endocept. The next important step in the development of symbolization occurs when an individual succeeds in equating an external

* For a more adequate discussion of this subject the reader is referred to Cassirer,[26] Langer,[57] and, in relation to schizophrenia, Arieti.[4, 18]

event or thing for something that is not present. (A sound or a thing [fetish] or a gesture may be equivalent for the object that is not present.) The thing that is taken as equivalent of the absent object is originally perceived as part or predicate of the missing object and becomes a paleosymbol. But paleosymbols, too, are individualistic and private. Paleosymbols (and the higher types of symbols) may be auditory, visual, tactile, etc., but, for the sake of simplification, we shall consider only the auditory.

When an auditory paleosymbol, for instance the sound *ma-ma*, uttered casually or accidentally by a primitive man in connection with his mother, is understood by a second man (for instance, a sibling) as referring to the mother, we have the occurrence of a *verbal symbol* (called also *common* or *social symbol*). The verbal symbol evokes in the person who pronounces it the same reaction that it evokes in others, it elicits "consensual validation."

The verbal symbol not only replaces the missing object but also is shared by many people. Thus, it is no longer a paleosymbol, even for the person who used it for the first time, because the person now knows the reaction that the symbol will elicit from others, and knows that this reaction is approximately similar to his own.

The evolution of the word from the paleosymbol to the most abstract levels cannot be described here in detail, but a brief summary will be presented. A word, when it is created by primitive men, has at least two characteristics: first of all, *denotation*. The denotation is the object meant. The denotation of the word *ma-ma* is the mother of the primordial siblings. Second, it has *verbalization*. The verbalization is the word applied to the object; it is the word as a word, that is, as a verbal entity, independent of its symbolic value. In primitive societies, the emphasis is on these two aspects of terms. The word is so strictly tied to the object it denotes that it is often confused with that object. We have thus "word magic:" the word applied to an object assumes the same quality that the object itself has. A great deal of attention is paid to the

word, from the point of view of sound, rhythm, rhyme, assonance, homonymy, etc.

Later on, however, the word acquires *connotation* (or enlarges the primitive connotation); that is, it represents the concept of the object it stands for. It refers not only to a particular embodiment of the object but to the whole category of the object. Thus, in the example given, the sound *ma-ma* came to refer not only to the particular mother of the primordial siblings but to any mother, and came to assume the meaning, "female who begets offspring."

At high levels of development new symbols and roles are continuously created. The child is immediately exposed not only to many already made words, which have denotations and connotations, but to groups or configurations of words which reproduce or represent concepts and roles.

At the same time that he learns new words, he learns new relationships and concepts and the roles that he must assume. The image of himself, which consists predominantly of the body image, self-esteem, and self-identification, needs words, concepts, and roles reflected to the self from the human environment.

In schizophrenia, we have an approximate reproduction in reverse order of all the stages of symbolization and socialization. Furthermore, all of these stages may overlap and mix in several proportions, so that what results is a very confusing picture.

The process of desocialization starts first with the progressive loss of those organizations of symbols that are referred to the self. There is thus a tendency to reject, or to divest the self of, those attitudes and tendencies that were reflected from others and became part of the self, and a tendency also to project, or give back the introjected attitudes. For example, the nagging, scolding attitude of the parent is originally introjected by the child who will acquire a critical, condemnatory attitude toward himself. When the patient becomes psychotic, this attitude is projected, or given back to a parent-substitute—an authority or a person paleologically conceived as a persecutor because he seems to have one of the persecuting traits of the parent.

Thus, projection is not only attributing an idea to others but also giving back, restoring to the people who the patient believes have contributed to the building of an unpleasant part of his self. The patient no longer accepts self-condemnation as a part of the self; condemnation now comes from the persecutor. This mechanism is greatly complicated and obscured by the fact that what is given back is returned not to the original givers but to persons who symbolize them. Thus, paleologic mechanisms will transform the condemnatory quality of a parent into the persecutory actions of an FBI agent.

We may distinguish three successive stages: First, the stage of introjection where the action or attitude of the parent is still external, actual, and is being introjected. Second, the stage of assimilation where the child has distorted and then accepted the attitude of the parent, which has become his own attitude toward himself. He accuses, hates, or controls himself, as he believes the parents did. Third, the stage of projection (the psychotic stage) where the patient projects back to symbolic parents those attitudes toward himself that he now rejects.

This mechanism of projection may be viewed as the expression of a changing interpersonal relation between the I (the patient) and the Thou. At first, the Thou is the parent or parent-substitute; then, the Thou, after undergoing some distortions, becomes that component of the patient himself which may be called superego, if we adopt Freud's terminology. Eventually, when psychosis occurs, the Thou is the persecutor.

We have seen earlier how basic introjections occurred early in childhood when the unpleasant experiences took place. These unpleasant experiences are repressed, but continue to act on the patient during the second and third periods of development by unconsciously motivating him toward awkward actions and distorted interpersonal relations. They participate in making the derogatory self-image much more pronounced and more

difficult to tolerate. During the fourth period, the psychosis tries to eliminate this self-image.

At the same time that delusional formations occur, or later, other processes take place which are more directly related to language. Although the healthy person in a wakened state is concerned mainly with connotation and denotation of a symbol, he can shift his attention from one to another of its three aspects; the regressing schizophrenic, however, is concerned more and more with denotation and verbalization, and experiences a partial or total impairment of his ability to connote. This is what I have called *reduction of the connotation power*. For example, when regressed schizophrenics are asked to interpret proverbs, they do so literally. (A patient, asked to explain the proverb, "When the cat's away, the mice will play," replied that the mice felt free to play when the cat was away. He could not give to the word "cat" the special connotation, "a cruel person in authority.")

At the same time that the connotation power is decreased, denotation and verbalization become more important.

The verbal characteristics of schizophrenics are well known. The patients pay much attention to the sound, alliteration, and repetition of words. They seem to enjoy writing or pronouncing words that have sound associations —as, for instance, in the following series of words written by patients: "C, see, sea." "I know it, you know it. Chuck, luck, luck, Buck. True-two. These are it. I know it. I know it, you know it." "Are you pure? Sure? Yes! Yes! Yes! Frame! Name! Same! Same! Same! Came."

In the course of the illness, the patient gradually relinquishes common symbols and reverts to paleosymbols—that is, to symbols which he himself creates and which have no consensual validation. The paleosymbols represent a return to the level of the autistic expression of the child. As it happens in children, however, these paleosymbolic expressions are not completely original and private, but use remnants of common symbols. Often, we recognize in neologisms common symbols that have undergone autistic or paleosymbolic distortions.

This process of desocialization and desymbolization is sometimes delayed or arrested by restitutive phenomena.[4,18] With the progression of the schizophrenic process, however, the process of desocialization increasingly impoverishes the patient's repertory of common symbols. With the advancing impoverishment of common symbols it becomes progressively more difficult for the patient to assume his own role and to visualize the roles of others. This process reveals how much of man is actually made of social life. When what was obtained from others is eliminated, man remains an insignificant residue of what he used to be.

⟨ Causality and Action: Motor Dysfunctions

Man uses two forms of causality to explain the universe and himself. The first is mechanical or deterministic causality: "Each cause has an effect." The necessary antecedent A is the cause of a necessary consequent B. The second is teleologic (or psychological) causality. Things occur because of their purpose. B (reading a book) takes place because of A, the reader's *purpose* (learning a subject). Psychological causality is a variety of teleologic causality.

In pathological conditions or primitive thinking, mechanical causality plays a very small role. Instead of finding a physical explanation for an event, the paleologic thinker looks for a cause in a personal motivation or an intention. Every act, every event, occurs because it is willed or wanted either by the person himself who seeks an explanation or by another person or by something which becomes personified. In other words, causality by logical deduction, often implying concepts involving the physical world, is replaced with causality by psychological explanation: *the necessary antecedent of any event is an act of will.* The study of primitive concepts of causality consists of the study of what is attrib-

uted to the will. This method of interpreting the world, *projected psychological causality*, is always found in paranoiacs and paranoids who interpret almost every occurrence as expressions of psychological intentions related to their delusional complexes.

More difficult to understand, perhaps, is the concept of *introjected psychological causality*, which is pronounced in catatonics. Although this type is psychological causality related to the thinker himself, and therefore not essentially dissimilar from projected psychological causality, it requires the study of other aspects of the problem. Here one's own will becomes the antecedent of events.

The symptomatology of catatonia consists not of motor disorders but of will disorders. The patient cannot move, not because he is paralyzed, but because he cannot will to move. The human action is not a simple motion, it is also an act of will. One of the first things primitive man became aware of was that he was able to will. He became aware of this long before he was able to evolve the concept of physical (deterministic) causality.

Human action is a very complicated phenomenon. Just as symbolism includes an elaborate transformation of what the posterior human brain (temporal, occipital, and pariental lobes) receives from the external world, willing and acting include the elaborate transformation of motor impulses, which take place in the anterior brain (frontal lobes). At the same time, of course, other noncortical mechanisms permit the precise execution of the movement as a neurological function.

What seems to be the first clear-cut manifestation of willed action is the inhibition of the reflex response. The toilet-trained baby is a clear example of this. Because of rectal distention, he has the impulse to defecate, but he learns to inhibit the response. He learns, by using cortical mechanisms, to control his sphincters. The will of the child is necessary: the child must want not to defecate. He develops the capacity and the will to resist. But if the child wants not to defecate, although it would be pleasant do so, it is because he learns to please his mother. Thus, even in the first volitional acts, which imply choices, a new dimension enters: the interpersonal (the Thou). From a philosophical point of view, it seems almost a contradiction in terms: The first acts of volition are acts of obedience, or of submission to the will of others. Choice, this new, portentous tool which emerges in phylogenesis with the human race, in the early ontogenetic stages requires support from others before it can be exercised independently.

Individual primitive man, as an independent doer, often feels guilty.[4,17,18] To do is to be potentially guilty, because, after all, you cannot know what event will follow what you are doing. It might have an effect on the whole tribe; its repercussions might be enormous, such as an epidemic or a drought. Kelsen[52] has illustrated well the relations between *to do* and *to be guilty* in the primitive. In order to diminish their feelings of guilt, primitive men refrain from acting freely; they perform only those acts that are accepted by the tribe. The tribe teaches the individual what act to perform for any desired effect. Ritualism and magic thus originate. By performing each act according to ritual, primitive man removes the anxiety that arises from the expectation of possible evil effects. The ritual ensures that the effect will be good.

From a certain point of view, the subsequent development of humanity can be seen largely as a gradual freedom from this reliance on the support of the group and as an expansion of the individual will. This act of liberation from the influence or suggestion of others ontogenetically is seen during the negativistic stage of children, when they refuse to do what they are told to do. By disobeying, they practice their newly acquired ability to will; but they do so with the most primitive method (volition of resistance).

The phylogenetic history of human action may be summarized diagrammatically, as shown in Figure 24–1. This is, of course, a simplified scheme, and many intermediate stages have probably been omitted. Furthermore, many stages overlap and coexist. In normal human beings, all possible stages are found, but in pathological conditions we find a preponderance of earlier stages and partial or total loss of others. For instance, in neurotic

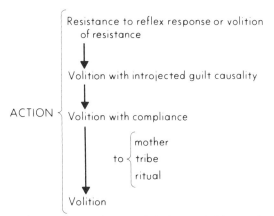

Figure 24–1.   Diagram of phylogenetic history of human action.

persons, neurotic compliance to others; in obsessive-compulsives, volition with compliance to ritual. But the most pathological forms of volition are found in catatonic patients.

Dynamic studies reported elsewhere[4,18] indicate that people who are apt to become catatonic are those who in their early childhood have been prevented from developing confidence in their own actions and reliance on their capacity to will. The parents or parent substitutes have forced these patients either not to will or to follow parental decisions. When the patients later had to make their own choices, they found themselves unable to act; if they acted, they were criticized and made to feel guilty. In catatonia, the typical schizophrenic childhood struggle with significant adults is connected particularly with the actions and choices of the patient.

The eventual catatonic may try to remove the anxiety which accompanies his actions by compliance or obsessive-compulsiveness. In precatatonic patients, in fact, we find strong ambivalent attitudes, pseudocompliance, and compulsions. But if the symptoms are not sufficient to protect the patient from excessive anxiety, or if they cannot be built up rapidly enough to dam the anxiety, catatonia develops. Catatonia is a removal of action in order to remove the panic connected with the willed action. Sometimes, this panic is generalized. When it is extended to every action, the patient may lapse into a state of complete immobility (stupor).

In less advanced cases, one clearly recognizes the impairment of the function to will. For instance, as an answer to an order, the patient starts a movement, but then stops, as if a counterorder had prevented him from completing the movement. Having decided to obey, he is then afraid to will the act involved, and he stops. At other times, there is a series of alternated opposite movements, rather like a cogwheel movement, superficially similar to that observed in postencephalitic patients affected by muscular rigidity. In the middle of a movement, the patient becomes afraid of willing the act, decides not to perform it, and arrests his arm. But to decide not to perform the act is also a volition. The patient becomes afraid of it and starts to make the movement again. To do this is also volition and he is again afraid. This series of attempted escapes from volition may go on for a long time; it is a horrifying experience, which only a few patients are able to relate.

This fear of volition accounts for other characteristics encountered in cases of catatonic schizophrenia. In order to avoid anxiety and guilt, the patient cannot will any act, but he may passively follow orders given by others because the responsibility will not be his—there is a complete substitution of someone else's will for his own. Waxy flexibility or the retention of body positions in which the patient is passively put, no matter how uncomfortable, can also be explained in this way. When the patient is put in a given position, the will or responsibility of someone else is involved. If he wants to change positions, he has to will the change, and this engenders anxiety or guilt.

Quite often, the reverse seems to occur. The patient will resist the order, or will do the opposite. This is the phenomenon of *negativism* which has baffled many investigators. This action of willed disobedience is sometimes present in the normal person and in the negativistic child, as if unwillingness to obey or to follow an order automatically engendered an action of resistance. Perhaps, we may understand this phenomenon of negativism if we interpret it as a return to the most primitive act of volition, or volition of resistance.

There seems to be a correlation, although not yet statistically proved, between the decline in the catatonic type of schizophrenia and the decline in manic-depressive psychosis. Perhaps, a cultural environment which emphasizes the concept of guilt predisposes to these two conditions. (See Chapter 21.) But, whereas generally the premanic-depressive feels guilty for not acting, the catatonic feels guilty for acting. Actually, this is not the only difference between the guilt of the manic-depressive and that of the catatonic. The guilt feeling of the catatonic is much more primitive; it is a syncretic feeling of guilt-fear and is associated with the elementary concept of action, rather than with the higher concepts of sin and atonement.

At times, the catatonic loses this inhibiting guilt-fear complex and acts in an opposite way—that is, as if he were not concerned at all with responsibility or as if he were defying previous feelings of fear and responsibility. His behavior manifests a manic-like sequence of aimless acts. He may become violent and homicidal. This is the state of *catatonic excitement*.

Other patients who remain in a catatonic stupor for a long time develop what I have called a feeling of *negative omnipotence* or an alleged expansion of will power. They feel that if they move, the whole world will collapse or all mankind will perish. In a case which I have reported elsewhere,[11] a patient experienced an unusual phenomenon. There was a discrepancy between the act he wanted to perform and the action that he really carried out. For instance, when he was undressing, he wanted to drop a shoe, and instead he dropped a piece of wool; he wanted to put something in a drawer, and instead he threw a stone away. However, there was a similarity between the act that he had wanted and anticipated and the act he actually performed. The two actions were analogic; they had become psychologically equivalent because they were similar or had something in common. This phenomenon is, in my opinion, of theoretical importance because it extends to the area of volition those characteristics mentioned in schizophrenic paleologic thinking.

❨ Progressive Teleologic Regression

If we view schizophrenia as a pathological release of a set of mechanisms, which in normal conditions is controlled by higher structures, we find this phenomenon similar to many others described in general medicine. For instance, in some pathological conditions of the heart, when the sino-auricular node is injured, the more ancient auriculo-ventricular bundles take over its functions. Like the auriculo-ventricular node, the primary process has normal functions in various activities of the mind, for instance in dreams.

If we accept this point of view, we still have to explain how the re-emergence of the primary process is to be reconciled with the psychodynamic formulations of schizophrenia, to which we strictly adhere. On one side, we deal with psychodynamic factors which eventually lead to the defeat of the self. On the other side, we deal with such phenomena as archaic mechanisms, less differentiated structures, paleologic thinking, concretization of the abstract. It seems almost as if we embraced two logical universes, two irreconcilable views of man and nature.

I have tried to interpret this passage from a psychodynamic to a psychostructural or formal frame of reference with the concept of *progressive teleologic regression*.[4,16] In my conceptualization, regression—more than being related to a return to earlier stages of fixation, as Freud saw it—means renewed availability of functions belonging to lower levels of integration. Whereas the *content* of symptoms may reproduce, in either identical or symbolic fashion, earlier ontogenetic experiences and their derivatives, the *forms* that the symptoms assume may use even mechanisms that appeared in earlier phylogenetic levels. In the schizophrenic's psychological structure, an attempt is made *to fit a higher content into a lower form*.

Hughlings Jackson's mechanisms of dissolution may still be considered as a heuristic frame of reference.[85] Jackson[45] demonstrated that when a high level of nervous integration (for instance, the cerebral cortex) is in a pathological condition, the functions of that level may be absent (negative symptoms), and the functions of a lower level, which are usually inhibited, re-emerge (positive symptoms). In other words, the symptoms would not be only the effect of pathology at higher levels, but also of a return to a lower level of functionality. In Jackson's view, regression (or, as he called it, dissolution) is completely a mechanistic or deterministic process. The higher level is eliminated by an organic disease, and the organism operates at the lower levels, which are still intact. This point of view does not provide for a psychodynamic understanding. We may build a bridge between determinism and psychodynamics if we view the psychiatric patient as channeling his conflicts through a form of teleologic regression.

The term "teleologic" implies that the regression is purposeful, having the purpose of removing excessive anxiety and re-establishing some kind of psychic equilibrium. This is not a completely vitalistic or animistic concept; it is an additional application of concepts developed in general medicine by Claude Bernard and in psychiatry by Freud. A teleological point of view is not a denial that psychological and psychopathological phenomena follow physical determinism (according to which, causes have effects), but an additional affirmation that the living organism, in health or disease, seems to be subject to both mechanical and teleologic causalities. An example from physical medicine may clarify the matter. An infective disease produces an invasion of foreign proteins in an organism, and foreign proteins bring about a temperature rise; that is, fever. All this follows mechanical causality. We know, however, that fever has a purpose: to combat the invasion of the foreign proteins. Here the organism seems to follow purposeful causality. Obviously, in the course of evolution only those organisms survived which had such inherited biochemical properties that enabled them to respond with fever to bacterial invasion. For us, who are interested in survival, the mechanism is teleological. It is teleological at the level of human values. In the same way, we may admit that when the evolution of the nervous system reached the human level, the psyche, in order to survive, had to develop the capacity of readjusting at least at some psychopathological levels. In Freudian language, we could say that the symptoms could not be just regressive but also restitutional. A psychological defense is a pathological readjustment, purposeful, although determined by previous causes.

Cybernetics also tries to find a reconciliation between a deterministic and a teleological interpretation of biological phenomena.

The phenomenon of teleologic regression can be formulated in the form of a principle: "If in a situation of severe anxiety, such as that provoked by deep injury to the self-image and to the self, the psyche cannot function at a certain level of integration and cannot attain the desired results, a strong tendency exists toward functioning at lower levels of integration in order to effect those results."[4,16] In schizophrenia, functioning at a lower level means functioning with the mechanisms of the primary process. It means fitting a higher content into a lower form, changing the abstract into the concrete, a general threat into a specific one, something that originates from the inner self into something that comes from the external world. For instance, the feeling of self-accusation is changed into an accusation that comes from other persons, the persecutors. The regression can thus be interpreted as purposeful or teleologic. This point of view is not irreconcilable with the point of view that a biological factor, constitutional or biochemical, predisposes some individuals to this type of regression, when the mentioned circumstances occur.

In schizophrenia, the regression is *progressive*, because, although it is purposeful, with few exceptions it fails of its purpose and tends to repeat itself. An individual who is deprived of the highest level of integration can be compared to an animal experimentally deprived of the cerebral cortex. This animal will not be in a physiological condition comparable to that of an organism of a low species which does not possess the cerebral cortex. Rather, it remains in an abnormal condition, because its whole organism is attuned to the cerebral cor-

tex, or integrated with the functions of the cerebral cortex.

In a similar way, the schizophrenic patient will *regress to*, but not *integrate at*, a lower level: He will remain disorganized. The organism then defends itself from this disorganization with further regression to an even lower level. The process repeats itself in a vicious circle that can lead to complete dilapidation. The situation is thus different from that occurring in other psychopathological conditions. For instance, the phobic patient also undergoes a regression. The phobic patient, however, as a rule remains arrested at a phobic level, without progression toward lower mechanisms.

A limited regression from the highest levels of functionality may be a preserver of normality in sleep, convalescence, neurotic conditions, and some overwhelming circumstances, but it is pathological in schizophrenia because it resorts to mechanisms usually repressed and discordant with the state of normality of the individual. When the regression continues, the patient proceeds to more severe stages: the second or advanced, the third or preterminal, the fourth or terminal.[4,18]

The description of the process of progressive teleologic regression in schizophrenia should not be interpreted as the description of an ineluctable unfolding of events. The process can be arrested, and, as Chapter 27 of this volume illustrates, even completely reversed, reaching results by far superior to the condition in which the patient was prior to the onset of the psychosis.

(Bibliography

1. ACKERMAN, N. W. "Interpersonal Disturbances in One Family: Some Unsolved Problems in Psychotherapy," *Psychiatry*, 17 (1954), 359–368.
2. ———. *The Psychodynamics of Family Life.* New York: Basic Books, 1958.
3. ARIETI, S. "Special Logic of Schizophrenic and Other Types of Autistic Thought," *Psychiatry*, 11 (1948), 325–338.
4. ———. *Interpretation of Schizophrenia.* New York: Brunner, 1955.

5. ———. "What is Effective in the Therapeutic Process," *American Journal of Psychoanalysis*, 17 (1957), 30.

6. ———. "Schizophrenic Thought," *American Journal of Psychotherapy*, 13 (1959), 537.

7. ———. "Schizophrenia," in S. Arieti, ed., *American Handbook of Psychiatry*, New York: Basic Books, 1959.

8. ———. "Some Socio-Cultural Aspects of Manic-Depressive Psychosis and Schizophrenia," in J. H. Masserman, and J. L. Moreno, eds., *Progress in Psychotherapy*, Vol. IV. New York: Grune & Stratton, 1959.

9. ———. "Recent Conceptions and Misconceptions of Schizophrenia," *American Journal of Psychotherapy*, 14 (1960), 1–29.

10. ———. "The Loss of Reality," *Psychoanalysis and Psychoanalytic Review*, 48 (1961), 3.

11. ———. "Volition and Value: A Study Based on Catatonic Schizophrenia," *Comprehensive Psychiatry*, 2 (1961), 74–82.

12. ———. "A Re-Examination of the Phobic Symptoms and of Symbolism in Psychopathology," *The American Journal of Psychiatry*, 118 (1961), 106–110.

13. ———. "The Microgeny of Thought and Perception," *Archives of General Psychiatry*, 6 (1962), 454.

14. ———. "Studies of Thought Processes in Contemporary Psychiatry," *The American Journal of Psychiatry*, 120 (1963), 58–64.

15. ———. "Contributions to Cognition from Psychoanalytic Theory," in J. Masserman, ed., *Science and Psychoanalysis*, Vol. 8. New York: Grune & Stratton, 1965.

16. ———. *The Intrapsychic Self: Feeling, Cognition and Creativity in Health and Mental Illness*. New York: Basic Books, 1967.

17. ———. *The Will to Be Human*. New York: Quadrangle Books, 1972.

18. ———. *Interpretation of Schizophrenia*, 2nd ed. New York: Basic Books (in preparation).

19. BATESON, G., D. D. JACKSON, J. HALEY, J. WEAKLAND. "Toward a Theory of Schizophrenia," *Behavioral Science*, 1 (1956), 251.

20. BERTALANFFY, L. VON. "General System Theory," in L. von Bertalanffy and A. Rapaport, *General Systems Yearbook of the Society for the Advancement of General Systems Theory*. Ann Arbor: University of Michigan Press, 1956.

21. ———. "General System Theory and Psychiatry," in S. Arieti, ed., *American Handbook of Psychiatry*, Vol. 3, 1st ed. New York: Basic Books, 1966.

22. ———. *General System Theory. Foundation, Development, Applications*. New York: Braziller, 1968.

23. BUBER, M. *I and Thou*, R. E. Smith, transl. Edinburgh: Clark, 1953.

24. CAMERON, N. "Reasoning, Regression and Communication in Schizophrenics," *Psychological Monographs*, 50 (1938), 1.

25. ———. *The Psychology of Behavior Disorders. A Biosocial Interpretation*. Cambridge: Houghton Mifflin Company, Riverside Press, 1947.

26. CASSIRER, E. *The Philosophy of Symbolic Forms*, Vols. 1, 2, 3. New Haven: Yale University Press, 1953, 1955, 1957.

27. CHAPMAN, J. "The Early Diagnosis of Schizophrenia," *British Journal of Psychiatry*, 112 (1966), 225–238.

28. CHAPMAN, L. J. "Intrusion of Associative Responses into Schizophrenic Conceptual Performance," *Journal of Abnormal Social Psychology*, 56 (1958), 374–379.

29. ———. "Confusion of Figurative and Literal Usages of Words by Schizophrenics and Brain-damaged Patients," *Journal of Abnormal Social Psychology*, 60 (1960), 412–416.

30. ———. "A Re-Interpretation of Some Pathological Disturbances in Conceptual Breadth," *Journal of Abnormal Social Psychology*, 62 (1961), 514–519.

31. CHAPMAN, L. J., J. P. CHAPMAN, and G. A. MILLER. "A Theory of Verbal Behavior in Schizophrenia," in B. Maher, *Progress in Experimental Personality Research*, Vol. 1. New York: Academic Press, 1964.

32. CHAPMAN, L. J., and J. P. CHAPMAN. "The Interpretation of Words in Schizophrenia," *Journal of Personality and Social Psychology*, 1 (1965), 135–146.

33. DOMARUS, E. VON. "*Über die Beziehung des Normalen zum Schizophrenen Denken*," *Archives of Psychiatry*, 74 (1925), 641.

34. ———. "The Specific Laws of Logic in Schizophrenia," in J. S. Kasanin, ed., *Language and Thought in Schizophrenia: Collected Papers*. Berkeley: University of California, 1944.

35. FODOR, N. "Prenatal Foundations of Psychotic Development," *Samiksa*, 11 (1957), 1.

36. FREUD, S. *The Interpretation of Dreams*. New York: Basic Books, 1960.

37. FROMM-REICHMANN, F. *Principles of Intensive Psychotherapy*. Chicago: University of Chicago Press, 1950.

38. GOLDSTEIN, K. *The Organism*. New York: American Book Company, 1939.

39. ――――. "The Significance of Psychological Research in Schizophrenia," *Journal of Nervous and Mental Disease*, 97 (1943), 261–279.

40. GUNTRIP, H. *Schizoid Phenomena, Object Relations and the Self*. New York: International Universities Press, 1968.

41. HILL, L. B. *Psychotherapeutic Intervention in Schizophrenia*. Chicago: University of Chicago Press, 1955.

42. HORNEY, K. *Our Inner Conflicts*. New York: W. W. Norton, 1943.

43. JACKSON, A. P. Comments in C. A. Whitaker, *Psychotherapy of Chronic Schizophrenic Patients*. Boston: Little, Brown, 1958.

44. JACKSON, D. D. "Schizophrenia, The Nosological Nexus," in J. Romano, ed., *The Origins of Schizophrenia*. Amsterdam: Excerpta Medica Foundation, 1968.

45. JACKSON, J. H. *Selected Writings*. London: Hodder and Stoughton, 1932.

46. KAGAN, J. "Do Infants Think?" *Scientific American*, 226(3) (1972), 74–83.

47. KANNER, L. "Early Infantile Autism," *Journal of Pediatrics*, 25 (1944), 211.

48. ――――. "Irrelevant and Metaphorical Language in Early Infantile Autism," *The American Journal of Psychiatry*, 103 (1946), 242.

49. ――――. "Problems of Nosology and Psychodynamics of Early Infantile Autism," *American Journal of Orthopsychiatry*, 19 (1949), 416.

50. ――――. "Infantile Autism and the Schizophrenias," *Behavioral Science*, 10 (1965), 412–420.

51. KANTOR, R. E., and W. G. HERRON. *Reactive and Process Schizophrenia*. Palo Alto: Science and Behavior Books, 1966.

52. KELSEN, H. *Society and Nature*. Chicago: University of Chicago Press, 1943.

53. KLÜVER, H. *Behavior Mechanisms in Monkeys*. Chicago: University of Chicago Press, 1933.

54. ――――. "The Study of Personality and the Method of Equivalent and Non-equivalent Stimuli," *Character and Personality*, 5 (1936), 91–112.

55. LAING, R. "Schizophrenia: Sickness or Strategy?" Lectures under the auspices of the William Alanson White Institute, New York City, January 1967.

56. ――――. *The Politics of Experience*. New York: Pantheon Books, 1967.

57. LANGER, S. K. *Philosophy in a New Key*. Cambridge: Harvard University Press, 1942.

58. LIDZ, T. "The Influence of Family Studies on the Treatment of Schizophrenics," *Psychiatry*, 32 (1969), 237–251.

59. LIDZ, T., A. R. CORNELISON, S. FLECK, and D. TERRY. "The Intrafamilial Environment of Schizophrenic Patients: II. Marital Schism and Marital Skew," *The American Journal of Psychiatry*, 144 (1957), 241.

60. ――――. "The Intrafamilial Environment of the Schizophrenic Patient: The Father," *Psychiatry*, 20 (1957), 329.

61. ――――. "Intrafamilial Environment of the Schizophrenic Patient: The Transmission of Irrationality," *Archives of Neurology and Psychiatry*, 79 (1958), 305.

62. LIDZ, T., and S. FLECK. "Family Studies and a Theory of Schizophrenia." Presented at the Annual Meeting of the American Psychiatric Association, 1964.

63. LIDZ, T., S. FLECK, and A. R. CORNELISON. *Schizophrenia and the Family*. New York: International University Press, 1965.

64. LIDZ, T., B. PARKER, and A. R. CORNELISON. "The Role of the Father in the Family Environment of the Schizophrenic Patient," *The American Journal of Psychiatry*, 113 (1956), 126.

65. LIMENTANI, D. "Symbiotic Identification in Schizophrenia," *Psychiatry*, 19 (1956), 231–236.

66. LU, Y. "Mother-Child Role Relations in Schizophrenia," *Psychiatry*, 24 (1961), 133–142.

67. McGHIE, A., and J. CHAPMAN. "Disorder of Attention and Perception in Early Schizophrenia," *British Journal of Medical Psychology*, 34 (1961), 103–116.

68. MEAD, G. H. *Mind, Self and Society*. Chicago: University of Chicago Press, 1934.

69. MEDNICK, S. A., and J. L. FREEDMAN. Stimulus Generalization," *Psychological Bulletin*, 57 (1960), 169–200.

70. MISHLER, E., and N. WAXLER, eds. *Family Processes and Schizophrenia*. New York: Science House, 1968.

71. NOY, P. Personal Communication, 1968.

72. PAYNE, R. W. "Cognitive Abnormalities," in H. J. Eysenck, ed., *Handbook of Abnormal Psychology.* New York: Basic Books, 1961.

73. PAYNE, R. W., P. MATTUSEK, and E. I. GEORGE. "An Experimental Study of Schizophrenic Thought Disorder," *Journal of Mental Science,* 105 (1959), 627.

74. PIRO, S. *Il Linguaggio Schizofrenico.* Milan: Feltrinelli, 1967.

75. ROSEN, J. N. *Direct Psychoanalytic Psychiatry.* New York: Grune & Stratton, 1962.

76. ———. *The Concept of Early Maternal Environment in Direct Psychoanalysis.* Doylestown: The Doylestown Foundation, 1963.

77. SCHUR, M. *The Id and the Regulatory Principles of Mental Functioning.* New York: International Universities Press, 1966.

78. SEARLES, H. *Collected Papers on Schizophrenia and Related Subjects.* New York: International Universities Press, 1965.

79. SIIRALA, M. *Die Schizophrenie—des Einzeln und der Allgemeinheit.* Göttingen: Vandenhoeck & Ruprecht, 1961.

80. ———. "Schizophrenia: A Human Situation," *American Journal of Psychoanalysis,* 23 (1963), 39.

81. STRUM, I. E. "Overinclusion and Concreteness among Pathological Groups," *Journal of Consulting Psychology,* 29 (1965), 9–18.

82. SULLIVAN, H. S. *Conceptions of Modern Psychiatry.* New York: W. W. Norton, 1953.

83. ———. *Schizophrenia as a Human Process.* New York: Norton, 1962.

84. SZASZ, T. "The Problem of Psychiatric Nosology. A Contribution to a Situational Analysis of Psychiatric Operations," *The American Journal of Psychiatry,* 114 (1957), 405.

85. TAYLOR, J., ed., *Selected Writings of John Hughlings Jackson.* London: Hodder and Stoughton, 1932.

86. VYGOTSKY, L. S. *Thought and Language.* Cambridge: M.I.T. Press, 1962.

87. WARING, M., and D. RICKS. "Family Patterns of Children Who Became Adult Schizophrenics," *Journal of Nervous and Mental Disease,* 140 (1965), 351–364.

88. WERNER, H. "Microgenesis and Aphasia," *Journal of Abnormal Social Psychology,* 52 (1956), 347.

89. ———. *Comparative Psychology of Mental Development.* New York: International Universities Press, 1957.

90. WILL, O. "Catatonic Behavior in Schizophrenia," *Contemporary Psychoanalysis,* 19 (1972), 29–58.

91. WOLMAN, B. B. *Vectoriasis Praecox or the Group of Schizophrenia.* Springfield: Thomas, 1966.

92. WYNNE, L. C., I. M. RYCKOFF, J. DAY, and S. HIRSCH. "Pseudomutuality in the Family Relations of Schizophrenics," *Psychiatry,* 21 (1958), 205–220.

93. WYNNE, L. C., and M. T. SINGER. "Thought Disorder and Family Relation of Schizophrenics. I. A Research Strategy. II. A Classification of Forms of Thinking," *Archives of General Psychiatry,* 9 (1963), 191–198, 199–206.

CHAPTER 25

THE GENETICS OF SCHIZOPHRENIA

David Rosenthal

IT SHOULD BE CLEAR at the outset that if we understand the genetics of schizophrenia, we are in a favorable position to develop optimal preventive and therapeutic measures with respect to this grave mental disturbance. The fact is that we do not understand the genetics of schizophrenia. In truth, the primary task of genetic research on this disorder over the past six decades has been to show that heredity has anything to do with schizophrenia at all. The burden of proof has not been borne easily, despite the fact that the conception of the disorder by its originators, Kraepelin[27] and Bleuler,[3] took place in an intellectual climate which assumed almost without question that the disorder was indeed inherited. In this article, we will review the main body of genetic evidence gathered to date and try to place a fair evaluation on it.

The opinions expressed herein are those of the author and do not necessarily express the position of the National Institute of Mental Health.

(Determining That a Disorder Is Genetic

First, the reader ought to be reminded of the kinds of information that permit us to make decisions about the role of genes in various disorders. The genetics issue is most readily resolved, and perhaps can only be resolved conclusively, if we can demonstrate that a disorder (the phenotype) follows a Mendelian distribution in families. To make such a demonstration requires that we examine at least two generations. Such research has been done extensively with regard to schizophrenia, and although theorists have advocated a single-gene theory, in the main, they have never been able to demonstrate a consistent, simple Mendelian distribution of the disorder within families, nor have they been able to agree on whether the postulated mode of genetic transmission follows a dominant or recessive pattern. In fact, investigators have been able to find families that simulated a pattern of dominance, recessiveness, or no pattern at all, and one investigator[36] has taken the view that the families in which the distribution of schizophrenia represents a dominant, recessive, or intermediate pattern actually constitute three different genetic disorders. This latter view—that there may be a number of major single genes, each of which can respectively be responsible for schizophrenic illness—is referred to as heterogeneity theory. In different forms, it is a view that is not uncommonly held, and indeed it was advocated by E. Bleuler[3] himself, who thought of the illness as a group of schizophrenias.

Failing to find evidence for a clear Mendelian distribution, we might advance our understanding of the genetics of schizophrenia if we could point to a specific metabolic disturbance that is clearly associated with the disorder. To date, however, no such finding has been made, although, as in most bodies of literature on schizophrenia, a large number of theories have been put forward over the years, some of them based on suggestive empirical findings. Until such a finding is forthcoming, our understanding of the genetics of schizophrenia must remain limited and questionable.

A third kind of information that could be helpful would derive from studies analogous to breeding experiments carried out with animals. In such studies the experimenter is able to develop different strains of a species and to inbreed or crossbreed them in various ways over several generations. Fortunately, scientists cannot exercise such controls with regard to humans who mate as they will. The best that the scientist can hope for is to find naturally transpiring matings that follow along the lines he would have chosen had he been able to control the matings in a laboratory-like situation. In fact, it is information from just such matings and from twin studies which provides us with whatever we do know about the genetics of schizophrenia. To demonstrate that genes have anything to do with schizophrenia, the investigator, lacking the desiderata noted above, must marshal the following group of statistical findings:

1. The frequency of schizophrenia must be greater in the families of schizophrenics than in the families of nonschizophrenic controls or in the population at large.
2. The frequency of schizophrenia in relatives of schizophrenics should be positively correlated with the degree of blood relationship to the schizophrenic index cases.
3. The concordance rate for schizophrenia must be higher in monozygotic than in dizygotic twins.

(Familial Evidence and Twin Studies

Table 25–1 indicates the expected rate of schizophrenia in the sibs of schizophrenic index cases and in the corresponding population at large. Clearly, the rates are always significantly higher for the sibs than for the general population, thus meeting the first criterion. With respect to the second criterion, a median risk value for second-degree relatives is about 2.1 percent, which is lower than the median risk value for sibs in Table 25–1, and a median risk value for third-degree relatives is about 1.65 percent, which is lower than the median rate for second-degree relatives and higher than the median rate for the populations shown in Table 25–1. Thus, the data provide support for the second criterion, but the differences between median values, once one moves beyond first-degree relatives, are slight indeed, and involve a fair amount of overlap when one looks at the individual studies separately.[46]

Table 25–2 presents the main studies regarding the third criterion. With the exception of one study, the concordance rate for MZ twins is always significantly higher than that for DZ twins, thus meeting the third criterion strongly.

Once we have met the primary three criteria, we can add a fourth. We may now make the reasonable tentative assumption that individuals who have the disorder also have the genotype that leads to that disorder. When

TABLE 25–1.   Morbidity Risk Estimates for Sibs of Schizophrenic
Index Cases and for the Population at Large

| Study | MORBIDITY RISK ESTIMATE IN PERCENT | |
	Sibs	General Population
Brugger, 1928	10.3	1.53
Schultz, 1932	6.7	0.76
Luxenburger, 1936	7.6	0.85
Strömgren, 1938	6.7	0.48
Kallmann, 1938	7.5	0.35
Bleuler, 1941	10.4	1.53
Böök, 1953	9.7	2.85
Hallgren & Sjögren, 1959	5.7	0.83
Garrone, 1962	8.6	2.40

TABLE 25–2.   Approximate Concordance Rates for Schizophrenia
in Monozygotic and Dizygotic Twins

| Study | ESTIMATED CONCORDANCE RATE IN PERCENT | |
	MZ Twins	DZ Twins
Luxenburger, 1928–1934	55	2.1
Rosanoff et al., 1934–1935	61	10.0
Essen-Möller, 1941	42	13.0
Kallmann, 1946	73	12.2
Slater, 1953	70	12.3
Inouye, 1961	48	9.0
Tienari, 1963, 1968	6	4.8
Gottesman and Shields, 1966	50	9.1
Kringlen, 1967	31	9.0
Fischer et al., 1969	37	9.5
Pollin et al., 1969	15.5	4.4

NOTE: These are not necessarily the rates reported by the investigators. They
indicate this author's estimate of the rate that might best represent the data in
each study, but the reader should know that a simply expressed concordance
can be misleading, that it masks or disregards much information necessary to
understand the basic data on which the rates are based.

they mate, they should pass this genetic loading on to their children in appreciable degree,
depending on the mode of genetic transmission. In fact, children who have a schizophrenic parent have about a 10 percent median risk of developing schizophrenia themselves.[46] With *both* parents schizophrenic, the
assumed genetic loading transmitted increases
proportionately, and the median risk of developing schizophrenia in children of such dual
matings increases to about 40 percent.[45] Thus,
these findings are also consistent with the
genetic hypothesis and provide additional
support for it.

❡ An Alternative Hypothesis

Nevertheless, it is time to pause in our discussion to look at the matter more broadly. It is
true that all the data mentioned are consistent
with what genetic theory predicts, but might
the data not be explained in some other way
as well? If schizophrenia runs in families,
could it be that there are certain behavioral
and psychological events that occur in these
families that induce schizophrenic symptoms
and behavior in some of their members? Investigators who have observed such families
intensively have long called attention to be-

havioral patterns in mothers whom they call "schizophrenogenic." Some have thought that families with strong mothers and weak, dependent fathers produce schizophrenic children.[12,26] Others have pointed to parents who "double-bind" their children[2] or who create an impalpable "rubber-fence" around the family, or nongenuine relationships among themselves called "pseudomutual",[64] or who fragment the child's foci of attention in various ways,[53] especially through loose or garbled forms of verbal communication,[63] or who create a family climate that has been called "skewed"[9] or chaotic,[1] and that such familial characteristics induce schizophrenic disorder in children subjected to them.[29] Some evidence suggests that families in the lowest socioeconomic status breed a disproportionately large number of schizophrenics.[25]

Let us then for the moment make another reasonable but tentative assumption, namely, that those observations listed above do indeed indicate that familial interaction patterns play a causal role in the development of schizophrenia. How could such an hypothesis account for the four groups of findings noted above?

First, the fact that sibs of schizophrenics develop schizophrenia more often than the population at large is not surprising, since the sibs grow up in the same family as the schizophrenic index cases. Both have been victimized by the same noxious influences, which in turn do not apply to the general population, at least not with the same intensity or frequency. The fact that there is a correlation between the rate of schizophrenia in relatives and the degree of blood relationship to schizophrenics might also be predicted by our tentative hypothesis. First-degree relatives should show the highest rate since all are subjected to the same noxious influences. Second-degree relatives, such as aunts or uncles, grew up in the same environment as the mothers and fathers of the schizophrenic cases, and may have developed behavioral patterns similar to those of the schizophrenics' parents, thus abetting the production of schizophrenia in their own children, but to a lesser extent. These shared environments occur to lesser extents as the de-

gree of blood relationship becomes further removed, thus accounting for the observed correlation.

A similar line of argument would apply to families in which one of the parents is schizophrenic. Of course, a psychotic parent will be more likely than a normal parent to produce a chaotic family, with increased schizophrenia among his offspring. When both parents are schizophrenic, conditions for complete familial chaos are ripe indeed, and it is no wonder that the rate of schizophrenia among their offspring increases about fourfold, a rate of increase not strictly predicted by genetic theory. It may be, too, that some of the children identify with the schizophrenic parent, see themselves as being like that parent or even being a "part" of her (which, genetically speaking, is true), and eventually come to a schizophrenic denouement in which the identification with the parent reaches its fullest expression.

Now, what about the MZ and DZ twins, in which both members of the pair grew up in the same home? Why should the concordance rate be higher for the MZ pairs? Well, the tentative hypothesis under scrutiny is a psychological one. Two people may grow up in the same home but have completely different psychological experiences in it. This point applies especially to twins. DZ twins should share experiences much as ordinary siblings do, although they also share some additional ones that have to do with the fact that they were born together and are the same age. However, MZ twins have a unique psychological experience which pervades their entire lives. Identification with another person reaches its strongest point in such genetically identical individuals. The literature on twins is replete with all kinds of experiences and lore that bear on this intense communality or psychological bond.[11,18,51] If one twin develops an illness, the other is likely to do so as well. This sharing of fates is an ongoing, integral part of their development and learning. Therefore, if one twin develops a schizophrenic illness, the likelihood of the second twin's developing that illness is increased inordinately, and the concordance rates for MZ pairs should be appreciably higher than that for DZ pairs, according to the tentative hypothesis.

(Studies Separating the Genetic and Rearing Variables

Thus, we see that the same basic data can be explained plausibly by at least two competing hypotheses which are completely different from one another, and which have vastly different implications with regard to our understanding, treatment, and research on schizophrenia. Such a situation is scientifically intolerable, and it becomes incumbent on scientists working on the problem to determine which hypothesis is correct. Resolution of the issue is no simple matter since both hypotheses depend on familial distributions to support their veridicality, and both the hypothesized genes and the reported behavioral-psychological factors are confounded in the same families. The scientist's task is to unconfound the two implicated variables, and this can best be done by taking advantage of naturally occurring adoptions.

In a study carried out in western U.S.A. by Heston,[16] the index cases were adults who had been born of hospitalized, actively schizophrenic women and who had been placed at birth in foundling homes or in the care of paternal relatives, or adopted away. A matched control group consisted of subjects who had been placed in the same foundling homes. Of the forty-seven index cases five, or 16.6 percent, were hospitalized chronic schizophrenics, but none of the controls was schizophrenic.

Karlsson,[22] in a study done in Iceland, compared the biologic and foster sibs of schizophrenics who had been adopted in their first year of life. Six of twenty-nine biologic sibs (20.7 percent) were found to be schizophrenic, as compared to none of the twenty-eight foster sibs.

In an eastern U.S.A. study carried out by Wender et al.,[62] the index cases were adult schizophrenics who had been adopted by nonrelatives in their first year of life. One control group consisted of matched schizophrenics who were reared in the parental home, and a second control group consisted of matched adult adoptees who were psychiatrically normal. The adopting parents of the index cases had less severe psychopathology than the biologic parents of the schizophrenic controls, but more psychopathology than the adopting parents of normals.

In a study done in Denmark by Kety et al.,[24] the index cases were adults who had been given up for nonfamily adoption in their first four years of life and who were diagnosed as having a schizophrenic disorder. A control group consisted of matched adoptees who had had no known psychiatric admission. The adoptive and biologic parents, sibs and half-sibs of both groups were evaluated with respect to schizophrenia and schizophrenic disorders called acute, borderline, severely schizoid, paranoid, or inadequate. These diagnoses combined were called *the schizophrenia spectrum.* There was one case of chronic or process schizophrenia among 150 biologic relatives of the index cases and one among the 156 biologic relatives of the controls, but with regard to all schizophrenia spectrum disorders, thirteen occurred in relatives of index cases as compared to three of controls, a difference significant at the .01 level. No differences in such disorders occurred among the adoptive relatives of the index and control subjects.

A second study carried out in Denmark by Rosenthal[47] selected adult index cases who had had a schizophrenic biologic parent but who had been adopted away in the first four years of life. A control group consisted of matched adoptees whose biologic parents had never had a psychiatric admission for a schizophrenia spectrum disorder. Both groups of adoptees were examined in an interview lasting three to five hours by a psychiatrist who did not know if the subject was an index or control case. Among the index cases, three were diagnosed as schizophrenic, only one of whom had been hospitalized, but none of the controls was so diagnosed. With respect to all schizophrenia spectrum diagnoses combined, the rate was almost twice as high in the index cases as in the controls, the difference being statistically significant.

([Problems in the "Unconfounding" Studies

Thus, we now have five independent studies in which the genetic and rearing families have been unconfounded. All five point strongly to the conclusion that genes do in fact determine to an appreciable extent whether schizophrenic types of disorder will or will not occur.

Nevertheless, each of the five studies leaves some lingering questions. In the Heston study,[16] the biologic mothers were actively schizophrenic, and were hospitalized and treated while pregnant with the index cases. Could such prenatal influences foster a schizophrenic outcome? Also, many of the rearing families knew about the schizophrenic mother, and conceivably some may have had the common expectation of "like parent, like child," and may have communicated this expectation to the child in various ways and behaved toward him accordingly. Could such factors have been implicated in the index case disorders observed?

In the Karlsson study,[22] we are provided with too little information about the methodological details, expecially in regard to diagnosis. Moreover, among the separated biologic sibs of his index cases he finds 20.7 percent schizophrenic. A glance at Table 25–1 will show that this rate is twice as high as the highest rates shown in the table. Why should this be so, especially when the index cases and their sibs are *not* reared together?

In the Wender et al. study,[62] the number of subjects was smaller than one would like, and the major examiner was not blind with respect to which parents being interviewed were related to which proband group. This study has been repeated with a new sample to address itself to these problems, but the data are not yet available.

In the Kety et al. study,[24] there was no significant difference between the biologic and adoptive relatives of index and control subjects with regard to clear-cut schizophrenia. Perhaps, this result could be traced to the fact that the number of clear-cut schizophrenic index cases was relatively small. This study has been expanded and additional findings may change this statistical picture. The findings that did discriminate the biologic relatives of index and control subjects depended on mental disturbances tentatively assumed to be milder forms of schizophrenic disorder that are genetically linked to process schizophrenia. This assumption of a genetically unified spectrum of disorders needs further testing and clarification, and indeed these investigators are working to provide it.

In the Rosenthal study,[47] only one index case was a hospitalized schizophrenic. Two additional index cases diagnosed schizophrenic by the examining psychiatrist were managing their lives in the community and never required hospitalization. Of the offspring of thirty process schizophrenics, not one was hospitalized for schizophrenia, and only one was diagnosed schizophrenic (3.3 percent, not age corrected, as compared to Heston's 16.6 percent, corrected for age). Among offspring of a schizophrenic generally, the median rate of schizophrenia reported is approximately 10 percent. Thus, a possible interpretation of the Rosenthal finding is that rearing in an adoptive home may indeed protect children of a schizophrenic parent from developing the disorder themselves.

With respect to twins, the best way to unconfound the genetic and psychological variables that may account for the high concordance rates in MZ pairs is to separate them early in life. Although this obviously cannot be done in any systematic way, Slater[56] has compiled from eight sources a series of MZ pairs in which the twins were separated early in life and at least one was schizophrenic. Of the sixteen twin pairs compiled, ten were concordant and six were discordant. The concordance rate of 62.5 percent may be compared with the rates for MZ twins in Table 25–2, in which the median concordance rate is 48 percent. As a matter of fact, only two of the eleven rates in Table 25–2 are higher than the rate for the separated twins.

This finding again points to the importance of genetic factors in schizophrenia and certainly indicates that at least not all instances of concordance in MZ twins arise from psychological factors unique to such twins. Does not the high concordance rate of 62.5 percent indicate that such psychological factors are really irrelevant? No, because the twin pairs do not constitute a systematic sample. For example, the first five pairs of separated twins reported were *all* concordant. Among the eleven pairs reported later, when sampling problems in genetic studies were being discussed with increased concern,[39,43] five pairs were found to be concordant and six pairs were discordant. We do not know what the concordance rate would be for a systematically collected sample of separated twins, and indeed it might be an insuperable task to try to collect such a sample. Of the three pairs found through birth registers, all were discordant. Thus, the high rate of 62.5 percent might simply reflect the fact that concordant pairs were more likely than discordant pairs to find their way into samples, a factor that might also have accounted in part for the three highest MZ concordance rates in Table 25–2. If the true concordance rate for separated MZ twins could be shown to be less than the rate for reared-together MZ twins from the same population, the rate increment among the together-reared twins could reflect the influence of the psychological factors common to MZ twinship.

❲ Summing the Major Evidence

What conclusions can we draw from such research findings with respect to the genetics of schizophrenia? Most important is the fact that all statistical findings are consistent with a genetic hypothesis, whether they derive from studies of two-generation families, of first-, second- or third-degree relatives, of twins reared together or apart, or of studies in which the principally implicated variables of heredity and rearing are separated or unconfounded. In fact, if we were asked to foretell which persons are most likely to become schizophrenic, the best predictor now available to us is the simple fact of blood relationship to another schizophrenic: The more genes the individual shares with a schizophrenic, the greater is the probability that he will become schizophrenic. Our predictive success may not be great, except in the case of MZ twins, but it will be the best we can do. Since no other predictive criterion can presently approach blood relationship as a predictor of schizophrenia, almost all investigators who embark on so-called high risk longitudinal studies to explore the precursors of schizophrenia, even those who favor environmentalist explanations of the disorder, prefer to have index cases who are children of schizophrenics.

For such reasons, it seems reasonable to make the operating or working assumption that the case for considering a hereditary factor in the etiology of schizophrenia has been sufficiently demonstrated, and that further research will continue to support this assumption.[48] Such a position does not by any means imply that we should rule out the possible contribution of environmental factors to the disorder. In fact, we know that such factors must play a role in schizophrenia because among all MZ twin pairs in which one twin is schizophrenic, in as many as half the pairs, or sometimes more, the co-twin, who has exactly the same genes, may not be clinically schizophrenic. Unfortunately, we have up till now only crudely formulated notions of what some of these nongenetic factors may be, but knowledge of them will surely increase.

On the other hand, our operating assumption amounts to an open admission that we understand very little about the genetics of schizophrenia. True enough, we have an abundance of genetic theories that try to account for the statistical distributions obtained in a large number of studies that vary appreciably among themselves in many ways, but we are not yet in a position to make a clear choice among these theories. As a matter of fact, it may be that we should not really be talking about the genetics of schizophrenia at all, but about the genetics of schizophrenic disorders, a point that is implied in the studies that concern themselves with a broader spectrum of possibly schizophrenia-related disorders.

(The Genetic Unity of Schizophrenic Disorders

The term "schizophrenia" has been applied to a wide variety of behavioral disorders that differ clinically to an appreciable extent, although they also share a number of common features or symptoms. Some of these disorders are represented by the classical Kraepelinian subtypes: simplex, catatonia, hebephrenia, and paranoia. Others are designated borderline, pseudoneurotic, or pseudopsychopathic. Some make a distinction between process and reactive, or nuclear and peripheral forms of schizophrenia. Some disorders labeled symptomatic, atypical, or schizophreniform, are sometimes thought not to be true schizophrenia. Many people are called schizoid, many schizoaffective. Some age-related disorders such as preadolescent schizophrenia or early infantile autism are often thought to be variant forms of schizophrenia. Can there be a simple genetic explanation for all these forms of clinical disorder? Is it possible that some are genetically related and that some are not, and if so, how can we tell?

This is a key problem which we must resolve if we are to obtain any real understanding about the genetics of schizophrenic disorders. The topic and the research done on it are too extensive to review in appreciable detail here, but it has been thoroughly reviewed and evaluated elsewhere.[46] We may state briefly, however, that decisions about whether two different forms of illness are genetically related are based on the finding that both occur in families and in twinships at a greater than chance frequency. On this basis, we may tentatively draw the following conclusions from the known literature:

1. The classical subtypes, catatonia, hebephrenia, and paranoia, are genetically related. Not enough research has been done with regard to the simplex form, which is appar-

ently diagnosed with very low frequency, to draw any conclusion about its genetic relatedness to the other subtypes.

2. The process-reactive delineation is based primarily on a continuum of severity with regard to the clinical outcome of schizophrenic disorders. Clearly, outcomes can be graded in many ways, all of which may have a dimensional character. In the main, it appears that most forms of schizophrenic disorder intermediate between the most hapless outcomes and those in which the subject eventually manages to achieve a fair to good level of social and occupational adjustment in the community are genetically related. However, the cases at the extreme end of the reactive continuum, those who have a good premorbid social, sexual, and personality history, who have a single schizophrenic-like episode of modest duration, and who make a full and relatively rapid recovery with no indication of residual integrative defects, probably do not share the genetic background that is implicated in other schizophrenic disorders.

3. Cases called borderline, pseudoneurotic, or severely schizoid or paranoid, are probably genetically related to cases with full-blown schizophrenia.

4. Preadolescent forms of schizophrenia are probably genetically related to adult forms of schizophrenia, but the literature on early infantile autism is too sparse and contradictory to permit any conclusions about its etiology or its possible genetic relatedness to schizophrenia.

5. To complicate the matter even further, there is some evidence to suggest that some other types of disorder, not usually thought of as being in the schizophrenia spectrum, may also be related to schizophrenia. These include some forms of neurosis, especially certain severe obsessive-compulsives, and the disorder called depersonalization neurosis; some forms of personality, e.g., those called odd or eccentric, cold and schizoid, or paranoid; some forms of psychopathy, including those with prison psychosis, cases called pseudopsychopathic schizophrenia, and cases called schizoid psychopathy. There is even some suggestion of genetic overlap between schizophrenia and

manic-depressive psychosis. Some investigators have also linked schizophrenia with epilepsy and mental deficiency.

Clearly, this morass must be straightened out. Some influential psychiatrists and most clinical psychologists have proposed that we throw out the genetic hypothesis altogether, as well as all diagnostic labels,[34] and the whole concept of mental illness to boot.[58] However, proponents of such views are merely turning their backs on all the evidence for a genetic factor in schizophrenic disorder. Moreover, traditional psychiatric nosology, if it is to have any meaning at all, will probably best find vitality and real psychiatric relevance when at least some of the currently accepted diagnostic categories are grouped according to whether they share a common genetic etiological basis or not.

(Genetic Theories of Schizophrenia

Modern theorizing about the genetics of schizophrenia began in 1916.[50] Since then, we have never had a dearth of such theories and new ones continue to turn up regularly. Rosenthal[44] grouped them all into two main classes which he called monogenic-biochemical and diathesis-stress theories. These were in turn counterposed to a class of theories that assumed no genetic basis at all for schizophrenia, and which he called life-experience theories. Monogenic-biochemical theories assume that a single pathological gene is necessary, if not sufficient, to produce schizophrenia. The schizophrenic phenotype itself may be dominant, recessive, or intermediate. The genotype is responsible for a specific metabolic error that produces the patterns of behavior that are pathognomonic of schizophrenia. Theories that invoke two single major genes in the etiology of the illness really belong in the monogenic-biochemical class as well, because they, too, assume that the two genes in combination produce a particular biochemical abnormality that causes the illness and its lingering psychological defects. It

is such theories, and the research material on which they are based, that lead many scientists to devote their professional lives to search for *the* metabolic error in schizophrenia and the chain of biochemical aberrations it is assumed to produce.

According to diathesis-stress theories, what is inherited in schizophrenia is a predisposition to develop the illness. The nature of the assumed predisposition is usually vaguely conceived. Most often, it is formulated in terms of personality characteristics manifested early in life, such as social avoidance behavior, high anxiety, unusual habits or predilections, lack of interests, self-preoccupation, or some other characteristics thought to be signs of deviance. However, since some hereditary deviation is postulated as an essential contributor to the illness, some metabolic digression must be assumed to have taken place. In diathesis-stress theory, however, this digression is usually thought to have manifested itself prenatally in some structural anomaly in the central nervous system itself, primarily in the form of a neural integrative defect.[33] Thus, a diathesis-stress theorist would hold out little hope of finding a particular abnormal metabolite whose ebb and flow make for lesser or greater manifestation of schizophrenic pathology. Instead, he would be more concerned with trying to find aberrations in CNS neurophysiology.[35] But he also would be especially interested in life stresses, biological or psychological, which he assumes are necessary to precipitate the schizophrenic psychopathology. Thus, this class of theories invokes a model of heredity-environment interactionism, as contrasted with monogenic-biochemical theory in which the role of environmental factors is thought to be minimal, or even in some instances, nonexistent. The implicated diathesis could result from a single gene, but most likely it involves a sizeable number of genes of small effect, called polygenes, whose combined effects are accumulative or additive, i.e., the more of these genes the individual harbors, the more vulnerable he is to stresses that trigger schizophrenic manifestations, and the more psychopathology he is likely to show.

Theories of genetic heterogeneity are difficult to fit into any particular model. Such theories hold that there may be several major single genes which are not alleles of one another, each of which may underlie schizophrenia. The concept has a kind of attractiveness in a clinical sense, since the range of clinical manifestations in schizophrenia is wide indeed, especially, for example, as compared to manic-depressive psychosis, and it is tempting to postulate a different gene for each different type of clinical manifestation. However, it will be difficult enough to show that even one major gene lies at the roots of schizophrenia. To demonstrate that there are *n* such genes will require an extraordinary research effort. Moreover, as has been pointed out above, the available literature on this problem provides considerable support for the view of genetic homogeneity (or unity) with respect to most forms of schizophrenic disorder. Vartanyan and Gindilis,[61] however, cite evidence to support the view that chronic, deteriorating forms, and periodic forms with temporally discrete, acute attacks and complete recession of symptoms during remission, with only slight personality changes, are two genetically different forms (morphisms) of schizophrenia. In further support of heterogeneity theory, it should be noted that recent findings have turned up a greater than chance frequency of chromosomal abnormalities in schizophrenic populations.[21,61] However, it may well be that the chromosomal abnormality does not provide any specific *Anlage* for schizophrenia, but rather that it imposes an unusual degree of psychological stress on the affected individual, and that this increased stress makes for heightened vulnerability to the illness. This would be especially true of XXY phenotypic males (Klinefelter's syndrome) who suffer prolonged intense crises around their sex role and identity, and who may tend to develop schizophrenic disorders at a frequency greater than that of the population at large.[46] Moreover, the possibility exists that some aneuploidic schizophrenics may represent phenocopies of the illness, in the same sense that some cases of Huntington's disease, lues, temporal lobe epilepsy, head injury, or amphetamine toxication, may present clinical pictures that simulate schizophrenia.

Which genetic theory is the most plausible, in the light of all the evidence to date? Actually, there are four competing theories that need to be mentioned.

In the 1940s, Kallmann's[19] influence was at its height and his theory was the most highly regarded. He postulated a single recessive gene in a typical monogenic-biochemical model to account for his research findings. Thus, a schizophrenic had to receive one pathological allele from each parent. However, to account for deviations from expected Mendelian ratios, he postulated polygenic modifiers which made for more or less resistance to clinical manifestation. Most homozygotes—who carried the pathological gene in double dose—would develop schizophrenia, but those whose resistance to manifestation was high would have a mild form of the illness, or would merely be schizoid. Some homozygotes, with very high constitutional resistance would even be clinically normal. Heterozygotes who carried only one allele would be schizoid or normal, depending on their degree of resistance.

In the 1950s, Böök[5] introduced a theory in which the major gene was a partial dominant. This theory, as reformulated by Slater,[55] attempted to account for data obtained in several studies. It was statistically more sophisticated and elegant than Kallmann's, and supplanted it in general favor. The theory assumes that only relatively few individuals are homozygous for the pathological gene, but that all these homozygotes become schizophrenic. Assuming an estimated 0.8 percent frequency of the illness in the population, Slater was able to show the rate of schizophrenia expected in sibs and children of a schizophrenic, as well as in children with both parents schizophrenic, with varying degrees of the gene frequency in the population and varying degrees of gene penetrance. A best fit to the selected known data indicated a gene frequency of fifteen per thousand, and a manifestation rate of 26 percent in heterozygotes who accounted for 97 percent of all schizophrenics, the other 3 percent being homozygous.

In the 1960s, two noteworthy theories appeared. One, by Karlsson,[22] has not caught on, but it is interesting in that it assumes two separate major genes in the causation of schizophrenia, one recessive, the other dominant, and attempts to account genetically for schizophrenics' relatives who are productive leaders, gifted and creative. Along with the theories of Kallmann, Böök, and Slater, it is essentially a monogenic-biochemical theory.

The second genetic theory to be launched successfully in the 1960s[14,23] is the one most widely accepted today, not only by genetically minded psychiatrists, but by many investigators who had previously rejected any genetic role in schizophrenia.[48] It is a simple polygenic theory that also postulates a threshold effect in regard to process schizophrenia. It is a model that is prototypical for diathesis-stress theories and it accounts most readily for all the known statistical distributions regarding schizophrenic disorders without postulating such variables as genetic modifiers, constitutional resistance, manifestation rate, or penetrance. It also accounts nicely for the gradation of disorders subsumed in the schizophrenia spectrum and for the relatively important role played by nongenetic factors in the etiology of clinical schizophrenia. The threshold effect implies that process schizophrenics harbor relatively more of the polygenes and/or are subjected to greater life stresses, the latter potentiating the former, so that latent biological capacities for the development of secondary and gross primary Bleulerian signs are unleashed. The task for adherents of this theory is to identify the implicated genes and their number, to determine how they achieve the quality of additivity, and to understand how environmental factors trigger the threshold effect that culminates so often in chronic schizophrenia.

It is to be hoped that the 1970s will be the decade in which clear and irrefutable findings will settle at least some of the issues regarding this fundamental psychiatric problem. Despite all the statistical evidence to support their position, proponents of the genetic viewpoint will probably not be able to maintain the high credibility of their position in the long run, unless the implicated biological defect is finally discovered and elucidated. At the present time, many laboratories and independent investigators are searching for the presumed metabolic or enzymatic abnormality that they believe must be present in schizophrenia, but as of this writing the most provocative findings are only suggestive. With respect to a possible neurological integrative defect, in a study as yet unpublished but described briefly by Rosenthal et al.,[49] Marcus was able to discriminate children who had a schizophrenic parent, and matched controls with normal parents on the basis of a neurological examination. This finding is promising but needs to be replicated. Many researchers and theoreticians are optimistic about a breakthrough in the 1970s. We can only wait and see.

(Bibliography

1. ALANEN, Y. O., with J. K. REKOLA, A. STEWEN, K. TAKALA, and M. TUOVINEN. "The Family in the Pathogenesis of Schizophrenic and Neurotic Disorders," *Acta Psychiatrica Scandinavica*, Suppl. 189 (1966), 42.

2. BATESON, G., D. JACKSON, J. HALEY, and J. WEAKLAND. "Toward a Theory of Schizophrenia," *Behavioral Science*, 1 (1956), 251–264.

3. BLEULER, E. *Dementia Praecox or the Group of Schizophrenias*. New York: International Universities Press, Inc., 1950.

4. BLEULER, M. "*Krankheitsverlauf, Persönlichkeit und Verwandtschaft Schizophrener und ihre gegenseitigen Beziehungen*," in *Sammlung Psychiatrischer und Neurologischer Einzeldarstellungen*, Vol. 16. Leipzig: Georg Thieme Verlag, 1941.

5. BÖÖK, J. A. "A Genetic and Neuropsychiatric Investigation of a North-Swedish Population with Special Regard to Schizophrenia and Mental Deficiency," *Acta Genetica*, 4 (1953), 1–139.

6. BRUGGER, C. "*Die Erbbiologische Stellung der Propfschizophrenie*," *Z. Ges. Neurol Psychiat.*, 113 (1928), 348.

7. ESSEN-MÖLLER, E. *Psychiatrische Untersuchungen an einer Serie von Zwillingen*. Copenhagen: Munksgaard, 1941.

8. FISCHER, M., B. HARVALD, and M. HAUGE.

"Neuropsychological Bases of Schizophrenia," in P. H. Mussen, and M. R. Rosenzweig, eds., *Annual Review of Psychology*, 20 (1969), 321–348.

9. FLECK, S., T. LIDZ, and A. CORNELISON. "Comparison of Parent-Child Relationships of Male and Female Schizophrenic Patients," *Archives of General Psychiatry*, 8 (1963), 1–7.

10. GARRONE, G. "*Étude Statistique et genetique de la Schizophrenie á Génève de 1901 á 1950*," *J. Genet. Humaine*, 11 (1962), 89–219.

11. GEDDA, L. *Twins in History and Science*. Springfield: Charles C. Thomas, 1961.

12. GERARD, D. L., and J. SIEGAL. "The Family Background of Schizophrenia," *Psychiatric Quarterly*, 24 (1950), 47–73.

13. GOTTESMAN, I. I., and J. SHIELDS. "Schizophrenia in Twins: 16 Years' Consecutive Admissions to a Psychiatric Clinic," *British Journal of Psychiatry*, 112 (1966), 809–818.

14. ———. "A Polygenic Theory of Schizophrenia," in L. Erlenmeyer-Kimling, ed., *Genetics and Mental Disorders, International Journal of Mental Health*, 1 (1971), 107–115.

15. HALLGREN, B., and T. SJÖGREN. "A Clinical and Genetico-Statistical Study of Schizophrenia and Low-Grade Mental Deficiency in a Large Swedish Rural Population," *Acta Psychiatrica et Neurologica Scandinavica*, Suppl. 140 (1959).

16. HESTON, L. L. "Psychiatric Disorders in Foster Home Reared Children of Schizophrenic Mothers," *British Journal of Psychiatry*, 112 (1966), 819–825.

17. INOUYE, E. "Similarity and Dissimilarity of Schizophrenia in Twins," in *Proceedings of Third World Congress of Psychiatry, Montreal*. Toronto: University of Toronto Press, 1961.

18. JACKSON, D. D. "A Critique of the Literature on the Genetics of Schizophrenia," in D. D. Jackson, ed., *The Study of Schizophrenia*. New York: Basic Books, Inc., 1959.

19. KALLMANN, F. J. *The Genetics of Schizophrenia*. Locust Valley: J. J. Augustin, 1938.

20. ———. "The Genetic Theory of Schizophrenia," *The American Journal of Psychiatry*, 103 (1946), 309–322.

21. KAPLAN, A. R. "Association of Schizophrenia with Non-Mendelian Genetic Anomalies," in A. R. Kaplan, ed., *Genetic Factors in Schizophrenia*. Springfield: Charles C. Thomas, 1971.

22. KARLSSON, J. L. *The Biologic Basis of Schizophrenia*. Springfield: Charles C. Thomas, 1966.

23. KAY, D. W. K. "Late Paraphrenia and Its Bearing on the Aetiology of Schizophrenia," *Acta Psychiatrica Scandinavica*, 39 (1963), 159–169.

24. KETY, S. S., D. ROSENTHAL, P. H. WENDER, and F. SCHULSINGER. "The Types and Prevalence of Mental Illness in the Biological and Adoptive Families of Adopted Schizophrenics," in D. Rosenthal and S. S. Kety, eds., *The Transmission of Schizophrenia*. London: Pergamon Press, 1968.

25. KOHN, M. "Social Class and Schizophrenia: A Critical Review," in D. Rosenthal and S. S. Kety, eds., *The Transmission of Schizophrenia*. London: Pergamon Press, 1968.

26. KOHN, M., and J. A. CLAUSEN. "Parental Authority Behavior and Schizophrenia," *American Journal of Orthopsychiatry*, 26 (1956), 297–313.

27. KRAEPELIN, E. *Psychiatrie*, 5th ed. Leipzig: Johann Ambrosius Barth, 1896.

28. KRINGLEN, E. "Hereditary and Social Factors in Schizophrenic Twins: An Epidemiological-Clinical Study," in J. Romano, ed., *The Origins of Schizophrenia*. Amsterdam: Excerpta Medica Foundation, 1967.

29. LIDZ, T. "The Family, Personality Development, and Schizophrenia," in J. Romano, ed., *The Origins of Schizophrenia*. Amsterdam: Excerpta Medica Foundation, 1967.

30. LUXENBURGER, H. "*Vorläufiger Bericht über Psychiatrische Sereinuntersuchungen an Zwillingen*," *Z. Ges. Neurol. Psychiat.*, 116 (1928), 297–347.

31. ———. "*Die Manifestationswahrscheinlichkeit der Schizophrenie im Lichte der Zwillingsforschung*," *Z. Psychol. Hyg.*, 7 (1934), 174–184.

32. ———. "*Zur frage der Erbberatung in den Familien Schizophrener*," *Med. Klin.*, 32 (1936), 1136–1138.

33. MEEHL, P. E. "Schizotaxia, Schizotypy, Schizophrenia," *American Psychologist*, 17 (1962), 827–838.

34. MENNINGER, K., with M. MAYMAN and P. PRUYSER. *The Vital Balance*. New York: The Viking Press, 1963.

35. MIRSKY, A. F. "Neuropsychological Bases of

Schizophrenia," in P. H. Mussen and M. R. Rosenzweig, eds., *Annual Review of Psychology*, 20 (1969), 321–348.

36. MITSUDA, H. "A Clinico-genetic Study of Schizophrenia," in H. Mitsuda, ed., *Clinical Genetics in Psychiatry*. Tokyo: Igaku Shoin, 1967.

37. POLLIN, W., M. G. ALLEN, A. HOFFER, J. R. STABENAU, and Z. HRUBEC. "Psychopathology in 15,909 Pairs of Veteran Twins," *The American Journal of Psychiatry*, 126 (1969), 597–609.

38. ROSANOFF, A. J., L. M. HANDY, I. R. PLESSET, and S. BRUSH. "The Etiology of So-called Schizophrenic Psychoses," *The American Journal of Psychiatry*, 91 (1934–1935), 247–286.

39. ROSENTHAL, D. "Some Factors Associated With Concordance and Discordance With Respect to Schizophrenia in Monozygotic Twins," *Journal of Nervous and Mental Disease*, 129 (1959), 1–10.

40. ———. "Confusion of Identity and the Frequency of Schizophrenia in Twins," *Archives of General Psychiatry*, 3 (1960), 297–304.

41. ———. "Sex Distribution and the Severity of Illness Among Samples of Schizophrenic Twins," *Journal of Psychiatric Research*, 1 (1961), 26–36.

42. ———. "Problems of Sampling and Diagnosis in the Major Twin Studies of Schizophrenia," *Journal of Psychiatric Research*, 1 (1962a), 116–134.

43. ———. "Familial Concordance by Sex With Respect to Schizophrenia," *Psychological Bulletin*, 59 (1962b), 401–421.

44. ———, ed. *The Genain Quadruplets*. New York: Basic Books, Inc., 1963.

45. ———. "The Offspring of Schizophrenic Couples," *Journal of Psychiatric Research*, 4 (1966), 169–188.

46. ———. *Genetic Theory and Abnormal Behavior*. New York: McGraw-Hill, 1970.

47. ———. "A Program of Research on Heredity in Schizophrenia," *Behavioral Science*, 16 (1971), 191–201.

48. ROSENTHAL, D., and S. S. KETY, eds. *The Transmission of Schizophrenia*. London: Pergamon Press, 1968.

49. ROSENTHAL, D., P. H. WENDER, S. S. KETY, J. WELNER, and F. SCHULSINGER. "The Adopted-Away Offspring of Schizophrenics," *The American Journal of Psychiatry*, 128 (1971), 307–311.

50. RÜDIN, E. *Zur Vererbung und Neuentstehung der Dementia Praecox*. Berlin: Springer Verlag OHG, 1916.

51. SCHEINFELD, A. *Twins and Supertwins*. Philadelphia: J. B. Lippincott Co., 1967.

52. SCHULTZ, B. "Zur Erbpathologie der Schizophrenie," *Z. Ges. Neurol. Psychiat.*, 143 (1932), 175–293.

53. SINGER, M. T. "Family Transactions and Schizophrenia: I," in J. Romano, ed., *The Origins of Schizophrenia*. Amsterdam: Excerpta Medica Foundation, 1967.

54. SLATER, E. *Psychotic and Neurotic Illnesses in Twins*. London: Her Majesty's Stationery Office, 1953.

55. ———. "The Monogenic Theory of Schizophrenia," *Acta Genetica*, 8 (1958), 50–56.

56. ———. "A Review of Earlier Evidence on Genetic Factors in Schizophrenia," in D. Rosenthal and S. S. Kety, eds., *The Transmission of Schizophrenia*. London: Pergamon Press, 1968.

57. STRÖMGREN, E. *Beiträge zur Psychiatrischen Erblehre*. Copenhagen: Munksgaard, 1938.

58. SZASZ, T. *The Myth of Mental Illness*. New York: Harper's, 1961.

59. TIENARI, P. "Psychiatric Illness in Identical Twins," *Acta Psychiatrica et Neurologica Scandinavica*, Suppl. 171 (1963).

60. ———. "Schizophrenia in Monozygotic Male Twins," in D. Rosenthal and S. S. Kety, eds., *The Transmission of Schizophrenia*. London: Pergamon Press, 1968.

61. VARTANYAN, M. E., and V. M. GINDILIS. "The Role of Chromosomal Aberrations in the Clinical Polymorphism of Schizophrenia," in L. Erlenmeyer-Kimbling, ed., *Genetics and Mental Disorders, International Journal of Mental Health*, 1 (1971), 93–106.

62. WENDER, P. H., D. ROSENTHAL, and S. S. KETY. "A Psychiatric Assessment of the Adoptive Parents of Schizophrenics," in D. Rosenthal and S. S. Kety, eds., *The Transmission of Schizophrenia*. London: Pergamon Press, 1968.

63. WYNNE, L. C. "Family Transactions and Schizophrenia: II," in J. Romano, ed., *The Origins of Schizophrenia*. Amsterdam: Excerpta Medica Foundation, 1967.

64. WYNNE, L. C., I. M. RYCKOFF, J. DAY, and S. I. HIRSCH. "Pseudomutuality in the Family Relations of Schizophrenics," *Psychiatry*, 22 (1958), 205–220.

CHAPTER 26

THE BIOCHEMISTRY OF SCHIZOPHRENIA

Charles E. Frohman and Jacques S. Gottlieb

IN DISCUSSING research in schizophrenia, D. W. Woolley once wrote that "new and revolutionary scientific discoveries do not leap into the world complete and final as Athene was said to have sprung, mature and fully armed, from the head of Zeus. Instead, they come stumbling into view not fully formed nor completely ready to defend themselves from any possible attack. They come to full stature only as the result of modifications to meet their shortcomings."[179] Our knowledge of the biology of schizophrenia most certainly is not complete or final. Many interesting discoveries have been made but they are just beginning to form an intelligible picture. It may well be that in the next few years these ideas will come to full stature and that then we will have a complete understanding of the biology of this disease. At the present time, only some very interesting research trends and numerous unconnected bits of information can be presented.

(Plasma Proteins

Many workers have speculated on the possibility that a toxic factor is present in the blood of schizophrenic patients. One of the earliest reports was that of Macht.[119] He showed that human serum retarded plant growth and that the retardation was greatest when serum from schizophrenic patients was used. Rieder[142] showed that serum from schizophrenic patients caused spiders to spin bizarre webs and again attributed this to a toxic substance in the blood. Bishop[20] showed that, in rats, reward learning was severely retarded by the administration of serum from schizophrenic patients but that avoidance learning was hardly affected at all. Winter and Flataker,[178] using the reward system, showed that the material affecting rat behavior was a protein. Bergen et al.[14] carried this work further and were able to separate and characterize the protein. Two other groups (Frohman[63] and Lozovsky[116]) have confirmed the work of

Bergen[11] and have been studying the same protein. These three groups have produced many similar findings on this protein. All three groups used different isolation techniques. Bergen et al. used a zinc-EDTA complex to isolate their protein. This protein when injected into rats caused a reduction of the rat's ability to perform a simple learned task, i.e., climbing a rope to receive a reward. Frohman et al.[72] isolated the protein by means of DEAE cellulose chromatography followed by electrophoresis and finally ultracentrifugation with a sucrose gradient. They tested the protein by its effect on the ratio of lactic acid to pyruvic acid (L/P ratio) in chicken erythrocytes incubated with the protein. The protein from the schizophrenic patients caused a higher L/P ratio. Later, as an indicator, they used the protein's ability to increase the uptake of tryptophan by cells.[74] Through a series of studies in which factors were exchanged on a blind basis, it was shown that the protein factors that the two groups[14,72] were working on were identical.[13] Samples isolated by Bergen et al., using their isolation procedures and known to affect their rat climbing-time measure, also affected the L/P ratio in chicken erythrocytes and the uptake of tryptophan by the cell (the measures used by Frohman et al.). Samples isolated by Frohman et al. and found active by their methods also affected rat climbing-time when tested by Bergen et al. The group headed by Lozovsky[116] has isolated the same protein. They used a modification of Frohman's method for the isolation of their protein and the same technique as Frohman for detecting it. In all likelihood, these methods have yielded the same protein. Frohman and the Lafayette Clinic group[64] found that their protein was an a-2-globulin as did Pennell[136] on the fraction isolated by the Worcester group. The Russians, however, reported that their protein was a β globulin.[116] This apparent difference in electrophoretic mobility probably arises from the use of two different electrophoretic systems (the Spinco CP electrophoretic apparatus used by the Lafayette Clinic and the Russian-made apparatus of the Academy of Science) and certainly does not suggest that

the two groups are working on different proteins. Quite the contrary, the similarity between the biological effects reported by the different groups working on the factor would indicate that all are working on the same protein.

In studying the plasma protein further, the Lafayette Clinic[74] found that it significantly increased the ratio of intracellular to extracellular tryptophan and 5-hydroxytryptophan while that of most other amino acids is affected only slightly. Further work[73] has shown that bovine brain incubated with the protein from patients produced more dimethyltryptamine (DMT) than bovine brain incubated with the same protein isolated from nonschizophrenic subjects. The effect of increased production of DMT will be discussed in the section on indole amines. Many other attributes of this protein have been investigated. The Russian Institute[116] claims that complement enhanced the activity of the a-2-globulin. The Worcester Foundation group[14] showed that the protein decreased the amplitude, increased the latency and increased the variability of photically evoked EEG responses in the rabbit. The Lafayette Clinic group[38] has found that when the protein is injected into the lateral sinus of a rat's brain it decreased the rate at which the animal will press a bar to receive pleasureable sensations from stimulation of the medial forebrain bundle. This possibly may mean that the protein blocks the enjoyment of pleasure stimulations in the rats. Using a clinical classification system which differs from that used in the United States, Lozovsky[116] has demonstrated that the activity of the a-2-globulin is related to the malignancy of the disorder. The more rapidly the patient deteriorates, the more active is the a-2-globulin. By measuring the activity of the protein upon admission to the hospital and at bimonthly intervals afterwards, they have been able to demonstrate that the activity of the factor is high on admission, that it increases for about two years, then levels off. The activity of the plasma diminishes only after ten or more years. The Russians interpret this as an indication of a relationship between the active process and the protein. Thus, at two years after the start of the disease, the process is at its most active stage, and after ten years or more the process has discontinued and the patient has entered a chronic deteriorated level of the disorder.

Other groups have isolated a protein from the blood of schizophrenic patients similar to and possibly identical to the α-2-globulin. Walaas and co-workers[86] have isolated a protein which affects the uptake of glucose by rat hemidiaphragm and have indicated that it is a β-globulin, and Ehrensvaard[54] has isolated a protein which affects the oxidation of an aromatic amine.

As mentioned previously, Bergen[14] found that the α-2-globulin affected evoked potentials. A labile serum factor which decreases the amplitude of evoked potentials recorded from the cerebral cortex and limbic system structures of cats has also been described by Fayvishevsky and Nemtsov.[57] Another serum neurotropic factor is said by Fayvishevsky to affect the spontaneous electroencephalogram and to be stable during storage. Until protein fractionation techniques are applied to purify these latter two neurotropic factors, one can only speculate about their possible relationships to the α-2-globulin.

Biochemical and Biophysical Nature of the α-2-globulin

All three groups (the Worcester Foundation, the Lafayette Clinic, and the Russians) agree that the protein has quite a high molecular weight, the Lafayette Clinic group placing the molecular weight around 400,000. All agree that the molecule contains a great deal of lipid (about 80 per cent lipid, according to the Lafayette Clinic group). They also agree that the activity is quite labile and the protein can be inactivated by heating, freezing, or aging, and that it can be protected with compounds which inhibit sulfhydryl oxidation such as ascorbic acid, mercaptoethanol, and sucrose. The activity is preserved best if the protein solution is adjusted to pH 6–8 and stored at about 4° C. The protein appears to bind large amounts of ethylenediaminetetraacetic acid (EDTA).[137] Pennell felt that this

indicated that the protein might also bind a metal. His careful and thorough analysis for metal in the protein showed that the protein contained only trace amounts of any metals believed to be involved with biologically active proteins. Consequently, he discarded the idea that a metallic ion was involved with the protein. Nevertheless, Bergen[11] demonstrated that the activity of the protein could, through double dialysis, be transferred from an active protein to an inactive one. This indicates that the activity of the protein could be contained in a small molecule attached to the protein. As a possible aid to the identification of this small molecule Pennell[136] demonstrated that a portion of the protein was chromogenic; upon heating, it formed a red pigment with an absorption spectrum consistent with a quinone derivative of a catecholamine or indole.

The Lafayette Clinic group[69] has isolated the α-2-globulin in relatively pure form; they refer to it as the S-protein. Examination by disc gel electrophoresis, analytical ultracentrifugation, and DEAE cellulose chromatography revealed only a single component. Using this homogeneous protein, further careful studies became possible. Earlier, it was believed that the level of the S-protein was higher in schizophrenic patients than in control subjects, but following the isolation of pure fractions, it could be shown that there was no difference in the level of this protein between the blood of control subjects and schizophrenic patients.

Other properties of the S-protein were investigated in an effort to explain the difference in effect of this protein in plasma from schizophrenic patients and control subjects upon tryptophan accumulation in cells. This difference of the effect of the S-protein must be the result of some difference within the protein molecule isolated from the two types of subjects. Amino acid content of the protein isolated from control subjects and that of the protein isolated from schizophrenic patients were the same. In addition, the levels of cholesterol and of fatty acid were the same in both samples so that the difference in activity could not be attributed to a difference in the lipid content.

The tertiary structure of the S-protein was investigated by means of optical rotatory dispersion. In this procedure, the rotation of polarized light at various wavelengths is indicative of certain organized structures. The protein isolated from schizophrenic patients was found by Harmison and Frohman[88] to be primarily in the α-helical conformation. They found that the inactive protein from control subjects had little or no α-helical conformation, and was primarily in the β and/or random chain form (Figure 26–1). In other

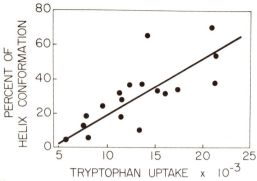

Figure 26–2.   Correlation between tryptophan uptake and percentage of α-helix in the molecule of S-protein.

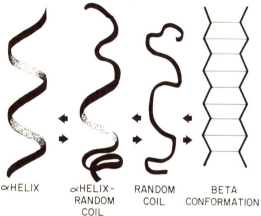

α HELIX   α HELIX - RANDOM COIL   RANDOM COIL   BETA CONFORMATION

Figure 26–1.   Graphic representation of three conformations which the tertiary structure of a protein can assume.

words the shape of the protein molecule isolated from plasma from schizophrenic patients is very different from the shape of the one isolated from the control subjects.

It has been known for some time that the shape of some proteins is intimately related to their biological activity, although laboratory evidence from work with purified proteins has been relatively scarce. Definite proof has now been presented that this is the case with the S-protein. Figure 26–2 shows the correlation between tryptophan uptake and the percentage of α-helix in the molecule. The correlation coefficient is 0.84 (P < 0.01). From this correlation, it can be postulated that the α-helical form of this protein is responsible for its effect on tryptophan accumulation.

Frohman and co-workers[66] have isolated a second protein which counteracts the effect of the S-protein. This anti-S-protein is present in both human and animal tissue.[74] It is purified by starch block electrophoresis followed by

DEAE cellulose chromatography. The activity is enhanced by administering norepinephrine to the animal before the tissue is removed. There is four times as much activity in brain as in erythrocytes. It has been demonstrated that the α-helical form of the S-protein is converted to the random chain conformation when incubated with the anti-S-protein. At the same time the effect of the S-protein on tryptophan levels in the cell is negated. Levels of the anti-S-protein have been measured in the human brain from both schizophrenic and nonschizophrenic patients and are almost four times as high in the nonschizophrenic patients.[74] It is suggested that the large amount of the α-helical form of the S-protein in the schizophrenic patients could result from the lack of anti-S-protein in brains of schizophrenic patients, and that the excess of the α-helical form of the S-protein results in the changes observed in tryptophan metabolism.

⟨ Biologically Active Amines

Much work concerning the biochemistry of schizophrenia has focused upon indole amines and catecholamines. This occurred after the discovery of how the action of reserpine, the earliest tranquilizing drug used to treat schizophrenia, is related to the binding of catechol and indole amines. These two classes of compounds, both believed to be involved in nerve transmission, came under systematic study. Since reserpine releases some of the bound serotonin and bound norepinephrine present in the brain,[28] thereby lowering the amount of serotonin and norepinephrine available for nerve transmission in the midbrain, it is probable that the tranquilizing action of this drug involved depletion of one or both of these neurotransmitters in the midbrain.

Indole Amines

The observation that some naturally occurring analogs of serotonin (e.g., LSD and bufotenine) could cause symptoms which resembled some of those found in schizophrenia made work with the indoles even more intriguing. Since lowered serotonin apparently caused improvement of symptoms, administration of these structural analogs probably increases the apparent level of serotonin through some sort of agonistic action. Woolley[180] predicted that synthetic analogs of serotonin would cause hallucinations when given to humans, and then actually proved that this was the case with the benzyl analog of serotonin. The interest in serotonin spread to other physiological indoles and to their precursor in mammalian metabolism, the aromatic amino acid, tryptophan. Figure 26-3

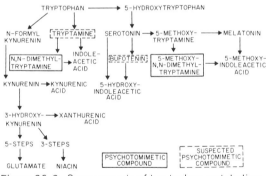

Figure 26-3. Some aspects of tryptophan metabolism.

shows several of the pathways by which tryptophan is metabolized in the body. It can be hydroxylated to 5-hydroxytryptophan which then can be converted to serotonin. A limiting step in this conversion is the 5-hydroxylation to 5-hydroxytryptophan.[124] Serotonin (a neurotransmitter) can be O-methylated and N-acetylated to form melatonin (a compound closely connected with sleep and diurnal rhythm). Serotonin can also be N-

methylated to form bufotenine. O-methylated serotonin can be N-methylated to form N,N-dimethyl-5-methoxytryptamine. Both bufotenine and N,N-dimethyl-5-methoxytryptamine are reputed to be psychotomimetic. Serotonin and melatonin are also oxidized to 5-hydroxyindoleacetic acid, the normal excretion product. On the other side of the scheme, tryptophan can be decarboxylated to form tryptamine. If an excess of tryptophan is present, most of the excess is likely to be disposed of in this manner since the 5-hydroxylation is the rate-limiting step. Tryptamine can then be methylated to N,N-dimethyltryptamine (another psychotomimetic compound) or oxidized to indoleacetic acid (an excretion product). In addition, tryptophan can be converted to kynurenine and ultimately to niacin. All of these pathways could be involved in some way in schizophrenia.

Many workers[143,183] have shown that loading the diet with tryptophan results in a number of abnormal indole metabolites appearing in the urine of schizophrenic patients, suggesting the possibility that deviant indole metabolism may play a significant role in schizophrenia. However, the presence of some of these abnormal metabolites has not always been confirmed when other laboratories repeated the original studies.

Studies that are more sophisticated seem to indicate that indoles may play a role in producing the symptoms of schizophrenia. Much attention has been centered on the methylation of both indole and catecholamines. Pollin and co-workers[140] caused exacerbation of schizophrenic symptoms by feeding methionine and a monoamine oxidase inhibitor simultaneously. Substituting tryptophan for the methionine produced some effect on symptoms but not as great an effect as with methionine. This would indicate that increased methylation of indoles may be related to exacerbation of schizophrenic symptoms. Alexander et al.[3] were able to repeat the study of Pollin with the same results. Kakimoto[103] also administered methionine and a MAO inhibitor and caused symptoms to worsen. After administration, an increase of methylcatecholamines and indoles was found in the urine of the patients. In a similar experiment by Jus et al.,[101] tryptamine was found to increase in urine of the patients before exacerbation occurred. Administration of α-methyldopamine by Herkert and co-workers[95] also caused exacerbation of symptoms. He reported a decrease in the excretion of 5-hydroxyindoleacetic acid and an increase in urinary tryptamine, possibly suggesting that the exacerbation was the result of a block in the conversion of tryptophan to 5-hydroxytryptophan. Spaide et al.[160] substituted cysteine for methionine. Again, behavior worsened and indole excretion increased. The behavioral worsening appeared to correlate very closely with the excretion of the indole amines, many of which were not those usually found in normal urine. However, Feldstein[58] reported that the excretion of indoles was probably more closely related to urine volume than to symptoms, but in his experiment he did not make clear whether the urine volume increased because of the extra indoles or whether the reverse was true. In another series of experiments,[59] he administered labeled serotonin to schizophrenic patients and control subjects and found no difference in the conversion of serotonin to 5-hydroxyindoleacetic acid in the two groups. Therefore, he hypothesized that serotonin was not involved in schizophrenia. From the data of others indicating increased tryptamine excretion during exacerbation of schizophrenic symptoms, it would be logical to expect that the conversion of tryptophan to 5-hydroxytryptophan was the faulty step. Under the circumstances, one would not expect much effect on the metabolism of serotonin. A better approach would have been to study excretory products, particularly tryptamine, indoleacetic acid, 5-hydroxytryptamine, and 5-hydroxyindoleacetic acid, following administration of labeled tryptophan. According to Naneishvili,[128] plasma from schizophrenic patients, especially from the acutely ill, elevated the blood levels of serotonin when administered to dogs. The elevation was reported to be accompanied by a corresponding fall in the excretion of the serotonin metabolite, 5-hydroxyindoleacetic acid. This, of course, is the oppo-

site of the results described by Feldstein.

If tryptophan metabolism is particularly responsible for some of the symptoms of schizophrenia, one would expect that a decrease of the indole content of the diet might cause amelioration of the symptoms. Berlet et al.,[16] however, have shown that a decrease of indoles in the diet causes no improvement in schizophrenic patients. On the other hand, Dohan[51] claims that schizophrenic patients do improve on a gluten-free diet. Gluten is unusually low in tryptophan but extremely high in glutamic acid. This result is very difficult to reconcile with other evidence.

Not only are there more indole amines excreted during the exacerbation of schizophrenic symptoms but these indole amines contain more methylated products than those found in urine of nonschizophrenic subjects.[31,33] Berlet et al.[15] have now identified two of those methylated products as N,N-dimethyltryptamine (DMT) and 5-methoxy-N,N-dimethyltryptamine (5-methoxy-DMT). Fischer[61] has confirmed that there are methylated indoles in urine from schizophrenic patients. He identified the indole as bufotenine but it is questionable whether his method could differentiate between bufotenine and DMT. Even more to the point, Heller et al.[92] have found DMT and 5-methoxy-DMT in the blood of acute schizophrenic patients but not in the blood of control subjects.

The presence of methylated indoles in the body fluids of schizophrenic patients is very interesting and important indeed. Most of these compounds are known to be potent psychotomimetic agents. If these compounds are present in the schizophrenic patients, then it could be possible that they are responsible for some of the symptoms of schizophrenia. The behavioral effects of administering methylated indoles to humans have been thoroughly described.[182] To be sure, these effects are quite different from the symptoms of schizophrenia. However, this does not necessarily mean that these indoles are not responsible for the symptoms of schizophrenia since the acute effects of a drug (as in the case of administering a single dose) can be quite different from the chronic effect (as the result of the presence of the compound over periods of years in the schizophrenic patient if produced *in vivo*).

Unless enzymes capable of converting indoles to methylated derivatives can be found in human tissue, a theory involving production of methylated indoles would not be of much value. Such an enzyme has been isolated from the human brain.[125] As mentioned previously, Frohman and co-workers[69] demonstrated that the a-helical form of the S-protein increased the uptake of 5-hydroxytryptophan and tryptophan by cells. This excess in the cell might then be converted to methylated derivatives. In a study of the effect of the S-protein on bovine hypothalamus it has been shown that in the presence of the a-helical S-protein, bovine hypothalamus produces almost two and one-half times as much DMT as it does in the presence of the nonhelical protein.[73] Further evidence that indoles enter the cell in greater amounts in schizophrenic patients was presented by Polishchuk,[139] who found that oral administration of 10 gm. of tryptophan caused a much larger increase in urinary indicans, anthranilic acid, kynurenine and 5-hydroxyindoleacetic acid from the patients than from control subjects.

Methylated indole amines could be at higher levels in the schizophrenic patient for several reasons: (1) increased methylation due to more active N-methyl transferase, (2) increased amounts of methylating agents such as methionine, (3) increased amounts of tryptophan and other indoles in the cell. The work of Frohman would indicate the latter is true. The experiments on methionine feeding lend some credence to the increased methylation hypotheses. However, an increased level of methionine has never been found in schizophrenia and the work of Frohman has shown that the a-helical S-protein has no effect on the uptake of methionine by the cell. There still remains the possibility that the brain of the schizophrenic patient could have a highly increased N-methyl transferase activity. This hypothesis is very attractive and has been proposed by many workers.[7,36,158] Recent work by Domino,[52] however, has failed to reveal any difference in N-methyl transferase activity between brains from nonschizophrenic and schizophrenic patients.

Regardless of how the methylated indoles are formed, the evidence indicates that they may play an important role in the production of schizophrenia. There is a possibility that there is also a change in serotonin level which could be related in some way to the schizophrenic process. Both the serotonin level and the level of methylated indoles could be affected by an increase of tryptophan in the cell, but since the 5-hydroxylation of tryptophan is the limiting reaction in the scheme (Figure 26–3), the effect of excess tryptophan would have a more pronounced effect on DMT production than it would on serotonin production.

Other studies indicating that tryptophan metabolism through the kynurenine pathway is somewhat different in schizophrenia have been performed by Brown and co-workers[31] who found a decrease in the excretion in kynurenine metabolites in schizophrenia. However, Benassi[9] found the opposite result i.e., that the metabolites of the kynurenine pathway were increased, especially 3-hydroxykynurenine which was increased threefold. On the other hand, Faurbye[55] reports that the excretion of kynurenine metabolites is completely normal in schizophrenia. It does not appear that any definite information has been gained from study of the kynurenine pathway to date.

Catecholamines

Besides serotonin, a second compound released by reserpine and also active in nerve transmission is norepinephrine, a demethylated epinephrine derivative. Norepinephrine and its analogs belong to a class of compounds called catecholamines, characterized chemically by an alkyl amine group attached to a dihydroxy phenol. Hoffer[97] first suggested that adrenochrome, an oxidation product of epinephrine, might be responsible for psychotic symptoms. He synthesized adrenochrome, administered it to volunteers, and claimed that they then showed psychotic symptoms. Attempts by others to repeat this were unsuccessful. Axelrod[5] demonstrated that epinephrine was disposed of not only by oxidation but by methylation of the hydroxyl groups on the phenol portion of the molecule. The previously described experiments of Pollin et al.,[140] in which they administered methionine and iproniazid, were primarily designed to determine if methylated catecholamines could cause exacerbation of symptoms, and the results they obtained could equally implicate catecholamines as well as indoles.

Figure 26–4 shows the metabolism of catecholamines in the body.

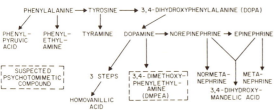

Figure 26–4. Some aspects of catecholamine metabolism.

Phenylalanine is converted to tyrosine which accepts a second hydroxyl group to form dihydroxyphenylalanine (DOPA). This is then decarboxylated to form dopamine. Dopamine can be O-methylated to form 3,4-dimethoxyphenylethylamine (DMPEA). Dopamine can also be hydroxylated to form norepinephrine, which in some portions of the body, but not to any appreciable extent in the brain, is N-methylated to form epinephrine. Inside the cell, norepinephrine and epinephrine are oxidized to 3,4-dihydroxymandelic acid, while outside the cell in the synaptic cleft they are O-methylated to form normetanephrine and metanephrine respectively. The strong parallels between catechol metabolism and indole metabolism can be seen immediately. In many steps, the same or similar enzymes catalyze the reactions involved in the anabolism and catabolism of both the catecholamines and indole amines.

Just as in the case of the indole amines, there are reports of increased catecholamines being excreted in the urine during exacerbation of schizophrenic symptoms.[129] Himwich

has proposed that the increase of catecholamines and derivatives in the urine during exacerbation of schizophrenic symptoms is the result of increased activity in the patient and is not related to the symptoms of the disease. Some of the methylated metabolites of catecholamines are psychotomimetic. As stated previously, among the methylated indoles DMT is psychotomimetic. In a parallel manner, mescaline is a prime example of a methylated catecholamine which is psychotomimetic.

Smythies[157] has shown that all 4-methoxy catecholamines are hallucinogenic and that the most potent is the 2,4,5-methoxy compound. Hall[87] demonstrated that administration of O-methyltransferase, the enzyme which forms O-methyl catecholamines, caused exacerbation of schizophrenic symptoms. Friedhoff[62] demonstrated that discernible amounts of a 4-methylated catecholamine, DMPEA, were found in urine from acute schizophrenic patients but not from control subjects. This work has been confirmed by others.[25] However, two other groups[56,164] were unable to confirm it. Barbeau[8] showed that injection of DMPEA in the rat caused increased dopamine level in tissue and proposed that it may block dopaminergic nerve endings while Hoffer[96] claimed that dopamine is elevated in schizophrenia. Upon administering DMPEA to trained rats, Bergen[10] found that it produced marked behavioral effects which resembled very closely the effects of the α-helical S protein. However, Wagner[175] has shown that tissue from schizophrenic patients is incapable of synthesizing DMPEA. More recently, Siegel and Tefft[154] have shown that part of the chromatographic spot that was previously believed to be DMPEA was due to metabolites of tranquilizing drugs and that when this portion was subtracted the amount of DMPEA in urine from control subjects and schizophrenic patients was the same.

If norepinephrine were involved in schizophrenia, it would seem reasonable that administering α-methyl-p-tyrosine, which blocks norepinephrine synthesis, would affect schizophrenic symptoms. Two different groups[43,79] have shown that this compound has no effect at all on behavior of schizophrenic patients.

(Abnormal Antibodies

Malis,[120] in 1959, claimed to have found a specific antigen from schizophrenic patients. He demonstrated the presence of this antibody both by complement fixation and anaphylaxis in guinea pigs. Semenov and collaborators[152] reported that they were able to detect brain antigen in serum and cerebrospinal fluid in schizophrenic patients during the period of exacerbation of symptoms. At a later stage in the course of the illness, after the appearance of brain antigen, antibrain antibodies were discovered. For those patients who developed antibrain antibodies, a significantly greater familial incidence of psychoses was found; as a rule, the mothers of these patients suffered from various neuropsychiatric disorders, including schizophrenia. The possibility is under consideration by Semenov that the central nervous system of the child may be subjected to immunopathological effects that will cause the child to manifest the disease later.

Heath[110] has presented evidence that schizophrenia may be the result of an antigen-antibody disturbance. For many years, he has been working with a plasma protein factor which he named taraxein. Recently, he has discovered that this γ-globulin is an antibody.[90] Previously, Heath had been able to demonstrate that injection of this protein into normal human volunteers could give rise to the symptoms of schizophrenia.[91] By using fluorescein-tagged anti-human γ-globulin along with taraxein, Heath was also able to demonstrate *in vitro* attachment of taraxein to neural cell nuclei in the septal region of the patient's brain.[90] This protein did not attach itself to any other area of the brain, therefore he claimed it must be considered a specific antibody to the septal region. Heath had previously shown that in schizophrenia, subjects

often show abnormal EEG spiking and slow wave activity in the septal region of the brain. His conclusion therefore was that this antibody, taraxein, caused abnormal functioning of the septal area. In order to determine if such a situation could give rise to schizophrenic symptoms, Heath produced antiseptal antibody by injecting septal tissue into sheep and isolating the antibodies produced. These antibodies when administered to monkeys did give rise to focal abnormal EEG's from the septal region and led to catatonic behavior. Sheep γ-immunoglobulin reactive to parts other than the septal region of monkey and human brains caused no discernible changes in EEG's or behavior of test monkeys. To this extent, Heath claims to have proved his point that schizophrenia is a disease involving damage to a specific area of the brain by an antibody. It should be added that full confirmation of this work has not yet been achieved. Logan and Deodhar[114] were unable to repeat Heath and Krupp's work, reporting only negative results. Whittingham and co-workers[177] were also unable to repeat Heath's work. In fact, the work with the technique of using fluorescein-tagged anti-human γ-globulin is certainly open to question since this type of process usually stains cytoplasm not nuclei. Bergen has partially confirmed Heath's work by showing that injection of taraxein from schizophrenic patients was more likely to cause focal abnormal EEG's than the same protein fraction from control subjects, but the results were inconsistent.[12]

Kuznetsova[109] also reported antibrain antibody in serum from schizophrenic patients but these were antibodies to brain mitochondria rather than to nuclei. Stoimenov,[162] using complement fixation methods, reported that 79 percent of the paranoid schizophrenic patients had antibody to white matter and subcortical nuclei. Kolyaskina[107] also showed antibrain antibodies in the serum of more schizophrenic patients than control subjects. She found, however, that after stress, the antibrain antibodies rose in the control subjects to the point where there was a higher percentage of control subjects than schizophrenic patients with these antibodies. In order to study the mechanism of this process, rabbits were given electroshock treatment to cause the production of the antibrain antibodies. Kolyaskina theorized that stress or electric shock or both affected the permeability of the blood-brain barrier, causing brain proteins and plasma to come in close contact and in turn producing the antibrain antibodies. The activity of the S-protein previously discussed has been shown to increase following stress.[71] It is only a short step then to reason that since the S-protein affects membrane permeability, the presence of antibrain antibodies could be a result of this protein, and the mechanism of action of the a-helical S-protein may be through the production of antibodies which affect the functioning of the brain. There are other indications that membrane permeability is affected in schizophrenia. Meltzer[123] has shown that two enzymes, creatine phosphokinase and aldolase, are both circulating in plasma at higher levels than would be expected unless membrane damage had taken place. Lozovsky[117] reports that lactic dehydrogenase (LDH) is elevated in serum from schizophrenic patients. The LDH is apparently from brain cells as shown by a study of the distribution of the isoenzymes. He attributes it almost completely to the damaging action of the previously described S-protein on the cell membrane.

Many workers have reported abnormal immunoglobulin levels in schizophrenia; none of them, however, report the same immunoglobulin to be abnormal. Strahilevitz[163] reported increased IgA but normal levels of IgG and IgM. Bock and co-workers[21] reported IgA and IgG normal with IgM slightly lowered.

Gosheva[84] has investigated the morphological features of lymphocytes from schizophrenic patients. *In vitro*, lymphocytes from schizophrenic patients underwent spontaneous blast-transformation. The neuroblasts appeared to connect themselves to normal lymphocytes by means of plasmatic bridges. DNA granules have been seen in these plasmatic bridges, suggesting that the neuroblasts are able to pass information to the target cells

they contact by means of nuclear substances. Many additional changes took place in the leukocytes, such as vacuolization, granular decomposition of the cytoplasm, picnosis, and nuclear lysis. The changes described above all could be attributed to an immune reaction so that this effect may be related to antibody production in schizophrenia. Knowles and co-workers,[106] however, demonstrated that blast formation in leukocytes in schizophrenia is the result of administering phenothiazines and not of the disease.

In addition to the change in appearance of these cells, Glazov[82] has shown that the metabolism of the leukocytes is abnormal in schizophrenic patients. This abnormality is a diffuse effect in which the activity of practically all oxidative enzymes is decreased. Even more interesting is the increase he reported in sulfhydryl groups in the leukocytes. This was confirmed by Chalisov[42] who also showed an increase in sulfhydryl groups in the protein-free filtrate of blood serum from patients. He also reported a difference in the level of several metallic ions between the blood of schizophrenic patients and control subjects. This has not as yet been confirmed.

Because of the many claims of elevated antibodies, Solomon[159] used antimetabolites to change γ-globulin levels in subjects in an attempt to influence their behavior. He was unsuccessful. To make things even more complicated, Fessel[60] reported that psychotics, especially schizophrenics, had higher serum levels of S_{19} macroglobulin as compared to control subjects. This is an a-globulin which is different from the one Frohman reported. Zahradnicka[181] reported a decrease in albumin and an increase in a-globulin in schizophrenia, while Kopeloff[108] reported that schizophrenic patients have higher β- and a-globulin, but there was no indication that immunoglobulins are higher.

Through all the confusion involving the various changes of levels of antibodies, there is a strong possibility that all of the results reported are nonspecific effects more closely related to hospitalization than to schizophrenia. No consistent pattern has developed concerning elevated antibodies in schizophrenia.

From all of this, it is quite clear that a definitive experiment linking immunoglobulins with schizophrenia has not been performed and it is doubtful if it ever will be.

❰ Hemolytic Factors

Many groups of workers have reported the hemolytic effect of plasma from schizophrenic patients on erythrocytes of humans, chickens, and rabbits. Durell and co-workers[144] at the National Institutes of Health have reported a hemolysin present in the blood of schizophrenic patients. They have theorized that the hemolysin and the S-protein are one and the same and that the previously described biochemical effects of the S-protein are merely the result of hemolysis. They arrived at this conclusion after observing that the rate of hemolysis of chicken erythrocytes incubated in plasma from schizophrenic patients correlated with the increase in L/P ratio of the same cells. Also, in a study of red cells from schizophrenic patients, Lideman[112] found that the red cells from the patients were significantly more prone to hemolysis by 0.004N HCL than those of control subjects, and that cells from the patients with a more malignant form of the disease were significantly more prone to hemolysis than cells from patients with a sluggish form. His thorough study of the kinetics of the hemolysis led him to conclude that the action of the hemolysin was not an antibody reaction but probably a reaction with a lipid peroxide. As did Durell, Lideman attributed the action of the S-protein to the effects of the hemolysin.

Neither Lozovsky[116] nor Frohman[64] is in agreement with the above conclusion. The Russian Institute and the Lafayette Clinic group have reported that hemolysis of chicken erythrocytes correlates with the effect of the S-protein on the L/P ratio but both groups have shown that the hemolytic effect and the metabolic effect are separable. The Russian Institute demonstrated that heating the serum caused the loss of metabolic activity before hemolytic activity was lost, and the Lafayette Clinic group separated two distinct proteins responsible for the two effects. The Lafayette Clinic group have shown the hemolysin to be a β-2-globulin instead of an α-globulin. In view of this, it is impossible that the hemolysin and the S-protein are identical. It is possible that the hemolysin is the result of the long hospitalization connected with schizophrenia and is not related to the etiology of the disease. It is equally possible that damage to the red cell membrane by the S-protein permits the production of the hemolysin. The α-helical form of the S-protein probably increases the intracellular tryptophan and 5-hydroxytryptophan concentration through a change in cell membrane permeability. An alteration of this sort could possibly permit extracellular protein to come in contact with intracellular protein, thus leading to the production of an antibody to the intracellular protein. Most hemolysins are antibodies to intracellular proteins.

Uzunov and co-workers[170,171] have shown that a factor affects the permeability of the erythrocyte membrane to $P^{32}O_4$. When cells are treated with chlorpromazine, trifluoperazine, or insulin, less radioactive phosphate is taken up by the cells in the presence of this protein factor. This effect is the greatest with cells from schizophrenic patients. They therefore hypothesize that a factor present in the blood of schizophrenic subjects reduces permeability of the erythrocytes to $P^{32}O_4$. Moreover, they have isolated proteins that have this activity from the spinal fluid of schizophrenic patients. After protein electrophoresis most activity was in the pre-albumin fraction, distinguishing this factor from the S-protein and from the hemolysin which appears to be a β-2-globulin.

❰ Carbohydrate Metabolism

Carbohydrate metabolism is one of the earliest topics studied by workers in schizophrenia. Many have tried to determine glucose tolerance in schizophrenic patients.[6] Some have reported abnormal glucose tolerance following oral administration of glucose. Both the nutritional condition and physical condition of patients in hospitals probably have more to do with the abnormal glucose tolerance results than does schizophrenia. In fact, in many of the reports all mental patients are reported to have abnormal tolerance test results rather than just schizophrenic patients. If the patients are prepared by feeding high carbohydrate diets for three days before the test, the abnormality usually disappears, indicating that subclinical malnutrition probably is the biggest factor in producing abnormal glucose tolerance.[153] While oral glucose tolerances are quite often abnormal, rapid intravenous glucose tolerance tests never show this abnormality.[94] This might, of course, indicate some abnormality in transport of glucose across membranes even though malnutrition may play a large role. It is somewhat surprising how often membrane transport appears to be involved in deficiencies in schizophrenia. To bolster somewhat the idea that membrane transport might be involved here, one can cite the work of Walaas and co-workers[86] in which they showed that glucose uptake by rat hemidiaphragm is impaired by serum from schizophrenic patients. Later, these workers were able to isolate a plasma protein which was responsible for this. This protein may be identical to the S-protein. The metabolism of glucose by the cell is shown in Figure 26–5.

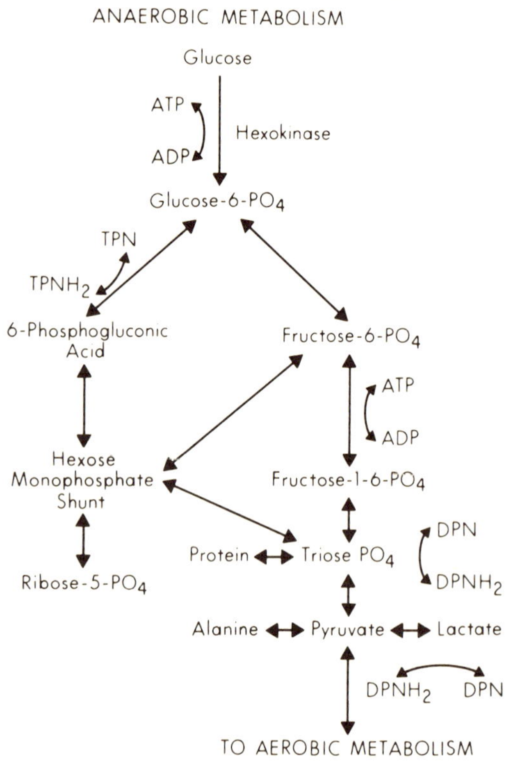

Glucose may be converted by means of the Embden-Meyerhof scheme to the hexosephosphates and triosephosphates, then to lactic and pyruvic acids. It may be oxidized to glucuronic acid and passed through the hexosemonophosphate shunt forming pentose phosphate, and then pyruvate. Pyruvate is oxidized to carbon dioxide and water by means of the tricarboxylic acid cycle. It is first converted to acetyl coenzyme A which is then combined with oxalacetic acid to form citric acid. Citrate is converted in turn to cis-aconitate, isocitrate, a-ketoglutarate, succinate, fumarate, malate, and finally back to oxalacetate. During one turn of the cycle one molecule of pyruvate is oxidized to carbon dioxide and water and the energy is stored in ATP.

Upon administering glucose to schizophrenic patients, blood lactate and pyruvate

Figure 26–5.   An abbreviated representation of the scheme of anaerobic metabolism of glucose.

increase abnormally.[94] This is the opposite response to that obtained in diabetes.[17] In addition, a-ketoglutarate levels are increased. Experiments indicating that blood lactate and pyruvate concentration increase after exercise in schizophrenia probably demonstrate the poor physical conditioning of a patient rather than some metabolic deficiency in schizophrenia.[53,115] The pile-up of a-ketoglutarate has been interpreted as inability of the patients to oxidize a-ketoglutaric acid. However, it has been demonstrated that serum from schizophrenic patients has no effect on the oxidation of a-ketoglutarate.[111] On the other hand, when chicken erythrocytes were incubated with serum from schizophrenic patients and labeled acetate, the levels of a-ketoglutarate were significantly higher than when serum from control subjects was used.[65] However, the specific activity of a-ketoglutarate was lower in the samples incubated with the serum from schizophrenic patients than in the samples incubated with serum from control subjects. This would indicate that the a-ketoglutarate was being formed from some substance other than acetate. Since it has been shown that in addition to tryptophan the α-2-globulin causes glutamic acid to enter the cell,[64] it can be proposed that the excess of α-ketoglutarate arises from transamination or deamination of glutamic acid.

Frohman[67] has shown that when chicken erythrocytes are incubated with the α-helical S-protein or with serum from schizophrenic patients, the L/P ratio is higher than when incubated with the nonhelical S-protein or serum from normal subjects. This could indicate a deficiency in the hydrogen transport system, but all attempts to find such a defect resulted in failure.[111] The real problem may result from flooding the hydrogen transport system with amino acids, namely tryptophan and glutamic acid, because of the effect of the α-helical form of the S-protein.

Most attempts to find abnormality in enzymes affecting carbohydrate metabolism have failed. Lactic dehydrogenase activity is normal,[4] as is activity of malic dehydrogenase and the transaminases. Dern[50] reported that glucose-6-phosphate dehydrogenase activity was related to the type of symptoms manifested in schizophrenia, but not to the disease itself. Some studies have been performed on the operation of the hexosemonophosphate shunt. The results from such experiments are conflicting. One group[146] reported that more glucose was metabolized by the shunt in schizophrenia, while the other[70] reported that less glucose was oxidized.

There are indications that some abnormalities in carbohydrate chemistry exist in schizophrenia, but most data suggest that these irregularities merely reflect abnormality in other phases of metabolism.

Both the oxidation of glucose and the operation of the tricarboxylic acid cycle lead to the production of energy in the form of ATP. The conversion of ADP to ATP to produce stored energy is shown in Figure 26–6.

Because the clinical appearance of the typical schizophrenic patient would lead one to believe that the manifestations of energy may be disturbed, the metabolism of phosphate has been of interest to many workers. Upon the

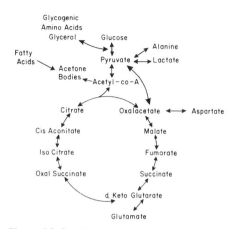

Figure 26–6.   The tricarboxylic acid cycle.

ingestion of glucose, serum inorganic phosphate drops much more in patients with schizophrenia than in control subjects.[176]

The phosphate on ATP is hydrolyzed by 1N HCL in seven minutes at 100° C and therefore is called Δ7 phosphate. It was reported that the formation of Δ7 phosphate in the erythrocytes of schizophrenic patients is quite different from that of normal individuals.[22,23,24] In these experiments, insulin pre-treatment of red blood cells from normal subjects inhibited formation of ATP when the cells were incubated with pyruvate and hexosediphosphate. This insulin depression did not occur with erythrocytes from schizophrenic subjects. Skaug[132,133] also reported that ATP turnover was lower in schizophrenic subjects, and also reported an accumulation of phosphoglycolic acid. The concentration of riboflavin phosphate, but not that of riboflavin, was found to be lower in schizophrenic patients.[104] This would indicate again an interference in the utilization of ATP. Many studies have been performed on the formation of ATP by blood from schizophrenic patients. Burnsohn[35] reported an increase in ATP formation while others[167] could not find any. Studies by Frohman and co-workers[85] demonstrated that insulin increased the rate of ATP turnover in the blood of normal subjects, but had no such effect in the blood of chronic schizophrenic patients. These results could be caused either by a defect in an energy production system or by a lack of response to insulin. (The lack of the effect of insulin will be discussed in another section.) In addition to ATP formation there was a differential in the effect of insulin in the formation of fructose-1,6-diphosphate. Other abnormalities in ATP formation by erythrocytes, following stress with a large dose of succinate, are reported by Hofmann and Arnold.[98] Both the ATP/ADP ratio and the fructose-1,6-diphosphate level were quite different in erythrocytes from schizophrenic patients than in erythrocytes from control subjects. The authors present evidence that the defects are genetically linked. In general, evidence seems to indicate that some defect does exist in energy metabolism in schizophrenia. However, whether this is a primary defect or the result of some other defect still remains to be determined.

Seeman and O'Brien[151] reported that sodium- and potassium-activated adenosine triphosphatase activity was increased in erythrocytes of schizophrenic patients, finding that these erythrocytes split 79.1 mμ mole of ATP per hour per mg. of dry weight while erythrocytes from control subjects only split 35.2 mμ mole. Parker and Hoffman[134] were unable to confirm this finding.

(Hormones

A huge number of studies have been concerned with the levels and the effects of hormones in schizophrenia. Because of the wide variation of levels of most hormones from hour to hour and even minute to minute, only the most careful control can produce meaningful results. The time of day of specimen withdrawal, the environmental conditions surrounding the patient, and the mental and physical state of the patient at the time of drawing the specimen must all be controlled. In many studies, the need for these controls has not been stringently observed. In addition, many reports of lack of response to hormone administration may be merely manifestations of general lack of responsivity of the schizophrenic patient to any stress.

Funkenstein[75] devised a test which predicted fairly well the clinical effect of electroshock treatment in schizophrenia. If, after the

patient was injected with methacholine, his blood pressure increased 50 mm. of mercury or more, or if the patient experienced a chill, the prognosis for electroshock therapy was good. If neither of these conditions existed, the prognosis was poor. This test, however, does not appear to be related to long-term prognosis since only 42 percent of the patients who had positive Funkenstein tests and who recovered following electroshock stayed out of the hospital for the next fourteen years.[172] In any case, administration of epinephrine-like compounds does appear to have a different effect in schizophrenia. Cardon[40] reported that injection of norepinephrine caused a smaller increase in blood pressure and glucose, but a larger increase in free fatty acids in schizophrenic patients as compared with control subjects.

It has long been known that many schizophrenic patients have an abnormal response to the administration of insulin. They are usually considered to be insulin resistant. Meduna[122] first described a diminished response in the decrease of blood glucose level after the administration of insulin. Lingjaerde[113] also described a diminished response of blood glucose following administration of insulin in schizophrenia. In addition this decreased response of glucose was followed by a prolonged hypoglycemic period. The deviation from the expected response was corrected if the carbohydrate intake of the patient was increased for several days prior to insulin administration. However, in the opinion of Lingjaerde, this increase in carbohydrate intake needed to be huge and above and beyond any physiological level. Insulin is also reported to cause a greater increase of cortisone after the hypoglycemic period in schizophrenic subjects.[105]

Gjessing[81] has shown some relationship between the thyroid hormone and schizophrenic symptomatology. The level of thyroid hormone increased during the catatonic phase of periodic catatonia and then returned to normal following the phase. During exacerbation of symptoms of this disease, excretion of hydroxymandelic acids also increased. However, as explained earlier, this probably is more closely related to the patient's emotional state than to the disease.[80] There are also large changes in urine volume reported in periodic catatonia.[81] Simpson[155] reports that 28 percent of schizophrenic patients are hypothyroid and that there is decreased I^{131} uptake in 93 percent. The protein carriers of thyroxine are increased in schizophrenia without any symptoms of hyperthyroidism being present.[48] It has been suggested that the thyroid defect in schizophrenia might be the result of abnormally high thyroid antibody; however, Goodman[83] reported that thyroid antibodies are not abnormal in schizophrenic patients.

Stabenau and Pollin[161] have also suggested a link between schizophrenia and thyroid hormone in their study of monozygotic twins discordant for schizophrenia. They demonstrated that the schizophrenic twin almost invariably had a lower birth weight and a lower PBI than the normal twin. The difference was significant at the 1 percent level of significance.

Hollister[99] has demonstrated that the plasma levels and urinary excretion of steroids in schizophrenia are normal. Other workers have shown increased corticosteroid excretion, but usually only during acute psychotic turmoil. When organized psychotic symptoms are re-established, the excretion of corticosteroids returns to normal.[145] Probably such a change in steroid excretion is the result of the acute agitation of the patient rather than of schizophrenia. Chulkov[45] reported an increase in excretion of sodium and potassium in schizophrenic patients and interpreted this as a mineral corticosteroid insufficiency. In general, however, no definitive studies have shown a difference in corticosteroids in schizophrenic patients, with the exception of Cookson's work[46] with periodic catatonic patients. In one female with periodic catatonia having a 36-day rhythm, the stuporous phase coincided with cyclic excretion of 17-ketosteroids and 17-hydroxysteroids. The 17-hydroxysteroid cycle occurred four days later than that of the 17-ketosteroids. This periodicity was not related to the menstrual cycle because it continued after the menstrual cycle had been interrupted by administration of Enovid.

Orlovskaya and co-workers[131] apparently have discovered a factor in the blood of schizophrenic patients which has an effect on the response to stress. When serum from a normal individual is injected into a rabbit, the rabbit produces a stress response characterized by an increase in the level of circulating corticosteroids, a decrease in eosinophils, and an increase in blood glucose level. This is a typical response to a stress situation. In experiments performed by Orlovskaya, serum was used from three groups of subjects—control, periodic schizophrenic, and nuclear schizophrenic. When serum from the control subjects or periodic schizophrenic patients was injected, a normal stress reaction followed. However, when serum from nuclear schizophrenic patients was injected, the stress reaction was either diminished or absent completely. These workers have been able to show that a protein component in the serum blocks the response to stress; however, this factor intensified the cellular damage resulting from such an injection. Whenever serum from one species is injected into another species, massive damage to cellular components can be expected. In this study, hyperemia, stasis, and petechial hemorrhages were noted. When serum from nuclear schizophrenic patients was used, the cellular damage became much more severe. This might indicate that the protein factor of Orlovskaya was acting upon adrenocortical hormones. In a later experiment, rabbits were stressed by applying electroshock, causing a change in the electrical activity of both the hypothalamus and cerebral cortex. This, in turn, affected the level of corticosteroids, lymphocytes, and blood glucose, in the same manner as in the previous experiment. When serum from schizophrenic patients was administered beforehand, the cerebrocortical electrical activity was affected by the shock, but there was no effect on the hypothalamus. Without the change in the electrical activity in the hypothalamus, there was no change in corticosteroids, lymphocytes, or blood glucose.[76] From this, Gerber[77,78] proposed that in schizophrenia there were pathological alterations in the hypothalamo-hypophyseal-adrenal system, causing a long-term decrease in activity. If such is the case, many of the hormonal changes reported could be a result of change in the hypothalamus. Since many of the nerve pathways in the hypothalamus are serotonergic, disturbed tryptophan metabolism could be the basis of all the above described defects.

Schizophrenia is characterized by a number of psychosexual disturbances.[168] This has led many workers to believe that something is abnormal in the production of sex hormones. Very early, Hoskins[100] reported a reduced androgen-estrogen ratio for male schizophrenic subjects, but this work did not have the benefit of modern methods. The excretion of 17-ketosteroids by male schizophrenic patients is apparently normal.[47] However, as previously mentioned, there was a change in 17-ketosteroid excretion in one female patient with periodic catatonia.[46] Despite a great deal of work on sex hormones in schizophrenia, very little has been accomplished. Brambilla[27] reported a decrease in pituitary gonadotropins in schizophrenia, while Brooksbank[30] found lower excretion of 16-androsten-3ᵃ-ol. Finally, Tourney[169] has reported that dehydroepiandrosterone is significantly lower in chronic schizophrenic subjects. Since this is a cortical androgen, it may be the result of a selectively reduced adrenocortical function in chronic schizophrenia. With the emergence of methods for determination of individual sex hormones, much more work should be done in this area.

Taylor[165,166] has observed that if a pregnant woman has a schizophrenic episode within one month of conception, any live offspring was likely to be female, and that if a mother has a schizophrenic episode within one month after delivery, the offspring was likely to have been male. He interpreted his data as indicating that the male sex hormone offered the mother some protection against some other factor involved in the production of schizophrenia. Thus, the drop in androgens following the birth of a male precipitated the exacerbation of schizophrenic symptoms. Other investigators[149] could not confirm his findings.

From the above it can be seen that very little sound evidence is available at the present time that hormones are involved in schizophrenia in other than a secondary manner. However, as methodology continues to develop in the study of individual hormones, clearer relationships may be found.

❲ Vitamins

To study vitamins in schizophrenia, the investigator must start with the assumption that hospitalized schizophrenic patients will probably be deficient in one or more vitamins as a result of the disease or the confinement. Nutritionally, many schizophrenic patients are in notoriously poor condition, and any study comparing schizophrenic patients and outside controls without first investigating the nutritional state of the patients is invalid. Much research suffers from this defect.

Attempts have been made from time to time to implicate vitamin C in schizophrenia. The work of Akerfeldt[2] indicated that the oxidation of ethylenediamine by plasma from schizophrenic patients was slower because of the lack of vitamin C. Slowik[156] reported lower vitamin C levels in patients with schizophrenia. He found that it took 6.2 days to saturate patients with vitamin C while it only took 3.2 days to saturate controls. Vanderkamp[173] claims that tissue from schizophrenic patients destroys ten times as much vitamin C as that from control subjects and suggested that excess dietary vitamin C caused patients to improve. Binette[19] did not find low vitamin C levels in schizophrenic patients. He did, however, report a decrease in the permeability of the blood-CSF barrier to vitamin C.[18] More recently, Pitt,[138] using nonschizophrenic hospitalized controls found that the level of ascorbic acid was actually higher in schizophrenic patients than in other patients. He measured the vitamin C level in the buffy coat layer of the patient's blood. He also found that there was no difference in the length of time required to saturate the schizophrenic patients and the other patients with vitamin C.

Hoffer[96] has claimed that niacin causes dramatic improvement in schizophrenic patients and his work has led to the contemporary megavitamin therapy for schizophrenic patients. In this treatment, huge unphysiological amounts of a number of vitamins are administered daily for long periods of time. The megavitamin therapy for schizophrenic patients has become quite popular with some physicians. Others believe that this type of therapy is completely useless. Other workers[7] have not been able to confirm Hoffer's findings. In fact, there have been reports of niacin actually exacerbating symptoms in some schizophrenic patients.[93] Hawkins[89] claims that the relapse rate is better with megavitamin therapy than without it. It would appear, however, that the fact that there is still a substantial relapse rate would indicate that niacin is not a cure-all for schizophrenia. Pauling,[135] after studying the claims for vitamin C and niacin in schizophrenia, proposed a broad, all-inclusive theory of molecular psychiatry in which he states that each individual has a different requirement for various vitamins and that by properly satisfying this requirement many psychiatric illnesses could be avoided. Oken[130] has taken Pauling severely to task for this viewpoint, stating that such a theory would only impede progress in biological psychiatry.

Other vitamins have been mentioned in connection with schizophrenia. Several workers[49,126,174] have claimed that pyridoxine, a vitamin involved in the metabolism of indole and catecholamines, causes improvement of schizophrenic symptoms. It is claimed that pyridoxine particularly improved the thought-degenerative symptoms, the affective symptoms, and the difficulty in concentrating. Because folic acid may be intimately involved in some forms of temporal lobe epilepsy, it has been proposed that it may also be involved in schizophrenia.[39]

Much controversy, it is true, exists concerning the relationship of vitamins and schizophrenia. It would appear, however, that much more positive data must be presented before vitamins can be shown to play anything but a secondary role in the schizophrenic process.

Inorganic Ions

Considerable controversy existed for a time concerning the copper-containing protein, ceruloplasmin, and schizophrenia. Akerfeldt[2] found that serum from schizophrenic patients oxidized N,N-dimethyl-p-phenylenediamine more rapidly than serum from controls, and claimed that this was due to increased ceruloplasmin "activity." (Ceruloplasmin is known to act on this amine as its principal "substrate.") Abood[1] also claimed that ceruloplasmin "activity" was increased. This was confirmed by a number of other workers.[44,141] At the time much of this work was done, it was not taken into consideration that ceruloplasmin activity was inhibited by vitamin C, and that vitamin C was often quite low in schizophrenic patients. This alone explained much of the difference in ceruloplasmin "activity" found in schizophrenia.

However, the whole concept that an enzyme called ceruloplasmin is abnormal in schizophrenia should be examined from another direction. The protein, ceruloplasmin, itself is probably not an enzyme, and the term ceruloplasmin "activity" probably describes an artifact related to ceruloplasmin's role as a transport protein carrying a prosthetic group for cytochrome oxidase. Since ceruloplasmin is not an enzyme,[29] the term "activity" is completely inappropriate in referring to its physiological function. It does not seem logical to base a theory of schizophrenia on ceruloplasmin activity if that activity is an artifact. When ceruloplasmin level is directly measured, no increase is found.[68,118] In addition, Frohman could not find an elevated level of copper in schizophrenic subjects. When all other conditions are controlled, no significant elevation of ceruloplasmin "activity" is found in schizophrenic patients, either.[148] The conclusion must be that neither copper nor ceruloplasmin are abnormal in schizophrenia.

It has been demonstrated that Ca++, Na+, and K+ are normal in schizophrenic patients, as are also Fe++ and $PO_4^{\equiv}$.[41,102] Burdeinyi[34] found that Zn++ was elevated in uninterrupted schizophrenia but was normal in the remitted and interrupted types. Cade[37] found that schizophrenia was associated with raised plasma Mg++ levels. In his patients, Mg++ was almost 20 percent higher than in controls. This was also reported by Brackenridge.[26] However, Seal[150] reports that serum Mg++ is normal in schizophrenia.

Many investigations have been performed involving inorganic ions and schizophrenia, and as yet there is no clear indication that abnormal levels of inorganic ions are involved in any way in the disease.

❨ Conclusion

Over the many years that biological phenomena have been investigated in schizophrenia, almost every phase of biochemistry has been studied. Many defects have been discovered. Some of these are undoubtedly artifacts resulting from abnormal diet and the underactivity that most schizophrenic patients exhibit. However, there remain many atypical findings that indicate real biochemical deficiencies. Most notable of these are an abnormal plasma protein, abnormal amines (particularly catechol and indole amines), abnormal carbohydrate metabolism, abnormal energy metabolism, and increased antibodies in the blood. One is, of course, tempted to search for a common underlying cause to which all of these defects could be related. It may be too soon in the course of events to find such a common factor, or no such factor may exist. Yet, with all the information now available, one could offer a guess as to what the defect might be. Most of the positive findings in schizophrenia could be related in one way or another to a functional defect in the cell membrane system. Thus, the finding of decreased glucose uptake by rat hemidiaphragm in the presence of plasma from schizophrenic patients[86] could be attributed to a membranal phenomenon. The lack of response of the ATP-producing system to insulin stress[85] could be attributed to the lack of response of the cell membrane to insulin. The numerous abnormalities in catechol and indole amines[160] could be the result of altered membrane transport of tryptophan and other amino acids. The effects on cell membranes,[117] and the numerous S-protein has been reported to have profound autoantibodies and hemolysins could all result from altered membrane permeability, which would allow intracellular proteins to mingle freely with plasma globulins.[107] While it is much too soon to attribute biochemical defects in schizophrenia to a single factor, it would appear to be very rewarding in the future for workers in the field to expend their effort studying the biochemistry and biophysics of cell membrane function in schizophrenic patients.

❨ Bibliography

1. ABOOD, L. G., F. A. GIBBS, and E. GIBBS. "Comparative Study of Blood Ceruloplasmin in Schizophrenia and Other Disorders," *Archives of Neurology and Psychiatry*, 77 (1957), 643.

2. AKERFELDT, S. "Oxidation of N,N'-Dimethyl-*p*-phenylenediamine by Serum from Patients with Mental Disease," *Science*, 125 (1957), 117.

3. ALEXANDER, F., G. C. CURTIS III, H. SPRINCE, and A. P. CROSLEY, JR. "L-Methionine and L-Tryptophan Feedings in Non-Psychotic and Schizophrenic Patients with and without Tranylcypromine," *Journal of Nervous and Mental Disease*, 137 (1963), 135–142.

4. ANTEBI, R. N., and J. KING. "Serum Enzyme Activity in Chronic Schizophrenia," *Journal of Mental Science*, 108 (1962), 75–79.

5. AXELROD, J., and R. TOMCHICK. "Enzymatic O-Methylation of Epinephrine and Other Catechols," *Journal of Biological Chemistry*, 233 (1958), 702.

6. BALTER, A. M. "Glucose Tolerance Curves in Neuropsychiatric Patients," *Diabetes*, 10 (1961), 100–105.

7. BAN, T. A. "On-Going National Collaborative Studies in Canada: Niacin in the Treatment of Schizophrenias," *Psychopharmacology Bulletin*, 5 (1969), 5–20.

8. BARBEAU, A., P. SINGH, P. GAUDREAU, and M. JOUBERT. "Effect of 3,4-Dimethoxy-

phenylethylamine Injections on the Concentration of Catecholamines in the Rat Brain," *Review of Canadian Biology*, 24 (1965), 229–232.

9. BENASSI, C. A., G. ALLEGRI, P. BENASSI, and A. RABASSINI. "Tryptophan Metabolism in Special Pairs of Twins," *Clinica Chimica Acta*, 9 (1964), 101–105.

10. BERGEN, J. "Schizophrenia Studies: A Possibly Related Blood Factor," in M. Vartanian, ed., *Biological Research in Schizophrenia*. Moscow: Ordina Lennia, 1967.

11. ———. "Possible Relationship of Plasma Factors to Schizophrenia," in O. Walaas, ed., *Molecular Basis of Some Aspects of Mental Activity*, Vol. 2. New York: Academic Press, 1967.

12. ———. Personal Communication (1971).

13. BERGEN, J., T. W. MITTAG, C. E. FROHMAN, R. E. ARTHUR, K. A. WARNER, L. GRINSPOON, and H. FREEMAN. "Plasma Factors in Schizophrenia," *Archives of General Psychiatry*, 18 (1968), 471–476.

14. BERGER, J., R. B. PENNELL, C. A. SARAVIS, and H. HOAGLAND. "Further Experiments with Plasma Proteins from Schizophrenics," in R. G. Heath, ed., *Serological Fractions in Schizophrenia*. New York: Hoeber, 1963.

15. BERLET, H. H., C. BULL, H. E. HIMWICH, H. KOHL, K. MATSUMOTO, G. R. PSCHEIDT, J. SPAIDE, T. T. TOURLENTES, and J. M. VALVERDE. "Endogenous Metabolic Factor in Schizophrenic Behavior," *Science*, 144 (1964), 311–312.

16. BERLET, H. H., J. SPAIDE, H. KOHL, C. BULL, and H. E. HIMWICH. "Effects of Reduction of Tryptophan and Methionine Intake on Urinary Indole Compounds and Schizophrenic Behavior," *Journal of Nervous and Mental Disease*, 140 (1965), 297–304.

17. BEUDING, E., H. I. WORTIS, H. D. FEIN, and D. ESTURONNE. "Pyruvic Acid Metabolism in Diabetes Mellitus," *American Journal of Medical Science*, 204 (1942), 838–845.

18. BINETTE, Y., L. P. FERRON, G. GRAVEL, O. HAMEL, G. LAMARRE, R. LEGAULT, L. MORIN, and M. BERTHIAUME. "Schizophrenia, Absorption Spectra of the Cerebrospinal Fluid and Ascorbic Acid," *Union Médicale du Canada*, 93 (1964), 270–275.

19. ———. "Study of Vitamin C in Schizophrenics," *Union Médicale du Canada*, 94 (1965), 1272–1275.

20. BISHOP, M. P. "Effects of Plasma from Schizophrenic Subjects upon Learning and Retention in the Rat," in R. G. Heath, ed., *Serological Fractions in Schizophrenia*. New York: Hoeber, 1963.

21. BOCK, E., B. WEEKE, and O. J. RAFAELSEN. "Immunoglobulins in Schizophrenic Patients," *Lancet*, 2 (1970), 523.

22. BÖSZÖRMÉNYI-NAGY, I., and F. J. GERTY. "Diagnostic Aspects of a Study of Intracellular Phosphorylations in Schizophrenia," *The American Journal of Psychiatry*, 112 (1955), 11–17.

23. ———. "Differences between the Phosphorus Metabolism of Erythrocytes of Normals and of Patients with Schizophrenia," *Journal of Nervous and Mental Disease*, 121 (1955), 53–58.

24. BÖSZÖRMÉNYI-NAGY, I., F. J. GERTY, and J. KUEBER. "Correlation between an Anomaly of the Intracellular Metabolism of Adenosine Nucleotides and Schizophrenia," *Journal of Nervous and Mental Disease*, 124 (1957), 143–149.

25. BOURDILLON, R. E., and A. P. RIDGES. "3,4-Dimethoxyphenylethylamine in Schizophrenia?" in H. E. Himwich, S. S. Kety, and J. R. Smythies, eds., *Amines and Schizophrenia*. Oxford: Pergamon Press, 1967.

26. BRACKENRIDGE, C. J., and C. McDONALD. "The Concentrations of Magnesium and Potassium in Erythrocytes and Plasma of Geriatric Patients with Psychiatric Disorders," *Medical Journal of Australia*, 2 (1969), 390–394.

27. BRAMBILLA, F., C. L. CAZZULLO, and F. RIGGI. "Endocrinology in Chronic Schizophrenia," *Diseases of the Nervous System*, 28 (1967), 745–748.

28. BRODIE, B. B., M. S. COMER, E. COSTE, and A. DLABAC. "Role of Brain Serotonin in the Mechanism of the Central Action of Reserpine," *Journal of Pharmacology and Experimental Therapeutics*, 152 (1966), 340–349.

29. BROMAN, L. "The Function of Ceruloplasmin—A Moot Question," in O. Walaas, ed., *Molecular Basis of Some Aspects of Mental Activity*, Vol. 2. New York: Academic Press, 1967.

30. BROOKSBANK, B. W. L., and W. PRYSE-PHILLIPS. "Urinary Δ^{16}-Androsten-3-α-ol, 17-Oxosteroids and Mental Illness," *British Medical Journal*, 1 (1964), 1602–1606.

31. BROWN, F. C., J. B. WHITE, and J. K. KENNEDY. "Urinary Excretion of Tryptophan Metabolites in Schizophrenic Individuals," *The American Journal of Psychiatry*, 117 (1960), 63–65.

32. BRUNE, G. G., H. H. KOHL, and H. E. HIMWICH. "Urinary Excretion of Bufotenin-like Substance in Psychotic Patients," *Journal of Neuropsychiatry*, 5 (1963), 14–17.

33. BUENO, J. R., and H. E. HIMWICH. "Excretion of Indoleamines in Schizophrenia," *International Journal of Neurology*, 6 (1967), 65–76.

34. BURDEINYI, A. F. "Levels of Copper and Zinc in the Blood of Patients with Various Types of Schizophrenia," *Zhurnal Nevropatologii i Psikhiatrii imeni S. S. Korsakova*, 67 (1967), 1041–1043.

35. BURNSOHN, J., J. T. CUSTOD, A. P. REMENCHIK, and P. J. TALSO. "High Energy Phosphate Compounds in Erythrocytes from Schizophrenic and Non-Schizophrenic Subjects." *Journal of Neuropsychiatry*, 4 (1962), 22–27.

36. BUSCAINO, G. A., V. SPADETTA, and A. CARELLA. "Methylation Test in Schizophrenia: Considerations on 500 Experimental Cases," *Acta Neurologica*, 24 (1969), 113–118.

37. CADE, J. F. J. "The Biochemistry of Schizophrenic and Affective Psychoses," *Medical Journal of Australia*, 1 (1964), 878–881.

38. CALDWELL, D. F. Personal Communication (1972).

39. CALLAGHAN, N., R. MITCHELL, and P. COTTER. "The Relationship of Serum Folic Acid and Vitamin B 12 Levels to Psychosis in Epilepsy," *Irish Journal of Medical Science*, 2 (1969), 497–505.

40. CARDON, P. V., JR., and P. S. MUELLER. "Effects of Norepinephrine on the Blood Pressure, Glucose, and Free Fatty Acids of Normal and Schizophrenic Men, with Reference to Heart Rate and to Indices of Physical Fitness and of Thyroid and Adrenal Cortical Function," *Journal of Psychiatric Research*, 2 (1964), 11–23.

41. CASEY, A. E., F. GILBERT, E. L. DOWNEY, J. FERGUSON, and S. THOMASON. "Interpretation of Electrolytes in the Metabolic Profile. II. Chloride, Carbon Dioxide, and Potassium," *Southern Medical Journal*, 64 (1971), 342–348.

42. CHALISOV, M. "Concerning the Pathogenesis of Schizophrenia," in M. Vartanian, ed., *Biological Research in Schizophrenia*. Moscow: Ordina Lennia, 1967.

43. CHARALAMPOUS, K. D., and S. BROWN. "A Clinical Trial of a-Methyl-Para-Tyrosine in Mentally Ill Patients," *Psychopharmacologia*, 11 (1967), 422–429.

44. CHITRE, V. S., and B. D. PUNEKAR. "Changes in Serum Copper and PPD-Oxidase in Different Diseases. Part II. Comparative Studies in Wilson's Disease, Schizophrenia, and Parkinsonism," *Indian Journal of Medical Research*, 58 (1970), 563–573.

45. CHULKOV, N. Z. "On the State of Electrolyte Metabolism in Schizophrenia," *Zhurnal Nevropatologii i Psikhiatrii imeni S. S. Korsakova*, 69 (1969), 97–102.

46. COOKSON, B. A., B. QUARRINGTON, and L. HUSZKA. "Longitudinal Study of Periodic Catatonia: Long-Term Clinical and Biochemical Study of a Woman with Periodic Catatonia," *Journal of Psychiatric Research*, 5 (1967), 15–38.

47. COPPEN, A., T. JULIAN, D. E. FRY, and V. MARKS. "Body Build and Urinary Steroid Excretion in Mental Illness," *British Journal of Psychiatry*, 113 (1967), 269–275.

48. CRANSWICK, E. H., and T. B. COOPER. "Thyroxine Serum Protein Complexes in Schizophrenia," *Journal of Clinical Endocrinology and Metabolism*, 25 (1965), 177–180.

49. DELAY, J., T. LEMPERIÈRE, and A. FELINE. "Trials of Piridoxilate in Psychiatric Therapy," *Annales Médico-Psychologiques*, 2 (1970), 606-613.

50. DERN, R. J., M. F. GLYNN, and G. J. BREWER. "Studies on the Correlation of the Genetically Determined Trait, Glucose-6-phosphate Dehydrogenase Deficiency, with Behavioral Manifestations of Schizophrenia," *Journal of Laboratory and Clinical Medicine*, 62 (1963), 319–329.

51. DOHAN, F. C. "Is Celiac Disease a Clue to the Pathogenesis of Schizophrenia?" *Mental Hygiene*, 53 (1969), 525–529.

52. DOMINO, E. F. Personal Communication (1972).

53. EASTERDAY, O. D., R. M. FEATHERSTONE, J. S. GOTTLIEB, M. L. NUSSER, and R. V. HOGG. "Blood Glutathione, Lactic Acid, and Pyruvic Acid Relationships in Schizophrenia," *Archives of Neurology and Psychiatry*, 68 (1953), 48–57.

54. EHRENSVAARD, G. "Some Observations on Serum Constituents in Relation to Schizo-

phrenia," in M. Rinkel, ed., *Biological Treatment of Mental Illness*, New York: L. C. Page and Co., 1966.

55. FAURBYE, A., and K. PIND. "Investigations on the Tryptophan Metabolism (via Kynurenine) in Schizophrenic Patients," *Acta Psychiatrica Scandinavica*, 40 (1964), 244–248.

56. ———. "Failure to Detect 3,4-Dimethoxyphenyl-ethylamine in the Urine of Psychotic Children," *Acta Psychiatrica Scandinavica*, 42 Suppl. 191 (1966), 136.

57. FAYVISHEVSKY, V. A., and A. V. NEMTSOV. "The Effect of Blood Serum of Patients with Schizophrenia on the Electrical Activity of the Cerebrum of Experimental Animals," *Zhurnal Nevropatologii i Psikhiatrii imeni S. S. Korsakova*, 65 (1965), 247–250.

58. FELDSTEIN, A., H. HOAGLAND, and H. FREEMAN. "Schizophrenic Behavior and Urinary 5-HIAA," *International Journal of Neuropsychiatry*, 1 (1965), 41–45.

59. FELDSTEIN, A., K. K. WONG, and H. FREEMAN. "The Metabolism of Serotonin Administered by the Intramuscular and Intravenous Routes in Normal Subjects and Chronic Schizophrenic Patients," *Journal of Psychiatric Research*, 2 (1964), 41–49.

60. FESSEL, W. J. "Blood Proteins in Functional Psychoses: a Review of the Literature and Unifying Hypothesis," *Archives of General Psychiatry*, 6 (1962), 132–148.

61. FISCHER, E. and H. SPATZ. "Determination of Bufotenin in the Urine of Schizophrenics," *International Journal of Neuropsychiatry*, 3 (1967), 226–228.

62. FRIEDHOFF, A. J. and E. VAN WINKLE. "Isolation and Characterization of a Compound from the Urine of Schizophrenics," *Nature*, 194 (1962), 897–898.

63. FROHMAN, C. "A Study of a Protein Factor in Schizophrenia," in M. Vartanian, ed., *Biological Research in Schizophrenia*. Moscow: Ordina Lennia, 1967.

64. ———. "Studies on the Plasma Factors in Schizophrenia," in C. Rupp, ed., *Mind as a Tissue*. New York: Hoeber, 1968.

65. ———. "Biochemical Mechanisms," in G. Tourney and J. S. Gottlieb, eds., *Lafayette Clinic Studies on Schizophrenia*. Detroit: Wayne State University Press, 1971.

66. FROHMAN, C., P. G. S. BECKETT, and J. S. GOTTLIEB. "Control of the Plasma Factor in Schizophrenia," in J. Wortis, ed., *Recent Advances in Biological Psychiatry*, Vol. 7. New York: Plenum Press, 1964.

67. FROHMAN, C., N. CZAJKOWSKI, E. D. LUBY, J. S. GOTTLIEB, and R. SENF. "Further Evidence of a Plasma Factor in Schizophrenia," *Archives of General Psychiatry*, 2 (1960), 263–267.

68. FROHMAN, C., M. GOODMAN, E. D. LUBY, P. G. S. BECKETT, and R. SENF. "Ceruloplasmin, Transferrin, and Tryptophan in Schizophrenia," *Archives of Neurology and Psychiatry*, 79 (1958), 730–734.

69. FROHMAN, C., C. R. HARMISON, R. E. ARTHUR, and J. S. GOTTLIEB. "Conformation of a Unique Plasma Protein in Schizophrenia," *Biological Psychiatry*, 3 (1971), 113–121.

70. FROHMAN, C., L. K. LATHAM, P. G. S. BECKETT, and J. S. GOTTLIEB. "Evidence of a Plasma Factor in Schizophrenia," *Archives of General Psychiatry*, 2 (1960), 255–261.

71. FROHMAN, C., L. K. LATHAM, K. A. WARNER, C. O. BROSIUS, P. G. S. BECKETT, and J. S. GOTTLIEB. "Motor Activity in Schizophrenia: Effect on Plasma Factor," *Archives of General Psychiatry*, 9 (1963), 83–88.

72. FROHMAN, C., E. D. LUBY, G. TOURNEY, P. G. S. BECKETT, and J. S. GOTTLIEB. "Steps Toward the Isolation of a Serum Factor in Schizophrenia," *The American Journal of Psychiatry*, 117 (1960), 401–408.

73. FROHMAN, C., K. A. WARNER, and J. JUNTUNEN. In preparation.

74. FROHMAN, C., K. A. WARNER, H. S. YOON, R. E. ARTHUR, and J. S. GOTTLIEB. "The Plasma Factor and Transport of Indoleamino Acids," *Biological Psychiatry*, 1 (1969), 377–385.

75. FUNKENSTEIN, D. H., M. J. GREENBLATT, and H. C. SOLOMON. "A Test Which Predicts the Clinical Effects of Electric Shock Treatment on Schizophrenic Patients," *The American Journal of Psychiatry*, 106 (1950), 889.

76. GASKIN, L. Z., E. I. MINSKER, D. D. ORLOVSKAYA, and V. A. FAYVISHEVSKY. "The Central Mechanisms of the Stress Effect of Schizophrenic Patient Serum," *Zhurnal Nevropatologii i Psikhiatrii imeni S. S. Korsakova*, 70 (1970), 576–581.

77. GERBER, E. L. "Histopathology of Neurosecretory Nuclei in Different Types of

Schizophrenia," *Vestnik Akademii Meditsinskikh Nauk SSSR*, 21 (1966), 37–44.

78. GERBER, E. L., and M. B. NIKOLAEVA. "Pathomorphological Changes of the Hypothalamo-Hypophyseal-Adrenal System of Rats Injected with the Blood of Schizophrenics," *Zhurnal Nevropatologii i Psikhiatrii imeni S. S. Korsakova*, 68 (1968), 90–95.

79. GERSHON, S., L. J. HEKIMIAN, A. FLOYD, JR., and L. E. HOLLISTER. "Alpha-Methyl-p-Tyrosine (AMT) in Schizophrenia," *Psychopharmacologia*, 11 (1967), 189–194.

80. GJESSING, L. R. "Studies of Periodic Catatonia. I. Blood Levels of Protein-Bound Iodine and Urinary Excretion of Vanillyl-Mandelic Acid in Relation to Clinical Course," *Journal of Psychiatric Research*, 2 (1964), 123–134.

81. GJESSING, R. "Disturbance of Somatic Functions in Catatonia with Periodic Course, and Their Compensation," *Journal of Mental Science*, 84 (1938), 608–621.

82. GLAZOV, V. "Certain Features of the Metabolism of Leucocytes in Nuclear Schizophrenia," in M. Vartanian, ed., *Biological Research in Schizophrenia*. Moscow: Ordina Lennia, 1967.

83. GOODMAN, M., M. ROSENBLATT, J. S. GOTTLIEB, J. MILLER, and C. H. CHEN. "Effect of Age, Sex, and Schizophrenia on Thyroid Autoantibody Production," *Archives of General Psychiatry*, 8 (1963), 518–526.

84. GOSHEVA, A. E., and N. P. PODOZEROVA. "On the Effect of the Lymphocytes of Patients with Schizophrenia on Tissue Cultures of Human Embryonic Brain and Brains of Newborn Rats," *Zhurnal Nervopatologii i Psikhiatrii imeni S. S. Korsakova*, 67 (1967), 1352–1355.

85. GOTTLIEB, J. S., C. E. FROHMAN, G. TOURNEY, and P. G. S. BECKETT. "Energy Transfer Systems in Schizophrenia: Adenosinetriphosphate (ATP)," *Archives of Neurology and Psychiatry*, 81 (1959), 504–508.

86. HAAVALDSEN, R., O. LINGJAERDE, and O. WALAAS. "Disturbances of Carbohydrate Metabolism in Schizophrenics. The Effect of Serum Fractions from Schizophrenics on Glucose Uptake of Rat Diaphragm in Vitro," *Confinia Neurologica*, 18 (1958), 270–279.

87. HALL, P., G. HARTRIDGE, and G. H. VAN LEEUWEN. "Effect of Catechol O-Methyl Transferase in Schizophrenia," *Archives of General Psychiatry*, 20 (1969), 573–575.

88. HARMISON, C. R., and C. E. FROHMAN. "Conformational Variation in a Human Plasma Lipoprotein." *Biochemistry*, 11 (1972), 4985–4993.

89. HAWKINS, D. R., A. W. BORTIN, and R. P. RUNYON. "Orthomolecular Psychiatry: Niacin and Megavitamin Therapy," *Psychosomatics*, 11 (1970), 517–521.

90. HEATH, R. G., and I. M. KRUPP. "Schizophrenia as an Immunologic Disorder. I. Demonstration of Antibrain Globulins by Fluorescent Antibody Techniques," *Archives of General Psychiatry*, 16 (1967), 1–9.

91. HEATH, R. G., S. MARTENS, B. E. LEACH, M. COHEN, and C. A. FEIGLEY. "Behavioral Changes in Nonpsychotic Volunteers Following the Administration of Taraxein, the Substance Obtained from Serum of Schizophrenic Patients," *The American Journal of Psychiatry*, 114 (1958), 917–920.

92. HELLER, B., N. NARASIMHACHARI, J. SPAIDE, L. HASKOVEC, and H. E. HIMWICH. "N-Dimethylated Indoleamines in Blood of Acute Schizophrenics," *Experientia*, 26 (1970), 503–504.

93. HENINGER, G. R., and M. B. BOWERS. "Adverse Effects of Niacin in Emergent Psychosis," *Journal of the AMA*, 204 (1968), 1010–1011.

94. HENNEMAN, D. H., M. D. ALTSCHULE, and R. M. GONCZ. "Carbohydrate Metabolism in Brain Disease. II. Glucose Metabolism in Schizophrenic, Manic-Depressive, and Involutional Psychoses," *Archives of Neurology and Psychiatry*, 72 (1954), 696–704.

95. HERKERT, E. E., and W. KEUP. "Excretion Patterns of Tryptamine, Indoleacetic Acid, and 5-Hydroxyindoleacetic Acid, and Their Correlation with Mental Changes in Schizophrenic Patients under Medication with Alpha-Methyldopa," *Psychopharmacologia*, 15 (1969), 48–59.

96. HOFFER, A. "Treatment of Schizophrenia with a Therapeutic Program Based upon Nicotinic Acid as the Main Variable," in O. Walaas, ed., *Molecular Basis of Some Aspects of Mental Activity*, Vol. 2. New York: Academic Press, 1967.

97. HOFFER, A., H. OSMOND, and J. SMYTHIES. "Schizophrenia: New Approach; Result of Year's Research," *Journal of Mental Science*, 100 (1954), 29.

98. HOFMANN, G., and O. H. ARNOLD. "Results of Biochemical Investigations in Schizophrenics," in O. Walaas, ed., *Molecular Basis of Some Aspects of Mental Activity*, Vol. 2. New York: Academic Press, 1967.

99. HOLLISTER, L. E. "Steroids and Moods: Correlations in Schizophrenics and Subjects Treated with Lysergic Acid Diethylamide (LSD), Mescaline, Tetrahydrocannabinol, and Synhexyl," *Journal of Clinical Pharmacology*, 9 (1969), 24–29.

100. HOSKINS, R. G. *Biology of Schizophrenia*. New York: W. W. Norton, 1946.

101. JUS, A., H. ROSENGARTEN, H. WARDASZKO-LYSKOWSKA, A. SZEMIS, I. WLOSINSKA, J. KRZYZOWSKI, K. STENCKA, and K. KOWALSKA. "Correlations between Disturbances of Tryptophan Metabolism Induced by Methionine and Nialamide Administration and Changes of the Mental State in Chronic Schizophrenic Patients," *Psychiatria Polska*, 4 (1970), 365–371.

102. KACZYNSKI, M., E. BERNASKIEWICZ, M. WYPYCH, and H. WOJNICKA. "Levels of Sialic Acid, Cholinesterase and Some Electrolytes in Treated Early Schizophrenia," *Polski Tygodnik Lekarski*, 19 (1964), 1074–1075.

103. KAKIMOTO, Y., I. SANO, A. KANAZAWA, T. TSUJIO, and Z. KANEKO. "Metabolic Effects of Methionine in Schizophrenic Patients Pretreated with a Monoamine Oxidase Inhibitor," *Nature*, 216 (1967), 1110–1111.

104. KERPPOLA, W. "The Content of Riboflavin and Riboflavin-Containing Co-enzymes in the Blood in Health and in Various Disease in Particular Schizophrenia, Neurocirculatory Asthenia and Tuberculosis," *Acta Medica Scandinavica*, 153 (1955), 33–48.

105. KISTLER, C. R., N. F. BESCH, G. R. VAN SICKLE, R. H. McCLUER, and D. B. JACKSON. "Epinephrine and Insulin Effects. II. ACTH and Cortisol," *Archives of General Psychiatry*, 14 (1966), 287–290.

106. KNOWLES, M., M. SAUNDERS, and H. A. McCLELLAND. "The Effects of Phenothiazine Therapy on Lymphocyte Transformation in Schizophrenia," *Acta Psychiatrica Scandinavica*, 46 (1970), 64–70.

107. KOLYASKINA, G. "A Study of the Immunological Reactions of the Delayed Type in Schizophrenic Patients," in M. Vartanian, ed., *Biological Research in Schizophrenia*. Moscow: Ordina Lennia, 1967.

108. KOPELOFF, L. M., and E. FISCHEL. "Serum Levels of Bactericidin and Globulin in Schizophrenia," *Archives of General Psychiatry*, 9 (1963), 524–528.

109. KUZNETSOVA, N. "Some Data Concerning the Immunological Properties of Brain Mitochondria," in M. Vartanian, ed., *Biological Research in Schizophrenia*. Moscow: Ordina Lennia, 1967.

110. LEACH, B. E., L. W. BYERS, and R. G. HEATH. "Methods for Isolating Taraxein," in R. Heath, ed., *Serological Fractions in Schizophrenia*. New York: Hoeber, 1963.

111. LEES, H., D. J. GREENWOOD, C. E. FROHMAN, P. G. S. BECKETT, and J. S. GOTTLIEB. "The Effects of Sera from Schizophrenic Subjects on the Oxidation of Succinate and Alpha-Ketoglutarate," *Journal of Neuropsychiatry*, 5 (1964), 534–538.

112. LIDEMAN, R. R., and YU I. IRYANOV. "The Hemolytic Stability of Erythrocytes of Patients Having Schizophrenia," *Zhurnal Nevropatologii i Psikhiatrii imeni S. S. Korsakova*, 65 (1965), 1201–1205.

113. LINGJAERDE, O. "Contributions to the Study of the Schizophrenias and the Acute, Malignant Deliria: A Survey of Forty Years' Research," *Journal of the Oslo City Hospitals*, 14 (1964), 41–83.

114. LOGAN, D. G., and S. D. DEODHAR. "Schizophrenia, an Immunologic Disorder?" *Journal of the AMA*, 212 (1970), 1703–1704.

115. LOONEY, J. M. "Changes in Lactic Acid, pH and Gases Produced in the Blood of Normal and Schizophrenic Subjects by Exercise," *American Journal of Medical Science*, 198 (1939), 57–66.

116. LOZOVSKY, D., A. KRASNOVA, M. FACTOR, N. POLYANSKAYA, and N. POPOVA. "The Effect of the Serum of Schizophrenic Patients upon Certain Glucose Transformation Indices in Experiment," in M. Vartanian, ed., *Biological Research in Schizophrenia*. Moscow: Ordina Lennia, 1967.

117. LOZOVSKY, D. B., and B. P. MUSCHENKO. "Damaging Membranotropic Effect in Schizophrenia," *Zhurnal Nevropatologii i Psikhiatrii imeni S. S. Korsakova*, 71 (1971), 711–717.

118. LYKO, J. "Serum Ceruloplasmin Levels in Healthy Persons and in Certain Pathologic Conditions," *Acta Medica Polona*, 8 (1967), 269–277.

119. MACHT, D. I. "Phytotoxic Blood Sera in Medicine," *Bulletin of the Torrey Botanical Club*, 76 (1949), 235–243.

120. MALIS, G. U. *Concerning the Etiology of Schizophrenia.* Moscow: Medgiz, 1959.

121. MATTOK, G. L., D. L. WILSON, and A. HOFFER. "Catecholamine Metabolism in Schizophrenia," *Nature,* 213 (1967), 1189–1190.

122. MEDUNA, L. J. *Oneirophrenia.* Urbana: University of Illinois Press, 1950.

123. MELTZER, H. Y. "Muscle Enzyme Release in the Acute Psychoses," *Archives of General Psychiatry,* 21 (1969), 102–112.

124. MOIR, A. T. B., and D. ECCLESTON. "The Effects of Precursor Loading in the Cerebral Metabolism of 5-Hydroxyindoles," *Journal of Neurochemistry,* 15 (1968), 1093–1108.

125. MORGAN, M., and A. J. MANDELL. "Indole(ethyl)amine N-Methyltransferase in the Brain," *Science,* 165 (1969), 492–493.

126. MORRONI, O. B. "Immediate Clinical Results with Gamma Aminobutyric Acid B6 in Schizophrenias and Deliriums," *Semina Medica,* 123 (1963), 892–900.

127. MUSAJO, L., and C. A. BENASSI. "Aspects of Disorders of the Kynurenine Pathway of Tryptophan Metabolism in Man," *Advances in Clinical Chemistry,* 7 (1964), 63–135.

128. NANEISHVILI, B., A. SIHARULIDZE, and Z. ZURABASHVILI. "Some Data on the Study of the Biological Properties of Blood Plasma of Schizophrenic Patients," in M. Vartanian, ed., *Biological Research in Schizophrenia.* Moscow: Ordina Lennia, 1967.

129. NELSON, G. N., M. MASUDA, and T. H. HOLMES. "Correlation of Behavior and Catecholamine Metabolite Excretion," *Psychosomatic Medicine,* 28 (1966), 216–226.

130. OKEN, D. "Vitamin Therapy: Treatment for the Mentally Ill," *Science,* 160 (1968), 1181.

131. ORLOVSKAYA, D., L. GASKIN, and E. MINSKER. "Certain Features of the Biological Activity of Blood Serum of Schizophrenic Patients and the Problem of Stress," in M. Vartanian, ed., *Biological Research in Schizophrenia.* Moscow: Ordina Lennia, 1967.

132. ORSTROM, A. "Isolation of Phosphoglycolic Acid from Human Erythrocytes," *Archives of Biochemistry and Biophysics,* 33 (1951), 484–485.

133. ORSTROM, A., and O. SKAUG. "Isolation from Blood of Chronic Schizophrenic Patients of Compounds Active in Radioactive Phosphate Turnover," *Acta Psychiatrica et Neurologica Scandinavica,* 25 (1950), 437–441.

134. PARKER, J. C., and J. F. HOFFMAN. "Failure to Find Increased Sodium, Potassium-ATPase in Red Cell Ghosts of Schizophrenics," *Nature,* 201 (1964), 823.

135. PAULING, L., "Orthomolecular Psychiatry," *Science,* 160 (1968), 265–271.

136. PENNELL, R. "Biological Properties of the Blood Serum of Schizophrenic Patients," in M. Vartanian, ed., *Biological Research in Schizophrenia.* Moscow: Ordina Lennia, 1967.

137. PENNELL, R., C. PAWLUS, C. A. SARAVIS, and G. SCRIMSHAW. "Chemical Characteristics of a Plasma Fraction which Influences Animal Behavior," in O. Walaas, ed., *Molecular Basis of Some Aspects of Mental Activity,* Vol. 2. New York: Academic Press, 1967.

138. PITT, B., and N. POLLITT. "Ascorbic Acid and Chronic Schizophrenia," *British Journal of Psychiatry,* 118 (1971), 227–228.

139. POLISHCHUK, I. "On the Character and Pathogenesis of Biochemical Disturbances in Schizophrenia," in M. Vartanian, ed., *Biological Research in Schizophrenia.* Moscow: Ordina Lennia, 1967.

140. POLLIN, W., P. V. CARDON, and S. S. KETY. "Effects of Amino Acid Feedings in Schizophrenic Patients Treated with Iproniazid," *Science,* 133 (1961), 104–105.

141. PUZYNSKI, S. "Studies on Ceruloplasmin in Chronic Schizophrenia," *Neurologia, Neurochirurgia i Psychiatria Polska,* 6 (1966), 131–137.

142. RIEDER, H. P. "Biological Determination of the Toxicity of Pathological Body Fluids. III. Testing of Urine Extracts of Mental Patients by Means of the Spider's Web Test." *Psychiatrie et Neurologie,* 134 (1957), 378–396.

143. RIEGELHAUPT, L. M., "Investigation on Glyoxylic Acid Reaction on Urine from Schizophrenic and Other Psychotic Patients," *Journal of Nervous and Mental Disease,* 123 (1956), 383.

144. RYAN, J. W., J. D. BROWN, and J. DURELL. "Antibodies Affecting Metabolism of Chicken Erythrocytes: Examination of Schizophrenic and Other Subjects," *Science,* 151 (1966), 1408–1410.

145. SACHAR, E. J. "Psychological Factors Re-

lating to Activation and Inhibition of the Adrenocortical Stress Response in Man: A Review," *Progress in Brain Research*, 32 (1970), 316–324.

146. SACKS, W. "Cerebral Metabolism of Isotopic Glucose in Chronic Mental Disease," *Journal of Applied Physiology*, 14 (1959), 849–854.

147. SAI HALAZ, A., G. BRUNECKER, and S. SZARA. "Dimethyltryptamine: A New Psychotic Agent," *Psychiatrie et Neurologie*, 135 (1958), 285–301.

148. SCHEINBERG, I. H., A. G. MORELL, R. S. HARRIS, and A. BERGER. "Concentration of Ceruloplasmin in Plasma of Schizophrenic Patients," *Science*, 126 (1957), 925.

149. SCHORER, C. E. Unpublished Data.

150. SEAL, U. S., and H. EIST. "Serum Magnesium Concentration in Schizophrenia and Epilepsy," *Clinical Chemistry*, 13 (1967), 1021–1023.

151. SEEMAN, P. M., and E. O'BRIEN. "Sodium-Potassium-Activated Adenosine Triphosphatase in Schizophrenic Erythrocytes," *Nature*, 200 (1963), 263–264.

152. SEMENOV, S. F. "Some Clinical Characteristics and Course of Schizophrenia with Signs of Autoimmunization with Brain Antigens," *Zhurnal Nevropatologii i Psikhiatrii imeni S. S. Korsakova*, 64 (1964), 398–403.

153. SHARP, H. C., and C. N. BAGANZ. "A Study of the Problem of Malnutrition in Institutionalized Psychotic Patients," *The American Journal of Psychiatry*, 97 (1956), 650–656.

154. SIEGEL, M., and H. TEFFT. "'Pink Spot' and Its Components in Normal and Schizophrenic Urine," *Journal of Nervous and Mental Disease*, 152 (1971), 412–426.

155. SIMPSON, G. M., E. H. CRANSWICK, and J. H. BLAIR. "Thyroid Indices in Chronic Schizophrenia," *Journal of Nervous and Mental Disease*, 137 (1963), 582–590.

156. SLOWIK, S. "Study of the L-Ascorbic Acid Level in Body Fluids of Patients with Chronic Schizophrenia," *Neurologia, Neurochirurgia i Psychiatria Polska*, 15 (1965), 881–887.

157. SMYTHIES, J. "The Essential Hallucinogenic Molecule," in M. Vartanian, ed., *Biological Research in Schizophrenia*, Moscow: Ordina Lennia, 1967.

158. ———. "The Skeleton Structure of a Hallucinogenic Molecule," *Vestnik Akademii Meditsinskikh Nauk SSSR*, 24 (1969), 41–44.

159. SOLOMON, G. F., R. H. MOOS, W. J. FESSEL, and E. E. MORGAN. "Globulins and Behavior in Schizophrenia," *International Journal of Neuropsychiatry*, 2 (1966), 20–25.

160. SPAIDE, J., H. TANIMUKAI, R. GINTHER, J. BUENO, and H. E. HIMWICH. "Schizophrenic Behavior and Urinary Tryptophan Metabolites Associated with Cysteine Given with and without a Monoamine Oxidase Inhibitor (Tranylcypromine)," *Life Sciences*, 6 (1967), 551–560.

161. STABENAU, J. R., and W. POLLIN. "Maturity at Birth and Adult Protein Bound Iodine," *Nature*, 215 (1967), 996–997.

162. STOIMENOV, I. A. "Relationship between Forms and Symptoms of Schizophrenia and Presence of Brain Antibodies in the Blood Serum," *Vestnik Akademii Meditsinskikh Nauk SSSR*, 24 (1969), 67–70.

163. STRAHILEVITZ, M., and S. D. DAVIS. "Increased IgA in Schizophrenic Patients," *Lancet*, 2 (1970), 370.

164. TAKESADA, M., E. MIYAMOTO, Y. KAKIMOTO, I. SANO, and Z. KANEKO. "Phenolic and Indole Amines in the Urine of Schizophrenics," *Nature*, 207 (1965), 1199–1200.

165. TAYLOR, M. A. "Sex Ratios of Newborns: Associated with Prepartum and Postpartum Schizophrenia," *Science*, 164 (1969), 723–724.

166. TAYLOR, M. A., and R. LEVINE. "The Interactive Effects of Maternal Schizophrenia and Offspring Sex," *Biological Psychiatry*, 2 (1970), 279–284.

167. THELLE, P. "Investigations in vitro of the Turnover of Acid Labile Phosphate in Blood Corpuscles of Schizophrenic and Normal Persons," *Acta Psychiatrica et Neurologica Scandinavica*, 28 (1953), 213–218.

168. TOURNEY, G. "Psychosexual Factors in Schizophrenia," in G. Tourney, and J. S. Gottlieb, eds., *Lafayette Clinic Studies on Schizophrenia*. Detroit: Wayne State University Press, 1971.

169. ———. "Androgen Metabolism in Schizophrenics, Homosexuals and Normal Controls." *Biological Psychiatry*. 6 (1973), 23–26.

170. UZUNOV, G., B. IORDANOV, and I. DOSEVA. "Cellular Membrane Permeability in Schizophrenia. I. Effect of Various 'Labilisers'

and 'Stabilisers' on Erythrocyte Membrane Permeability in Schizophrenia," in M. Vartanian, ed., *Biological Research in Schizophrenia*. Moscow: Ordina Lennia, 1967.

171. ———. "Cellular Membrane Permeability in Schizophrenia. II. Effect upon Erythrocyte Membrane Permeability of Various Protein Fractions Isolated from Cerebrospinal Fluid of Schizophrenic Patients," in M. Vartanian, ed., *Biological Research in Schizophrenia*. Moscow: Ordina Lennia, 1967.

172. VAILLIANT, G. E., and D. H. FUNKENSTEIN. "Long-Term Follow-Up (10-15 Years) of Schizophrenic Patients with Funkenstein (Adrenalin-Mecholyl) Tests," *Proceedings of the American Psychopathological Association*, 54 (1966), 244–251.

173. VANDERKAMP, H. "A Biochemical Abnormality in Schizophrenia Involving Ascorbic Acid," *International Journal of Neuropsychiatry*, 2 (1966), 204–206.

174. VERGA, G. "Pyridoxine in the Pathogenesis and Therapy of Neurologic and Psychiatric Diseases," *Acta Vitaminologica*, 17 (1963), 239–254.

175. WAGNER, A. F., V. J. CIRILLO, M. A. P. MEISINGER, R. E. ORMOND, F. A. KUEHL, JR., and N. G. BRINK. "A Further Study of Catecholamine O-Methylation in Schizophrenia," *Nature*, 211 (1966), 604–605.

176. WHITEHORN, J. C. "The Effect of Glucose upon Blood Phosphate in Schizophrenia,"

Research Publications of the Association for Research in Nervous and Mental Disease, 5 (1928), 257–261.

177. WHITTINGHAM, S., I. R. MacKAY, I. H. JONES, and B. DAVIES. "Absence of Brain Antibodies in Patients with Schizophrenia," *British Medical Journal*, 1 (1968), 347–348.

178. WINTER, C. A., and L. FLATAKER. "Effect of Blood Plasma from Psychotic Patients upon Performance of Trained Rats," *Archives of Neurology and Psychiatry*, 80 (1958), 441–449.

179. WOOLLEY, D. W. "Biochemical Theories of Schizophrenia," *International Journal of Psychiatry*, 1 (1965), 436–437.

180. WOOLLEY, D. W., and E. SHAW. "A Biochemical and Pharmacological Suggestion about Certain Mental Disorders," *Science*, 119 (1954), 587.

181. ZAHRADNICKA, J. M. "Dynamics of Changes in Blood Globulins in the Course of Schizophrenia," *Activitas Nervosa Superior*, 7 (1965), 204–205.

182. ZARA, S. "Dimethyltryptamine: Its Metabolism in Man; the Relation of Its Psychotic Effect to the Serotonin Metabolism," *Experientia*, 12 (1956), 441–442.

183. ZELLER, E. A., J. BERNSOHN, W. M. INSKIP, and J. W. LAUER. "On the Effect of a Monoamine Oxidase Inhibitor on the Behavior of Tryptophan Metabolism of Schizophrenic Patients," *Naturwissenschaften*, 44 (1957), 427.

CHAPTER 27

INDIVIDUAL PSYCHOTHERAPY OF SCHIZOPHRENIA

Silvano Arieti

THERE ARE MARKED DISAGREEMENTS as to the treatment of choice in schizophrenia. Many psychiatrists prefer physical therapies, especially drug therapy; in recalcitrant cases, convulsive shock treatment or insulin therapy; and, in some especially difficult cases some use of psychosurgery.

My own marked preference in the average case is individual psychotherapy, although with numerous patients I use a mixed psychotherapy and drug therapy. My "bias" is based on the belief that physical therapies, as far as we know or can infer, produce only a symptomatic improvement, whereas psychotherapy tends to (1) remove the basic conflicts which are important and necessary causative elements of the disorder; (2) correct the psychopathologic patterns; (3) change the self-image of the patient and therefore make him less vulnerable; and (4) permit the regenerative

psychological powers of the organism to regain the lost ground.

These assertions should not be interpreted as a condemnation of physical therapies. On the contrary, I have found physical therapies, with the exception of psychosurgery, useful at times in a variety of situations:

1. When psychotherapy for psychotic patients is not available (and, unfortunately, it is not available to by far the majority of patients), physical therapies should be administered.

2. Psychotherapy is not effective in every case. Although in the last two decades we have made great progress in this field, our technique is still not completely satisfactory. We often encounter patients (fortunately, in decreasing number) who do not improve. In rare cases, every interpersonal relation, even

that with the experienced therapist, increases the anxiety of the patient to such a point as to enhance his psychological disintegration. Perhaps, with the refinement of technique, such cases will eventually disappear; but, for the time being, if more than a few therapists have been unsuccessful and the condition is worsening (especially, in cases of rapid disintegration or those in which no contact at all is made), an attempt should be made to arrest the process, at least in a symptomatic way.

3. Finally, drug and even shock therapies must be used in cases which are urgent because of a concurrent physical illness. Here, quick results must be obtained before they could be achieved with the long psychotherapeutic procedure.

Even when shock or drug therapy is used with apparently successful results, psychotherapy is important in order to prevent relapses.

An increasing number of patients today are being treated with a combination of drug therapy and psychotherapy. The drug therapy decreases the anxiety and makes them more accessible to (or less fearful of) the interpersonal contact. In my experience, this combination does not shorten the treatment but does have the advantage of making hospitalization unnecessary for many patients. In many cases, a full-fledged schizophrenic is transformed into an ambulatory schizophrenic. This transformation is not to be disregarded, as many patients are kept in the community in this way and are able to work while undergoing effective treatment. Drug therapy establishes a certain distance between the patient and his distressing symptoms, which may be welcome for therapeutic reasons as well. On the other hand, if the patient who receives drug therapy experiences less anxiety, he becomes somewhat less sensitive to psychotherapy, too. Thus, each case has to be evaluated individually. We have to decide in each instance whether we gain or lose more with adjuvant drug therapy. In a considerable number of cases the gain is greater than the loss.

No matter which treatment for schizo-

phrenia a psychiatrist prefers, he cannot ignore psychotherapy, nor can he escape practicing psychotherapy with schizophrenics even if he is determined to do so. Even a psychiatrist whose practice consists predominantly in administering phenothiazines cannot help inquiring about the dynamics of the patient's anguish and conflict, cannot help observing and interpreting what happens between the patient and himself. He may not apply all the insights that people who have specialized in the psychotherapy of schizophrenia have revealed; he may not follow all their recommendations, but some of them have been assimilated by him, even if in diluted forms. Moreover, even those who have enlarged the field of psychotherapy of schizophrenia to include family therapy, group therapy, and community psychiatry, have built upon the foundations laid by individual psychotherapy.

A historical review of the development of this type of treatment will reveal that each method adopted was the clinical expression or the therapeutic realization of one or a few underlying principles held by its originator. Often, the principle was deduced from the clinical experiences of the therapist; in several instances it was a preconceived theoretical view which oriented the therapist in certain directions.

(A Historical Survey

Freud and the Freudian School

Any review of the psychotherapy of schizophrenia must start with Freud.[35] And yet, paradoxically, Freud, to whom we owe so much for the understanding of many aspects of this disorder, discouraged psychotherapy with schizophrenics. To be exact, as early as 1905, he did not consider the obstacles to remain insurmountable in the future and did not exclude the possibility that some techniques would be devised which would permit the psychoanalytic treatment of the psychoses. Later, however, Freud assumed a more pessimistic attitude. He felt that the psychosis could be compared to a dream and understood as a dream, but not cured.

An underlying principle was at the basis of this pessimism. Freud believed that in schizophrenia there is a withdrawal of libido from the objects into the self; therefore, no transference can take place, and without transference no treatment is possible.

One of Freud's first and famous pupils, Federn,[34] made repeated and successful attempts in the treatment of schizophrenic patients, in spite of the prevailing discouraging theories. One of Federn's underlying principles was based on the concept of ego-feeling, that is, an autonomous reservoir of libido in the ego. He felt that the ego of the schizophrenic is poorer, not richer, in libido as Freud's theories implied. He also felt that transference with the schizophrenic was possible. As a matter of fact, he succeeded in establishing it.

Another tenet of Federn (of the ego boundaries), however, limited his therapeutic aims. Federn believed that in the schizophrenic "the boundaries" separating the areas of the psyche (the id from the ego and the ego from the external world) are defective, so that material from the id may invade the ego and even be projected to the external world. The most important goal of therapy should be that of establishing normal boundaries. Reversing a famous sentence of Freud, Federn said that, as a result of therapy in the schizophrenic, "There, where ego was, id must be."

Federn stressed the fact that it is possible to establish transference with the part of the patient that has remained healthy, and strongly suggested that the therapist have a helper to be with the patient in the intervals between sessions. Fundamentally, in Federn's method, the patient is guided to understand that a part of his ego is sick and that that part is not trustworthy.

Gertrude Schwing,[76] a nurse who was analyzed by Federn, applied her analyst's concepts to hospitalized patients. In a straightforward and honest but not fully convincing little book, *A Way to the Soul of the Mentally Ill*, she describes the schizophrenic as a person who has been deprived of the experience of having a real mother, one who loves her child at any cost. The psychiatric nurse must offer that love to the patient. She described several techniques that establish continuity of contact with the patient and stressed the point that the patient must have the feeling that this new mother is there and does not intend to abandon him. Schwing considers her treatment a preliminary one, to be followed by Federn's method.

Hinsie[50] is one of the American pioneers in the psychotherapy of schizophrenia. As early as 1930, he published a book devoted to this topic. He studied patients in the adolescent period who voluntarily sought treatment, had insight into the fact that they were sick, and were communicative and willing to follow the directions of the therapist. Thus, Hinsie selected the easiest patients to treat. He relied predominantly on the clinical psychoanalytic method of "free association."

Eissler[30,3] has stressed the importance of early psychotherapy during the acute episode. The way in which the case is handled at the beginning, he claims, often determines the whole course of the illness. He distinguishes the acute phase from "the phase of relative clinical muteness."

Wexler[88] reported the successful treatment of a patient whom he treated by assuming the role of a tyrannical superego.

Bychowski[29] has provided, in addition to important studies on schizophrenic thinking, important details on the manifestations, dynamics, and therapeutic handling of hostility.

Hill,[49] again, emphasized the crucial role of the mother in the development of schizophrenia and gave details of technique in handling patients.

Within the Freudian school, noteworthy also are the contributions of Arlow and Brenner[17,18] and Jacobson.[52]

The ego psychologists of the Freudian school (Hartmann,[43–47] Rapoport,[64,65,66] and Hartmann, Kris, and Lowenstein[48]) have acknowledged that schizophrenia is predominantly a disorder of the ego, but their practical impact on the psychotherapy of schizo-phrenia is not discernible so far.

The Kleinian School

The theories of Melanie Klein have been applied by many authors to the treatment of schizophrenia. According to Klein, very early in life the ego develops the capacity to intro-ject and project as a defense against an over-whelming anxiety of annihilation. In the para-noid-schizoid position, which occurs during the first four or six months of life, anxiety is experienced as persecutory in nature. Accord-ing to Rosenfeld,[74] this way of experiencing anxiety contributes to certain defenses, "such as splitting off good and bad parts of the self and projecting them into objects which, through projective identification, become identified with these parts of the self." This process is the basis of narcissistic object rela-tionships, which prevail in psychoses.

The fundamental point of view, advocated by Klein's pupils, Rosenfeld,[72,73,74] Segal,[82] Bion,[23,24] and early Winnicott,[90] is that no modification in the classic Freudian psycho-analytic technique is needed in the treatment of psychotics. Winnicott later changed his views, and came to attribute great importance to environmental factors. Rosenfeld, Segal, and Bion have maintained adherence to Klein-ian theory and to the classic psychoanalytic technique. They continue to use the couch, to rely on free association and interpretation.

In 1954, Rosenfeld[72] reported "that the psychotic manifestations attached themselves to the transference in both acute and chronic conditions, so that what might be called a transference psychosis develops." The concept of transference psychosis had already been introduced by Federn. But contrary to Federn, Rosenfeld felt that the transference psychosis should not be avoided, is indeed analyzable, and should be worked through by means of interpretation. In 1969, Rosenfeld[74] described a number of projective identifications which occur in the treatment of psychotics. He stressed that it is essential to differentiate

these projective parts of the self from the saner parts, which are less dominated by pro-jective identification. These saner parts are in danger of submitting to the persuasion of the delusional self.

On the whole, the theory and methodology of the Kleinian school have received moderate acceptance in England but little acceptance in the United States. It is in South America, espe-cially in Argentina, that they have attained the most prominent role among the various psy-choanalytic orientations.

Methods Based on Participation in Patients' Vision of Reality

Some significant psychotherapeutic meth-ods, although originated from quite different theoretical premises, have the common aim of making the therapist enter and share the pa-tient's vision of reality.

Rosen[68-71] originated his method in 1943. At the suggestion of Federn, he called it "di-rect psychoanalysis." Whereas the usual or indirect psychoanalytic approach establishes communication with the patient through the ego, Rosen's treatment aims at communicating directly with the unconscious, presumably with the id, or with the "ego-states of infancy and childhood" (Federn[33]). As we have al-ready mentioned, Federn also thought that a transference psychosis may occur in the treat-ment of the psychotic, but whereas Federn felt that it had to be avoided, Rosen makes of it the major tool of therapy. In his early writ-ings, Rosen[68,69] described his technique with-out giving theoretical explanations. He gave abundant interpretations to the patient in a vivid and shocking language purported to re-veal what Freud's early works attributed to the unconscious. Such explanations as, "You want to fuck your mother," or "You wish to kill your father," "You want to suck my cock" or "sleep with me," were quite frequent. The explanations were thus based on the concept of repressed sexuality, oedipal in origin.

Rosen believed also that the schizophrenic is the victim of a mother who had suffered from "a perversion of maternal love," and tried to offer to the patient what he did not have. The patient must experience in the therapist a powerful, protective, benevolent person, as he wished his mother would have been in his early childhood. The analyst must spend a long time with the patient—up to sixteen hours a day—and, like Federn, must often resort to an assistant. The patient is showered or shocked with the interpretations, which explain the classic Freudian mechanisms. Such overwhelming, all-embracing treatment would often solve the acute episode in a few weeks and would have to be continued by the second stage of treatment, which follows a technique more similar to classic psychoanalysis.

During the treatment, the analyst enters the psychotic world of the patient, who immediately feels better because he is finally understood. The therapist should not even avoid becoming one of the imaginary persons who appear in the delusions. At times he assumes the role of the persecutor and tries to convince the patient that he will have a beneficial rather than a persecuting effect.

It is worthwhile to take a rapid look at Rosen's theories, developed after his first therapeutic efforts. After the first period of his therapeutic evolution, during which sexuality played the preponderant role, he developed the concept of "early maternal environment." According to Rosen, for the child "mother" equals "environment." "Mother" is an entity that includes not only the mother herself and what she does or fails to do in her maternal role, but also other people, what they do or fail to do. This concept of early maternal environment expands the concept of the "perversion of the maternal instinct" in the etiology of schizophrenia. If this early maternal environment possesses many negative qualities, it may become the chief cause of the disorder.[70]

Another important concept of Rosen is his own modification of the Freudian superego. The superego is "the psychical representative" of the whole early maternal environment. The whole early maternal environment may be worse than the patient's parents. Rosen does not seem, however, to attribute any role to the child in experiencing the environment in a worse manner than it really is.*

Rosen's third important concept is, "You seek the mother you knew," that is, the individual unconsciously selects in his present environment the original characteristics of the early maternal environment. He tries consciously and unconsciously to make a mother out of anybody or anything in his surroundings. "His need for mother is so great that he continues to project maternal attributes upon persons or things which are manifestly not maternal in relation to him."

Rosen's fourth basic concept is that of transference, which is different from the classic Freudian concept. For Rosen, transference is a variety of the tendency to "seek the mother you knew." It is a "transformation of the nonmaternal into the maternal," a projection into the person the patient is involved with of the qualities and attributes he is seeking.

Whereas early in his career Rosen seemed to rely more on the shocking effect of his interpretations, later he came to see the role of the therapist predominantly as one of "foster parent." The unit where the patient lives during the treatment is a foster home. There, the patient will find compensation for the inadequacies of the early maternal environment.

Rosen's method has been the object of much criticism. Even his early admirers pointed out the fragility of his theoretical framework when he had not yet developed his late theories. These admirers attributed his therapeutic successes to his personal qualities: lack of hostility, in spite of some apparently hostile attitudes, straightforwardness, perseverance, physical endurance, etc. Others felt that the interpretations he gave the patients were arbitrary, not even necessary, and that his success was due simply to the fact that he was able in some way to establish contact with the patient. Others[51] doubted even his results. They stated that his claims of many recoveries were exaggerated; that some of his patients were misdiagnosed; that others who were undoubtedly schizophrenic had relapses and

* In this connection, see Arieti, [10, 11, 12, 16] and also Chapter 24 of this volume.

were later treated with physical therapies.

I, too, feel that Rosen's early assertions, like those of many pioneers, suffered from the enthusiasm of their advocate. Also, some of the theoretical bases of his techniques seem unsubstantiated. Nevertheless, it is beyond question that Rosen obtained at least temporary results and that he was able to inject enthusiasm into many workers at a time when the prevalent opinion was that psychotherapy with schizophrenics was an impossibility.

In addition to Rosen's own works on the method of direct analysis are the writings by Brody,[26] English et al.,[32] and Scheflen.[75]

The Swiss psychologist Sechehaye also believed that the world of psychosis can be entered by the therapist with her method of "symbolic realization."[79,80,81] She accepted much of the classic psychoanalytic and existentialist approaches, but added many innovations. In her method, the actions and manifestations of the patient are not interpreted to him but *shared* with him. Of course, by resorting to his psychoanalytic training, knowledge of the patient's life history, and his own intuition, the therapist must in his own mind interpret what the patient experiences and means. Sechehaye's method aims at helping the patient to overcome the initial traumata of his life by offering him a level of interpersonal relations which is corrected and adjusted to the weak state of the psychotic ego. The patient is able to relive the unsolved conflicts of his early life and to solve them, or at least he becomes able to gratify some of his primitive needs. For instance, by giving her patient Renée apples (symbols of the maternal breast), Sechehaye allowed the patient to relive an early trauma and permitted a magical gratification of an oral need. Once the meaning of the patient's symbols is understood by the therapist, he uses them repeatedly in order to establish communication and also to transform reality to a level which the patient can accept without being hurt or traumatized.

What Sechehaye tried to accomplish can be seen as the staging of a dream in waking life. As in dreams, symbols replace the objects which appear in the state of being awake.

Gratification of primitive needs thus can take place. Sechehaye's method aims at entering the dream of the psychosis by creating an artificial and curative dream which eventually will lead to a healthy awakening.

Sechehaye's technique is difficult to practice. Is it possible in the majority of cases to set up an artificial dream which uses the symbols that belong only to a specific patient? A certain capacity for intuition is necessary, which manifests itself after contact is made with the inner core of the patient. Such capacity is not reducible to, or deducible from, rules or instructions or theoretical premises to be found in Sechehaye's method.

Laing's method is difficult to describe, because in spite of the author's many writings it has never been reported in the literature. In his first book, *The Divided Self*,[54] he insists on examining the existential despair, the division of the patient's psyche, his "ontologic insecurity." In his later writings, Laing not only shares the psychotic world of the patient but embraces it. He feels that the patient is correct in blaming his family and the environment. He had to live in an unlivable situation; he really was persecuted, was labeled "psychotic," dismissed from the human community. The method helps the patient to reassert and accept himself, and re-evaluate his position with the society in which he lives. Laing relies very much also on family therapy.[55]

Frieda Fromm-Reichmann and Her School

In contrast with the three previous authors, Harry Stack Sullivan and Frieda Fromm-Reichmann tried to reach the patient not by entering or sharing the psychotic world but by remaining in the world of reality.

Sullivan[85,86] is very well known for his theoretical innovations in psychiatry in general and schizophrenia in particular. People who have worked with him have attested to his therapeutic successes. Unfortunately, his premature death has prevented Sullivan from reporting in writing his technique. Mullahy[59,60] has reported Sullivan's hospital therapy. Mullahy writes that Sullivan attempted a direct and thorough approach, chiefly by reconstructing the actual chronology of the psychosis. Sullivan impressed on the patient that whatever had befallen him was related to his life experience with a small number of people.

Fromm-Reichmann worked closely with Sullivan. Unlike him, she became better known for her therapeutic work than for her theoretical contributions. The value of her therapy received wide recognition. Fromm-Reichmann named her treatment "psychoanalytically oriented psychotherapy," and not "psychoanalytic treatment," to emphasize that it constituted a departure from the classic Freudian psychoanalytic procedure.

Fromm-Reichmann's courage in treating difficult patients, the qualities of her personality—her genuine warmth, humility, and exquisite psychological intuition—certainly played an important role in establishing a milieu of therapeutic acceptance of the schizophrenic and in stimulating others toward similar pursuits. In addition to a very insightful book on psychotherapy,[39] she wrote many papers,[36,37,38,41,42] which have been collected and published by Bullard.[28] Nevertheless, her basic ideas on the therapy of schizophrenia have never been integrated in a systematic whole, perhaps because of a lack of an original theoretical system. For theoretical foundations she leaned on Freud and to a larger extent on Sullivan. Sullivan's idea,[85] that some degree of interpersonal relatedness is maintained throughout life by everyone, including the schizophrenic, was a basic prerequisite of her attempts to establish transference with the psychotic. Fromm-Reichmann stressed that it is very hard for the patient to trust anyone, even the therapist; and if the latter disappoints him in any way, the disappointment is experienced as a repetition of early traumas, and anger and intense hostility result.

Fromm-Reichmann treated the patient with daily sessions, did not make use of the couch or of the method of free association. She relied much less than other authors on the therapeutic effect of interpretations. She made a cautious use of them, however, and emphasized that the symptomatology is susceptible of many interpretations, all correct, and that

at times it is useful to give even partial interpretation.

Fromm-Reichmann was among the first to emphasize that the schizophrenic is not only alone in his world but also lonely. His loneliness has a long and sad history. Contrary to what many observers believe, the patient is not happy with his withdrawal, but is ready to resume interpersonal relations, provided he finds a person who is capable of removing that suspiciousness and distrust which originated with the first interpersonal relations and made him follow a solitary path. In order to establish an atmosphere of trust, the therapist must treat the patient with kindness, understanding, and consideration, but not with condescending or smothering attitudes as if he were a baby. Profession of love or of exaggerated friendship is also out of place. These would be considered by the patient bribery and exploitation of dependency attitudes.

Fromm-Reichmann tried to explain to the patient that his symptoms are ways of remodeling his life experiences in consequence of or in accordance with his thwarted past or present interpersonal relations. She wanted the patient to become aware of the losses he sustained early in life, but he must become aware of them on a realistic level. That is, he must not distort or transform symbolically these losses, but must accept the fact that they can never be made up and that he is nevertheless capable of becoming integrated with the interpersonal world. It will be easier for him to integrate when he recognizes his fear of closeness and even more so his fear of his own hostility.

Fromm-Reichmann inspired many people, not only as a therapist but also as a teacher. Many of her pupils, although maintaining her general therapeutic orientation, have made important contributions. Prominent among them are Otto Will[89] and Harold Searles.[77,78]

Among Will's major points are his insistence that the therapist "define his relationship with his patient, refusing the patient's attempts to avoid such definition by his withdrawal or his insistence that he can never change, that there is nothing the matter, and that the therapist is of no significance to him." In addition to reporting vivid case presentations of patients treated in a hospital setting, Will has given useful instructions about what he calls "the development of relational bond" between the patient and the therapist. Such development requires (a) recurrent meetings of the participants, (b) contact of the participants with each other—verbal, visual, tactile, aural, etc., and (c) emotional arousal.

Searles has written many insightful papers, which have been collected in one volume.[78] They make very rewarding reading, especially for some aspects of the psychodynamics of schizophrenia and of the phenomenon of transference. Searles has described the difficulties of the transference situation: how the patient fights dependence that would compel him to give up fantasies of omnipotence. He has also shown how the transference situation leads the patient to additional projections. In an important paper,[77] he clearly differentiates between concrete and metaphorical thinking in the recovering schizophrenic patient, although he makes no use of the studies done by other authors on this important subject.

Miscellaneous Contributions

Bowers[25] applied hyponosis to the treatment of schizophrenia, although the general opinion is that such treatment is not suitable for psychotics. She hypothesizes that in hypnosis the therapist rapidly establishes contact "with the repressed, healthy core of the patient." She points out that the problems of resolution of the symbiotic relationship require the utmost skill, but long remissions have been secured. A successful hypnotized schizophrenic is moving toward recovery, as he is able to reincorporate the other, the therapist, and thus re-establish interpersonal relations.

Benedetti,[19,20,21] an Italian psychiatrist who studied with Rosen and now teaches and practices in Switzerland, accepts a great deal of Sullivan and Fromm-Reichmann, as well as some existentialist concepts. He feels that the two basic tools in the treatment of schizophrenics are sharing of the feeling of the patient and interpretation. Benedetti feels that

high sensitivity, extraordinary need for love, and reactivity above the average level, make the patient very vulnerable to schizophrenia. The therapist must understand the request inherent in the suffering of the patient.[22] The patient wants the therapist to understand his essence, his being the way he is, even if at the same time he rejects the therapist. Society, including therapists, tends to evade the patient's request by objectifying his symptoms and by not permitting him to make claims.

From an Adlerian point of view, Shulman[84] has described very useful procedures. The therapist must help the patient to make a better rapprochement with life, to avoid the use of psychotic mechanisms, to change mistaken assumptions. In a very human and compassionate way, Shulman describes in specific details how to help the patient through these therapeutic procedures.

❪ Psychotherapy in Practice

In the rest of this chapter an account will be given of psychotherapy of schizophrenics as practiced by the author. Much more extensive accounts of this technique, covering special situations and paradigmatic reports, are reported elsewhere.[4,5,6,7,8,15,16] For didactic purposes, the author's approach can be considered as consisting of four aspects: (1) establishment of relatedness; (2) treatment of the psychotic symptomatology; (3) psychodynamic analysis, that is, acquisition of awareness of unconscious motivation and insight into the origin and development of the disorder; (4) general participation in patient's life. We shall examine these four aspects separately, although they occur simultaneously in various degrees.

Establishment of Relatedness (Transference and Countertransference)

We must frankly acknowledge that, contrary to the other aspects of this type of therapy, establishment of relatedness is at a pre-scientific level of development. Szalita[87] wrote that the therapist must still resort to a large extent to his own intuition. On the other hand, we should not be discouraged or exaggerate the difficulties of this treatment. Even the sickest patient can reacquire the wish to rejoin the human community, which is never completely extinguished. And yet, when we see the patient for the first time, he may have cut all human contacts or may retain only paranoid ties with the world. He feels unaccepted and unacceptable, afraid to communicate, and at times even unable to communicate, having lost the usual ways by which people express themselves. How can we break his isolation, aloneness, overcome the barrier of incommunicability, the uniqueness of his thought sequences?[4,6,8] The therapist's attitude must vary according to the condition of the patient. With patients who are in the prepsychotic panic or who have already entered the psychosis and are acutely decompensating, we must assume an attitude of active and intense intervention. A sincere, strong, and healthy person enters the life of the patient and conveys a feeling of basic trust. From the very beginning, the therapist participates in the struggle which goes on; he does not listen passively to dissociated ideas. With his facial expression, gestures, voice, and attitude of informality and general demeanor, he must do whatever he can to remove the fear which is automatically aroused by the fact that a human being (the therapist) wants to establish contact.

In the confused, unstable, and fluctuating world of the patient, the therapist establishes himself as a person who emerges as a clear and distinct entity, somebody on whom the patient can sustain himself. The therapist must clarify his identity as an unsophisticated, straightforward, simple person who has no façade to put on, who can accept a state of nonunderstanding, who wants to help, though he may be the target of mistrust and hostility, and who has unconditional regard for the dignity of a human being, no matter what his predicament is. An atmosphere of reassurance is at least attempted, and the patient recognizes it. Clarifications are given immediately. The therapist enters the picture, not as an examiner who is going to dissect psychologi-

cally the patient, but as one who immediately participates in what seems an inaccessible situation. To a male patient in panic, I said, "You are afraid of me, of everybody, scared stiff. I am not going to hurt you." To a woman who had given birth recently, I said, holding her hand, "You are going to be a good mother. I am here with you. I trust you."

These statements are "passing remarks" or "appropriate comments"[83] and not detailed interpretations. They are formulations the therapist makes at once, during his first contacts with the patient. They must be given in short, incisive sentences. Their importance lies in conveying to the patient the feeling that somebody understands he is in trouble and feels with him. They should not be confused with deeper interpretations given later.

Some nonverbal, meaningful actions, such as touching the patient, holding his hand, walking together, etc., may be useful in several cases. The therapist must keep in mind, however, that this procedure may be dangerous with some patients. For instance, a catatonic stupor may be transformed into a frightening catatonic excitement.

This attitude of active intervention is not only not indicated in some acutely disintegrating cases, but can be harmful. It may be experienced as an intrusion, and even more than that, as an attack. The patient may be scared, withdraw, and disintegrate even more.

In these cases, we have to resort to an approach similar to the one used with patients who are withdrawn, or barricaded behind autistic detachment. The therapist must be prepared to face negative attitudes and not to experience them as a rebuff. For instance, the withdrawn patient finds it unbearable to look at the therapist's face. He may close his eyes, or turn his face in a diametrically opposite direction. The therapist should not interpret this behavior as rejection of the treatment or of himself, but as ways to reduce to a less intolerable degree the frightening aspect of the interpersonal contact. If the patient is in an acute condition, frightened, and wanting to tell his troubles, the therapist must listen patiently and reassure him warmly. But if the patient does not desire to talk about himself or anything else, he should not be asked questions. Each question is experienced by the schizophrenic as an imposition, or an intrusion into his private life, and will increase his anxiety, his hostility, and his desire to desocialize. The request for information is often interpreted by the patient as "an attempt to take away something from him." Even the therapist seems to him "to take away," not to give. And yet we must convince him of our desire to give to him because he is so much in need.

This technique of not asking questions is a difficult one, especially for a therapist who has been trained in a hospital where patients must be legally committed. The administration of the hospital requires that information be collected directly from the patient which will show that the patient is psychotic and legally detained. The administration also requires a complete physical examination to exclude infective or other acute conditions. Of course, these procedures are necessary, but I feel that the therapist should not carry them out. Perhaps, another physician could take care of these physical and legal requirements before the patient is assigned to a therapist. Although there may be some disadvantages to such a procedure and some physicians might resent the division of jobs, this is, as a rule, the best way to avoid the negative feelings that the patient would immediately develop for the therapist. Whenever it is possible, the contemporaneous treatment of a nonpsychotic member of the family (sibling or parent) can lead to a fuller understanding of the family constellation.

If the therapist is not supposed to ask questions of a reluctant patient, what is he to do? Again, various techniques are indicated according to the various cases:

1. It may be advisable for the therapist to take the initiative and talk about neutral subjects, conveying to the patient the feeling that a sincere effort is being made to reach him, without any strings attached.

2. If the patient is mute, almost mute, or catatonic, the therapist, expressing sympathy and a desire to break the incommunicability

must talk to him. He must tell the patient that he (the therapist) realizes that the patient, though he feels and understands, is so frightened that he cannot talk. At times, however, it is better not to talk at all to the catatonic, if he seems to resent talking and withdraws more. The therapist must then "share" a state of silence without being disturbed by it. Even a simple state of proximity without any talk may disclose to the sensitive therapist almost imperceptible ways of nonverbal communication which are specific for each patient and therefore impossible to report.

3. If the patient is very disturbed, or incoherent, and his speech consists of word-salad, the therapist should not pretend to understand him when he does not, but listen patiently. Soon, it will be realized that the word-salad, too, makes some sense. Some themes recur frequently, and the atmospheric quality of the patient's preoccupations is transmitted.

4. At a more advanced stage of treatment, the patient will be able to talk more freely about himself and about his life. The gaps that still exist either in the knowledge of his life history or in the understanding of his production are often filled in easily by the therapist's knowledge of the psychodynamics of schizophrenia and its formal mechanisms. The therapist must, however, always be alert to the possibility of uncommon and unpredictable dynamic and formal mechanisms.

5. If the patient is a verbose, apparently well-systematized paranoid who fanatically speaks about his delusions, an attempt must be made to detour his attention and re-establish his interest in the other aspects of life.

When the patient speaks to the therapist about his delusions and hallucinations, the latter must not pretend that he accepts them, but must explain to the patient that there must be reasons why he sees or hears or interprets things in a different way.[41]

There are many patients who present active psychotic symptoms, like hallucinations, delusions, or ideas of reference, but have no difficulty in communicating. The more preserved is the bulk of the personality of the patient, the more we can depart from the above recommendations. We may even ask questions and direct the patients to explain their obscure experiences. In these cases, too, the dialogue between the therapist and the patient should not be diagnostic or predominantly exploratory. The emphasis should be on giving and sharing. As a rule, free association, which was impossible with poorly communicating patients, should be discouraged with these relatively integrated patients, as it can promote scattering of thoughts. However, in some mildly psychotic patients free association can be occasionally resorted to when we feel that an attempt to repress important material is more dangerous than the risk of provoking regressive features.

There is a relatively large group of schizophrenics, especially those who had a prepsychotic stormy personality (see Chapter 24), with whom it is very easy to establish some contacts. These patients are hungry for contacts of any kind; they ask questions repeatedly and cling tenaciously to the therapist. The verbal contacts, however, are brittle. They consist of extremely anxious, superficial, and self-contradicting statements. The therapist should not try to force these tenuous contacts to a breaking point. He should realize that at this stage the patient is capable of only this type of communication. The therapist should focus on a few issues which the patient is able to face.

What we have so far described demonstrates that we can indeed talk of transference and countertransference in the treatment of schizophrenics, but not in the same sense as in classic psychoanalysis. As we have seen in Chapter 24, the patient has never had a solid sense of basic trust, and after his break with reality, his mistrust reached gigantic proportions. The ferocious imprinting of early life and the resurgence of the primary process give monstrous shapes to whatever is experienced. The therapist, too, is part of a world of hostility, persecution, and desolation for the patient. In this world, it is easy to feel that it is better to have nothing, not even hope or any positive feeling for other human beings, because if you have them, you are bound to lose them.

The therapist must not fit into this world of unrelatedness, autism, distrust, and suspiciousness. It is by not fitting this world, by escaping from the category of malevolent forces, that the therapist will open a window, facing new, unfamiliar, but promising vistas.

The therapist must play what at first seems a dual and therefore difficult role: He must be a companion of the patient in his journey in the world of unreality, and at the same time he must remain in the realm of a reality shared with the human community. If the therapeutic effort is successful, the distance between these two roles will decrease. With the methods to be described, the unreality of the patient will lose its uniqueness, because it will be partially shared by the therapist, at least emotionally, if not in its symbolic or cognitive elements. The patient will be more willing to return to reality if the anxiety caused by the realistic appreciation of his life's predicament is understood and shared by the therapist. In other words, an interpersonal tie must be established between therapist and patient, which I call *relatedness*. Relatedness includes transference and countertransference. It is the simultaneous occurrence, interplay, and merging of all the transferential and countertransferential feelings and attitudes. The feeling that the patient has for the therapist and the feeling that the therapist has for the patient, elicit other feelings about each other's feelings, in a self-perpetuating reciprocal situation. Although relatedness includes the classic psychoanalytic concept of object relation, it is not only a centrifugal force emanating from each of the two partners in the therapeutic situation, but also an interrelation between at least two persons, more an I-Thou relationship in Buber's sense,[27] an entity whose intrapsychic and interpersonal parts could not exist without the other. At a theoretical level, the ideal goal of any psychotherapy would be the establishment of a state of communion among human beings, but this state is almost always impossible to achieve even among normal people. We must be content with a state of relatedness where an exchange of trust, warmth, and desire to share and help exist.

The relatedness goes through several

stages, which generally follow one another slowly and gradually, but in some cases rapidly and dramatically. From a state of autistic alienation the patient may pass into a state of genuine relatedness. This "breaking through" may be an extremely important episode, experienced at times with great intensity. In some instances, it is remembered by the patient with an emotional outlet reminiscent of the Freudian abreaction. However, "breaking through" in this context does not have the usual psychoanalytic meaning. It does not refer to the breaking of resistances and repressive forces, so that abreaction is possible and what was repressed is now remembered. It means only breaking the barrier of autism, the incommunicability, and the state of desocialization. A human bond between two persons who are important to each other is re-established. Although the therapist must avoid the mistakes the parent has made, the relationship must at first bear some resemblance to the parent-child relationship. Although the therapist, like the parent, is willing to give much more than he receives, a reciprocal concern develops. One fundamental point is that at the stage of treatment in which the establishment of relatedness is the primary goal, this relatedness must be *lived* by the patient as a new experience, and should not be taken into consideration as something to be psychodynamically interpreted, unless some complication necessitates doing this at once. Transference and countertransference are obviously very important as objects of interpretation, but in this respect they must, as a rule, be examined later in the treatment.

Unfortunately, in a considerable number of cases, several and at times contradictory complications may jeopardize relatedness. We shall examine here the most common ones individually, although in several cases they occur in united forms. (For a more elaborated description of these complications, the reader is referred elsewhere.[16]) The complications may necessitate an otherwise premature psychodynamic interpretation of the transferential situation. In many cases, the patient cannot stand too much closeness; he anticipates rejection and fears that rejection after so much

closeness will be more painful, and he wants to be the one who rejects and hurts. These feelings are not fully conscious and put paranoid mechanisms into operation again. The patient tries to place the therapist, too, in the system of delusions, or will test him in many ways, in an attempt to prove that he, too, is not trustworthy. The mistrust may cover any aspect of the relatedness. Manifestations of warmth, interest, participation, sharing, may be viewed by the patient as having ulterior motives, as proofs of the therapist's intent to exploit the patient for heterosexual or homosexual gratification, or for purposes of experimentation, or in order to make a profit of some kind. Whenever tendencies of this type develop, they have to be corrected immediately, before they acquire a degree of strength which may jeopardize the treatment.

Hostility is to be found sooner or later in every schizophrenic. Whenever possible, one should explain to the patient that the hostility is misdirected, and that he is acting as if situations that have long since disappeared were still in existence. When it has proven to be impossible to handle the hostility, the therapist may allow another person to be present at the interview. The patient will not resent this person as an intruder if he understands that this is being done to protect him, too, from the expression of his own hostility.

Some patients, once some elementary relatedness is established, develop an attitude of total dependency on the therapist. They act like babies, trying to reproduce the parasitic or symbiotic attitude they once had toward their mother.[56] The patient must soon realize that the relationship with the therapist is not just a repetition of the old bond with mother, but a new type of close relationship. The new important person in the patient's life is a person who *cares* for him, not only *takes care* of him.

There is an additional type of transference the patient may develop, which also reveals a psychotic structure or understructure. The patient may develop "positive" feelings and concepts for the therapist which are so intense as to achieve unrealistically grandiose proportions and characteristics. The therapist becomes omniscient, omnipotent, a genius, a prophet, a benefactor of the highest rank, a superb lover, etc. This type of relatedness is an exaggeration of the psychotic distortion that certain psychoneurotic patients experience. At times, it reaches comic proportions: The therapist is literally considered an angel or a divinity. The inexperienced therapist may, especially if the distortions are not too obviously psychotic, tolerate this relation and in some cases even receive from it narcissistic gratification.

It is possible to understand such an attitude, even if it is inappropriate. The therapist is the only person with whom the patient relates well; he is the only person who presently counts in the life of the patient, and therefore the only representative of what is good in the universe. If the therapist is of the opposite sex, a romantic element may enter and make the relation more intense. In spite of the fact that the intensity of feeling can be understood, the transferential relation is obviously abnormal. Primary-process cognition distorts the images the patient had once conceived of the good mother and of the ideal lover, and confuses them with the person of the therapist.

The proper procedure consists in correcting these distortions from the very beginning. The therapist must convey the feeling to the patient that he cares for him and that he is very important to him, even if his idealized position has to be dismantled.

We have so far discussed mainly that part of the relatedness which is usually called transference. The countertransference also plays a very important role in the psychotherapy of the schizophrenic. By countertransference we must not mean only identifying the patient with a figure of the therapist's past life or with the therapist himself as he was in his early life, although these identifications play a definite role. The therapist may experience an unusual motivation. Eissler[31] felt that while he was treating schizophrenics his childhood fantasy of wanting to rescue people was reactivated. Rosen[69] wrote that in the treatment of schizophrenics the countertransference must be similar to the feelings that a good parent would have for a highly disturbed

child. Rosen expressed the idea extremely well when he said that the therapist must identify with the unhappy patient, as the good parent identifies with the unhappy child, and be so disturbed by the unhappiness of the patient that he himself cannot rest until the patient is at peace.

If, because of his own problems, the therapist identifies with the patient or even sees in the patient a psychotic transformation of his own problems, he may be helped in his therapeutic efforts rather than hindered.

At an advanced stage of treatment, the therapist loses the parent-like role. The two persons involved in the therapeutic situation become more like peers. We do not mean that they develop a relation similar to the one generally occurring between two young schoolmates, but something reminiscent of the peer-relationship that good parents establish with their adult children.

We often read that termination of the treatment should occur only when the transference and the countertransference are solved. But, if with these terms we mean strong reciprocal feelings, transference and countertransference are hardly ever solved in the treatment of psychoses. The patient cannot cease to have positive feelings for his former therapist, just as a child does not cease to love his parents when he grows and does not need them any longer. Conversely, the therapist cannot forget a patient with whom he had such a long and close relation—a person with whom he shed "blood, sweat, and tears." Therapists remember with great pleasure the feeling of joy and the atmosphere of festivity created when former schizophrenic patients come to visit them years after the end of the treatment. Former psychotic patients never become index cards or collections of old data on yellowed medical records. They remain very much alive in the therapist's inner life to the end of his days.

Treatment of the Psychotic Symptomatology

Some therapists rely only on the establishment of relatedness in the treatment of schizophrenia, especially in very acute cases. The manifest symptoms drop at times as soon as relatedness is established. In this author's experience, although loss of symptoms occurs in some cases, in the majority of cases the symptoms persist or return if the patient has not acquired insight into his psychological mechanisms, and has not changed his vision of himself, the others, life, and the world. Although psychodynamic interpretations are more widely known, interpretations concerning mechanisms and forms are also important, especially in an early phase of the treatment, and we shall devote most of this section to that topic.

Since Jung's formulations, schizophrenic symptoms have been compared to dreams of normal and neurotic persons, and have been interpreted similarly. However, whereas dreams are interpreted while the patient is awake and has reacquired the normal cognitive functions, the schizophrenic has to be treated while he is still in "the dream" of the psychosis.

In several writings,[2,4,5,6,7,8,16] I have described in detail the technical procedures that I have devised to help the patient become aware of the ways in which he converts his psychodynamic conflicts into psychotic symptoms. Whereas the benefit from traditional interpretations is due, or believed to be due, to acquisition of insight into repressed experiences and to the accompanying abreaction, and therefore is supposed to be immediate, the effectiveness of the second type of interpretation consists in the acquisition of methods with which the patient can work at his problems. It does not consist exclusively of insights passively received, but predominantly of tools with which the patient has to operate actively.

We shall discuss this type of treatment in regard to such symptoms as hallucinations, delusions, ideas of reference, and related manifestations. Before doing so, however, we must clarify some issues. Insistence on attacking the schizophrenic symptoms and not the foundations of the disorder may seem advocating only a symptomatic or secondary type of treatment. In the most serious psychiatric conditions, however, we find ourselves in unusual circumstances. The symptom is more than a symptom. Often, it is a maneuver that tends to make consensus with others impossible, or at least to maintain interpersonal distance. What may have originated as a defense makes the position of the patient more precarious and may enhance regression.

Secondly, the symptom, by building a symbolic barricade around the core of anxiety, does not permit us to touch the genuine anxiety. Let us take the typical example of the patient who has an olfactory hallucination: he smells a bad odor emanating from his body. On a deeper level, the patient feels he has a rotten personality; he "stinks" as a person. A schizophrenic process of concretization takes place and an olfactory hallucination results. The patient, by virtue of the symptoms, stops worrying about his personality and worries only about his allegedly stinking body. As long as he talks only about the odor that emanates from him, he will not permit us to affect the focus of his anxiety.

But, if the symptom is needed to cover up or convert the anxiety, why do we want to remove it? Isn't removal of the symptom dangerous? It is dangerous unless we offer something in return which is more valuable. With the establishment of relatedness we offer a great deal to the patient: the realization that a person is there to share the uncovered anxiety and to make an attempt together with the patient to overcome it.

In this spirit of relatedness, the patient is now willing to adopt methods with which he can conquer his symptoms. We shall start with the treatment of hallucinations, which are perhaps the most typical schizophrenic symptoms.

Until recently, the opinion prevailed that incorrigibility was one of the fundamental characteristics of hallucinations. That is, until the symptom disappeared altogether, either through treatment or spontaneously, it would be impossible for the schizophrenic patient to become aware of the unreality of the phenomenon and to correct it. I have found that this is not necessarily so.[4,5,6,7] Only auditory hallucinations will be taken into consideration here, but the same procedures could be applied to other types of hallucination after the proper modifications have been made.

With the exception of patients who are at a very advanced state of the illness, or with whom no relatedness can be reached, it is possible to recognize that the hallucinatory voices occur only in particular situations, that is, *when the patient expects to hear them.*

For instance, a patient goes home, after a day's work, and expects the neighbors to talk about him. As soon as he expects to hear them, he hears them. In other words, he puts himself in what I have called *the listening attitude.*

If we have been able to establish not only contact but relatedness with the patient, he will be able under our direction to distinguish two stages: that of the listening attitude, and that of the hallucinatory experience. At first, he may protest vigorously and deny the existence of the two stages, but later he may make a little concession. He will say, "I happened to think that they would talk, and I proved to be right. They were really talking."

A few sessions later, however, another step forward will be made. The patient will be able to recognize and admit that there was a brief interval between the expectation of the voices and the voices themselves. He will still insist that this sequence is purely coincidental, but eventually he will see a connection between his putting himself into the listening attitude and his actually hearing. Then, he will recognize that he puts himself into this attitude when he is in a particular situation or in a particular mood—for instance, in a mood that causes him to perceive hostility in the air, as it were. He has the feeling that everybody has a disparaging attitude toward him; he finds corroboration for this attitude of the others in hearing them making unpleasant remarks about him. At times, he feels inadequate and worthless, but he does not sustain this feeling for more than a fraction of a second. The self-condemnation almost automatically induces him to put himself into the listening attitude, and then he hears other people condemning him.

When the patient is able to recognize the relation between the mood and putting himself in the listening attitude, a great step has

been accomplished. He will not see himself any longer as a passive agent, as the victim of a strange phenomenon or of persecutors, but as somebody who still has a great deal to do with what he experiences. Moreover, if he catches himself in the listening attitude, he has not yet descended to, or is not yet using, abnormal or paleologic ways of thinking from which it will be difficult to escape. He is still in the process of falling into the seductive trap of the world of psychosis, but may still resist the seduction.

I have found that if an atmosphere of relatedness and understanding has been established, patients learn with not too much difficulty to catch themselves in the act of putting themselves into the listening attitude at the least disturbance, several times during the day. At times, although they recognize the phenomenon, they feel that it is almost an automatic mechanism, which they cannot prevent. Eventually, however, they will be able to control it more and more. Even then, however, there will be a tendency to resort again to the listening attitude and to the hallucinatory experiences in situations of stress. The therapist should never be tired of explaining the mechanism to the patient again and again, even when such explanation seems redundant. It is seldom redundant, as the symptoms may reacquire an almost irresistible attraction.

Now, that we have deprived the patient of his hallucinations, how will he be able to manage with his anxiety? How can we help him to bear his burden or a heavier but less unrealistic cross? An example will perhaps clarify this matter. A woman used to hear a hallucinatory voice calling her a prostitute. Now, with the method I have described, we have deprived her of this hallucination. Nevertheless, she experiences a feeling, almost an abstract feeling, coming from the external environment, of being discriminated against, considered inferior, looked upon as a bad woman, etc. She has almost the wish to crystallize or concretize again this feeling into a hallucination. If we leave her alone, she will hallucinate again. If we tell her that she projects into the environment her own feelings about herself, she may become infuriated. She says, "The voices I used to hear were telling me I am a bad woman, a prostitute, but I never had such a feeling about myself. I am a good woman." The patient, of course, is right, because when she hears a disparaging voice, or when she is experiencing the vague feeling of being disparaged, she no longer has a disparaging opinion of herself. The projective mechanism saves her from self-disparagement. We must, instead, point out to the patient that there was one time when she had a bad opinion of herself. Even then, she did not think she was a prostitute but had a low self-esteem, such as she probably thought a prostitute would have about herself. In other words, we must try to re-enlarge the patient's psychotemporal field. As long as he attributes everything to the present, he cannot escape from the symptoms. Whereas the world of psychosis has only one temporal dimension—present— the world of reality has three—past, present, and future. Although at this point of the illness the patient already tends to live exclusively in the present, he retains a conception of the past, and such conception must be exploited. We direct the patient to face longitudinally his deep feeling of inadequacy. At the same time, the therapist with his general attitude, firm reassurance, and sincere interest, will be able to share the burden. At this point, the therapeutic assistant may be very useful.

What we said about hallucinations could be repeated with the proper modifications for ideas of reference and delusions. Before the delusions or ideas of reference are well formulated, the patient must learn to recognize that he is in what I call the *referential attitude*. Let us take the example of a patient who tells us that while he was in the subway he observed peculiar faces, some gestures that some people made, an unusual crowd at a certain station, and how all this is part of a plot to kidnap and kill him. It is useless to reply to him that these are imaginary or false interpretations of certain occurrences. At this point, he is forced to believe that these events refer to him. We must, instead, help the patient to recapture the mood and attitude which he had prior to those experiences, that is, to become aware of his referential attitude. He will be able to remember that before he went into the subway, he looked for the evidence, he almost hoped to find it, because if he found that evidence, he would be able to explain the indefinite mood of being threatened that he was experiencing. He had the impelling need to transform a vague, huge menace into a concrete threat. The vague menace is the anxiety of the interpersonal world, which, in one way or another, constantly reaffirms the failure of his life.

The patient is then made aware of his tendency to concretize the vague threat. The feelings of hostility and inadequacy he experienced before the onset of the psychosis have become concretized, not to the point of becoming hallucinations, but to the point of delusions, or ideas of reference. No longer does the patient feel surrounded by an abstract world-wide hostility. It is no longer the whole world that considers him a failure; now "they" are against him, "they" call him a failure, a homosexual, a spy. This concretization is gradual. The "they" obviously refers to some human beings who are not better defined.

Not only do we make the patient aware of his referential and delusional attitude, but also of his concretizing attitude. In other words, although the delusions and referential thoughts are symbolic, at this stage of treatment we avoid complicated explanations of symbols. Instead, we help the patient to become aware of his own concretizing, of substituting some ideas and feelings for others that are easier to cope with. For instance, the patient will be helped to recognize that it is easier for him to think that his wife poisons his food than to think she poisons his life. He may also recognize that the feeling he has that some people control his thoughts is a reactivation and concretization of the way he once felt that his parents were controlling or trying to direct his life and his way of thinking. If relatedness is achieved, the patient becomes gradually aware of the almost incessant process of converting the abstract part of his life into concrete representations.

Some of this active concretizing may be difficult for some patients to understand, especially in some manifestations. However, a large number of patients will eventually understand it with great benefit. One of the most obscure and yet most important manifestations of this process of concretization is a phenomenon that has baffled not only patients but psychiatrists as well. A patient happens to think, let us say, that dead relatives are coming to visit him in the hospital. As soon as such thought occurs, it becomes a reality! He believes that the relatives are already there in the hospital. Thoughts are immediately translated into the real facts they represent, just as in hallucinations and dreams they are transformed into perceptions. A thought that represents a possibility cannot be sustained. Schizophrenics are still capable of conceiving and even sustaining thoughts of possibilities when they do not involve their complexes. However, possibilities concerning anxiety-provoking situations are conceived but not sustained for a long time: They are translated into actuality.

The patient is made aware of this tendency, and although at the beginning of the treatment he may not be able to arrest the process, he becomes familiar with what he himself is doing to bring about the delusional world.

The concretizing attitude is expressed not only by ideas and delusions, but also by bizarre behavior. Some patients always stand close to a wall, away from the center of the room. The habit is so common and so well known that we are not liable to make a mistake if we say to the patient, "You want the wall to protect you from the threatening feelings you sense all around. I am here with you. Nothing will attack us. Nothing will injure us. We need no walls. Let's walk together."

To some patients who injure themselves to substitute a physical pain for an emotional one, we may say, "you want to hurt yourself to remove your anguish. If you talk to me about it, we may share the anguish; the pain may diminish." This explanation has to be given with some caution, because self-injury is not always an attempted concretization of mental pain. At other times, it is exclusively or predominantly an expression of need for punishment, or a way to achieve change in gender, or bodily disfigurations that have a symbolic meaning.

A frequent symptom is screaming, at times occurring abruptly, loudly, and in a terrifying manner. Screaming is a way of expressing sorrow, powerlessness, and protest in a way more primitive than even the crying of the sufferer. Crying, as a baby would do, has an appealing quality, which the scream does not possess. The patient feels he cannot appeal to anybody. His life-long whimpering was never heard, and he must scream now. But the therapist must perceive the scream as a lifetime of whimpering and suffering in desolate solitude. He must let the patient know that he has received the message and is ready to answer it.

Different, although related, is the apparently inappropriate hebephrenic smile or, less frequently, the almost spasmodic laughter. The patient laughs at it all, or laughs the world off. The trouble is too big, too lurid; not only must you keep distance, not only must you have nothing to do with it, but you must laugh at it. The therapist must receive the hebephrenic message of defiance and rejection of the world, and help him to find at least a small part of this big world at which he does not need to laugh.

All interpretations discussed in this section require a knowledge of the abnormal cognition of the schizophrenic. The therapist must be able to recognize the special thinking and logic used by the patient and explain it to him. However, if the patient is very regressed, he will not benefit from any direct explanation. There are, however, some abnormal ways of thinking which are not too dissimilar from those of the normal person and can be easily explained.[8,16]

Many other techniques, such as the acquisition of punctiform insight, cannot be reported here for lack of space, and the reader is referred to other writings.[5,16]

Psychodynamic Analysis

Psychodynamic treatment aims at the acquisition on the part of the patient of awareness of his unconscious motivation and of insight into the psychological components of the disorder.

Psychodynamic treatment starts at the beginning of therapy but expands when relatedness has been established and at least some of the prevailing psychotic mechanisms have abated or disappeared. Contrary to what is believed by many, schizophrenics have no insight into the psychodynamic meaning of most of their symptoms. Interpretations are thus necessary when patients are ready to accept them.

A detailed analysis of psychodynamic therapy would require repetition of a great part of the substance of Chapter 24. We shall focus here on some of the fundamental points. In the beginning of treatment, the parental role is generally shifted in a distorted way to the persecutors. In a minority of cases, it is shifted not to persecutors, but to supernatural, royal, or divine benefactors who, in these grandiose delusions, represent figures antithetical to the parents. When the patient re-establishes relatedness and discovers the importance of childhood and his relations with his parents, he goes through another stage. The original parental image comes to the surface and he attributes to the parents full responsibility for his illness and despair. As we have seen in Chapter 24, even many analysts and psychiatrists accept these explanations given by patients as real insights and as accurate accounts of historical events. It is easy to believe in the accuracy of the patients' accounts, first of all because some parents seem to fit this nonparental image; secondly, because the patients who have shifted their target from persecutors to parents have made considerable improvement, are no longer delusional or only to a minimal degree, and seem to a large extent reliable. The therapist must be careful. In a minority of cases, the parents have really been as the patient has depicted them, but in by far the great majority of cases, the patient who comes to recognize a role played by his parents exaggerates and deforms that role. He is not able to see his own deformations until the therapist points them out to him. Fortunately, some circumstances may help. In this newly developed antiparental zeal, the patient goes on a campaign to distort even what the parent does and says *now*. Incidentally, this tendency

is present not only in schizophrenics, but also in some preschizophrenics who never become full-fledged psychotics. By being fixated in an antiparental frame of reference they may not need to become delusional and psychotic. To a much less unrealistic extent, this tendency occurs in some neurotics, too. At times, the antiparental campaign is enlarged to include parents-in-law and other people who have a quasiparental role.

The therapist has to help in many ways. First, he points out how the patient distorts or exaggerates. For instance, a white lie by the parent is transformed into the worst mendacity, tactlessness into falsity or perversion. These deformations are caused by the need to reproduce a pattern established in childhood, a pattern that was the result of not only what historically happened but also of the patient's immaturity, ignorance, and misperception. At times, these deformations are easy to correct. For instance, once the mother of a patient told her, "Your mother-in-law is sick." The patient interpreted her mother's words to mean, "With your perverse qualities you have made your mother-in-law sick, as you made me sick once." On still another occasion, the mother spoke about the beautiful apartment that the patient's newly married younger sister had just furnished. The patient who, incidentally, was jealous of the mother's attention to her sister, interpreted this remark as meaning, "Your sister has much better taste than you." The patient must be brought to realize that the negative traits of parents or other important people are not necessarily arrows or weapons used purposely to hurt the patient. They are merely characteristics of these people and should not be considered qualities involving the total personality.

For instance, there might have been some elements of hostility in the remarks of the mother of the patient, which we have just reported. In every human relation and communication, in every social event, there are many dimensions and meanings, not only in the so-called double-bind talk of the so-called schizophrenogenic mother. But the patient focuses on this negative trend or aspect, and neglects all the other dimensions of the rich and multifaceted communication. The patient is unable to tolerate any ambivalence, any plurality of dimensions.

Most importantly, the original parental introject must lose importance. The patient is an adult now; it is up to the patient to provide for himself or to search out for himself what once he expected to get from his parents.

Whereas at an earlier stage of treatment relatedness (with its transference and countertransference components) was a lived experience, at a more advanced stage of therapy it becomes one of the main objects of interpretation. Whereas earlier in life the patient molded his relations with the world according to a deformed pattern established with the parents or other people, now he has to revise these relations because of the influence of the transferential pattern. Interpretations lead the patient to understand the need for old patterns in his past life and for new ways now.

As we have already mentioned, the general attitude of the therapist will change gradually from one that could be called maternal to one that is paternal at first and later a peer-relation.

Two possible types of countertransference must be recognized and combated. The therapist may have become so used to treating the patient that he is not aware of his improvement. The other type of countertransference is almost the opposite. The therapist has become so familiar with the patient's ways that he no longer recognizes the patient's pathology as such, especially if he has a strong liking for him. He may consider the patient improved when he is not.

Unless the patient changes his self-image, he is not likely to lose his psychosis or potentiality for psychosis. Some symptoms which are generally very resistant to treatment and persist even after long therapy are dismorphophobic delusions, such as the feeling of being very little or deformed, having changed the aspect of one's face, one's head having become flat or empty. These delusions are concrete representations of the distorted image of one's personality. The self-image is so unacceptable

to the patient that he does not want to reveal it. When these dismorphophobic delusions and hallucinations have been lost, the patient has to face what he thinks of himself as a person, not as a body. But now, as we have already mentioned, he will know that the anxiety caused by this confrontation with himself will be shared by the therapist. Moreover, the patient knows by now that his human dignity has been recognized by the therapist, that he is not a specimen in an insane asylum. The therapist has become his peer; the therapist shares values with him.

The therapist eventually makes it clear to the patient that his difficulty to adapt to the environment is not necessarily a negative characteristic from a moral point of view, even if it is from the point of view of practicality and comfort. Normality, or what we call normality, may require mental mechanisms and attitudes that are not so positive or admirable from a point of view that transcends adjustment. Often, what is demanded of the normal person is callousness to noxious stimuli. Normal people protect themselves by denying these stimuli, by hiding them, becoming insensitive, or finding a thousand ways of rationalizing them or adjusting to them. By being so vulnerable and so sensitive the patient may teach us to counteract our callousness, to strive to become the sovereigns of our own will.[14]

Interpretation of dreams plays an important role also in the psychotherapy of schizophrenia. As a rule of thumb, we may say that schizophrenics and nonschizophrenics differ much less in their dreams than in their waking life. However, if we examine a large number of dreams of schizophrenics, we may recognize the following characteristics (valid only statistically, but not necessarily for a single dream):

1. The element of bizarreness is more pronounced.
2. Secondary-process mechanisms hide the latent content less.
3. There is often an element of despair or a crescendo of anxiety, with no resolution.

For other studies of dreams of schizophrenics see Noble,[61] Kant,[53] Richardson and Moore,[67] and Arieti.[7,16]

General Participation in Patient's Life

The treatment of the schizophrenic cannot consist only of the sessions, but an active participation in his life is necessary.

When the patient is very sick and his requirements are immense, I have resorted to the help of a therapeutic assistant.[15] A psychiatrically trained nurse or a former patient, when a nurse cannot be found, are the best qualified to act as therapeutic assistants. Federn[34] and Rosen[69] were the first to report this procedure. If the patient is hospitalized, a nurse assigned especially to him may be very useful to the patient when the latter is not in session with the therapist. A former patient who has been successfully treated and has a fresh memory of the experiences he went through may have a feeling of empathy and understanding difficult to match.[58]

It is particularly at a certain stage of the treatment that the therapeutic assistant is valuable. When the patient has lost concrete delusions and hallucinations, he may nevertheless retain a vague feeling of being threatened, which is abstract, diffuse, and from which he tries to defend himself by withdrawing. The assistant is there to dispel that feeling. That common exploration of the inner life in which the patient and therapist are engaged is now complemented by an exploration of the external life, made together with the therapeutic assistant. The therapeutic assistant helps the patient to decrease his fears in the act of living. Peplau[62,63] thinks that the nurse (or attendant) can accomplish that by establishing a feeling of "thereness." (For many details concerning the relation between the patient and the therapeutic assistant, the reader is referred elsewhere.[16])

At this stage, the patient wants tasks to be given to him and demands to be made on him contrary to the way he felt at the beginning of the treatment. By fulfilling these tasks, the patient will make gains in self-evaluation.

Advanced Stage of Treatment

At an advanced stage of treatment, the patient becomes increasingly similar to a neurotic patient. The therapist should not be overly impressed with the change and should remember that the recovering psychotic always remains more vulnerable and unstable than the neurotic and that some relapses are liable to occur. Conversely, if minor relapses occur, the therapist should not feel unduly discouraged. Their occurrence and their relative mildness in comparison to the initial stages of the illness should be explained to the patient and his family in reassuring terms.

One of the difficulties encountered at a late stage of treatment is fear of improvement. This fear may be caused by many factors. One of the most common is the fear of having to face life again and not succeeding. Being healthy implies responsibility. Again, the fear of life should be analyzed and reduced to normal proportions.

In other cases, in the process of reassuring himself the patient may re-experience that feeling which tormented him in his prepsychotic stage, when he thought that to be himself meant to be odd, and that therefore it was advisable for him to be as others wanted him to be. Actually, this feeling will not last a long time because the patient has learned to accept himself as a person in his own right.

For the handling of the patient in case of separation from his family, the reader is referred to other writings.[16,39]

Several important complications may occur at an advanced stage of treatment. We shall mention here only one: the occurrence of depression, while the patient is improving from schizophrenic symptoms. At times, the reason for the depression is a relatively simple one. By losing the symptoms, especially of the paranoid type, the patient is deprived of something that he may consider valuable. Although manifestations of pathology, the symptoms permitted a certain tie or involvement with the world. Now, the patient feels he has sustained a loss, is empty, more alone and lonely than before. However, the recovering schizophrenic often feels depressed on account of a much more complicated mechanism. When he was paranoid, he projected the bad image of himself to the external world. The persecutors were accusing him, but he felt he was an innocent victim, and his self-esteem apparently benefited. When, as a result of treatment, he is deprived of these paranoid mechanisms, he may tend to reintroject the bad image of himself, to consider himself worthless, guilty, and consequently feels depressed. Generally, in these cases tendencies toward retention of a bad self-image and strong depressive overtones existed even before the psychosis started, but when the psychosis occurred, schizophrenic projective mechanisms prevailed. The self-accusing tendencies have to be analyzed, discussed, traced to their origin, and corrected.

Another idea that may bring about depression or discourage the patient from improving is the thought of getting well for somebody else's sake, not for his own. The idea of submitting again to others, or to the world, is not appealing to the patient. This feeling also will be temporary if the patient now accepts himself and has learned to assert himself.

Criteria for Termination— Concept of Cure

Psychotherapy of the psychotic involves many important considerations, and the reader is again referred elsewhere[16] for such important topics as precautionary measures, legal responsibilities, relations of the therapist with the family of the patient, and rehabilitation of the former psychotic.

When can a patient be considered ready for termination? Loss of symptoms is not enough. End of treatment has to be considered when the patient has modified his self-image, his vision of life and of the world. Self-identity must be more definable and awareness of inner worth must have increased. Reality must be experienced as less frightening and less impinging. The patient no longer experiences a sense of passivity, that is, he does not see himself any longer purely as the object of fate, chance, nature, persecutors, spouse, parents, children, etc., but as somebody who thinks and acts as independently as the other members of society do. He must have succeeded in maintaining an active and satisfactory role in his work, interpersonal relations in general, and intimacy.

Is schizophrenia curable? Before attempting an answer we must define the word "cure." Traditional medicine considered cure a *restitutio ad integrum* or to the *statu quo ante,* that is, a return to the state that existed prior to the onset of the illness. The concept loses some of its significance in psychiatry because in many psychiatric conditions the so-called premorbid state was already morbid and very much related to the subsequent condition. If by cure we mean simply loss of manifest schizophrenic symptomology, the answer is definitely yes. But we have already seen that no psychotherapist should be satisfied with this type of recovery.

If by cure we mean the return to the premorbid state or to an equivalent condition, the answer is still yes. But, again, we cannot be satisfied with a return to a prepsychotic personality. If by cure we mean the re-establishment of relatedness with others, satisfactory intimacy with a few human beings, and reorganization of the personality, which includes a definite self-identity, a feeling of fulfillment or of purpose and hope—and this is the cure we want—in my opinion the answer is still yes. In my experience, we can obtain these results in a considerable number of cases. As a result of psychotherapy, many patients have achieved a degree of psychological maturity far superior to the one that existed prior to the illness.

If by cure we mean a state of immunity, with no possibility of recurrence later in life, my reply is that we are not yet in a position to give an absolute guarantee. Not enough years have passed since intensive psychotherapy has been applied to schizophrenia and the cases are not yet so numerous as to permit reliable statistics.

In reviewing the cases that have been treated satisfactorily with intensive psychotherapy, I have come to the conclusion that my optimistic predictions of no recurrence proved to be accurate in the great majority of cases, but not in all. To my regret, I remember patients whom I treated to a degree that I deemed satisfactory and who nevertheless had relapses. I must stress, however, that in most of these cases the relapses were moderate in intensity and the patients promptly recovered.

In cases in which we cannot obtain a complete cure, we nevertheless achieve a level of living where social relations, conjugal rapport, and work activities are possible to a level matching or surpassing the one prevailing prior to the psychosis. In some less successful cases, the patients learned to recognize situations to which they were vulnerable. By avoiding them, they were able to live an acceptable life.

Many patients whom I consider cured have achieved important positions and a maturity in their personal life that would have been difficult to envision and predict in people who were so ill.

(Bibliography

1. ARIETI, S. "Special Logic of Schizophrenic and Other Types of Autistic Thought," *Psychiatry*, 11 (1948), 325–338.
2. ———. *Interpretation of Schizophrenia.* New York: Brunner, 1955.
3. ———. "The Two Aspects of Schizophrenia," *Psychiatric Quarterly*, 31 (1957), 403–416.
4. ———. "Introductory Notes on the Psychoanalytic Therapy of Schizophrenia," in A. Burton, ed., *Psychotherapy of the Psychoses.* New York: Basic Books, 1961.
5. ———. "Hallucinations, Delusions and Ideas of Reference Treated with Psychotherapy," *American Journal of Psychotherapy*, 16 (1962), 52–60.
6. ———. "Psychotherapy of Schizophrenia," *Archives of General Psychiatry*, 6 (1962), 112–122.
7. ———. *The Psychotherapy of Schizophrenia in Theory and Practice.* American Psychiatric Association Psychiatric Research Report 17, 1963.
8. ———. "The Schizophrenic Patient in Office Treatment," in *Psychotherapy, Schizophrenia, 3rd International Symposium, Lausanne 1964.* Basel: Kargel, 1965.
9. ———. "New Views on the Psychodynamics of Schizophrenia," *The American Journal of Psychiatry*, 124 (1968), 453–458.
10. ———. "The Psychodynamics of Schizophrenia: A Reconsideration," *American Journal of Psychotherapy*, 22 (1968), 366–381.
11. ———. "Current Ideas on the Problem of Psychosis," *Excerpta Medica International Congress, Series No. 194*, 1969.
12. ———. "The Origins and Development of the Psychopathology of Schizophrenia," in M. Bleuler, and J. Angst, eds., *Die Entstehung der Schizophrenie.* Bern: Huber, 1971.
13. ———. "Schizophrenia," *The American Journal of Psychiatry*, 128 (1971), 348–350.
14. ———. *The Will To Be Human.* New York: Quadrangle Books, 1972.
15. ———. "The Therapeutic Assistant in Treating the Psychotic," *International Journal of Psychiatry*, 10 (1972), 7–11.
16. ———. *Interpretation of Schizophrenia*, 2nd Ed. New York: Basic Books, 1974.
17. ARLOW, J., and C. BRENNER. "The Psychopathology of the Psychoses: A Proposed Revision," *International Journal of Psycho-Analysis*, 50 (1969), 5–14.
18. ———. *Psychoanalytic Concepts and the Structural Theory.* New York: International Universities Press, 1964.
19. BENEDETTI, G. "Il Problema della Coscienza nelle Allucinazioni degli Schizofrenici," *Archivio di Psicologia, Neurologia e Psichiatria*, 16 (1955), 287.
20. ———. "Analisi dei Processi di Miglioramento e di Guarigone nel Corso della Psicoterapia." *Archivio di Psicologia, Neurologia e Psichiatria*, 17 (1956), 1971.
21. ———. "Ich-Stourkturierung und Psychodynamik in der Schizophrenie," in M. Bleuler, and J. Angst, eds., *Die Entstehung der Schizophrenie.* Bern: Huber, 1971.
22. ———. Response to Frieda Fromm-Reichmann Award Presentation. Meeting of American Academy of Psychoanalysis, May 1972.
23. BION, W. R. "Notes on the Theory of Schizophrenia," in *Second Thoughts.* London: Heinemann, 1954.
24. ———. "Differentiation of the Psychotic from the Non-psychotic Personalities," in *Second Thoughts.* London: Heinemann, 1957.
25. BOWERS, M. K. "Theoretical Considerations in the Use of Hypnosis in the Treatment of

Schizophrenia," *International Journal of Clinical and Experimental Hypnosis*, 9 (1961), 39–46.

26. BRODY, M. W. *Observations on "Direct Analysis," The Therapeutic Technique of Dr. John N. Rosen*. New York: Vantage Press, 1959.

27. BUBER, M. *I and Thou*, R. G. Smith, transl. Edinburgh: Clark, 1953.

28. BULLARD, D. M. *Psychoanalysis and Psychotherapy: Selected Papers of Frieda Fromm-Reichmann*. Chicago: University of Chicago Press, 1959.

29. BYCHOWSKI, G. *Psychotherapy of Psychosis*. New York: Grune and Stratton, 1952.

30. EISSLER, K. R. "Remarks on the Psychoanalysis of Schizophrenia," *International Journal of Psycho-Analysis*, 32 (1951), 139.

31. ———. "Remarks on the Psychoanalysis of Schizophrenia," in E. B. Brody and F. C. Redlich, eds., *Psychotherapy with Schizophrenics*. New York: International Universities Press, 1952.

32. ENGLISH, O. S., W. W. HAMPE, C. L. BACON, and C. F. SETTLAGE. *Direct Analysis and Schizophrenia: Clinical Observations and Evaluations*. New York: Grune and Stratton, 1961.

33. FEDERN, P. "Discussion of Rosen's Paper," *Psychiatric Quarterly*, 21 (1947), 23–26.

34. ———. *Ego Psychology and the Psychoses*. New York: Basic Books, 1952.

35. FREUD, S. "On Psychotherapy" (1905), in *Collected Papers*, Vol. 1. London: Hogarth Press, 1946.

36. FROMM-REICHMANN, F. "Transference Problems in Schizophrenia," *The Psychoanalytic Quarterly*, 8 (1939), 412.

37. ———. "A Preliminary Note on the Emotional Significance of Stereotypes in Schizophrenics," *Bulletin of the Forest Sanitarium*, 1 (1942), 17–21. (Reprinted in Bullard, Ref. #28.)

38. ———. "Notes on the Development of Treatment of Schizophrenia by Psychoanalytic Psychotherapy," *Psychiatry*, 11 (1948), 263–273.

39. ———. *Principles of Intensive Psychotherapy*. Chicago: University of Chicago Press, 1950.

40. ———. "Some Aspects of Psychoanalytic Psychotherapy with Schizophrenics," in E. B. Brody and F. C. Redlich, eds., *Psychotherapy with Schizophrenics*. New

York: International Universities Press, 1952.

41. ———. "Psychotherapy of Schizophrenia," *The American Journal of Psychiatry*, 111 (1954), 410.

42. ———. "Basic Problems in the Psychotherapy of Schizophrenia," *Psychiatry*, 21 (1958), 1.

43. HARTMANN, H. "Comments on the Psychoanalytic Theory of the Ego," in *The Psychoanalytic Study of the Child*, Vol. 5. New York: International Universities Press, 1950.

44. ———. "Psychoanalysis and Developmental Psychology," in *The Psychoanalytic Study of the Child*, Vol. 5. New York: International Universities Press, 1950.

45. ———. "The Metapsychology of Schizophrenia," in *The Psychoanalytic Study of the Child*, Vol. 8. New York: International Universities Press, 1953.

46. ———. "Notes on the Reality of Principle," *The Psychoanalytic Study of the Child*, Vol. 11, 1956.

47. ———. *Essays on Ego Psychology*. New York: International Universities Press, 1964.

48. HARTMANN, H., E. KRIS, and R. M. LOEWENSTEIN. "Comments on the Formation of Psychic Structure," *The Psychoanalytic Study of the Child*, Vol. 2. New York: International Universities Press, 1945.

49. HILL, L. B. *Psychotherapeutic Intervention in Schizophrenia*. Chicago: University of Chicago Press, 1955.

50. HINSIE, L. E. *The Treatment of Schizophrenia*. Baltimore: Williams and Wilkins, 1930.

51. HORWITZ, W. A., P. POLATIN, L. C. KOLB, and P. H. HOCH. "A Study of Cases of Schizophrenia Treated by 'Direct Analysis,'" *The American Journal of Psychiatry*, 114 (1958), 780.

52. JACOBSON, E. *Psychotic Conflict and Reality*. New York: International Universities Press, 1967.

53. KANT, O. "Dreams of Schizophrenic Patients," *Journal of Nervous and Mental Disease*, 95 (1952), 335–347.

54. LAING, R. D. *The Divided Self*. London: Tavistock, 1960.

55. LAING, R. D., and A. ESTERSON. *Sanity, Madness and the Family*, Vol. 1: *Families of Schizophrenics*. New York: Basic Books, 1965.

56. LIDZ, R. W., and T. LIDZ. "Therapeutic Considerations Arising from the Intense Symbiotic Needs of Schizophrenic Patients," in E. B. Brody and F. C. Redlich, eds., *Psychotherapy with Schizophrenics*. New York: International Universities Press, 1952.

57. LIDZ, T., S. FLECK, and A. R. CORNELISON. *Schizophrenia and the Family*. New York: International Universities Press, 1965.

58. LORRAINE, S. "The Therapeutic Assistant in Treating the Psychotic; Case Report," *International Journal of Psychiatry*, 10 (1972), 11–22.

59. MULLAHY, P. "Harry Stack Sullivan's Theory of Schizophrenia," *International Journal of Psychiatry*, 4 (1967), 492–521.

60. ———. *Psychoanalysis and Interpersonal Psychiatry*. New York: Science House, 1968.

61. NOBLE, D. "A Study of Dreams in Schizophrenia and Allied States," 107 (1950), 612–616.

62. PEPLAU, H. E. *Interpersonal Relations in Nursing*. New York: G. P. Putnam's Sons, 1952.

63. ———. "Principles of Psychiatric Nursing," in S. Arieti, ed., *American Handbook of Psychiatry*, Vol. 2, 1st ed., New York: Basic Books, 1959.

64. RAPOPORT, D. *Organization and Pathology of Thought*. New York: Columbia University Press, 1951.

65. ———. "The Theory of Ego Autonomy: A Generalization," *Bulletin of the Menninger Clinic*, 22 (1958), 13.

66. ———. *The Structure of Psychoanalytic Theory*. New York: International Universities Press, 1960.

67. RICHARDSON, G. A., and R. A. MOORE. "On the Manifest Dream in Schizophrenia," *Journal of the American Psychoanalytic Association*, 11 (1963), 281–302.

68. ROSEN, J. N. "The Treatment of Schizophrenic Psychosis by Direct Analytic Therapy," *Psychiatric Quarterly*, 2 (1947), 3.

69. ———. *Direct Analysis: Selected Papers*. New York: Grune and Stratton, 1953.

70. ———. *Direct Psychoanalytic Psychiatry*. New York: Grune and Stratton, 1962.

71. ———. "The Study of Direct Psychoanalysis," in P. Solomon and B. C. Glueck, eds., *Recent Research on Schizophrenia*. Report 19, Psychiatric Research Reports of the American Psychiatric Association, 1964.

72. ROSENFELD, H. A. "Considerations Regarding the Psycho-analytic Approach to Acute and Chronic Schizophrenia," in *Psychotic States: A Psychoanalytic Approach*. New York: International Universities Press, 1965.

73. ———. *Psychotic States: A Psychoanalytic Approach*. New York: International Universities Press, 1965.

74. ———. "On the Treatment of Psychotic States by Psychoanalysis: An Historical Approach," *International Journal of Psycho-Analysis*, 50 (1969), 615–631.

75. SCHEFLEN, A. *A Psychotherapy of Schizophrenia: Direct Analysis*. Springfield: Thomas, 1961.

76. SCHWING, G. *A Way to the Soul of the Mentally Ill*. New York: International Universities Press, 1954.

77. SEARLES, H. F. "The Differentiation Between Concrete and Metaphorical Thinking in the Recovering Schizophrenic," *Journal of the American Psychoanalytic Association*, 10 (1962), 22–49.

78. ———. *Collected Papers on Schizophrenia and Related Subjects*. New York: International Universities Press, 1965.

79. SECHEHAYE, M. A. *Symbolic Realization*. New York: International Universities Press, 1951.

80. ———. *Autobiography of a Schizophrenic Girl*. New York: Grune and Stratton, 1951.

81. ———. *A New Psychotherapy in Schizophrenia*. New York: Grune and Stratton, 1956.

82. SEGAL, H. "Some Aspects of the Analysis of a Schizophrenic," *International Journal of Psycho-Analysis*, 31 (1950), 268–278.

83. SEMRAD, E. J. "Discussion of Dr. Frank's Paper," in E. B. Brody and F. C. Redlich, eds., *Psychotherapy with Schizophrenics*. New York: International Universities Press, 1952.

84. SHULMAN, B. H. *Essays in Schizophrenia*. Baltimore: Williams and Wilkins, 1968.

85. SULLIVAN, H. S. *Conceptions of Modern Psychiatry*. New York: Norton, 1953.

86. ———. *Schizophrenia as a Human Process*. New York: Norton, 1962.

87. SZALITZ-PEMOW, A. B. "The 'Intuitive Process' and Its Relation to Work with Schizophrenics," *Journal of the American Psychoanalytic Association*, 3 (1955), 7.

88. WEXLER, M. "The Structural Problem in

Schizophrenia: The Role of the Internal Object," in E. B. Brody and F. C. Redlich, eds., *Psychotherapy with Schizophrenics*. New York: International Universities Press, 1952.

89. WILL, O. A. "The Psychotherapeutic Center and Schizophrenia," in B. Cancro, ed., *The Schizophrenic Reactions*. New York: Brunner-Mazel, 1970.

90. WINNICOTT, D. W. "Primitive Emotional Development," in *Collected Papers*. London: Tavistock, 1958.

CHAPTER 28

PHYSICAL THERAPIES OF SCHIZOPHRENIA

H. E. Lehmann

(Historical Introduction

ONCE DEMENTIA PRAECOX had been established as a nosological entity by Kraepelin,[84] an entity which was later extended by Bleuler[14] to encompass the whole concept of the schizophrenias, the search for some physical treatment of this condition began in earnest. Since no single cause of schizophrenia has ever been found, no systematic, rationally focused research in this field could be mounted, except for some isolated attempts to test certain hypotheses. As a result, empirical experiments with a very large number of treatments were conducted by many clinicians all over the world, involving such varied approaches as the administration of manganese*,[118] or the production of sterile abscesses, and such heroic procedures as the artificial induction of aseptic meningitis.

* Although this treatment was unsuccessful and soon abandoned, it is interesting to note that manganese will, in toxic amounts, produce extrapyramidal symptoms, and in this unusual aspect resembles all those drugs which until now have been shown to be effective in the treatment of schizophrenia.

Six physical treatment methods of schizophrenia proved eventually to be at least partially effective, and all were, in fact, developed on a trial-and-error basis, sometimes supported by theoretical speculations or generalizations and sometimes only by chance observations. These six treatment methods were, in chronological order:

1. *Fever,* induced either by typhoid vaccine, foreign protein (milk), or sulphur injections. It was tried, with varied temporary success, by many investigators who were encouraged to attempt this approach following Wagner-Jauregg's successful malaria treatment of dementia paralytica.[127]

2. *Continuous sleep,* induced and sustained by a variety of hypnotic and sedative substances, and introduced as a somewhat risky, but nevertheless sometimes successful, treatment by Klaesi,[80] at a time when no other equally effective treatment of schizophrenia was known.

3. *Hypoglycemic coma,* induced by insulin, and introduced as the first dramatically effec-

tive treatment of schizophrenia by Sakel,[121] after he had observed that the accidental occurrence of hypoglycemic coma in drug addicts was sometimes followed by improvement of their mental state.

4. *Convulsions*, induced first by camphor and later metrazol, and introduced as an effective treatment into psychiatry by Meduna[95] who—incorrectly—speculated that there was biological antagonism between epilepsy and schizophrenia. Convulsive therapy was later improved in its clinical application by Cerletti and Bini,[25] who developed an electrical method of producing convulsions (ECT).

5. *Psychiatric surgery*, first consisting in the surgical serverance of the cerebral tracts between frontal lobes and thalamus (prefrontal lobotomy), after Moniz[97] had learned of certain behavioral observations following experimental neurosurgical interventions in monkeys. Since then, many varieties of the neurosurgical procedures which characterize this treatment modality have been developed.

6. *Systematic pharmacotherapy*, the most successful single treatment of schizophrenia to date, which was introduced into psychiatry by Delay and Deniker[33] in 1952, after they had observed the parmacological action of a newly developed class of psychotropic drugs, i.e., the neuroleptics, on psychiatric patients.

Hyperpyrexia and continuous sleep therapy have now become obsolete as treatments for schizophrenia. Insulin coma therapy is only rarely used today, since electroconvulsive treatment is equally effective for the production of temporary remissions, but simpler, shorter, less hazardous, and less expensive in its application. ECT is still used widely in the treatment of schizophrenia, although mainly in special cases and in combination with pharmacotherapy; but psychosurgery is only very occasionally employed, when all other treatments have failed. The physical treatment of choice in acute and chronic schizophrenia today is pharmacotherapy. It is not equaled by any other treatment in effectiveness, reliability, simplicity, availability, and relative absence of major risks.

Some new physical therapies have been proposed in recent years, e.g., high-dose nicotinic acid and multiple megavitamin treatment, based on the so-called orthomolecular approach.[63,109] Although controlled studies have not yet produced convincing evidence that these treatments are specifically effective, they have been so widely publicized in the professional and lay press that a lively controversy has arisen around them; and for this reason, they will be discussed in some detail.

In this chapter, these physical treatment modalities of schizophrenia which are currently in general use—or, at least, are claimed to have some clinical validity—will be divided into four categories and dealt with under the headings: (1) Pharmacological treatment; (2) metabolic treatment; (3) hypoglycemic coma treatment; (4) neurophysiological treatment; and (5) psychiatric surgery.

(Pharmacological Treatment

There are today ten different chemical groups of drugs that have been shown in clinical trials to effectively reduce schizophrenic symptomology. All of them belong to the pharmacological class of neuroleptics, also often referred to as major tranquilizers and, occasionally, as antipsychotics. These groups are: the phenothiazines, the thioxanthenes, the butyrophenones, the rauwolfia alkaloids, the benzoquinolines, the benzothiazines, the acridanes, the diphenylbutylpiperidines, the phenylpiperazines and the indolic derivatives.[10]

Only compounds belonging to the first four of these chemical groups are in clinical use today, but drugs belonging to some of the other known, or still undiscovered, chemical groups will probably be marketed and find clinical application in the near future. Some of the more promising candidates for future use will be referred to later in the text.

The first two drugs that were developed in this new pharmacological class were chlorpromazine and reserpine, and their most prominent action appeared to be sedation. This fact accounts for their designation as "tranquilizers," although some of the subsequently developed drugs of this type did not produce primary sedation and were, in fact, weak stimulants. To distinguish these substances from the old-type sedatives, which do not possess any specific antipsychotic potential, they are now usually referred to as "major tranquilizers," while the traditional sedatives are called "minor tranquilizers" or "anxiolytics."

All major tranquilizers are characterized by their neuroleptic effects and thus are also frequently classified as neuroleptics. Neuroleptic effects are of three types: (1) on the extrapyramidal system (globus pallidus and corpus striatum), often resulting in a variety of extrapyramidal symptoms, such as Parkinsonism, akathisia, or dystonia; (2) on hippocampus and amygdala, resulting in a lowering of the convulsive threshold; (3) on the reticular formation and the hypothalamus, resulting in a reduction of perceptual input, as well as psychomotor excitement and emotional tension, and in the occurrence of varied changes in the functioning of the autonomic nervous system.

Mechanisms of Action

No definitive account can be given of the way in which neuroleptic drugs bring about their antipsychotic effects, but several theories exist. Neurophysiologically, the drugs diminish activation (arousal) of the CNS without producing significant inhibition of cortical functioning and thus, in contrast to the minor (anxiolytic) tranquilizers, they do not induce disinhibition of behavior and affect, nor significant impairment of the higher functions of the CNS, e.g., impairment of the processes of rational abstraction and synthesis. The reduction of excessive perceptual input and psychomotor output serves as a therapeutic intervention in conditions where "jamming" of the CNS, through disproportionate input and arousal, has resulted in psychotic disintegration of functioning.[87]

Most neuroleptic drugs possess a strong sympatholytic action which is probably mediated through a blocking of adrenergic and dopaminergic receptor sites in the neurones.

Mobilized by this blockade, compensatory feedback mechanisms call forth an accelerated production of catecholamines, with the result that dopamine levels in the brain are increased following the administration of neuroleptic drugs, despite the fact that systemic adrenergic effects are diminished.[130,114,38]

Metabolically, the major tranquilizers seem to exert a sparing action, which manifests itself in increased cerebral levels of the high-energy phosphate ATP.[55]

Finally, there is considerable evidence that neuroleptic drugs interfere with the functioning of cellular membranes and thus with the exchange of electrolytes at the neuronal level.[58]

Clinical Application

The use of neuroleptic drugs in the treatment of schizophrenia may be considered under four headings:

1. As *symptomatic treatment* of acute psychomotor agitation, aggression, or chronic tension.
2. As the principal therapeutic agent in the management of *acute schizophrenic* breakdowns.
3. As a major single treatment factor in the management of *chronic schizophrenic* conditions.
4. As *maintenance therapy* for patients in remission, in whom the recurrence of schizophrenic symptoms must be prevented.

Prior to 1952, no drugs were known which could deal effectively with psychotic symptoms indicating a severe disturbance of a patient's contact with reality, such as hallucinations, delusions, and autistic thought disorders; nor was there any effective way of preventing psychotic relapses of a patient in remission. Now, there is a wide choice of pharmacological agents which can help the psychiatrist to control both of these special problems.

Table 28–1 lists the neuroleptic drugs that are currently available in the United States and Canada. Figures 28–1 to 28–4 show the

TABLE 28–1. **Different Neuropleptic Drugs Available in the United States and/or Canada and Their Estimated Equivalence in Milligrams When Compared to Chlorpromazine**

GENERIC NAMES	TRADE NAMES *United States*	*Canada*	ESTIMATED EQUIVALENT POTENCY
PHENOTHIAZINES			
Aliphatic Derivatives			
Chlorpromazine	Thorazine	Largactil	1
Methotrimeprazine	Levoprome	Nozinan	1.5
Promazine	Sparine	Sparine	0.5
Triflupromazine	Vesprin	Vesprin	4
Piperazine Derivatives			
Acetophenazine	Tindal	Notensil	6
Butaperazine	Repoise	Randolectil	10
Carphenazine	Proketazine	N.A.	4
Fluphenazine	Prolixin	Moditen	50
Perphenazine	Trilafon	Trilafon	10
Prochlorperazine	Compazine	Stemetil	6
Thiopropazate	Dartal	Dartal	10
Thioproperazine	N.A.	Majeptil	40
Trifluoperazine	Stelazine	Stelazine	20
Piperidine Derivatives			
Mesoridazine	Serentil	Serentil	1.5
Piperacetazine	Quide	Quide	10
Propericiazine	N.A.	Neuleptil	3
Thioridazine	Mellaril	Mellaril	1
THIOXANTHENES			
Chlorprothixene	Taractan	Tarasan	1
Thiothixene	Navane	Navane	50
BUTYROPHENONE			
Haloperidol	Haldol	Haldol	70
RAUWOLFIA ALKALOID			
Reserpine	Serpasil	Serpasil	60

chemical structure of some representative compounds of the four groups of the neuroleptics which are now in clinical use, i.e., the rauwolfia alkaloids, the phenothiazines, the thioxanthenes, and butyrophenones.

The active principle of the rauwolfia plant, which had been used for centuries in India as a treatment for various mental and emotional ills, was isolated in the form of reserpine.

The first derivative of the phenothiazine group which proved to be effective in the treatment of psychotic symptoms was chlor-promazine; it was the synthetic product of a pharmacological search for a tranquilizing substance to be used in anesthesia.

The thioxanthenes were the result of a systematic modification of the phenothiazine nucleus, once its therapeutic potential had been discovered.

The first butyrophenone derivative with good therapeutic action in psychotic conditions was haloperidol. This drug was the result of a deliberate search for new chemical compounds with antipsychotic properties, such as

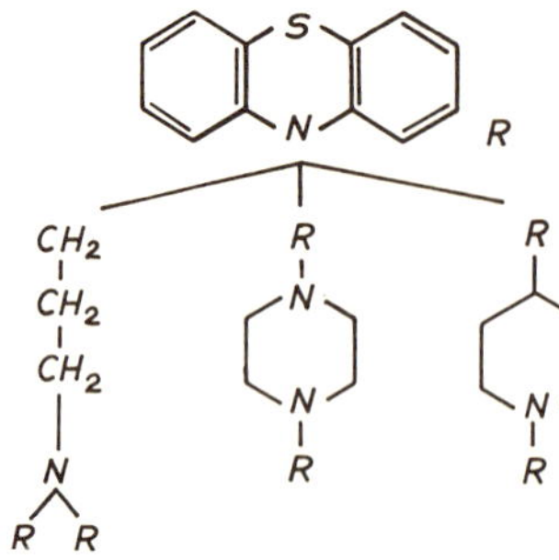

DIMETHYL   PIPERAZINE   PIPERIDINE

Figure 28–1.   Phenothiazine structure.

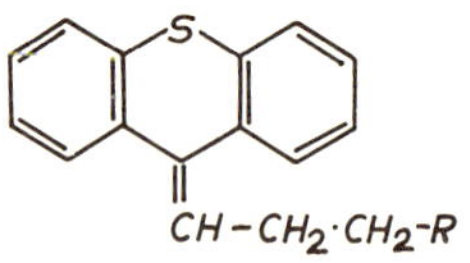

Figure 28–2.   Thioxanthene structure.

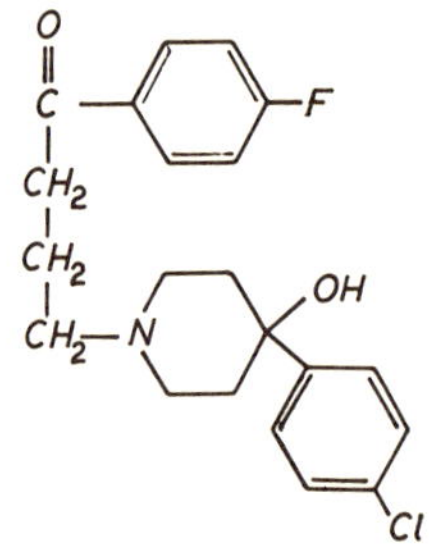

HALOPERIDOL

Figure 28–3.   Butyrophenone derivative.

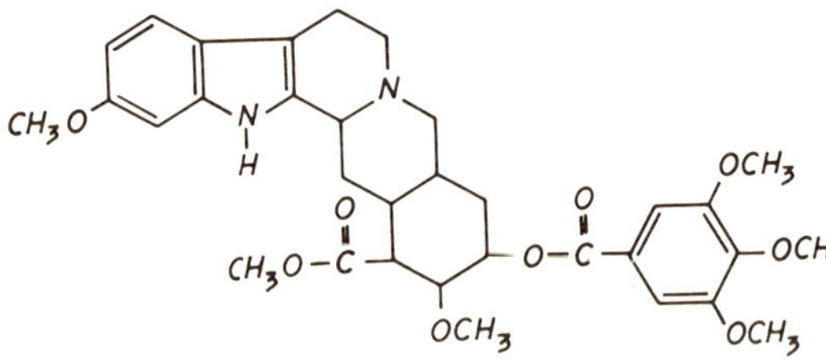

RESERPINE

Figure 28–4.   Rauwolfia derivative.

had been discovered in the rauwolfia and phenothiazine derivatives.

RAUWOLFIA ALKALOIDS

Reserpine and other rauwolfia preparations are prescribed today only infrequently in the treatment of schizophrenia. They act more slowly than phenothiazines and butyrophenones, and their side-effects are often more disturbing. However, in a small number of cases which have been relatively refractory to treatment with other antipsychotic agents, the rauwolfia derivatives are still prescribed occasionally.

A specific effect of reserpine is the release of stored neurohormones, e.g., serotonin and norepinephrine, from brain cells. Related to this effect is probably the observation that a certain proportion of patients receiving reserpine may develop depressive conditions. Rauwolfia derivatives are incompatible with monoamine-oxidase inhibitors and should not be prescribed simultaneously with them. It has also been shown that electroconvulsive therapy must not be administered while patients are on reserpine medication. At least a week should elapse between discontinuation of reserpine therapy and the first electroconvulsive treatment.

PHENOTHIAZINES

The most widely employed drugs in the management of schizophrenia are the phenothiazines. Common to all of them is the phenothiazine nucleus. However, the various phenothiazine derivatives differ in the structure of their side chains. Almost all of the currently used preparations with good antipsychotic action present a straight chain of three carbon atoms attached to the nitrogen of the phenothiazine nucleus, but in other respects the side chains may differ considerably (Figure 28–1).

Phenothiazine compounds with a *dimethyl* or *aliphatic* side chain tend to evoke drowsiness and various autonomic symptoms.

The *piperazine derivatives* do not produce drowsiness as a rule, and might, in fact, be mildly stimulating in their pharmacological action. However, since many schizophrenic patients are agitated, owing to their particular psychopathology, the secondary and global effect of these drugs might, nevertheless, be tranquilization, because the drugs reduce psychotic tension or other psychopathological manifestations, such as hallucinations and delusions. While less likely than the aliphatic derivatives to produce sedation and autonomic effects, phenothiazine derivatives with a piperazine structure are characterized by a much greater likelihood to evoke extrapyramidal symptoms than the phenothiazines with an aliphatic side chain, and milligram for milligram, they possess greater pharmacological potency than the latter.

The *piperidine derivatives* currently in clinical use are characterized by the lowest incidence of extrapyramidal symptoms and also, like the group with an aliphatic side chain, by a tendency to produce somnolence and more autonomic symptoms.

THIOXANTHENES

The thioxanthene derivatives are tricyclic neuroleptics with a modified phenothiazine nucleus: The nitrogen in the middle ring is missing. Only two drugs of this category are on the market now, and most of what has been stated about the structure-response relationships in phenothiazines, depending on the nature of the side chains, applies also to the thioxanthenes.

BUTYROPHENONES

Butyrophenones differ in their chemical structure from reserpine, the phenothiazines, and thioxanthenes. Pharmacologically, they resemble the piperazine group of phenothiazines, in that they are effective in small doses and provoke extrapyramidal symptoms in a high proportion of cases.

DIFFERENTIAL ACTION OF DRUGS

Which of the many neuroleptic drugs should one prescribe in a given case? If the use of reserpine today is limited because of the reasons given above, what about the choice between the different phenothiazines, thioxanthenes, and butyrophenones? For some time, it was thought that phenothiazines with predominantly sedative properties—for instance, chlorpromazine and thioridazine—would be indicated in the excited schizophrenic, but would be contraindicated in the withdrawn or stuporous one. It has been shown, however, that a stuporous catatonic patient might respond with an increase of spontaneity and activity to chlorpromazine just as rapidly as he might respond to one of the more stimulating phenothiazines, for instance, perphenazine or trifluoperazine. Most clinicians prefer, nevertheless, to prescribe one

of the more sedating phenothiazines for the excited schizophrenic, and one of the piperazine derivatives, which have a mildly stimulating effect, for the chronically inert patients. While this is the general practice, the fact remains that there is no persuasive evidence that the reasoning behind this choice is valid.[103]

Some authors were able to reveal certain differential effects of one phenothiazine or another, and the findings—while significant more in the statistical than in the clinical sense—were based on carefully designed and well-controlled multihospital studies and on relatively large samples of patients.[*][102,82,48] However, when trying to replicate their findings in follow-up studies, two investigators could not crossvalidate their original results.[45,47] Others have been unable to detect any differential pattern of response to haloperidol, a butyrophenone, or perphenazine, a phenothiazine.[50]

For clinical purposes, it may thus be concluded that all neuroleptic drugs are of approximately equal therapeutic efficacy in the treatment of schizophrenia.[26] Their chief differences are to be found in the dosages they require and in the side-effects they produce. Of course, another difference to be considered, particularly with drugs which may have to be used for a long time, is the economic differential—the price of each drug.

DOSAGE

Dose requirements for neuroleptic drugs vary according to the following factors: (1) Type of drug; (2) stage of the illness; (3) therapeutic goals, e.g., suppression of symptoms or preventive maintenance treatment; (4) individual differences.

* For instance, in one large NIMH collaborative study with acute schizophrenic patients, the investigators concluded, from regression equations based on symptoms present before treatment, that chlorpromazine was most effective for "core" symptoms of schizophrenia (e.g., slowness of speech, poor self-care, indifference to environment), acetophenazine for "bizarre," and fluphenazine for "depressive" symptoms.[102] Casework interviews with these same patients later revealed that fluphenazine was relatively more effective in patients whose premorbid history would suggest a poor prognosis, and less effective in patients where good prognostic conditions existed; in this latter case, acetophenazine appeared to cause greater improvement.[122]

In discussing dosage, it is convenient to reduce the dose requirements for different drugs to standard "chlorpromazine units," or the milligram for milligram potency of other neuroleptics relative to chlorpromazine. Table 28–1 gives this ratio by showing the approximate potency (in milligrams) of various neuroleptic drugs in comparison to chlorpromazine. For example, perphenazine being ten times as potent as chlorpromazine, one milligram of perphenazine is roughly equivalent to 10 mg. of chlorpromazine. As a rule of thumb, it may be assumed that neuroleptic drugs which are administered intramuscularly—they should never be given intravenously—are about three times as effective as orally administered drugs.

An informative review by Klein and Davis[81] has shown that in a large number of placebo-controlled studies, the cutting point for effective doses of neuroleptics in the treatment of acute schizophrenic conditions was at a daily dose of about 300–500 mg. of chlorpromazine. We consider a daily dose range of *300-1000 mg.* as indicated for the treatment of *acute schizophrenic conditions.* In certain patients, these daily doses may have to be increased to 2000–3000 mg. of chlorpromazine, or the equivalent dose of another neuroleptic. When the acute symptoms have been brought under control, a gradual reduction of dose should be attempted to prepare the patient for *maintenance therapy,* which usually employs daily doses of *100–500 mg.* of chlorpromazine, or its equivalent.

While it is a good general rule to gradually increase the dose of drugs which may cause systemic effects, one will often have to proceed more rapidly in the case of an acutely disturbed schizophrenic patient. It is advisable to initiate treatment in an agitated patient with a 50 mg. dose of chlorpromazine, or its equivalent, given intramuscularly (or 100 to 150 mg. by mouth), and then give subsequent doses at thirty-minute intervals—if necessary, doubling the initial dose—until the patient's most disturbing symptoms are controlled. It may thus be necessary to reach a dose of 500–600 mg. in staggered increments during the first day.

Once the optimal daily dose has been established, it may be divided into three or four daily doses during the acute stage, but when the subacute or chronic stage of the illness prevails, there will be no need to exceed twice-a-day medication, as has been demonstrated in recent studies. During maintenance treatment, it is advisable to restrict the patient's drug-taking to once—certainly not more than twice—a day.[36]

Neuroleptic drugs have relatively low toxicity, which allows for a large therapeutic margin. It is not well understood why dose requirements of neuroleptic drugs often vary widely in different individuals, but some recent work indicates that different ways of metabolizing drugs characterize different individuals, and genetic-constitutional differences of enzymatic breakdown mechanisms and protein binding are probably responsible for the fact that identical doses of neuroleptics may produce greatly different plasma levels in different subjects. Although no clear correlation between plasma levels and therapeutic outcome has been established so far, plasma levels do correlate with the occurrence of side-effects.[52,30,31]

What is an adequate dose? There is a clinical relation between the time of disappearance of certain symptoms and dosage, which can be helpful in determining whether a particular dosage schedule is effective. It has been observed that symptoms belonging to the parameter of arousal, e.g., excitement, restlessness, irritability, and insomnia, tend to be the first ones to be controlled by effective doses of neuroleptic drugs, i.e., after two to four weeks of pharmacotherapy. Symptoms related to perceptual and cognitive functions, e.g., hallucinations, delusions, and thought disorder, disappear last, i.e., in many cases, only after a treatment period of four to eight weeks.[87]

Observing this "timetable" of therapeutic responses to neuroleptic therapy will enable the physician to determine whether the dose of the drug he is prescribing is adequate for a given patient. There may be need to increase the dose if the patient is still restless, irritable sleepless, anxious, and withdrawn four weeks after drug treatment was started; on the other hand, dosage may be adequate if after six weeks of therapy the patient is quiet, friendly and co-operative, although in a psychiatric examination he may still show evidence of hallucinations, delusions, and thought disorder, which may not disappear for another few weeks.

Maintenance Treatment

It is now well established that medication must be continued for some time after the schizophrenic patient has become symptom-free, or an optimal level of symptom control has been reached. Since pharmacotherapy can not cure schizophrenia—not any more than insulin can cure diabetes or digitalis congestive failure—but only suppresses its symptomatic manifestations, maintenance medication must be continued indefinitely, if no spontaneous remission of the basic pathology occurs. Unfortunately, there is as yet no way to select those patients in whom spontaneous remission in the natural course of schizophrenia would make it unnecessary to continue with maintenance medication. This means that one either has to accept the risk of a psychotic relapse, or the patient must continue, perhaps unnecessarily, on maintenance medication for an undetermined period of time.

Just how great is the risk of relapse? There are many studies, some controlled, some uncontrolled, all of which tend to indicate that the risk of recurrence of a schizophrenic attack is at least twice as great for patients on no maintenance drug or on placebo, as it is for those on active maintenance drug therapy.[85,115,128,57, 23,106,124,49,40]

Relapse rates reported in these studies vary widely, from 7 percent (in a one-year follow-up) of patients on maintenance drug in uncontrolled studies, to 33 percent in controlled trials; and from about 20 percent to more than 70 percent for patients not taking neuroleptics. In one of the best recent controlled studies, which was carried out simultaneously in three different clinics, Hogarty and his co-workers[74] found a 72.5 percent relapse rate of schizophrenic patients at the end of twelve months

in patients receiving only placebo, and a 32.6 percent relapse rate of schizophrenic patients receiving an active drug (chlorpromazine). These results were somewhat improved when social therapy was combined with placebo or drug; the relapse rates were then 62.65 percent with placebo and 25.74 percent with drugs. The investigators point out that 30 percent of their patients did well on placebo for a period of ten months, and then rather suddenly relapsed without having given warning. It was not possible to determine any criteria by which these late relapsers could have been identified earlier. The research team also felt that the relapse rate of the patients on drug would have been lower, 20 percent or less, if all patients would have taken their drug regularly.

It is, however, well known that many patients are very unreliable about following a maintenance drug regime. One study[60] in Britain reports that almost 40 percent of patients on maintenance treatment were irregular drug-takers or stopped taking their medication altogether. How to induce patients—and their families, who are often opposed to the "doping" of a relative in remission—to take their maintenance treatment seriously, is a difficult problem in motivation, a problem which is frequently much more difficult to resolve than the one presented by the treatment of an acute schizophrenic breakdown.

Long-acting neuroleptics are now available, for instance, fluphenazine enanthate or fluphenazine decanoate, which can be injected intramuscularly every two weeks (in doses from 25 to 50 mg.) and remain effective for that fifteen-day period. A new butyrophenone derivative—penfluridol—is now being studied and may soon be available for clinical purposes; this drug may be given orally and retains its effectiveness for five to seven days.[12] The potential impact of long-acting drug therapy on the management of the unreliable or possibly dangerous patient in remission is being widely discussed.[88]

Adverse Reactions

Although the neuroleptics have a remarkably low toxicity and unusually wide therapeutic margin, they also have a broad range of unpleasant side-effects. Most of these do not constitute serious complications, and many can be effectively counteracted with other drugs or through simple reduction of dosage.

However, the inconveniences they cause for the patient may become important obstacles to the proper and consistent application of pharmacotherapy in some schizophrenics. It is, therefore, important to anticipate the occurrence of such side-effects, so that the patient may be reassured if they make their appearance.

Table 28–2 (adapted and extended from *Medical Letter*) lists some of the most important adverse reactions and their frequency of occurrence.

Oversedation, particularly frequent with the aliphatic and piperidine phenothiazines and thioxanthenes, usually disappears after about two weeks, when tolerance to this reaction develops.

Extrapyramidal symptoms occur in about 30 percent of patients receiving aliphatic or piperidine phenothiazines or thioxanthenes, and in more than 50 percent of those receiving other neuroleptics. Antiparkinsonism drugs counteract these reactions effectively. How-

TABLE 28–2.   Nature and Frequency of Adverse Reactions to Various Types of Neuroleptic Drugs

| | PHENOTHIAZINES | | | THIOXAN-THENES | BUTYRO-PHENONES |
	Aliphatic Derivatives	*Piperazine Derivatives*	*Piperidine Derivatives*		
Behavioral					
Oversedation	+++	−	+++	+++	−
Extrapyramidal					
Parkinson's Syndrome	++	+++	+	++	+++
Akathisia	++	+++	++	++	+++
Dystonic reactions	++	+++	++	++	+++
Autonomic					
Postural hypotension	+++	+	+++	++	++
Anticholinergic effects	+++	++	+++	++	+
Genito-Urinary					
Inhibition of Ejaculation	++	++	+++	−	−
Cardio-vascular					
ECG abnormalities	+	+	++	−	−
Hepatic					
Cholestatic Jaundice	++	+	+	+	+
Hematological					
Blood dyscrasias	++	+	+	+	++
Ophthalmological					
Lenticular pigmentation	++	+	−	−	−
Pigmentary retinopathy	−	−	++	−	−
Dermatological					
Allergic skin reaction	++	+	+	+	+
Photosensitivity reaction	++	+	++	+	+
Skin Pigmentation	++	−	−	−	−

KEY: +++, Common   ++, Uncommon   +, Rare

ever, it has recently been shown that in many patients antiparkinsonism drugs have to be administered only for a few weeks; they may then be withdrawn without a recurrence of extrapyramidal symptoms. Because most antiparkinsonism drugs have a powerful anticholinergic action and thus often produce complications of their own, it has been recommended that these drugs should not be prescribed routinely for prophylactic purposes, but used mainly to counteract extrapyramidal symptoms after they have appeared, and withdrawal should be tried after a few weeks.[37,110]

Tardive dyskinesia is an extrapyramidal syndrome that occurs in about 7–15 percent of patients who have been exposed to long-term treatment with neuroleptics. So far, the syndrome has been most frequently observed in patients on piperazine phenothiazines; but this may be because not sufficient observations on cases who are treated with newer neuroleptics have been accumulated as yet. This syndrome, which is most likely to appear in elderly patients, is characterized by involuntary movements of the oral region of the face, mostly of the lips and tongue, and sometimes also by chorea-like movements of other muscle groups. What makes this drug-induced condition more serious is the fact that these late-occurring involuntary movements, unlike the earlier-appearing drug-induced extrapyramidal symptoms, are seldom reversible. However, they often appear only after the neuroleptic medication has been reduced or discontinued, since the same drugs that are causing the extrapyramidal damage underlying tardive dyskinesia are also capable of inhibiting its symptomatic manifestations. Until now, these complications have mostly been observed in aged, chronic, often institutionalized patients who seem to be little distressed by it. However, there is now some evidence that children who have been treated for a long time with neuroleptic drugs may develop a similar condition.[32,59,28,39]

It may be possible eventually to develop antipsychotic drugs that do not produce extrapyramidal symptoms, which are the most troublesome of all neuroleptic side-effects. As an example, a recently developed drug (clozapine), which has not yet been released for general use, has shown good antipsychotic properties in clinical trials and appears to be free from extrapyramidal reactions.[4]

Anticholinergic effects are usually restricted to constipation, dryness of the mouth, and, in some cases, to difficulties with visual accommodation. More severe reactions of this type, e.g., toxic psychotic states or adynamic ileus, are, as a rule, the result of a combination of neuroleptics, particularly phenothiazines, with antiparkinsonism drugs and/or tricyclic antidepressants.[131,132]

Inhibition of ejaculation may cause the patient some anxiety if he has not been warned of the possible occurrence of this symptom; reduction of dosage is usually all that is necessary to control this side-effect.

ECG abnormalities, consisting of a prolongation of the QRS complex and changes in the T-wave, are due to faulty repolarization in the myocard; they resemble the abnormalities seen in potassium deficiency and are fully reversible. They occur most frequently with thioridazine and are probably of little clinical significance, except in patients who have some pre-existing cardiac impairment or are in electrolyte imbalance.[8]

Cholestatic jaundice used to occur much more frequently when chlorpromazine was first introduced, but, for reasons not fully understood, is a comparatively rare occurrence today. When it occurs, it ends almost invariably in spontaneous recovery after a few days or weeks.

Of the *blood dyscrasias*, temporary leucopenia may occur rather frequently, but agranulocytosis only once in every 1500 to 5000 cases. It has been observed most frequently with the aliphatic phenothiazines. Routine blood counts are of little help in predicting agranulocytosis; only continuous clinical vigilance can discover the appearance of this complication early enough to control it successfully with immediate, energetic, therapeutic measures.[75,7,113,91]

Lenticular pigmentation, in the form of stellate cataracts and pigment deposits in the posterior wall of the cornea, is seen almost exclusively after long-term treatment with chlorpromazine. They can be detected by slit-lamp examination. Fortunately, they usually do not interfere significantly with visual acuity, even when they are present to considerable degree. *Pigmentary retinopathy* has only been observed with large doses (over 900 mg./day) of thioridazine. It is a serious complication, because it impairs visual function and is often irreversible.

Allergic skin reactions usually respond promptly to antihistaminics, a reduction of dosage, or a change to another neuroleptic. *Photosensitivity* is most pronounced with chlorpromazine; but every person taking a neuroleptic drug should guard against exposing unprotected skin to sunlight. Persistent purple *pigmentation of the face* has been observed in a small proportion of patients who had been exposed to large doses (over 500 mg./day) of chlorpromazine for extended periods of time (longer than twelve months).

A number of *sudden, often unexplained and autopsy-negative deaths* occurring in patients receiving neuroleptics, more particularly phenothiazines, have been attributed by several authors to certain adverse effects of these drugs on the cardiovascular or respiratory system, or on autonomic regulation mechanisms. This conjecture has recently been challenged by two investigators who surveyed the literature on such cases in several countries and concluded that many of the "sudden phenothiazine deaths" may have been cases of "lethal catatonia," or the result of some other unexplained factors which are also operating in drug-free subjects in the general population.[111]

A survey of 4,625 patients, half of them on neuroleptics, showed that the mortality of patients on neuroleptic drugs was not higher than of hospitalized schizophrenic patients who were not on drugs.[126]

A study in a Canadian mental hospital compared the death rates in several patient groups prior to and after the introduction of neuroleptic drugs and concluded that mortality in hospitalized patients under sixty-five years of age was actually significantly de-

creased in the years following the introduction and general use of these drugs.[10]

Neuroleptic drugs have been administered to thousands of *pregnant women*, and except for a few isolated, and unconfirmed, reports of malformed children born to those mothers, one is probably safe to assume that neuroleptic drugs are not teratogenic, although the usual precautions during the first trimester of pregnancy should be observed as with any other medication. It has been reported that a newborn infant whose mother had been on a neuroleptic regimen right up to delivery showed signs of extrapyramidal dysfunction, which disappeared rapidly and completely with conservative management.[64]

Efficacy

How effective are neuroleptic drugs in the treatment of schizophrenia? Extensive and carefully controlled multihospital studies, carried out by the Veterans Administration and later by the National Institute of Mental Health, have established, beyond any doubt, the superiority of all phenothiazines tested over phenobarbital and placebo in chronic and acute schizophrenics.[24,102] Klein and Davis[8] reviewed 118 placebo-controlled studies and found that in 101 the neuroleptic drugs were definitely superior to placebo. Whenever chlorpromazine or another neuroleptic was not found to be superior to placebo, it was almost always due to inadequate doses (less than 500 mg./day) or insufficient time of treatment (less than two months).

An informative study by Prien and Cole[116] showed that higher than usual doses, i.e., 1000–2000 mg./day of chlorpromazine or the equivalent, were effective in a proportion of patients who had remained refractory to lower doses, if the patients were under forty years of age and had been hospitalized for less than ten years.

Neuroleptic drugs can be safely combined with each other, as well as with anxiolytic sedatives, tricyclic antidepressants, and MAO inhibitors. However, except for the practice of combining neuroleptics with antidepressants for schizophrenic patients who are also clearly depressed, there is no good evidence that such combinations are more effective than a single neuroleptic drug by itself.

In comparison with insulin coma therapy, neuroleptic treatment has consistently been shown to be at least equally effective—and, of course, simpler, less expensive, and less hazardous—but Kelly and Sargant[78] demonstrated convincingly the superiority of neuroleptic pharmacotherapy over insulin coma treatment.

Similarly, ECT was shown to be as effective as pharmacotherapy or somewhat less effective than neuroleptic drugs.[94]

In a frequently quoted paper, Brill and Patton[18] reported a decrease of 500 hospital patients in the State of New York—instead of an increase of 2,000–2,500 patients, anticipated on the basis of previous yearly increases—following the first year of large-scale neuroleptic treatment. Battegay and Gehring,[13] in Switzerland, compared the average duration of hospitalization before and after the introduction of neuroleptic drugs, and found a marked shortening of hospital stay for patients in the post-neuroleptic era. Even if new social attitudes and practices, not directly related to drug therapy, might have been responsible for some of these changes, as British and Scandinavian authors point out, there is no doubt that pharmacotherapy has played an important role in reducing the duration of hospitalization of many schizophrenics.[65,105]

Forty years ago, 60 percent of schizophrenic admissions were expected to remain in hospital indefinitely, only 20 percent made a good remission, and another 20 percent, still symptomatic, nevertheless also had a chance to get out of the hospital.[92,62,19] Following insulin therapy, between 1945 and 1950, only 34 percent of a group of schizophrenic patients in Britain were still hospitalized after five years, while 45 percent had made a good social remission, and 21 percent were still showing symptoms, but lived in the community.[61] Finally, after the introduction of neuroleptic pharmacotherapy, a five-year follow-up study of another group of schizophrenic patients in Britain revealed only 11 percent to be still

hospitalized, 56 percent as socially recovered, and 34 percent as showing symptoms, but living in the community.[20] These figures also reflect the general clinical impression that modern pharmacotherapy has been instrumental in increasing the proportion of schizophrenic patients who, although still showing residual symptoms of their disease, can be managed in the community; but, at the same time, drug treatment seems to have substantially increased the number of schizophrenics who make a good social remission.

Well-designed studies, comparing neuroleptic pharmacotherapy with milieu therapy, group therapy, or individual psychotherapy, in schizophrenic patients, report the greatest improvement with pharmacotherapy.[94] That drug treatment did not impede progress of individual psychotherapy in schizophrenics was demonstrated in a placebo-controlled two-year study by Grinspoon and Ewalt;[56] on the contrary, the neuroleptic (thioridazine) seemed to increase the effectiveness of psychotherapeutic communication.

Several studies have suggested that the combination of psychotherapy, milieu therapy, or other social therapies with pharmacotherapy may increase the effectiveness of the latter.[54,15,94] Similarly, Hogarty[74] et al. observed that patients in remission who receive drug maintenance treatment combined with social therapy tend to do better after six months than patients on drugs alone.

CONCLUSION

Pharmacotherapy has clearly emerged today as the most important and most widely used single treatment of schizophrenia. It is simpler, much more available, more effective, less hazardous, and less expensive than insulin therapy. It is simpler and more effective than ECT, at least over extended periods of time. It is simpler, much more reliable, briefer, and, as May[94] has shown in an interesting analysis, considerably less expensive than psychotherapy or milieu therapy. The effectiveness of megavitamin therapy has by no means been convincingly demonstrated, and psychosurgery is no longer considered a serious therapeutic choice for any but the most exceptional schizophrenic patient.

Perhaps the most significant achievement of pharmacotherapy has been its impact on the uncertainty that used to surround the schizophrenic patient in remission; whether he recovered spontaneously or in response to treatment, he always carried a relapse risk of at least 50 percent within the next twelve months. Twenty years ago, there was still nothing anyone could do to effectively reduce this threat. Today, neuroleptic drugs allow the psychiatrist to control and decrease this risk to a considerable extent, if his clinical judgment tells him that constitutional, social, or psychological factors—or the natural history of schizophrenia—seems to make such pharmacological control desirable.

(Metabolic Treatment

In 1954, Hoffer et al.[69] proposed large doses of nicotinic acid (niacin or Vitamin B$_3$), and later of nicotinamide, as a new treatment for schizophrenia. At that time, he gave 3000 mg. of niacin per day; lately, he has been recommending doses of up to 30,000 mg. of niacin per day in unresponsive cases. Ascorbic acid (Vitamin C) in doses of 3000 mg. per day, and pyridoxine in doses of 150 mg. might be added to this regimen.[68]

In 1968, Pauling[109]—not a behavioral or biological scientist, but a Nobel laureate in chemistry—published his theory of orthomolecular psychiatry, which postulates that certain individuals, because of constitutional deficiencies, may need much larger quantities of vitamins than the average person.

In one of his latest publications, Hoffer[68] recommends a therapeutic program approach to schizophrenia that makes use of all available treatment modalities in addition to high-dose vitamin (megavitamin) treatment. He claims that his therapeutic program gives results that are superior to other treatments—in particular to pharmacotherapy, if it is used as the principal treatment—in terms of general functioning and time out of hospital.

Mechanisms of Action

The original theory, proposed by Osmond and Smythies,[107] assumed that in schizophrenic patients the physiological N-methylation of noradrenaline to adrenaline is replaced by pathological O-methylation. This metabolic fault would then result in the production of 3,4-dimethoxyphenylethylamine (DMPEA), which had been shown in animals to produce experimental catatonia. Later, other psychotoxic metabolites of adrenaline (e.g., adrenochrome or adrenolutin) were postulated to be responsible for the pathological manifestations of schizophrenia, as a reaction to excessive stress.

Nicotinic acid was thought to act as a methyl-acceptor that would trap errant methyl-groups and thus prevent the formation of potentially toxic compounds. Nicotinamide—and later nicotinamide adenine nucleotide (NAD)—were also proposed by Hoffer for the correction of the assumed metabolic defect.[73] Large doses of these substances would be necessary to counterbalance the daily normal intake of methionine, an amino-acid which serves as one of the chief methyl-donors in the human organism.

In support of the theory of disturbed transmethylation in schizophrenia has been the finding of a "pink spot" in the urine chromatogram of schizophrenic patients by Friedhoff and Van Winkle,[44] who thought to have demonstrated that the substance responsible for the "pink spot" was DMPEA. This claim has since been challenged by a number of investigators, and the controversy about the identity of the spot and the association of DMPEA with schizophrenia has continued, almost unabated, for ten years.[41,123,104, 16,112,133]

Further support for the "transmethylation hypothesis" of schizophrenia has come from several clinical experiments which showed that the administration of methyl-donors, such as methionine and betaine, consistently aggravated the psychotic manifestations of schizophrenic patients.[27,108,2]

Another hypothesis assumes that in schizophrenics there is a metabolic impairment in the pathway from tryptophan to nicotinic acid, leading to a deficiency of nicotinic acid and to a surplus of methylated indole-metabolites, which have psychotoxic effects. The administration of nicotinic acid might then correct this deficiency and also prevent the excessive production of noxious methylated substances.[22]

While all these hypotheses are imaginative and intriguing, because they are based on interesting observations, it must be understood that none of them has been experimentally proven beyond a great deal of reasonable doubt.

Clinical Application

In a recent paper, Hoffer[73] describes his two-phase approach to megavitamin B$_3$ therapy in schizophrenia. In phase I, co-operative patients with acute symptoms are started on either nicotinamide or nicotinic acid, 3 grams per day. Sometimes ascorbic acid, 3 grams per day, is added, to reduce the danger of viral infections. Sucrose intake should be restricted. If improvement on this program is unsatisfactory after one month, the patients are then given any of the current drug therapies.

Phase II is entered when the patient is unable to follow this regimen and must be admitted to hospital, where he may be given ECT plus pharmacotherapy. The dose of nicotinic acid may be increased up to 30 grams per day, with a mode of 6 to 9 grams. The dose range of nicotinamide would lie between 3 and 9 grams.

After a patient has left the hospital, he is continued on outpatient therapy. If necessary, he may be brought back to the hospital at intervals of six to twelve months for another brief series of ECT. This entire program will be continued for at least five years.

ADVERSE REACTIONS

Nicotinic acid, particularly in high doses, is not as innocuous as had been thought for some time. Side-effects and complications with this substance include flushing, skin rashes, and lesions resembling acanthosis nigricans.

Nausea, vomiting, diarrhea, and activation of peptic ulcers have been observed, as well as increases in transaminase values, jaundice, and hypoalbuminemia. Other side-effects include hyperglycemia, hypotension, tachycardia, and headache.[98,10]

EFFICACY

Most of the positive reports on megavitamin therapy have been published by Hoffer and his co-workers.[66,67,68,69,70,71,72,73] However, others, too, have reported good results, sometimes with great enthusiasm. Not many of these studies were designed and conducted according to the standards that might be expected in modern clinical trials.[35,1,27,63,100,101,120]

Negative results with megavitamin therapy were also published by a number of authors, as well as inconclusive or negative results of treatment with NAD.[6,117,129,3,89,11,46,83,96]

Lately, Hoffer[68] has reported good results with nicotinamide, 3 to 6 grams, and ascorbic acid therapy, 3 grams per day, in mentally disturbed children. Favorable results have also been obtained with megavitamin treatment in children by Green[52] and Rimland,[119] while Greenbaum[53] did not observe any significant improvement in the children he treated.

CONCLUSION

The conflicting reports on the efficacy of megavitamin therapy have been presented in some detail, because of the public controversy that has developed around this particular treatment modality in recent years. The underlying rationale has neither been proved nor disproved. Negative results of the clinical treatment have so far been reported more frequently than positive ones, when controlled clinical trials were designed so as to meet current research standards. However, the possibility that certain schizophrenic patients may benefit from megavitamin therapy can not be entirely excluded, in view of a great number of enthusiastic, though uncontrolled, clinical reports. Unfortunately, at this time we do not know any criterion that would reliably select those schizophrenic individuals who might possibly be helped by magavitamin treatment.

Although many conscientious clinicians might feel that under these circumstances the treatment should not be given until its efficacy has been proven, this author is taking the stand that the plausible theories behind the treatment, the existing reports of its positive results, even if largely unconfirmed, and finally, the potentially powerful placebo effect resulting from the publicity surrounding megavitamin treatment today, must not be altogether disregarded. There does not seem to be sufficient evidence at this time to initiate megavitamin therapy on clinical grounds alone, but its possible negative effects are probably not serious enough to refuse treating a patient with megavitamins—in addition to the generally accepted physical therapeutic approaches in schizophrenia, e.g., pharmacotherapy—if the patient or his family insists on it. Such a compromise must, of course, always remain the personal decision of the psychiatrist in the context of his clinical judgment about the best possible over-all management of his schizophrenic patients.

❰ Hypoglycemic Coma Treatment

This particular form of treatment is only very rarely administered today. It was, however, the first treatment ever to achieve reliable therapeutic results in schizophrenic patients and in that capacity deserves at least more than ordinary historical interest. Its technique has been described in detail in many publications, and for these reasons, reference to it here will be very brief.[77]

The treatment aims at the reduction of cerebral metabolism through the production of insulin-induced hypoglycemia until the patient has reached coma. This state is allowed to last for approximately one hour, after which time the patient is awakened with a sucrose solution, administered by gavage, or with an intravenous injection of glucose, or an intramuscular injection of the hormone glucagon. The treatment is given five times a week, over a period of two to four months.

Mechanisms of Action

It is probable that a combination of factors is responsible for the beneficial effects of insulin coma therapy in schizophrenia. These factors include cerebral hypoxia and multiple physiological defense mechanisms which are being mobilized by the unspecific, systemic shock, as well as probably important psychological effects. The latter are associated with rendering the patient completely dependent on the nurses and physicians involved in this treatment and then exposing him in this anaclitic situation to a therapeutic re-enactment of early infantile dependence and mothering, but, in contrast to the original real situation, this time with the possibility of therapeutically controlling the "maternal" care given by the nursing and medical personnel.[76]

Clinical Application

The treatment is administered in very few places today. It has been claimed that it is particularly indicated in the management of schizophrenic patients who belong to the simple or hebephrenic subtypes and whose deficit symptoms have failed to respond to pharmacotherapy.[76]

ADVERSE REACTIONS

Hypoglycemic coma therapy is potentially more dangerous than most other physical treatments of schizophrenia, since death or permanent brain damage may supervene if the patient is permitted to reach a state of irreversible coma.

EFFICACY

As mentioned earlier, it has been shown that hypoglycemic coma treatment is less effective than pharmacotherapy in unselected schizophrenics[78]. Successes that have been claimed for it in certain patients who were refractory to pharmacotherapy have not been confirmed in controlled studies.[76,77]

CONCLUSION

There seems to be little justification for a psychiatric treatment center today to maintain the special facilities and the highly trained staff that would be required for the administration of this type of therapy.

(Neurophysiological Treatment

The effective treatment modalities which fall into this category are all characterized by the induction of convulsions. This may be achieved by the intravenous injection of metrazol, or by the inhalation of flurothyl (indoclon), or by the application of an electric current to the head region. The various forms of convulsive therapy have been discussed in detail in another volume of this edition of the Handbook; some of them are mainly of historical interest today. For these reasons, this discussion will be brief and restrict itself to those types of convulsive therapy which still find fairly widespread application in schizophrenia.

Electro-Convulsive Therapy (ECT)

In the standard form of this treatment, electrodes are applied bilaterally to the patient's head, he is given an intravenous injection of a muscle relaxant—usually succinyl chloride—together with an ultra-short-acting barbiturate, and an alternating current of about 120 Volts and 300 milliamperes is then switched on for a period of 0.1 to 1.0 seconds. If necessary, the application of the current may be repeated once or several times within the next minute, until a convulsive reaction has occurred. The peripheral manifestations of the convulsion are, of course, greatly attenuated by the muscle relaxant.

Two modifications of this standard form of ECT have been developed in recent years: unilateral ECT and multiple monitored ECT.

In unilateral ECT both electrodes are placed on the nondominant side (left in right-handed and right in left-handed persons) of the head. Advantages claimed for this form of treatment include less memory disturbance following a series of treatments, more particularly, less impairment of learning and recall, and less retrograde amnesia, as well as a shorter period of confusion following each seizure.[34]

Multiple monitored ECT involves the administration of several electric stimuli during one treatment session while the patient's EEG and ECG are being monitored continuously. From three to five seizures may be produced in 30–45 minutes. This makes it possible to reduce the time required for a full course of treatment.[17]

Mechanisms of Action

Although ECT has now been in use for more than thirty years, its mechanism of action is virtually unknown. Cerebral hypoxia, systemic "alarm" reaction, psychodynamic speculations about experiencing symbolic death and revival, have all been proposed as explanations of the dramatic effects of ECT on mental processes, but little evidence has been provided for these or any of the many other theories that have been suggested. Kety and his co-workers[79,99] have shown in animals that electrically induced convulsions increase the turnover rate of biogenic amines in the brain, and a similar mechanism in man may be related to the normalizing effects of ECT in depression or acute psychotic disorders.

Clinical Application

The principal indication for ECT is severe and persistent depression; however, the first successful trials with convulsive treatment were performed on schizophrenic patients, and—after pharmacotherapy—ECT is still the most reliable and most widely accepted physical treatment modality used in the management of schizophrenia. Today, standard ECT, or one of its modifications, is mainly used in schizophrenic patients who have failed to respond to pharmacotherapy, or when severe agitation and very acute symptoms must be rapidly controlled. Several authors[78,134] recommend a combination of ECT with pharmacotherapy as the best approach to schizophrenia, and point out that ECT often breaks through a therapeutic block in drug therapy and makes it possible to reduce the doses of drugs needed to maintain the patient in remission.

ADVERSE REACTIONS

The memory disorder occurring with ECT is its most disturbing side-effect. It is in almost every case fully reversible after the treatment has been discontinued for a few weeks, but the patient's improved affect may conceal a still existing objective memory defect for some time, and, particularly in elderly patients, a permanent loss of memory may ensue.[29] Fractures and dislocations were frequent prior to the routine use of muscle relaxants, but can be avoided today. Cardiovascular and respiratory accidents are uncommon. There are no confirmed reports of teratogenic effects of ECT, and its use in pregnant women seems to be relatively safe.[42,86]

EFFICACY

Kalinowsky and Hippius[77] report 68.3 percent remissions in institutionalized schizophrenic patients who had been ill for less than six months, if treated with a minimum of twenty convulsions, but only 9.2 percent in those ill for more than two years. They feel that pharmacotherapy in acutely ill patients may be attempted, but should be tentatively discontinued after several weeks or months; if the patient relapses, he should then be treated with ECT. It should be noted, however, that relapse rates following ECT are about the same as those following the discontinuation of pharmacotherapy, i.e., about 50 percent in twelve months.

CONCLUSION

ECT results in schizophrenia are often dramatic, but all too often only short-lived. This author's clinical experience has led him to employ pharmacotherapy as the first treatment of choice in acute as well as chronic schizophrenics. Only if the patient's psychotic symptoms have not significantly improved after three months in acute patients or after six months in chronic ones should ECT be given a therapeutic trial. Frequently, six to ten seizures suffice to activate the patient's response to neuroleptics, and he may then be maintained on pharmacotherapy. In more refractory cases, a longer course of up to twenty-five or thirty ECT may be indicated, if the response to pharmacotherapy is unsatisfactory.

❨ Psychosurgery

Psychosurgery is a badly chosen name for the kind of brain surgery which is being performed for the treatment of certain functional psychotic disorders. It is likely that the term "psychosurgery" will be exchanged for "psychiatric surgery" in the future, since the term designates, of course, not surgery performed on the psyche but on the psychiatric patient.

This kind of treatment has had a bad press for a long time, and merely mentioning its name—or, even more so, that of lobotomy—evokes almost violent emotional reactions in many people. Nevertheless, it may be an effective last resort when every other treatment has failed.

In schizophrenia, psychosurgery enjoyed a brief popularity between 1940 and 1950, when thousands of acute and chronic patients were lobotomized. But the results were often disappointing, because the selection of patients had been inadequate and surgical procedures were still crude.

Today, the development of many refined surgical approaches has reduced adverse reactions and improved therapeutic efficacy; at the same time, much has been learned about selection of appropriate patients for this treatment. All psychosurgical procedures, whether they be frontal lobotomies, cingulotomies, thalamotomies, hypothalamotomies, or any other of the many available techniques, aim at a leveling of emotional responsivity, but also at minimal interference with higher nervous functions and basic personality structure.

The operation must be chosen and performed by a neurosurgeon, while the diagnosis and recommendation for psychosurgery are the responsibility of a psychiatrist.[89]

Mechanisms of Action

How improvement of psychiatric disorders may be brought about by surgical interference with cerebral structures is very poorly understood. On the other hand, this type of treatment is the only one which was originally based on theoretical extrapolations of observations made in experimental studies on animals. Admittedly somewhat simplistic, the hypothesis was that a consistent calming effect, which was observed following certain neurosurgical procedures performed on the frontal thalamic or limbic systems in animals, e.g., a reduction of anxiety or aggressive responses, without significant interference with cognitive and perceptual functions, might also occur in man and would reduce psychotic manifestations, if they were present.

Clinical Applications

Any psychosurgical procedure should be considered only as the last resort in those exceptional cases where all other treatments have failed and the patient has been ill for at least two years without remission. When these conditions are fulfilled, this form of treatment is frequently successful in states of severe, chronic anxiety, depression, or obsessive-compulsive pathology. Its indications in schizophrenia are questionable, because acute schizophrenic patients who may respond well to psychosurgery are also excellent prospects for pharmacotherapy; and chronic schizophrenics have a much poorer record of success. One group of patients in whom psychosurgery has shown good results is that of the pseudoneurotic schizophrenics.[93] The only other indication for psychosurgery in schizophrenia today might exist in those extremely rare cases where severe agitation, anxiety, or aggression has consistently failed to respond to energetic treatment with neuroleptic drugs and ECT.

Adverse Reactions

Mortality, which was comparatively high in the early operations, has today been very considerably reduced and must no longer be considered a serious risk of psychosurgery. The same is true for the incidence of convulsions in the post-treatment phase. Likewise, the gross and unfavorable personality changes, which were not uncommon following the early frontal lobotomies and are responsible for the bad image psychosurgery has acquired, are almost never seen any more.

Nevertheless, psychosurgery is the only psychiatric treatment that aims at the production of irreversible changes in the central nervous system, and permanent neurological deficits or undesirable psychological changes may remain as sequelae of the treatment.

Efficacy

A recent follow-up survey of 210 patients suffering from long-standing, intractable psychiatric illness after bifrontal stereotactic tractotomy reports no favorable results in the chronic schizophrenic patients of this population.[125] But a short-term study of nine treatment-resistant, chronic schizophrenics after stereotactic cingulotomy reports at least gratifying reduction of anxiety and a positive activating effect.[5] Freeman,[43] reporting up to thirty-year follow-ups on 415 *early* schizophrenics (less than one year hospitalized) whom he treated with frontal lobotomy, found that 57.4 percent were employed or keeping house, 24.5 percent were living at home unemployed, and only 18.2 percent were in hospital.[43]

Conclusion

Psychosurgery in schizophrenic patients has only very limited application. It may be considered in pseudoneurotic schizophrenia if the patient is greatly distressed, has shown no spontaneous remission for at least two years, and has failed to respond to adequate trials with every other accepted treatment method, including psychotherapy. In rare cases, psychosurgery may be indicated for chronic schizophrenics whose anxiety and agitation

have remained refractory to adequate pharmacotherapy and ECT.

⟨ Bibliography

1. ALVAREZ, W. C. "A Chemical Treatment for
    Schizophrenia," *Geriatrics*, 22 (1967),
    111–112.

2. ANANTH, J. V., T. A. BAN, H. E. LEHMANN,
    and J. BENNETT. "Nicotinic Acid in the
    Prevention and Treatment of Methionine-
    induced Exacerbation of Psychopathology
    in Schizophrenics," *Canadian Psychiatric
    Association Journal*, 15 (1970), 3–14.

3. ANANTH, J. V., L. VACAFLOR, G. KEKHWA,
    C. STERLING, and T. A. BAN. "Nicotinic
    Acid in the Treatment of Newly Admitted
    Schizophrenics," *Canadian Psychiatric As-
    sociation Journal*, 15 (1972), 15–19.

4. ANGST, J., D. BENTE, P. BERNER, et al. "Clin-
    ical Effect of Clozapine (Study with the
    AMP System)," *Pharmakopsychiat. Neuro-
    psychopharm.* 4(4) (1971), 201–211.

5. APO, J., L. LAITINEN, and J. VILKKI. "Stereo-
    tactic Cingulotomy in Schizophrenia: In-
    troduction," *Psychiatria Fennica*, (1971),
    105.

6. ASHBY, W. R., G. H. COLLINS, and M. BASS-
    ETT. "The Effect of Nicotinamide and
    Placebo on the Chronic Schizophrenic,"
    Journal of Mental Science, 106 (1960),
    1555–1559.

7. AYD, F. J., JR. "Phenothiazine-induced
    Agranulocytosis: the 'at-Risk' Patient," *Int.
    Drug Therap. Newsletter* No.4 & 5 (1969).

8. BAN, T. A. *Psychopharmacology*. Baltimore:
    Williams and Wilkins, 1969.

9. BAN, T. A. *Schizophrenia—A Psycho-
    Pharmacological Approach*. Springfield:
    Thomas, 1972.

10. BAN, T. A., and H. E. LEHMANN. "Nicotinic
    Acid in the Treatment of Schizophrenia.
    Canadian Mental Health Association Col-
    laborative Study—Progress Report I."
    Toronto: *Canadian Mental Health Associa-
    tion*, 1970.

11. ———. "Niacin in the Treatment of Schizo-
    phrenias: Alone and in Combination".
    Presented at the 8th Congress of the
    College of International Psychopharma-
    cology, Copenhagen, August 7-14, 1972.

12. BARO, R., J. BRUGMANS, R. DOM, and R.
    VAN LOMMEL. "Maintenance Therapy of

13. BATTEGAY, R., and R. GEHRING. "*Vergleich-
    ende Untersuchungen an Schizophrenen
    der präneuroleptischen und der postneuro-
    leptischen ära.*" *Pharmakopsychiatrie-Neu-
    ropsychopharmakologie*, 2 (1968), 107–
    122.

14. BLEULER, E. *Dementia Praecox or the
    Group of Schizophrenias*. New York: Inter-
    national Universities Press, 1950.

15. BOROWSKI, T., and T. TOLWINSI. "Treatment
    of paranoid schizophrenics with chlorprom-
    azine and group therapy," *Disease of the
    Nervous System*, 30 (1969), 201–202.

16. BOURDILLON, R. E. and A. P. RIDGES. "3,4-
    dimethoxyphenylethylamine in schizophre-
    nia," H. E. Himwich, S. S. Kety, and J. R.
    Smythies, eds., in *Amines and Schizo-
    phrenia*, Oxford: Pergamon Press, 1967.

17. BRIDENBAUGH, R. H., F. R. DRAKE, and T. J.
    O'REGAN. "Multiple Monitored Electrocon-
    vulsive Treatment of Schizophrenia," *Com-
    prehensive Psychiatry*, 13 (1972), 9–17.

18. BRILL, H., and R. PATTON. "Analysis of
    1955-1956 population fall in New York
    State Mental Hospitals in first year of
    large scale use of tranquilizing drugs," *The
    American Journal of Psychiatry*, 114
    (1957-1958), 509.

19. BROWN, G. W. "Length of hospital stay and
    schizophrenia," *Acta Psychiatrica Neuro-
    logica Scandinavica*, 35 (1960), 414–430.

20. BROWN, G. W., M. BONE, B. DALISON, and
    J. K. WING. *Schizophrenia and social care*.
    London: Oxford University Press, 1966.

21. BRUNE, G. G. "Tryptophan metabolism in
    psychoses," in H. E. Himwich, S. S. Kety,
    and J. R. Smythies, eds., *Amines and
    Schizophrenia*. Oxford: Pergamon Press,
    1967.

22. BRUNE, G. G., and H. E. HIMWICH. "Effects
    of methionine loading on the behavior of
    schizophrenic patients," *Journal of Nervous
    and Mental Disease*, 134 (1962), 447–
    450.

23. CAFFEY, E. M., L. S. DIAMOND, T. V.
    FRANK, J. C. GRASBERGER, L. HERMAN,
    C. J. KLETT, and C. ROTHSTEIN. "Discon-
    tinuation or reduction of chemotherapy in
    chronic schizophrenics," *Journal of Chronic
    Diseases*, 17 (1964), 347–348.

24. CASEY, J., J. LASKY, C. KLETT, and L.

HOLLISTER. "Treatment of schizophrenic patients with phenothiazine derivatives," *The American Journal of Psychiatry*, 117 (1960), 2, 97.

25. CERLETTI, U., and L. BINI. "'*L*' Elettroshock," *Arch. Psicol. Neurol. e Psichiat.*, 19 (1938), 266.

26. COLE, J. O., S. GOLDBERG, and J. DAVIES. "Drugs in the treatment of psychosis: controlled studies," in P. Solomon, ed., *Psychiatric Drugs*. New York: Grune and Stratton, 1966.

27. COTT, A. A. "Treatment of ambulant schizophrenics with vitamin B3 and relative hypoglycemic diets," *Journal of Schizophrenia*, 1 (1967), 189–196.

28. CRANE, G. E. "Prevention and Management of Tardive Dyskinesia," *The American Journal of Psychiatry*, 129 (1972), 466–467.

29. CRONHOLM, B., and J. O. OTTOSON. "The Experience of Memory Function after Electroconvulsive Therapy," *British Journal of Psychiatry*, 109 (1963), 251–258.

30. CURRY, S., J. DAVIS, D. JANOWSKY, and J. MARSHALL. "Factors effecting chlorpromazine plasma levels in psychiatric patients," *General Psychiatry*, 22 (1970), 209.

31. CURRY, S., J. MARSHALL, J. DAVIS, and D. JANOWSKY. "Chlorpromazine plasma levels and effects," *Archives of General Psychiatry*, 22 (1970), 289–296.

32. DEGKWITZ, R., W. WENZEL, K. R. BINSACK, H. HERKERT, and O. LUXEMBURGER. "*Zum Probleme der terminalen extrapyramidalen Hyperkinesen an Hand von 1600 langfristig mit Neuroleptica Behandelten.*" *Arzneimittelforschung*, 16 (1966), 276–279.

33. DELAY, J., and P. DENIKER. "38 cases of psychoses under prolonged and continuous R.P. 4560 treatment," *Compt. Rend. Congr. Méd. Alien. Neurol.*, July 21 (1952), 7.

34. D'ELIA, G. *Unilateral Electroconvulsive Therapy*. Copenhagen: Munksgaard, 1970.

35. DENSON, R. "Nicotinamide in the treatment of schizophrenia," *Diseases of the Nervous System*, 23 (1962), 167–172.

36. DIMASCIO, A. "Dosage scheduling," in A. Dimascio, and R. I. Shader, eds., *Clinical Handbook of Psychopharmacology*. New York: Science House, 1970.

37. DIMASCIO, A., and E. DEMIRGIAN. "Antiparkinsonian drug overuse," *Scientific Proceedings of APA*, May 1970.

38. DOMINO, E. F. "Pharmacological analysis of the pathobiology of schizophrenia," in D. V. Silva Sankar, ed., *Schizophrenia— Current Concepts and Research*. Hicksville: P.J.D., 1969.

39. ENGLEHARDT, D. M. Personal communication.

40. ENGLEHARDT, D. M., et. al. "Phenothiazine in prevention of psychiatric hospitalization: III. Delay or prevention of hospitalization —a re-evaluation," *Archives of General Psychiatry*, 6 (1967), 98–101.

41. FAURBYE, A., and K. PINK. "Investigation of the occurrence of the dopamine metabolite 3,4-dimethoxyphenylethylamine in the urine of schizophrenics," *Acta Psychiatrica Scandinavica*, 40 (1964), 240–243.

42. FORSSMAN, H. "Follow-up study of sixteen children whose mothers were given electric convulsive therapy during gestation," *Acta Psychiatrica et Neurologica Scandinavica*, 3 (1955), 436–441.

43. FREEMAN, W. "Frontal lobotomy in early schizophrenia; long follow-up in 415 cases," *British Journal of Psychiatry*, 119 (1971), 621–624.

44. FRIEDHOFF, A. J., and E. VAN WINKLE. "Isolation and Characterization of a compound from the urine of the schizophrenic," *Nature*, 194 (1963), 1271–1272.

45. GALBRECHT, C., and C. KLETT. "Predicting response of phenothiazines: The right drug for the right patient," *Journal of Nervous and Mental Disease*, 147 (1968), 2.

46. GALLANT, D. M., M. P. BISHOP, and C. A. STEELE. "DPN (NAD-oxidized form): A preliminary evaluation in chronic schizophrenic patients," *Current Therapeutic Research*, 8 (1966), 542–547.

47. GOLDBERG, S. "Prediction of response to antipsychotic drugs," in D. H. Efron, ed., *Psychopharmacology: A Review of Progress, 1957–1967. PHSP No. 1836*. Washington: U. S. Government Printing Office, 1968.

48. GOLDBERG, S., H. MATTSON, J. COLE, and G. KLERMAN. "Prediction of improvement in schizophrenia under four phenothiazines," *Archives of General Psychiatry*, 16 (1967), 107.

49. GOLDMAN, D. "Drugs in treatment of psychosis: Clinical Studies," in P. Solomon, ed., *Psychiatric Drugs*. New York: Grune & Stratton, 1966.

50. GOLDSTEIN, B., B. BRAUZER, and J. CALD-

WELL. *The differential patterns of response to haloperidol and perphenazine in psychopharmacology and the individual patient.* New York: Raven Press, 1970.

51. GREEN, D. E., and I. FORREST. "In vivo metabolism of chlorpromazine," *Canadian Psychiatric Association Journal*, 11 (1966), 299–302.

52. GREEN, P. G. "Subclinical pellagra: Its diagnosis and treatment," *Schizophrenia*, 2 (1970), 70–79.

53. GREENBAUM, G. H. C. "An evaluation of niacinamide in the treatment of childhood schizophrenia," *The American Journal of Psychiatry*, 127 (1970), 89–92.

54. GREENBLATT, M., M. H. SOLOMON, A. S. EVANS, and G. W. BROOKS. *"Drug and social therapy in chronic schizophrenia."* Springfield: Thomas, 1965.

55. GRENELL, R. B. "Effect of chlorpromazine on brain metabolism," *Archives of Neurology and Psychiatry*, 73 (1955), 347.

56. GRINSPOON, L., J. R. EWALT, and R. SHADER. "Psychotherapy and pharmacotherapy in chronic schizophrenia," *The American Journal of Psychiatry*, 124 (1968), 1945–52.

57. GROSS, M., "Discontinuation of treatment with ataractic drugs," J. Wartis, ed., in *Recent Advances in Biological Psychiatry.* New York: Grune & Stratton, 1961.

58. GUTH, P. "The mode of action of chlorpromazine (CPZ): A review," *The Bulletin of the Tulane University Medical Faculty*, 24 (1964), 36–42.

59. GUTTMAN, H., H. E. LEHMANN, and T. A. BAN. "A survey of extrapyramidal manifestations in patients attending an aftercare clinic of a psychiatric hospital," *Laval Médical*, 41 (1970), 450–455.

60. HARE, E. H., and D. WILCOX. "Do psychiatric inpatients take their pills?" *British Journal of Psychiatry*, 113 (1967), 1435–1439.

61. HARRIS, A., I. LINKER, V. NORRIS, and M. SHEPHERD. "Schizophrenia: a prognostic and social study," *British Journal of Preventive and Social Medicine*, 10 (1956), 107–114.

62. HASTINGS, D. W. "Follow-up results in psychiatric illness," *The American Journal of Psychiatry*, 114 (1958), 12.

63. HERJANIC, M., J. L. HERJANIC, and W. K. PAUL. "Treatment of schizophrenia with nicotinic acid," *Journal of Schizophrenia*, 1 (1967), 197–199.

64. HILL, R. M., M. M. DESMOND, and T. L. KAY. "Extrapyramidal dysfunction in an infant of a schizophrenic mother," *Journal of Pediatrics*, 69 (1966), 589–595.

65. HOENIG, J. "The prognosis of schizophrenia," in A. Coppen, and A. Walk, eds., *Recent Developments in Schizophrenia.* Ashford: Headley Brothers, 1967.

66. HOFFER, A. "Nicotinic acid: An adjunct in the treatment of schizophrenia," *The American Journal of Psychiatry*, 120 (1963), 171–173.

67. ———. "The effect of nicotinic acid on the frequency and duration of rehospitalization of schizophrenic patients: A Controlled comparison study," *International Journal of Neurology*, 2 (1969), 78–87.

68. ———. "Megavitamin B$_3$ therapy for schizophrenia," *Canadian Psychiatric Association Journal*, 16 (1971), 499.

69. HOFFER, A., H. OSMOND, and J. SMYTHIES. "Schizophrenia: A new approach," *Journal of Mental Science*, 100 (1954), 29–54.

70. HOFFER, A., H. OSMOND, M. J. CALLBECK, and I. KAHAN. "Treatment of schizophrenia with nicotinic acid and nicotinamide," *Journal of Clinical and Experimental Therapeutics*, 18 (1957), 131–158.

71. HOFFER, A., and H. OSMOND. "Some schizophrenic recoveries," *Diseases of the Nervous System,* 2 3 (1962), 204–210.

72. ———. "Treatment of schizophrenia with nicotinic acid," *Acta Psychiatric Scandinavica*, 40 (1964), 171–189.

73. HOFFER, A., and H. OSMOND. "Nicotinamide adenine dinucleotide (NAD) as a treatment for schizophrenia." *Journal of Psychopharmacology*, 1 (1966), 79.

74. HOGARTY, G. E., S. D. GOLDBERG, and the Collaborative Study Group. "Drug and sociotherapy in the Post Hospital Maintenance of schizophrenic patients: One year relapse rates," *Archives of General Psychiatry*, in press.

75. HOLLISTER, L. E. "Complications from psychotherapeutic drugs," *Clinical Pharmacology and Therapeutics*, 5 (1964), 322–333.

76. JUILLET, P. *"Traitements insuliniques et méthodes de choc dans la schizophrénie,"* *Confrontations Psychiatriques*, 2 (1968), 107–120.

77. KALINOWSKY, L. B., and H. HIPPIUS. *Phar-*

macological, Convulsive and other Somatic Treatments in Psychiatry. New York: Grune & Stratton, 1969.

78. KELLY, D., and W. SARGANT. "Present treatment of schizophrenia—a controlled follow-up study," *British Medical Journal*, 5428 (1965), 147–150.

79. KETY, S. S., F. JAVOY, A. M. THIERRY, L. JULOU, and J. GLOWINSKI. "Sustained effects of electroconvulsive shock on turnover of norepinephrine in central nervous system of rat," *Proceedings of National Academy of Science*, 58 (1967), 1249–1254.

80. KLAESI, J. "*Dauernarkose mittels Somnifen bei Schizophrenen,*" *Ztschr. Ges. Neurol. Psychiat.*, 74 (1922), 557–592.

81. KLEIN, D., and J. DAVIS. *Diagnosis and Drug Treatment of Psychiatric Disorders.* Baltimore: Williams & Wilkins, 1969.

82. KLETT, C., and E. MOSELEY. "The right drug for the right patients," *Journal of Consulting Psychology*, 29 (1965), 546–551.

83. KLINE, H. S., G. L. BARCLAY, J. O. COLE, A. H. ESSER, H. E. LEHMANN, and J. R. WHITTENBORN. "Diphosphopyridine nucleotide in the treatment of schizophrenia," *Journal of the AMA*, 200 (1967), 881–882.

84. KRAEPELIN, E. *Psychiatrie. Ein Lehrbuch für Studierende und Aerzte.* 3 vols. Leipzig: Barth, 1909–1913.

85. KRIS, E. B., and D. M. CARMICHAEL. "Follow-up study on thorazine treated patients," *The American Journal of Psychiatry*, 114 (1957), 449–452.

86. LAIRD, M. "Convulsive therapy in psychoses accompanying pregnancy," *New England Journal of Medicine*, 252 (1955), 934–936.

87. LEHMANN, H. E. *Pharmacotherapy of Schizophrenia*, in P. Hoch and J. Zubin, eds., *Psychopathology of Schizophrenia.* New York: Grune & Stratton, 1966.

88. ———. "The philosophy of long-acting medication in Psychiatry," *Dis. Nerv. Syst.*, 31 (1970), 7–9.

89. ———. "Perspectives in Psychosurgery." Presented at the Hahnemann Symposium of Psychosurgery. June 17, 1972, Philadelphia.

90. LEHMANN, H. E., T. A. BAN, and J. V. ANANTH. "Nicotinic acid and the trans-

methylation hypothesis of schizophrenia." Presented at the Sixty-Second Annual Meeting of The American Psychopathological Association, March 3-4, 1972, New York City.

91. LITBACK, R., and R. KAELBLING. "Agranulocytosis, Leukopenia and Psychotropic Drugs," *Archives of General Psychiatry*, 24 (1971), 265–267.

92. MALAMUD, W., and I. N. RENDER. "Course and prognosis in schizophrenia," *The American Journal of Psychiatry*, 95 (1939), 1039–1057.

93. MALITZ, S., V. LOZZI, and M. KANZLER. "Lobotomy in schizophrenia: A review," in D. V. Siva Sankar, ed., *Schizophrenia: Current Concepts and Research.* Hicksville: P.J.D., 1969.

94. MAY, P. R. A. *Treatment of schizophrenia: A comparative study of five treatment methods.* New York: Science House, 1968.

95. MEDUNA, L. J. *Die Konvulsionstherapie der Schizophrenie.* Halle: Marhold, 1936.

96. MELTZER, H., R. SHADER, and L. GRINSPOON. "The behavioral effects of nicotinamide adenine dinucleotide in chronic schizophrenia," *Psychopharmacologia*, 15 (1969), 144–152.

97. MONIZ, E. "*Tentatives opératoires dans le traitement de certaines psychoses.*" Paris: Masson, 1936.

98. MOSHER, L. R. "Nicotinic acid side effects and toxicity: A review," *The American Journal of Psychiatry*, 126 (1970), 129–196.

99. MUSACCHIO, J. M., L. JULOU, S. S. KETY, and J. GLOWINSKI. "Increase in rat brain tyrosine hydroxylase activity produced by electroconvulsive shock," *Proceedings of National Academy of Science*, 63 (1969), 1117–1119.

100. NEUMANN, H. "*Klinische und pathophysiologische Aspekte der Therapie schizophrener Kernpsychosen mit Nicoinsaureamid,*" *Nervenarzt*, 38 (1967), 511–514.

101. NEWBOLD, H. L. "Niacin and the schizophrenic patient," *The American Journal of Psychiatry*, 127 (1970), 535–536.

102. National Institute of Mental Health, Psychopharmacology, Collaborative Study. "Phenothiazine Treatment in Acute Schizophrenia," *Archives of Gen. Psychiatry*, 10 (1964), 246.

103. ———. "Difference in clinical effects of

three phenothiazines in 'acute' schizo-phrenia," *Diseases of the Nervous System*, 28 (1967), 369–383.

104. NISHIMURA, T., and L. G. GJESSING. "Failure to detect 3,4-dimethoxyphenylethylamine and bufotenin in the urine from a case of Periodic catatonia," *Nature*, 206 (1965), 963.

105. ØDEGARD, Ø. "Changes in the prognosis of functional psychoses since the days of Kraepelin," *British Journal of Psychiatry*, 113 (1967), 813–822.

106. ORLINSKY, N., and E. D'ELIA. "Rehospitalization of the schizophrenic patient," *Archives of General Psychiatry*, 10 (1964), 47–54.

107. OSMOND, H., and J. SMYTHIES. "Schizophrenia: A new approach," *Journal of Mental Science*, 98 (1952), 309–315.

108. PARK, L., R. BALDESSARINI, and S. S. KETY, "Methionine effects on chronic schizophrenics," *Archives of General Psychiatry*, 12 (1965), 340–351.

109. PAULING, L. "Orthomolecular Psychiatry," *Science*, 160 (1968), 265.

110. PECKNOLD, J. C., J. V. ANANTH, T. A. BAN, and H. E. LEHMANN. "Lack of indication for the use of antiparkinson medication—A follow-up study," *Diseases of the Nervous System*, 32 (1971), 538–541.

111. PEELE, R., and I. S. VON LOETZEN. "Phenothiazine deaths: A clinical review." Presented at APA Annual Meeting, May 1-5, 1972, Dallas, Texas.

112. PERRY, T. L., S. HANSON, L. MacCOUGALL, and C. J. SCHWARTZ. "Studies of amines in normal and schizophrenic subjects," in H. E. Himwich, S. S. Ketty and J. R. Smythies, eds., *Amines and Schizophrenia*. Oxford: Pergamon Press, 1967.

113. PISCIOTTE, A. V. "Drug-induced leukopenia and aplastic anemia," *Clinical Pharmacology and Therapeutics*, 12 (1970), 13–43.

114. PLETSCHER, A. "Pharmacologic and biochemical basis of some somatic side effects of psychotropic drugs," H. Brill, ed. New York: *Excerpta Medica*, 129 (1966).

115. POLLACK, B. "The effect of chlorpromazine in reducing the relapse rate in 716 released patients." *The American Journal of Psychiatry*, 114 (1958), 749–751.

116. PRIEN, R. F., and J. COLE. "High dose chlorpromazine therapy in chronic schizophrenia," *Archives of General Psychiatry*, 18 (1968), 482–495.

117. RAMSAY, R. A., T. A. BAN, H. E. LEHMANN, B. M. SAXENA, and J. BENNETT. "Nicotinic acid as adjuvant therapy in newly admitted schizophrenic patients," *Canadian Medical Association Journal*, 102 (1970), 939–942.

118. REED, G. E. "The use of manganese chloride in dementia praecox," *Canadian Medical Association Journal*, 21 (1929), 46–49.

119. RIMLAND, B. "High dosage levels of certain vitamins in the treatment of children with severe mental disorders," in L. Pauling and D. Hawkins, eds., *Orthomolecular Psychiatry*. San Francisco: Freeman Press. In press.

120. ROBIE, T. R. "The rewards of research—a new clarification of schizophrenia by the term 'Metabolic Dysperception,'" *Schizophrenia*, 3 (1971), 168–176.

121. SAKEL, M. "Zur Methodik der Hypoglykamiebehandlung von Psychosen," *Wien. Klin. Wchncshr.* 49 (1936), 1278–1822.

122. SCHOOLER, H. R., H. BOOTHE, S. GOLDBERG, and C. CHASE. "Life history and symptoms in schizophrenia: Severity at hospitalization and response to phenothiazines," *Archives of General Psychiatry*, 25 (1971), 138–147.

123. SEN, N. P., and P. L. McGEER. "3,4-dimethosythenylethylamine in human urine," *Biochem. Biophys. Res. Commun.*, 14 (1964), 227–232.

124. SIMON, W. "Long-term follow-up of schizophrenic patients," *Archives of General Psychiatry*, 12 (1965), 510–515.

125. STROM-OLSEN, R., and S. CARLISLE. "Bifrontal stereotactic tractotomy," *British Journal of Psychiatry*, 118 (1971), 141–154.

126. TURUNEN, S., and J. SALMINEN. "Neuroleptic treatment and mortality," *Diseases of the Nervous System*, 29 (1968), 474–477.

127. TUSQUES, J. "Sulfur pyretotherapy alone or associated with chrysotherapy in so-called dementia praecox or schizophrenia," *Semaine d'hôpital de Paris*, 13 (1937), 109–111.

128. TUTEUR, W. "The discharged mental hospital chlorpromazine patient," *Diseases of the Nervous System*, 20 (1959), 512–517.

129. VALLEY, J., T. D. LOVEGROVE, and G. E. HOBBS. "Nicotinic acid and nicotinamide in the treatment of chronic schizophrenia," *Canadian Psychiatric Association Journal*, 16 (1971), 433–435.

130. VAN ROSSUM, T. M. "The significance of Dopamine—Receptor blockade for the action of neuroleptic drugs," H. Brill, ed. New York: Excerpta Medica, 1966.

131. WARNES, H. "Toxic psychosis due to antiparkinsonian drugs," *Canadian Psychiatric Association Journal*, 2 (1967), 323.

132. WARNES, H., H. E. LEHMANN, and T. A. BAN. "Adynamic ileus during psychoactive medication: a report of three fatal and five severe cases," *Canadian Medical Association Journal*, 96 (1967), 1112.

133. WATT, J., G. ASHCROFT, R. DALY, and J. SMYTHIES. "Urine volume and pink spots in schizophrenia and health," *Nature*, 221 (1969), 971–972.

134. WEINSTEIN, M. R., and A. FISCHER. "Combined treatment with ECT and Antipsychotic drugs in schizophrenia," *Diseases of the Nervous System*, 12 (1971), 801–808.

CHAPTER 29

PARANOID CONDITIONS AND PARANOIA

Norman A. Cameron

T HE TERM "PARANOIA" WAS coined in ancient Greece, no one knows when; it appears in the works attributed to Hippocrates as a word already in current use. It was probably used to mean what the lay public and the legal profession call "insanity." After disappearing from the literature and occasionally reappearing for centuries, it was revived in the eighteenth and nineteenth centuries to designate a number of different severe mental disorders. For a time, in the nineteenth century, it covered delusional and delirious syndromes, a confusion easy to understand when one realizes that the French, who then led the field, employ the term "*délire*" for both delirium and delusion.

Toward the end of the century, Kraepelin began his renowned work on classification, which mushroomed through successive editions until it became the standard text for most of Europe. In his 1915 edition of a four-volume work,[58] he devoted more than seventy pages to detailed descriptions of a variety of paranoic forms, some of which merged gradu-ally into his descriptions of dementia praecox and some into manic-depressive psychoses. He followed Kahlbaum in recommending also the term "paraphrenia." Even Bleuler, when he wrote his compendious monograph on what he called the group of schizophrenias,[7] could not break away from Kraepelin's classification with its multitudinous subdivisions. This is in marked contrast to the situation today when paranoid conditions and paranoia appear only sporadically as separate entities in the current literature.

An independent new spirit entered medical psychology when Freud formulated paranoia as a neuro-psychosis of defense in 1896,[25] and followed up with a series of papers that ulti-mately established paranoid conditions and paranoia as psychodynamic phenomena with an ontogenetic development. He depicted this as a gradual weakening of defenses against self-reproaches, which were projected, but returned to consciousness in a delusional form, ascribed now to other persons and not to the self. His novel concept of *projection* and his interpretations of delusions as attempts at self-cure, as reconstructions of external reality to embrace the distortions of inner reality also, have dominated psychiatry ever since.

Freud's formulation of paranoia as the result of a failure to maintain homosexual wishes under repression[29] has given rise to considerable controversy, still not wholly resolved, to which I shall return later. There is a widespread misconception to the effect that Freud based this hypothesis upon his famous analysis of the autobiography of the talented jurist, Daniel Paul Schreber[72]. Actually, Freud had arrived at this formulation much earlier; his paper on the Schreber case gave him the opportunity to enunciate and document his theory.

During the past decades, *paranoia* has been reserved for a rare syndrome in which an elaborate delusional system becomes firmly rooted in a person's thinking, while the rest of his personality may remain relatively well-preserved. The much more numerous paranoia-like clinical syndromes, which shade over into schizophrenia or depression, are designated *paranoid states* or *paranoid conditions*.[2] A growing contemporary trend treats paranoid conditions as variants of schizophrenia or of depression. The revised official classification still retains the older distinctions, but with outspoken evidence of uncertainty as to their validity.

❲ Official Classification

The revised edition of the official manual prepared by a committee of the American Psychiatric Association[18] defines *paranoid states* as psychotic disorders in which the essential abnormality is a delusion, usually persecutory or grandiose. Whatever disturbances in mood, behavior, and thinking occur, including hallucinations, are said to derive from the basic delusion. A proviso is added that most authorities today question whether paranoid states are distinct clinical entities, whether they are not just variants of schizophrenia or paranoid personality.

Paranoia is defined as an exceedingly rare condition in which an intricate, complex, elaborate delusional system develops logically out of some misinterpretation of an actual event. The patient often believes that he possesses unique and superior ability. His condition, in spite of a chronic course or a static balance, appears not to interfere with the rest of his thinking and general personality.

Involutional paranoid state (*involutional paraphrenia*) refers to delusion formation with onset in the involutional period. It is to be distinguished from schizophrenia by an absence of conspicuous thought disorders. The whole concept of involutional psychoses loses much of its usefulness when it is recommended, as in a recent article, that *any* psychosis appearing at age forty be considered involutional.

Paranoid personality is listed separately among personality disorders that are not psychotic. It consists of deeply ingrained maladaptive behavioral patterns usually recognizable at adolescence or earlier. It is characterized by hypersensitivity, rigidity, unwarranted suspiciousness, jealousy, excessive self-importance, envy, and a tendency to blame others and ascribe evil motives to them. Interpersonal relationships are maintained with difficulty.

❲ Paranoid Conditions

Since paranoia is only a rare and extreme form of *paranoid condition*, we shall focus upon the far more common paranoid conditions, and give a nod to history by adding a brief statement about *classical paranoia* toward the end. It should be clearly understood from the start that pure paranoid conditions, with no sign of schizophrenia, no taint of depression or manic grandiosity and aggression, no evidence of neurotic defense, are rarely if ever found. This is obviously true of all forms of classification of human experience and behavior; none of the classes excludes traces, or even major contaminations, of the symptoms of other disorders. Most of what we shall be describing—

the defensive organization, ego adaptations, the half-real, half-imaginary pseudo-community reconstructions, the paranoid behavior—will be found entering into paranoid trends in all psychoses, including brain disorders, in some neuroses, and in more than a single personality disorder. Nonetheless, we cannot get along without some form of classification, for the sake of communication with colleagues, teaching students, and clarifying certain basic issues. It is only necessary to guard against taking our artificial groupings too literally or resisting change when they prove contrary to clinical experience.[2]

Incidence

The incidence of paranoid conditions, within the meaning of DSM-II, the revised official classification of 1968,[18] is generally believed to be high in the population. Unfortunately, there is no reliable way to estimate the actual incidence for a number of reasons. For one thing, clinical and incidental observation suggests that paranoid trends are widely distributed; yet only a fraction of mildly and moderately paranoid persons ever seek help. Usually, paranoid trends are uncovered in the course of medical, paramedical, psychological, and legal situations, or in personal encounter, almost by accident.

I have emphasized elsewhere in some[16] detail the attitudes of belief, disbelief, trust and suspicion, expectation and apprehension, that are integral components of everyone's daily mood and thought. It is normal and essential to proceed with our everyday life by utilizing perceptions that reveal only fragments of objects, the beginnings of action and bits of conversation, inferences as to another's intent, and, as a rule, only a sketchy knowledge of his background. Such incompleteness of input leaves large areas of potential uncertainty. At times, it places a strain upon confidence and credibility and it may set the stage even in normal people for a haunting suspicion that something evil may be afoot. It is not really a great jump from suspicion and mistrust to a transitory paranoid fear. This happens on a large scale in disaster and threats of extinction.

Defenses such as *projection* and *denial*,[1,45] whose exaggerated use is basic to paranoid delusions, are also a part of normal ego defenses and adaptations, from infancy to old age. It is largely a question of the degree to which such maneuvers become dominant and pervasive, of the ease of regression under stress, and the readiness of any given person to correct his misinterpretations through further communication, mutual exchange, trust, and consensual validation. And even these criteria are not infallible. Irrational beliefs that resist corrective emotional experience and contradict the evidence are common in many treasured human institutions. We are witnessing today in our own culture a striking rise in mysticism among the highly educated, as well as among those less well equipped to think logically. But to call all such widespread and expanding unwarranted credulity *paranoid* would be to reduce an already overworked concept to mere nonsense.

A further impediment to accurate estimates of the incidence of paranoid conditions is that even definitely paranoid persons rarely recognize their delusions as pathological. Thus, in every community there are chronically suspicious individuals, who understand neither the motives of others nor their own, who cannot really trust anyone enough to confide freely and ask for help. The reaction of the common man to suspicious, wary "loners" is seldom one to encourage frankness and trust. Besides all this, even psychotic paranoid persons may be in better contact with their personal surroundings and appear more competent than equally disturbed depressive and schizophrenic persons. Pinderhughes[69] has contributed original contributions to the presence of much paranoid violence among both pathological and "normal" persons in our contemporary culture.

Heredity

In spite of great advances in the fields of genetics, twin studies, perinatal stress, individual differences at birth, and longitudinal studies, there is still no conclusive evidence to refute Miller's[61] classical review of four hundred hospitalized patients, which included all psychotic persons with marked paranoid trends. He could unearth clear evidence of paranoid illness among the ancestors of only eight patients, or 2 percent. Only forty–four, or 11 percent, were direct descendants of ancestors who had suffered from "nervous or mental illness" of any description. On the other hand, observations of neonates and young infants reveal wide differences in sensitivity to external stimulation and internal stress, and a wide range in tension, restlessness, and quiescence.[4,9,23] There is no doubt that such individual differences may conceivably be linked to later hypersensitivities in adult life.[18,19] We have the right to speculate that the more sensitive and tense infants might react later in life, or even throughout life, more maladaptively than average under the impact of life stresses. But for the present these are speculations, conceivable but not demonstrated preludes to adult paranoid developments. Ongoing intensive studies of infancy, and the continuance of longitudinal research, may some day throw much needed light upon our problems.

Sex and Marital Status

What data we have in this area come from perusal of hospital records also. Tyhurst[79] reported an actual lack of reliable evidence concerning sex distribution of paranoid conditions. Kolb[57] asserts that an abnormally high percentage of psychotic paranoid persons has never married. He attributes this to their basically homosexual orientation and chronic hostility, which make them unacceptable partners.

Age

Paranoid psychoses occur more frequently in adulthood than during adolescence or postadolescence. There are special sources of anxiety, frustration, conflict, and personal insecurity during the fifth decade and later. Waning youth and attractiveness in a youth-oriented culture are no light matters, neither is a decrease in vigor and flexibility of adaptation, progressive deafness, or diminished acuity of sight and other senses. Age brings with it an inevitable accumulation of disappointments; opportunities for new ventures usually fall off sharply in the elderly. Thus, a person with compensated life-long paranoid trends may grow less and less able to cope with such losses. He may react to ordinary neglect and social isolation with frank delusions of persecution, jealousy, and sometimes with compensatory delusions of grandeur.[16]

Social Milieu

There is nothing to indicate valid differences in the incidence of paranoid conditions among different socioeconomic groups. We may speculate that, even before middle life and old age, an adult with an unstable or inflexible personality organization, and with poor interpersonal relations, must face special difficulties as his achievements fall farther and farther short of expectation and desire. This is especially true of the underprivileged who are being studied today more extensively in psychiatry than ever before. A dissatisfied, insecure, neglected person at any socioeconomic level is likely—if he does not simply give up—to redouble his efforts, try aggressively to meet challenges, overcome obstacles, and prove himself. He may also spur himself on in his sex life, or seek new and untried sources of gratification. If his efforts in any human endeavor fail, the temptation to look outside himself for explanations may be irresistible. Then his habitual denial and projection may lead him to construct delusions that seem to provide explanations and protect him from having to acknowledge painful, humiliating defeat.

A basically paranoid person who becomes disheartened, and feels moved to submit to failure, risks the revival of primitive fears for his own bodily intactness and his psychological integrity, which may have lain dormant within him for decades. The world around him will then seem full of threat. At this point, it is most useful to focus our attention upon by far the commonest form of paranoid conditions, upon the development of persecutory delusions.

❨ Persecutory Paranoid Development

Personality Background

What characteristics in the premorbid personality of persons who develop delusions of persecutions must we look for, and how do these operate in precipitating such disasters? A simple answer is impossible. The potentially paranoid person, before frank illness, may have been utilizing any one or any combination of a variety of ego defenses and adaptations.[42] The search for simplistic cause-and-effect cannot succeed; we have to think in terms of complex matrices out of which persecutory convictions may emerge. Until a great deal more is known about the origins of these matrices, we must content ourselves with noting certain characteristics that seem to emerge with considerable regularity from the background of vulnerable individuals.

To begin with, persons who develop persistent, pervasive paranoid delusions have always been tense, insecure, and fearful, operating at high levels of general anxiety, which is often discharged as overactivity, aggression, or chronic anger. They easily become suspicious and distrustful under ordinary living conditions, have difficulty in confiding, and when they do confide, they expect to be betrayed.[47] What genuinely close and reciprocal relationships they have are limited to a very few individuals; and even such ties may not survive an interpersonal crisis. What past histories can be obtained reveal almost life-long tendencies toward secretiveness, seclusiveness, and solitary rumination. These may be hidden behind a brittle façade of superficial give-and-take.

The world in which such a person lives is dangerous; he must always be on the lookout for attack. He finds people unpredictable and untrustworthy, because he is relatively incapable of taking the role of other persons and viewing things from their different perspectives. This concept is derived from George

Herbert Mead's *generalized other*.[60] The paranoid person, who needs more than an ordinary degree of understanding of others' motives, because he is so fearful and uneasy, has developed next to none. Therefore, he is easily exposed to surprise and suffers hurts and humiliations which more socially adept people foresee, discount, or ignore. He is often relatively incompetent in everyday situations of co-operative, competitive, and complementary relationships. He lives with endless tensions over mutual misunderstandings and misinterpretations; he is plagued by ideas of *self-reference*.

Mild, harmless ideas of self-reference are familiar to everyone. An occasional mistake in assuming that a critical remark or a compliment is meant for oneself, when actually it is not, lies within everyone's range, no matter how revealing it sometimes is. Persons with well-compensated paranoid trends may be especially prone to self-reference without being in danger of psychosis. It is only when, in the face of exceptional stress, their self-reference focuses upon a particular theme, or singles out certain individuals who seem banded together, that a threat of decompensation looms.

The apparent *self-sufficiency* that many aggressive or pseudo-autonomous paranoids exhibit is a screen that hides their weakness. They are actually always overconcerned about what others think and feel in relation to them, and less able than the average to satisfy their need to know. When stress increases their need, without increasing their ability to meet it, they tend to increase vigilance and look for signs that confirm their suspicions. This in turn heightens general anxiety, reduces still further a less than normal trust, and stimulates *basic distrust*.

It has frequently been pointed out that persecutory paranoid persons are fundamentally hostile.[54,69] Their organization includes major fixations at sadistic levels, a preponderance of disowning projective aggression, and an ease of ego-regression. The aggressiveness is rarely aimless; it is almost always *reaction-sensitive*. The paranoid's special sensitivities correspond to some of his outstanding weaknesses—his fears, frustrations, guilt, or ego-alien impulses. In short, each paranoid has an exceptional readiness to overreact with counteraggression to whatever he personally misconceives as a threat to his vulnerable *security system*. He may unconsciously fear bodily attack or the loss of something vital to him—the residual of his early unresolved castration fears.

Premorbid Personality Stresses

It is well established that *denial* and *projection* occur most often at completely unconscious levels,[16] so that a paranoid person is entirely unaware of exactly what he is defending against and what he is doing. His misfortune is that he unwittingly creates around him an atmosphere of uneasiness and resentment, which makes others avoid his company and actually increases his social isolation. He feels more and more misunderstood and threatened, unwanted, unloved, and discriminated against; yet, his multiple frustrations push him continually to overcome the hostility gathering around him, and this, too, is experienced by others as stepped-up aggression.

To offset his gnawing sense of being constantly misunderstood, he develops further ego defenses and adaptations in an attempt to strengthen his position vis-à-vis other persons. This is often accomplished at the cost of increasing his characteristic rigidity. It is easy to see why anyone who must rigidly defend his vulnerable personality organization should have to be insistent upon his opinions as the only possible interpretations, unable to allow the possibility of uncertainties or contradictions into his established ways of thinking.[2] The alternative would be to invite an already potential disorganization. Without in the least realizing it consciously, he is staving off a threat, however dimly felt, of precipitating a disastrous experience that might lead to eventual decompensation. He is the little boy holding his fingers of primitive defenses in the dike, to protect himself from being being overwhelmed by the dammed-up waters of his repressed urges and fears.

What paranoid persons rarely recognize is that their own hostile aggression nurtures the very hostility that they correctly perceive in their human surroundings. As Pinderhughes[69] has pointed out in several recent studies, the paranoid unknowingly *stimulates violence* in others by his own unconscious urges to defensive violence. When he can no longer otherwise guard against his threats of personal failure, inferiority, temptation, or misdeed, he is forced to call in such secondary defenses as rationalization, misunderstanding, and distortions of recall—as indeed *normal persons* also do under comparable circumstances—but with far greater single-mindedness and determination. It is essential for every therapist to remind himself that all paranoid maneuvers are not products of personal malice, but reactions to intolerable pressures of urgent necessity—the necessity to preserve and shore up an unstable personality structure, to discharge excessive libidinal and aggressive impulses which the person cannot channel or control by any other means.

It must be said that most paranoids do not fail. Fortune smiles on some, while others show creativity in evolving effective compensatory adaptations. The more fortunate succeed in discharging their intolerable energies in socially acceptable action, or in marketable fantasies—as we often witness in literary creations and the arts—or in setting up self-protective systems of reaction formation that withstand their life stresses. Many succeed in ridding themselves constantly of otherwise inadmissible impulses by entering upon crusades, for example, against socially condemned forms of sexuality, against the hostile encroachment of oppressors, against cruelty, depravity, and crime. Many are able to line themselves up beside normal persons in promoting the constructive uses of brotherly love.[43]

We are here concerned, of course, with the paranoids who fail. Among these, three characteristics are outstanding: (1) An extreme sensitivity to certain unconscious trends in others, with a remarkable insensitivity to similar trends in themselves; (2) a marked tendency to self-reference, and an incapacity for correcting their false self-reference by empirical, objective reality-testing; and (3) the already mentioned severe defects in reciprocal role representation, by which ordinary people manage to view things from others' perspectives. It must not be forgotten that there is nearly always a core of truth in paranoid accusations; and this alone accounts for the defensive resentment and hostility which they arouse in normal persons, a resentment toward someone who is unintentionally stirring up their own unconscious guilt. This all sounds very intricate and complex; but it is really only the description of common interactions between unrecognized trends in paranoids and corresponding unrecognized trends in normal persons. Familiarity with such patterns makes them readily intelligible.

Precipitating Factors

The single most general factor in precipitating paranoid attacks is stimulation, internal or external, to a traumatic discharge of hostile and erotic impulses when frustration provokes intolerable overexcitation.[16,69] The upsurge of impulse may result from the loss, or threats of loss, of major sources of gratification. It may come as an overcompensatory reaction to the dangers of a person's unrecognized passive wishes or fears of impotence, or as a vigorous defense against temptation. In this regard, the paranoid is often exceptionally vulnerable to ego disruption from his own superego assaults, and once more these may be experienced consciously or unconsciously as a sudden increased sense of guilt. The concept of unconscious guilt is easiest to demonstrate in dreams, where the guilt that is ignored completely during the day comes out clearly in ˙accusations against the self, which are represented in the dream as stemming from others.

Paradoxically, both rivalry and isolation can be dangerous for a potential paranoid even in the presence of success. Close competitive situations not only stimulate an oversensitive person to hostile counteraggression, they also harbor homoerotic temptation in everyday contests as to who shall dominate and who shall submit. Similar threats arise, even in the absence of competition, when a vulnerable person is thrown into close quarters with like-sexed individuals for long periods of time.

Increased isolation can have comparable effects for different reasons. Isolation leaves a person at the mercy of his private daydreams, without the safeguard of countervailing external contacts, without the corrective effects that the talk and action of others normally provide. Experimental work in sensory deprivation with normal subjects,[11] and recent extensive studies of dreams and daydreams,[22] have brought such factors into new prominence.

Internal stresses can become unbearable when a paranoid person suffers humiliation in actual failure or feels belittled by public setback. He has habitually relied for narcissistic support upon extravagant hopes and imaginings to offset a hidden pervasive sense of inadequacy. Again, the overreactions are not simply the product of thwarted ambition and wounded pride; they arise out of serious threats to an ego integrity that is in fragile balance.

Hypochondriacal anxieties are common in preparanoid personalities. These often express an unconscious suspicion of bodily defect, fears of damage, and vulnerabilities, that have personal symbolic meanings. Accident and physical illness, including intoxication and brain damage,[10] can have similar results, especially when they involve helplessness, dependence, and a somewhat infantile position.

In this section, we have considered mainly external reality situations and influences. This does not mean that paranoid conditions are produced by rivalry, erotic temptation, actual failure and defeat, or sudden close contact, or social isolation, or even solely by major losses in security and gratification. These are often the precipitating factors. They tip the balance of a chronically unstable personality organization, one dependent upon primitive defenses, defective in interpersonal reality-testing, hypersensitive to unconscious processes in others, and burdened by irresistible pressures to deny, project, and form pseudo-communities.[14,15,16] Nonetheless, these precipitating factors are both dynamically and clinically crucial, since they start off a paranoid development that may lead to decompensation.

Onset

The earliest phase of a psychotic paranoid attack may be quite indistinguishable from the ordinary fluctuations of a hypersensitive person's life. It may be only in retrospect that one can say when the habitual suspiciousness, blaming others, and self-reference blossom as outright delusion.[15] Even the most abrupt onset is often analogous to sudden cardiac decompensation. Outwardly, a person seems to be functioning well; and then decompensation comes without warning. The precipitating stress is sometimes proportionately severe and suddenly applied; sometimes, the new stress is only the last straw.

Early Phases

In most psychotic paranoid developments there is a prodromal phase in which interest is withdrawn from real interpersonal events. Preoccupation ensues and partial ego regression. But even while preoccupied and still regressing in some respects, the patient begins making his first step toward a reconstruction ("restitution"), toward regaining contact with his social environment, but now on a *delusional basis*. In the initial steps, a paranoid may be aware only of feelings of estrangement and puzzlement. Things have changed for him inexplicably; and he tries to understand what is happening. He scrutinizes his surroundings uneasily, engages in solitary observations, and looks for hidden meanings. He watches the little things people do and say, their glances and gestures, their frowns, smiles, and laughter. He listens to conversations, asks leading questions, and ponders over it all like a detective.[2,15,48]

Finding a Focus: Preliminary Crystallizations

If the situation is too unstructured, too anxiety-laden, the paranoid is driven irresistibly to form hypotheses, as normals do in unintelligible situations. But, here, paranoid defects in valid reality-testing and in tolerating

uncertainty trip him up. He cannot turn to someone else confidently; and he cannot just give up his projected fears and retrace his path. His projection and regression are necessary components of his whole defensive maneuver against being overwhelmed by a disintegrating hostility. Thus, while he goes on projecting, he moves toward a reconstructed "reality" that incorporates his pathological urges, his defenses, his inner misinterpretations and adaptations, with whatever he can accept of his external surroundings.

Final Crystallization: The Paranoid Pseudo-Community

Up to this point the projections, although by no means random, have still lacked a fixed focus—a specifically recognizable danger coming from a particular source. It remains now for the patient to conceptualize the dangerous "others" as a unified group with some definite plot, of which he is center.[16] This he achieves by organizing a well-structured pseudo-community, with all his projections and misinterpretations operating intelligibly within it.

The paranoid pseudo-community is an imaginary organization; but it includes some real persons with real functions, as well as persons whom the patient misidentifies, and some wholly imagined persons who serve to complete and justify the complex imaginary community of conspirators. All these real, misidentified, and imagined persons seem united for the express purpose of acting aggressively toward the paranoid, who is the focus of everything.[14,15] The pseudo-community often seems well-co-ordinated, with specific plans, like the fictional gangs in mystery stories. Pseudo-communities are not limited to paranoid psychoses; they have been described in psychotic depressions[46] and in schizophrenia.[51]

Once formed, the pseudo-community may move irresistibly along drive-determined vectors, picking up momentum as it goes. Real happenings are distorted and remolded to feed the ongoing process; vague and trivial incidents are endowed with significance; contrary winds of evidence are transformed into components of the rising delusional tempest. Because of the overinclusion of so much environmental material, the patient's attempts to come to grips with his seeming predicament are doomed to failure. The pseudo-community is closely related to the concept of *overinclusion*, originally formulated by this writer[12] to describe cognitive processes in schizophrenia, but since then found valid for other psychotic confusions.

Many paranoids do not carry their delusional systems over into overt action. Some remain chronically fixed at a pseudo-community level in an otherwise passive state; and some are able to replace at least part of the unrealistic reconstruction, their delusion, with more realistic components. The rare few go on to elaborate a classical paranoia.

Paranoid Action

In many, perhaps most psychotic paranoids, action amounts to no more than a morose, resentful, suspicious, or hostile attitude toward the world, behind which delusional convictions of being badly treated or maligned are concealed. Occasional phases of openly hostile accusation or threat may appear from time to time.[60] But if a paranoid acts out publicly his aggression, which to him seems justified and completely reasonable, he is usually met by some social sanction. To the patient any counteraggression seems the final confirmation of his delusional expectation of hostile attack. Thus, in the end, he unintentionally *brings about* a social reality situation that corresponds to his psychotic, angry, frightened reconstruction. An excerpt from a case will serve here as an illustration.

Charles G., an unmarried man of forty-nine, was persuaded to enter the clinic on a voluntary basis, after admitting suicidal plans to avoid being kidnapped and tortured to death. He was polite and superficially co-operative, but basically distrustful and uncommunicative. He had been living in idleness on a private income, when he suddenly got into a situation where he felt cheated. He became enraged and threatened to assault the man he accused. After thinking this over alone, he

went into a panic because he "realized" that the man he had threatened might have gangster protection. Under cover of darkness, he fled in his car to relatives he had in the West. As he drove west, across country, he became quickly convinced that he was being followed, and that even the police were in on the imagined plot. He slept in the back of his car under a pile of clothing to avoid detection. Arriving at last at his relatives' home, he was found to have made preparations for suicide, including writing a farewell note.

His childhood had given Charles no adequate basis for developing basic trust. After his mother's death, when he was a small child, his father did not remarry, but boarded his children in the homes of various relatives or friends, moving them about the country as his work moved him, and often putting each in a separate home. Charles often lived with strangers, separated from his siblings, and shifted somewhere else without advance warning. He had no chance to develop meaningful relations with anyone; and, as children often do, he blamed himself for his plight that seemed to him evidence that he was guilty of something.

Charles continued this pattern of life as an adult, leading a solitary life as a realtor, shifting his place of employment, developing no friendships, and confiding in no one. In telling his story at the clinic, it was striking how he slipped from probable fact to palpable inference in constructing chains of pseudo-logic, which satisfied his need for certainty, even while it frightened him. In the clinic, he even repeated his life pattern by declining to confide—while saying that he had something he wanted to tell someone—and by finding grounds for suspicion in other patients, the staff, and some visitors. One day, he went into another panic after a visitor whom he himself had invited by telephone had gone. He suddenly "realized" that the man was a gangster in disguise; he made an impulsive suicidal attempt, and then demanded transfer at once to a Veterans' Hospital. There we lost track of him. (See Ref. 16 in Bibliography for a more detailed account of this case.)

With such a life history, which denied him

even ordinary opportunities for affectionate acceptance and interchange, the wonder is not that he developed a paranoid psychosis at forty-nine, but rather that he had managed reasonably well for so many decades on such meager resources. It was the same cluster of personality defects that faulted his life and defeated him and us in attempts at therapy—his utter loneliness, his sweeping distrust, his unsupported inferences in terms of life-long fears and guilt, and his incapacity for sharing in anyone else's perspective, once he had reached his frightening conclusions.

(Other Psychotic Paranoid Reactions

Delusional Jealousy

As Freud[32] pointed out half a century ago even normal jealousy is by no means rational; it is neither under conscious control nor proportional to the situation in external shared reality. Its constituents are: grief over loss or threats of loss of love; hostility toward both a love-object and a rival; and a narcissistic injury which painfully lowers self-esteem. Jealousy becomes delusional when it shows the characteristics already described for delusions of persecution, i. e., when it leads to excessive projection, regression, and a renewed contact with external reality achieved through distortions. Here, too, unfounded beliefs become fixed, contradictory evidence is scorned or ignored, and the most trivial or irrelevant incident is mistaken for confirming validation. The jealous paranoid watches vigilantly for signs that he is right and misinterprets minimal signs of unconscious attitudes in others (the "core" of truth), while remaining blind to his own corresponding unconscious trends. The primitive ego defenses of denial and projection are as striking as they are in persecutory delusions. A brief case excerpt will illustrate delusional jealousy.

Peter J., a lawyer, became convinced that he had been duped by his wife and her obstetrician, both of whom belonged to a dark-skinned minority. His jealousy was aroused by

her praise of her obstetrician and by her seeming pleased at going for frequent check-ups. The newborn baby was also dark-skinned; and when the obstetrician sent Peter an unexpectedly small bill for the delivery, he was certain that the baby was not his own.

The childhood background of this man makes his delusional jealousy intelligible, though no less pathological. His parents were passionately devoted to appearances, conformity, and status, but not to affection for their son. He married into an immigrant family against their violent objections, and despite his own dislike for his wife's family and friends. His own disdain made him feel like an outsider from the start. During his wife's pregnancy, he augmented his own anxiety and sense of wrongdoing by having an extramarital affair. His experiences reinforced his suspicions of his wife's "infidelity," a clear case of projection of his own guilt. His delusion seemed to justify his own unfaithfulness; it was a new construction of reality which ascribed his own infidelity to his innocent wife.

In therapy, Peter was able to work through some of the background of his paranoid jealousy and, although he retained a small residue of suspicion, he gained enough insight and objectivity to make a recurrence unlikely. One interesting development was his spontaneous recognition that he had identified with his wife in the obstetrical situation and secretly envied her. He laughed this off after he had revealed it; and since he was seeking only ameliorative therapy, there was no need to explore his identification or his envy. Freud's original accounts emphasized unconscious homoerotic fantasies in the background of both delusions of jealousy and of persecution.

Erotic Delusions

In erotic delusions, a person, usually a woman, believes that she is beloved sexually by a man who, for some unknown reason, does not make an open avowal of love, but does give little signs of his affection.[16,31,62] Passive men sometimes have a corresponding erotic delusion. The supposed lover is often a public figure—in politics, on stage or lecture platform, in the movies or on television. Since such deluded persons sometimes pester the object of their affections with letters, pay them visits, or demand a public avowal, they may drive their target to seek police intervention.

The love involved may be narcissistic self-love projected in fantasy and ascribed to the target person. It may be a defensive maneuver, as Freud maintained, which substitutes a delusional heterosexual attachment for denied unconscious homosexual wishes. Fenichel[21] wrote that the sex of the imaginary lover was unimportant in borderline erotic delusional men. These sense vaguely an imminent object loss, and cling frantically to at least some love-object. Many persons with erotic delusions experience pleasure from their imagined predicament; but some feel "persecuted by love" and protest indignantly.

Paranoid Grandiosity

Grandiose delusions are met less frequently than those of persecution; but when they do occur, they are usually more intractable than any others. Manifest grandiose delusions range in complexity from relatively simple convictions that one is enormously talented, attractive, or inspired, all the way to intricately systematized beliefs that one is about to revolutionize the life of man, as a prophet, reformer, scientist, or great inventor. Many such delusions are stable, persistent, and even well-organized. Occasionally, a grandiose delusional person is able to play a significant part in some realistic social, artistic, or scientific movement; and in rare instances, he initiates and carries through reforms.[43] Delusions of grandeur are attempts to recapture lost object relationships. Their higher incidence among severe, rather than mild, paranoid conditions, points to the greater denial of consensual reality demanded. It is no surprise that they are common in classical paranoia.

Classical Paranoia

The rare classical paranoia represents only the ultimate in elaborate systematization and fixity of delusional reconstruction. Some persons with such severe paranoia may still be able to conduct their own affairs in spite of harboring an intricate, complex, unmodifiable delusional system, without disorganizing or desocializing. The delusions seem more or less isolated from the rest of the personality organization in such cases, almost like a foreign body reaction, leaving large areas of thinking and action free to operate normally. One of the most extraordinary examples of this was the case of Schreber, whose behavior and conversation were almost without exception outwardly normal for several years, even though at the same time he maintained incredible delusions.[72]

What has already been said of persecutory, erotic, and grandiose delusions applies to classical paranoia. It is generally regarded as untreatable. However, if one avoids the trap of equating treatability with complete recovery, there is no reason to conclude in advance that no amelioration is possible, even though the delusions remain fixed. There is no reason why psychiatrists and psychologists should make such an equation when medicine and surgery have long ago discarded it. The healing arts have as their goal the improvement of a person's life, and the relief of unnecessary suffering, and no more.

Folie à Deux

More than a century ago, Baillarger reported the admission on the same day of two relatives with the same delusions. The term later adopted, *folie à deux*, has led to a needless multiplication of terms, such as *folie à trois*, *folie à cing*, and even *folie à douze*.[40] The typical setup is that of a dominant delusional person who induces a parallel delusional development in a dependent one. If the two are separated, the dependent one recovers quickly, but not the dominant one. A majority exhibit persecutory paranoid delusions.

In his classical case reports, Gralnick[39] points out the preponderance of persons living in intimate contact, and lists the frequency of each relationship in 103 cases. He ascribes the greater susceptibility of women to their being obliged to play a somewhat restricted, submissive role. Sex role differences may also be invoked.

([Psychodynamics and Early Childhood

What are the psychodynamics of paranoid conditions, and what congenital and early childhood experiences predispose a person to become seriously paranoid? Since paranoid thinking is almost universal, and appears even when defective communication occurs in normal people, no simple cause-and-effect relationship can be invoked. There are interesting possibilities in the results of direct observation of neonates; they reveal striking differences in sensitivities to environmental stimulation, and in relative tolerance for delays in satisfying such simple needs as nourishment, warmth, and general comfort.

Is the hypersensitive neonate more vulnerable than others to later stress? Probably so, but we really do not know for sure. Some hypersensitive infants remain consistently hypersensitive and some do not; some placid newborns become hypersensitive later.[19,20] One must always remember that enormous internal physiological readjustments follow birth, and we have very little idea as to what these portend. Is there a genetic factor involved? Undoubtedly, but here also the vicissitudes of embryonic and fetal development, the process of birth and of perinatal stresses, form an extremely complex matrix. A great deal more is known today than twenty years ago, but not yet enough for final conclusions to be drawn.

The early handling of infants presents such a multitude of potentialities in itself that it may be decades before we can be sure how much weight to give any infant's experiences during the first few weeks or months. The reports of the many who observe infants directly, and such speculations as, for example, Melanie Klein's[53,55] contention that every infant passes through an early paranoid and a later depressive "position," are still as tentative as the genetic conclusions repeating a very old tradition that people are "just born that way."[53,55] We must always bear in mind that each approach to the thorny question of the infantile origins of paranoid disorders is also a quest for certainty by students of behavior, experience, and genetics. It is easy to be seduced by an elegant hypothesis and by impressive accumulations of data; but there is no justification in 1973 for dogmatic assertions. For even if we knew far more than we now do about genetic loading, perinatal stress, and the patterns of child-rearing and mothering, we would still be a long way from being able to link such data with paranoid development twenty or thirty years later.[4,8,9,80]

As for the psychodynamics of paranoid development, these, too, must depend at least to some extent upon the innate biology of the individual infant, upon the early defensive and adaptive maneuvers he develops, upon his success in forming a symbiotic unit with his mother, and his success in dissolving the symbiosis to become a more or less autonomous individual. No professional person conversant with the current status of these factors is likely to ignore any one of them. (This writer has discussed these problems in some detail elsewhere, and has set forth the probable, but still speculative, background of persons especially vulnerable to paranoid development.[16] These accounts are obviously too long to be included here. Although they make every effort to present a coherent picture in terms of contemporary knowledge, they remain in part hypothetical, since our knowledge is uncertain and there are many gaps.)

The probable origins of paranoid conditions, both ontogenetic and biosocial, have already been indicated in the case illustrations sketched in this chapter, and they are representative of the direct clinical observations to others, as the citations imply. Whether these can be considered universal is a question that only the future can answer. As others have found, in addition to this writer, some of the most "typical" paranoid delusions appear in classical manic-depressive, schizophrenic, and organic brain damage syndromes.[46] One must learn to avoid dogmatic assertion and remain receptive to the ongoing changes in theoretical orientations that point toward a different future.

In addition to the current literature already cited, a recent treatise by Swanson et al.[78] deserves mention. It gives a partial history of the paranoid concept, takes a position on the basic nature of the paranoid person, and gives summary accounts of problems arising in the paranoid's family and community, and of the importance of paranoid trends in government, industry, law, and religion. An extensive bibliography is usefully arranged by topic. (A special chapter on international political attitudes might be added after the startling and welcomed reversal of Chinese-American relations has been assayed.)

The chief weaknesses of this treatise are the attempt to cover too much in too short a space, and a relative neglect of dynamics. For example, the authors seem to discount Freud's fundamental contributions on grounds that he was inexperienced in working with psychotics, although he explicitly stated that he had had considerable contact in this area.[29] They call attention clearly, as does Pinderhughes,[69] to the enormous potential dangers of having paranoid personalities in positions of power, dangers that have been realized in our own time and throughout history.

A major controversy, that exemplifies dominant interpretations of the whole paranoid concept during the past two or three decades, centers around Freud's insistence that paranoid conditions grow out of failures in ego defense against previously repressed homosexual wishes. This claim has never been disproved. It is significant for today's situation that Freud himself published[26,27,28] convincing evidence of prevalent procreative fantasies and beliefs in small children at the same time that he wrote his famous critique of the Schreber case.[29] It is these two seemingly opposed revelations—actually, not mutually exclusive—that continue as dominant themes up to the present. Arguments over whether to place Schreber's diagnosis in the official box marked "paranoid state" or in the more popular one labeled "paranoid schizophrenia" are immaterial, since what we are considering is the paranoid modes of thought and feeling, in whatever combination they occur.[2]

Theories and Observations Since Freud: Homosexual Origins

In the mainstream of professional concern, homosexual origins have received the most support.[6,34,36,44,48,70] Only a few examples, out of hundreds, will be cited here. The whole situation is currently complicated by a longstanding conviction that paranoid delusions are nearly always components of schizophrenia, and the more recent emphasis upon their presence in mania and depressions.[46] During the 1940s, a number of variations appeared on the homosexual theme. There were then, and still are, occasional publications with opposed findings, as, for example, that male paranoids tend more to homosexual delusions (even when overtly homosexual), whereas females believe themselves accused of being prostitutes. Knight[56] stressed intense homosexual love that needed hatred to counteract it, while Bak[3] emphasized delusional masochism, against which the paranoid tried vainly to defend himself.

Klein[53,55] postulated normal infant sadism, and referred predisposition to paranoia to arrested development beyond a phase in which a terrifying superego reigned. Segal[14] has written a lucid introduction to Klein's work. Jaffe[48] and Frosch[34,35] have further advanced the homosexual hypothesis. The doubt cast upon this interpretation by reports of overt homosexuals being paranoid has been countered by a claim that overt and repressed impulses can operate at the same time in the same person.

More recently, hatred has again been highlighted in paranoid developments, notably by Pinderhughes,[69] and Carr et al.[52] The important researches of Baumeyer,[5] Katan,[49,50,51] and Carr, et al. have spelled out the actual sadistic treatment that Schreber experienced at his own famous father's hands, which is clearly represented in his distorted delusions. Freud knew nothing of all of this. Niederland[63-67] researches continue and promise future enrichment. Two especially significant new findings are: (1) that Schreber's older brother was also a jurist, was also named Daniel, and committed suicide in the face of success, just as the younger Daniel was engulfed by psychosis in the face of his success; and (2) that Schreber's mother was of great importance in his life, although this possibility seems to have been neglected even by Freud.[52] Obviously, the whole issue of homosexuality in paranoia needs overhauling, in spite of abundant clinical evidence of feminine homosexual attitudes in Schreber's illness.

Procreation Fantasies and Deep Regression

Although Freud urged everyone to go to the original autobiography of Schreber,[72] his advice was followed only in exceptional instances, for example, by Katan and Niederland. Since its translation into English in 1955, interest has rapidly increased in its restudy. The translators, MacAlpine and Hunter, have been criticized for being unsympathetic to Freud. Be that as it may, their comments in their Introduction and Discussion included with the translation raise valuable questions, which deserve, at least, not to be ignored. For example, they state: "Neither in theory nor in therapy is projection of and conflict over unconscious homosexuality as firmly established as the cause of paranoid illness . . . as is generally believed and stated." And: "Schreber fell ill when a wish-fantasy that he could, would or should have children became pathogenic. Simultaneously he became doubtful of his own sex."[59]

They seem to be implying that Schreber's paranoia arose from his repressed infantile procreation fantasies. If one rereads Schreber's *Memoirs*, there is plenty of evidence for such fantasies in the fusion of God, Flechsig, and Schreber père, as well as strong hints that not only the older brother but Schreber's mother also played leading roles in the delusional systems. It is ironic that Freud's delightful contributions to infantile procreation fantasies, especially in the "Little Hans" case,[28] should now be used to refute his other interpretation. Actually, the two approaches supplement each other. Katan[51] has recently tried an integration, with clarity and restraint, in which he designates paranoia as a special form of schizophrenia. It is safe to conclude that, whatever the controversies, paranoid thinking will always be with us,[16,69] because it is a variant of normal experiences.

(Individual Psychotherapy of Paranoid Conditions and Paranoia

An immediate goal in the treatment of paranoid persons, including paranoia, is reduction of anxiety and development of trust. This is not easy to achieve, since the patient is highly suspicious of everyone, and cannot be won over by words of reassurance or advice. The therapist must be relaxed, and neither inquisitive nor indifferent; he must keep his distance and not be dismayed by apparent lack of progress or even the prospect of ultimate failure. He needs to practice suspended judgment as much as his patient does. Whatever reassurance and emotional support he gives must be only in an unfeigned attitude of respect, acceptance, and concern, never expressed in words and never encroaching upon the paranoid's excessive need for privacy and concealment. It is essential to keep in mind that paranoid delusions may be indispensable protective devices, security operations that keep a patient in some effective contact with his surroundings, and allow him to reconstruct his conceptions of his social environment while providing a tolerable harmony with his conscious and unconscious inner desires, fears, hates, and hope.[16] To attack delusions may be to precipitate an immediate sweeping regression into panic or an undifferentiated state.

Niederland[68] has recently suggested touching upon the ambulatory paranoid's distrust of his therapist from the start, and continuing to explore it throughout treatment. This must be done, of course, with circumspection and as unobtrusively as possible, to avoid giving the slightest impression of blaming the patient, which he will always be overready to infer because of his pathological unconscious hostility and his superego projections. The paranoid is exquisitely sensitive to traces of unconscious aggression in others, to any hint of interference in his affairs, and to threatened restrictions of his liberty of thought, feeling, and action, which he experiences as intentional humiliation. Only the therapist who has learned to walk on eggs with comfort, skill, and self-assurance should treat seriously paranoid persons, unless he does so under the supervision of someone experienced in this area of treatment.

This writer has suggested that in all paranoid psychoses there is an active nucleus of neurotic conflict which in itself helps keep the patient from deeper regression.[16] The therapist who is reasonably comfortable in the presence of psychosis can approach neurotic components with techniques usually employed in working with neurotics. This general approach has received further support in the recent literature.

If the general tension of a paranoid subsides, communication markedly improves, and he becomes able to express underlying fears, anger, and a sense of being ostracized. What Freud said about "deep interpretation" in the therapy of psychoses is as true today as when he wrote it.[33] A psychotic is often able to interpret unconscious meanings more immediately and significantly than his therapist can. Such special insight may be a gift; but it is an expensive one and usually a misfortune. Obviously, therapy of paranoid persons involves something quite different from even the most intelligent common sense. It demands therapist attitudes unique in the patient's life experience—completely non-judgmental ones which avoid both premature agreement and unwanted explanation, as well as intolerable contradiction. There is always a core of truth in every delusion; and therapists must never forget it.

There is no exclusive technique for the treatment of paranoia. Some therapists succeed with a naturally warm, kindly, but not too familiar and never condescending approach. A paranoid patient may be superior in mental ability and achievement to his therapist; and even when the opposite is true, he

has had experiences that may be richer than his therapist's, as well as different. One might as well be condescending to his own dreams—which many naïve normal persons are—as to the daytime delusions of a patient. Other therapists enter into the paranoid delusions deliberately, but with caution, and with a clear understanding that they do not accept the patient's paranoid beliefs as social fact. Some therapists keep rigorously out of delusional systems without making an open issue of acceptance or rejection.

This writer favors an interested, attentive, relaxed, and unaffected attitude, with an unfeigned air of detachment and suspended judgment. This avoids stimulating suspicions and fears by avoiding any hint of intrusion or overt friendliness that might be mistaken for intimacy. Suspended judgment is essential, since a therapist cannot know how much of what he hears is social fact and how much fantasy. Many paranoid complaints are justified, and the most fantastic things happen in real life, as one quickly learns. If a therapist's feelings are genuine, any patient will feel this at nonverbal and unconscious levels; if they are false, he will readily sense deceit behind the most clever mask of feigned friendliness and fair words.

There is no difference of opinion about the necessity for scrupulous but not cruel honesty, for respect, truthfulness, and steadfastness. What the patient needs is not merely a chance to talk and "ventilate" his feelings; he needs to break out of his isolation, and share his fright, anger, and resentments with someone who does not take sides or pretend to know everything. The therapist must become what one of my own patients called "a new point of reference,"[17] a person who gives the patient the chance to catch glimpses of his own personal world from another's perspective. An indispensable therapeutic goal is that of replacing a pervasive, uneasy suspicion and mistrust with a specific confidence, which then forms a new base for further explorations by the patient. One must always remember that it is not the delusion that calls for therapy, but the frightened person;[48,70] sometimes, a paranoid regains effective social health without entirely giving up his delusional beliefs. This is as real a recovery as that of a diabetic who learns to regulate his life independently without ever losing his original vulnerability to diabetes.

Progress in paranoid conditions must always be guarded. The most important limiting factors are the basic ego-adaptive and -defensive organization, its potentialities for flexibility and change, and its capacity for forming new ego and superego identifications. There are wide differences among paranoid persons in these dimensions, which must be recognized and dealt with as therapy progresses. It is fortunate that today attention is focused upon the human setting in which the patient lives, or if he has been hospitalized, the setting to which he will return. It is here that the social worker is the most significant person, not the psychiatrist, the psychologist, or the nurse. As an expert in community attitudes and resources, he can make the difference between success and failure, as individual psychotherapy tapers off and terminates. His therapy deals as much with the community as with the recovered or recovering patient. He must understand the patient's internal dynamics, his group and general social behavior, the structure of the minicommunity of his immediate associates, and the total effective environment to which an ex-patient must adapt himself, without losing his individuality and identity.

(Bibliography

1. ALTSCHUL, D. "Denial and Ego Arrest," *Journal of American Psychoanalytic Association*, 16 (1968), 301.
2. ARIETI, S. *The Intrapsychic Self: Feeling, Cognition and Creativity in Health and Mental Illness*. New York: Basic Books, 1967.
3. BAK, R. "Masochism in Paranoia," *Psychoanalytic Quarterly*, 15 (1946), 285.
4. BARGLOW, R., and L. SADOW. "Visual Perception: Its Development from Birth to Adulthood," *Journal of American Psychoanalytic Association*, 19 (1971), 433.
5. BAUMEYER, F. "The Schreber Case," *International Journal of Psycho-Analysis*, 37 (1956), 61.
6. BIEBER, I., et al. *Homosexuality: A Psychoanalytic Study*. New York: Basic Books, 1962.
7. BLEULER, E. *Dementia Praecox or the Group of Schizophrenias*, J. Zinkin, transl. New York: International Universities Press, 1950.
8. BRODY, S. *Patterns of Motherhood: Maternal Influences During Infancy*. New York: International Universities Press, 1956.
9. BRODY, S., and S. AXELROD. "Anxiety, Socialization and Ego Formation: An Historical Approach," *International Journal of Psycho-Analysis*, 47 (1966), 218.
10. BROSIN, H. W. "Contributions of Psychoanalysis to the Study of Organic Cerebral Disorders," in F. Alexander and H. Ross, eds., *Dynamic Psychiatry*. Chicago: University of Chicago Press, 1952.
11. BROWNFIELD, C. *Isolation: Clinical and Experimental Approaches*. New York: Random House, 1970.
12. CAMERON, N. "Schizophrenic Thinking in a Problem-Solving Situation," *Journal of Mental Science*, 85 (1939), 1012.
13. ———. "The Development of Paranoic Thinking," *Psychology Review*, 50 (1943), 219.
14. ———. "The Paranoid Pseudo-Community," *American Journal of Sociology*, 49 (1943), 32.
15. ———. "The Paranoid Pseudo-Community Revisited," *American Journal of Sociology*, 64 (1959), 52.
16. ———. *Personality Development and Psychopathology: A Dynamic Approach*. Boston: Houghton, Mifflin, 1963.
17. ———. *Varieties of Inner Turmoil*. (Submitted for publication.)
18. *Diagnostic and Statistical Manual*, 2nd ed. Washington: American Psychiatric Association, 1968.
19. ESCALONA, S. *Prediction and Outcome: A Study in Child Development*. New York: Basic Books, 1959.
20. ———. "Patterns of Infantile Experience and the Developmental Process," in *The Psychoanalytic Study of the Child*, Vol. 18. New York: International Universities Press, 1963.
21. FENICHEL, O. *The Psychoanalytic Theory of the Neuroses*. New York: W. W. Norton, 1945.
22. FOULKES, D. *The Psychology of Sleep*. New York: Scribner's, 1966.

23. FREUD, A. *Normality and Pathology in Childhood: An Assessment of Development.* New York: International Universities Press, 1965.

24. FREUD, S. "The Neuro-Psychoses of Defence (1894)," in Standard Edition, Vol. 3. London: Hogarth Press, 1962.

25. ———. "Further Remarks on the Neuro-Psychoses of Defence (1896)," in Standard Edition, Vol. 3. London: Hogarth Press, 1962.

26. ———. "Three Essays on the Theory of Sexuality (1905)," in Standard Edition, Vol. 7. London: Hogarth Press, 1953.

27. ———. "On the Sexual Theories of Children (1908)," in Standard Edition, Vol. 9. London: Hogarth Press, 1959.

28. ———. "Analysis of a Phobia in a Five-Year-Old Boy (1909)," in Standard Edition, Vol. 10. London: Hogarth Press, 1955.

29. ———. "Psycho-Analytic Notes on an Autobiographical Account of a Case of Paranoia (Dementia Paranoides) (1911)," in Standard Edition, Vol. 12. London: Hogarth Press, 1958.

30. ———. "A Case of Paranoia Running Counter to the Psycho-Analytic Theory of the Disease (1915)," in Standard Edition, Vol. 14. London: Hogarth Press, 1957.

31. ———. "The Psychogenesis of a Case of Homosexuality in a Woman (1920)," in Standard Edition, Vol. 18. London: Hogarth Press, 1955.

32. ———. "Some Neurotic Mechanisms in Jealousy, Paranoia and Homosexuality (1922)," in Standard Edition, Vol. 18. London: Hogarth Press, 1955.

33. ———. "Analysis Terminable and Interminable (1937)," in Standard Edition, Vol. 23. London: Hogarth Press, 1964.

34. FROSCH, J. "Delusional Fixation, Sense of Conviction and the Psychotic Conflict," *International Journal of Psycho-Analysis*, 48 (1967), 475.

35. ———. "Psychoanalytic Consideration of the Psychotic Character," *Journal of American Psychoanalytic Association*, 18 (1970), 24.

36. GERSHMAN, H. "The Use of the Dream in the Treatment of Homosexuality," *American Journal of Psychoanalysis*, 31 (1971), 80.

37. GLOVER, E. *Psycho-Analysis: A Handbook for Medical Practitioners and Students of Comparative Psychology.* London: Staples, 1949.

38. ———. *The Technique of Psycho-Analysis.* New York: International Universities Press, 1955.

39. GRALNICK, A. "Folie à deux: The Psychosis of Association," *Psychiatric Quarterly*, 16 (1942), 230.

40. GREENBERG, H. "Crime and Folie à deux: A Review and Case History," *Journal of Mental Science*, 102 (1956), 772.

41. GREENSON, R. *The Technique and Practice of Psychoanalysis.* New York: International Universities Press, 1967.

42. HARTMANN, H. *Ego Psychology and the Problem of Adaptation.* New York: International Universities Press, 1958.

43. HOFFER, E. *The True Believer.* New York: Harper and Row, 1951.

44. HORNSTRA, L. "Homosexuality," *International Journal of Psycho-Analysis*, 48 (1967), 397.

45. JACOBSON, E. *The Self and the Object World.* New York: International Universities Press, 1964.

46. ———. "Problems in the Differentiation Between Schizophrenic and Melancholic States of Depression," in R. Loewenstein, L. Newman, M. Schur, and A. Solnit, eds., *Psychoanalysis: A General Psychology.* New York: International Universities Press, 1966.

47. ———. "Acting Out and the Urge to Betray in Paranoid Patients," in *Depression: Comparative Studies of Normal, Neurotic and Psychotic Conditions.* New York: International Universities Press, 1971.

48. JAFFE, D. "The Mechanism of Paranoia," *International Journal of Psycho-Analysis*, 49 (1968), 662.

49. KATAN, M. "Schreber's Hallucinations About the 'Little Men,'" *International Journal of Psycho-Analysis*, 21 (1950), 32.

50. ———. "Schreber's Prepsychotic Phase," *International Journal of Psycho-Analysis*, 34 (1953), 43.

51. ———. "A Psychoanalytic Approach to the Diagnosis of Paranoia," *The Psychoanalytic Study of the Child*, Vol. 24. New York: International Universities Press, 1969.

52. KITAY, P., A. CARR, W. NIEDERLAND, J. NYDES, R. WHITE. "Symposium on 'Reinterpretations of the Schreber Case: Freud's Theory of Paranoia,'" *International Journal of Psycho-Analysis*, 44 (1963), 191.

53. KLEIN, M. *Contributions to Psycho-Analysis.* London: Hogarth Press, 1948.

54. ———. "Love, Guilt and Reparation," in M. Klein, and J. Riviere, *Love, Hate and Reparation*. London: Hogarth Press, 1027.

55. KLEIN, M. P. HEIMANN, R. MONEY-KYRLE, eds., *New Directions in Psycho-Analysis: The Significance of Infant Conflict in the Patterning of Adult Behavior*. New York: Basic Books, 1955.

56. KNIGHT, R. "The Relationship of Latent Homosexuality to the Mechanism of Paranoid Delusions," *Bulletin of Menninger Clinic*, 4 (1940), 149.

57. KOLB, L. *Noyes' Modern Clinical Psychiatry*, 7th ed. Philadelphia: Saunders, 1968.

58. KRAEPELIN, E. *Psychiatrie: Ein Lehrbuch für Studierenden und Ärzte*. Leipzig: Barth, 1915.

59. MACALPINE, I., and R. HUNTER. "Introduction" and "Discussion," in D. P. Schreber, Ref. 72.

60. MEAD, G. H. *Mind, Self and Society*. Chicago: University of Chicago Press, 1934.

61. MILLER, C. "The Paranoid Syndrome," *Archives of Neurology and Psychiatry*, 49 (1941), 953.

62. MODLIN, H. "Psychodynamics and Management of Paranoid States in Women," *Archives of General Psychiatry*, 8 (1963), 263.

63. NIEDERLAND, W. "Schreber: Father and Son," *Psychoanalytic Quarterly*, 28 (1959), 151.

64. ———. "The 'Miracled-Up' World of Schreber's Childhood," *The Psychoanalytic Study of the Child*, Vol. 14. New York: International Universities Press, 1959.

65. ———. "Schreber's Father," *Journal of American Psychoanalytic Association*, 8 (1960), 492.

66. ———. "Further Data and Documentation in the Schreber Case," *International Journal of Psycho-Analysis*, 44 (1963), 201.

67. ———. "Schreber and Flechsig," *Journal of American Psychoanalytic Association*, 16 (1968), 740.

68. ———. "Paranoia: Theory and Therapy," *Psychiatry and Social Science Review*, 4 (1970), 2.

69. PINDERHUGHES, C. A. "Managing Paranoia in Violent Relationships," in G. Usdin, ed., *Perspectives on Violence*. New York: Bruner/Mazel, 1972.

70. ROSENFELD, H. "On the Treatment of Psychotic States in Psychoanalysis: An Historical Approach," *International Journal of Psycho-Analysis*, 50 (1969), 615.

71. SCHAFER, R. *Aspects of Internalization*. New York: International Universities Press, 1968.

72. SCHREBER, D. P. *Memoirs of My Nervous Illness*, I. MacAlpine, and R. Hunter, transl. London: Dawson, 1955.

73. SCHWARTZ, D. "A Re-View of Paranoia," *Archives of General Psychiatry*, 8 (1963), 349.

74. SEGAL, H. *Introduction to the Work of Melanie Klein*. New York: Basic Books, 1964.

75. SHAPIRO, D. *Neurotic Styles*. New York: Basic Books, 1965.

76. SHIBUTANI, T. *Society and Personality*. New York: Prentice-Hall, 1961.

77. SPITZ, R. *The First Year: A Psychoanalytic Study of Normal and Deviant Development of Object-Relations*. New York: International Universities Press, 1965.

78. SWANSON, D., P. BOHNERT, and J. SMITH. *The Paranoid*. Boston: Little, Brown, 1970.

79. TYHURST, J. "Paranoid Patterns," in A. Leighton, J. Claus, and R. Wilson, eds., *Explorations in Social Psychiatry*. New York: Basic Books, 1958.

80. WOLFF, P. "Review of Psychoanalytic Theory in the Light of Current Research in Child Development," *Journal of American Psychoanalytic Association*, 19 (1971), 565.

CHAPTER 30

INVOLUTIONAL DEPRESSION

Saul H. Rosenthal

SOME MATERIAL in this chapter is modified from my paper, "The Involutional Depressive Syndrome," which appeared in the *American Journal of Psychiatry*, 124 (May 1968) Supplement, pp. 21–35, and is used with permission of the *American Journal of Psychiatry*.

Involutional melancholia has developed an anomalous position in psychiatry. It is an illness that is described in almost all of the textbooks and is maintained in the classification systems; however, the diagnosis is rarely used. Involutional melancholia apparently was encountered fairly frequently in the past, and was described as a quite clear-cut psychiatric illness. Today, however, one rarely encounters a "classical case" of the full-blown involutional melancholia syndrome.

Partially because of this, involutional melancholia has become a questionable illness. Many writers today feel that it is undistinguishable from other depressive syndromes. The APA *Diagnostic and Statistical Manual of Mental Disorders* (DSM-II)[12] reflects this ambivalence. It defines involutional melancholia as a disorder occurring in the involutional period, which is characterized by worry, anxiety, agitation, and severe insomnia, with guilt and somatic preoccupation. Involutional melancholia is included with manic-depressive illness under the category of major affective disorders as a psychosis not directly related to precipitating life experience. DSM-II goes on to note that opinion is divided as to whether involutional melancholia can be distinguished from other depressions, and advises that one not use this diagnosis, unless all other affective disorders have been ruled out.

In DSM-I, involutional melancholia and involutional paranoid disorders were combined together under the diagnosis of "involutional psychotic reaction." The current splitting of the two categories probably reflects the impression that involutional melancholia may be etiologically related to other depressive disorders, while the paranoid reactions of the involutional years may be more clearly related to schizophrenic disorders.

⟦ The Classical Picture

Although there is a good deal of mixed opinion as to whether involutional melancholia does shade off into other depressions, or whether it is a separate entity, there is remarkably little controversy about the description of the classical picture. That is to say, it is a well-defined syndrome, and most psychiatrists have the same picture in mind when they use the term "involutional melancholia," whether they believe in it or not. I will summarize the textbook picture here to clarify what is being discussed:

Involutional melancholia is a depressive episode of major proportion occurring *for the first time* in the involutional age without a prior history of manic-depressive illness. The involutional age generally refers to ages 40-55 for women and 50-65 for men. Involutional depressions are more common in women, as are most depressive illnesses.

The *premorbid personality* is often described as rigid, overconscientious, and restricted. Superego domination is stressed, with life-long repression of sexual and aggressive drives, in an anal-erotic personality utilizing primarily obsessive-compulsive defenses. The illness is seen as decompensation of the obsessional defensive life pattern.

The *genetic background* has been in question, with a few early studies indicating a relationship to schizophrenia. Modern studies tend to consider involutional melancholia in the context of a late onset unipolar depression, and find some genetic relationship to other depressive disorders.

Although involutional melancholia in women tends to occur approximately at the time of the menopause, it is now felt that the psychological impact of the menopause has more effect on symptom formation than does its direct physiologic action. It is also felt that aging per se, rather than the specific changes around the climacterium, is probably a major factor in determining a particular pattern of symptoms.

The *onset* is gradual, with the slow buildup of hypochondriasis, pessimism, and irritability finally flowering into full-blown depressive syndrome. The most prominent features are motor agitation and restlessness, a prevailing affect of anxiety and apprehension, an exaggerated hypochondriasis (sometimes with bizarre delusions), and occasional paranoid ideation which infrequently dominates. These distinguishing symptoms may be thought of as superimposed on a basic depressive substrate with insomnia, anorexia, and weight loss, and feelings of guilt and worthlessness. The depressed affect is described by some as shallow, as compared to that seen in other depressive patients. Retardation is often described as absent or masked by agitation.

The untreated *course* was felt to be quite long and, in the days before electroconvulsive therapy, was estimated at one to five years for the 30–60 percent of patients who recovered spontaneously. For example, Huston and Locker[26] reported a retrospective study in 1948, following up patients hospitalized between 1930 and 1939 at Iowa Psychopathic Hospital. They found that only 46 percent of the patients recovered spontaneously and for those recovered patients the average course of the illness was forty-nine months with a median duration of thirty-one months. Eighteen percent of the patients did not recover and, interestingly, 36 percent died. This included 13 percent who suicided (usually within two years of the onset of the illness); 10 percent who died directly due to the illness, from exhaustion and malnutrition; and 13 percent who died from intercurrent medical illnesses, of whom half were perhaps indirectly due to the depression. Treatment with electroconvulsive therapy changed this picture markedly; involutional agitated depressions are noted to have an excellent response to ECT[6,8,26,67] and the duration of the illness is shortened to three to six weeks in many cases. For example, Huston's group reported that 84 percent of his patients with melancholia treated with ECT between 1941 and 1943 had complete recovery or pronounced improvement, which was maintained for at least thirty-six months of follow-up. The median time in the hospital fell from seven months untreated, to one-and-a-half months with ECT. Three-fourths of those patients who failed to respond, or who relapsed, responded to a second series.[26]

(The Controversy

Some writers feel that involutional melancholia can be distinguished from other depressions on multiple grounds. They usually make their distinction between involutional melancholia and manic depressive illness. The criteria include: a history lacking previous episodes of depression; a rigid, obsessive premorbid personality, rather than a cyclothymic one; a gradual rather than abrupt onset; a clinical picture dominated by agitation and hypochondriasis, rather than by sadness and retardation; the absence of manic symptoms; and a poor prognosis without treatment with a longer course and fewer recoveries.

The problem is that this is a comparison against the classical manic-depressive picture. It is a vestige of the psychiatric era when it was assumed that all depressed patients fit into either one or the other category. The epidemiological picture has changed tremendously, and with changing attitudes towards psychiatry and psychiatric hospitalization, both involutional melancholia and manic-depressive illness have been submerged in a sea of patients with milder neurotic depressions or depressive reactions.

A second problem is that the classic contrasts do not take into account the vast number of patients with intermediate or mixed pictures. Involutional melancholia seems to shade off on a continuum of mixed clinical pictures into other depressive conditions. We are unfortunate in psychiatry in that our diagnoses are, for the most part, made on the basis of clinical picture and clinical course alone. We do not have the reassuring laboratory tests that are available in medicine and provide firm end points by which one can say that a patient "has" one illness or another. Diagnoses made on clinical picture alone can be quite frustrating and the lack of firm end points has caused some writers to essentially abandon the struggle and subsume all depressions under a unitary category of "depression" or "affective disorders," and one frequently runs across studies that simply refer to populations of "depressed patients."

Among those who take either a unitary point of view or a view including involutional melancholia with other depressions, Lewis,[39,40] in an influential series of papers reviewing the case histories of a large number of psychiatric patients, felt that involutional

depression should be included in the general category of affective disorders. He pointed out that the same symptoms may be seen at an earlier age and that many types of premorbid personality may be found. Roth[58] asserted that "The concept of a specific involutional pattern of endogenous depression . . . is no longer tenable." Stenback,[62] after reviewing the syndrome, found that there is no characteristic ideology, syndrome, or course for involutional depression. More recently, Beck[3] reviewed the evidence in his monograph on depression and concluded, ". . . there is no more justification for allocating a special diagnostic label to depressions in the involutional period, than there is for setting up other age specific categories. . . ." Similarly, Mendels[43] sees little rational basis for using a separate diagnostic category. He feels that involutional melancholia is probably a variety of depression whose clinical presentation has been affected by age and life situations.

Further towards a middle ground, Lehmann[37] pointed out that while there is some supporting evidence for involutional melancholia as independent entity, it is not direct or definitive. Redlich and Friedman[50] take the view that without any specific knowledge of the etiology, diagnostic disputes are unprofitable; they conclude that "at present, there is no good nosological or etiological reason to recognize involutional disorders as specific entities." This probably represents the informal opinion of a great many present-day psychiatrists.

Other textbooks tend to be more conservative and still describe involutional melancholia as a separate entity to more or less extent. Ford,[17] writing in Freedman and Kaplan's textbook, acknowledges the controversy but considers and describes involutional psychotic reaction as a clear-cut separate disorder. Slater and Roth,[61] in Mayer-Gross' textbook, include involutional melancholia as a subheading in a chapter primarily devoted to manic-depressive illness. They feel that depressions in this age group may be related to functional or organic changes, but exactly what endocrine or metabolical alterations are responsible are currently unknown. They feel that some of the involutional depressive patients are manic-depressives, but that not all are, as there seems to be a different heredity, personality, prognosis, and response to treatment. They feel that the differences in symptoms are only partly atributable to influences of age.

Other texts maintain that involutional melancholia is clearly a distinct entity, and that it differs from other depressions, specifically from manic-depressive illness, in many ways. Kolb,[35] writing in the new edition of Noyes' textbook, asserts, "In spite of the feature of depression common to both manic-depressive and involutional reactions, there are such special physiological and psychological factors in the latter, that it is no longer considered to be a modified manic-depressive reaction occurring at a particular physiological epoch". Batchelor,[2] in Henderson and Gillespie's textbook, takes basically the same point of view as does English and Finch's[14] textbook.

The problem is thus complicated by a phenomenon whereby textbooks pass on clinical descriptions as stereotypes without validation at the same time when most clinicians and clinical writers do not believe that the syndromes have any validity. An additional problem is that clinical description in psychiatry, and involutional melancholia as a syndrome, have both fallen into relative disrepute in the United States, and this has discouraged further re-evaluation. It is complicated by the fact that attention in psychiatry in the past twenty years has shifted markedly away from older psychotic patients and toward young, verbal psychotherapy candidates on the one hand, and community and social issues on the other. These may be quite beneficial changes for psychiatry, but have contributed to the lack of investigational interest in involutional depressive disorders.

(Early History

Kraepelin,[36] in the fifth edition of his textbook, *Psychiatrie* (1896), divided the functional psychosis into three major groups:

dementia praecox, manic-depressive psychosis, and involution psychoses, with the last including melancholia. Kraepelin indicated that:

Melancholia is restricted to certain conditions of mental depression occurring during the period of involution. It includes all of the morbidly anxious states not represented in other forms of insanity, and is characterized by uniform despondency with fear, various delusions of self accusation, of persecution, and of a hypochondriacal nature, with moderate clouding of consciousness, leading in the greater number of cases, after a prolonged course, to moderate mental deterioration.

It was distinguished from manic-depressive illness by being an acquired condition in which external influences played an important etiological role, while manic-depressive illness was considered to be constitutionally determined.

Kraepelin included little discussion of premorbid personality, or what we would refer to as "psychodynamics." He noted that the condition apparently had some relation to the climacterium, but this was mentioned only in passing. Therapy was supportive, with emphasis on bed rest, nutrition, isolation from the family, and prevention of suicide.

As with many Kraepelinean syndromes, prognosis was an important part of the diagnosis. The poor prognosis and prolonged course were important diagnostic criteria. If the patient recovered, the diagnosis became doubtful and the patient might be considered to have been manic-depressive all along. Dreyfus,[13] a student of Kraepelin, took up this issue and in 1907 published an extensive follow-up of eighty-five of Kraepelin's cases diagnosed as melancholia at the Heidelberg Clinic since 1892. Dreyfus found a history of previous manic-depressive psychosis in 54 percent and a high eventual recovery rate of 66 percent (although sometimes after a course as long as ten years). He thus concluded, since the patients recovered and had had previous episodes of illness, that they were late manifestations of manic-depressive disease and that involutional melancholia was not a distinct entity.

Rather surprisingly, Kraepelin came to

agree with Dreyfus and between his seventh and eighth editions he changed his classification to include involutional depressions and involutional anxiety states in the category of manic-depressive psychosis. This change carried a good deal of weight in German psychiatry, but was not generally accepted in English-speaking countries. Most texts and classification systems, as noted above, still describe involutional melancholia as a separate illness some sixty years later.

Dreyfus' work was soon attacked by Kirby,[33] who felt that Dreyfus' conclusion that previous manic-depressive episodes had been present in these patients was based on very meager data in many cases. Many more scathing attacks followed, such as that by Hoch and MacCurdy,[23] who commented that "Dreyfus' zeal outran his judgment." They stated that while looking for evidence of manic-depressive psychosis, "He ferreted out a history of depressions so mild as to seem to be neurosis or merely more or less normal mood swings . . . they should not be called 'psychoses' . . . otherwise, nearly the whole world is, or has been, insane."

As during these years the term "melancholia" was used interchangeably with "involutional melancholia," it was probably patients in this group that Freud[18] described in 1917 in "Mourning and Melancholia." Freud made initial investigations into the psychodynamics of melancholia and emphasized unconscious processes.

The question of the relationship of prognosis to diagnosis was approached in a different way in the discussion of involutional melancholia by Hoch and McCurdy[23] in 1922. While Kraepelin had simply included deterioration as one of the criteria for the diagnosis of melancholia, these authors attempted to discover what specific clinical features could be used to predict whether or not the patient would deteriorate. They used the Kraepelinean reasoning of prognosis as an aid in diagnosis, but with an empirical twist. They retrospectively divided their involutional-age patients into recovered cases (who they felt were probably manic-depressives) and the unrecovered (who were felt to be melan-

cholics), and then they tried to find the clinical characteristics that had distinguished them. Poor prognostic signs (or signs of melancholia) were found to include severe hypochondriasis with delusions often related to the alimentary canal, and a restriction of interests and affect. The authors found that if no improvement occurred in four years, the patients would probably remain chronic.

Bleuler's[9] textbook in 1924 showed the confusion that existed even then about the diagnosis of melancholia. Bleuler obviously did not entirely agree with Kraepelin's decision to include melancholia under the diagnosis of manic-depressive disease: "It does not seem reasonable to bunch all the apparently independent depressions of the period of involution and class them with manic-depressive insanity." He defers, however, to Kraepelin and states that the original nosologic independence can no longer be sustained. He seems rather ambivalent, as he continues by saying, "But the reasons for the separation were, nevertheless, weighty." He then gives the distinguishing characteristics of melancholia as a more protracted course, with a slow onset and recession, retardation concealed by restlessness, frequent agitation, and usually single attacks. It is interesting that deterioration and chronicity, which were two of the cardinal points in Kraepelin's original formulation, were no longer considered criteria. Predisposing personality has not yet been mentioned.

In the late 1920s and early 1930s, a major issue of debate in the study of depression was the proposed distinction between reactive and autonomous or endogenous depressions. In 1929, Gillespie[19] made an important distinction between "reactive" and "autonomous" depressions. He included involutional depressions as a subgroup of autonomous depression in which hypochondriacal preoccupations were prominent and in which there was less depth of affect and a poor prognosis. It is of significance that he described the personalities of his four subjects as timid, quiet, unambitious, worrying, hypochondriacal, and overconscientious.

In their textbook of psychiatry, in 1932, Henderson and Gillespie[22] described involutional melancholia as a separate entity, as did other texts of the time, such as Noyes[47] and Strecker and Ebaugh.[64] Henderson and Gillespie's clinical description became a classic and was often quoted: "Depression without retardation, anxiety, a feeling of unreality, and hypochondriacal delusions."

As noted above, Lewis reviewed the literature on melancholia in an influential series of papers commencing in 1934. After extensively examining a large number of patients, he concluded that depressive syndromes could not be validly distinguished on clinical grounds, but rather formed a continuum. He pointed out that symptoms of agitation and hypochondriasis were found in younger age groups, as well as in involutional age patients.[39,40]

(Premorbid Personality

In the early writings, there was very little discussion of premorbid personality specifically related to involutional melancholia. Freud did not emphasize it but commented that a good, capable, conscientious woman was more likely to develop melancholia than one who is actually worthless, and he emphasized narcissistic object choice as a predisposing factor. Abraham emphasized obsessive-compulsive personalities before and between depressive attacks, but he was referring specifically to manic-depressive patients. Gillespie, as noted above, described the worrying, overconscientious personality, but on a basis of very few subjects.

In the 1930s, however, interest in premorbid personality was growing throughout psychiatry. This interest came from many sources, ranging from the analytic writings of Abraham and others to the work by Kretchmer attempting to relate character type and physique to psychiatric diagnostic groups.

Titley[68] was the first to make an extensive description of premorbid character in "involutional depression" (which was at that time replacing "involutional melancholia" as the name given to the syndrome). He compared ten involutional depressive (five men and five women) with ten manic-depressives and ten normals on twenty-two character traits, of which fifteen were found to discriminate between the groups. The character profile of involutional depressives was found to be markedly different from that of either the manic-depressives or the normals. It included rigid adherence to a high ethical code, a narrow range of interests, overmeticulousness and overconscientiousness, stubornness, anxiety, and poor sexual adjustment. Titley noted that Noyes had given the same description, based on clinical impressions, three years before in his textbook, and that the same character type was described by analytic authors as the anal-erotic personality.

There were some obvious flaws in Titley's study. The most glaring was that the average age of his involutional patients was fifty-six, while the average age of his manic-depressive patients was twenty-nine. It is hard to imagine that this did not account for some of the differences between these groups.

Palmer and Sherman,[48] compared fifty melancholics and fifty manic-depressives and confirmed the findings of a rigid premorbid character in melancholia. They emphasized obsessional traits, strong repression, sadomasochism, introverted personality, sexual maladjustment, and (citing the psychoanalytic contributions of Freud, Rado, and Abraham) they saw the obsessional character as a reaction formation against repressed anal tendencies with regression to oral-sadism and narcissism. They felt that involutional melancholia could be clearly differentiated from manic-depressive psychosis by personality, history of previous attacks, course, symptoms, and prognosis. They also emphasized the high incidence of paranoid trends in involutional melancholia.

Palmer and Sherman presented no data in any kind of tabular form to justify their conclusions, did no organized rating, and did no tests of any kind of statistical significance. It is also possible that the patients' self-perception of their previous personality may have been distorted by their illnesses.

The premorbid personality described above was printed in the textbooks of the 1940s with references back to these two studies. Since then, it has been widely accepted and is referred to in almost all psychiatric texts that discuss involutional depression. Although it is now usually presented without citing the above studies, it is still based on these two small studies constructed without blind techniques, with impressionistic ratings, and with little confirmation. One is hard-pressed to find any recent studies that confirm these findings with more sophisticated statistical techniques.

Relation of the Menopause and Climacterium to Involutional Depression

A distinction is made between the menopause, which refers to the cessation of menses, and the climacterium, which refers to the adaptational period lasting a number of years during which there are physiological, psychological, and social role changes. Thus, the distinction between menopause and climacterium is roughly equivalent to the distinction between menarche and adolescence.

In approximately 25 percent of women, following the menopause, decreasing estrogen deduction causes widespread atrophic changes.[46] The average age of onset of this physiologic menopause has gradually increased and it is currently in the late forties. Vasomotor, somatic, depressive, and anxiety symptoms often occur concomitantly. It is felt that the speed of the decrease in estrogen levels is responsible in part for the severity of the symptoms.[27] Approximately 25 to 30 percent of women have symptoms severe enough to have to go to a physician.[46,27] The relationship between menopause and more severe involutional depressions has long been a question of controversy. The discussion is centered on conceptions of estrogen deficiency as the primary etiology of involutional depressions and on estrogen as a specific treatment for these depressions.

In the 1920s, therapeutic enthusiasts reported excellent treatment results with whole ovary and corpus luteum extracts, which in later years were shown to have been inert.[7,45] In 1930, however, estrogens became available and the next ten years produced a new enthusiasm for the treatment of involutional depressions with estrogens. The initial reports were quite favorable and led Werner et al.[69,70] to conclude that "So-called involutional melancholia is only an extreme manifestation of the symptomatology of the menopause," and that estrogen was a specific treatment.

As so often happens, these glowing reports were followed by a contrasting series of studies reporting little or no improvement of involutional depressed patients when treated with estrogens.[45,51,72] Ripley et al.,[51] for example, found the only improvement to be the relief of vasomotor symptoms and an increased feeling of well-being. This was useful in mild reactive depressions, but caused no significant improvement in severe involutional depressions. Wittson[72] noted that in his series of 100 patients the psychosis was clearly related temporally to the menopause in less than 50 percent. In other patients, it came either before the menopause or more than five years after it. Novak,[45] a prominent gynecologist, reviewing the menopause, pointed out that many symptoms that were thought to arise from the menopause may come ten years before the cessation of menses. He asserted that the only symptoms that are definitely hormone-related are the vasomotor symptoms, which are objective and which respond to estrogen treatment.

Malamud et al.[42] reviewed the evidence and concluded that there was no foundation for considering involutional psychosis as primarily an estrogen deficiency, nor is there any proof that it can be treated successfully by gonadotropic agents. He felt that the menopause was an important factor, but not the cause of the condition. The depression was basically due to the stresses of involution on a personality with prominent features of rigidity, lack of plasticity, and restriction of interests. Bennett and Wilbur[6] showed the new impact of electroconvulsive therapy on the treatment of involutional depression. They reported on a series of seventy-five patients who had not responded to various doses of estrogen but who showed a high percentage of rapid recovery with ECT. The new emphasis on ECT, which was developing at this time, cast estrogen treatment further into the background.[6]

Thus, most investigators have accepted the conclusion that the hormonal change is not the physiologic cause of involutional depression, but only a contributing factor. The predominant current feeling is that only vasomotor symptoms react significantly to estrogen and, specifically, that major depressive symptoms are not improved.[52]

It should be noted that by present-day standards the studies investigating the use of estrogens in involutional melancholia were not adequately designed. The samples were small, there was little apparent attempt at achieving a nonbiased population, and there was no double blind. This was as true for the studies debunking estrogen therapy, as for those with enthusiastic positive results. For instance, one study, which was quoted over and over again as demonstrating the ineffectiveness of estrogens, achieved its results in a population of only ten patients, six women and four men![59] It is hard to see now how this could have been accepted at the time as disproving the effect of anything.

Another problem is that most of the studies reported patients who had been "psychotic" for one to nine years at the time of treatment. These chronic patients are certainly a different population from that which we are now primarily concerned with, and they might be more resistant to any treatment. Some of the questions raised with regard to estrogens might, therefore, warrant reinvestigation.

As noted above, about 25 percent of women have physical signs of estrogen deficiency at menopause with vasomotor symptoms, atrophy of vaginal mucosa, etc. It has never been clearly established whether those women who develop severe depressions come from this group primarily, or are scattered throughout the population.

In recent years, findings that estrogen deficiency may cause an increase in symptoms of arteriosclerosis and osteoporosis, in addition to the vasomotor symptoms, have caused a num-

ber of gynecologists to consider the endocrinologic involution to be a pathologic state of estrogen deficiency, rather than a physiologic one.[20,34] Some investigators feel that nearly all post-menopausal women should have estrogen replacement. Continued estrogen maintenance could prevent a cessation of menses and decrease physical atrophic changes. Thus, while estrogens are not commonly used to treat already formed depressive syndromes, replacement therapy might be a different question. Whether the subsequent maintenance of physical self-image would act to decrease the incidence of milder depressions in the involutional years has not been definitively tested in a large population.

There is a second question that would be useful to consider. If one considers, as many people do, that the full involutional psychotic depressions are either late-onset manic-depressive illnesses, or late-onset unipolar depressions, studies demonstrating that estrogens are not an effective treatment for these severe depressions are really irrelevant. Few people would expect them to be an effective treatment. The issue is not whether estrogens are effective treatment for psychotic depressions of whatever etiology, or whether lack of estrogens are the cause of the depression, but rather, would estrogens help the far more common mild or early depressions of the climacterium, which are often associated with vasomotor symptoms and changes in the patient's psychosocial situation.

(Psychopharmacology

While in the past ten years there has been a great deal of interest in the role of catecholamines, serotonin, and steroid metabolism in the etiology and development of depression, there has been little effort to investigate involutional depression specifically from this point of view. The major reviews of the role of catecholamines and indolamines in depression usually do not even mention involutional depression as a separate entity. Similarly, studies of corticosteroid function and depression ignore the question of involutional depression as a separate entity.

⟮ Genetics

The role of heredity has always been felt to be less prominent in involutional depression than in schizophrenia or manic-depressive illness. Kraepelin noted that defective heredity occurred in only a little more than half of his cases, but that relatives of melancholics often suffered from apoplexy, senile dementia, or alcoholism.

Two early modern researchers in the 1940s and 1950s, Kallmann[28,29,30] and Stenstedt,[63] took opposing points of view. In his early studies, Kallmann found a relatively high incidence of schizophrenics in families of involutional psychotics, and found no relationship to manic-depressive illness. He concluded that involutional psychosis is pluridimensional and partly nonspecific with multiple factors of causation. He felt that while there is no single-factor genetic mechanism, the people most likely to break down under the emotional impact of involutional stresses were those with schizoid personalities (under which he included the traits of rigidity, compulsiveness, and oversensitivity). These he considered heterozygous carriers of schizophrenia, which he felt explained the higher incidence of schizophrenia in their families.

Stenstedt, on the other hand, in a large genetic study from Swedish hospitals, made an effort to exclude paranoids and schizophrenics from his probands (and criticized Kallmann for including paranoid cases). Stenstedt found relatives of his probands with involutional melancholia, manic-depressive illness, and endogenous depression, but found no relationship to schizophrenia. He found that the risk of all affective disorders in the relatives of his patients was about twice that of the general population. He concluded that his probands were etiologically heterogeneous and that involutional depression probably consisted of some cases of late manic-depressive illness and others of exogenous or reactive depression.

Hopkinson[24] studied 100 patients aged over fifty who were admitted depressed. He divided them into "early onset" (those who had had previous attacks before they were fifty) and "late onset" (whose first depressive episode was past fifty). He found little difference in the symptomatology between early-onset and late-onset patients although, perhaps somewhat surprisingly, he found less agitation in late-onset patients. When examining the relatives of his patient population he found that late-onset patients had fewer relatives with a history of depression than had early-onset patients. The age of onset of depression, however, for affected relatives of late-onset patients were the same as the age of onset for relatives of early-onset patients. That is to say, the type of depressive illnesses of the relatives of late-onset patients was the same as of relatives of early-onset patients, and the depressive illnesses of the relatives of late-onset patients were not of late onset themselves. He concluded, as had Stenstedt before him, that his population was heterogeneous and nonspecific. He also agreed with Stenstedt in finding no increase in schizophrenia in the relatives of his patients.

Hopkinson and Ley[25] reported on 182 patients of all ages. They found that there was a marked drop in the number of affected relatives for patients whose age of onset was more than thirty-nine. They concluded that late-onset patients may be different nosologically with fewer recurrences, less mania, and less family history; although their final common pathway clinically was the same with similar depressive symptoms.

Most other modern genetics studies use a distinction between bipolar affective disorder (in which the patients have had episodes of mania as well as depression), and unipolar depression in which there have been no episodes of mania.[60] (Involutional melancholia is thus considered as late-onset unipolar depression.) The unipolar-bipolar distinction was introduced by Leonhard in 1959,[38] and expanded in a monograph by Perris.[49] Perris found that affected relatives of patients with bipolar depressions were mainly bipolar, and vice-versa.

Angst,[1] in a major monograph, concluded that cycloid (bipolar) and monophasic (unipolar) syndromes were genetically distinct. He felt that there was a major autosomogene in the bipolar depressions and a multifactorial etiology in the unipolar depressions.

Winokur et al.[71] reported a study comparing early-onset unipolar depressions with late-onset unipolar depressions. He confirmed Hopkinson's results, finding that there were more relatives of early-onset patients affected than of late-onset patients, and especially more female relatives. Woodruff et al.[73] also used the distinction between unipolar and bipolar depressions. He confirmed that late-onset unipolar patients had less family history of psychiatric hospitalizations, suicide attempts, and family alcoholism.

Thus, from the genetic point of view, involutional depression is now considered as late-onset unipolar depression with fewer affected relatives than early-onset depression or bipolar depression, but with no relationship to schizophrenia. It is usually not considered a genetically distinct illness.

(Psychological Aspects of Depressions of the Involutional Years

In "Mourning and Melancholia," Freud[18] discussed a small number of cases of melancholia with "indisputable" psychogenic etiology and warned against assuming general validity for his findings. Nonetheless, the conclusions of his paper are widely held to represent the psychodynamics of depression in general. Freud emphasized the similarity of melancholia to mourning, with the addition of a marked tendency to self-reproach and a fall in self-esteem. He noted that in grief the world becomes empty, while in melancholia it is the ego which becomes empty. He also found an inability, in some cases, to discover what object has been lost and concluded that in these cases there has been an unconscious loss.

Freud concluded that part of the disposition to succumb to melancholia comes from a narcissistic object choice, which regresses to narcissism. This entails the introjection of an ambivalently held object; the self-reproaches are directed at this introjected part of the ego. Thus, the reproaches fit someone "whom the patient loves, has loved, or ought to love." He also noted the sadistic aspects of the self-punishment as the patient torments the original love object with the illness, while avoiding the direct expression of hostility.

Although Freud was not pessimistic, psychoanalytic writers were reluctant to treat involutional psychotics, both because of their age and because of the psychotic nature of their illness. This neglect by psychoanalysis meant that the psychodynamics of the involutional period received little attention. Fenichel's[15] encyclopedic monograph of psychoanalytic theory devoted only one short paragraph to involutional melancholia and acknowledged: "Psychoanalytically, not much is known about the structure and mechanisms of involutional melancholias." However, he described the mechanism of melancholia as the failure of a rigid, compulsive defensive system with oral regression.

By the 1940s, there was a new interest in the meaning of involution to the patient and especially to women. This included speculation about the possible relationship of the psychological aspects of involution to the etiology of involutional psychosis.

Deutsch,[10] in her classic study of the psychology of women, emphasized that dealing with the organic decline was one of the most difficult tasks of a woman's life. Old oedipal relationships and problems, worked out a second time in puberty, are faced a third time in the climacterium. The symptoms seen in puberty in any given patient may thus be similar to those seen in the climacterium, and a stormy puberty may warn of a stormy involution.

Benedek[5] emphasized the climacterium in women as a developmental period in the sense that it is a period of intrapersonal reorganization. She also noted the similarity of the climacterium to puberty and the menarche, and the repetition of problems faced in assuming the female identity. She felt that, if handled in a healthy way, the decrease in hormonal action and desexualization of emotional needs may release psychic energy for sublimation and further integration of the personality.

Fessler[16] emphasized a premorbid hysterical character in women with involutional "nonendogenous" depressions. She theorized that to a woman the ability to have a child is her compensation for not having a penis. Menstruation is the constant reminder of this and is thus a penis substitute and implies female completeness. The cessation of menses therefore may cause regression and penis envy.

Szalita[65] related involutional depressions to an oral fixation and stated rather unequivocably that persons who develop involutional disorders can be assumed to have been crippled by a period of oral deprivation at an early age.

The dynamics of depression have been reevaluated in recent years from an ego-psychological point of view. Some of these re-evaluations are quite applicable to involutional depressions. Bibring[7] felt that depression occurs when "A blow is dealt to the person's self-esteem, on whatever grounds such self-esteem may have been founded." It thus represents "the emotional expression of a state of helplessness and powerlessness of the ego." It occurs in situations beyond the power of the ego, when narcissistically important goals seem beyond reach. Thus, using Bibring's formulation, it can be seen that in patients to whom the involutional years represent a loss of self-esteem, change in body image, and possible loss of narcissistically held objects, due either to organic decline or to change in social roles, a depression may be the natural response.

Bemporad[4] emphasizes that guilt is no longer seen as often in depressions as it used to be described, and that this may relate to social changes. He feels that the entire concept of introjection in depression is in need of clarification.

It would appear that depression is brought about by a sense of helplessness to alter oneself or one's environment, together with a future devoid of meaning and gratification . . . depression has been considered here as an affective reaction, elicited by the individual's realization that an important source of self-esteem and meaning is lost . . . whereas, for some the relationship with the environmental object is crucial, for others a specific cause, social position, or definite self-image may be important.

Both Bemporad and Bibring emphasized the loss of self-esteem and disappointment at the real and prospective nonattainment of goals. Thus, they seem quite applicable to the prospects and disappointment of the involutional years.

Modern textbooks emphasize more sociocultural aspects of the involutional period for women. McCandless[41] refers to anthropologic studies showing major shifts in identity, social role, and role expectations at the time of climacterium that are seen in many cultures. Our own society places great cultural emphasis on youth, attractiveness, and sexuality. At the same time, it has placed a strong positive evaluation on the role of motherhood. Both of these areas of woman's identification and self-esteem suffer losses at the time of the menopause. At menopause, the woman may feel that she is losing her youth and sexual attractiveness. Aging is seen as imminent, and a preoccupation with death may occur. Atrophic changes throughout the body are felt as a loss not only of sexual desirability, but of femininity as well, and a woman may feel that she has lost a part of herself.

The role of motherhood is lost in a double sense: The child-bearing capacity is lost on the one hand, and the growing children are leaving home on the other.[11] Even if the woman had long ago decided against having more children, the menopause signals the irrevocability of the decision, a sign that the opportunity has passed. For the unmarried woman or the childless woman, the menopause may imply a recognition of nonfulfillment of hopes for marriage, child-bearing, and family.

It has been noted that involutional depressions are seen in women in their middle and late forties and early fifties, while in men they are not seen until the decade later. In the past, this has been because at an age when the woman was losing her cultural role most men were just moving into their peak years of economic role accomplishment, with years ahead before retirement. In recent years, however, there has been a shift in emphasis in the role of women, with less emphasis on motherhood and homemaking and more emphasis on fulfillment through other channels, including economic and other forms of creativity. The effects of such a shift will probably be gradual, but should be interesting to observe.

At any rate, there are major similarities for both men and women in some of the effects of the involutional years. These years represent an inevitable awareness of the nonachievement of some of life's cherished goals. They may also be a time of loneliness. Children are leaving home. Ties with friends of adolescence and early adulthood are loosening. Friends may be dying, with the inevitable reminder that the person himself is aging. These are also years of practical difficulties, of increasing physical disease and disability, and possibly of unemployment or forced retirement.

(Symptomatology

Recent studies of the symptomatology of depression in general have not borne out a clear-cut clinical distinction between the depressions of involutional years and those of earlier years.

Tait and associates[66] studied fifty-four women in the involutional age group who were first-admission psychiatric patients. The authors used a free interview technique without rating scales. After excluding hysterics, anxiety states, alcoholics, and late schizophrenics, they were left with only twenty-nine patients whom they considered as having "endogenous depressive psychotic illnesses." They noted that "These depressions did not seem markedly distinct, symptomatically, from psychotic depressions appearing at other ages," and that "the typical features of traditional or developed involutional melancholia were remarkable in this material only for their almost complete absence." Bizarre hypochondriasis, nihilistic delusions, and great agitation were confined to a handful of cases. The authors suggested the interesting thought that perhaps these are secondary symptoms which in the past have developed with chronicity, but now are aborted by early therapy.

Kendall's[31] study showed that patients with a diagnosis of involutional melancholia have the same symptoms and the same outcome with treatment as do psychotic depressive patients, but differed from neurotic depressives. He concluded that involutional depression differs in no fundamental way from other psychotic depressions.

More recently, a series of studies[21,32,54-57] attempted to use the correlational device of factor analysis to find subsyndromes in depression. These studies have freely included depressed patients of the involutional age range. Factor analytic studies in general terms rate depressed patients on symptom rating scales and attempt to group together those symptoms that are co-variant and those that tend to be present or absent together. These studies have all been remarkable by the absence of any pattern that clearly represented an agitated involutional depression.

Failure of these correlational techniques to demonstrate the classical involutional pattern is not conclusive evidence that it does not exist, but that in the depressive population studied it is not common enough to be demonstrated by these methods.

(Conclusion

We are thus left with involutional melancholia as a clinical psychiatric illness cited by the textbooks and the classification systems, and with a fairly well-defined symptom pattern, premorbid personality, onset, course, prognosis, and response to therapy. The puzzle is, however, whether it really exists as a clinical entity. As Tait[66] stated, ". . . while most of us still carry in our minds the Gestalt of a classical involutional melancholia, we may confess that such pictures are increasingly rare, or alternatively are swamped by the larger mass of mild depressions of the involution which therapy has given us the encouragement to discover." Thus, we all know a classical case of involutional melancholia when we see one, but it is not clear whether this is a distinct syndrome with its own ideology, natural history, and clinical picture, or whether it is a severe depression of the involutional years which shades off continuously with mildly menopausal neuroses on a vertical severity axis, and with other psychotic depressions on a horizontal descriptive axis.

The old debate as to whether involutional melancholia is a subtype of manic-depressive disease seems fairly irrelevant today. Involutional melancholia is probably best thought of in the terms introduced by psychiatric genetics, as a late-onset unipolar depression, which in practice is not clinically distinguishable from other unipolar depressions.

A more relevant question is the relationship between the classical involutional melancholia syndrome and the multitudinous mild depressions and mixed depression and anxiety states of the climacterium. Part of the problem is dilution. As recently as twenty years ago, psychiatric hospitals were populated primarily by psychotic and organic patients. Patients described as involutional melancholics made up a small but appreciable percentage of these patients. Studies dealing with involutional melancholics primarily dealt with these hospitalized patients. In recent years, with the reorientation of psychiatric practice and facilities, and with the change in public attitudes towards mental hospitalization, there has been a flood of youthful patients with nonpsychotic, voluntary hospitalizations.[53]

As a second consideration, the symptoms of involutional melancholia may have been secondary symptoms, or the accretions of chronicity. In the past, patients waited longer before coming for psychiatric care, remained a longer time, became more psychotic, and developed a full flowering of symptoms. Now, they may be treated earlier by their family physician, psychiatrist, or outpatient clinic, with antidepressant medications, or ECT. The onset of the old involutional melancholia syndrome was noted as being gradual, and if seen early in the course the patients probably would be diagnosed as depressive neurotics. It is probably that the syndrome is now aborted at this stage in most patients.

Most of the studies done in the past, whether from a point of view of the effect of estrogens, clinical symptomatology, or course of the illness, dealt with those patients who had progressed to major psychotic depressions. Thus, the results of these studies may have very little to do with the large number of mild depressions that develop under the psychological and social stresses of the climacterium. Under these stresses, it is probable that depressive illness may emerge in many different kinds of patients and in varying degrees of severity. These might include patients with obsessive, hypochondriacal, and hysterical life patterns, those with depressive reactions to loss, and others with possible first or recurrent episodes of manic-depressive illness. The full-fledged involutional depression may have represented the untreated course of only a small part of the minor depressive illness seen during the climacterium. It may have represented a variant of the basic "endogenous" depressive pattern, and whatever specific symptomatology was present was possibly shaped by factors of age and cultural setting.

It is now the predominant opinion that involutional depression probably does not represent a specific syndrome. It is clear, however, that the whole subject of depressions in the involutional years has become a relatively stagnant subject with little research work being done. As patients with mild or moderate depressive illness during this period make up a fairly large population, further studies of this area would be warranted.

(Bibliography

1. ANGST, J. Zur Aetiologie und Nosologie Endogener Depressiver Psychosen. Berlin: Springer, 1966.

2. BATCHELOR, I. R. C. Henderson and Gillespie's Textbook of Psychiatry, 10th Ed. New York: Oxford University Press, 1969.

3. BECK, A. T. "Involutional Psychotic Reaction," in *Depression*. New York: Harper & Row, 1967.

4. BEMPORAD, J. R. "New Views on the Psychodynamics of the Depressive Character," in S. Arieti, ed., *The World Biennial of Psychiatry and Psychotherapy*. New York: Basic Books, 1970.

5. BENEDEK, T. "Climacterium: A Developmental Phase," *Psychoanalytic Quarterly*, 19 (1950), 1–27.

6. BENNETT, A. E., and C. B. WILBUR. "Convulsive Shock Therapy in Involutional States After Complete Failure with Previous Estrogenic Treatment," *American Journal of Medical Science*, 208 (1944), 170–176.

7. BIBRING, E. "The Mechanism of Depression," in P. Greenacre, ed., *Affective Disorders*. New York: International Universities Press, 1953.

8. BIGELOW, N. "The Involutional Psychoses," in S. Arieti, ed., *American Handbook of Psychiatry*, Vol. 1. New York: Basic Books, 1959.

9. BLEULER, E. P. *Textbook of Psychiatry*, A. A. Brill, transl. New York: Macmillan Co., 1924.

10. DEUTSCH, H. *The Psychology of Women*, Vol. 2. New York: Grune & Stratton, 1945.

11. DEYNIN, E. V., S. JACOBSON, G. KLERMANN, and M. SOLOMON. " 'The Empty Nest'—Psychosocial Aspects of Conflict Between Depressed Women and Their Grown Children," *The American Journal of Psychiatry*, 122 (1966), 1422–1426.

12. *Diagnostic and Statistical Manual of Mental Disorders*, 2nd Ed. Washington: American Psychiatric Association, 1968.

13. DREYFUS, G. L. *Die Melancholia*. Jena: Fischer, 1907.

14. ENGLISH, O. S., and S. M. FINCH. *Introduction to Psychiatry*, 3rd ed. New York: W. W. Norton & Co., 1964.

15. FENICHEL, O. *The Psychoanalytic Theory of Neurosis*. New York: W. W. Norton & Co., 1945.

16. FESSLER, L. "The Psychopathology of Climacteric Depression," *Psychoanalytic Quarterly*, 19 (1950), 28–42.

17. FORD, H. "Involutional Psychotic Reaction," in A. M. Freedman, and H. I. Kaplan, eds., *Comprehensive Textbook of Psychiatry*. Baltimore: Williams & Wilkins, 1967.

18. FREUD, S. "Mourning and Melancholia" (1917), in *Collected Papers*, Vol. 4. London: Hogarth Press, 1953.

19. GILLESPIE, R. D. "The Clinical Differentiation of Types of Depression," *Guy Hospital Reports*, 79 (1929), 306–344.

20. GREENBLATT, R. B. "Current Concepts: Estrogen Therapy for Post-menopausal Females," *New England Journal of Medicine*, 272 (1965), 305–308.

21. HAMILTON, M. "A Rating Scale for Depressions," *Journal of Neurology and Neurosurgical Psychiatry*, 23 (1960), 56–62.

22. HENDERSON, D. K., and R. D. GILLESPIE. *A Textbook of Psychiatry for Students and Practitioners*, 3rd ed. New York: Oxford University Press, 1932.

23. HOCH, A., and J. T. MacCURDY. "The Prognosis of Involutional Melancholia," *Archives of Neurology and Psychiatry*, 7 (1922), 1–17.

24. HOPKINSON, G. "A Genetic Study of Affective Illness in Patients Over 50," *British Journal of Psychiatry*, 110 (1964), 244–254.

25. HOPKINSON, G., and P. LEY. "A Genetic Study of Affective Disorders," *British Journal of Psychiatry*, 115 (1969), 917–22.

26. HUSTON, P. E., and L. M. LOCKER. "Involutional Psychosis," *Archives of Neurology and Psychiatry*, 59 (1948), 385–94.

27. ISRAEL, S. L. *Menstrual Disorders and Sterility*, 5th ed. New York: Harper & Row, 1967.

28. KALLMANN, F. J. *Heredity in Health and Mental Disorder*. New York: W. W. Norton & Co., 1953.

29. ———. "Genetic Aspects of Mental Disorders in Later Life," in O. J. Kaplan, ed., *Mental Disorders in Later Life*, 2nd ed. Stanford: Stanford University Press, 1956.

30. ———. "The Genetics of Mental Illness," in S. Arieti, ed., *American Handbook of Psychiatry*, Vol. I. New York: Basic Books, 1959.

31. KENDALL, R. E. "The Problem of Classification," in A. Coppen, and A. Welk, eds., *Recent Developments in Affective Disorders*. Ashford, Kent: Headly Bros. Ltd., 1968.

32. KILOH, L. G., and R. F. GARSIDE. "The Independence of Neurotic Depression and Endogenous Depression," *British Journal of Psychiatry*, 109 (1963), 451–463.

33. KIRBY, G. H. Cited in Titley, W. B., Ref. 68.

34. KISTNER, R. W. *Gynecology*. Chicago: Year Book Medical Publishers, 1969.

35. KOLB, L. C. *Noyes' Modern Clinical Psychiatry*, 7th ed. Philadelphia: W. B. Saunders Co. 1968.

36. KRAEPELIN, E. *Clinical Psychiatry*, A. R. Diefendorf, transl. New York: Macmillan Co., 1907.

37. LEHMANN, H. E. Psychiatric Concepts of Depression: Nomenclature and Classification," *Canadian Psychiatric Association Journal*, 4 (Suppl.) (1959), 1–12.

38. LEONHARD, K. *Aufteilung der endogenen Psychosen*. Berlin: Akademie Verlag, 1959.

39. LEWIS, A. J. "Melancholia: A Historical Review," *Journal of Mental Science*, 80 (1934), 1–42.

40. ———. "Melancholia: A Clinical Survey of Depressive States," *Journal of Mental Science*, 80 (1934), 277–378.

41. McCANDLESS, F. D. "Emotional Problems of the Climacteric," *Clinical Obstetrics and Gynecology*, 7 (1964), 489–503.

42. MALAMUD, W., S. L. SANDS, and I. MALAMUD. "The Involutional Psychoses: A Socio-Psychiatric Study," *Psychosomatic Medicine*, 3 (1941), 410–426.

43. MENDELS, J. *Concepts of Depression*. New York: John Wiley & Sons, 1970.

44. NOTKIN, J., B. DENNIS, and V. HUDDART. "Folliculin Menformon (Theelin) Treatment of Involutional Melancholia," *Psychiatry Quarterly*, 14 (1940), 157–166.

45. NOVAK, E. "The Management of the Menopause," *American Journal of Obstetrics and Gynecology*, 40 (1940), 589–595.

46. NOVAK, E. R., et al. *Novak's Textbook of Gynecology*, 8th ed. Baltimore: Williams & Wilkins, 1970.

47. NOYES, A. P. *Modern Clinical Psychiatry*. Philadelphia: W. B. Saunders Co., 1934.

48. PALMER, H. D., and S. H. SHERMAN. "The Involutional Melancholia Process," *Archives of Neurology and Psychiatry*, 40 (1938), 762–788.

49. PERRIS, C. "A Study of Bipolar (Manic-Depressive) and Unipolar (Recurrent Depressive) Psychoses," *Acta Psychiatrica Scandinavica*, Suppl. 194, 1966.

50. REDLICH, F. C., and D. X. FRIEDMAN. *The Theory and Practice of Psychiatry*. New York: Basic Books, 1966.

51. RIPLEY, H. S., E. SHORR, and G. N. PAPANILOLAOU. "The Effect of Treatment of Depression in the Menopause with Estrogenic Hormone," *The American Journal of Psychiatry*, 96 (1940), 905–911.

52. ROGERS, J.: "The Menopause," *New England Journal of Medicine*, 254 (1956), 697–703, 750–756.

53. ROSENTHAL, S. H. "Changes in a Population of Hospitalized Patients with Affective Disorders," *The American Journal of Psychiatry*, 123 (1966), 671–681.

54. ROSENTHAL, S. H., and J. E. GUDEMAN. "The Endogenous Depressive Pattern: An Empirical Investigation," *Archives of General Psychiatry*, 16 (1967), 241–249.

55. ———. "The Self-Pitying Constellation in Depression," *British Journal of Psychiatry*, 113 (1967), 485–489.

56. ROSENTHAL, S. H., and G. L. KLERMANN. "Content and Consistency in the Endogenous Depressive Pattern," *British Journal of Psychiatry*, 112 (1966), 471–484.

57. ———. "Endogenous Features of Depression in Women," *Canadian Psychiatric Association Journal*, 11 (Suppl.) (1966), 11–16.

58. ROTH, M. "The Phenomenology of Depressive States," *Canadian Psychiatric Association Journal*, 4 (Suppl.) (1959), 32–54.

59. SCHUBE, P. G., M. D. McMANAMY, C. E. TRAPP, and G. F. HOUSER. "Involutional Melancholia: Treatment with Theelin," *Archives of Neurology and Psychiatry*, 38 (1937), 505–512.

60. SLATER, E., and V. COWIE. *The Genetics of Mental Disorders*. London: Oxford University Press, 1971.

61. SLATER, E., and M. ROTH. *"Mayer Gross Clinical Psychiatry"*. Baltimore: Williams & Wilkins, 1969.

62. STENBACK, A. "On Involutional and Middle-Age Depressions," *Acta Psychiatrica Scandinavica*, 169 (1963), 14–32.

63. STENSTEDT, A. "Involutional Melancholia," *Acta Psychiatrica et Neurologica Scandinavica*, 127 (1959), 1–79.

64. STRECKER, E. A., and F. G. EBAUGH. *Clinical Psychiatry*, 4th ed. Philadelphia: P. Blakiston & Son, 1935.

65. SZALITA, A. B. "Psychodynamics of Disorders of the Involutional Age," in S. Arieti, ed., *American Handbook of Psychiatry*, Vol. 3. New York: Basic Books, 1966.

66. TAIT, A. C., J. HARPER, and W. T. McCLATCHEY. "Initial Psychiatric Illness in

Involutional Women. I. Clinical Aspects," *Journal of Mental Science*, 103 (1957), 132–145.

67. TAIT, C. S., and G. C. BURNS. "Involutional Illnesses," *The American Journal of Psychiatry.* 108 (1951), 27–36.

68. TITLEY, W. B. "Prepsychotic Personality of Involutional Melancholia," *Archives of Neurology and Psychiatry*, 36 (1936), 19–33.

69. WERNER, A. A., G. A. JOHNS, E. F. HOCTOR, C. C. AULT, L. H. KOHLER, and M. W. WEIS, "Involutional Melancholia: Probable Etiology and Treatment," *Journal of the AMA*, 103 (1934), 13–16.

70. WERNER, A. A., L. H. KOHLER, C. C. AULT, and E. F. HOCTOR. "Involutional Melancholia: Probable Etiology and Treatment," *Archives of Neurology and Psychiatry*, 35 (1936), 1076–1080.

71. WINOKUR, G. et al. "Depressive Disease: A Genetic Study," *Archives of General Psychiatry*, 24 (1971), 135–144.

72. WITTSON, C. L. "Involutional Melancholia," *Psychiatric Quarterly*, 14 (1940), 167–184.

73. WOODRUFF, B. A., et al. "Unipolar and Bipolar Primary Affective Disorder," *British Journal of Psychiatry*, 119 (1971), 33–38.

CHAPTER 31

RARE, UNCLASSIFIABLE AND COLLECTIVE PSYCHIATRIC SYNDROMES

Silvano Arieti and Jules R. Bemporad

IN THE FIRST EDITION of the Handbook, hesitation was expressed over including a chapter on rare, unclassifiable, collective, and exotic* psychotic syndromes. Time has shown that the inclusion of such material was beneficial to the student and researcher, as well as the practitioner, of psychiatry in that the stated chapter has frequently been cited in the subsequent literature. While single case reports of these syndromes are occasionally reported in various journals, there appears to be a continuing need for a description of these disorders, as well as a review of the pertinent literature that is readily accessible. As stated previously, another reason for including these rare syndromes is that they pose interesting problems in terms of theory and it is hoped that by presenting them here, it may be possible to stimulate further work that may be applicable to other areas of psychiatry. The

* See Chapter 32 for exotic psychiatric syndromes.

majority of these syndromes are of especial interest in that although they are not psychoses in the usual sense, peculiar distortions of reality are manifested, as well as a rigidity of the symptomatology that is reminiscent of psychotic disorders.

⟨ Rare and Unclassifiable Syndromes

Ganser's Syndrome

The essence of this disorder consists of the patient giving approximate or inexact answers to the simplest questions imaginable. The answers are not totally random but bear some relationship to the question asked; they are slightly off the mark. Although Moeli[43] first described the symptom of *vorbeireden*, or "talking past the point" (i.e., giving slightly incorrect responses) in 1888,[2] Ganser[26] fully described the syndrome ten years later.* Ganser specified four major features of this syndrome: (1) the giving of approximate answers, (2) a clouding of consciousness, (3) somatic or conversion symptoms, and (4) hallucinations. While all features are occasionally found, the first symptom is considered essential to the Ganser syndrome. It may be of interest that this syndrome has been more frequently reported in the European than the American literature.

Although relatively rare, the Ganser syndrome is interesting from psychopathological and legal points of view. It is generally encountered in prisoners who have to face trial but also, occasionally, in patients in the general population who have to face unpleasant conditions. Jolly[33] reported that one third of his cases were noncriminal civilians. Of the six cases reported by Weiner and Braiman,[59] only one was a prisoner. Dogliani[22] reported one case occurring after a relatively minor automobile accident. It has also been reported as not infrequent among Negro soldiers in Africa.[13]

One finds in the Ganser syndrome a more or less acute loss of the capacity to reason normally. Many cases present total or partial amnesia. The patient is disoriented as to time and space and gives absurd answers to questions. Often, he claims he does not know who he is, where he comes from, or where he is. When he is asked to do simple calculations, he makes obvious mistakes—for instance, giving 5 as the sum of 2 plus 2. When he is asked to identify objects, he gives the name of a related object. Upon being shown scissors, the patient may say that they are knives; a picture of a dog may be identified as a cat, a yellow object may be called red, and so on. If he is asked what a hammer is used for, he may reply, to cut wood. If he is shown a dime, he may state that it is a half dollar, and so on. If he is asked how many legs a horse has, he may reply, six.

---

* Older psychiatric works, such as Bucknill and Tuke's textbook published in 1862, also report cases where patients under stress gave nonsensical yet approximate answers when interviewed. See Enoch et al.[23] for a review of the early literature.

At times, almost a game seems to go on between the examiner and the patient. The examiner asks questions that are almost silly in their simplicity, but the patient succeeds in giving a sillier answer. And yet, it seems that the patient understands the question, because the answer, although wrong, is related to the question. Often, if pressed, the patient will begin to answer, "I don't know," until he refuses to answer at all, lapsing into a state of lethargy or stupor.

Of the other features mentioned by Ganser, conversion reactions are occasionally seen, but headache is the most frequent somatic complaint. Hallucinations, when present, may often be of a fantastic nature such as those reported by a patient cited by MacDonald.[39] This individual claimed he saw red horses, partially dressed in human clothing, sitting atop lamp posts. In their review of the syndrome, Ingraham and Moriarity[31] specified visual hallucinations, as well as clouding of consciousness, disorientation of time and space, amnesia, and lack of insight, as prominent features of the Ganser's syndrome.

DIAGNOSIS

Ganser's syndrome may be confused with voluntary malingering in prisoners who want to escape indictment. In some cases, the diagnosis is difficult. The malingerer will at times lose the air of bewilderment and confusion when he is not watched, whereas the Ganserian patient remains in that state all the time. The malingerer is watchful, suspicious, and (although he appears indifferent) ill-at-ease all the time, being conscious of the unreality of his symptoms.

The syndrome can also be confused with schizophrenia. The answers of the Ganserian patient are reminiscent of those given by schizophrenics, the productions Cameron calls "metonymic distortions." The answers given by the Ganserian seem even sillier, however, almost as if a voluntary effort had been made to say something ridiculously inappropriate. Even the most deteriorated schizophrenic will not lose his memory for simple everyday behavior, such as how to unlock a door or how to use eating utensils. Also, unlike schizophrenics, some of the patients with Ganser syndrome recover in a few days if withdrawn from stress, although recurrences are common.

A third misdiagnosis easily made is one of mental deficiency or organic conditions. But a mental deficiency of a degree that would explain such absurd answers would have been known prior to the onset of the disorder. Similarly, an organic condition that might lead to these symptoms would have to be at a very advanced stage; again, there would be no difficulty in making the diagnosis.

INTERPRETATION

Is the Ganser syndrome a psychosis? Ganser himself, Kraepelin, Bumke,[7] Henderson and Gillespie,[30] and MacDonald,[39] felt that it is a psychoneurosis, similar to what Wernicke called "hysterical pseudodementia," and should be included in the group of hysterias. The conversion syndrome would consist in the patient's acting as if he had lost his rationality. The secondary gain, of course, would be the avoidance of the indictment or whatever unpleasant situation he has to face.

Other authors felt, instead, that the condition is a psychotic one (Moeli,[43] Weiner and Braiman,[59] Dogliani,[22] Whitlock[61]). We must say that the syndrome indeed presents a psychotic flavor not usually found in psychoneuroses. The psychodynamic mechanism also seems surprisingly simple: It is obvious that the patient wants to avoid the unpleasant situation and the burden of responsibility. Perhaps, as Weiner and Braiman state, he wants to do more than that. By unconsciously selecting symptoms which make him lose his rationality and often forget his personal identity and his past, he wants to reject his whole self, his whole life history—a denial of his total self. While many reported cases have demonstrated accompanying psychotic symptoms, other patients have shown this syndrome in "pure form," without psychotic contamination, leading to the opinion that the Ganser syndrome may be encountered in a number of psychopathological states.

We encounter difficulties when we try to explain the symptoms from a formal point of view. The answers of the patient are related to the questions, although inappropriately, and are reminiscent of the metonymic distortions of the schizophrenic, and in particular of the negativistic answers of some catatonics. The similarity is, however, only apparent. The Ganserian seems almost to make an effort to give a silly answer; a catatonic would not say that a horse has six legs.

Many authors have reported that this condition occurs mostly among people who, although not mentally defective, were at least dull adults of borderline intelligence, or high-level morons. It has never occurred in a person who was of superior intelligence prior to the disorder. This fact suggests the possibility that the low mentality of these people had made them aware of one thing: that at times in life it was convenient not to be smart. The mental defect, although not present, was within grasp or could be exaggerated.

Capgras' Syndrome

Capgras' syndrome is a condition that has received considerable attention in the European literature, especially the French and Italian. In the American literature, Davidson,[20] Stern and MacNaughton,[54] and Todd[55] have published articles on the subject. Recently three cases have been reported in the Australian literature.[5,28,42]

In 1923, the French psychiatrist Capgras, in collaboration first with Reboul-Lachaux and later with several others, started a series of articles on what he called "L'illusion des sosies."[8,9,10] Sosie means "double," a person who looks exactly like another one, just as an identical twin would resemble the other twin.

The phenomenon (or syndrome) described by Capgras is the following: The patient will claim, on meeting someone he knows well, that the person is a double or an impostor who has assumed this person's appearance. For example, the mother of a female patient comes to visit the patient at the hospital. The patient claims that this visitor is not her mother, but either a double or an impostor who has tried to assume the appearance of the mother in order to deceive the patient. This phenemenon is thus a complicated type of misidentification, much more characteristic and specific than the usual misidentification occurring in schizophrenia.

Although the first publications reported cases of female patients only, a few cases among males have recently been described.

Is this condition, described by Capgras, a special syndrome, or just a symptom occurring in one of the well-known clinical entities? The problem is controversial. Generally, French authors tend to give Capgras' syndrome a special place in psychiatric nosology, whereas German authors tend to see it as a symptom. From the cases reported in the literature, however, it is obvious that, although the patients presented other symptoms, this particular delusion of the double was the center of the symptomatology.

The authors of this chapter have never seen a case as typical as those described in the literature. The senior author, however, has seen two patients, paranoids with almost completely well-organized delusions, who doubted that their parents were their real parents. One of them felt that most probably her parents had died a short time before (that is, at the onset of her illness) and the persons who acted as her parents were either impostors or reincarnations of her parents. The writer considered this delusion part of a paranoid condition (bordering on paranoia). The second patient, together with the typical picture of paranoid schizophrenia, had the idea that her mother was an impostor. The senior author has also seen Capgras-like syndromes in elderly patients.

From an examination of the literature one gets the impression that the patients described could be classified under either paranoid schizophrenia or paranoid states. Capgras' syndrome thus should be more properly called Capgras symptom. As a matter of fact, similar phenomena are described in the European literature in even rarer syndromes: for instance, the illusion of Fregoli, described by Courbon and Fail.[17] The patient identifies the persecutor successively in several persons—the doctor, an attendant, a neighbor, a mailman, etc. The persecutor allegedly changes faces, as the

famous European actor, Fregoli, used to do on the stage. Courbon and Tusques[18] have also described the delusion of intermetamorphoses. The patient believes that the persons in his environment change with one another: A becomes B, B becomes C, C becomes A, etc.

But, going back to Capgras' syndrome, several authors report that they have found the syndrome not only in schizophrenic-like or paranoid patients, but also in manic-depressives.[54,55]

Many patients reported recently in the literature have been treated with insulin or electric shock treatments, apparently with good results. Others retained their delusions and illusions or had relapses.

Recently Moskowitz[44] reported the successful treatment of a twelve-year-old boy with Capgras' syndrome by psychotherapy. Perhaps due to the young age of this patient, paranoid elements were not as prominent as in other reported cases.

INTERPRETATION

Even if we deny recognition as a clinical entity to the Capgras phenomenon, it deserves further study from dynamic and formal points of view. The already abundant literature seems to be preoccupied almost exclusively with classificatory controversies.

Cargnello and Della Beffa,[12] reporting on existentialist analysis of the phenomenon, write that in the delusional experience of the patient three persons enter: the patient, the *alter* (the other, the person who was well known to the patient), and the *alius* (the double or the impostor). They conclude that actually it is the *alius* who is lived intensely in the *Erlebnis* of the patient and, although misidentified, is the closest to the ego of the patient.

A few things seem obvious in this syndrome. First, the person whose existence is denied is a very important person in the life of the patient —for instance, the mother. The patient rejects the mother, actually attributes very bad traits to her, but cannot allow herself to become conscious of this rejection because of concomitant guilt feelings or other ambivalent attitudes. What the patient feels about the

mother is thus displaced to the double or impostor who allegedly assumes her appearance.
Often, the idea that the misidentified person is
a double or an impostor occurs to the patient
as a sudden illumination or "psychotic insight."

Capgras' syndrome thus may be seen as an
unusual form of psychotic displacement. All
gradations of displacement occur from normal
states to neuroses and psychoses. In private
practice, we often see how the young wife's
resentment toward her own mother is freely
displaced and freely expressed to the mother-
in-law, for whom she has no ambivalent feelings.

In Capgras' syndrome the real person is
spared the hate of the patient—even becomes
sanctified, a model of virtue—and the impostor made the target. But the real person, the
person whom Cargnello and Della Beffa
called the *alter*, becomes a pale, peripheral
figure. The patient is really concerned with
the *alius*, the impostor.

More difficult than the dynamic is the formal understanding of the Capgras phenomenon. Often, in schizophrenia, the opposite
process takes place: Persons and things which,
in thinking processes, should only be associated, are identified. In the Capgras phenomenon, not only is there no increased tendency to
identify, but a person who should be easily
identified is not.

The real person is almost divided into two
parts (the *alter* or the good part, and the *alius*,
the bad part), as it often happens in dreams.
In the Capgras phenomenon, the persons are
different, but the body has the same appearance. There is thus not only a denial of the
Aristotelian first law of logic (law of identity),
but also a denial of von Domarus' principle
(for instance, in spite of characteristics in
common, the visitor is not the mother but an
impostor). Obviously, the mother is identified
with the impostor, but this identification remains unconscious.

This syndrome seems to represent in a dramatic fashion what Melanie Klein proposed as
the early infantile solution to ambivalence, the
"splitting" of the parent into good and bad

imagos. Moskowitz' case,[44] whose therapy is
described in detail, recounted how he began
to believe that his parents were being imper-
sonated by aliens after he realized that they
preferred his brother and that they had
treated him unfairly. He could not believe
that his real parents could act in such a fashion, nor could he tolerate the anger he began
to feel toward them. By creating the impersonation fantasy, he was able to continue to
love the idealized image of his parents while
transferring his hatred to the supposed imper-
sonators.

Autoscopic Syndrome

CLINICAL PICTURE

Like Capgras' syndrome, the autoscopic
syndrome consists of the delusional experience
of a double. In the autoscopic syndrome,
however, the double is not a person from the
patient's environment but the patient himself.
The patient sees a person nearby who looks
exactly like himself, talks, dresses, and acts as
he does. Quite often, this double seems exactly
like a mirror image of the patient. Lukianowicz[37] reported an excellent study of this
syndrome. Other important reports are those
of Lippman,[36] Lhermitte,[35] Pearson and
Dewhurst,[46] and Todd and Dewhurst.[56]

The double may appear suddenly and without warning; at other times, there are aural
warnings. It generally appears in gray, or
black and white, like images in dreams. Colors
are seldom perceived. The patient occasionally
reacts to the discovery of the presence of the
double with sadness and amazement, but
more often seems indifferent or even happy
about it. In a few cases, the double is constantly present; in the majority of instances,
however, the appearance of the double lasts
only a few seconds. Some patients have the
experience of the double only once in their
life; others repeatedly or constantly, after an
important event has occurred. Many patients
experience the phenemonon only in the evening, at night, or at dawn. Although occasional instances of autoscopic syndrome have

been reported in schizophrenia and in depressions, the majority of cases occur in patients suffering from migraine and epilepsy.

Numerous works of fiction have dealt with the theme of a person encountering his double. In some cases (Hoffmann's *The Devil's Elixir* or Poe's *William Wilson*), the two protagonists represent the good and evil sides of man. Perhaps the best known of such stories is Dostoevski's *The Double*, in which Golyatkin, a petty bureaucrat, meets his exact double who increasingly takes over his life until Golyatkin is sent to a mental hospital, helped into the carriage by his double. This story may be loosely interpreted as the struggle between the benign and malicious aspects of the same person. It is questionable, however, how much value these literary works offer in terms of explaining the condition as it occurs in psychiatric practice. Rogers[50] has written a valuable summary of the use of the "doubles" as a literary device and presents an interesting psychoanalytic interpretation.

INTERPRETATION

Autoscopic manifestations may be remotely related to, but certainly are not identical with, others which are encountered more often in psychiatric practice, such as eidetic images, hypnagogic hallucinations, or those imaginary companions about whom some patients, especially children, have enduring fantasies.

The term "autoscopy" was used by Schilder[51] to describe the process by which the individual is capable of doubling his body image and projecting it into the outside world. As used by Lukianowicz,[37] the term refers to hallucinatory phenomena, predominantly visual. These hallucinatory phenomena have only a remote resemblance to those found in schizophrenia; they have a much stronger resemblance to the phenomena found in organic conditions, especially those involving the parietal and temporal lobes (Critchley,[19] Penfield and Rasmussen,[47] Gerstman[27]), and in some cases of epilepsy. Sperber[52] has mentioned the possibility of sensory deprivation in some cases of autoscopic illusions.

The greatest resemblance is to those conditions in which a psychological picture is superimposed on an original organ condition, such as symptomatic epilepsy, cases of phantom limb,[34] duplications of parts of body, and denial of illness.[60]

There seem to be indications, however, that the psychogenic element is important in some cases. For instance, one of the cases reported by Lukianowicz was that of a fifty-six-year-old woman who experienced autoscopic phenomena upon returning from her husband's funeral. These phenomena continued thereafter. Lukianowicz does not attempt a dynamic interpretation of the case, although no organic findings are reported. One could speculate that the hidden purpose of the symptom was to make the patient aware that, although the husband was dead, she did not need to feel alone; she could be her own companion.

Wagner[58] has described the case of a twenty-one-year-old woman who, after being rejected by her fiancé, started to complain that her friends were persecuting her by telling her about having encountered a married couple whose description exactly fit that of herself and her former lover. In this instance, the patient did not hallucinate a double, but rather created one as part of a delusional system. Wagner found that many of his patient's Rorschach responses consisted of bilateral identical figures looking at each other, so that he concluded that her cognitive set partially predisposed toward the creation of a double. In this case, as in that described by Lukianowicz, the creation of a double appears to serve as a reparative process after a loss.

Ostow[45] has reported two patients who experienced autoscopic phenomena during the course of psychoanalysis. Both patients had a tendency to "split" themselves into acting and self-observing parts, and both patients experienced the phenomeon at a time of self-depreciation and disappointment. Ostow interprets the disorder as "an attempt to fracture off from the suffering ego the fragment which is felt to be the source of pain." On a deeper level, Ostow believes, that the autoscopic phenomenon represents a wish for the death and rebirth of an unacceptable part of the self.

Todd and Dewhurst[56] have attempted to delineate these factors that seem to predispose to autoscopic phenomena. General factors are a state of fatigue and above-average powers of visualization. A specific factor of psychogenic origin is an extreme narcissism and self-preoccupation. In defense of this, Todd and Dewhurst cite many authors who have experienced autoscopic phenomena. They believe this is because a writer always pictures himself in situations in order to create works of literature. An organic specific factor is damage to the parietal lobes, and they present a case who experienced autoscopic phenomena after injury to this area. A general factor that is mentioned is the use of archetypal or paleologic thought, which allows for concretization of an idea into a visual image. In his presentation of a case, McConnell[38] states that the most important psychogenic factors are excessive narcissism, a tendency toward wish fulfilment, and the use of visual imagery.

Cotard's Syndrome

In 1880, at the meeting of the Societé Médico-Psychologique in Paris, the French psychiatrist Cotard reported cases of what he called "délire de negation," or delusional state of negation. Since that time, controversy has continued as to whether this syndrome deserves a special place in the psychiatric classification or whether it should be included among recognized entities.

In 1892, a congress of neurologists, which took place in France, devoted itself to this topic, but no definite conclusions were reached. At the present time, it is only in France and in Italy that the condition continues to be described as a separate entity, but even in these countries there are many psychiatrists who deny its existence. In the United States, the condition would probably be included in the paranoid type of involutional psychosis. This symptomatology is in fact somewhat rare in the United States. A brief description follows:

After an interval of anxiety, the patient, generally a woman in the involutional age, but at times even men and younger or older women, denies any existence to the surrounding reality. Nothing exists; the world has disappeared. After the cosmic reality is denied, the physical reality of the patient himself is denied. At first, the patient claims that he has lost all sensation throughout his body; in some cases, he later claims that he does not exist. Everything is denied in this overwhelming delusional state. At times, even the possibility of death is denied—the patient considers himself immortal. Other symptoms resemble the picture of involutional psychosis—the patient is depressed, may refuse food, has ideas of having been condemned by God. He may also hallucinate. He retains, however, the capacity to talk freely in spite of the depression, and often is given to philosophical contemplations about his own life, life in general, and the world.

In the past few years, additional cases of Cotard's syndrome have been described in the Italian literature. Ahlheid[1] states that the nihilistic experience is common to many psychotic states and cites three cases, an arteriosclerotic, a syphilitic, and an alcoholic, with incomplete Cotard's syndrome. His point is that these symptoms can be seen in a number of conditions. Vitello[57] reports a case of paranoid schizophrenia who demonstrated excessive negation. These recent articles further question the validity of separating Cotard's syndrome as a specific diagnostic entity.

For further study, the reader is referred to Cotard,[16] Ey,[24] Capgras and Daumezon,[11] Perris,[48] and De Martis.[21]

"Psychose Passionelle" of Clérambault

In the French literature and to a lesser degree in the Italian, the so-called "psychose passionelle," or "pure erotomania," is still given a distinct nosologic place by some psychiatrists. It is sometimes called Clérambault's syndrome, after the author who devoted many studies to it.[15]

The condition is not too rare, even in the United States, and the senior author has seen several cases of it. In the United States, however, the condition is generally classified as a paranoid condition, paranoia, or paranoid type of schizophrenia. A brief description is reported here of the symptoms, which in some European psychiatric schools are generally considered part of Clérambault's syndrome.

The patient, generally a woman, claims that a man is very much in love with her. The man is generally of a social rank superior to hers, at times very wealthy, or a prominent actor, lawyer, physician, etc. The patient would like to reciprocate this love, but the world does not permit her to do so.

In other instances, the patient is convinced that the rebuffs or lack of interest on the part of the alleged lover are only pretenses, and that he is hiding his love for some hidden motive. The patient's love becomes the purpose of the existence of the patient, and everything else in her life revolves around it. The patient starts to interpret everything as a proof of the love this man has for her, and a delusional system is thus built. For instance, one patient, the wife of a successful storekeeper, considered the business success of her husband as a proof of the other man's love for her. Because of his love, he was directing many customers into the husband's store, so that the husband would make a lot of money. Any gift the husband bought for the patient was interpreted as an indirect gift from the other man.

Despite the persistence of this irrational belief of being loved, some patients may function normally in other areas. Enoch et al.[23] have reported the case of a forty-one-year-old spinster who, although convinced that she was secretly loved by an older professor, was able to carry on her work as a university lecturer.

In general, patients with this syndrome cling stubbornly to their delusion, despite all sorts of proof to the contrary. Even repeated confrontations with the alleged lover, during which he disclaims any feeling for the patient, are interepreted as his having been forced to "pretend" not to love her. Usually, the illness is chronic, with little change in the delusional system, despite various forms of treatment. For further study, the reader is referred to Clérambault[15] and Balduzzi.[4]

Munchausen's Syndrome

While this syndrome has been recognized for decades and has plagued innumerable physicians in the past, it was not until 1951 that Asher[3] formally described this condition and termed it "Munchausen's syndrome." This eponym was based on Baron Munchausen who lived in the eighteenth century, traveled widely, and was fond of telling fantastic tales. Raspe[49] portrayed the Baron in a somewhat fanciful biography, inventing even more fantastic adventures and anecdotes. The similarities between the legendary Baron and the patients described by Asher rest on both being compulsive travelers and both telling somewhat believable yet fantastic stories. More specifically, Asher's patients used their stories to gain admission to hospitals for factitious illnesses. Usually, these individuals will present themselves at emergency rooms late at night or on weekends when admission is easier. They will present themselves with dramatic symptoms which, however, are medically plausible.

Those patients who have been followed up or whose histories have been traced reveal that they have deceived numerous doctors by feigning serious illness, often to the point of undergoing surgery or other complex procedures. More commonly, however, once admitted to a hospital, these individuals tend to be argumentative and demanding, antagonize the staff, and ultimately sign themselves out against medical advice. While in hospital, they often assume dramatic impostures, such as war heroes, or other esteemed personages.

Since Asher's initial description, about forty cases have been reported, but these have been primarily in the nonpsychiatric literature. In fact, few patients have been studied by psychiatrists, because these patients appear skillful in avoiding psychiatric examination, and, also, since they present plausible medical histories and symptoms, psychiatric consultation is rarely sought. In reviewing the literature, caution is needed to make sure that the various articles do not refer to the same patient in a different guise. For example, one individual was responsible for no less than seven publications.[14] On the whole, however, the following generalizations may be considered. Munchausen's syndrome usually presents in three forms: (1) the acute abdominal type, in which the patient complains of severe abdominal cramps, often requiring emergency laparotomy; (2) the hemorrhagic type, in which the patient induces bleeding from various orifices; and (3) the neurologic types, in which mysterious yet striking neurologic symptoms are manifested. Cardiac and dermatologic symptoms have also been reported.

The syndrome appears more frequently in men than in women. Among the latter, hysteria is the most frequent psychiatric diagnosis, while among men there is an equal mixture of psychopathic personality and chronic undifferentiated schizophrenia. Because of the notoriety that this disorder has received, there is the danger of overdiagnosis, and Jensen[32] has reported the death of two patients believed to have Munchausen's syndrome because surgery was deferred. One of the present authors is familiar with an unfortunate woman who was repeatedly turned away from emergency rooms where she presented with abdominal pain, unusual neurologic symptoms, and mental confusion. Eventually, she was properly diagnosed as suffering from acute intermittent porphyria.

Spiro[53] has reported one of the few cases that was studied in detail from a psychiatric point of view. This patient was a thirty-year-old man who had repeatedly sought and obtained admission to hospitals because of abdominal pain. In addition to his feigned illness, the patient was unable to hold a job, frequently assumed false roles, and was a heavy drinker. Past history was significant, in that he was the second of ten children and was subjected to early deprivation. At age four, he was hit by a car and had both legs broken. This incident began a series of hospitalizations, during which the patient was the center of attention. His earliest memory, in fact, was of this initial hospitalization which

was remembered as extremely pleasant. After a prolonged and complicated recovery from his injury, he continued to use somatic symptoms, such as leg cramps, for secondary gain.

His later symptom of abdominal pain began when he could not cope with the rigors of military life. He was discharged from the service on the grounds of "unadaptability," and for years drifted from job to job. Gradually, he began to seek hospital admission following life stresses, such as the break-up of his first marriage, so that by the time he was thirty years old he had been hospitalized for feigned illnesses no less than fifty-three times. Once admitted, he was hostile and demanding of the staff, made fun of other patients, and assumed imagined identities. Despite attempts at psychotherapy, Spiro notes that a year after terminating treatment he was informed that the patient had been admitted to yet another hospital and had undergone a partial gastrectomy.

In his discussion of this patient, Spiro notes the early deprivation, the positive memory of hospitalization, leading to an effort to parentify hospital staff and create a hostile-dependent relationship in times of stress. Barker[6] believes that such patients harbor a grudge against the medical profession for real or imagined past mismanagement. Menninger,[41] while not referring to Munchausen's syndrome, per se, describes instances where individuals seek surgery as a means of punishment or as a way of escaping an imagined greater disaster by sacrificing part of themselves. In these cases, the individual sets himself as the passive victim of the doctor or surgeon to whom he has transferred responsibility for self-punishment. Most probably, different motives are active in various patients with this syndrome. The features that seem to stand out, however, are a need for dependency on a hospital in time of stress, and the use of illness to express anger at authority figures without threat of retaliation. The frequent use of assumed roles points out the severe lack of self-esteem in these patients, as well as the marked degree of psychopathology. At present, additional detailed psychiatric studies of such patients are needed to explain the use of self-mutilation or feigned illness as a prime symptom.

(Collective Psychoses

In old books of psychiatry, one can find reports of collective psychoses or "psychic epidemics" occurring in Europe, from the eleventh to the seventeenth centuries. These reports have to be read with more than a grain of salt, as they lack scientific rigor, although Hecker's volume,[29] published in 1832, is a valuable study.

We believe that many cases dealt not with real psychoses or neuroses, but with collective manifestations of fanaticism in members of particular religious sects. The Flagellants of the plague epidemics in the thirteenth and fourteenth centuries, trying to atone their sins, the Palamites who tried to touch the umbilicus with their head in order to see the glory of the Divinity, the Adamites who walked naked, can hardly be called "psychotic" in a medical sense.

Nevertheless, one gets the impression that actual "collective psychoses" or psychic epidemics occurred at times in the Middle Ages. In our opinion, these were not psychoses, but psychoneuroses of hysterical nature which were induced by the effect the crowd had on the predisposed person. The atmosphere of superstition, ignorance, and intense religiosity, predisposed unstable individuals to this form of collective hypnosis. Perhaps, a type of society that Riesman has called "group-directed" is necessary for the occurrence of such epidemics.

Ferrio,[25] from whom most of this information is taken, reports that between the eleventh and the fifteenth centuries a psychic epidemic of St. Vitus' dance occurred, especially in the German and Flemish countries. People affected by the disease gathered together in the vicinity of churches, dancing and singing for several days and nights until they lost consciousness. Many of them had convulsive seizures. In the midst of this excitement, some women were made pregnant. In the year 1278, when two hundred afflicted people gathered on a bridge on the Rhine at Utrecht, the bridge collapsed and many of them perished. According to Ferrio, it seems that the name of "St. Vitus' dance" comes from the fact that some of the afflicted were kept for treatment in a chapel dedicated to St. Vitus, in Zabern.

A similar epidemic occurred in the south of Italy in the fifteenth century. According to Zilboorg,[62] it was first described scientifically by Gaglivi, under the name "tarantism" or "tarantulism." The name has nothing to do with the Italian city Taranto, as some believe, but with the fact that the sick were thought to have been bitten by a particular spider, Lycosa tarantula. The patients presented convulsions and general excitement. It was also believed that music would be an effective treatment for it—thus, the melody "tarantella" was created, a popular dance music still played in Italy.

Perhaps, of all the collective psychoses, the most important is lycanthropy, some cases of which are said to occur even now in some mountain villages of Italy. According to Zilboorg, lycanthropy has been described and reported in the medical literature by Marcellus in the third century, by Paré, Pomponazzi, Leloyer, Weyer in the sixteenth century, and by Sennert in the seventeenth century (all quoted by Zilboorg). People affected by this condition considered themselves transformed into animals, especially wolves. They saw themselves as animals and acted as such. Many of them committed crimes while they were in this state. People recognized as affected by this condition were often arrested and executed. According to Ferrio, a French judge named Boguet prided himself on having condemned to death about six hundred people suffering from lycanthropy during an epidemic that occurred in France in the department of Giura.

Although some of these lycanthropous were probably schizophrenics, it seems possible that the majority of them were suffering from some kind of collective hysteria. The conviction that men could be transformed into animals is described in the myths and literature of various peoples. Nebuchadnezzar, King of Babylon, thought he was a wolf, and St. Patrick is reported to have transformed Veneticus, King of Gallia, into a wolf.

A strong feeling of guilt and unworthiness, experienced so deeply as to make the individual feel that he did not deserve to belong to the human race, found this concrete expression in a suitable cultural atmosphere. In a certain way, lycanthropy is a counterpart of other neurotic symptoms, such as phobias, obsessions, etc. In phobias, the patient is apparently afraid of a danger coming from the outside world, in lycanthropy he is afraid of undergoing a metamorphosis. Later, the patient must act out the metamorphosis by behaving like an animal. He acts hysterically or impulsively, rather than compulsively, but in order to do so he must receive the assent of a group of people who behave as he does. This group replaces his usual social self or superego.

Today, lycanthropy is a term reserved to describe the delusions appearing in isolated cases of schizophrenia and paranoia of having been transformed into animals.

Other collective epidemics are said to have occurred in convents where all the nuns would suddenly become possessed by the illness, abandon the religious discipline, and give vent to hysterical and bizarre actions. Ferrio reports that around the year 1700 the nuns of a convent near Paris started to mew as if they had been transformed into cats.

A similar event, described by Mackay,[40] occurred at a girl's school in Lille in the seventeenth century. The headmistress imagined that she saw black angels flying over the heads of her pupils. In her alarm, she warned them to be on guard against the devil. The girls reinforced the hysteria among themselves until all fifty confessed that they were witches and that they had attended a meeting of fiends, could ride through the air on broomsticks, and feasted on the flesh of infants. These forms of collective psychoses or hysteria seem predisposed by certain factors. Usually, the affected members of a group live in close proximity with each other but are isolated from society at large. The group is arranged into a repressive, authoritarian hierarchy that discourages independent thought or inquiry.

These factors reduce the individual ability to test reality and are conducive to suggestion, especially when sanctioned by authority figures, and when the pathologic behavior allows expression of repressed desires.

(Bibliography

1. AHLHEID, A. "Considerations on Nihilistic Experience and on Cotard's Syndrome on the Organic and Symptomatic Psychoses," *Lav. Neuropsichiat*, 43 (1968), 927.

2. ANDERSON, E., W. H. TRETHOWAN, and J. KENNA. "An Experimental Investigation of Simulation and Pseudo-dementia," *Acta Psychiatrica Scandinavica*, 34 (Supp. 132):1 (1959).

3. ASHER, R. "Munchausen's Syndrome," *Lancet*, 1 (1951), 339.

4. BALDUZZI, E. "Un Caso di Erotomania Passionata Pura Secondo Clérambault," *Riv. sperim. di freniatria*, 80 (1956), 407.

5. BALL, J. R. B., and M. A. KIDSON. "The Capgras Syndrome—A Rarity?" *Aust. N.Z.J. Psychiat*, 2 (1968), 49.

6. BARKER, J. C. "The Syndrome of Hospital Addiction (Munchausen Syndrome)," *Journal of Mental Science*, 108 (1962), 167.

7. BUMKE, O. *Handbuch der Geisteskrankheiten.* Berlin: Springer, 1932.

8. CAPGRAS, J., and P. CARRETTE. *"L'Illusion des Sosies et Complexe d'Oedipe,"* Ann. méd.-psych., 82 (1924), 48.

9. CAPGRAS, J., and J. REBOUL-LACHAUX. *"L'Illusion des Sosies dans un Délire Systematisé Chronique,"* Soc. Clin. Méd. Psych., 81 (1923), 186.

10. CAPGRAS, J., P. LUCETTINI, and P. SCHIFF. *"Du Sentiment d'Estrangeté à l'Illusion des Sosies,"* Ann. méd.-psych., 83 (1925), 93.

11. CAPGRAS, J. and J. DAUMEZON. *"Syndrome de Cotard Atypique,"* Ann. méd.-psych., 94 (1936), 806.

12. CARGNELLO, D., and A. A. DELLA BEFFA. *"L'Illusione del Sosia,"* Arch. Psicol. neurol. e psichiat., 16 (1955), 173.

13. CAROTHERS, J. C. *The African Mind in Health and Disease. A Study in Ethnopsychiatry.* Geneva: World Health Organization Monograph Series, 1953.

14. CHAPMAN, J. S. "Peregrinating Problem Patients—Munchausen Syndrome," *Journal of the AMA*, 165 (1957), 927.

15. CLÉRAMBAULT, G. G. DE. *Oeuvre Psychiatrique*. Paris: Presses Universitaires, 1942.

16. COTARD, J. *Maladies cérébrales*. Paris, 1891.

17. COURBON P., and J. FAIL. "*Syndrome de Fregoli et Schizophrenie*," *Soc. Clin Med. Ment.*, July, 1927; quoted in Ref. 15.

18. COURBON, P., and J. TUSQUES. "*Illusion d'Intermetamorphose et de Charme*," *Ann. méd.-psych.*, 90 (1932), 401.

19. CRITCHLEY, M. *The Parietal Lobes*. London: Arnold, 1953.

20. DAVIDSON, G. M. "The Syndrome of Capgras," *Psychiatric Quarterly*, 15 (1941), 513.

21. DE MARTIS, D. "*Un Caso di Sindrome di Cotard*," *Riv. sperim. di freniatria*, 80 (1956), 491.

22. DOGLIANI, P. "*Su di un Caso di Psicose di Ganser*," *Nevrasse*, 6 (1956), 12.

23. ENOCH, M. D., W. H. TRETHOWAN, and J. C. BARKER. *Some Uncommon Psychiatric Syndromes*. Baltimore: Williams and Wilkins, 1967.

24. EY, H. *Études Psychiatriques*. Paris: Desclee de Brouwer, 1954.

25. FERRIO, C. *La Psiche e i Nervi*, Turin: Utet, 1948.

26. GANSER, S. "*Ueber einen Eigenartigen Hysterischen Dammerzustand*," *Arch. Psychiat.*, 30 (1898), 633,

27. GERSTMANN, J. "Psychological and Phenoneurological Aspects of Disorders of the Body Image," *Journal of Nervous and Mental Disease*, 126 (1958), 499,

28. GLUCKMAN, L. K. "A Case of Capgras Syndrome," *Aust. N.Z.J. Psychiat.*, 2 (1968), 39,

29. HECKER, J. F. C. *Die Tanzwuth: eine Volkskrankheit im Mittelalter*. Berlin: 1832.

30. HENDERSON, D. K., and R. D. GILLESPIE. *A Text-Book of Psychiatry*. New York: Oxford University Press, 1941.

31. INGRAHAM, M. R., and D. M. MORIARTY. "A Contribution for the Understanding of the Ganser Syndrome," *Comprehensive Psychiatry*, 8 (1967), 35,

32. JENSEN, S. E. "The Indications for Abdominal Surgery in Psychiatric Patients," *Canadian Psychiatric Association Journal*, 8 (1963), 267,

33. JOLLY, F. Quoted in Ref. 59.

34. KOLB, L. C. *The Painful Phantom. Psy-*

35. LHERMITTE, J. "Visual Hallucination of the Self," *British Medical Journal*, 1 (1951), 431.

36. LIPPMAN, C. W. Hallucinations of Physical Quality in Migraine," *Journal of Nervous and Mental Disease*, 117 (1953), 345,

37. LUKIANOWICZ, N. "Autoscopic Phenomena," *Archives of Neurology and Psychiatry*, 80 (1958), 199,

38. McCONNELL, W. B. "The Phantom Double in Pregnancy," *British Journal of Psychiatry*, 111 (1964), 67,

39. MacDONALD, J. J. *Psychiatry and the Criminal*. Springfield: Thomas, 1958.

40. MACKAY, C. *Extraordinary Popular Delusions*. New York: Noonday, 1966.

41. MENNINGER, K. A. *Man Against Himself*. New York: Harcourt, Brace & World, 1938.

42. MINNS, R. A. J. "A Case of Capgras Syndrome," *Medical Journal of Australia*, 57 (1970), 239,

43. MOELI, C. Quoted in Ref. 59.

44. MOSKOWITZ, J. A. "Capgras Syndrome in Modern Dress," *International Journal of Child Psychotherapy*, 2 (1972), 45,

45. OSTOW, M. "The Metapsychology of Autoscopic Phenomena," *International Journal of Psycho-Analysis*, 41 (1960), 619,

46. PEARSON, J., and K. DEWHURST. "*Sur Deux Cas de Phenomènes Autoscopiques Consecutifs a des Lesions Organiques*," *L'Encéphale*, 43 (1954), 166,

47. PENFIELD, W., and T. RASMUSSEN. *The Cerebral Cortex of Man*. New York: Macmillan, 1952.

48. PERRIS, C. "*Sul Delirio Cronico Di Negazione (Sindrome di Cotard)*," *Neuropsichiatria*, 11 (1955), 175,

49. RASPE, R. E. *Baron Munchausen*. New York: Dover, 1960.

50. ROGERS, R. *The Double in Literature*. Detroit: Wayne State University Press, 1970.

51. SCHILDER, P. *Mind, Perception and Thought*. New York: Columbia University Press, 1942.

52. SPERBER, M. A. "Sensory Deprivation in Autonopic Illusion and Joseph Conrad's 'The Secret Sharer,'" *Psychiatric Quarterly*, 43 (1969), 711.

53. SPIRO, H. R. "Chronic Factitious Illness," *Archives of General Psychiatry*, 18 (1969), 569.

54. STERN, K., and D. MacNAUGHTON. "Cap-

gras' Syndrome, a Peculiar Illusionary Phenomenon, Considered with Special Reference to the Rorschach Findings," *Psychiatric Quarterly*, 19 (1949), 139,

55. TODD, J. "The Syndrome of Capgras," *Psychiatric Quarterly*, 31 (1957), 250,

56. TODD, J., and K. DEWHURST. "The Double: Its Psychopathology and Psychophysiology," *Journal of Nervous and Mental Disease*, 122 (1955), 47,

57. VITELLO, A. "Cotard's Syndrome in Schizoid Paranoia," *Rass. Studi. Psychiat.*, 59 (1970), 195,

58. WAGNER, E. E. "The Imaginary Lover's De-

lusion," *J. Proj. Tech. Personal Assos.*, 4 (1966), 394,

59. WEINER H., and A. BRAIMAN. "The Ganser Syndrome: A Review and Addition of Some Unusual Cases," *The American Journal of Psychiatry*, 111 (1955), 767,

60. WEINSTEIN, E. A., and R. L. KAHN. *Denial of Illness*. Springfield: Thomas, 1955.

61. WHITLOCK, F. A. "The Ganser Syndrome," *British Journal of Psychiatry*, 113 (1967), 19,

62. ZILBOORG, G., and G. W. HENRY. *A History of Medical Psychology*. New York: W. W. Norton, 1941.

CHAPTER 32

EXOTIC PSYCHIATRIC
SYNDROMES

Johannes M. Meth

SOMATIC PATHOLOGY IS UNIVERSAL and so is psychopathology, and what is more, psychopathology appears in basically identical clinical forms, wherever it occurs in the world. According to Forster:[44]

Psychiatric syndromes or reactions, by and large, are similar in all races throughout the world. The mental reactions seen in our African patients can be diagnosed according to Western textbook standards. The basic illness and reaction types are the same. Environmental, constitutional, and tribal cultural background merely modify the symptom constellation. Basically, the disorders of thinking, feeling, willing, and knowing are the same.

And Edgerton[41] writes:

It is remarkable how alike the African conceptions of psychosis are to the Western-European psychoses. The Africans of the four tribes do not regard a single behavior as psychotic which could not be so regarded in the West. That is, they do not produce symptoms which are understandable as psychotic only within the context of their own cultures. What is psychotic for them would be psychotic for us.

This uniformity of psychopathology is puzzling, particularly for those of us who have accepted Horney's[62] and other "cultural psychiatrists'" theory of the pathogenetic role of the environment. How could as different a culture as that of a Stone-Age Arauca produce the same clinical picture as that of a highly industrialized society? In somatic medicine, we accept, as a matter of course, that a trauma produces a fracture in an Arauca, as well as in an astronaut. What does differ, may be the cause of the trauma: The Arauca may fall from a tree, the astronaut may have a flying accident. The repertoire of psychological responses is as biologically limited as that of somatic responses. Fear, anger, sadness, joy, and anxiety resulting from inner conflicts are universal. The cause of the conflicts may differ; but transgression of a taboo creates anxiety in the same way as transgression of one of our society's standards.

Furthermore, the most incisive psychological influence occurs in early childhood. Stone-age parents may be affectionate or hostile, accepting or rejecting of their children, as are our parents. Technological advancement is no guarantee of healthy emotional parent-child relationships. Kubie[76] expresses this idea in the following manner:

We must consider the interactions of developmental *universals* and of cultural *variables* of those ingredients of the neurotic process which are unique for human kind. . . . The neurotic potential is universal in all human beings, partly inherent in the biological character of development and partly in the universal relationship of infancy.

The uniformity of psychopathology is not absolute. Deviations occur in the following areas: morbidity (psychiatric epidemiology);* relative frequency of the various diagnostic categories; existence of a group of psychiatric syndromes which are limited both geographically as well as in their occurrence in only few population groups. The morbidity varies greatly even within racially, ecologically, and economically similar populations. For example, the Iatmul and the Arapesh are two tribes who live near each other in New Guinea. The morbidity among the Iatmul is considerably higher than among the Arapesh. There is a high incidence of severe mental disorders among the Ojibwas and Aiviliks, as high as in any technologically advanced society. It is, therefore, not true that psychopathology increases with the increase of complexity of a society. The relative frequency of different diagnostic categories varies not only among different nations or societies, but changes may occur in the same population group. Manic states appear definitely more often in African cyclothymic patients than in ours; affective disorders are more frequent in Italy than in the USA. However, manic-depressive psychoses are observed less often in Italy now than only a decade ago.[6] Suicidal rates differ widely in different countries and/or different

* Psychiatric statistics are notoriously unreliable. In addition to the usual difficulties of diagnostic criteria and of communication, mental illness is considered in some cultures to be shameful to the patient, his family, and even to his tribe, and is therefore kept hidden. In other cultures, there may be a remarkable tolerance for deviant behavior, so that patients are not reported unless they become grossly unmanageable.[15, 21, 23, 72, 79]

population groups of the same country.[9,15,23] [38,58,98] Finally, another deviation from the global universality and uniformity of psychopathology is represented by a group of psychiatric syndromes, which Arieti and I called "exotic psychiatric syndromes" in the first edition of this Handbook. Yap[154-158] used the term, "culture-bound reactive syndromes," Weidman and Sussex,[149] "culture-bound responses to culturally patterned stresses," Enoch et al.[42] simply, "some unknown psychiatric syndromes." This group of syndromes has in common only—aside from their geographical and cultural limitations—that they are not observed in the West and that they have a bizarre, psychosis-like flavor, though most of them are to be classified as neuroses. They present fascinating clinical pictures, but even more importantly, they offer to the student of cross-cultural psychiatry a rich source of investigation. Sapir[130] exhorts us:

Perhaps it is not too much to expect that a number of gifted psychiatrists may take up the serious study of exotic and primitive cultures in order to learn to understand more fully than we can out of the resources of our own culture the development of ideas and symbols and their relevance for the problem of personality.

Before I go on to describe the various syndromes, I want to caution Western-trained psychiatrists about some diagnostic pitfalls.

1. Most of us have abandoned the definition of psychiatry as the science of abnormal behavior as too limited. However, psychiatric diagnosis is still based to a great extent on the observation of deviant behavior. But what is *normal* for us, may be *abnormal* in other cultures, and vice versa. Here are some examples. In the West, suicide is considered a sign of emotional disorder. In Japan, it is expected behavior under certain circumstances.[9,64] No sane woman on the island of Dobu (Melanesia) would have left her cooking pots unguarded for fear of being poisoned.[45,108] We would suspect paranoia. Eskimo mothers used to accept, as a matter of course, the killers of their sons in their son's stead. Homosexual practices between uncles and nephews are

expected and normal behavior among some Papuan tribes. In Tibet, a father's second wife is inherited by his sons, when he gets old. Arapesh males may marry simultaneously a mother and her daughter. A Navajo may marry a widow; later on, he discards her and marries her daughter. The Urubus of the Brazilian jungle feel fully dressed with a string around their penises as their only garment; they feel naked and terribly embarrassed when they lose the string.[11,14,36,45] Chinese and East Indian males may attribute their discomfort to semen having gone up to their brains.[122,151]

In the West, hallucinations are considered almost pathognomonic for the diagnosis of psychosis. In non-Western countries hallucinations are a normal requirement for priests and shamans during their religious or healing rituals. In fact, priests and shamans are often chosen for their ability to hallucinate and to fall into states of altered consciousness. These hallucinations differ, however, from those of psychotics, since they begin and end with the religious ceremonies, since the visions and voices are usually benign, not threatening, and since they require, to be induced, monotonous repetitive sounds or continuous rhythmic movements.

To illustrate the difficulty of differential diagnosis in a culture in which hallucinations and religious beliefs, similar to delusions, are normal, I cite the occasion when A. H. Leighton asked T. A. Baasher of the Clinic for Nervous Diseases in Khartoum, Sudan, how he would distinguish religious beliefs from delusions. Baasher told him of a Sudanese member of a religious sect who began hearing voices, telling him to kill his leader's rival. He went from village to village to find the rival whom he did not know personally. After a long search, his voices told him that *there* was his man. In spite of the man's protestations that he was no religious leader, the hallucinating Sudanese speared him. According to Baasher, it was in keeping with the Sudanese culture and considered normal to hallucinate and even to kill on one's master's behalf. But the composite of all the elements in this case made no sense even from the particular culture's point of view. So, Baasher diagnosed the murderer as a case of paranoid schizophrenia. In other words, the diagnosis of mental disease in primitive societies cannot be made by observing behavior that is abnormal according to our standards; even behavior patterns that are normal in the culture in which they occur are no proof of mental health. We must apply the same criteria that we use in our patients with due regard for cultural peculiarities.

2. Another diagnostic pitfall, particularly in tropical and semitropical countries, is the simulation of functional psychiatric disorders by infectious diseases. It must be kept in mind that positive laboratory findings are not decisive in populations in which these infections are endemic. The most important conditions to rule out are:

(a) Malaria, particularly the pernicious type caused by the Plasmodium Falciparum, can produce psychiatric symptoms, such as confusional states with excitement or stupor, an amok-like syndrome, epileptiform attacks. According to Carothers,[23] malaria accounts for 3.4 percent of first admissions to mental hospitals in Kenya.

(b) Trypanosomiasis (sleeping sickness) was according to Tooth[145] the "commonest cause of mental derangement throughout large areas of West Africa." Whereas malaria has been eradicated in many parts of the world, sleeping sickness is still a scourge of many parts of Africa.

   The first symptom is usually a change of habits; the patient becomes increasingly irritable, then apathetic and morose; the speech is slow and tremulous; sleep disturbances occur in 60-70 percent of the cases. Delusions, hallucinations, and manic attacks are not rare. According to Tooth, every type of schizophrenia may be simulated. The end stage consists of a euphoric dementia, punctuated by episodes of irrational and impulsive behavior.[23,46,145,149]

(c) Ankylostomiasis (hookworm disease) may appear at first as a depression, sometimes of a severe degree, until the profound anemia and the positive laboratory findings together with the reversal of the psychological symptoms, when the patient is treated for hookworms, confirm the diagnosis.

(d) Massive infestation with Ascaris lumbricoides in children. I have observed several cases in Ecuador with initial symptoms of confusion, epileptiform attacks, carpo-pedal spasms in children between four and six years of age. In two of the children, the confusion disappeared dramatically after the patients vomited clumps of the parasites.

(e) Syphilis is very common in many underdeveloped populations, although a positive Wassermann cannot be taken as a sure indication of the disease. Yaws is frequent in tropical countries and can be responsible for the positive serology.

General paresis, once believed to be rare among non-Western people,[75] occurs usually without the complete deterioration and dementia seen in the West. Carothers[23] has seen a fair number of cases in Kenya. The most prominent symptom was that of manic excitement.

3. Nutritional deficiencies are common among underdeveloped populations and may simulate or be accompanied by psychiatric disorders. The deficiencies which produce psychological symptoms most frequently are pellagra and kwashiokor.[49,137,142]

Pellagra may be difficult to diagnose, in spite of the classical triad: dermatitis, diarrhea, and dementia. The dermatitis may be absent or hard to recognize in colored people; diarrhea is frequent in hot climates for causes other than pellagra; dementia is an end stage. Initially, the patient shows sudden irrational mood changes; or he may be constantly irritable, has paranoid delusions, and may even hallucinate.

Kwashiokor is a disease caused by protein deficiency. It is unknown in populations whose food contains certain amino acids, either through animal proteins (meat, fish, or milk) or through vegetal proteins (beans). Infants develop normally at first, that is as long as they are nursed. After weaning, they lose their previous liveliness, become apathetic, morose, growth is retarded, skin lesions appear, and the children succumb often to an intervening infection.

4. A fourth class of diagnostic difficulties for Western psychiatrists are drug-induced psychiatric symptoms. The use of certain mushrooms or leaves in order to produce psychological effects is very widespread. They are taken during religious ceremonies or, sometimes, to increase endurance for particularly strenuous tasks. Most of these drugs alter the state of consciousness. Their effect lasts usually only a few hours, but at times it persists and, as in some of our patients on LSD, a latent psychosis may become apparent.

The psychologically most destructive drug, aside from opium and its derivatives, is alcohol, a Western import to most primitive people. During my years among the Indians in Ecuador, I saw violent crimes committed almost exclusively under the influence of alcohol.

Not all primitive people use drugs. It seems that they are used mostly by peoples who live under particularly harsh natural or man-made conditions in an attempt to escape into an illusory paradise.

The healing practices of primitive populations, long neglected, have recently attracted considerable interest. In the West, we pride ourselves in our rationality. We strive to recognize the etiology and pathogenesis of an illness. We expect to discover the underlying unresolved conflicts and to help our patients to take responsibility for their thoughts, feelings, and behavior. We hope that our patients will thereby feel less helpless and inadequate and be able to cope with the vicissitudes of their lives. The native healer starts out from the same premise. He, too, tries to understand the cause of his patient's illness which he may attribute to the transgression of a taboo, in an affront to a deity or spirit, in the malevolence of supernatural forces, or in the witchcraft of a sorcerer. The etiological agents are assumed to produce their pathogenetic effect by either introjecting evil objects into the patient's body or by depriving him of his soul, sexual powers, normal intelligence, etc. Native healers have keenly observed what re-establishes happiness to a child who has fallen from the good graces of his mother. He runs to her, hides his face in her lap, and therefore submits to her mercy. This show of submission may be enough to win back mother's acceptance. Sometimes, mother must prove her power by punishing the child, before she can forgive him. But then atonement, the acceptance of the punishment, frees the child of all guilt feelings. These observations of basic human behavior are applied as treatment methods. The shaman finds out where and when his patient has been "bad." He then makes the patient admit and helps the patient to a cathartic confession. The offended powers may be mollified by this act of submission alone or the shaman, as mediator of the deity or spirit, subjects the patient to punishment in form of physical, psychological, or economical pain.

Another healing method, also derived from the observation of basic human needs, is the Shaman's permission, as representative of the group, for the patient to let go of his repressed feelings. For example, the native healer may allow a male patient, whose culture demands complete denial of dependency needs, to indulge in these otherwise unacceptable feelings or he will encourage a female patient to vent her hostility, if her group's standards expect self-effacement for women.

In other words, native therapy is not as senseless as it has arrogantly been claimed in the West, but it is an often effective way to help patients by furthering self and group acceptance. Native technique usually involves the mobilization of intense emotions. The shaman has an advantage over us, since his patients have usually absolute faith in his healing powers. I believe that the shaman's trances and hallucinations are one way to demonstrate his powers and also a way to show to his pa-

tients that it is possible to get out of these states.

⟨ Latah

Latah is a syndrome, first described in Malaya, but recognized later on in many parts of the world. The etymology of the word "latah" is not known. It may derive from the Malayan words for love-making, tickling, or creeping. In Malaya, this syndrome has been known for many centuries and is regarded more as an eccentricity than a disease. It occurs mostly in middle-aged or elderly women. In other parts of the world, it is equally as frequent in men. Sometimes, it has assumed epidemic proportions.

Similar syndromes have been described in Siberia under the names of "myriachit" and "tara;" among the Ainu of Hokkaido, Northern Japan, as "inu"; in Siam as "bahtschi"; in Burma as "yuan"; in the Philippines as "mali-mali"; in Madagascar as "ramenajana"; in Nyasaland as "misala"; and as "banga" in Zaire. It has also been reported from Somaliland, the southern part of the Sahara, and from Tierra del Fuego without any particular name. Some authors believe that Gilles de la Tourette's disease and the syndrome called by Beard "Jumping Frenchmen of Maine" belong to the same psychiatric category.

Clinical Picture

The patients in Malaya are usually middle-aged or elderly women of dull intelligence and of compliant character in low socioeconomic positions. They become increasingly fearful and seclusive. The disorder may start with a sudden fright. Among the Ainu, the illness begins when the patient has seen or imagines having seen, or stepped on, a snake. At first, the patient repeats the words or sentences of other people, specially of persons in authority. Then, the patient imitates, in pantomime fashion, the gestures and acts of other people or does the exact opposite of what other people do or expect her to do. Later, the patient starts to mumble incomprehensible sounds which, still later, become clearly curses or obscenities, words hitherto alien to the patient. The echolalia, echopraxia, and coprolalia appear to be uncontrollable by the patient who, as soon as she has pronounced the curse words, gives signs of feeling utterly embarrassed and frightened. Latah patients are often subjected to ridicule. Adults and children may tease them unmercifully until they beg their tormentors to leave them in peace or until, less often, they become violent.

In other parts of the world, latah patients may present additional symptoms. In Africa, they may run into the forests; in Tierra del Fuego, they may climb dangerous cliffs without regard to their safety. During these fugues, the patients, who are most often males, become violent and present a picture similar to "running amok."

The "Jumping Frenchmen of Maine" belong to a sect—The United Society of Believers in the Second Appearing of Christ—which came to the United States from Wales in the eighteenth century and settled along the eastern coast. During their rites and at the height of their religious ecstasy, one member starts to jump, roll around on the ground, and utter barking sounds. The others follow suit. Most of them stop this behavior at the end of the religious ceremony. A few, however, remain in this state or begin to jump and shake again if a sharp command is directed at them, or even if someone just points a finger at them.

I don't believe that the "Jumping Frenchmen of Maine" should be included in the latah syndrome. One essential feature of latah, coprolalia, is absent, which in psychodynamic terms is as important as the echolalia and echopraxia, as we shall see. Gilles de la Tourette's disease (also called *Tic de Guinon, maladie des tics impulsifs, myospasia impulsiva*, multiple tics with coprolalia, or *imbacco*) begins in children between the ages of five and fifteen years with spasms of the orbicularis oculi. Later, it spreads to other muscles of the face, then neck, upper extremities, and at times, to the muscles of the whole body. At the same time or somewhat after the appearance of the tics, all the symptoms of the latah

syndrome are added. The course of the disease is unpredictable. It may become progressively worse, ending in a severe obsessive-compulsive neurosis or even in a psychosis. In other cases, the symptomatology remains stationary or the disease may run a paroxysmal course, the paroxysms lasting for weeks or months.

One of my patients showed first symptoms at the age of eight years. Coprolalia appeared several years later and was particularly hard to understand in this very gentle, compliant boy. At twelve, he developed a frank psychosis. He stopped hallucinating at twenty-one and has remained severely obsessive-compulsive ever since. The patient is now forty-three years old. Sometimes, signs of his old disease break through. He starts to stutter, repeats his last words and those of the persons whom he talks with, and finally lets go of a barrage of obscenities which are very much out of keeping with his usual vocabulary.

Pibloktok, also spelled Pibloktoq, or called Pibloktoq hysteria, or the "copying mania," or amurakh, are the names of latah-like syndromes, occurring among Polar Eskimos. These are paroxysmic states of excitement, some lasting just a few minutes, others for hours. The patients disrobe themselves or tear off their clothes, run away, roll in the snow, jump into the icy waters of a lake, or try other unusual acts, and grimace. Glossolalia (mimicking animal sounds or pronouncing meaningless neologisms) and coprophagia are common.[105]

In *amurakh*, or "copying mania," which occurs in Siberian women, the mimicking of other people's words or acts is the main symptom.

Menerik is a syndrome which has been observed in Eskimos of both sexes. It manifests itself in paroxysms of wild screaming and dancing and may culminate in epileptiform seizures.

Interpretation

The latah patient is a compliant, self-effacing person who, before becoming ill, has tried to blot out all aggressiveness, so as not to feel the conflict between her compliance and aggression. The latah symptoms appear when these attempts at repression fail. Her hostility breaks through and shows in her curses and obscenities. She still tries desperately to check this breakthrough by obliterating her spontaneity—saying and doing only what others have said or done before her. I consider the appearance of coprolalia as an essential symptom of latah and would therefore not include the "Jumping Frenchmen of Maine" syndrome.

This interpretation, obviously, does not tell us why latah patients choose their particular symptoms and not those presented by our patients with similar psychodynamics. Mimicking and the expression of obscene words must have a meaning in the cultures in which latah occurs, which they do not have in other cultures, and only a very intimate knowledge of cultural peculiarities and idiosyncrasies will allow a full understanding of the symptom choices. I have often marveled about the frequency with which psychotic episodes in Latin-Americans begin with a homosexual panic, until I understood that the word *maricón* (homosexual) is the most derogatory term, used constantly in Spanish-America. Contempt and self-contempt has no parallel or equally meaningful word in Spanish.

(Amok

Amok or running amok is another syndrome first described in Malaya, but also found in many other parts of the world, for example in the Philippines, in Africa, in the Caribbean, in Tierra del Fuego, etc. The "going berserk" of the old Vikings was probably similar to running amok. It used to be common in Malaya until the beginning of this century. According to van Wilfften Palthe,[151] it was observed with regularity among the patients of the old Batavia Hospital until the old building was replaced by a modern structure and until modern medical care was instituted in 1914. Since then, amok has become rare among the hospital's patients. Van Wilfften Palthe claims that he has never observed or heard about a

case of amok among the many Malayans living in European countries.

In the early days of American occupation of the Philippines, a number of American soldiers became victims of amok Moros, a Moslem tribe. When the Moros' level of education was raised, amok disappeared. Maguigad[102] claims that amok is still quite frequent in the Philippines. It also appears to be fairly common among the Papuans of New Guinea under the name of "Negi-negi" or "Lulu," and in Melanesia.

The "Puerto Rican Syndrome," or *Mal de Pelea* is, in my opinion, similar to amok, although the outcome is usually less gruesome. As in amok, the patient withdraws at first and gets into a brooding mood. All of a sudden and without any recognizable provocation, he becomes violent and strikes out at anyone near him.[43]

According to Zaguirre[159] and Kline,[74] the premorbid personality is impulsive, emotionally hyper-reactive, according to other authors schizoid. However, the psychodynamic interpretation is probably the same. The patient's attempt at conflict-solution by repressing his hostility is failing. He makes a last desperate attempt by withdrawing within himself. According to Maguigad, amok derives from the Malayan word "amoq," which means engaging furiously in battle. It is a life or death battle against a feeling of complete disintegration. I have sometimes sensed this feeling in a patient who from a catatonic stupor suddenly switched to catatonic excitement. It is a last-ditch attempt at survival against the inner forces which are about to disintegrate him.

The Bantus express this idea in their belief that a person destined to die may escape death by killing someone else in his stead.

In other words, the amok patient externalizes his desperate need to destroy the death-bringing inner conflict by killing other persons. The most violent cases of amok seem to occur in cultures which demand repression of hostility, as in Malaya, Bandung, and the Philippines. In Puerto Rico, violence is more acceptable, and, in fact, expected of males under certain circumstances. The investment of energy in the repression of hostility is not large and therefore the violence—once repression fails—is of a lesser degree.[43]

The multiple violent acts occasionally committed in Western countries by persons with a schizoid personality resemble the clinical picture of running amok and may be due to similar psychodynamic mechanisms. These acts have been the subject of several novels by authors like Camus and D'Annunzio. The differential diagnosis between the violent acts of paranoid or catatonic schizophrenics and of amok patients is helped both by the history—since amok patients did not show any delusions or hallucinations—and by the lack of amnesia in schizophrenic patients.

Pseudo-amok is a syndrome in which the patients seem to simulate all the symptoms present in amok, except that they do not hurt anybody and that they give themselves up meekly once cornered—a situation which does not occur in real amok. Pseudo-amok is probably a hysterical syndrome.

⟨ Koro[*]

The origin of the word "koro" is not clear. It may stem from the Malayan word "kuru," shake; the Javanese word "keruk," shrink; or according to Yap,[153] from the Javanese word for tortoise. The Chinese and Southeast Asians call the glans penis tortoise.

The Chinese name for the syndrome is "shook yong." It has been known in China for

centuries. One of their emperors died supposedly of shook yong. The Chinese author Pao described it in 1834. He claimed that it is precipitated by exposure to cold or by the ingestion of cold or raw food. It starts out with abdominal pain, spasms, and cyanosis of the limbs, retraction of the penis and scrotum into the abdomen; then, there is trismus, and finally death. It is a serious emergency. According to Chinese folk medicine, it is related to the middle female meridian which is supposedly governed by the liver—the organ most susceptible to worry, fear, and anger. One of the triggering causes is believed to be excessive intercourse or improper sexual relations.

The symptoms usually start without warning. The patient, usually between thirty and forty years of age, is suddenly worried that his penis will disappear into his abdomen and that he will die. To prevent this from happening, the patient has to grip his penis firmly; when he becomes tired, his wife, relatives, or friends help him. The Chinese constructed a special wooden clasp for this purpose. At times, fellatio, practiced immediately by the patient's wife, can stop the phobia, otherwise it can last for days, or even weeks. Linton[97] describes a female equivalent of koro in Borneo where the patient is afraid that her breasts are shrinking as well as her labia, which would lead to the disappearance of important female characteristics.

The Chinese believe that shook yong is caused by an imbalance of yin and yan. The prevalence of the female factor yin must be counteracted by the administration of a drug which increases yan, for example, powdered rhinoceros horn.

Our male patients, afflicted by castration anxiety, choose different symbols to express their fears. They may be worried about the length of their penises, of being homosexual, etc. What makes Southeast Asian or Chinese patients adopt their particular symbolism is impossible to say without intimate knowledge of their cultures. However, a recent outbreak of a koro epidemic might give us some hints.

For about ten years prior to 1967, rumors circulated that males who ate chickens injected with hormone pellets developed large

---

[*] The psychiatric syndrome "koro" must not be mistaken for the familiar central nervous disorder, also called "koro" or "kuru," which has been observed in a very limited area of the eastern highlands of New Guinea. The disease begins with tremors, which spread all over the body and become progressively worse, muscle inco-ordination, dysarthria. Death follows within three months to one year. At autopsy, a severe cerebellar degeneration is found. This disease occurs almost exclusively in children and women. Intense investigation in the late 1950s led to the discovery that the disease is caused by a slow-acting virus which is transmitted when the children and women eat the livers of killed members of neighboring tribes. The virus concentrates in the liver. The male adults eat other parts of the body which contain much less virus and therefore are less massively infected. This discovery led the editor of the *Journal of the American Medical Association* to write an editorial on "On Not Eating Your Neighbor."[4, 13, 47, 94, 104]

breasts and became impotent. In July 1967, an outbreak of swine fever in Singapore was stopped through vaccination. The injection of the vaccine was equated with the injection of hormones with the disastrous effects mentioned above, in those who had eaten inoculated pork. It is possible that a few people of the poorer class who could afford to buy only chicken necks (the hormone pellets are injected in the necks) developed gynecomastia and that this change in secondary sexual character signified decreased masculinity.

Susto and Espanto

"Susto" and "espanto" are two Spanish words which can be translated as fright or fear, but in this context refer to names used throughout Central and South America for psychiatric syndromes. They are used for a number of clinical pictures which have in common only that they occur most frequently in small children, and are characterized by an intense fear or anxiety. Somatic pathology is also rather common.

The affected child becomes tearful, easily frightened, loathes to be left alone, loses his appetite or acquires strange appetites, and is irritable. This clinical picture may have started after a fall, after encountering a snake or other frightening animals or situations, or for no apparent reason. In some countries, the terms "susto" and "espanto" are used interchangeably, and in others "espanto" is reserved for the more severe cases.

The popular explanation holds the loss of soul responsible for the syndrome. The soul flees and seeks shelter in caves or trees, particularly at night, at which point the child wakes up frightened and crying and cannot be consoled.

It is up to the shaman to identify the reason for the soul's flight. It may be because of a parent's neglect or the malevolence of spirits or a witch. I believe that in every case of susto in children which I have seen in Ecuador, an organic cause was present, either malnutrition or infectious diseases or parasitoses. These somatic ailments often made the par-

ents irritable with their children and this led to the children's fears and anxiety. In the few cases of susto in adults, we may recognize diagnoses from anxiety neurosis to acute schizophrenic panic.

Whitico Psychosis

This syndrome has been observed among the Eskimos who live in the Hudson Bay area, particularly among the Cree Eskimos. The Ojibwas of Southeastern Ontario call this syndrome "windigo."

Clinical Picture

The first symptoms may be anorexia, nausea, vomiting, and diarrhea. The patient falls into a brooding mood, fearing that he has been bewitched, that he will become a "whitico." A whitico is a supernatural figure, a giant skeleton, made of ice, which devours human beings. The patient withdraws more and more, is sleepless, refuses to eat, and sinks into deeper and deeper melancholia. The frightened family calls on a good shaman to counteract the witch's or bad shaman's spell. Most often, the patient improves after appropriate magic is applied. But, at times, particularly in remote areas where no "good" shaman is available, the patient may coldly kill one or more members of his family and eat them. Cannibalism has been a recognized extreme means of survival among the Eskimos. The occurrence of cannibalism in their phobias or delusions is, therefore, not surprising.

The whitico patient, who acts out his fears, mistakenly believes that the life-saving effect of cannibalism during a realistic emergency (extreme famine), will save him from suffering in an emotional emergency, too. Another motive of the whitico patient may be the use of a folklore tale to realize his sadistic desires. Finally, the stark, cruel Arctic environment must create a feeling of utter isolation in its inhabitants who must crave for the relief of their loneliness, and what could offer greater closeness than the incorporation of another human being?

(Voodoo Death (Thanatomania)

Voodoo death has been observed among most primitive peoples. The patient dies without any discernible organic cause when he becomes aware of having transgressed a taboo or when he fears having been bewitched. The following is a typical case report. A sorcerer in New Guinea had been offended by a young Papuan. In revenge, he told the young, healthy man that a few days ago he had put a *bofiet* (an object poisoned by witchcraft) into the young man's path. The young Papuan appeared immediately extremely ill; he did not talk and seemed completely removed from his environment. Within two days he was dead. The sorcerer was indicted by a Dutch court which, recognizing the bewitchment as cause of death, condemned the sorcerer—who, by the way, admitted his guilt freely—to several years' imprisonment.

Our language is aware of the possible connection between extreme fear and death; we say "frightened to death." But we in the West would expect death to occur only in very rare cases of the most extreme fright, and not for apparently trifling reasons, as happened in the case mentioned above. We ought not to forget, however, that the transgression of a taboo or the feeling of being bewitched is no less trifling for primitive peoples as those symbols which have become charged with explosive meaning in our culture.

In the Bible (II: Sam. 6:6–8), it is reported that Uzzah accidentally touched the ark of God while it was shaken by the oxen which were carrying it. Touching of the ark was strictly forbidden and Uzzah is reported to have died immediately, because of the "anger of the Lord." This account is hardly reconcilable with other statements in the Bible where great care is taken to differentiate voluntary from involuntary crimes (Numbers, Ch. 35; Joshua, Ch. 20). The interpretation that Uzzah died a voodoo death is more likely, since to him the touching of the ark must have meant the transgression of one of the most stringent taboos.

In the West, dying from the fear of, or the expectancy of, death, may not be rare. Arieti has heard from reliable witnesses the case of an elderly man, of the village of Pomerance, Italy who used to say that he would die only when the several-centuries-old tower of the village fell, meaning that he would live for a long time. During a storm, the tower was hit by lightning and did fall. Shortly after hearing the news, the old man died.

Experienced surgeons and anesthetists know that some very frightened patients die during or shortly after an operation for no discernible organic reason. The usual explanation is that the patient went into shock. At the autopsy, only signs of vasomotor paralysis are found, the same as in voodoo deaths.

Actually, voodoo death is only one of the many ways in which emotions act on the organism. We still do not know whether death occurs because Selye's[133] reaction to stress fails or because it involves the vital vascular systems.

(Final Remarks

In the preceding pages, I have pointed to a paradoxical dichotomy: On the one hand, there is by now a consensus that mental disorders exist in very much the same form everywhere in the world. No group of human beings is known in which every member can cope with life without the need for neurotic or psychotic defenses. On the other hand, I described a number of psychiatric syndromes which occur only in a few societies and which are not observed in the West.

Two facts account mainly for the universality of psychopathology: (1) The repertoire of psychological responses to psychological stresses is biologically limited. (2) The parent-child relationship is universal; it does not change with technological advances.

Psychological responses to psychological stresses—anxiety, anger, sadness, etc.—call forth in all human races defense constructs against the disintegrating forces of conflict, for example, externalizations, repressions, phobias —in other words, neuroses and psychoses.

But differences in psychiatric pathology exist; they are:

1. Quantitative, epidemiological differences;
2. Variations of the proportions of the various psychiatric entities: More obsessive-compulsiveness in some groups, more phobias in others, more or less depressions or manic states, more or less schizophrenic reactions, etc.
3. Variations in content: Our patients' delusions talk of radar waves, whereas a Papuan may be afraid to end up in his neighbor's cooking pot. It is hardly surprising that castration fear is externalized to the shrinkage of secondary sexual characteristics in a member of a culture in which little boys are constantly threatened to have their penises cut, even for minor infractions; or that mimicking is resorted to as a defense mechanism in cultures which demand that a social inferior agree to every word and deed of his superior.

Is culture also responsible for the quantitative epidemiological differences and the relative variations of the various psychiatric entities among different groups?

Lesbianism[51] was unknown among the Maoris in Australia until new restrictive sexual mores were introduced by missionaries. A previously conflict-free psychological area then became laden with anxiety; when the former sexual freedom ended, a new sexual outlet was found. Sexual psychopathology[25] is rare in societies which do not surround sex with threatening taboos. (For example, among the Trobrianders, and most tribes in East Africa.)

On the other hand, in cultures which regulate their members' daily life by strict rules, obsessive-compulsive neuroses seem to be infrequent, as if the need for this particular defense mechanism had been satisfied by the compulsiveness of the culture, whereas it is more common in societies which allow greater freedom of choice. This raises the interesting question whether our pursuit of ever greater freedom does not exact the tremendous price of more psychopathology.

Arieti,[6] in a paper about the relative frequency of affective disorders and schizophrenic reactions, found a remarkable decrease of the former, which he attributes to cultural changes.

Some authors[56,60,66,89,90,91,123,149] claim that cultural changes lead always to greater psychopathology. I believe this to be true only when these changes bring about new conflicts (for example, the Maoris mentioned above), when old value systems are destroyed without replacing them with new ones, when a previous group cohesion disappears, when old preferred positions within the group have to be given up (for example, the loss of status of the males among the Yemeni Jews in Israel). However, when the cultural changes help to alleviate old stressful conditions (e.g., the prohibition of cannibalism by Western powers in New Guinea and some South Sea Islands), psychiatric morbidity diminishes.

So far, we have explored whether culture increases the incidence of psychopathology. Can it encourage mental health?

I mentioned already the favorable changes wrought by the abolition of cannibalism, but there is a more basic influence, postulated by some authors, like Roheim[127] and Bertalanffy.[16,17] Roheim spent several years among the Papuans of Eastern New Guinea. He came to the conclusion that culture is *the* main defensive institution created by man against the onslaught of anxiety. Bertalanffy calls culture a "psychohygienic" factor; by providing standards of behavior, particularly of interpersonal relationships, it helps to diminish conflict-promoting situations which otherwise would tear apart the fabric of any human group.

❨ Bibliography

1. ABERLE, D. F. "Arctic Hysteria and Latah in Mongolia," *Transactions of the New York Academy of Science*, 2 (1952), 291–294.
2. ABRAHAM, J. J. "Latah and Amok," *The British Medical Journal*, (1912), 438–439.

3. ACKERKNECHT, E. H. "Psychopathology, Primitive Medicine and Primitive Culture," *Bull. Hist. Med.*, 14 (1930), 30.

4. ALPERS, M. "Changing Patterns of Kuru," *Amer. J. Trop. Med.*, 14 (1965), 852–879.

5. ARIETI, S. "Histopathologic Changes in Cerebral Malaria and Their Relation to Psychotic Sequels," *Arch. Neurol. and Psych.*, 56 (1946), 56–79.

6. ———. "Manic-Depressive Psychosis," in *American Handbook of Psychiatry*, 1st ed. S. Arieti ed., New York: Basic Books, 1959, 419–454.

7. ASCHER, E. "Psychodynamic Considerations in Gilles de la Tourette's Disease (Maladie des Tics)," *Amer. J. Psych.*, 105 (1948), 267–276.

8. ———. "Motor Syndromes of Functional or Undetermined Origin: Tics, Cramps, Gilles de la Tourette's Disease and Others," in *American Handbook of Psychiatry*, 1st. ed. Vol. III, S. Arieti ed., New York: Basic Books, 1966, 148–157.

9. BEALL, L. "The Psychopathology of Suicide in Japan," *Intern. J. Soc. Psychol.*, 15 (1968), 213–225.

10. BECKER, E. "The Relevance to Psychiatry of Recent Research in Anthropology," *Amer. J. Psychother.*, 15 (1962), 600–617.

11. BENEDICT, R. F. "Anthropology and the Abnormal," *J. Gen. Psychol.*, 10 (1934), 59.

12. ———. "Some Comparative Data on Culture and Personality With Reference to the Promotion of Mental Health," *Ment. Health*, 9 (1939), 245.

13. BENNETT, J. H. "Further Changes of Pattern in Kuru," *Med. J. Austr.*, 1 (1968), 379–386.

14. BERNDT, R. N., and C. BERNDT. "The Concept of Abnormality in an Australian Aboriginal Society," in *Psychoanalysis and Culture*, G. B Wilbur and W. Muensterberger eds., New York: International Universities Press, 1951, 75–89.

15. BERNE, E. A. "A Psychiatric Census of the South Pacific," *Amer. J. Psych.*, 117 (1960), 44–47.

16. BERTALANFFY, L. VON. "The Theory of Open Systems in Physics and Biology," *Science*, III (1950), 23.

17. ———. "General System Theory and Psychiatry, in *American Handbook of Psychiatry*, S. Arieti ed., Vol. III, New York: Basic Books, 1966, 705–721.

18. BRILL, A. A. "Piblokto or Hysteria Among Pear's Eskimos," *J. Nerv. and Ment. Dis.*, 40 (1913), 514–520.

19. BURTON-BRADLEY, B. G. "The Amok Syndrome in Papua and New Guinea," *Med. J. Psych.*, 1 (1968), 252.

20. ———. "Papua and New Guinea Transcultural Psychiatry: Some Hazards of the Mixed-Blood Marginal Situation," *Austr. and New Zeal. J. Psych.*, 1 (1967), 40.

21. ———. "Papua and New Guinea Transcultural Psychiatry: The First One Thousand Referrals," *Austr. and New Zeal. J. Psych.*, 3 (1969), 130–136.

22. CANNON, W. B. "Voodoo Death," *Amer. Anthropol.*, 44 (1942), 169.

23. CAROTHERS, J. C. "The African Mind in Health and Disease—A Study in Ethnopsychiatry," World Health Organization, Monograph series, Geneva, 1953.

24. CARPENTER, E. S. "Witch Fear Among the Aivilik Eskimos," *Amer. J. Psych.*, 110 (1953), 194.

25. CARSTAIRS, G. M. "Cultural Differences and Social Deviation," in *Pathology and Treatment of Sexual Deviations*, I. Rosen ed., London: Oxford University Press, 1964, 419–434.

26. CAWTE, J. E. "Ethnopsychiatry in Central Australia: I. Transitional Illnesses in the Eastern Aranda People," *Brit. J. Psych.*, 111 (1965), 1069.

27. CAWTE, J. E., G. N. BIANCHI, and L. G. KILOH. "Personal Discomfort in Australian Aborigines," *Austr. and New Zeal. J. Psych.* 2, (1968), 68.

28. CAWTE, J. E. and M. A. KIDSON. "Ethnopsychiatry in Central Australia: II. The Evolution of Illness in a Walbiri Lineage," *Brit. J. Psych.*, 111 (1964), 1079.

29. ———. "Australian Ethnopsychiatry: The Walbiri Doctor," *Med. J. Australia*, 2 (1969), 977.

30. CHANCE, N. A. "Conceptual and Methodological Problems in Crosscultural Health Research," *Amer. J. Publ. Health*, 52 (1961), 410–417.

31. ———. "A Crosscultural Study of Social Cohesion and Depression," rev. in *Transcult. Psych. Res.*, I (1964), 19–22.

32. CHIN, T. L., J. E. TONG, and K. E. SCHMIDT. "A Clinical and Survey Study of Latah in Sarawak, Malaysia," rev. in *Transcult. Psych. Res.*, VIII (1971), 134.

33. COOPER, J. M. "The Cree Witiko Psychosis," *Primitive Man*, 6 (1933), 24.

34. CORIAT, J. H., "Psychoneuroses Among Primitive Tribes," *J. Abnorm. and Soc. Psychol.*, 10 (1915), 201.

35. DEVEREUX, G. "Psychiatry and Anthropology: Some Research Objectives," *Bull. Menninger Clin.*, 16 (1952), 167.

36. ———. "Normal and Abnormal: The Key Problem of Psychiatric Anthropology," in *Some Uses of Anthropology: Theoretical and Applied*, Washington, D.C.: The Anthropol. Soc. of Washington, 1956.

37. ———. "Cultural Thought Models in Primitive and Modern Psychiatric Theories," *Psychiatry*, 21 (1958), 359–374.

38. ———. "Mohave Ethnopsychiatry and Suicide: The Psychiatric Knowledge and the Psychiatric Disturbances of an Indian Tribe," Bull. 175, Smithsonian Inst., Bur. Amer. Ethnology, Washington, D.C., 1961.

39. DOHRENWEND, B. P. and B. S. DOHRENWEND. *Social Status and Psychological Disorder*, New York: John Wiley and Sons, 1969.

40. DU BOIS, C. *The People of Alor*; A Social-Psychological Study of an East Indian Island, Minneapolis: Minneapolis University Press, 1944.

41. EDGERTON, E. R. "Conceptions of Psychosis in Four East African Societies," *Amer. Anthropol.*, 68 (1966), 408–425.

42. ENOCH, M. D., W. H. TRETHOWAN, and J. C. BARKER. "Some Unknown Psychiatric Syndromes," Bristol: John Wright and Sons, 1967.

43. FERNANDEZ-MARINA, R. "The Puerto Rican Syndrome," *Psychiatry*, 24 (1961), 79–82.

44. FORSTER, E. B. "The Theory and Practice of Psychiatry in Ghana," *Amer. J. Psychother.*, 16 (1962), 7–51.

45. FORTUNE, R. *The Sorcerers of Dobu*, London: G. Routledge and Sons, 1932.

46. FREITAS, J. L. P. DE, and R. T. MENDES. "Serological Study of Chronic Nervous Forms of Chagas Disease in Patients of a Psychiatric Hospital," *Rev. Paulista Med.*, 46 (1955), 123.

47. GAJDUSEK, J. "Slow-acting Virus Implicated in Kuru," *J. Am. Med. Assoc.*, 199 (1967), 34.

48. GAULT, E. I., J. KRUPINSKI, and A. STOLLER. "Psychological Problems of Aboriginal Adolescents and Their Socio-cultural Environment," *Austr. and New Zeal. J. Psych.*, 4 (1970), 174–182.

49. GEBER, M. and R. F. DEAN. "Psychological Factors in the Etiology of Kwashiokor," Bull. World Health Organiz., 11 (1954), 471.

50. GILLIN, J. "Magical Fright," *Psychiatry*, 11 (1948), 387–400.

51. GLUCKMAN, L. K. "Lesbianism in the Maori," *Austr. and New Zeal. J. Psych.*, 1 (1967), 98–103.

52. ———. "Drau Ni Kau, The Ethnopsychiatry of Fiji in Historical and Clinical Perspective," *Austr. and New Zeal. J. Psych.*, 3 (1969), 152.

53. GUSSOW, Z. "Pibloktoq (Hysteria) Among the Polar Eskimo: An Ethno-Psychiatric Study," in *Psychoanalysis and the Social Sciences* VI, W. Muensterberger and S. Axelrad eds., New York: International Univers. Press, 1960.

54. GWEE, AH-LENG. "Koro: Its Origin and Nature as a Disease Entity," *Singap. Med. J.*, 9 (1968), 3–6.

55. ———. "Koro," paper read at the World Feder. Ment. Health, Singapore, 1970.

56. HALEVI, H. S. "Frequency of Mental Illness Among Jews in Israel," *Internat. J. Soc. Psychol.*, 9 (1963), 268–282.

57. HALLOWELL, A. I. "Culture and Mental Disorders," *J. Abnorm. and Soc. Psychol.*, 29 (1934), 1.

58. ———. "The Social Function of Anxiety in a Primitive Society," *Amer. Sociol. Rev.*, 6 (1941), 869–881.

59. ———. "Myth, Culture and Personality," *Amer. Anthropol.*, 49 (1947), 544–556.

60. ———. "Values, Acculturation and Mental Health," *Amer. J. Orthopsych.* (1950), 732–743.

61. HOEVEN, J. A., VAN DER. "Psychiatrisch-neurologische Beobachtungen bei Papuans in Neu Guinea," *Arch. Psychiatr.*, 194 (1956), 415.

62. HORNEY, K. *The Neurotic Personality of Our Time*, New York: Norton, 1937.

63. HOSKIN, J. O. and A. VENESS. "Psychiatry in New Britain," *Austr. and New Zeal. J. Psych.*, 1 (1967), 35.

64. JACOBSON, A. and A. B. BERENBERG. "Japanese Psychiatry and Psychotherapy," *Amer. J. Psych.*, 109 (1952), 321.

65. KIDSON, M. A. "Psychiatric Disorders in the

Walbiri, Central Australia," *Austr. and New Zeal. J. Psych.*, 1 (1967), 14.

66. KIEV, A. "Beliefs and Delusions Among West Indian Immigrants to London," *Brit. J. Psych.*, 109 (1962), 356–363.

67. ———. "Primitive Therapy: A Cross-cultural Study of the Relationship Between Child Training and Therapeutic Practices Related to Illness," in *Psychoanalytic Study of Society*, Muensterberger and Axelrad eds., New York: International Univers. Press, 1964, 185–217.

68. ———. *Magic, Faith and Healing*, A. Kiev ed., New York: The Free Press of Glencoe, 1964.

69. ———. "Prescientific Psychiatry," in *American Handbook of Psychiatry*, 1st. ed. S. Arieti ed., New York: Basic Books, Vol. III, 1966, 166–179.

70. ———. *Transcultural Psychiatry*, London: The Free Press, Collier-Macmillan, 1972.

71. KIMURA, B., "Vergleichende Untersuchungen über Depressive Erkrankungen in Japan und in Deutschland," *Fortschr. Neurol. Psychiatr.*, 1 (1965), 14.

72. KLINE, N. S. "Psychiatry in the Underdeveloped Countries," Report of Roundtable Meetings, 116th Ann. Meet. Am. Psych. Assoc., Atlantic City, 1960.

73. ———. "Psychiatry in Kuwait," *Brit. J. Psych.*, 109 (1963), 766–774.

74. ———. "Psychiatry in Indonesia," *Am. J. Psych.*, 119 (1963), 809.

75. KRAEPELIN, E. "Vergleichende Psychiatrie," *Zentralbl. Nervenh. u. Psych.*, 27 (1904), 433.

76. KUBIE, L. S. "Social Forces and the Neurotic Process," in *Explorations in Social Psychiatry*, A. H. Leighton ed., New York: Basic Books, 1957, 98.

77. KUNITZ, S. J. "Equilibrium Theory in Social Psychiatry: The Work of the Leightons," *Psychiatry*, 33 (1970), 312–328.

78. LA BARRE, W. "Confession as Cathartic Therapy in American Indian Tribes," in *Magic, Faith and Healing*, A. Kiev ed., New York: The Free Press of Glencoe, 1964, 36–49.

79. LAMBO, T. A. "A Form of Social Psychiatry in Africa," *World Mental Health*, 13 (1961), 190.

80. ———. "Malignant Anxiety," *J. Ment. Sci.*, 108 (1962), 256–264.

81. ———. "Patterns of Psychiatric Care in Developing African Countries," in *Magic, Faith and Healing*, A. Kiev ed., New York: The Free Press of Glencoe, 1964, 443–453.

82. LAMONT, A. M., and W. J. BLIGNAULT. "A Study of Male Bantu Admissions at Weskoppies During 1952," *South Afric. Med. J.*, 27 (1953), 637.

83. LANDES, R. "The Abnormal Among the Ojibwa Indians," *J. Abnorm. and Soc. Psychol.*, 33 (1938), 14.

84. LANGER, T. S. and S. T. MICHAEL. "Life, Stress and Mental Health: The Midtown Manhattan Study," London: Collier-Macmillan, 1963.

85. LANGNESS, L. L. "Hysterical Psychoses in the New Guinea Highlands: A Benabena Example," *Psychiatry*, 28 (1965), 258–277.

86. ———. "Hysterical Psychosis: The Cross-cultural Evidence," *Amer. J. Psych.*, 124 (1967), 143.

87. LEIGHTON, A. H. "My Name is Legion: Foundations for a Theory of Man in Relation to Culture," vol. I, The Sterling County Study of Psychiatric Disorder and Socio-cultural Environment, New York: Basic Books, 1959.

88. ———. "Mental Illness and Acculturation," in *Medicine and Anthropology*, J. Galdstone, ed., New York: International Universities Press, 1959, 108–128.

89. ———. "Causes of Mental Disorder: A Review of Epidemiological Knowledge," Proceed. Roundtable Discuss. Arden House, Harriman, N.Y., Milbank Memorial Fund, 1959.

90. LEIGHTON, A. H., and J. M. MURPHY. "Cultures as Causative of Mental Disorder," *Milbank Memorial Fund Quarterly*, 39 (1961).

91. ———. *Psychiatric Disorders Among the Yoruba*, Ithaca: Cornell University Press, 1963.

92. LEIGHTON, D. C. "The Distribution of Psychiatric Symptoms in a Small Town," *Amer. J. Psych.*, 112 (1956), 716.

93. ———. *The Character of Danger: Psychiatric Symptoms in Selected Communities*, New York: Basic Books, 1963.

94. LENG, G. A. "Koro: Its Origin and Nature as a Disease entity," *Singapore Med. J.*, 9 (1968), 3–6.

95. LEON, D. A. "El Espanto," 2nd Latin-American Congress Psiquiatría, Mexico,

1962, rev. in *Transcult. Psych. Res.*, II (1965), 45–48.

96. LIN, T-Y. "Anthropological Study of the Incidence of Mental Disorders in the Chinese and Other Cultures," *Psychiatry*, 16 (1953), 313.

97. LINTON, R. *Culture and Mental Disorder*, Springfield, Ill.: Charles C Thomas, 1956.

98. LOPES, C. "Ethnographische Betrachtungen Über Die Schizophrenie," *Ztschr. f. d. Ges. Neurol. u. Psych.*, 142 (1932), 706.

99. LUBCHANSKY, I., G. EGRI and J. STOKES. "Puerto Rican Spiritualists View Mental Illness: The Faithhealer as a Paraprofessional," *Am. J. Psych.* 127 (1970), 312–321.

100. MacDONALD, I. J. "A Case of Gilles de la Tourette's Syndrome with some Aetiological Observations," *Brit. J. Psych.*, 109 (1963), 206–210.

101. McKEEL, H. S., "Clinic and Culture," *J. Abnorm. and Soc. Psych.*, 30 (1935), 292.

102. MAGUIGAD, E. L. "Psychiatry in the Philippines," *Am. J. Psych.*, 121 (1964), 21–25.

103. MARGETTS, E. L. in *Ciba Foundation Symposium on Crosscultural Psychiatry*. A. V. S. De Renck and R. Porter eds., Boston: Little, Brown and Co., (1965).

104. MATHEWS, J. D. "A Transmission Model for Kuru," *Lancet*, 1 (1967), 821–825.

105. MAY, L. C. "A Survey of Glossolalia and Related Phenomena in Non-Christian Religions," *Amer. Anthropol.*, 58 (1956), 75–86.

106. MAZUR, W. P. "Gilles de la Tourette's Syndrome," *Canad. M. J.*, 69 (1953), 520.

107. ———. "Gilles de la Tourette's Syndrome," *Edinburgh M. J.*, 60 (1953), 427.

108. MEAD, M. "Some Relationships Between Social Anthropology and Psychiatry," in F. Alexander and H. Ross eds., *Dynamic Psychiatry*, Chicago: University of Chicago Press, (1952), 401.

109. ———. "Illness as a Psychological Defense," in J. E. Fairchild ed., *Personal Problems and Psychological Frontiers*, New York: Sheridan, (1957).

110. MOFFSON, A. "A Study of 400 Consecutive Male Bantu Admissions in Weskoppies Mental Hospital," *South Afric. M. J.*, 291 (1955), 681.

111. MURPHY, H. B. M. "Culture and Mental Disorders in Singapore," in *Culture and Mental Health*, M. K. Opler ed., New York: The Macmillan Co., (1959).

112. MURPHY, H. B. M., E. D. WITTKOWER, and A. N. CHANCE. "Crosscultural Inquiry into the Symptomatology of Depression: A Preliminary Report," *Intern. J. Psych.*, 3 (1967), 6–15.

113. MURPHY, J. M. "Psychotherapeutic Aspects of Shamanism," in *Magic, Faith and Healing*, A. Kiev ed., New York: The Free Press of Glencoe, 1964.

114. MURPHY, J. M. and A. H. LEIGHTON. *Approaches to Cross-cultural Psychiatry*, Ithaca: Cornell University Press, 1965.

115. NEWMAN, P. L. "Wild Man Behavior in a New Guinea Community." *Amer. Anthro.*, 66 (1964), 1–19.

116. NGUI, P. W. "The Koro Epidemic in Singapore," *Austr. and New Zeal. J. Psych.*, II (1969), 263–266.

117. OPLER, M. E. "Some Points of Comparison and Contrast Between the Treatment of Functional Disorders by Apache Shamans and Modern Psychiatric Practice," *Amer. J. Psych.*, 92 (1935), 1371–1387.

118. OZTURK, O. M. "Folk Treatment in Turkey," in *Magic, Faith, and Healing*, A. Kiev ed., New York: The Free Press of Glencoe, 1964, 343–363.

119. PANDE, S. K. "The Mystique of 'Western' Psychotherapy: An Eastern Interpretation," *J. Nerv. and Ment. Dis.*, 146 (1968), 425–432.

120. PARKER, S. "Eskimo Psychopathology in the Context of Eskimo Personality and Culture," *Amer. Anthro.*, 64 (1962), 76–96.

121. PFEIFFER, W. M. *Transkulturelle Psychiatrie—Ergebnisse und Probleme*, Stuttgart: G. Thieme Verlag, 1970.

122. ———. "Die Stellung des Psychisch Kranken in Aussereuropäischen Kulturen," Paper presented at Kongress der Deutschen Gesellschaft für Psych. u. Nervenheilk., Bad Nauheim, West Germany, October 1970.

123. PFLANZ, M. and L. LAMBELET. "Zivilisationskrankheiten und Psychosomatische Probleme im Ländlichen Indien," *Münch. Med. Wschr.* (1965), 1493–1502.

124. PIDOUX. C. "Les États de Possession Rituelle Chez les Mélano-Africains: Eléments d'une Étude Psychosociologique de Leur Manifestations," *Evolution Psychiatr.*, 2 (1955), 271.

125. PLANQUES, L. and H. COLLOMB. "Les Psychoses des Noires," *Rev. du Corps de Santé Milit.*, 13 (1957), 194.

126. RAWNSLEY, K. and J. B. LONDON. "Epidemiology of Mental Disorders in a Closed Community," *Brit. J. Psych.*, 110 (1964), 830–839.

127. ROHEIM, G. "The Origin and Function of Culture," *Nerv. and Ment. Dis. Monographs*, 1943.

128. RUBEL, A. J. "The Epidemiology of a Folk Illness: Susto in Hispano-America," *Ethnology*, 3 (1964), 268–283.

129. SAPIR, E. "Cultural Anthropology and Psychiatry," *J. Abnorm. and Soc. Psychol.*, 27 (1932), 229.

130. ———. "Culture and Personality," in *Selected Writings of E. Sapir in Language, Culture, and Personality*, D. G. Mandelbaum ed., Berkeley, Cal.: University of California Press, 1951.

131. SCHNECK, J. M. "Gilles de la Tourette's Disease," *Am. J. Psych.*, 120 (1963), 78.

132. SELIGMAN, C. G. "Temperament, Conflict and Psychosis in a Stone-age Population," *Brit. J. Med. Psychol.*, 4 (1929), 195.

133. SELYE, H. *The Stress of Life*, New York: McGraw Hill, 1956.

134. SHELLEY, H. M. and W. H. WATSON. "An Investigation Concerning Mental Disorders in the Nyasaland Natives," *J. Ment. Sci.*, 87 (1936), 701.

135. SINGER, K. "Gilles de la Tourette's Disease," *Am. J. Psych.*, 117 (1963), 80–81.

136. SPIES, T. "Nutrition and Disease, Pellagrous Psychosis," *Postgrad. Med. J.*, 17 (1955), 70.

137. SPIRO, M. E. "A Psychotic Personality in the South Seas," *Psychiatry*, vol. 13, (1950), 189–204.

138. ———. "The Psychological Function of Witchcraft: The Burmese Case," Paper presented at Conference on Mental Health in Asia and the Pacific, Honolulu, 1966, rev. in *Transcult. Psych. Res.*, III (1966), 127.

139. STAINBROOK, E. "Some Characteristics of the Psychopathology of Schizophrenic Behavior in Bahian Society," *Am. J. Psych.*, 109 (1952), 330.

140. STANLEY, D. R. and D. THONG. "Shamanism Versus Psychiatry in Bali, 'Isle of Gods': Some Modern Implications," *Am. J. Psych.*, 129 (1972), 59–62.

141. STEVENS, H. "Jumping Frenchmen of Maine," *Arch. Neurol.*, 12 (1965), 311.

142. STITT, E. R. and R. STRONG. *Diagnosis, Prevention and Treatment of Tropical Diseases*, New York: Blakiston, 1945.

143. TENZEL, J. H. "Shamanism and Concepts of Disease in a Mayan Indian Community," *Psychiatry*, 33 (1970), 372–380.

144. TOBIN, W. G. and J. B. REINHART. "Tic de Gilles de la Tourette," *Amer. J. Dis. Chilr.*, 101 (1961), 778–783.

145. TOOTH, G. C. "Studies in Mental Illness in the Gold Coast," London, Her Majesty's Stationery Office, 1950, Colonial Research Papers, no. 6.

146. TOURETTE, de la G. "Jumping, Latah, Myriachit," *Arch. de Neurol.* (1884), 68.

147. WALLACE, A. E., and R. E. ACKERMAN. "An Interdisciplinary Approach to Mental Disorder Among the Polar Eskimos of Northwest Greenland," *Anthropologica*, 11 (1960), 1–12.

148. WEDGE, B. M. "Occurrence of Psychoses Among Okinawans in Hawaii," *Am. J. Psych.*, 109 (1952), 255.

149. WEIDMAN, H. H. and J. N. SUSSEX. "Cultural Values and Egofunctioning in Relation to the Atypical Culture-bound Reactive Syndromes," Paper read at the Second Intern. Congr. Soc. Psych., London, 1969.

150. WESTBROOK, C. H. "Psychiatry and Mental Hygiene in Shanghai: Historical Sketch," *Am. J. Psych.*, 110 (1953), 301.

151. WILFFTEN PALTHE, P. VAN. "Psychiatry and Neurology in the Tropics," in A. Liechtenstein, *A Clinical Textbook of Tropical Medicine*, Batavia: De Langen, 1936.

152. WITTKOWER, E. D. and J. FRIED. "Some Problems of Transcultural Psychiatry," in *Culture and Mental Health*, K. M. Opler ed., New York.: Macmillan, 1959.

153. YAP, P. M. "Mental Diseases Peculiar to Certain Cultures: A Survey of Comparative Psychiatry," *J. Ment. Sci.*, 97 (1951), 313.

154. ———. "The Latah Reaction: Its Pathodynamics and Nosological Position," *J. Ment. Sci.*, 98 (1952), 515.

155. ———. "Words and Things in Comparative Psychiatry, with Special Reference to the Exotic Psychoses," *Acta Psych. Scandin.*, 38 (1962), 163.

156. ———. "Koro—A Culture-bound Depersonilization Syndrome," *Brit. J. Psych.*, 111 (1965), 43.

157. ———. "The Culture-bound Reactive Syn-

dromes," in *Mental Health Research in Asia and the Pacific*, W. Caudill and T. Lin eds., Honolulu: East-West Center Press, 33–53.

158. ———. "Classification of the Culture-bound Reactive Syndromes," *Austr. and New Zeal. J. Psych.*, 3 (1969), 172–179.

159. ZAGUIRRE, J. C. "Amok in the Philippines," *J. Philippin. Fed. Priv. Med. Pract.*, 8 (1957), 1338.

PART SEVEN

Unclassified Behavior and Syndromes and Those Intermediate between Neurosis and Psychosis

CHAPTER 33

SUICIDE

James M. A. Weiss

THE SUICIDE OF A PATIENT, because of its finality, is perhaps the most devastating experience in the practice of psychiatry. And suicide, considered as a sign of mental disorder, is a prime cause of death among psychiatric patients. Inextricably involved with the attitudes, folkways, mores, taboos, and laws of culture and subculture, with tragedy for the person and the group, with emotions and values, suicide is a sociopsychiatric phenomenon about which much confusion exists. The nature of this phenomenon is complex, and its scientific study is difficult, in part for the obvious reason that persons who have committed suicide successfully are no longer available for psychological or psychiatric study. The universal fascination of the study of suicide, however, is reflected in the great bulk of literature concerning this subject. There are now more than 7000 books and articles about suicide (exemplified by Farberow's extensive bibliography[25] and an American journal—the *Bulletin of Suicidology*—devoted solely to this topic). But much prior research into suicide and attempted suicide has tended to be either actuarial and at times

somewhat superficial, or clinical and often anecdotal, or oriented to depth psychology and rather speculative.

It does seem evident that there are three chief etiological factors in suicide: the group attitudes in each particular society, the adverse extraneous situations that each person must meet, and the interaction of these with his character and personality. This last single variable appears to be the most important one. Obviously, different persons meet adversity differently. One whose personality is poorly integrated may respond to stress by taking or attempting to take his own life. Yet anthropologists and epidemiologists have demonstrated that suicide may be completely unknown among certain primitive tribes, that suicide rates are extremely low in certain countries, and, alternatively, that suicide is not only acceptable but obligatory as a consequence of certain specified activities or happenings in certain other cultures. The ancient warrior people of Germany and Scandinavia, as well as the Greek Stoics, approved of suicide, Oriental and Hindu cultures sanctioned it under specified conditions, and in some

South Sea Islands it is looked upon even today as an honorable act.[22] However, as cultural patterns affect large numbers of people who do not always act similarly, and as every person must meet difficult and dangerous situations in an environment that can never be "sterilized" psychologically, it appears likely that some degree of personality disintegration is the most important single variable in the etiology of suicide. The psychiatric concept applies, that external tensions are reacted to in proportion to the amount of internal tension already existing.

❲ Definitions and Types

Even the definition of suicide presents difficulties. The "suicidal patient" may be one who successfully commits suicide, unsuccessfully attempts suicide, threatens suicide, demonstrates suicidal ideation, or behaves in generally self-destructive patterns. "The expression 'suicidal act' is used . . . [by the World Health Organization[133]] to denote the self-infliction of injury with varying degrees of lethal intent and awareness of motive. . . . 'Suicide' means a suicidal act with fatal outcome, 'attempted suicide' one with non-fatal outcome." Operationally, some possibility of self-inflicted fatal termination is most commonly the distinguishing criterion of the term "suicidal." Thus, most investigators define successful or committed suicide as a violent self-inflicted destructive action resulting in death. Attempted suicide is usually defined similarly, except that there is no fatal termination; but, as Stengel[111] has pointed out, the action must have a "self-destructive intention, however vague and ambiguous. Sometimes this intention has to be inferred from the patient's behavior." The suicidal gesture is similar except that persons performing such an action neither intend to end life nor expect to die as a result of their action, although the action is performed in a manner that other persons might interpret as suicidal in purpose. In suicidal threats, the intention is expressed, but no relevant action is performed; in suicidal ideation, the person thinks or talks or writes about suicide without expressing any definite intent or performing any relevant action. (The term "parasuicide," to designate attempted suicide and related actions, has recently come into vogue. That term is, however, both ambiguous and a solecism, and should be deleted.)

The problem is further complicated by persons in the category termed by Farberow and Shneidman[27] the "submeditated death group," in whom unconscious or preconscious motivation to die or be killed is such that a large number of conditions (purposive accidents, provoked homicides, neglected personal health care, involvement in dangerous activities, and even severe psychosomatic disorders) might be considered suicidal equivalents. Whether such acts, as well as one-car accidents, voluntary overwork, drug addiction, chain-smoking, and alcoholism, are in fact "partial" or "chronic" suicidal attempts is debatable. Tabachnick[120] found that "suicidal and self-destructive factors which we tested for do *not* play a significant role in the general [automobile] accident picture." Choron[16] stated, "One could maintain that it is the lesser evil to drown one's sorrows in alcohol than to drown one's self," and suggested that such behavior might actually be a defense against suicide.

Actually, all medical-legal definitions of "suicide" or "attempted suicide" do include the concept that the person played a major role in bringing about, or trying to bring about, his own demise, and that his conscious intention in his behavior was to die. However, increasing evidence indicates that successful suicide and unsuccessful suicidal attempts represent two different kinds of acts performed in different ways for different reasons by different groups of people, although there is some overlapping. For example, successful suicides are more common among older people, males, and single, divorced, or widowed persons; reported unsuccessful suicidal attempts are more likely to occur among younger people, females, and the married population. In the United States during the past fifty years, about two-thirds of the persons who successfully committed suicide used the two methods of shooting or hanging; most persons reported to have attempted suicide unsuccessfully used ingestion of poison, cutting or slashing, or inhalation of gas—all less efficient than shooting and hanging, which only rarely fail to cause death. Several studies[27,67] have indicated that the success of the suicidal attempt varies markedly with the reported conscious "motive." Thus, for the modal committer of suicide the motive is most likely to be judged as "concern about ill health" or "loss of a loved one," as compared to the modal attempter of suicide for whom the motive is most likely to be "domestic or family worries" or "difficulties in love affairs."

Stengel and Cook[116] have reviewed the confusion that exists in the psychiatric literature relating to evaluation of the seriousness of suicidal attempts, and concluded that to understand such phenomena it is necessary to consider separately the degree of psychological intent and the degree of medical injury. Stengel,[115] Weiss et al.,[128] and other investigators have therefore rated cases as "serious" in psychological intent when an unambiguous impulse to suicide is admitted by the patient and also borne out by the patient's behavior before, during, and after the attempt. In such cases, the patient does not inform anyone else of the attempt in order to effect a rescue, does not make the attempt when other persons are present or nearby or likely to arrive in time to prevent death, and expects that he or she will certainly die as a result of the act. Attempts are rated as "gestures" when the patient clearly does not expect to die, as evidenced by his overt admission and behavior. Such gestures seem to be made most often to gain attention or to influence other persons, and the attempter often takes considerable precaution to make sure of remaining alive by making the attempt with other persons present, informing someone of the attempt, or initiating his own rescue. Suicidal attempts that are neither serious nor gestures have been defined by Weiss[125] as "gambles," insofar as the patient is uncertain about the possible consequences of the act or does not know for sure whether

he can expect certain death as a result of the act but believes there is some chance (even a good chance) of dying, as evidenced by his overt admission and behavior.

As to the medical consequences, suicidal attempts are rated as "absolutely dangerous" when the act results in severe danger to life with a very high probability that the patient will die, except for timely medical intervention. Generally, such acts produce such consequences as coma, bloody diarrhoea, penetrating injuries, fracture of a major bone, or laceration of a major artery. Cases are rated as "absolutely harmless" when there is no chance that the act will cause death under any foreseeable circumstances. "Somewhat dangerous" serves as an in-between category.

Weiss et al.[128] have termed the medically dangerous, psychologically serious attempts "aborted successful suicidal attempts," since these attempts were found to be qualitatively different from all others, and attempters in this group appeared to be epidemiologically more similar to persons who successfully committed suicide than to other classes of attempters. Probably, most persons who make such aborted successful suicidal attempts are brought to the attention of police, physicians, or hospitals, and are included in the statistical reporting of suicidal attempts. At the other end of the continuum are the persons who make medically harmless suicidal gestures, who are only rarely brought to the attention of reporting agencies. The remaining suicidal gambles, with varying severity of medical consequences, might be termed "true suicidal attempts," in the sense that persons making this sort of attempt appear to perform a violent, self-inflicted, destructive action with ambiguous intent, but with some chance of fatal termination. Of course, in some of these true suicidal attempts the gamble with death is undoubtedly lost—the attempter dies and the attempt is counted as a completed successful suicide. Many true suicidal attempts may not be brought to the attention of the authorities, but the large numbers that are made known to them appear to comprise the major segment of all reported cases of suicidal attempts.

❦ Basic Etiological Approaches

Dublin's[22] comprehensive review of the history of suicide indicates a marked interest in the subject since ancient times, but the scientific study of this phenomenon began only toward the end of the nineteenth century. In 1897, Emile Durkheim[23] published his famous monograph, "*Le Suicide*," an exhaustive statistical and sociological examination of the problem. Durkheim concluded that the common factor in all suicide patterns was the increasing alienation between the person and the social group to which he belonged. He suggested that a basic element, *anomie*—a sort of psychosocial isolatedness that occurs whenever the links that unite individual human beings into consolidated groups are weakened—is primary in the understanding of suicide in modern society.* Other ecological studies have provided important information to this end. Cavan[15] related the suicide rates in urban districts of Chicago to the degree of social disorganization in those areas. Gruhle[41] demonstrated how suicide rates were altered with social and cultural variations in different geographic sections of pre-World War II Germany. Sainsbury,[96] in a study of suicide in London, found that measures of social isolation correlated significantly with suicide rates. Yap's[134] report on suicide in Hong Kong also indicated the importance of the social matrix, noting especially high rates among immigrants from rural areas.

Most psychiatrists and psychoanalysts have identified suicide with self-directed aggressive

* In an attempt to explain the statistical facts as they were then known, Durkheim divided suicide into three social categories—anomic, egoistic, and altruistic. He postulated that "anomic" suicide results from a severe disorder in the equilibrium of society, disturbing the balance of a person's integration with his culture and leaving him without his customary norms of behavior. "Egoistic" suicide results from a lack of integration of the individual with other members of the group, and infrequently "altruistic" suicide results from "insufficient individuation," when proneness to suicide stems, rather, from excessive integration into a group that might at times require an individual to sacrifice his life (as in the case of the old person who has become a financial burden to his family).

tendencies. Freud[35] emphasized that melancholy and subsequent suicide are often the result of aggression directed at least partially toward an introjected love object, that is, a love object with whom the subject had previously identified himself. Later, Freud[34] established suicide as the extreme manifestation of the active component of the death instinct directed against the self. Schilder,[97] writing alone, and with Bromberg,[11] believed that "suicide is obviously merely a symptom and not a clinical entity"[97] and that, although suicide can serve as a form of self-aggression or as self-punishment for aggressive behavior previously directed toward another (loved) person, it may also serve as a form of punishment for a person who earlier may have denied love to the subject, or as a form of peace (or reunion with a love object), or certainly as an escape from insupportable difficulties.

Bernfeld's[8] classic formulation of the basic mental mechanisms underlying suicide was this: A person committing suicide does so because of strong, unconscious murderous impulses against another person, but the committer must also unconsciously identify himself with the hated (previously loved) object, so that he kills that object in killing himself. Since the committer usually feels guilty because of his murderous impulses, a tendency to self-punishment is commonly involved, and the choice of the method of suicide may have symbolic significance. Menninger[64,65] has elaborated these mechanisms in his well-known statement that the true suicide must expect to kill, be killed, and die, as well as in his discussions of "partial" or "chronic" tendencies to self-destruction. Menninger saw suicide in any form as the result of the struggle between Thanatos and Eros, with the former winning. All varieties of physical and psychological self-damage can be subsumed under his definition, with the suicidal act arising out of the conflict between an aggressive drive directed toward the self and the countering tendency toward both the preservation of the self and the restoration of the self's relations with other (loved) human beings. Jung[50] stressed unconscious wishes for a spiritual rebirth in a person who has a strong feeling that life has lost all its meaning, and Adler[1] emphasized inferiority, narcissism, and low self-esteem, as the characteristics of the potential suicide victim. Sullivan[118] regarded suicide as evidence of a failure arising out of unresolved interpersonal conflicts, and according to Horney[46] it occurs within a context of extreme alienation of the self resulting from great disparity between the idealized self and the perceived psychosocial self-entity (a formulation that becomes more attractive the longer one studies this subject).

In one symposium, Lindemann[39] suggested that the "state of readiness for violent behavior," the form of aggression that may or may not end in suicide, be termed "hypereridism" (from *Eris*, the Greek goddess of wrath and anger). Fenichel[31] summed up the psychoanalytic characteristics of this state as "an ambivalent dependence on a sadistic superego and the necessity to get rid of an unbearable guilt tension at any cost." The person submits to punishment and to the superego's cruelty, and may express the passive thought of giving up any active fighting; more actively, and at the same time, there is a turning of sadism against the person himself, a rebellion against the punishing superego. The intensity of this struggle is reflected in the depressed patient's strong tendency toward suicide. The ego, trying to appease the superego by submissiveness, has erred. The hoped-for forgiveness cannot be achieved because the courted part of the personality, through regression, has become sadistic, and, from the standpoint of the superego, the suicide of the depressed patient results from a turning of this sadism against the person himself. On the other hand, from the standpoint of the ego, suicide is an expression of the fact that the tension induced by the pressure of the superego has become unbearable. Frequently, the loss of self-esteem is so complete that any hope of regaining it is abandoned. As Fenichel wrote, "To have a desire to live evidently means to feel a certain self-esteem, to feel supported by the protective forces of a superego. When this feeling vanishes, the original annihilation of the deserted hungry baby reappears."

Other suicidal acts may have a far more active character, for they are simultaneously extreme acts of submission and extreme acts of rebellion (that is, murder of the original objects whose incorporation created the superego). Psychoanalyses of persons attempting suicide have frequently demonstrated that ideas of a relaxing gratification, or hopeful and pleasurable fantasies, may be connected with the idea of suicide. Such ideation is unconsciously related to hopes of forgiveness and reconciliation, with a simultaneous killing of the *punishing* superego and reunion with the *protecting* superego—thus putting an end to all losses of self-esteem by bringing back original fantasies of omnipotence.

These and similar psychodynamic theories of suicide may be valid, but they may also contain inherent methodological errors. They are based on data derived either from persons who, during or after a period of psychoanalytic scrutiny, have committed suicide successfully, or from persons who attempted suicide unsuccessfully. Generalizing from the few cases of the former type may be incorrect, for it is certainly possible that new dynamic forces —occurring between the last interview and the time of the actual suicide, and therefore unavailable for analysis—played a part. The relevance of premortem idiographic data to an understanding of the actual crisis that resulted in any particular successful suicide is therefore open to some question. And, since current data make it clear that successful suicide is not simply an exaggerated or completed form of attempted suicide, formulation of dynamic theories about successful suicide by extrapolation from what has been learned in clinical studies of patients who have attempted suicide is hardly justified.

However, the basic psychoanalytic concept involving self-directed aggression appears to hold, since suicide rates and homicide rates are often inversely related by cities and other regions, probably by countries, among certain racial and ethnic groups, and in periods of prosperity and depression. As Henry and Short[45] noted, "When behavior is required to conform rigidly to the demands and expectations of other persons, the probability of suicide as a response to frustration is low and the probability of homicide as a response to frustration is high. . . ." and vice versa. The often surprisingly low suicide rates among persons living under grim conditions—concentration camps, for instance, or really bad slums, or front-line combat—seem to support this observation. West[130] studied murderers in England and found that about one-third of them killed themselves after killing their victims. (About two-fifths of the suicidal murderers in this group were women.) Such suicidal murders were more likely to be involved in killing a spouse, lover, or child, and there was some evidence indicating that motivation may have been more related to despair than aggression.

The psychoanalytical point of view therefore may be as valid as the sociological theory stressing *anomie* and the lack of integration within human groups as etiological, but some synthesis of the two points of view is possible and should prove more comprehensive. The most frequently cited common characteristic of persons who later kill themselves is loneliness, or psychosocial isolation. Many investigations have pointed to a disruption of close personal relationships, particularly bereavement or loss, as being a main precipitating factor in suicidal behavior.[70,133] Such isolating factors as broken homes, unemployment, and old age have been noted. Weiss[127] found the major factor in the high suicide rates among older people to be such isolation along with depreciating sociocultural attitudes, low socioeconomic status with loss of psychologically and socially rewarding occupation, biological decline, and clinically recognizable psychiatric disorder. Psychological inability, refusal, or lack of opportunity to relate to others is clearly important, but many people continue living under such conditions. To precipitate a crisis, something more is necessary. Alvarez[2] (like West) indicated that this "something more" is despair. The victim sees no hope; when some possibilities exist, he denies or overlooks them. He turns to suicide, then, not because of any positive desire for death, but because he no longer can hope.

Zilboorg,[135,136] Andics,[4] and others have pointed out that persons who were denied in childhood a normal loving relationship with their parents or parental surrogates are likely to feel unloved and unwanted in later life, and therefore to develop suicidal tendencies. Hendin[44] found differential suicide rates in three Scandinavian countries to be related to child-rearing patterns. High rates in Sweden and Denmark were associated with rigid self-demands for superior performance (with subsequent self-hate for failure) in the former, and a "dependency loss" dynamic in the latter. The lower rates in Norway, on the other hand, were associated with persons reared to be externally aggressive who only become suicidal when that aggression is inverted toward the self. Hendin's methodology has been criticized, but other investigators have found that suicidal acts among children, although rare, are related to a need for love and at the same time to a desire to punish both the self and the human environment. Paffenbarger's[75,76] and his colleagues' studies of 40,000 American male former university students (with examination of records of fifteen to forty years previous) revealed that early loss or absence of the father was the dominant distinguishing characteristic of their subjects who committed suicide. Such developmental patterns may well provide a common etiological factor, since they are also likely to lead to social isolation, a hypothesis substantiated in part by the studies of Walton.[124]

Comprehensive psychosocial studies of the etiology of attempted suicide (rather than successful suicide) have been somewhat more common. In Stengel and Cook's[116] extensive investigations, attempted suicide was studied as a meaningful and momentous event in the person's life with special consideration of its effects on the social environment. Their chief conclusions were: (1) that the suicidal attempt is a phenomenon different from the successful suicide, one that should be studied as a behavior pattern of its own; (2) that an appeal to the human environment is a primary function of the suicidal attempt; and (3) that the suicidal attempt has a variety of social effects, especially on interpersonal relations, which may determine the eventual result of the attempt. Stengel and Cook declared that "in our society every suicidal warning or attempt has an appeal function whatever the mental state in which it is made." Their evidence supporting this statement is strong (although it may not apply to the limited group of aborted successful suicidal attempts), and their work makes it clear that attempted suicide does not represent a simple dynamic or even diagnostic pattern but is usually overdetermined behavior, involving both the person himself and the social environment in which he functions.

In contrast to this point of view, many persons still regard attempted suicide simply as a gesture to bring another person to terms. Although this secondary gain probably motivates the suicidal gesture per se, Weiss[125] demonstrated that the dynamics of the true suicidal attempt are more complicated, and involve in all cases a discharge of self-directed aggressive tendencies through a gamble with death (of varying lethal probability), in most cases an appeal for help, and in some cases a need for punishment and a trial by ordeal. First of all, true suicidal attempts are consciously or unconsciously arranged in such a manner that the lethal probability may vary from almost certain survival to almost certain death, and "fate"—or at least some force external to the conscious choice of the person— is compelled in some perhaps magical way to make the final decision. This appears to hold for the attempts of hysteric and psychopathic patients, as well as for those of schizophrenic and depressed psychotics.[115] The psychodynamic factors involved in such suicidal attempts are probably not unlike those involved in gambling itself, as described, for example, by Fenichel.[31] There is evidence that the true suicidal attempt does serve to discharge aggressive tendencies directed against the self or against introjected parental figures—self-mutilation may play a part in this. Both Stengel and Weiss have noted that patients who had made true suicidal attempts, whether or not they were then treated in any psychotherapeutic manner, demonstrated considerable subsequent improvement in affective state and general outlook. In some cases, improvement following the attempt appeared to be related to a guilt-relieving mechanism; the patients felt that in the very attempt, and in the associated gamble with death, they were punished for whatever acts committed or fantasies entertained that had contributed to their feelings of guilt. Stengel and Cook[117] noted that the outcome of the attempt "is almost invariably accepted for the time being and further attempts are rarely made immediately, even if there is no lack of opportunity. The outcome of the attempt is accepted like that of a trial by ordeal in mediaeval times."

In most true suicidal attempts, there is also discernible an effect of hidden or overt appeal to society, a "cry for help." The attempts are causally related to difficulties with interpersonal relationships and the social environment, but most attempters manage to maintain some contact with other persons, so that the call for help may be recognized. Stengel and Cook,[116] and later Farberow and Shneidman,[27] have demonstrated that such an appeal is inherent in most true suicidal attempts, irrespective of the mental state and the personality of the attempter. Evoking some change in the social situation, through the responses of individuals or groups to this conscious or unconscious appeal for help, is, then, one of the primary functions of such attempts. In the unreported cases, the person's difficulties are probably so modified as a consequence of the suicidal attempt that no immediate further action is required. Many people, whether responding as friends, policemen, or physicians, do not consciously recognize this appeal; nevertheless, they are shocked and interested by the fact that some human being was so disturbed as to attempt to take his own life. The suicidal act, although taboo in Judaeo-Christian culture, usually arouses sufficient sympathy to bring about some change in the circumstances surrounding the person who makes the attempt.

Often, the relationship of the patient to other persons, or to groups, undergoes marked changes as the consequences of a suicidal attempt. These changes are not usually consciously planned. Some relationships are strengthened, some terminated, but almost always the true suicidal attempt results in some immediate change in the constellation of relationships of the person to other persons or to the whole social group (although these changes may not be lasting). The fact that as a consequence of the attempt many persons are admitted to a hospital, there to remain for varying lengths of time, in itself often effects proximate changes. The patient is ready to accept these changes, for he has (it might be said) listened to the demands of a severe superego, atoned for his sins by attempting suicide in such a manner that he gambled with death, and accepted the outcome—life— as the answer (or perhaps reward), in a general sense, of fate or a divine judgment, or, more specifically, of the superego.

Since Weiss et al.[128] found the relatively small but important group of aborted successful suicidal attempters to be epidemiologically and clinically more similar to successful than to other nonsuccessful attempters, it seems likely that those persons whose attempts are both medically dangerous and psychologically serious may be differentiated psychodynamically as well from those whose attempts are not, and will in fact demonstrate patterns similar to those whose attempts are successful. Custer and Weiss[18] found that the dynamics of the aborted successful suicidal attempters were similar to those of a matched group of clinically depressed patients who had not evidenced suicidal behavior, but the attempters in addition had been predisposed both by a family history of suicide and by loss of one or both parents before age fifteen. With a past history of prior attempts, these suicidal persons then made the index serious attempt, precipitated in most cases by loss of a loved one within three months prior to the act.

It should be noted that the psychodynamics of suicidal attempts among children and adolescents may be somewhat different from those of adults. Many studies have indicated that the risk of attempted suicide with nonfatal outcome may be very high in the younger age groups, particularly among females and in the lower socioeconomic classes. In contrast with the older age groups, personal and domestic problems appear to predominate as causes and several investigators have found a high incidence of broken homes in early youth.[53,54,133] Schrut[101] noted that such younger attempters often have been involved in a series of various self-destructive acts. Such acts appear to arise from feelings of anxiety and helplessness which may be reduced by arousing parental concern. Jacobs[47] interviewed fifty adolescent suicide attempters, examined in detail their life histories, and compared them with those of a matched control group. The resulting data indicated that adolescent suicide attempters, as compared to the control nonattempters, demonstrated long-standing psychological problems, which escalated rapidly and to a marked degree after the onset of puberty. With subsequent progressive failure of available coping techniques, these adolescents then became more and more socially isolated. Finally, in the weeks and days preceding the suicide attempt, there appeared to be a chain-reaction dissolution of any meaningful social relationships which might have helped the subject deal with both old and increasing new problems.*

⟦ Basic Epidemiological Patterns

Since the classic research of Durkheim, the frequent occurrence of certain statistical trends and personality characteristics among persons who have attempted or committed suicide has been noted in a number of large-scale studies (reviewed by Dahlgren,[19] Dublin,[22] Farberow and Shneidman,[27] Rost,[92] Sainsbury,[96] Stengel,[115,116] and Weiss[126]). Such investigations have indicated that the more serious or successful suicidal attempts are most likely to occur among older persons, males, divorced, widowed, single, or married persons without children, persons isolated socially, persons with one or more close relatives dead or who have a history of suicide in the immediate family, persons who have made prior suicidal attempts, persons who use shoot-

* Jacobs drew some questionable inferences from these data regarding the nature of successful suicide, but his basic findings related to attempted suicide among adolescents appear to be valid.

ing or hanging as the attempted or considered method, persons who attribute the act to "concern about ill health" or "loss of a loved one," and persons suffering from affective psychoses, schizophrenic reactions, delirious states, chronic brain syndromes, or chronic alcoholism, or persons who appear clinically depressed regardless of diagnosis.*

The validity and importance of epidemiological studies as an adjunct to clinical analyses have been discussed and justified by numerous authors, Dublin[22] in particular. At one conference,[39] Faris cited the case of a scientist who made a newspaper statement to the effect that the marked decrease in United States suicide rates in the decade from 1937 to 1947 was undoubtedly due to the great popularity during that period of electric shock treatment of the mentally ill. The cited scientist was unaware, apparently, that suicide rates almost invariably decrease in periods (as in the decade noted) of war or prosperity. Suicide rates do vary from year to year: The rate in the United States at the beginning of the century was 10.2 suicides per 100,000 persons per year, and by 1915 it had increased to 16.2. The number of people taking their own lives decreased sharply in 1916 and continued to decline through the war years and immediate post-war years until, in 1920, the rate had returned to 10.2 per 100,000. By 1921, the rate had risen to 12.4, remaining near this level for the next five years. After 1925, it climbed steadily upward, reaching its maximum of 17.4 in 1932. In the later depression years, the rate dropped slowly to about 10 during World War II; thereafter, it has remained fairly constant between 10 and 12 per 100,000, although the lowest rate since 1900 has been 9.8, reached in 1957.[71]

More than 20,000 suicides now are recorded each year in the United States, and Dublin[22] has estimated that the true number is no less than 25,000 (more recently, Choron[16] suggested at least 30,000). Death by suicide thus represents about 1 to 2 percent of all deaths occurring in the United States during the year. An average of at least 1,000 persons each day commit suicide throughout the world, 80 of these in the United States. Thus, perhaps half a million persons in the world die by their own hand each year, and suicide has ranked among the first twelve causes of death in most European countries and in North America for many years. If these trends continue, out of every 1,000 white male infants, at least fifteen will eventually take their own lives; out of every 1,000 white female infants, four will do so, according to Dublin.

Many countries have higher suicide rates than the United States, especially Hungary, Finland, Austria, Czechoslovakia, Japan, Denmark, Germany, Switzerland, Sweden, France, and Australia. In striking contrast, suicide rates for Israel, Norway, the Netherlands, and Italy are low, and those for Ireland and Spain are extremely low, as are those in several South American countries. Sweden's rate is still roughly what it was before implementation of extensive welfare programs. Recent investigations have shown that suicide in developing countries is a more important problem than was formerly suspected.[133]

It is notable that suicide in white America is concentrated among older people: The rates for white males increase consistently with each advancing age group, while for white females they do so until the mid-fifties or early sixties, after which they tend to level or begin some decline. (Rates for nonwhite persons show somewhat different and less decided patterns.) Children rarely kill themselves, although, because of the often spectacular and tragic nature of the act, successful suicides of children and adolescents are sometimes thought to be quite frequent. Recent age-specific rates do show upward trends for the younger and middle ages, with a slightly downward trend for the older ages.[71] There has been a marked rise in successful suicide among adolescents aged from fifteen to nineteen, and suicide is now the third-ranking cause of death in this age group. In college

---

* Although persons who die from indirect "suicidal equivalents" or from premeditated "accidents," or whose deaths from obvious suicide are misreported, may not be included in suicide statistics, these sources of error seem to be rather constant, and the statistics for successful suicide in the United States for the past half-century appear relatively consistent from time to time and place to place.

students, suicide is the second-ranking cause of death (after accidents). However, in the United States, among adolescents and young adults, the suicide rate still runs only from about 4 to 6 per 100,000, but the successive increment in each succeeding age group imposes a maximum rate of 25 to 33 per 100,000 by the age period of seventy-five years and over. This correlation with age is especially marked for white males: At the younger ages, the rates for males are about three times those for females, but among the aged the ratio is ten to one, or more. In almost all European countries as well, about two to three males commit suicide for every female who does, although rates for females are increasing in many countries.

The suicide rate of foreign-born American men is significantly higher than that of the native-born, and the differences among the foreign-born population are similar to those found in their respective homelands. The Negro in this country is far less likely to commit suicide than the white, although rates among blacks are increasing, especially in the cities, and Hendin[43] found that young urban Negro males have a suicide rate that is probably higher than that for white men of the same age. Nonwhites other than Negroes generally have higher rates than white persons.* These differences, however, should not suggest that predisposition to suicide is inherited. Kallmann and Anastasio,[51] studying suicide in twins, found no evidence to implicate definite hereditary factors. But the work of Pitts and Winokur[81] indicates that at least a tendency to affective disorder and associated suicide may be related to familial patterns, especially in males.

Suicide has been more common in urban than in rural areas, but, as the United States has become more urbanized, the gap in suicide rates has been greatly narrowed. Suicide rates also vary among the major centers of population, and tend to be highest in the Western states and lowest in the Southern (except Florida and Virginia). Six metropolitan areas have very high rates: Tampa-St.

* All such rates are statistically adjusted for age, sex, and other relevant factors, when appropriate.

Petersburg, San Francisco-Oakland, Los Angeles-Long Beach, Seattle, Sacramento, and Miami. Other cities (including such very large centers as New York and Chicago) have moderate or even low rates. West Berlin is said to have the highest rate of any city in the world. In general, the incidence of suicide is not significantly related to climate, although in the great majority of countries suicide rates follow a certain rhythm with the changing seasons of the year, a maximum incidence occurring in springtime.[58] In the United States, April nearly always has the highest daily average number and December the lowest.[71]

Although there is no simple causal relation between economic factors and suicide, suicide rates do tend to decrease in times of prosperity and increase during depression. The relation between suicide rates and socioeconomic status is somewhat contradictory, although there is good evidence that members of the lower socioeconomic classes have lower suicide rates than do members of the upper socioeconomic classes, except after the age of sixty-five, when the rate for lower-class males becomes considerably higher than that for upper-class males.[126] Suicide rates among physicians are three times the national average, and among these psychiatrists may have even higher rates.[9] Age-adjusted suicide rates are highest for divorced persons, next for widowed, next for single, and lowest for married persons.

Suicide rates also decrease during war, apparently a universal phenomenon that has been reported in all wartime countries and has even been observed in some neutral nations during wartime. This latter phenomenon is always more marked among men than among women, and, in this country, among white than among black persons. It is difficult to measure statistically the influence of religion on the suicide rate, but suicide mortality is generally (although certainly not uniformly) lower in countries where a large proportion of the population is Catholic; however, suicide rates among Catholics living in non-Catholic countries may not be significantly lower than among Protestants living in the same countries. The rates among Jews have been variable, but, particularly in recent years in the United States and Israel, have tended to be low.

Early in the nineteenth century, one Matthew Lovat, an Italian shoemaker in Venice, attempted to commit suicide by nailing himself to a cross. Other fantastic suicide methods in history have included swallowing red-hot coals, self-suspension from a bell clapper in a village church, and beheading with a self-made guillotine. Most people, however, choose one of a very few common suicide methods. Almost nine-tenths of all successful suicides in the United States involve shooting, hanging, poisoning, or asphyxiation. Since the beginning of the century, shooting has increased in frequency and now accounts for almost half of all U.S. suicides, whereas poisoning and asphyxiation by gas (by far the leading methods in 1900) declined in popularity for some years but—in the form of ingestion of analgesic and/or soporific substances or asphyxiation by motor vehicle exhaust gas—are again being used more frequently. Cases of self-poisoning have constituted 4 to 7 percent of admissions to the medical wards of general hospitals in Great Britain. Dublin[22] suggested that the choice of method is in part determined by availability and accessibility of the agent, but he pointed out the multitude of means available to any determined seeker of suicide, noting that persons intent on self-destruction have used any method conveniently at hand, even crashing one's head against a wall or drowning in a few inches of water.

Another factor involved in the choice of a specific method may be related to suggestibility. Although suicides actually have occurred in epidemic form (in the United States in 1930, in Copenhagen during World War II), they are not generally manifested as such violent reactions under such singular circumstances. A "law of series" in suicides, claiming a high probability that after one suicide at a given location more will follow, has been mentioned in some earlier works. Modern data indicate, however, that such "series" usually consist of only a few cases, employing similar methods, which, although widely publicized,

occur but rarely. Dublin emphasized that individual psychological factors are most important: "The mental economy of the suicide is such that he sometimes will go to great lengths to kill himself in a particular manner that satisfies some personal or symbolic requirement." A case in point is that of the would-be suicide who some years ago jumped from the Brooklyn Bridge. Conscious after hitting the water, he refused to grab a rope lowered to him by a nearby policeman—refused, that is, until the policeman threatened to shoot him.

Epidemiological patterns of *attempted suicide* are far more difficult to analyze than those of successful suicide, because reports of the rates of suicidal attempts represent only a fraction of the real incidence of all suicidal attempts among the general population. To be included in any statistical study, a suicidal attempt must result in the person's being brought to the attention of a physician, a policeman, or some similar authority; and that authority must report the attempt. For a variety of reasons, most suicidal attempts are not so registered; moreover, there is some evidence that those attempts that are reported involve specially selected groups and that the selective factor varies in different places at different times. Such samples are, then, almost always unrepresentative.*

In many statistical reports, the number of suicidal attempts is listed as less than the number of successful suicides. The Metropolitan Life Insurance Company[66] has ventured the educated but conservative estimate that the real rate of suicidal attempts is at least six or seven times as great as that of successful suicides; Farberow and Shneidman[27] reported a ratio of eight attempted suicides to one successful suicide in Los Angeles—a figure that Stengel[111] has suggested as probably appropriate for at least the urban populations in the United States and England. Parkin and Stengel[77] found the actual ratio between at-

---

* Stengel[115] has suggested that reports of suicidal attempts indicate as much about their real occurrence as the number of divorces granted on the grounds of adultery reveal about the actual incidence of marital infidelity.

tempted suicide and suicide (in England) to be 9.7 to 1, and thought this was an underestimate. Choron[16] has calculated that between six and seven million U.S. residents have attempted suicide. Paykel et al.[78] conducted an extensive and careful survey of 720 subjects in the general population of New Haven, Connecticut. They found a ratio of thirty-two suicidal attempts to every one expected completed suicide for their subjects, with 0.6 percent of the total group reporting having made a suicidal attempt *during the previous year*, 1.5 percent having seriously considered suicide, and approximately 9 percent having had some sort of suicidal thoughts during the same period. These suicidal feelings were reported more by females than males, but otherwise appeared largely independent of sociodemographic status. They were strongly associated with other indices of psychiatric problems, social isolation, and life stress.

Certain facts are known about such unsuccessful attempts: They are more common among females than males, especially in the population group under thirty years of age. In a very detailed survey conducted in Edinburgh, Kessel[53] found very high rates of attempted suicide among teenage girls and women in their early twenties. The author suggested that these young women who attempt suicide, even though married and possibly looking after children, tend to be emotionally isolated. The peak for both sexes in Kessel's study was in the twenty-four to thirty-four age group, and in that age group the rates for widowed and divorced persons were especially high. The percentage of successful attempts becomes greater with increased age; attempted suicides among the young are the least successful. The socioeconomic class distribution among persons reported as attempting suicide tends to correspond to that of the general population, although some recent studies indicate a disproportionate concentration in the lower classes. The most efficient suicide methods (shooting, hanging, drowning, jumping from high places) are generally more common among men, whereas females

are more likely to use poison, the least efficient method.

If those who attempt suicide and those who successfully commit suicide do represent two different, but overlapping, populations, one would expect that the number of persons later committing suicide who have made earlier unsuccessful attempts would be proportionately small. Although difficult to collect, there are some limited data to this point. The studies of Sainsbury[96] and Stengel and Cook[117] suggest that about one-tenth of all persons who commit suicide have made one or more prior suicidal attempts. Other investigators have found a somewhat higher fraction—up to one-quarter.[133] Dorpat and Ripley[21] reviewed twenty-four published studies bearing on the relationship between attempted and committed suicide and reported that the incidence of prior suicidal attempts among those who completed suicide and the incidence of completed suicide among attempters were both much higher than that of the general population.

Since such reported suicidal attempts probably represent only a small sample of all suicidal attempts, both reported and unreported, information gathered to indicate just how many of those who attempt suicide finally do kill themselves also may be only approximate. But several such studies have been made and show surprisingly consistent results, despite reference to different countries and different times. In the comprehensive review by the World Health Organization,[133] some twenty investigators (including Dahlgren,[19] Ringel,[86] Schmidt et al.,[98] Schneider,[100] and Stengel[113,116]) conducting various types of frequently extensive follow-up studies of persons attempting suicide found that from about 2 percent in less than a year to about 10 percent in ten years subsequently killed themselves. Schmidt et al.,[98] Rosen,[91] Greer and Lee,[40] and Weiss and associates[128,129] all found definitely higher rates of subsequent committed suicide among those who made "serious" attempts, and in the WHO study it is noted that "if there have been two previous attempts, the subsequent risk of suicide is considerably increased." Therefore, although the total number of persons who finally commit suicide after a previous suicidal attempt obviously increases as the period following the attempt lengthens—at least up to ten years—it can be seen that only a limited proportion of those reported as having attempted suicide finally kill themselves, and that the proportion of all persons attempting suicide who finally kill themselves is probably quite small. However, it should be apparent that the risk of eventual successful suicide is still far higher among those persons who have attempted suicide than among the general population, and that those persons who have made one or more medically dangerous, psychologically serious prior attempts are at far higher risk of committing subsequent successful suicide than those whose prior attempts were of lesser medical danger and/or psychological seriousness.

(Relationships to Clinical Entities

It is also difficult to determine the quantitative relationship between categorical psychiatric disorders and suicide rates. Most such information is based on records of patients in hospitals. Kraepelin[55] indicated that psychiatric disorder was a factor in at least one-third of all successful suicides, and other early studies provided similar evidence to this effect. Jamieson,[49] Norris,[73] and Raines and Thompson[84] have all analyzed numerous case records, pointing out that suicide is most common among persons diagnosed as suffering from the affective psychotic disorders but is not uncommon among schizophrenics, and noting cases in which unplanned suicides have resulted from patients' confused states in delirium. Malzberg (cited by Dublin[22]) found an annual rate of 34 suicides per 100,000 resident patients per year, for New York State's mental hospitals in the two-year period from 1957 to 1959. Suicide was most common among patients suffering from manic-depressive and involutional disorders, and next most common among patients with cerebral arteriosclerosis

and those suffering from schizophrenia. Shneidman et al.[107] found that successful suicide among schizophrenic patients in psychiatric hospitals occurred in almost all cases after there had been a remission of illness, rather than in the depths of the psychotic process.

Sletten et al.[109] studied patients who had committed suicide in hospital or on one-year convalescent leave, and found that the rate was much higher for this group than for the general population. Rates among these subjects were higher for men than for women, for white than black, for married than single, and for Catholic than Protestant, but did not regularly go up with age. In decreasing order, rates were highest for those patients with a diagnosis of depresson, schizophrenia, and personality disorder. Rates were also highest during the first months after admission to the hospital.

The difficulties in diagnosis, particularly among nonhospitalized suicide victims, have led to several extreme points of view. Zilboorg[136] believed that most suicides are committed by persons considered "normal" before the act. Lewis,[59] on the other hand, considered that all persons who either commit suicide or make serious attempts are, by virtue of the act, essentially psychotic. Stengel,[115] after reviewing the literature, concluded that suicidal acts—successful or not—may be associated with almost any clinical psychiatric disorder. Seager and Flood's[102] study of 325 suicides in Bristol, England, over a five-year period, indicated that a family history of mental illness was present in 10 percent, a previous suicidal attempt in 16 percent, a disabling physical illness in 20 percent, and previous psychiatric illness requiring specialized treatment in 30 percent. There was evidence of mental illness of some kind in over two-thirds of the cases. Sainsbury's[95] investigations of persons who had committed suicide in England also demonstrated a psychiatric diagnosis of serious depressive illness in a large majority of cases, and reports from several major studies on the relationship between psychiatric disorders and ultimate death from suicide reveal that about 15 percent of persons found suffering from depressive illness will ultimately die by suicide[133] (as compared to probably 1 percent of the general population). Osmond and Hoffer[74] followed for twenty-five years 3,521 patients diagnosed as schizophrenic and found a suicide rate among these patients much higher than the normal rate of the countries concerned. These authors believe that the rate of suicide among schizophrenics at least approaches that among manic-depressives. Numerous investigators have also reported a high frequency of suicide among alcoholics, and of alcoholics among samples of persons who have committed or attempted suicide.[133] A large number of alcoholic fathers among young people attempting suicide has been noted,[119] and Murphy and Robins[70] found that among alcoholics per se who committed suicide, almost one-third had experienced disruption of affectional relationships within six weeks prior to the act.

Probably the most rigorous study relating clinical entities to suicide was made by Robins' group in St. Louis.[88] These investigators studied 134 consecutive successful suicides, including systematic interviews with family, in-laws, friends, job associates, physicians, ministers, and others, a short time after the suicide act. Using careful and well-defined criteria for illness, their results indicated that 94 percent of those committing successful suicide had been psychiatrically ill, with 68 percent of the total group suffering from one of two disorders: manic-depressive depression or chronic alcoholism. (If one summarizes other international cross-study data, it seems probable that of those persons who commit suicide, about half are suffering from serious depressive illness, perhaps one-fifth to one-quarter from some degree of chronic alcoholism, and a significant but smaller number from schizophrenia.) These results should be compared with those in an earlier study of 109 patients who *attempted suicide*, in which Schmidt et al.[98] found that the psychiatric disorders represented could be classified into nine different diagnostic categories; no attempter was thought to be "normal" prior to the attempt. Thus, attempted suicide is most likely a symp-

tom or sign associated with a large variety of clinical psychiatric disorders, whereas successful suicide (probably including the aborted successful suicidal attempt) is most likely to be associated with depressive disorder of psychotic proportions and chronic alcoholism, and probably, to a lesser degree, with schizophrenia and organic brain disorder.

Indicators of Suicide Potential: Implications for Prevention

Recent studies have indicated that successful suicide is far less often an impulsive act without prior indicators than had previously been supposed. Robins et al.[88] found that in their series a majority of the persons committing suicide had been under medical or psychiatric care, or both, within one year preceding the act, many of them within one month. In another paper,[87] Robins and his colleagues noted a high frequency among persons who later committed suicide of the communication of suicidal ideas, by specific statements of intent to commit suicide, by statements concerning preoccupation with death and desire to die, and by communications associated with unsuccessful attempts. These statements were made to family, friends, job associates, and many others, and were repeatedly verbalized, by well over half of those who did later kill themselves. Rudestam[93] also found that 60 percent of his fifty consecutive cases of confirmed suicide in both Stockholm, Sweden, and Los Angeles had made direct verbal threats prior to taking their lives, while more than 80 percent had voiced either direct or indirect threats.

Although many people who communicate suicidal intention may not commit suicide, it is clear from such studies and those of Shneidman and Farberow[105] that most people who actually commit suicide communicate their intention beforehand. Gardner et al.[36] also noted that in the high-frequency, successful suicide groups of older patients with depression, chronic alcoholism, or paranoid schizophrenia, there is a tendency to deny illness and to communicate any suicidal intention or need for help in an indirect, distorted manner. Shneidman and Farberow[106] found a critical period of about three months following a severe emotional crisis during which persons are most likely to commit suicide. An increase in psychomotor activity, therefore, does not necessarily indicate "improvement" in the long run.

Litman and Farberow[62] have noted that the potential for successful suicide increases specifically with age, prior suicidal behavior, loss of a loved person, clinically recognizable psychiatric disorder, physical health problems, and lowered interpersonal, social, and financial resources. They emphasize as warning signs withdrawal from and rejection of loved ones, suicide threats (particularly those giving details of time and place), and overt expressions of suicidal intention, plus such behavior as putting effects in order, making out a will, and writing notes and letters with specific instructions. They suggested: "The most serious suicidal potential is associated with feelings of helplessness and hopelessness, exhaustion and failure, and the feeling 'I just want out.'" Others have stressed that the feeling of "being a burden" to one's family or friends is also a special danger sign.

However, the intensive small-N investigation by Weiss et al.[128] has indicated that the many social, ecological, and personality factors that appear to relate to the seriousness of suicidal attempts in large-scale nomothetic studies do not for the most part seem to be useful for prediction with limited samples or individual patients. The only statistically significant indicators of the gravity or danger of the suicidal attempt for individual attempters appeared to be (a) attempts in which the psychological intent was "serious"; (b) attempts of older adults; (c) of those who attributed the act to concern about personal "mental illness"; and (d) of those who were diagnosed as suffering from a clinical psychotic process of any nature, but especially depression. In a ten-year follow-up study of the same patients, Weiss and Scott[129] found the risk of subsequent successful suicide to be much higher among those who had earlier made such serious attempts than among those who had made nonserious attempts, that persons who made any kind of attempt tended to have continuing psychosocial problems after the attempt, and that the lifestyle of suicide attempters generally showed little change when followed over that long period and no change significantly different from that evidenced by matched controls. The attempts of younger persons, of those whose method involved solely the ingestion of barbiturates or other substances of limited toxicity, and of those who attributed the act to the precipitating stress of "family trouble," were generally not psychologically serious or medically dangerous. The presence of a "death trend" (one or more close relatives of the attempter being dead) and the presence of nonpsychotic clinical depression appeared to be functions of increasing age rather than substantive indicators.

The WHO expert committee[133] stated, "Persons with [endogenous and involutional] depressive illness appear everywhere to constitute a high risk group. In suicide-prevention programmes, high priority should therefore be given to improvement in recognition and treatment of these conditions and organizations of after-care for treated cases." Rosen[91] noted that insomnia prior to the attempt is an additional sign of high risk. Sainsbury[95] also emphasized that suicidal risk is correlated with depression and with the primary medical symptom of insomnia, especially in the elderly.

Although such information provides a guide to probabilities, the fact remains that every emotionally disturbed person who indicates suicidal intent should be evaluated by a competent psychiatrist. Any depressive reaction may carry with it some danger of suicide, and no suicidal talk should be taken lightly. Almost all experienced clinicians indicate that, if there is any suspicion at all of suicidal intent, the patient should be questioned about it. Such a procedure will not give the patient any ideas of suicide that he does not already have, and his response will often help to determine his intent. If his response is bizarre, illogical, or delusional, or if it includes ideas of worthlessness or indicates a preoccupation with thoughts of suicide and with actual concrete procedures for carrying out the act, one should consider the danger of a serious or successful suicide attempt to be great.

Clinicians who deal with suicidal patients would, of course, find a valid and reliable screening test predictive of both the possibility of suicidal attempt and the degree of lethality of such attempt extremely useful. A considerable number of investigators have developed such suicide risk assessment schedules, indices, rating scales, and even biochemical tests (exemplified in Refs. 10, 12, 13, 17, 20, 26, 28, 60 62, 82, 85, 109, 122, and 123), but neither the specificity nor the sensitivity of such instruments has been adequate for general acceptance. Rosen[90] has pointed out the many limitations which make the prediction of infrequent events such as suicide so difficult. Perhaps the most promising technique to this end is being developed by Litman[60] and his colleagues, who are using actuarial methods to quantify the concept of suicidal risk as part of a mathematical model for predicting suicidal behavior. This model will assign a suicide probability both to individual subjects and to groups for any coming year, utilizing multiple factors input with an output providing an index of present risk and a guide for predicting future self-destructive behavior. Litman wrote, however, that "suicide probably is too complex and variable a problem to be handled by any general or unitary scale or testing device," that any such scale would need to be adapted to each different setting and utilized only to supplement the clinical judgment of professional workers with experience in that particular setting.

Many psychiatrists feel that, if suicidal intent is suspected, immediate hospitalization of the patient on a psychiatric inpatient service is mandatory. Other well-trained psychiatrists take a calculated risk with such patients and follow them as outpatients. Such a decision, however, must be made on the basis of special knowledge—knowledge of the probabilities and prognoses in similar cases, and knowledge of the particular patient, based on intensive interviews, psychological tests, social histories,

and similar data. It seems obvious that persons who express suicidal intentions or make suicidal attempts are so emotionally disordered that they are willing to consider risking their lives in a gamble with death, and it is the responsibility of physicians and other professional workers who come in contact with such persons to assess the meaning of each suicidal communication or attempt, with respect to how best to respond to the implied need for help.

In countries with highly developed and readily available health and welfare services, a variety of organizations exist for the prevention of suicide and the treatment of patients with suicidal behavior. These services vary from networks of general medical practitioners to general hospitals, and from outpatient clinics to specific psychiatric hospitals and community mental health centers. In some such countries, specialized institutions have been established to deal with suicidal patients and those who have already attempted suicide. A notable example is the Los Angeles Suicide Prevention Center, operated with the co-operation of available medical, psychological, welfare, pastoral, and other community resources. This agency maintains a telephone "hot-line," and referral in person may be made through medical or lay sources, or the patient may come on his own. More than 200 such centers have been established in other cities in the United States and also in other countries, such as Austria, France, Germany, and Switzerland. Lay organizations also offer help to suicidal persons who either do not regard their difficulties as medical problems or refuse to seek medical help. The best known is the Samaritans, which started in London but has become international. There are similar groups in several U.S. cities. They rely mainly on volunteers, who help to maintain full-time telephone services and offer useful advice and support, as well as referral to medical and welfare agencies. Former clients often cooperate in running such services.

Two major criticisms have been made of both the professional and lay suicide prevention services, namely, (1) that many of the patients evaluated and/or treated therein are not actually suicidal, and (2) that the services of such organizations cannot be proved to be effective. The first criticism is probably neither humane nor valid, since clients of such agencies would not be referred or seek aid voluntarily unless they perceived a need for help, and since Wold,[131] reviewing 26,000 Los Angeles SPC cases, found that 51 percent had made a suicidal attempt at some time in the past. The second criticism is refuted at least partially by Bagley's[5] study done in Great Britain, which provided evidence that recently instituted 24-hour telephone and other services, giving isolated, lonely, or desperate persons a chance to communicate with volunteer workers, were most probably related to a statistically significant drop in the suicide rate of 5 percent in the subject areas, compared to a rise of 20 percent in matched control areas without such services. And Barraclough[6] has reviewed evidence that institution of modern medical and psychiatric services is also likely (perhaps more likely) to be related to a drop in suicide rates.

The WHO expert committee[133] has recommended several guidelines for the establishment and development of suicide prevention services: (1) Local emergency services, accessible at all times, with skilled medical and nursing staff available, should be provided. (2) Adequate and prompt psychiatric consultation should be available to such treatment centers. (3) Emergency psychiatric services with easy access to care should also be continuously available where there is no other medical emergency service. Such emergency services should include facilities for immediate response to telephone calls or to patients who are referred or come of their own accord. Such services should focus on the handling of the crisis with which the person is immediately concerned, attempting to evaluate the suicide potential and to work out a treatment plan for the patient. Follow-up psychiatric care is highly desirable for many of the patients seen in emergency services, as well as for others identified as high-risk cases. Members of the same psychiatric team should work in both emergency and follow-up care.

The committee noted that many persons who have made suicidal attempts are found after screening not to need special psychiatric treatment but may require other help, such as that provided by social welfare agencies or voluntary groups. Measures taken to lower the incidence of suicide should have a four-fold aim: to deal with the desire to attempt suicide, to prevent the first attempt, to prevent repetition of suicidal acts, and to prevent fatal outcome of such acts. Education of both the general public and the possible providers of service, such as medical practitioners and social workers, thus becomes important, and both national and international associations of professional persons concerned with teaching, research, care, and prevention related to suicide have been organized.

(Treatment

Just as the suicidal act must be considered in terms of the psychological, clinical, and sociological aspects of the person involved, so must be his treatment. The therapy of the suicidal patient can be successful only if all these factors are investigated and the pertinent ones so modified that the self-destructive tendency—arising out of an acute emotional crisis, as well as a life-long accumulation of experience, a set of social circumstances, and most often a clinically recognizable psychiatric disorder—is reduced to nondeleterious proportions. Social measures and somatic therapies may be necessary in some cases and helpful in others, but psychotherapy directed toward understanding the need for a suicidal act appears to be a *sine qua non* in almost any rational treatment program for suicidal patients. Farberow and Shneidman[27] and their collaborators, in discussing the varieties of therapy useful in treating such patients, have noted that successful treatment may vary with the kind of patient, the nature of the suicidal attempt, the psychodynamic and psychosocial factors involved, the nature and degree of associated psychiatric disorder, and to some extent the theoretical framework within which the therapist operates.

Kessel[53] has stressed that there is considerable advantage in making a thorough psychiatric assessment of all suicidal cases admitted to emergency medical services as soon as possible, at least within a few hours of admission. At that time, inquiries are made into the situation while its impact is still very strong and before the family and patient attempt to cover up the underlying factors. And at that time, such patients can be screened and their further care discussed with the family and other persons most closely concerned. Frederick and Resnik[33] have developed a well-reasoned therapeutic approach based on evidence that many aspects of suicidal behaviors may be learned and that treatment techniques founded in general learning theory can be useful, and Frederick and Farberow[32] have also found that group psychotherapy can be very useful with suicidal persons, although some modifications of standard group methods are probably requisite. In dealing with suicidal behaviors in children, one should remember that the first goal is seldom prevention of death or injury (since completed suicides in young children are rare) but rather—according to Glaser[38]—assessment of the behavior as a sign of emotional disturbance. The presence of depression is not necessarily a prerequisite for suicidal acts in childhood, and persons other than the psychiatrist are most likely to be in a position first to deal with the problem. Whether one is treating children or adults, however, the clinician should note that almost all authors emphasize the importance of a therapist who manifests sensitivity, warmth, interest, concern, and consistency.

In the hospital environment, success in treating suicidal patients is more likely with a therapeutic milieu having easy lines of communication than with the previously utilized strictures of rigid "suicide precautions." As Stengel and Cook[116] pointed out, the suicide rates of the resident population of mental hospitals in England and Wales for the years 1920 to 1947 were about three to five times those among the general population, remaining steadily at about 50 per 100,000 patients per year. Those were the years when psychiatrists took away from their patients shoelaces, belts, safety razors, and any other articles that might conceivably be used for self-destruction. And yet, the rates remained consistently high within the closed doors of the mental hospitals of those days. The introduction of electroshock treatment in the late 1930s and 1940s had little or no direct influence on the frequency of successful suicidal acts per se in mental hospitals (although other studies clearly have indicated the clinical value of such therapy, especially in psychotically depressed older persons). In the 1945–1947 period, when EST was in widespread use, the suicide rates in mental hospitals in England actually increased slightly to 51.5. Surprisingly, in 1953 these in-hospital suicide rates dropped to 27.3, and have remained comparatively lower ever since. A significant decrease in suicide rates therefore occurred in a period when the English mental hospitals were adopting more liberal policies, including "open-door" and "therapeutic community," before the widespread use of the newer psychoactive drugs, and in spite of an increased admission rate during that period for patients with psychotic depression, as well as higher average ages of resident patients who therefore might be expected to be more suicide-prone.[94]

Other studies have indicated rather similar trends in mental hospitals in the United States and elsewhere. Petri's[79] work in Germany supports these findings, as does that of Kapamadzija[52] in Yugoslavia. The latter author suggested that the very humanization of the regimen of psychiatric hospitals and the abolition of the atmosphere of isolation and alienation are also the best means of prevention of suicide by the mentally ill in psychiatric units. Simply increasing the knowledge and sensitivity of all persons who are likely to come into contact with patients or with others who may be potentially suicidal has clearly proved of great importance, both in therapy and in prevention.[85,104,108]

Finally, as has been noted, the establishment of units either in categorical suicide prevention and treatment centers, comprehensive community mental health centers, or general hospitals and clinics, to provide well-publicized and easily available psychiatric first-aid, is already demonstrating marked value, both in rendering assistance to potentially suicidal persons and in collecting data that should add inestimable information to our body of knowledge. The evidence indicates that suicidal behavior is most often a symptom (or a terminating act) of biologically, psychologically, and culturally determined psychiatric disorder, not a free moral choice. As Freud wrote, "The moment one inquires about the meaning or value of life one is sick, since objectively neither of them has any existence." The prediction, prevention, and treatment of suicidal behavior is therefore a salient responsibility for the interacting efforts of the basic scientist, the behavioral investigator, the public health specialist, the social activist, and, not least, the clinician.

❙ Bibliography

1. ADLER, A. "*Selbstmord*," *Internationale Zeitschrift für Individualpsychologie*, 15 (1937) 49–52; *Journal of Individual Psychology*, 14 (1958), 57–61.

2. ALVAREZ, A. *The Savage God: A Study of Suicide*. New York: Random House, 1972.

3. ANDERSON, D. B., and L. J. McCLEAN, eds. *Identifying Suicide Potential*. New York: Behavioral Publications, 1971.

4. ANDICS, M. VON. *Suicide and the Meaning of Life*. London: Hodge, 1947.

5. BAGLEY, C. "The Evaluation of a Suicide Prevention Scheme by the Ecological Method," *Social Science and Medicine*, 2 (1968), 1–14.

6. BARRACLOUGH, B. M. "Doctors, Samaritans and Suicide," *British Journal of Psychiatry* (*News and Notes Supplement*), April (1972), 8–9.

7. BEALL, L. "The Dynamics of Suicide: A Review of the Literature, 1897–1965," *Bulletin of Suicidology*, March (1969), 2–16.

8. BERNFELD, S. "*Selbstmord*," *Zeitschrift für Psychoanalytische Pädagogik*, 3 (1929), 355–363.

9. BLACHLY, P. H., W. DISHER, and G. RODUNER. "Suicide by Physicians," *Bulletin of Suicidology*, December (1968), 1–18.

10. BOLIN, R. K., R. E. WRIGHT, M. N. WILKINSON, and C. K. LINDNER. "Survey of Suicide Among Patients on Home Leave from a Mental Hospital," *Psychiatric Quarterly*, 42 (1968), 81–89.

11. BROMBERG, W., and P. SCHILDER. "Death and Dying," *Psychoanalytic Review*, 20 (1933), 133.

12. BUGLASS, D. and J. W. McCULLOCH. "Further Suicidal Behavior: The Development and Validation of Predictive Scales," *British Journal of Psychiatry*, 116 (1970), 483–491.

13. BUNNEY, W. E., J. H. FAWCETT, J. M. DAVIES, and S. GIFFORD. "Further Evaluation of Urinary 17-Hydroxycorticosteroids in Suicide Patients," *Archives of General Psychiatry*, 21 (1969), 138–150.

14. CAIN, A. C., and I. FAST. "Children's Disturbed Reactions to Parents' Suicide," *American Journal of Orthopsychiatry*, 36 (1966), 873–880.

15. CAVAN, R. S. *Suicide*. Chicago: University of Chicago Press, 1926.

16. CHORON, J. *Suicide*. New York: Scribner's, 1972.

17. COHEN, E., J. A. MOTTO, and R. H. SEIDEN. "An Instrument for Evaluating Suicide Potential: A Preliminary Study," *The American Journal of Psychiatry*, 122 (1966), 886–891.

18. CUSTER, R. L., and J. M. A. WEISS. "The Aborted Successful Suicidal Attempt: Differential Patterns," *Journal of Operational Psychiatry*, 2 (1971), 29.

19. DAHLGREN, K. G. *On Suicide and Attempted Suicide*. Lund, Sweden: Lindstedts, 1945.

20. DEAN, R. A., W. MISKIMINS, R. DE COOK, L. T. WILSON, and R. F. MALEY. "Prediction of Suicide in a Psychiatric Hospital," *Journal of Clinical Psychology*, 23 (1967), 296–301.

21. DORPAT, T. L., and H. S. RIPLEY. "The Relationship Between Attempted Suicide and Committed Suicide," *Comprehensive Psychiatry*, 8 (1967), 74–79.

22. DUBLIN, L. I. *Suicide: A Sociological and Statistical Study*. New York: Ronald Press, 1963.

23. DURKHEIM, E. *Le Suicide*. New York: The Free Press, 1951.

24. ETTLINGER, R. W., and P. FLORDH. *Attempted Suicide: Experience of Five Hundred Cases at a General Hospital.*

Copenhagen: Acta Psychiatrica, Kbh. (Suppl. 103), 1955.

25. FARBEROW, N. L. *Bibliography on Suicide and Suicide Prevention.* Chevy Chase: National Institute of Mental Health, 1969.

26. FARBEROW, N. L., and A. G. DEVRIES. "An Item Differentiation Analysis of MMPIs of Suicidal Neuropsychiatric Hospital Patients," *Psychological Reports,* 20 (1967), 607–617.

27. FARBEROW, N. L. and E. S. SHNEIDMAN. *The Cry for Help.* New York: McGraw-Hill, 1961.

28. FARBEROW, N. L., E. S. SHNEIDMAN and C. NEURINGER. "Case History and Hospitalization Factors in Suicides of Neuropsychiatric Hospital Patients," *Journal of Nervous and Mental Disease,* 142 (1966), 32–44.

29. FEDERN, P. *"Diskussion über Selbstmord im Wiener Psychoanalytischem Verein,"* Zeitschrift für Psychoanalytische Pädagogik, 3 (1929), 333–344.

30. ———. "Reality of the Death Instinct, Especially in Melancholia," *Psychoanalytic Review,* 19 (1932), 129.

31. FENICHEL, O. *The Psychoanalytic Theory of Neurosis.* New York: Norton, 1945.

32. FREDERICK, C. J., and N. L. FARBEROW. "Group Psychotherapy with Suicidal Persons: A Comparison with Standard Group Methods," *International Journal of Social Psychiatry,* 16 (1970), 103–111.

33. FREDERICK, C. J. and H. L. P. RESNICK. "How Suicidal Behaviors are Learned," *American Journal of Psychotherapy,* 25 (1971), 37–55.

34. FREUD, S. "Beyond the Pleasure Principle" (1920), in Standard Edition, Vol. 18. London: Hogarth Press, 1957.

35. ———. "Mourning and Melancholia" (1917), in *Collected Papers,* Vol. 4. New York: Basic Books, 1959.

36. GARDNER, E. A., A. K. BAHN, and M. MACK. "Suicide and Psychiatric Care in Aging," *Archives of General Psychiatry,* 10 (1964), 547–553.

37. GIDDENS, A., ed. *The Sociology of Suicide.* London: Frank Cass, 1971.

38. GLASER, K. "Suicidal Children," *American Journal of Psychotherapy,* 25 (1971), 27–36.

39. GORDON, J. E., E. LINDEMANN, J. IPSEN, and W. T. VAUGHAN. "Epidemiologic Analysis of Suicide," in *Epidemiology of Men-*

tal Disorder. New York: Milbank Memorial Fund, 1950.

40. GREER, S., and H. A. LEE. "Subsequent Progress of Potentially Lethal Attempted Suicides," *Acta Psychiatrica Scandinavica,* 43 (1967), 361–371.

41. GRUHLE, H. W. *Selbstmord.* Leipzig: Theime, 1940.

42. HENDIN, H. "Attempted Suicide," *Psychiatric Quarterly,* 24 (1950), 39–46.

43. ———. *Black Suicide.* New York: Basic Books, 1969.

44. ———. *Suicide and Scandinavia.* New York: Grune and Stratton, 1964.

45. HENRY, A. F., and J. F. SHORT. *Suicide and Homicide: Some Economic, Sociological and Psychological Aspects of Aggression.* New York: The Free Press, 1954.

46. HORNEY, K. *Neurosis and Human Growth,* New York: Norton, 1950.

47. JACOBS, J. *Adolescent Suicide.* New York: Wiley-Interscience, 1971.

48. JACOBZINER, H. "Attempted Suicides in Children," *Journal of Pediatrics,* 56 (1960), 519–525.

49. JAMIESON, G. R. "Suicide and Mental Disease," *Archives of Neurology and Psychiatry,* 36 (1936), 1–12.

50. JUNG, C. G. "The Soul and Death," in H. Feifel, ed., *The Meaning of Death.* New York: McGraw-Hill, 1959.

51. KALLMANN, F. J., and M. M. ANASTASIO. "Twin Studies on the Psychopathology of Suicide," *Journal of Heredity,* 37 (1946), 171–180; *Journal of Nervous and Mental Disease,* 105 (1947), 40–55.

52. KAPAMADZIJA, B. "Suicide and Some Legal Problems," *Annals Bolnice Dr. M. Stojanovic,* 10 Supp. (1971), 50–55.

53. KESSEL, N. "Self-poisoning," *British Medical Journal,* 5473 (1965), 1265–1270, and 5474 (1965), 1336–1340.

54. KESSEL, N. and W. McCULLOCH. "Repeated Acts of Self-poisoning and Self-injury," *Proceedings of the Royal Society of Medicine,* 59 (1966), 89–92.

55. KRAEPELIN, E. *Lectures on Clinical Psychiatry.* New York: Wood, 1917.

56. KREITMAN, N. "Subcultural Aspects of Attempted Suicide," in E. H. Hare, and J. K. Wing, eds. *Psychiatric Epidemiology.* London: Oxford University Press, 1970.

57. LENDRUM, F. C. "A Thousand Cases of Attempted Suicide," *The American Journal of Psychiatry,* 13 (1933), 479–500.

58. LESTER, D. "Seasonal Variation in Suicidal Deaths," *British Journal of Psychiatry*, 118 (1971), 627–628.

59. LEWIS, N. D. C. "Studies on Suicide," *Psychoanalytic Review*, 20 (1933), 241–273, and 21 (1934), 146–153.

60. LITMAN, R. E. "Models for Predicting Suicidal Lethality," in *Resumenes—V. Congreso Mundial de Psiquiatria*. Mexico City: La Prensa Medica Mexicana, 1971.

61. ———. "When Patients Commit Suicide," *American Journal of Psychotherapy*, 19 (1965), 570–576.

62. LITMAN, R. E. and N. L. FARBEROW. "Emergency Evaluation of Self-destructive Potentiality," in N. L. Farberow, and E. S. Shneidman, eds. *The Cry For Help*. New York: McGraw-Hill, 1961.

63. MEERLOO, J. A. M. *Suicide and Mass Suicide*. New York: Grune and Stratton, 1962.

64. MENNINGER, K. A. *Man Against Himself*. New York: Harcourt, 1938.

65. ———. "Psychoanalytic Aspects of Suicide," *International Journal of Psychoanalysis*, 14 (1933), 376–390.

66. METROPOLITAN LIFE INSURANCE CO. "Suicides That Fail," *Statistical Bulletin* (May 1941).

67. ———. "Why Do People Kill Themselves?" *Statistical Bulletin* (February 1945).

68. MINTZ, R. S. "Basic Considerations in the Psychotherapy of the Depressed Suicidal Patient," *American Journal of Psychotherapy*, 25 (1971), 56–73.

69. MOTTO, J. A. "Suicide Attempts: A Longitudinal View," *Archives of General Psychiatry*, 13 (1965), 516–520.

70. MURPHY, G. E., and E. ROBINS. "Social Factors in Suicide," *Journal of the AMA*, 199 (1967), 303–308.

71. NATIONAL CENTER FOR HEALTH STATISTICS. *Suicide in the United States 1950–1964*. Washington: U.S. Department of Health, Education, and Welfare, 1967.

72. NEURINGER, C. "Methodological Problems in Suicide Research," *Journal of Consulting Psychology*, 26 (1962), 273–278.

73. NORRIS, V. *Mental Illness in London*. New York: Oxford University Press, 1959.

74. OSMOND, H., and A. HOFFER. "Schizophrenia and Suicide," *Journal of Schizophrenia*, 1 (1967), 54–64.

75. PAFFENBARGER, R. S., and D. P. ASNES. "Chronic Disease in Former College Students: III. Precursors of Suicide in Early and Middle Life," *American Journal of Public Health*, 56 (1966), 1026–1036.

76. PAFFENBARGER, R. S., H. KING, and A. L. WING. "Chronic Disease in Former College Students: IX. Characteristics of Youth Predisposed Suicide and Accidental Death in Later Life," *American Journal of Public Health*, 59 (1969), 900–908.

77. PARKIN, D., and E. STENGEL. "Incidence of Suicide Attempts in an Urban Community," *British Medical Journal*, 2 (1965), 133–138.

78. PAYKEL, E. S., J. K. MYERS, and J. J. LINDENTHAL. "Thoughts of Suicide: A General Population Survey," in *Resumenes—V. Congreso Mundial de Psiguiatria*. Mexico City: La Prensa Medica Mexicana, 1971.

79. PETRI, H. "The Problem of Suicide in Psychiatric Clinics," *Zeitschrift für Psychotherapie und Medizinische Psychologie*, 20 (1970), 10–19.

80. PIKER, P. "1817 Cases of Suicidal Attempt," *The American Journal of Psychiatry*, 95 (1938), 97–115.

81. PITTS, F. N., and G. WINOKUR. "Affective Disorder: III. Diagnostic Correlates and Incidence of Suicide," *Journal of Nervous and Mental Disease*, 139 (1964), 176–181.

82. PÖLDINGER, W. *"Psychologie und Prophylaxe des Suizids,"* *Monatskurse für die Ärztliche Fortbildung*, 3 (1967), 127–129.

83. PORTERFIELD, A. L., and R. H. TALBERT. *Crime, Suicide and Social Well-Being in Your State and City*. Fort Worth: Leo Potishman Foundation, 1948.

84. RAINES, G. N., and S. V. THOMPSON. "Suicide: Some Basic Considerations," *Digest of Neurology and Psychiatry*, 18 (1950), 97–107.

85. RESNICK, H. L. P., ed. *Suicidal Behaviors: Diagnosis and Management*. Boston: Little, Brown, 1968.

86. RINGEL, E. *Neue Untersuchungen zum Selbstmordproblem*. Vienna: Verlag Bruder Hollinek, 1961.

87. ROBINS, E., S. GASSNER, J. KAYES, R. H. WILKINSON, and G. E. MURPHY. "Communication of Suicidal Intent: A Study of 134 Cases of Successful (Completed) Suicide," *The American Journal of Psychiatry*, 115 (1959), 724–733.

88. ROBINS, E., G. E. MURPHY, R. H. WILKINSON, S. GASSNER, and J. KAYES. "Some Clinical Considerations in the Prevention

of Suicide Based on a Study of 134 Successful Suicides," *American Journal of Public Health*, 49 (1959), 888–899.

89. ROBINS, E., E. H. SCHMIDT, and P. O'NEAL. "Some Interrelations of Social Factors and Clinical Diagnosis in Attempted Suicide: A Study of 109 Patients," *The American Journal of Psychiatry*, 114 (1957), 221–231.

90. ROSEN, A. "Detection of Suicidal Patients: An Example of Some Limitations in the Prediction of Infrequent Events," *Journal of Consulting Psychology*, 18 (1954), 397–403.

91. ROSEN, D. H. "The Serious Suicide Attempt: Epidemiological and Follow-up Study of 886 Patients," *The American Journal of Psychiatry*, 127 (1970), 764–770.

92. ROST, H. *Bibliographie des Selbstmords*. Augsburg: Haas and Grabherr, 1927.

93. RUDESTAM, K. E. "Stockholm and Los Angeles: A Cross Cultural Study of the Communication of Suicidal Intent," *Journal of Consulting and Clinical Psychology*, 36 (1971), 82–90.

94. SAINSBURY, P. "Social and Epidemiological Aspects of Suicide with Special Reference to the Aged," in R. H. Williams, C. Tibbitts, and W. Donahue, eds., *Processes of Aging: Social and Psychological Perspectives*, Vol. 2. New York: Atherton Press, 1963.

95. ———. "Suicide and Depression," in A. Coppen, and A. Walk, eds., *Recent Developments in Affective Disorders*. London: Royal Medico-Psychological Association, 1968.

96. ———. *Suicide in London: An Ecological Study*. New York: Basic Books, 1956.

97. SCHILDER, P. *Psychotherapy*. New York: Norton, 1938, 1951.

98. SCHMIDT, E. H., P. O'NEAL, and E. ROBINS. "Evaluation of Suicide Attempts as Guide to Therapy," *Journal of the AMA*, 155 (1954), 549–557.

99. SCHNEER, H. I., P. KAY, and M. BROZOVSKY. "Events and Conscious Ideation Leading to Suicidal Behavior in Adolescence," *Psychiatric Quarterly*, 35 (1961), 507–515.

100. SCHNEIDER, P.-B. *La Tentative de Suicide*. Neuchatel-Paris: Delachaux et Niestlé, 1954.

101. SCHRUT, A. "Suicidal Adolescents and Children," *Journal of the AMA*, 188 (1964), 1103–1107.

102. SEAGER, C. P., and R. A. FLOOD. "Suicide in Bristol," *British Journal of Psychiatry*, 111 (1965), 919–932.

103. SEIDEN, R. H. *Suicide Among Youth: A Review of the Literature, 1900–1967*. (Supplement to the *Bulletin of Suicidology*.) Washington: National Clearinghouse for Mental Health Information, U.S. Department of Health, Education, and Welfare, 1969.

104. SHNEIDMAN, E. S., ed. *On the Nature of Suicide*. San Francisco: Jossey-Bass, 1969.

105. SHNEIDMAN, E. S. and N. L. FARBEROW, eds. *Clues to Suicide*. New York: McGraw-Hill, 1957.

106. ———. "Suicide—The Problem and Its Magnitude," *Veterans Administration Medical Bulletin*, MB-7 (March 1961).

107. SHNEIDMAN, E. S., N. L. FARBEROW, and C. V. LEONARD. "Suicide—Evaluation and Treatment of Suicidal Risk among Schizophrenic Patients in Psychiatric Hospitals," *Veterans Administration Medical Bulletin*, MB-8 (February 1962).

108. SHNEIDMAN, E. S., N. L. FARBEROW and R. E. LITMAN. *The Psychology of Suicide*. New York: Science House, 1970.

109. SLETTEN, I. W., M. L. BROWN, R. EVENSON, and H. ALTMAN. "Suicide in Mental Hospital Patients," *Diseases of the Nervous System*, 33 (1972), 328–334.

110. STEARNS, A. W. "Suicide," *New England Journal of Medicine*, 204 (1931), 9–11.

111. STENGEL, E. "Attempted Suicide: Its Management in the General Hospital," *Lancet* (February 2, 1963), 233–235.

112. ———. "Complexity of Motivations to Suicidal Attempts," *Journal of Mental Science*, 106 (1960), 1388–1393.

113. ———. "Enquiries into Attempted Suicide," *Proceedings of the Royal Society of Medicine*, 45 (1952), 613–620.

114. ———. "Old and New Trends in Suicide Research," *British Journal of Medical Psychology*, 33 (1960), 283–286.

115. ———. "Selbstmord und Selbstmordversuch," in *Psychiatrie der Gegenwart: Forschung und Praxis*, Band III. Berlin: Springer-Verlag, 1961.

116. STENGEL, E., and N. G. COOK. *Attempted Suicide: Its Social Significance and Effects*. New York: Basic Books, 1958.

117. ———. "Recent Research into Suicide and Attempted Suicide," *Journal of Forensic Medicine*, 1 (1954), 252–259.

118. SULLIVAN, H. S. *Clinical Studies in Psychiatry*. New York: Norton, 1956.

119. SZYMANSKA, Z., and S. ZELAZOWSKA. "Suicides et Tentatives de Suicide des Enfants et Adolescents," *Revue de Neuropsychiatrie Infantile*, 12 (1964), 715–740.

120. TABACHNICK, N. "Accident Victims: Self-Destructive or Not?" *Psychiatric News*, 7 (February 16, 1972), pp. 1, 28.

121. TOOLAN, J. M. "Suicide and Suicidal Attempts in Children and Adolescents," *The American Journal of Psychiatry*, 118 (1962), 719–724.

122. TUCKMAN, J., and W. F. YOUNGMAN. "Suicide Risk Among Persons Attempting Suicide," *Public Health Reports*, 78 (1963), 585–587.

123. ———. "Identifying Suicide Risk Groups Among Attempted Suicides," *Public Health Reports*, 78 (1963), 763–766.

124. WALTON, H. J. "Suicidal Behavior in Depressive Illness," *Journal of Mental Science*, 104 (1958), 884–891.

125. WEISS, J. M. A. "Gamble with Death in Attempted Suicide," *Psychiatry*, 20 (1957), 17–25.

126. ———. "Suicide: An Epidemiologic Analysis," *Psychiatric Quarterly*, 28 (1954), 225–252.

127. ———. "Suicide in the Aged," in H. L. P. Resnik, ed., *Suicidal Behaviors: Diagnosis and Management*. Boston: Little, Brown, 1968.

128. WEISS, J. M. A., N. NUNEZ, and K. W. SCHAIE. "Quantification of Certain Trends in Attempted Suicide," in *Proceedings of the Third World Congress of Psychiatry*. Montreal: University of Toronto Press and McGill University Press, 1961.

129. WEISS, J. M. A., and K. F. SCOTT. "Suicide Attempters Ten Years Later," in *Comprehensive Psychiatry*, in press (1973).

130. WEST, D. J. *Murder Followed by Suicide*. Boston: Harvard University Press, 1966.

131. WOLD, C. I. "Characteristics of 26,000 Suicide Prevention Center Patients," *Bulletin of Suicidology*, 6 (1970), 24–34.

132. WORLD HEALTH ORGANIZATION. "Mortality from Suicide," in *Epidemiological Vital Statistics, Report No. 9*. Geneva: WHO, 1956.

133. ———. *Prevention of Suicide*. Public Health Papers No. 35. Geneva: WHO, 1968.

134. YAP, P.-M. *Suicide in Hong Kong*. London: Oxford University Press, 1958.

135. ZILBOORG, G. "Considerations on Suicide, with Particular Reference to That of the Young," *American Journal of Orthopsychiatry*, 7 (1937), 15–31.

136. ———. "Differential Diagnostic Types of Suicide," *Archives of Neurology and Psychiatry*, 35 (1936), 270–291.

CHAPTER 34

DEPERSONALIZATION: PSYCHOLOGICAL AND SOCIAL PERSPECTIVES

James P. Cattell and Jane Schmahl Cattell

THIS IS A CHAPTER ON psychological and social theory concerning depersonalization. In the psychological analysis, we shall concentrate on solitary, individual behavior, motives and ideas which reflect rather than explain the general state of the contemporary American environment. In sociological analysis, we are interested in the process as it involves the individual in his role, and the reciprocal obligations that always come into play when two or more persons enter into relations with one another. Both levels of analysis consist of focusing on human behavior in interaction.

In our analysis, we shall tend to raise critical questions rather than attempt to provide

We gratefully acknowledge the constructive suggestions provided by: Sidney S. Goldensohn, M.D., Bernard Goldstein, Ph.D., Professor of Sociology, Rutgers University, and Esther Haar, M.D.

final answers. What is depersonalization? Under what circumstances does it occur? What are some of the factors that influence the onset of an episode of depersonalization? What types of relationships with significant others during developmental years may render the person vulnerable to depersonalization experiences? Some of the answers to these questions were explored in a survey of the literature prepared for Volume 3 of this *Handbook*[16] in 1965. That chapter, with some sixty references, was essentially a historical review.

Whether an individual will be healthy is largely out of his hands. It is influenced by the society in which he lives. A central proposition of this chapter is that depersonalization is influenced by manifestations of societal malintegration. How does one know how society makes a person sick? What is the relationship between a particular family social structure and the society of which the family is a part? What is the relationship between an individual who depersonalizes and the general condition of the society to which he belongs? What is the relationship between a person's loss of self-identity and the state of the social environment?

These questions point to the construction of a theory of depersonalization through the careful examination of the link between psychological and social concepts and social observations. This approach has influenced the method of presentation—the case method. It is particularly useful in both psychology and sociology because many of the concepts are of such a high level of abstraction that they tend to lose their connection with observation.

This chapter will focus on the following:

1. Definition and occurrence of depersonalization, citing certain recent literature.
2. The characteristics of contemporary America that lead to anomie, alienation, and social isolation.
3. The development of the self and the miscarriage that fosters depersonalization.
4. The role of the double bind in depersonalization, schizophrenia, and society.
5. Clinical vignettes from the lives and therapies of two such patients.

(Definition and Occurrence

The patient who has depersonalization experiences complains of having unpleasant feelings of unreality—of the self, the body, and the world. These feelings are not delusional, for the patient knows that reality has not changed. There is an attendant loss of affective response with complaints of no feeling for loved ones, no emotion, and no pleasure. There is loss of the ability to evoke visual imagery, to "picture" family and friends.

Depersonalization can occur in well-integrated individuals spontaneously, as well as in special circumstances or situations in which there is an alteration in the quantity and qual-

ity of input signals.[14,15] In a study of fifty-seven philosophy and psychology students, Roberts[54] found that twenty-three "showed past or present liability to brief periods of depersonalization." Contrary to the findings of others[1,42] that depersonalization occurs more commonly in women, Roberts found no sex differences. Alteration of input signals can occur through sensory deprivation or sleep deprivation, time changes with air flights, various states of altered physiological homeostasis, certain therapeutic drugs, and a number of psychotomimetic drugs,* thus jeopardizing reality sense.

The depersonalization experience is usually episodic, lasting from minutes to a few hours; conversely, on occasion, the condition is chronic and continues for months or years.[16]

Depersonalization occurs frequently in association with neuroses and psychoses, as well as with organic psychiatric syndromes. It is our clinical impression that patients experience depersonalization far more commonly than is generally recognized. Only anxiety and depression occur more frequently. It is difficult to determine the incidence of depersonalization experiences because of the relative strangeness of the symptoms and the attendant problems of patients communicating them to the psychiatrist.

A major portion of the literature on this subject has been devoted to a consideration of factors that predispose to and influence the onset of depersonalization. The contributions of Arlow,[69] Jacobson,[30] Rosen,[56] Sarlin,[58] Stewart,[69] Wittels,[78] and others, were enunciated in the earlier article. Bychowski[12] has chosen alienation as a term and concept that is more general and penetrating, for it also includes the way a person experiences his total reality including humanity at large. Bonime[10] described transitory feelings of depersonalization in a patient with personality change during the course of treatment. The patient had experienced growth and had the subjective

---

* The use of mind-expanding drugs has increased significantly in the past several years. Depersonalization is not a desired effect when one smokes marijuana, but is anticipated as part of the experience with psychotomimetic drugs.[9, 33, 37, 44, 48]

sensation that his personality was unfamiliar. Searles[62] also has noted that any change, even if it is clinically favorable, is an intense threat to the sense of identity and thus to one's perception of reality.

Characteristics of Contemporary America

In large part, the family is shaped by the industrial system. In this section, we shall examine the general state of contemporary American society to prepare the ground for exploring why the relations of family members are seen as the consequences of the dynamics of American society. First, we must look at the conditions of work and the self in America. Then, we shall examine fear in America as this refers particularly to acquiescence and conformity. Finally, we shall discuss anomie and alienation in relation to insatiability of social desires, social control and social change, loss of the self and social isolation.

Depersonalization has been defined as feelings of unreality. Thus, it is a subjective *experience*. In contrast, such behaviors as alcoholism, crime, divorce, drug addiction, psychoneurosis, and suicide are objective *actions*. They are difficulties of individuals, since we can always point to an individual alcoholic, criminal, drug addict, or divorcee. But, as has been demonstrated by Durkheim[21] in his study of suicide, the individual and his society are never independent of one another. In the study of social disorders, it becomes clear that a particularly large number of persons who suffer from behavior disorders are likely to appear in a society that shows certain other characteristics besides the individual incidences of the behavior disorder itself.

To further elaborate on this concept, personality development or socialization of a person occurs as a result of the interaction between the individual and his society. We cite Bredemeier's analogy which helps to clarify this relationship. On the one hand, personality needs can be likened to piano keys which have the potential for making music. Role, which refers to the way in which personality needs

are organized in terms of behavior, on the other hand, can be compared with the melody (or noise) that evolves. Like the co-ordination of the potential for music and the organization of tone, the individual and his society interpenetrate through role playing.*

A central purpose of this chapter is to demonstrate the relationship between our institutional structures and family values. Therefore, we shall outline some of our basic institutions and values. Through them, we shall interpret patterns of family life as these pertain to avenues to behavior disorders, generally, and to depersonalization specifically.

CONDITIONS OF WORK AND SELF

The worker does not own the product nor the tools of his production.[47] Centralized administrative decisions determine when men work and how fast. The product of man's labor is not a reflection of his imagination and dedication, nor is it an instrument through which he gains self-realization. People working under centralized bureaucracies are routinized, humiliated, and thereby dehumanized. The economic system prevents involvement and fosters detachment. It generates competition, creates feelings of inadequacy and fear of human obsolescence. It creates hostility and suspiciousness.

Personal Achievement. In contrast to some other societies, America's standard for personal excellence is occupational achievement. This emphasis on achievement is exclusively concerned with the objective results of man's activity, while man as a whole being is

---

* This dynamic analogy of the socialization process was given in a graduate course on contemporary sociological theory when the junior author was a doctoral student in sociology. The course was taught by Harry C. Bredemeier, Department of Sociology, Rutgers University, in 1965.

The term "role," as used in this chapter, represents a pattern of behavior of an individual by virtue of his *position* within a clearly defined division of labor, such as mother in a family, daughter, sister, wife, teacher, customer in a supermarket, or patient in a hospital. Shibutani[64] has stated, "The concept of role refers to the way in which the group norms apply to each of the participants. Each person is able to locate himself in the cast of the drama of which he is a part and thereby develops a working conception of what he should do."

minimized or even denigrated. Merton's[45] writing on anomie has highlighted the fact that the roots of alienation are evident in the widespread discrepancy between the universal need to achieve and the restricted means available to meet expectations of accomplishments. Consequently, there is a strong emphasis on the principle of individual competitiveness which frequently results in individual aggressiveness.

According to Beauvoir,[5] a basic characteristic of the American value orientation is that the source of one's value and truth is perceived in things and not in oneself. Consequently, craftsmanship has low value. Conversely, material comfort has a high place in the value hierarchy.[51] Success puts its emphasis on rewards. The success system, which William James has colorfully described as "the Bitch Goddess success," is comprised of money, prestige, power, and security. Mills[47] has expanded the concept of money as a medium of exchange. He has stated: "The intermediary becomes the real god since it is the real power which a person mediates to me. Money has omnipotence—the pander between need and object, between human life and the means of subsistence. What I am unable to do—what therefore all my individual faculties are unable to do is made possible by means of money."

The Corporate Structure and Bigness. Whyte[76] has stated that the shift from family-owned companies to management-run corporations has been a predominant influence on the movement from individual to group activities. The need to give priority to security over risk-taking has led to the emphasis on "bigness"—big business, big government, big unions.

In view of the humiliation and dehumanization of the individual, how does management bind him to the corporate structure? Management-run corporations, where most Americans work, offer job security through the establishment of guarantees, such as wage scales, bonuses, seniority rights and privileges, tenure, health insurance, sick leave, paid vacations, and retirement plans. The bureaucratic organization thereby binds the worker who is uninvolved in his work. In Becker's[6] terms, the corporation has thus bought the "commitment" of the worker through these "side bets."

FEAR IN AMERICA

The American man is a frightened individual. Fear, obsession, isolation, and suspicion are fostered by government, business. the press, school, the armed forces, and political reactionaries. The molding of the individual by these forces evolves from a specific concept of the human being. He must have a programmed view of the world: a national character who must be fearful and inclined to acquiesce.

There is a desire for security as opposed to risk-taking. There is a fear of becoming obsolete. The industrial system obliges too many people to devote their working hours to activities in which they have little interest. Change is rooted in obsolescence and both are basic to our industrial system.

The American is afraid of exploitation, competition, failure, and humiliation. Hence, one acts as if one were sincerely interested in others, but one is not. This "as if" behavior enables the individual to manipulate people, for he knows that manipulation is inherent in every human contact. Thus, there is a tendency to dismiss life as a dominance-submission struggle and to sacrifice tenderness and sensitivity to toughness and hardness. One result of dehumanization has been the development of countercultures. Some of these are the drug culture, drug-free communes, the "Jesus people," the worship of Satan with black masses, and the followers of gurus.

As with other cultures, the American is terrified of annihilation by unknown or foreign powers. According to Cook,[18] the American economy rests on fear generally, and particularly on America being a juggernaut state. Another sign of fear is the obsessional concern about the future. Emphasis on security and achievement lead to placing a high value on "side bets."

Acquiescence and Conformity. To want to be accepted by one's society is a universal phenomenon. As in most other cultures, to be accepted in contemporary American society a person must adopt an uncritical attitude toward its customs and fears. For example, one must hate and fear the Soviet Union, North Vietnam, Communist China, and Cuba (at least in some years). If he does not acquiesce, he isolates himself. As has been emphasized by Henry,[28] unthinking acquiescence results in "woolly-mindedness."

As has been noted by such foreign observers of the American social scene as Tocqueville[73] and Beauvoir,[5] the American values of equalitarianism, social mobility, and prestige underlie its stress on conformity. In buying patterns, fashion has acquired increasing influence over taste. By yielding to fashion, the consumer combines his need for both conformity and individuality. As analyzed by Simmel[66] in his classic paper on fashion, the fashionable individual derives the satisfaction of knowing that he represents something striking, while he feels inwardly supported by a set of persons who are striving for the same thing.

The impact of the changing occupational structure and bureaucratization (as a result of differentiation of labor, more education, and social mobility) is depicted as the collapse of individualism. The result, according to Riesman,[53] is movement from "inner-directed" man to "other-directed" man. He is characterized by (1) orientation toward situational rather than internalized goals; (2) extreme sensitivity to the opinion of others; (3) excessive need for approval; (4) conformity on internal experience as well as on externals; (5) loss of achievement orientation; and (6) loss of individualism.

The emptiness of values in a social system where life is lived in a mirror of how people evaluate an individual is exemplified in the Theater of the Absurd. In Arthur Miller's[46] *Death of a Salesman*, Willy Loman refers to the endless search for approval when he says that it is not enough to be just "liked," one must be "well liked." Like Freud's and Marx's ideas of decreased individuality and dignity making man the pawn of opposing forces from within and without, Samuel Beckett's[7] *Waiting for Godot* is primarily concerned with the basic problem of dualism whether it is psychic, religious, social, or economic. Despite

Vladimir's and Estragon's knowledge that each functions better separately, they find themselves bound together.

ANOMIE AND ALIENATION

According to Durkheim,[21] there are three conditions necessary for the development of anomie: insatiability of social desires, breakdown of collective order (social control), and social change. The loss of social control is the characteristic that gave the state of this society its name: anomie, a Greek word, meaning "lack of law."[29]

As a society, we are urban, democratic, bureaucratic, rationalized, large-scale, formal, open-class, geographically and occupationally mobile, secular, capitalistic, and technological.* These results of the French and Industrial Revolutions are fixed. They are irreversible. As a consequence, we propose that in various segments of contemporary America, the condition of *anomie* prevails.†

Insatiability, Collective Order, and Social Change. The purpose and mode of marketing is to create more and more desires, leading to an emphasis on consuming undurable goods. Durkheim has asked, "But how [do we] determine the quantity of well-being, comfort, or luxury legitimately to be craved by a human being? Nothing appears in a man's organic nor in his psychological constitution which sets

---

* The term "rationalization," as has been defined by Max Weber,[75] is a process of the conversion of social values and relationships from the primary communal and traditional shapes they once held to the larger, impersonal, and bureaucratic shapes of modern life. The concept of rationalization serves Weber exactly as equalitarianism serves Tocqueville.[73] In each, we see the historical tendency that can be understood only in relation to what happens to traditional society. Much of the emptiness of modern life is not so much a function of "commodity" production as of rationalization of life which has been developing at least since the seventeenth century.

† Since Durkheim has related the incidence of suicide to the state of anomie, it is of interest to note that the United States has had essentially the same incidence of suicide since 1900.[21] It falls in the middle of frequency of suicide in any consideration of world figures. The incidence is 10.5/100,000 and it has varied from 10.3 to 11—the extremes of the range. The incidence in the United States is about the same as in Great Britain. Sweden, Denmark, Japan, Austria, West Germany, and Hungary have an incidence of 15 to 23/100,000 that persists throughout the years.[27]

limits to such tendencies." Since the "sky is the limit," as far as man's social desires are concerned, a ceiling must be put on his passions so as to keep him from exploding. This ceiling consists of society which defines and regulates goals to which man should orient his behavior. When man's shared expectations of the "rules of the game" (expectations of the rights, obligations, and behavior of the other person) break down, it is as if the individual were stripped naked: A breakdown in collective man occurs. The shared meanings no longer serve as rules of a collective order. Action is no longer organized.

Social control breaks down under conditions of any sudden change, such as economic depression, or prosperity and extreme technological advance. Sudden change upsets the equilibrium and disturbs large numbers of people, thereby weakening the ruling forces of tradition (shared meanings and values).

To clarify these dynamics, we refer to the theoretical proposition of Strodtbeck and Short.[70] They have postulated that to the degree roles are not clearly defined by a social structure, the needs of the individual personality take precedence over playing the role (e.g., teacher or student) in a manner that meets the requirements of the social system (e.g., the university). When there is no conventional way to meet a situation satisfactorily, those who are involved are thrown back on their own resources. The result is either idiosyncratic or psychopathological behavior.

Loss of Self and Alienation. To be alienated is to be made alien—to be made strange and solitary, cut off from one's origin and history. Self-alienation might mean the loss of any of the three time dimensions, though loss of the past is the most frequent and important.[41] In Sartre's[59] *Nausea*, when Roquentin discovers that the past does not exist for him, he almost goes mad. Previously, Roquentin says the past to him "was another way of existing" and "each event, when it had played its part, put itself neatly into a box and became an honorary event." When he discovers he has no past, he is overwhelmed by "an immense sickness," and throughout the novel, he constantly insists that he really does exist.

Social Isolation. Empirically, alienation does not constitute an all-or-none dichotomy, but rather a continuum of relatedness. Such a continuum might consist of the following dimensions: (1) alienation from the Establishment —an individual voluntarily chooses to give up the society to which he belongs, because he does not find it intrinsically rewarding; for example, he withdraws from college, leaves home, to live in a commune-subculture; (2) alienation from others—the individual still hopes to be in the social system, but he has a feeling of being lost and he flounders rather than functions. He is estranged from others as each person secretly tries to make an instrument of the other, and a full circle is made— (3) he then makes an instrument of his self and is estranged from it also.[41] Thus, he has no sense of being and is in a state of despair.

We propose that the essence of social isolation is alienation from others and from the self. According to Fromm,[24] isolation is "moral aloneness." In May's[41] terms, isolation is defined as lack of a sense of being. In isolation, a person subordinates his existence to his functioning: a man knows himself not as a man but as a thing—the assembly-line worker in an automobile factory, the advertising executive, the post office employee, and so forth. We believe that the most destructive of all abuses that society inflicts upon the self or others is isolation.

In conclusion, in human history, there is one final conflict: man versus society. As has been emphasized by Norman Mailer,[39] "Society, which is necessary to enable men to grow, is also the prison whose walls he must perpetually enlarge." The relation between man and society is "half-wedding half-prison. Without man there cannot be a society, yet society must always seek to restrain man."

❲ The Self

The next sections of this paper are devoted to the consideration of the development of the self, the role of identity in the individual's interpersonal relationships, and how these can influence the development of depersonalization. These concepts are the common denominators in almost every relevant psychodynamic, sociological, and literary frame of reference. Even the language differences that once characterized various points of view are fading.

The definition and development of the self have been given wide attention in the literature. For example, Cooley,[19] Erikson,[23] May,[41] Mead,[43] Shibutani,[64] Sullivan,[71] and Winnicott[77] have formulated a developmental theory through which the self and identity emerge. They concur and emphasize that the self is to a large extent the product of culture, in that the individual picks up reactions of others and incorporates them into a meaningful, coherent self structure.

Sullivan's concept of the self dynamism has many similarities to those of Cooley and Mead. For example, Sullivan has defined the self as "the reflected appraisals of significant others."* This formulation closely approximates Cooley's concept of "the looking glass self"—the self is a mirror of how significant others have perceived the individual. In Mead's framework, the self is the capacity of a person to take the role of others, to see himself through their eyes. He has stated: "The individual experiences himself as such not directly, but only indirectly from the particular standpoints of other individual members of the same group or from the generalized standpoint of the social group as a whole to which he belongs."

Shibutani has described personal identity as one's only tie with society. Personal and social status are defined in terms of reciprocating relationships with people who recognize the individual as a specific being. It is this tie with society that is humanizing. According to May, self-identity is *being* (the potentiality of a person becoming what he truly is), and being is *becoming*. Being human is self-consciousness—to be aware of the self, to be responsi-

ble for himself if he is to become himself. Selfhood (identity) means having a history and knowing what that history is. The self lives in three time dimensions—past, present, and future—though the significant dimension for human beings is the future.

DEVELOPMENT OF THE SELF

Winnicott[77] has identified the main processes that take place in the emotional growth of the infant during early months as integration, personalization, and relating to objects.† The self comes into being in infancy through the good mother's response to the infant's gesture or spontaneous impulse. Through the mother's unconditionally meeting the infant's needs, the infant is able to identify and differentiate basic needs. This leads to the development of basic trust accompanied by satisfaction and security.‡ Any attendant anxiety is minimal. According to Winnicott, under optimal mothering circumstances, the "I" is experienced and differentiated from the "Not-Me." Add to this the basic perception: "I am seen or understood to exist by someone . . . I get back the evidence I need that I have been recognized as a being."

Erikson[23] and Shibutani[64] have observed that the feeling of being a distinct person also arises from one's sense of autonomy (versus shame and doubt), competency (industry versus inferiority) and the feeling of having some measure of control over one's destiny. In addition, Erikson has stated that the central task of the adolescent era of personality development is *role identity*, in contrast to role confusion.

According to the authors of this chapter, the issue of one's sexuality is implicit in the task of

---

* The term "significant others" refers to those persons who play a major role in the socialization process from infancy to maturity and to whom an individual relates in a meaningful manner, whether positively or negatively.[43, 71]

† The term "personalization," as used by Winnicott, describes the process of ego development, based on body ego, evolving as the self of the baby starts to be linked with the body and body functions, with the skin as limiting membrane. He has chosen this term because he defined "depersonalization" as a loss of firm union between ego and the body.

‡ Sullivan[72] clearly differentiates between needs which result in satisfaction and in security. He limits the term "satisfaction" to the infant's response to having his biological needs (feeding, bathing, and so forth) met. In contrast, he uses the term "security" to refer to the infant's need for the relief of anxiety. This need is met by the mother's unconditional nurturance, acceptance, recognition, tenderness, and support.

achieving identity. Thus, the concept of identity raises not only the question of "Who am I?" but also, more specifically, it raises the point of "What does it feel like to be a girl?" "A boy?" "Do I like being a boy?" Lidz et al.[35] have further commented: "Of all factors entering into the formation of personality characteristics, the sex of the child is most decisive; and security of sexual identity is a cardinal factor in the achievement of stable ego identity." As we have pointed out, probably all patients who depersonalize are seriously confused in their sexual identity. Frequently, a person may struggle to cope with a weak or lost self-identity by trying to belong to someone. Instead of resolving the problem of identity, he may shift his focus to achieving intimacy.[60] Erikson[22] has stated the dilemma succinctly, "You can't get your identity straightened out by trying to achieve intimacy ahead of identity."

As for the role of identity in depersonalization, Laing[34] has illustrated this in a statement of one of his patients: "It struck me that if I stared long enough at the environment that I would blend with it and disappear just as if the place was empty and I had disappeared. It is as if you get yourself to feel you don't know who you are or where you are . . . Then, you are scared of it (of disappearing) because it begins to come on without encouragement . . . I would get frightened and repeat my name over and over again to bring me back to life."

MISCARRIAGE IN THE DEVELOPMENT OF SELF

In view of the nature of the normal developmental process of the self, as well as its miscarriage, a crucial question with which this discussion must be concerned is: What is the process by which the development of the self and identity miscarry and lead to depersonalization?

Of particular relevance to our topic is the distorted message, the mixed message, or the nonmessage, and the relationships of the individual's perceptions of these to his concept of himself and the world. As has been pointed out by Roshco,[57] contact with reality depends on an objective perception of the self in relation to an objectively perceived external reality, i.e., the child's perceptions in relation to his mother. To the extent that there is a disturbance in the normal separation-individuation phase of development (sense of autonomy), the perception of the mother is distorted and, therefore, perception of the self is distorted. Thus, there is interference with reality contact—difficulty in distinguishing between self and objects.

Bettelheim[8] has cited a concrete example of miscarriage in development. He has stated: "Artificial feeding times dehumanize the infant and prevent him from feeling that his actions, cry or smile, are what bring about his being fed . . . When we feel that we cannot influence the important things that happen to us but that they follow the dictates of some inexorable power, then we give up trying to learn how to act or change them." The growth of the child is accompanied by the conviction that his personal efforts can influence a given chain of events providing the environment permits this. "If the infant's caretaker is not perceived as a human being, then neither can the infant grow up to be one."

In discussing the development of the self system, Laing,[34] Böszörményi-Nagy and Framo,[11] Shibutani,[64] and Winnicott[77] have emphasized that when such development miscarries, there is a split in the self. This results in two parts, the true self and the false self, or the subject and the object.

According to Laing, the true self is the unembodied self that functions as observer, controller, and critic of what the body is experiencing and doing. The true self translates into action what one wants to be. Winnicott has pointed out that in health, the true self remains dominant and perceives reality. He has emphasized that only the true self feels real.

As for the false self, both Laing and Winnicott have stressed that it is built on compliance. Laing has stated that there is a basic split in the individual along the line of cleavage between his outward compliance and his inner withholding of compliance. The false self arises in compliance with the intentions or expectations of the significant others or what one imagines these to be.

Laing has related the body to the false self. The body is perceived more as an object among other objects in the world than as the core of the individual's being. He has illustrated this perception in the following comment on one of his patients: "He found reassurance in the consideration that whatever he was doing, he was not being himself." This patient was always playing a part, usually the part of someone else but sometimes he played himself. Not that he was spontaneously himself, but he played a role depicting himself (as an intellectual, poet, or clown, for example). His goal was never to give his true self away.

In terms of perceiving the self as an object, Shibutani has stated that loss of identity means loss of humanness. The individual feels that he is a spectator observer of what his body is doing rather than a participant observer.* Winnicott has conceptualized the false self partly as having the function of defending the true self. When the false self becomes exploited in the extreme and is treated as real (as if it were the true self), there is a sense of futility and despair. This is the depersonalization experience which is terrifying.

Böszörményi-Nagy and Framo, Laing, Sullivan, and Winnicott agree that the occurrence of the "false self system" or "weak ego" or the "not me" emerges in response to deficiencies in the mothering of the infant. They have enunciated the fact that after the early months, the father often joins with the mothering one in the unconscious conspiracy of presenting the child with distortions in perceptions, identity, and interpersonal relationships.

* The term "participant observer," as used and defined by Sullivan,[71] refers first to the fact that a large part of mental disorder results from and is perpetuated by inadequate communication and that the communication process is being interfered with by anxiety. Second, the term means that each person in any two-person relationship is involved as a portion of an interpersonal field, rather than as a separate entity in processes which affect and are affected by the field. To illustrate, "participant observer" requires that one person not only observe the total behavior of the other person(s) in interaction, but also observe his own behavior—feelings, reactions, attitudes, thoughts, and so forth—and the impact of these on oneself and on whomever one is interacting with.

In this kind of total setting, the true self is sabotaged. It remains unformed, weak, easily disrupted, and not capable of moving through the evolutionary process of growth. Thus the dominating false self emerges in the child and he therefore becomes vulnerable to experiencing depersonalization at a later time in his life.

([Double Bind, Depersonalization, and Schizophrenia

According to Bateson et al.,[4] the double-bind situation is a necessary condition in the development of schizophrenia. It is of particular interest to note, however, that in most of the literature on depersonalization, double bind is a central, organizing concept. The occurrence of depersonalization and double bind together has been validated in our own clinical experiences and will be illustrated in the presentation of two clinical vignettes. Concerning the nature of the relationship between the depersonalization experience and the double-bind condition, we are faced with a critical theoretical question, namely: Does or can the double-bind situation occur in depersonalization without the development of schizophrenia?

In addressing this issue, Arieti[3] has pointed out that ". . . all of us would agree that our schizophrenic patients have been repeatedly exposed to this double-bind situation. But I think we would also agree that many neurotics were exposed, and many normal people, and we, too."

STRUCTURE OF THE DOUBLE BIND

For purposes of exploring the relationship between double bind and depersonalization, it is important to review the social structure of the double bind as analyzed by Bateson et al. In this creative work, the authors have identified five interacting parts that make up the structure of the double bind:

1. Two or more persons are involved, the child-victim and the mother alone, or in combination with father and/or siblings. The double bind, far from being a single traumatic

experience, is repeated so often that the double-bind structure comes to be a habitual experience.

2. There is a primary negative injunction based on avoidance of punishment. This injunction may have either of two forms: "Do not do so and so, or I will punish you," or "If you do not do so and so, I will punish you." The authors define the punishment as withdrawal of love, expressions of hate or anger, or the kind of abandonment that occurs when the parent expresses extreme helplessness.

3. There is a secondary injunction that conflicts with the first but at a more abstract level and again threatening punishment. In contrast to the direct verbalization that characterizes the primary injunction, the secondary one is communicated by posture, tone of voice, gesture, facial expression, or an indirect allusion to the primary injunction. For instance, "Do not submit to my prohibitions." "Do not see me as a punishing agent." "Do not see this as punishment." "Do not question my love of which the primary injunction is (or is not) an example." When the double bind is inflicted by two individuals, one parental partner may negate the injunctions of the other at a more abstract level.

4. There is a tertiary negative injunction that prohibits the victim from escaping from the field. If the double binds are imposed during infancy, escape is naturally impossible. In some instances, however, escape from the field is made impossible by certain devices which are not entirely negative. For instance, capricious promises of love.

5. Finally, the complete set of ingredients is not necessary once the individual has learned to perceive the universe in double-bind patterns. Almost any part of a double-bind sequence may then be sufficient to precipitate panic or rage. The pattern of conflicting injunctions may even be taken over by auditory hallucinations.

Even though the double-bind mode of communication has been identified as a core concept in the development of the schizophrenic process, depersonalization can occur under a wide variety of circumstances that have nothing to do with schizophrenia. However, deper-

sonalization experiences are common among those who have schizoid personalities and schizophrenia. Many of the distortions of perception and identity during early maturation that have been associated with depersonalization also obtain in the development of schizophrenia.

DOUBLE BIND IN SOCIETY

In view of our earlier question that pertained to the relationship between the individual who experiences depersonalization and the general conditions of the society to which he belongs, we raise the following question: What contributes to parents' expertise in using the double bind? Certainly, they developed some of their skills in this realm in their early relationships with their own parents. However, we suggest that in addition to such family determinants, there are cultural determinants.

Various organizations and cultural institutions disseminate double-bind messages. As an example, we shall focus on the plight of the faculty member in the university.

There are numerous illustrations of the double bind in the university setting, which may serve as a prototype for other bureaucratic organizations. The role of the university faculty member is formally defined as "teacher of students." The primary injunction, on the one hand, is, "Get close to the students," while on the other hand, the negative aspect of this injunction is, "Don't get too close to students, because if you do it means you no longer identify with us as faculty members and administration." The punishment for obeying either command is to be denied promotion and tenure. The teacher must demonstrate his loyalty to the university by doing so-called "research" and grinding out publications to the greater glory of the institution.

In another context, some universities have a policy of open admissions (every high-school graduate must be admitted, irrespective of grades). The positive aspect of the primary injunction is: "Be fair, but maintain reasonable standards of academic performance." This calls for an "as if" performance by the teacher in the face of the negative part of the injunction that states: "You, the teacher, are forbidden to fail any student." Thus, the administration obviates student demonstrations that might lead those in political power to question the ability of the leaders of the academic administration and the need to replace some of them. Thereby, the faculty member is encouraged to remain aloof from the student, to look down on him and to derogate him but is ordered to give him a passing grade.

The double bind communicated to the faculty member is inevitably passed on to the student. As a result, each is a pawn in an unfeeling system that dehumanizes people and creates "things." Finally, students who wish to become faculty members in a university setting are told that they are most welcome but that they must have a doctoral degree to achieve this high estate. Once the degree has been earned, frequently the message is different. The secondary injunction is that there are no jobs at the university level and the candidate is advised to apply for a teaching position in a junior college in Texas (if he is in New York, but the reverse formula is applied if he is in Texas).

It appears that the concepts of double bind and anomie may be positively correlated. In the situation we have described, there is a lack of an accepted standard for judging students', teachers', and administrators' role obligations. How can one person look down on someone who has acted wrongly if there is no clear definition of "wrong"? In this kind of situation in which roles, expectations, and norms are not clearly defined, there no longer can be inner cohesion. Thus, the entire university setting is anomic. There is mass indifference and the individuals who make up the university group are demoralized.

(Depersonalization and Family Structure

To illustrate the relationship between a person who depersonalizes and the small group, his family, we shall present clinical vignettes which include history, dynamics, and treatment of two patients.* In our presentation of

* Both patients were treated by the senior author.

the two family groups we shall scrutinize three elements of behavior: (1) individual activity —what Michelle Mahler and Nancy Cabot† do as members of the family group, as well as what other members of the family do; (2) feelings—the sum of internal feelings, whether physical or emotional, that a family member has in relation to what another member does;[29] (3) interaction—the relationship which the activity of one member of the group has to do with that of other members. In addition, we also shall examine these three elements of behavior in relation to significant others outside the family group, including the therapist.

Behavior disorders and psychoses are the final outcome of all that is wrong with a society. We shall focus on the parents, not as individuals, but on the individuals in their role in the social system. It is they who are the carriers of the culture and who transmit cultural ills and strengths, and thereby lay the foundation for sanity or madness.

(The Mahler Family

Michelle Mahler is a strikingly attractive girl of twenty-four. She is tall and shapely with a pretty face and finely chiseled features. She moves well and has an aristocratic air about her. Despite her foreign birth, she speaks English fluently and clearly.

Three years prior to seeking treatment with me, Michelle had begun treatment with a psychologist who was less than ten years her senior. She discontinued when she felt that he had become too involved with her personally. Next, she saw a psychiatrist who was old enough to be her father. He told her that she was inhibited and that this could be alleviated through personal contact with him. When he invited her to sit on his lap, she left.

† The names used are fictitious. The fact that both patients are women is fortuitous and is not meant to be a commentary on sexual incidence. Roberts[54] found no sex differences in depersonalization. In our study, it just happened that each of these patients was in treatment for more than two years and pertinent data could be collected.

Michelle wants treatment because of depression, depersonalization, painful self-consciousness, anxiety in many areas of behavior, migraine, nausea, and anorexia. Her depression is characterized by feelings of deep sadness, uncontrollable crying spells, withdrawal, suicidal ideation, and self-disparagement.

Before considering Michelle's social history and personality development, a consideration of her feelings of unreality and her sense of identity is in order.

Unreality Feelings and Sense of Identity

Speaking of her feelings of unreality, Michelle describes them as follows: "If anyone gets to know me really well, they and I would find out that there is nothing there, just hollow, rotten, crumby . . . A thing comes over me when I can't feel anything . . . As if I were living exclusively through my head with no real pleasure . . . A numb feeling, feeling really strange, as if the whole world were encompassed in a numb feeling . . . Feel there's nothing inside, a hole . . . A feeling I have to be acted upon in order to react. Otherwise, there is nothing. No outline of what kind of person I am. No shape, form, texture, just an amorphous blob . . . In arguments, words come out but I don't really feel anything inside . . . I have a tendency to feel that anything I say is not being heard by anyone . . . I mean what I say but it is as if someone else is saying it.

"A good friend from Boston is in New York, but I feel that I have nothing to contribute and she has so much vitality. It bothers me that I have no definite sense of who I am. I fear she'll be disappointed and that there's no me that exists for her to like. I don't feel this when I am with Derek (an old friend from Austria with whom she is comfortable). Then I feel my own self thrown into great relief and I can see myself and what I think."

Social History

Michelle's grandparents on both sides had been wealthy Protestant or Greek Orthodox aristocrats in Central Europe, with one excep-

tion. Her maternal great-grandfather had been Jewish, and her maternal grandfather had been a judge and an owner of factories. With the advent of Hitler, the latter was forced to give up everything because he was not pure Aryan. The maternal grandmother committed suicide.

Michelle's mother, Sigrid, grew up in a household that was run by a multitude of servants, and she had been cared for by governesses since infancy. She had never been in a kitchen until she was eighteen, when her social and economic status was devastated by the fact of her Jewish background. She had to go to work and people told her they could no longer speak to her. As long as Sigrid was married to Michelle's father, Hans, a wealthy landowner, the Jewish background was not a problem. However, the marriage was short-lived and was terminated before she brought Michelle to the United States.

PERSONALITY DEVELOPMENT

There are no specific data about Michelle before she was five. However, Sigrid's behavior in the past, and more recently, provides no evidence that she has changed in any way since Michelle was born. Having divorced her wealthy husband, it is quite likely that she came to the United States to seek her fortune. Thus, she brought Michelle to this country when she was five years old. Sigrid wanted to work and to find a new husband, so she placed her daughter in a series of foster homes for the next year. When Michelle was six and still had German as her principal language, her mother placed her in a boarding school for destitute children, where she remained for two years. In that setting, Michelle feels that she was dehumanized, as was the heroine of *Jane Eyre*.

When Michelle was eight years old, her mother married a second time, and the little girl lived in this household until she was sixteen and the parents were divorced. This eight-year period is the longest the patient has ever spent in any residence. For two years before going to college, she lived successively with the families of two high-school friends. The mother married her third husband during this period.

Mother-Daughter Relationship. In the following monologue, Michelle enunciates the essence of her relationship with her mother. "Mother is the key to me, not the fact of three different fathers . . . I have trouble believing she is not as nice as I thought when she does certain things. She used to say that I was the most fantastic thing ever created, beautiful, perfect. In contrast, she is opposed to another side of me and things that mean a lot to me, such as my working in the museum in the ghetto. She said I was selfish to do this, never thinking of her but surrounding myself with low-class people and dragging her down . . . I can never decide what to think of her. She says that she's the only one I can trust and that I can't trust my friends. She says she's right and my friends are wrong. Is she deliberately doing that or is it that she's just warped and can't help herself? She says things that aren't the truth. I could cope with her better if I could decide about these things.

"If I don't get love from my parents, then nothing else matters, though it does matter. I can't believe they are unloving people. Mother used to threaten me with having a lawyer take control of my affairs (a trust fund that will eventually become hers) or to put me in an institution. There were lots of such threats."

Father-Daughter Relationship. Beginning at the age of ten, Michelle visited her father, Hans Mahler, in Germany, once a year. These are some of her impressions of him and his way of life.

"Three years ago, when I was twenty-one, he was close to being an alcoholic when I visited. I'd have to sit up with him until 2 A.M. while he drank. He seemed very sexual, sensual. He was seductive verbally and I left. Now, he's more like a very old man and he no longer frightens me. He sculpts and paints fairly well. He tries to buy the love I'm incapable of giving him. He despises himself so it's difficult to love him. He's frustrated because he doesn't know who he is and he's done nothing with his life. I don't like him but I want to. I never know what to do when he's around. He's snide."

Relationships with Men. Initially in New York, Michelle lived alone. Later, she had a dour, young Jewish schoolteacher named Jacob move in with her. She subsequently joined him in an apartment nearer their places of work, but found their interests so far apart that, after much soul searching, she moved into her own apartment again. She expresses distress that she cannot seem to maintain a relationship with a young man for more than two months. She has continued relationships with one or two men who are her peers, such as Derek. She sees them from time to time, but does not find them attractive sexually. She has found herself attracted to emotionally unstable young men from disadvantaged backgrounds who exploit her and then repudiate her. Her sexual interests seem to focus on young black men who have had varying degrees of sociopathy. Michelle has done a kind of reversal of the Cinderella story, leaving the castle to go to the ghetto hearth and repudiating minor princes for relative paupers.

Dynamics of Feelings of Unreality and Confused Identity

Michelle's painful feelings of unreality have an "as if" quality. These feelings are not delusional for she speaks of *feeling* unreal in contrast to *being* unreal. She feels empty, numb, an amorphous blob. There is no feeling and no pleasure. These are the criteria for depersonalization that we have outlined.

She lacks the feeling of being a distinct person and of having the sense of autonomy and competency described by Erikson[23] and Shibutani.[64] She is a spectator observer in contrast to being a participant observer. In an argument, words come out, though she feels nothing, yet she means what she says, but repudiates the idea she is saying it. Thus, her sense of self or identity is very shaky and, for no apparent reason, it seems to come and go.

Michelle describes a feeling that she must be acted upon in order to react. The "personalization," described by Winnicott,[77] has never fully taken place. The experience of having been recognized as a separate being in infancy and having had her needs met unconditionally by the mothering one was deficient, and the opportunity for the development of the true self must have been less than optimal.

In addition, she notes that meeting someone she likes and respects paralyzes her functioning and she fears being judged and found wanting. Here is evidence of feeling compelled to adopt a compliant attitude, as enunciated by Winnicott, in the evolution of the self.

Interestingly enough, Michelle feels most comfortable and whole when she is with Derek, a peer and contemporary from her native land. This is one of the few such relationships she has permitted herself. He treats her with affection and respect. (This seeming paradox in her perception of herself will be considered later.)

Dynamics of Interaction

MARGINAL INDIVIDUAL

The concept of "marginal individual" was developed by Parks in the study of interethnic contacts. In the traditional sense, "marginal" means that a person stands on the border of two or more social worlds but is not accepted as a full participant in either. Marginality creates anxiety and can lead to feelings of alienation. A principal implication of marginality for this chapter is that the uprooting of the immigrant is a critical factor in determining the American character.

Marginal persons who develop emotional disturbances are those who attempt to improve their lot by identifying with the higher stratum (Michelle's pull to Germany, where her wealthy father resides), and to rebel when rejected. However, no necessary relationship between marginal status and personality disorder has been established.

The Mother. In several respects, Michelle's mother is a marginal woman, as this refers to being uprooted but not transplanted. First, at the age of eighteen, Sigrid was totally rejected by friends who could no longer speak to her because of her Jewish background. Second, her marriage ended in divorce, at which time she came to America. Third, she was compelled to work, though she was totally unprepared to do so.

Michelle. As Michelle grew up, she experienced a frightening quantity and quality of rootlessness, multiple identifications, and a lack of loving, consistent role models. She grew up in what was initially an alien culture with an alien language, and she has never regarded this country as her home. She is unclear about her nationality and language of choice. She expresses preference for Germany and the German language and feels alien to middle-class America. Yet, she seems content to limit her time in Germany to the annual visits. Her life has been that of a gypsy, in the sense of her moving frequently, except for the eight-year period when her mother was married to her first stepfather.

In the traditional sense, Michelle is a marginal woman, in that she maintains one foot in Germany and one foot in America. She has suffered from the inability to find integration of her self and society, and thus she is an alienated young woman.

PARENTAL-DAUGHTER INTERACTION

The mother is self-centered; she was more interested in finding a husband than in caring for Michelle. Frequently, she acts *as if* (the need to mask real feelings) she loved Michelle, when in fact she wishes the girl had never been born. Double binds are a central theme in the mother-daughter relationship. For example, on the one hand, she tells Michelle she is "the most fantastic, beautiful thing created," while on the other hand, she humiliates Michelle by telling her how ugly she is after plastic surgery and commanding her to cover her face with a handkerchief. Anyone who agrees to play the game of double bind can and does lose every time. Every reaction of Michelle elicits some form of punishment, rejection, further loss of self-esteem and self-reliance.

Michelle's mother uses terror as the instrument to obtain Michelle's acquiescence. To illustrate, the mother talks to Michelle about her "bad genes" and has threatened to place her in an institution if she does not acquiesce to her demands. She exploited and humiliated both her second husband and Michelle when she told her she had married a man "who was not interested in sex and was a manic-depressive" because her daughter needed a home. In conveying her dissatisfaction with this husband, she undermined his value to Michelle as a model for a love object.

Michelle was treated merely as an extension of her mother and thus was manipulated as a thing. She has had the perspicacity and detachment to question her mother's motives or illness: "Is she deliberately doing that or is it that she's just warped and can't help herself? . . . I could cope with her better if I could decide."

In infancy, Michelle did not have this objectivity and was subjected to an onslaught that wreaked havoc. This havoc could be defined in the language of any of several theoretical frameworks: Bettelheim's dehumanization, Erikson's lack of autonomy, Roshco's separation-individuation phase, or the failure of the development of the self, as described by Winnicott and Laing, respectively.

The father, though less prominent in her day-to-day life, has been her role model of a man. Michelle speaks of him as a man who is not a man and as a person who is empty and who lacks self-respect. He is difficult to love, yet he tries to buy Michelle's love. On the other hand, he tells her to do as she pleases and to live where she chooses. However, he promises to support her and her graduate education if she lives in Europe, but not if she lives in the United States, where she has a life of near-poverty. With this "very sexual, sensual, and verbally seductive behavior," Hans Mahler breaks the generation boundaries, in that he seeks emotional support and sense of completion from his daughter, rather than from his second wife.[35] Consequently, he confuses and humiliates Michelle and uses her as a pawn. He is impulse-driven. He is frustrated and despises himself, and so resorts to alcohol to assuage the pain of his feelings. This enigmatic man has been a very confusing influence in many areas, including Michelle's choice of men.

Michelle's penchant for selecting unstable young men has also been influenced by her need to rebel against parents and their way of life. However, her identity and conception of self are very shaky and she has doubts about her worthiness to live at a level consistent with her breeding, as well as doubts about her ability to cope with her peers. Ironically, she has chosen to work in one of the most difficult sociological areas imaginable in today's world. She has done very well in her occupational position despite the many problems inherent in it.

Michelle's mother, who has lived in America for twenty years, her father, and her stepfathers manifest American personality characteristics that are widespread. These are detachment, pathological "as if" behavior, a tendency to humiliate others, criticalness, and pecuniary motivations. Finally, there is the demand for acquiescence (through the threat of abandonment), which we have emphasized as the ultimate in conformity. Hand in hand with the use of terror is the illusory promise of forthcoming gratification. But whoever utilizes terror has no intention of gratifying anyone or anything but himself. The Mahlers have overtly terrorized Michelle and, to a point, she has acquiesced.

Perhaps the most remarkable aspect of this clinical vignette is that Michelle has not succumbed completely to her mother's domination or to a paralyzing schizophrenic reaction. It is a triumph for Michelle and a tribute to her that she has the strength and persistence to find the emerging potential of a true self and an identity. In addition, she has been able to make a significant contribution in her work, despite her talent for sabotaging her personal life.

The Cabot Family

Nancy Cabot is a blonde beauty of twenty. Her almond-shaped eyes are blue and she has the attractive figure of a young woman but the shyness and naïveté of an early adolescent. These are evident in her need to wear a trenchcoat on even the hottest days to hide herself, and in her frequently expressed wish to be a little girl and not a woman.

She had been referred by one of the deans at the college in New York City where she is a second-year student. Frequently, she is dominated by pervasive anxiety, depersonalization, obsession, phobias, depression with suicidal ideation and self-disparagement, as well as feelings of inadequacy and helplessness.

Unreality Feelings and Sense of Identity

Depersonalization feelings are recurring strands in the fabric of Nancy's symptomatology and are enunciated here for purposes of illustrating the phenomena. Her own descriptions of depersonalization gives us an additional perspective on her experiences. Her account is relatively characteristic and demonstrates the difficulties patients encounter in describing these strange and uncanny feelings.

"Sometimes, I feel foggy. Now, I feel disconnected, not foggy . . . At times, I know where I am but don't feel I'm really there . . . My head feels all cloudy. At times, I get so I can't think clearly or do my work. It is as if there's a big mass stuck in my head . . . Off and on during the past week I didn't feel real. Wherever I was, I just didn't feel I was there, just no place . . . Sometimes, on a bus, I feel like a stick, lose my balance . . . I get peppy and laugh but it doesn't feel like me laughing. It feels like something inside me is doing it . . . About half the time I feel real but with some blurring of vision . . . I'll sit for a long time doing nothing and just staring. It's as if someone had put Novocain in my brain."

Nancy's experiences become more meaningful when viewed in the context of her own symptoms and the interpersonal situation in which they occur.

If Nancy is in a public setting among strangers, the unreality feelings are accentuated. For example, she went to the library of the Academy of Medicine to prepare a paper for school but was very fearful. She felt awkward, bumped into things, feared the bookshelves would topple over on her—but once there she was afraid to leave. On her second visit there, she felt in a daze, was unable to concentrate and felt she was being watched all the time. "Every time I would look up, someone had their eyes on me." There probably is a reality basis for this perception, because attractive young women are conspicuous in such a setting.

When she was alone on the boardwalk in Atlantic City, she felt frightened of the crowds. "It was like a wall was there stopping me. I couldn't go on. This happened two times in Barbados. I couldn't go through the hotel gate to the street. My feet were like lead and I had to turn back."

These experiences of encountering a "wall," feeling paralyzed and unable to move forward and having to turn back, are disabling. However, her preoccupation with being watched by dead people is more pathological. When alone, she feels that dead people she has known are watching her. These include grandparents, friends of her mother, and others. At times, she feels they are judging her critically and at other times she feels they are neutral. This experience seems to vary between obsession and delusion. "They're watching you but you don't know they're there. They make you behave as you should and there's never any privacy. If they turn off, I wouldn't know what to do. They'd be pleased if I didn't do certain things, mainly go against my parents. When I die, I'll be able to see people on earth."

On many occasions when she feels depressed, she has obsessive thoughts about harming herself with medication or by cutting or burning herself. "Last night I called you because I felt futile and self-destructive, but less so now . . . This past week I've been feeling unreal much of the time. I made these cuts on my left wrist to hurt myself and I feel a little better when I do it. The cuts are not over the vein. I made some last week and some this week. I have to do it. I get so mad at myself for causing my parents concern. The feeling lifts several times a day and I'm able to function better than normally." On another occasion, she speaks of burning herself with a cigarette for that hurts more than a razor blade and would be less easy for her roommate and her friend Ruth to detect, though they have discovered it.

Social History

The social climate of the Cabot family is one of severe emotional deprivation and massive impoverishment. Nancy not only has numerous depersonalization experiences but also has had a schizoaffective episode for which she had to be hospitalized.

Nancy's mother, Elizabeth Whitney Cabot, comes from a wealthy, Social-Register family. She puts much emphasis on social position. Mrs. Cabot has had all the better things of life as defined by the American high-rising living standard. Her parental family is responsible for the trust funds that have been provided for her and her daughters. Nancy lives in an atmosphere of material indulgence.

Arthur Cabot, the father, was born in the South. He works in New York City, where he maintains a small apartment for himself; he commutes to the family home in exurbia only on weekends. Mr. Cabot drinks heavily, is frequently intoxicated, and regularly yields to uncontrolled impulse.

Nancy's two sisters, six and eight years her senior, are married, and each has a husband who is completing his professional training. One sister was taken to see a psychiatrist during adolescence, but there was an early termination of treatment by the parents whose opposition to psychiatric care persists in the present. Since Nancy is six years younger than the second daughter, one wonders if she may have been an unwanted child.

Ruth, whom the parents deeply resent, is a crucial figure in Nancy's life, filling the role of surrogate mother. She is the housemother of the boarding school that Nancy attended in New York City. Since the number of boarders was small, Ruth was able to give many of them a lot of individual attention and they, in turn, became attached to her. Nancy was one of several of these "poor little rich girls" who continued to see her after they had gone on to college and to spend all or parts of their holidays with her. Ruth was in her mid-thirties when Nancy came for treatment. Her personal life had been scarred by a number of tragedies, both in interpersonal relationships and physical health. During the period of Nancy's treatment, Ruth's time was devoted primarily to her job of caring for her "lost sheep."

PERSONALITY DEVELOPMENT

The parental home is in an exclusive section of exurbia where the married sisters and their families gather for Christmas each year. Details of Nancy's early developmental history are fragmentary, in view of the parents' aversion to psychiatrists and their reluctance to visit the senior author who treated Nancy. A good deal of material has been provided by Nancy's recollections and the parents' ongoing interactions with each other and with Nancy.

Nancy's developmental years have been marked by episodes of exposure to sexual stimulation and to periodic domestic violence. Both kinds of scenes continue to be familiar in current contacts with her parents.

Sexual Stimulation. When Nancy Cabot was young, theirs was a "nude household." She recalls having taken baths with her father when she was four and seeing him and others in the family running around nude. When she was five or six, her parents came home drunk one evening and got into a fight after they had taken their clothes off. Mother picked up a poker and the teen-aged daughter called the police. No one was seriously injured but some bruises were sustained.

Even then, Nancy feared the dark and would sleep with a sheet over her head. However, she rarely slept alone. Until she went to boarding school in her teens, she would sleep with her mother at times, but more often with her father. When they were in bed together, he would hold her in his arms, so she made him wear shorts under his pajamas. Occasionally, he would leave the bed and go to her mother's room for a half hour. When Nancy was ten, one of her sisters told her something about sexual intercourse. She then realized that this was the reason for her father's visits to her mother's bedroom. Subsequently, Nancy would feel angry and go to her own room.

From time to time, during the period of treatment, her father continued to touch her breasts, as well as those of her sisters and make a snide joke about it. A brother-in-law ignored or criticized Nancy on the one hand, while on the other hand he would grab her, kiss her, and grope at her breasts. Her mother and sisters tacitly disapproved of this behavior on the part of the men, but tolerated it.

Thomas, a sixty-two-year-old black, is the

man of all work in the parental household. He lives in a small house on the grounds with his young wife and small child. Nancy was devoted to them, felt safe with them, and enjoyed visiting their home and playing with the child. She was perplexed and alarmed that when they were alone together, Thomas grabbed her buttocks and breasts. He derided her by saying, "You've been asking for it." She was afraid to tell anyone and resolved never to be alone with him. Somehow, her mother found out. She told Nancy that Thomas' feelings were hurt because she was afraid of him and that he had cried. Her mother demanded that Nancy write to Thomas and apologize to him.

School Years. Nancy had been more assertive during childhood and preadolescence and there were frequent spankings for "talking back." She feels she may have been indulged by her mother, who defended her from her sisters' wrath when she teased them.

In school, Nancy's talkativeness provoked the teacher, who applied Scotch tape to her mouth and sent her to the principal's office for such misbehavior as kicking and scratching other children. The teacher kept a card on Nancy's desk and would paste a gold star on it in recognition of a week of good behavior. She fought a lot with peers and had few friends. Her two main playmates were younger than she.

After attending public school for five years, she was sent to a private day school for three years. She spent two of her high school years in a boarding school in a near-by state, and the final two years in the boarding school in New York City where she met Ruth. Following graduation, she went to a college in Florida, but left after two months, for she was lonely, frightened, and withdrawn. Subsequently, she entered the college she was attending at the time she began treatment.

Shortly after psychiatric treatment was initiated with the senior author, therapy became an area of controversy between Nancy and her parents, particularly the issue of three sessions a week. In addition, they were opposed to her spending time with Ruth, which limited Nancy's visits home to one or two weekends a month. It was not that they were eager to see her, but that they were jealous of her relationships with Ruth and the therapist.

A few months after starting treatment, Nancy earned an associate arts degree in June. She wished to return to college in the fall for a third year. However, her parents wanted her to spend a year living with a family in France and then return to the United States to work. Such a plan would effectively terminate both relationships they so vehemently opposed.

Family Violence. The Friday after graduation, Nancy returned home. After her parents' guests had left, she heard her intoxicated father yelling at her mother. When Nancy entered the room, the father turned on her and blasted her for not "controlling" her behavior and said there was no need for her to have treatment. He shouted that there was no hope for her amounting to anything and that she could leave home. He sneered, "As far as I'm concerned, you can go kill yourself." In addition, he accused her of not loving her mother because of her affection for Ruth. The mother defended Nancy, whereupon the father slapped his wife's face twice. Nancy slapped her father's face, then he grabbed her arms and bruised them. Elizabeth picked up a fireplace poker and threatened to call the police, but Nancy persuaded her to calm down. Arthur threatened to drive to the city, but since he was not sober enough to drive safely, Nancy hid the car keys.

The next day, Arthur behaved as if nothing had happened. Nancy felt her father had become angry at her in part "because he felt guilty that I am the way I am." It was not clear just how he felt responsible. He cried and reminded her he had given her things that should help solve any problem; he referred to a car he had given her for Christmas, even though she had not asked for it. He accused her of not enjoying anything he did for her and told her she was "driving him nuts."

Double-Bind Messages. Her parents had taken an adamant stand on Nancy's going to France in the fall. Then came a series of mixed messages and double binds.

If she wished to continue treatment, she must move out of the house, get a job, and live on her own. If she wished to return to college, she must live in her father's one-room apartment in the city, rather than in the college dormitory. Finally, permission was given for her to return to college for the fall semester, and the trip to France was postponed until the spring semester. This plan was contingent on Nancy's coming to treatment only once a week and seeing Ruth only once a month.

She was surprised at her parents' acquiescence. "They go along yet it seems like they never will. At times, they seem to give up on something like forbidding me to see Ruth, then they suddenly get mad about it. It's odd that they don't find out I see her more than once a month and you more than once a week. I don't understand why they never check up on me, but they never have. They just don't want to find out."

Dynamics of Feelings of Unreality and Confused Identity

Nancy's symptoms illustrate the occurrence of depersonalization in association with schizophrenia. By contrast, Michelle, who was not schizophrenic, nevertheless had depersonalization experiences.

In one sequence, Nancy speaks of feeling fuzzy and as if she did not have a head. "I get peppy and laugh, but it doesn't feel like me laughing. It feels like something inside me is doing it." These experiences have the "as if" quality and are alien to the self, thus representing depersonalization, not delusion. Her "as if" feelings develop further into ideas of reference and being influenced by some force outside herself (dead people). These feelings are held with conviction and are delusional.

Then, there are the somatic components of her unreality experiences, among which are blurring of vision, feeling like a stick, losing her balance, bumping into things, and feeling unable to bend her knees. There is a culmination in her "wall" experiences. Are we dealing with a continuum ranging from mild fleeting feelings of unreality to paralyzing catatonia? The literature notes that developmental experiences that precede and seem to predispose one to depersonalization experiences are similar to, or the same as, those antedating schizoid personality structure and schizophrenic reactions.[34,62,77]

Nancy's obsession-delusion that she is being watched by dead relatives becomes more meaningful in terms of Winnicott's formulation of the capacity to be alone.[77] He has stated that the basis for the ability to be alone is the experience of being alone in the presence of the ego-supporting mother during infancy. Gradually, the maternal support is incorporated and there develops the capacity to be alone. Nancy never had an adequate opportunity to develop this capacity, so she calls on beneficent spirits to be with her when no one else is around. This obviates her being alone.

Suicidal Ideation. Depression and thoughts of harming herself have been common in Nancy's life, particularly when she feels frustration and the threat of abandonment. However, on only a few occasions has she tried to damage herself. These occasions were overdetermined and represent a cry for help, expiation for sins, and ritual suicide, as well as the need to feel real pain and thus alleviate the pain of unreality feelings.

Winnicott has stated that if the balance between the true self and the false self is such that the true self cannot be realized, the outcome is suicide. The total self is destroyed in preference to annihilation of the true self. In Waltzer's[74] formulation of depersonalization, the individual acts as both participant and observer and responds as if his behavior were being carried out by another person. Thus, unacceptable impulses, such as suicide, often to escape panic, are more easily permitted partial or complete expression. Laing[34] has mentioned suicide as one outcome of the vicissitudes in the struggle between the real self and the false self. One is defensive: "If I'm dead, I can't be killed." The other is punitive, in the sense that one has no right to be alive because of one's guilt.

Dynamics of Interaction: The Family as a Social System

In exploring the dynamics that led to Nancy's futile attempts to cope, it is critical to view her as one part of the social system of the family. Although she was labeled as the "primary patient," her behavior cannot be understood outside the context of her family. From a theoretical point of view, the family is defined as a social system in which each member acts upon another. The various combinations and permutations of behavior define the social structure of the family.

THE MOTHER

Elizabeth Cabot has serious difficulty in differentiating Nancy from herself. She displays indifference. She is cold, detached, and uninvolved, despite the fact that on occasion she defends Nancy from her father. Elizabeth's defense of Nancy, rather than being an expression of love, is a way of retaliating against the husband. It is difficult for her to make decisions and she has seriously scattered thinking. Often, she is confused and vague. She, like her husband, drinks heavily and frequently is intoxicated.

Absence of Nurturance. The concept of "nurturance" or mothering is defined as *creating a climate for growth*. In Nancy's life, there was no real mothering. In the absence of nurturance, Nancy missed many of the child-centered rituals, such as those carried out at bedtime: bathing and playing in the water; being hugged and cuddled as she is being wrapped, mummy fashion, in a towel; a bedtime drink, a story, a song; and a goodnight kiss. These bedtime rituals are functional for both child and parent, for they coax the child to go to bed and make separation easier for parents and child.[28] "Any erosion or decay in ritual symbolizes a decay in the culture," and by this definition, the Cabot family is in decay, or worse, it has disintegrated.

"As If" Behavior. Elizabeth Cabot's relationship with Nancy is dominated by her need to mask reality through "as if" behavior. She acted *as if* she did not know of her husband's sexual exploitation of Nancy, but she does know. The mother has been aware of the father's behavior toward Nancy and her sisters throughout the years, since it was evident which beds had been slept in, but there was never any attempt to hide the wandering

hands. From time to time, she voiced disapproval but never really intervened or tried to protect Nancy. Instead of being mothered and nurtured, Nancy was offered to her father as a kind of sacrificial lamb. The result has been that Arthur's attention to Elizabeth has been minimized. Accordingly, when Nancy was sexually molested by Thomas, the houseman, Mrs. Cabot acted *as if* it was not Nancy who was suffering but rather the hired man.

Mrs. Cabot talked to Nancy *as if* she knew what she was talking about, but she did not know. With all of these *as if* behaviors, Elizabeth forces Nancy to deny her own perceptions, thereby adding to her confusion about her identity and about her worth as a person.

Violence and Humiliation. Mrs. Cabot apparently associated love with physical violence. She is a woman who feels dead. Thus, she has married a violent man who needs constantly to defend his own image as a male, perhaps because he is the only kind who can make her feel alive and arouse her sexually.

This is a household marked by massive humiliation. For example, when Nancy was humiliated by her brother-in-law's sexual advances, Mrs. Cabot never intervened. She thereby further humiliates Nancy, adding to her anguish. She ignores Nancy's emotional disturbance yet exaggerates trivia. Through humiliation, Mrs. Cabot saps any belief Nancy has in her self and thereby distorts her perceptions. Through this process, the mother turns Nancy into a *thing*.

THE FATHER

On the one hand, Arthur Cabot seeks admiration and attention that he has been unable to get from his wife. On the other hand, he has not maintained generation boundaries when he looks to Nancy for sexual and emotional support, rather than to his wife.[35] He has used Nancy as a pawn to purposely foster his wife's jealousy. Thus, Nancy has never been sure whether Arthur was father or lover. Consequently, she could not be clear about her own identity. Was she child, daughter, wife, lover? Or was she none of these and regarded merely as a sexual object?

Mr. Cabot is paranoid, inasmuch as he is

suspicious and feels persecuted by one family member or another much of the time. He shows open contempt of his wife in front of Nancy. At the same time, he pits Nancy against her mother when he flails her with the accusation, "You don't love your mother because you spend so much time with Ruth."

Double Binds, Violence and Humiliation. Nancy is exposed to constant double binds and humiliation. For example, the father requires Nancy's admiration and adulation and yet in an outburst of uncontained rage, he says, "You can go kill yourself." He is tough, violent, and insensitive, as illustrated when he blasted Nancy and slapped Mrs. Cabot in the face. He constantly tries to buy Nancy's love, while at the same time he is impervious to her emotional needs. He is bent on sacrificing tenderness to hardness.

He has weakened his role as a father through emotional withdrawal and physical absence from home. Although there are brief periods of affection (sexual), as when he holds Nancy in his arms, more often he is violent and humiliating.

MARITAL SCHISM

Lidz et al.[35] speak of the modes of interaction within a family that seem to lead to one member becoming schizophrenic. In particular, their discussion of the nature of the relationship of the marital pair has relevance for understanding Nancy's behavior and personality development.

Of the two types of marital relationships, they have characterized one as "marital schism." It is this mode of marital interaction that helps to clarify how and why Nancy became ill. According to Lidz et al., marital schism is a chronic, severe disequilibrium and discord in a couple's relationship. They have spoken of one partner's chronically "undercutting" the worth of the other in the eyes of the children and their competing for the children's affection and loyalty. One member of the couple may try to make a child a substitute to replace the affection missing from the spouse, or the motivation may be just to spite the marital partner. This description fits the relationship between Nancy's parents, including the

father trying to substitute daughters as sources of affection. He received little from his wife.

In the marital schism situation, the husband is said to retain little prestige in the home, for none is warranted by his behavior. "He becomes an outsider or a secondary figure who cannot assert his instrumental leadership and when he strives to dominate in tyrannical fashion, he eventually forces the family to conspire to circumvent him." When Nancy's father could not make his point by shouting, he would resort to muscular action that required police intervention or the threat of it. His subsequent petulant efforts to drive to the city were usually aborted by some family member making the car keys unavailable to him.

In the study of Lidz et al., communication between the partners was impeded by reciprocal withdrawal, as well as by scattered thinking by the wives and the husbands' rigidity and paranoid thinking. As has been emphasized, some of the mixed messages that Nancy received from her mother may well have been scattered. The father's wild accusations about Nancy's adversely affecting his health were certainly paranoid.

The Cabot couple falls into the category of the "woman-dominated competitive axes." "The outstanding feature is the wife's exclusion of the passive and masochistic husband from leadership and decision-making. She derogates him in work and in deed and is emotionally cold and distant to him. Her attention is focused on her narcissistic needs for competition and admiration. These wives are extremely castrating and their husbands are vulnerable. The husband withdraws from the relationship in an effort to preserve some integrity when defeated in the struggle, and may find solace in alcohol. The wife does not fill an expressive, supportive role to her husband and her expressive functions with the children are seriously distorted."[35]

This is a reasonably accurate description of Nancy's parental household. Her father's retreat to living in the city during the week was based on the withdrawal described above, not on the inconvenience of commuting. The same is true for his having a separate bedroom from his wife. This was withdrawal or banishment, not the fact of his snoring that was officially credited as the reason. He certainly sought solace in alcohol, but it is doubtful that he found it.

Lidz and his colleagues have stated that they do not seek to demonstrate a direct etiological relationship between marital discord and the appearance of schizophrenia in an offspring. However, the two phenomena occur together with striking frequency.

Nancy never knows how her parents will behave toward her. They are inconsistent and unpredictable. Nancy has always wondered whether they really care about her. She is puzzled that the only time they show emotion is when they are angry and condemnatory and that at other times they are more or less indifferent. They will continue to see her as a thing or as some extension of themselves and not as a person in her own right. To the extent that she has a relationship with Ruth or with the psychiatrist, the parents forbid such relationships, and having done so they refuse to see that any exist. Though they exercise denial on the one hand, they are capable of citing the relationships at any time for scapegoating purposes and as a basis for threats to demand that Nancy acquiesce to their wishes.

In conclusion, we will point out certain other dynamics of interaction that appear to have been operating in the Cabot household. We have previously mentioned that in the anguish of being unable to feel her self, Nancy slashes and burns her wrists. However, there is the problem of Nancy's repressed rage toward her mother. In addition to the above dynamic, does Nancy hurt herself *instead* of her mother?

Nancy tries to bridge the gap between her mother and father by playing the role of pseudo-wife and thereby gets caught in the schism, as for example, when she slapped her father's face. Despite all the violence in the Cabot household, both parents frequently acquiesce to Nancy's requests, e.g., they permitted her to return to college.

We have emphasized that the American characteristics of conformity and acquiescence are based on fear. What were Nancy's mother and father afraid of? Were they afraid they would lose her to the two most important people to Nancy—Ruth and the psychiatrist? Since Nancy was the scapegoat in this divisive marital pair, were the parents afraid that they would lose control with each other if they permitted Nancy to find her true self?

In view of another American characteristic, namely humiliation, it is critical to note that Nancy learned to enjoy the pleasures of humiliation. She found that humiliation brought some of its own reward. It was better for her to have her existence recognized even as a sexual plaything than not to have had her existence recognized at all.

(Treatment

Obviously there is no specific treatment for depersonalization any more than there is for any other constellation of psychiatric symptoms. However, there are special considerations in both the psychotherapeutic and the somatic approaches to patients who experience the depersonalization phenomena.

THE TASK OF THERAPY

The task of therapy is to help the patient recognize his stereotyped, anachronistic attitudes, concepts, and patterns of behavior, with their attendant anxiety and defensive maneuvers against anxiety. Then, alternative, flexible, contemporary reactions can be tested and facilitated and a dynamic growth process reinstituted.

Vulnerability to depersonalization comes about through deficiencies and distortions of the patient's experiences with nurturance in infancy and in subsequent stages of personality development. These include exposure to the double bind, rejection of the true self and fostering of the development of the false self. In essence, the infant is programmed to deny satisfaction of his needs, including the expression of his emotions, in order to avoid extreme anxiety. Such repudiation leads to repression so that the unacceptable needs and emotions are not consciously recognized. This is the intrapsychic programming that must be dealt with in treatment.

Why do depersonalization phenomena occur only episodically in the patient's daily living and why does a particular episode come about when it does? Some aspect of a present interpersonal relationship catalyzes the intrapsychic programming in such a way that depersonalization results. There is a meaningful sequence, of which the patient is unaware or only vaguely aware. The patient has an interpersonal experience that provokes anger, sexual interest, helplessness, or loneliness. Any one or all of these being unacceptable, it remains unrecognized. The effort to keep these feelings repressed is such that all feeling is nullified. Then, the patient reports that he feels nothing, that he feels unreal and that the world is unreal.

PSYCHOTHERAPEUTIC TECHNIQUE

Utilization of the couch is usually contraindicated in these patients. Their feelings of unreality about themselves and the world are such that lack of visual contact with the therapist can underline the symptomatology to the point of panic. It is very important for the patient to feel and see that he is "touching" the therapist with his eyes and his words. He perceives this through watching the therapist's eyes and facial expression and correlating these with the words that are spoken by therapist, as well as by patient.

Some of these patients are not able to free associate on request or demand. To the extent that they are dominated by the depersonalization experiences, there may be lapses in their ability to free associate or even to verbalize at all. There may be true blocking. In this kind of situation, it is not enough for the patient merely to see the therapist. It is incumbent on the therapist to "touch" the patient with appropriate verbalizations and to begin to bring the patient out of his paralysis of unreality and associated blocking.*

* Laing[34] has noted that the need to be perceived as a person is not purely a visual affair but extends to a general need to have one's presence confirmed by another. It includes the need to have one's total existence recognized and ultimately the need to be loved.

Does one really touch the patient in an effort to introduce a physical dimension of warmth and reality? Probably not, or only under unusual circumstances. Ordinarily, it is simpler to set the limit at no touching. Once touching is initiated, the patient may want more and more, and a line has to be drawn at some point. It is better to obviate physical touching in the beginning.

Neither Michelle nor Nancy has had much experience in being touched by someone who wanted to convey warmth and affection. Each has had her body used by men who wanted to titillate or satisfy their own lust. Each was extremely confused about her own sexual needs and their satisfaction; each was bewildered about the role of sex in love and love in sex. Each has attempted to arrange for recognition and affection by giving over her body to men. Michelle has had the wisdom twice to veto the possibility of this happening in an allegedly psychotherapeutic setting. Touching either of these girls, beyond the initial handshake, could have frightened them, on the one hand, and led to unconscious wishes for more contact, on the other hand. Such a development could have led to depersonalization experiences in the treatment session, or precipitated by the treatment. The complex transferential situation would have been further complicated.

Inasmuch as these patients have been subjected to manipulation and to the double bind for most of their lives, they in turn are usually expert in manipulation and in giving double-bind messages. Though scarcely aware of it, they enter treatment expecting the therapist to use the familiar, stereotyped parental techniques for controlling them. The patient more or less automatically responds with his own repertory of manipulative and double-binding techniques. Anticipating the likelihood of these developments, the therapist is better able to recognize them when they appear and to obviate the otherwise inevitable game-playing.

One must also be aware of parental efforts to manipulate the therapist or the therapy. Michelle's mother tried the former unsuccessfully. She called the therapist and tried to make him an instrument in her efforts to control Michelle. Once parents recognize that the therapist is an ally of the patient and of health, they try to sabotage treatment. This can be done by withholding or withdrawing financial support or by fostering plans that remove the patient from the city. Both ploys were undertaken by Michelle's and Nancy's parents, and Michelle's treatment was terminated because of lack of funds. Nancy used private income and her parents did not interfere though they voiced disapproval.

Michelle's Treatment. In treatment, it is crucial to delineate the sequences of events that lead to depersonalization experiences. For instance, Michelle would speak to her mother in a near-by city about once a week by telephone, the mother usually initiating the calls. She actively avoided any show of interest in Michelle's health and welfare. Rather, she criticized Michelle for the life she was leading because it was soiling the family escutcheon and also ruining her heath. Michelle would try either to endear herself to her mother, or become tearful, or both. Recognition and expression of rage, appropriate to the situation, never occurred to her. Each phone call was usually succeeded by depersonalization and an attack of migraine.

Conversely, her meetings with Derek, the contemporary and peer who had comparable European background, were marked by calm, comfort, and pleasure. There was never a hint of unreality feelings. However, she could not bring herself to allow the relationship to develop.

One of the focuses of Michelle's treatment was an ongoing review of her interpersonal encounters and her associated emotional reactions or their absence. Initially, Michelle regarded the therapist as a critical parent, a demanding authority, and an unfamiliar man who might have ulterior motives, as had her earlier therapists. On occasion, she would report having felt anger at the therapist after leaving a session, but she was not able to feel it, much less express it "on the spot." The therapist liked Michelle from the time she began treatment and felt warmth and compassion for her. It was important that he be her

ally in pursuit of health, rather than in condemning the "enemy," i.e., her mother, boyfriend, and others, who exploited her and demanded compliance to their wishes. The therapist's role was to emphasize the fact that she had alternative responses in a given situation to her usual stereotyped response that led to depersonalization. As therapy continued, she was gradually able to report feeling less unreal at the end of a treatment session. She began to experience positive feelings, including trust and warmth, in the treatment situation. Feelings of self-trust and self-respect began to emerge, i.e., a true self.

As the therapist became more familiar with her history, her attitudes, and patterns of behavior, it was possible to point out sequences leading to depersonalization. She began to recognize the appropriateness of a feeling in such a situation and then to identify the feeling itself.

The young man with whom she was living when she began treatment was remarkably like her mother in temperament and disposition, despite polar differences in background and breeding. Each had a remarkable talent for petulance, narcissism, and for demanding constant emotional feeding. Michelle came to recognize that living with him was some kind of replication of living with mother and that his presence was meant to obviate anticipated feelings of loneliness and helplessness. Realizing the price she was paying for this destructive companionship, she came to the point of challenging his demands and expressing her anger. Eventually, she developed the courage to move into her own apartment and to discontinue the relationship with him. In addition, she was able to be more assertive and to express anger in her daily work, which was filled with frustrating experiences.

Michelle's relationship to the therapist never had the depth and breadth of Nancy's. Several factors contributed to this difference. Nancy's three sessions a week permitted such a development. In contrast, Michelle had one or two weekly visits with increasingly numerous broken appointments, until she ceased coming. Nancy, as child-woman, was more able to accept nurturance and warmth from the therapist with less inclination to sexualize these than Michelle was. Most important, perhaps, was the fact that Nancy had grown up in a home and a family—however disruptive and chaotic. Michelle had never really had either.

Throughout most of her treatment, Michelle reiterated her concern that she would meet the therapist on the street and have no idea as to how to behave. She really preferred that the therapist have no existence, except during her hour in the office. She came to be able to report feeling anger at the therapist during a treatment session, but not to express it.

Over the two-year period of treatment, she was able to forego the need to dramatize the relationship with her parents in her day-to-day living and to obviate the development of depersonalization experiences in these relationships. Her terror of her mother persisted, however, and the sequence of unreality feelings followed phone calls and direct meetings. Anger toward the mother could be recognized more readily, but not expressed directly.

Michelle interrupted treatment because she barely had enough to live on. Characteristically, the mother had facilitated Michelle's entering treatment and had promised to pay all or half of the cost. She gave a series of double-bind messages that raised and lowered Michelle's hopes over some period of time. The ultimate message was that she and her third husband could not afford to provide financial assistance unless she (mother) obtained a job. However, her health was not sufficiently good for her to work and she attributed her ill health to concern about Michelle's way of life and need for treatment. Thus, Michelle was told that her need for treatment was the reason that her mother could not work and support treatment, a classical double-bind situation.

It is ironic that one of the principal areas of Michelle's growth—moving from Jacob's apartment where she lived rent-free—was the situation that made it financially unfeasible to continue treatment. Other substantial gains have been mentioned. However, there were many unresolved problems that made the interruption of treatment premature.

Nancy's Treatment. Though she was twenty years old when she came for treatment in the spring of 1963, Nancy was an early adolescent in many respects. Particularly in the earlier sessions, she was frightened and would sit and look at me wide-eyed as if she wanted to run away. She volunteered nothing, and on questioning she would respond by nodding or shaking her head as if that could suffice. If verbalization was necessary, her speech was so rapid and so low in volume that it was difficult to understand her. She was not accustomed to having adults pay any attention to what she said, or if they did, it was to respond with criticism or ridicule. The one exception was Ruth, her surrogate mother, who at times was interested and attentive.

The information in the clinical vignette about her feelings and fears, her family and developmental history, and her ongoing relationships, was gradually elicited. Treatment sessions were devoted to a review of her activities between visits: classes in school, her interpersonal contacts with her roommate, with Ruth, and two or three visits a month with her parents. In addition, we talked about her daytime fears and fantasies and her nightmarish dreams. She came to perceive the therapist as consistent and predictable and the office as a safe place where she would not be ridiculed, criticized, or ignored.

Treatment was interrupted during the summer when Nancy went as a junior counselor to a camp where Ruth was a senior counselor. Despite fears about coping with campers and with other counselors, and petulant demands on Ruth's time and attention, she survived the summer. After many mixed messages from her parents, they presented her with a package deal which allowed Nancy to resume college in the fall, but restricted her contacts with Ruth and the therapist. As already noted, Nancy did not abide by these restrictions. Parental quarreling continued during succeeding months, as did pressure on Nancy with threats that treatment would be discontinued.

Efforts to have her understand the role of unrecognized feeling in her depersonalization experiences met with success part of the time.

However, on one or two occasions the content of treatment sessions had a negative impact. She would remain in the waiting room for up to an hour after her session because she could not penetrate the "wall" at the street exit. She found safety in being in the waiting room and in proximity to the therapist, though she knew that he was with another patient. She was jealous of other patients, particularly young women, and wanted to be "the one and only and the favorite." After a period in the waiting room, her courage increased, or her fear of the street and possible loneliness in the dormitory decreased, and she was able to leave.

One evening, the therapist found her in the entrance foyer as he was leaving about an hour after she had finished her session. She was terrified of the "wall." He told her that he was going to attend a meeting near her dormitory, about ten blocks north of the office, and that they could walk together. She was grateful and relieved and, in contrast to Michelle, welcomed this opportunity to walk on the street with the therapist. They chatted as they went along and he invited her to look into shop windows and at the upper stories of buildings. She looked around a bit and seemed to like the experience. This was in sharp contrast to her usual pattern of scurrying along the avenue with downcast eyes that saw nothing and no one. When they reached the vicinity of her dormitory, she felt more calm and composed and able to travel the final half-block alone.

The therapist was fond of this girl and felt a good deal of compassion and protectiveness for her in her day-to-day living and her confrontations with her parents. He was the first male she had ever known who was attentive to her as a person and respected her. Other men had groped at her body, as if she were a toy or a thing for their pleasure. In contrast to her father, whose seductiveness helped maintain her infantile dependency on him, he was a surrogate who provided a growth-facilitating atmosphere. He provided a model for a male and a father that she could focus on in finding her way to individuation and a life and family of her own. In this setting, she could

gradually dissolve the symbiotic relationship with her mother and realize that her own growth in no way meant the simultaneous liquidation of mother.

During the course of treatment, there were inroads in these realms. However, at times the therapist despaired at Nancy's episodes of petulance with parents or with Ruth, and her inability or refusal to be as assertive as she might and to take a more active role in running her own life.

Ruth was a transitional object for Nancy. On the one hand, she repeated the mother's pattern at times by manipulating Nancy for her own needs. On the other hand, she was not Nancy's mother and thus was a positive resource in several ways. In addition, she shepherded other young women, as well as Nancy, on weekends to Nancy's chagrin. She would provoke Ruth by verbalizing her jealous feelings or by sulking.

There was a culmination of unpleasant experiences with her parents and with Ruth. Nancy's depersonalization and depression became more oppressive and she cut her wrist several times with a razor blade. Her condition was such that psychiatric hospitalization was required. Only then would the parents agree to discuss her illness and welfare with the therapist.

Following discharge from the hospital, Nancy resumed therapeutic sessions and undertook a typing course in a business school. Attendance and progress were impaired by her fears, shyness, and difficulties in concentrating. She lived in a YWCA residence facility for several weeks but spoke to no one and was afraid to enter the dining room. Subsequently, she found an apartment with another emotionally disturbed girl through Ruth. Despite the obstacles, the arrangement was somehow workable.

That summer, she again went to camp, this time as an arts and crafts counselor. She began writing letters, addressing the therapist as "Daddy Cattell." The content of the letters was not unlike that of her therapeutic sessions. The therapist's responses were intended to provide support and encouragement, and evidence of his interest in her and concern for her welfare. He typed his letters on his professional letterhead and signed them with his usual signature.

In the fall, she resumed courses in typing and shorthand. She lived with her roommate, saw Ruth as frequently as possible, and spent occasional weekends at her parents' home. Treatment sessions dealt with her feelings about herself, her relations with her parents and responses to their concocted crisis situations, to her feelings about Ruth, and about the therapist. Thus, the year passed, and she made little progress in business school. On her parents' initiative, there was discussion about Nancy's living away from the New York area. She was acquainted with the Stevensons, a family who operated summer cottages on the Jersey shore and lived in Florida during the winter. These people were Ruth's friends and Nancy had spent time with them at the shore. The Stevensons visited the therapist's office to discuss the feasibility of Nancy joining their family. He concurred. Therefore, in the summer of 1965 she joined the Stevenson family and helped in the summer cottage operation. She returned for a few weeks of treatment sessions in the fall and then went to Florida with them. She wrote about missing Ruth and the therapist, about her unhappiness, her lack of direction, and her collisions with Mrs. Stevenson. The latter was somewhat tyrannical in running her home and family. The therapist replied promptly and as helpfully as he could, pointing out her ambiguous position in the household—a combination of foster daughter, guest, and boarder. He noted that she had a choice to remain a rebel in the Stevenson family or to make other living arrangements. Unreality feelings were less marked at this time and she was aware of her anger and could express it in noisy temper tantrums and silent temper tantrums—periods of quiet sulking. The therapist suggested that these further incurred Mrs. Stevenson's displeasure and made Nancy's life that much more difficult.

She obtained work in a flower shop, where she showed a special proficiency in styrofoam creations and flower arrangements, but had little awareness of her own ability and minimum pleasure in utilizing it. Through 1967, the therapist kept abreast of developments through two or three sessions a year, when Nancy was in town, and occasional letters. Her devotion and trust were very real and she seemed to gain a kind of sustenance from the relationship.

Her contact with men had been minimal throughout this time. A young man's call for a date was a burden to her and she avoided social engagements when she could. In Florida, she began to have some social life. In 1967, she met a lawyer who was about to begin his judicial clerkship. He was a devoted member of a Protestant religious sect, which Nancy joined. This meant that she had to repudiate alcoholic beverages, cigarettes, coffee, and obey certain rules. They married and in due time had a son and a daughter. Nancy has been active in philanthropic organizations in the community where they are now living. Her endurance at jogging is greater than that of men her age. In all, she seems to be functioning in a healthy fashion consistent with her age.

RELEVANCE OF FAMILY THERAPY

It is important to re-emphasize that the family is more than a collection of individuals, it is a social system with a life, structure, and institutions of its own. Lidz et al.,[35] alluding to the contributions of several sociologists, have enunciated that within the family, the action of any member affects all, producing reactions, counterreactions, and shifts in the family's equilibrium. Furthermore, the member labeled as the primary patient is a profile or mirror of the various intricate interrelationships within the family. To treat one member of the social system outside the context of that system (the family) can be useful, but the alternative of treating the entire family is more relevant.

Theoretically, the treatment of the primary patient only leaves him with two options: to stay in the family or to remove himself from the family. In actuality, the third possibility is a combination of these two, as illustrated by Michelle and Nancy. That compromise is to remove oneself from the family, yet remain within it in spirit and through ongoing contact with the family and responding to its influences.

Family therapy in the case of Michelle would have involved two natural parents and three stepparents on two continents. Actually, the therapist was not in touch with her mother, who lived a few hundred miles away. She called him once and tried to engage him in her efforts to manipulate Michelle. He did not co-operate. Nancy's parents were hostile to psychiatric treatment, as already noted, and tolerated their daughter's therapy only because the college insisted. Following Nancy's hospitalization, each parent was seen individually on one or two occasions. They were disinclined to come together, since each one relegated responsibility for Nancy's problems to the other and to Ruth. They feared that joint sessions would disclose their own emotional problems.

Whatever the problems of logistics and cooperation in these families, family therapy was not indicated in the treatment of either patient. Family therapy is most relevant when the primary patient is living in the home and has no alternative possibility. Both Michelle and Nancy were living away from parents and joined them only for brief visits. The goal of therapy was to expedite each patient's living in the world, rather than to try to neutralize familial internecine warfare.

SOME LIMITATIONS OF
INDIVIDUAL PSYCHOTHERAPY

The patient who has depersonalization experiences may be inclined to isolate himself from the world of human relationships. Depersonalization can lead to divorcing oneself from reality and thus to underlying feelings of unreality. This fact, that in a sense depersonalization begets depersonalization, can be pointed out in therapy, as described above. The patient may agree to the correctness of the observation but, at the same time, be paralyzed to initiate any action to block or reverse the vicious cycle.

While Nancy was in college, much of her day was structured and she followed the schedule reasonably well, without too much discomfort. It was the unstructured time that panicked her. Ruth filled some of this time by having Nancy with her one evening a week and on most weekends. Nancy thrived on this, but was unhappy when she was not included or when she had to share Ruth with one or more other girls. Then, she became jealous, unhappy, panicky, and symptoms were exacerbated.

There were several disadvantages in this approach. Ruth was functioning as recreational director for these girls, rather than as leader and role model. She was entertaining them, rather than demonstrating to them how they could learn to entertain themselves through the use of more initiative. It is not our intention to criticize Ruth. She served a vital function to Nancy and to many girls in similar straits. Rather, we wish to point out some of the subtle difficulties and possible pitfalls in this kind of situation.

Though Ruth was providing structure for Nancy's leisure time, she was also providing structure for herself. She needed Nancy and the other girls at least as much as they needed her. When there is such need and dependency, the emotional involvements develop on a family level, rather than on a therapeutic level. Failing to realize countertransference phenomena, Ruth becomes the mother and reacts to her daughters as such, rather than as a therapist who maintains objectivity.

The extended amounts of time Ruth spent with Nancy made it extremely difficult for her to be objective, especially when she had no special training in therapy or psychiatric nursing, and all the clinical and dynamic insights that are included.

COTHERAPY

Both Michelle and Nancy have suffered from severe deprivation of parental nurturance. With certain selected patients whose overwhelming symptom is depersonalization, the authors recently have begun to collaborate as cotherapists. Our therapeutic model is based on Durkheim's[20] *Division of Labor* (the function of the division of labor is social, namely, *integration*) and on the social structure of the American family, as has been emphasized and clarified by Parsons and Bales.[50]

In applying concepts from these two frameworks, several critical principles will be enunciated.[35] First, it is through the gender-linked roles that parents transmit "the basic instrumental ways of their culture" to the child. Second, each child requires two parents: "A parent of the same sex with whom one can identify and who functions as a model to follow into adulthood and a parent of the opposite sex who becomes a basic love object." And third, there is a division of labor between the parents: They maintain their gender-linked roles. For example, the father's role is to provide masculine instrumental leadership; his concern is wih solving problems, completing tasks, setting directions and long-term goals which may conflict with giving immediate gratification to family members; and he paves the way for meeting the goals. The mother's role pertains to the expressive-affective functions: she provides nurturance to family members; she tends to be more concerned with immediate goals and gratification.

Implications of Theory. We have emphasized that the goal of therapy in situations of depersonalization is to help the individual to recognize his defensive maneuvers against the feelings of anger, sexuality, loneliness, and helplessness. In Laing's[34] and Winnicott's[77] frameworks, the task is to assist the patient to find his true self by building up his self-esteem. In more operational terms, the objective is to help the patient develop a pleasure economy so that he can *act* in terms of taking care of and giving to himself.

The assumption that underlies cotherapy is that a particular patient requires the therapist's participation in his whole life. The treatment of patients who are seriously disabled by depersonalization experiences requires more than the traditional, individual psychotherapeutic session. Rosen,[55] for example, has gone shopping with patients and has spent up to ten hours a day with them. Sechehaye's[63] only patient lived with her. Gertrude Schwing,[61] a psychiatric nurse, worked in cotherapy with Federn.

As in the case of the American nuclear family, the two therapists in cotherapy should be of a different sex. The therapy ("labor") is divided so that the female therapist takes the expressive-affectional role and the male therapist takes the instrumental-leadership role. To illustrate how we have applied the principles from the division of labor and the family structure to cotherapy, we shall give several illustrations that focus almost exclusively on the female expressive role of the therapist, simply because less has been written about it than about the traditional instrumental role in individual psychotherapy.

Alice Foster is twenty-five. She is very attractive, intellectually bright, and a skilled physiotherapist. She has had depersonalization experiences of a degree that have partially or totally incapacitated her episodically for several years. Her therapy schedule with the authors consists of seeing each of us individually once a week and, from time to time, seeing us together. The senior author sees her in his office, where she sits in a chair facing him. However, I conduct my therapy sessions with Alice mostly on the streets of New York.* My goal and function is to *reintroduce* Alice to the world.

For our first session together, I had planned to take Alice to Central Park. I had prepared two packages of bread and some nuts for us to feed birds and squirrels. When Alice arrived at my office, she slumped in a chair and said in an almost inaudible voice, "I don't want to go out." (I heard "I *won't* go out.") "I'm scared. I like it better here." As I put on my coat, I said "I know and that's just why we have planned this kind of therapy for you." As we walked into the park, she was very rigid, her head was down, her face was blank as if she were miles away; and she walked several steps ahead of me. After a long silence, I asked, "What are you feeling?" She responded, "Nothing." "Do you know where you are?" I asked. "Doesn't make any difference," she mumbled.

We walked for at least fifteen minutes in silence. Then, we came to a massive, magnificent oak tree. As I pointed to the tree, I asked,

* In the discussion of cotherapy, use of the personal pronoun refers to the junior author.

"Can you experience the tree?" She responded in a flat voice, "Nothing is real. I'm not real." I suggested that we go over to the tree and touch it. She walked beside me. I ran my hand up and down the trunk and described the texture. She made a motion with her hand as if to touch the tree. Gently, I took her hand, placed it on the bark and with my hand over hers, guided it up and down. Then, I took my hand away, but she continued to "feel" the tree. We walked away in silence. Suddenly she turned full face to me and said, "It's all right now. I'm back. I don't feel numb and empty like I did. I wonder why?" I withheld any interpretation, namely, that perhaps the fact that I had "touched" her physically and emotionally had brought her back to reality.

Operating on the principle that the development of the infant and young child is organized largely around feeding, I took Alice to a restaurant for lunch. Before she ordered, I told her, "Today, I am paying the check, so order whatever you like." Our luncheon "session" lasted for two hours, during which she poured out problems concerning her former therapist (she had begun the same discussion in her latest session with the senior author), who came from the same mold as her mother. After lunch, we visited several small art galleries for three hours. I shared some of my favorite artists with her. She mentioned one who has been her favorite. It was touching and exciting to observe Alice reaching out to a new world; to hear her laugh and set free her delightful sense of humor. Later, as she waited with me at the bus stop to return home, she told me, "You know this is the very first time in my life that I have looked into a shop window in the city. I always walk with my eyes on the sidewalk, because I feel people are staring at me and making odd remarks about me. But today this didn't happen."

After a few months of cotherapy, she blurted out to me, "I hate my mother; I could kill her." One or two sessions later, we were in my office, because it was raining. Alice sat in her usual chair and I sat on the sofa next to it, as I do when I am with her, rather than in my chair across from the patient. In this session, Alice stared blankly at the bookshelves and

smoked continuously. I waited. She straightened up and became rigid. "What is it?" I asked. She nodded her head and shrugged her shoulders, which told me she did not know. More silence. She said, "I feel so bad; I'll never get any better. I don't know what sends me into these spells." I responded, "You know you told me about hating your mother and wanting to kill her. I wonder if this might be bothering you now." She stared straight ahead, put down her cigarette, and for the first time I saw tears come to her eyes. I asked, "What is it?" She put her head in her lap over her hands and sobbed as her whole body shook. I said, "Give me your hand." She extended her hand and I held it in mine. She squeezed so hard that the ring on my finger dug into my flesh. I stroked her head with my free hand and said, "Go ahead. You have been keeping these feelings and tears bottled up for years." A lump stuck in my own throat and my eyes felt misty.

After some time, the sobs abated. With her head still in her lap, she said, "I feel calmer now." She lifted her head, looked at me squarely and asked, "Will you be my mother?" I felt like taking her in my arms. Instead, I responded, "Alice, I can't be your mother but I think I can give you the kind of *mothering* you need." She nodded with understanding.

The senior author and I have had two planned joint sessions with Alice. The first was at the time of her initial visit. About six weeks later, we had another. When, in our individual session, I asked Alice how she had felt about it, she spontaneously replied, "I felt you two had ganged up on me." The senior author and I discussed the matter and we agreed that we had been premature. Alice first had to identify with both of us individually. In many ways, I have served as a bridge to the senior author for Alice. For example, when she told me that she feels stupid when she cannot answer his questions, I urged her to discuss the matter with him. She did.

We have had several unscheduled joint sessions in our kitchen. On one particular occasion—it was a hot sticky day—I offered her a cold drink. We sat at the kitchen table across from each other. She acted as if she really belonged there. I asked her to help me repot a plant. "But I've never done it before," she replied. "So that makes two of us," I responded. I showed her how to break up some crockery with a hammer to use for drainage in the larger pot. I directed, "Hit harder—it's great for the hostility." She gritted her teeth and her eyes narrowed as she struck hard several times in obvious enjoyment. The senior author walked into the kitchen to get a cold drink. Alice beamed at him as he put an arm on my shoulder. The three of us chatted for about ten minutes. The family structure had been re-created, but in a different way than Alice had ever known. She saw her doctor relate affectionately to her female therapist. Neither the senior author or myself detected any jealousy —only unabashed pleasure in being part of the circle.

Alice has grown, particularly in using initiative and experiencing pleasure. She and two friends planned a camping trip over a three-day weekend. Until that time, we had never seen her register sheer joy, pleasure, and excitement. When she told each of us about this first camping trip, her face was radiant. She said, "I am really *excited*, so *excited* I can hardly wait." The trip went well and when she described it the words tumbled out. Another camping trip is pending.

She almost "lives" in Central Park and goes to concerts there with friends. She had become interested in art and sculpture and has visited several galleries. From time to time, we have talked about bicycling together, but Alice has never ridden a two-wheeler. I offered to get the name of a bicycle instructor for her. She readily accepted. Several weeks later, she bounced into my office and announced, "Guess what? I learned to ride a bike by myself. I just practiced with all the little kids in an empty parking lot."

It is important to point out that my role has not been limited to helping Alice experience the world and thus to find her true self solely through activities. Like the senior author, I have worked with Alice's transference to me and her various resistances.

To work effectively in cotherapy, just as in a marriage and a family, it is imperative for the cotherapists to have worked through problems of competition. Perhaps for one of the few times in her life, Alice has not been exploited and used as a pawn. Her gradual development of autonomy, initiative, and self-identity are emerging, because we have provided her with a new kind of "family setting" which has allowed her to grow.

SOMATIC TREATMENTS AS ADJUVANTS TO PSYCHOTHERAPY

The person who is dominated by depersonalization, anxiety, and depression, is unable to perceive the experiences of living in the world and is thus not able to really participate in psychotherapy. Freud alluded to anxiety as the motor that keeps treatment going, but a racing motor is useless unless the gears mesh.

The considered use of selected medications can obviate suicide, panic, and hospitalization, successively or simultaneously. Hospitalization for acute psychiatric conditions serves a most important role. However, in many instances, the essence of dynamic growth occurs in psychotherapy that takes place in a setting of day-to-day living. As we mentioned earlier, today's vicissitudes activate yesterday's programming of the individual. The problems are much more likely to be solved in the arena of everyday living than in some confined cloister.

We recommend the use, in selected cases, of a phenothiazine—chlorpromazine or prochlorperazine—in spansule form every twelve hours for twenty-four-hour coverage. Dosage should be tailored to the individual patient's needs and tolerance of side-effects. If side-effects outweigh therapeutic effects, as happens in a minority of patients, a minor tranquilizer, such as chlordiazepoxide or diazepam can be substituted in therapeutic doses consistent with the tolerance of the patient.

The combination of dextroamphetamine with amytal tends to neutralize the depersonalization experience in many instances. The twelve-hour extended release capsule taken upon arising provides coverage through the day. This in combination with one of the tranquilizers mentioned can facilitate the patient's coming to grips with his problems in psychotherapy.[16]

To the extent that electric treatment is indicated for depression, associated depersonalization will be relieved along with the depression. The outcome of such treatment of depressive patients is the same, whether depersonalization is present or absent.[2] In those instances in which depersonalization phenomena represent microcatatonic phenomena or alternate with delusional thinking, electric treatment can often be equally successful.[17]

In all instances, depersonalization must be dealt with, finally, by psychotherapeutic means.

(Conclusions

We have presented some of the psychological and sociological determinants of depersonalization and related psychopathology. To the extent that anomie exists in society, and adults are alienated from themselves, they are more inclined to treat their children as things and to demand their compliance. This is in contrast to providing nurturance and fostering their individual growth and development. Such children are rendered vulnerable to depersonalization and to schizophrenia.

Michelle and Nancy both complain that everything they do is incomprehensibly dead, empty, and meaningless, or even that it is not their own action but that of a stranger. This absence of meaning, lack of involvement (never developing feeling for anybody), is the essence of Meursault's existence in Camus'[13] *The Stranger*. He just allows things to happen to him because everything is the same; nothing matters. It is only when he is sentenced to death that he is compelled to take a look at himself. Kafka[31] also portrays the despairing dehumanized situation in society.

In this chapter, we have illustrated that there are many avenues to emotional illness—the final consequence of all that is wrong with society. In both the families presented, the parents are withdrawn from the children and engage in transforming them into nonhuman objects, and there is massive humiliation.

The central issue, however, is why does one child become psychotic and another not? Why did Nancy have a schizophrenic reaction and Michelle not? It is never a single episode or one ongoing abuse that results in a child's becoming psychotic. Rather, it is a climate of living, an accumulation of abuses, especially, *social isolation*, which we see as being the most destructive. The parents who inflict these abuses have several characteristics: They are disoriented in terms of being adrift in time, unable to differentiate one's self from the person acted upon;[28] they mask reality (as-if behavior) and give double-bind messages.

And what are the future prospects for Michelle and Nancy? Both young women have physically extricated themselves from their parents. Michelle is still emotionally tied to her mother and has many other unresolved problems. Her life chances are less favorable than Nancy's. She certainly needs more treatment. Nancy will continue to have her ups and downs. However, her growth has led to what appears to be a stable marriage and she seems to thrive on the responsibility of caring for two children.

(Bibliography

1. ACKNER, B. "Depersonalization: I. Aetiology and Phenomenology," *Journal of Mental Science*, 100 (1954), 838.

2. ACKNER, B., and Q. F. A. R. GRANT. "The Prognostic Significance of Depersonalization in Depressive Illnesses Treated with Electro-Convulsive Therapy," *Journal of Neurology, Neurosurgery and Psychiatry*, 23 (1960), 242.

3. ARIETI, S. *Interpretation of Schizophrenia*. New York: Brunner, 1955.

4. BATESON, G., D. D. JACKSON, J. HALEY, and J. H. WEAKLAND. "Toward a Theory of Schizophrenia." *Behavioral Science*, I (1956), 251–264.

5. BEAUVOIR, S. DE. *America Day by Day*, P. Dudley, transl. New York: Grove Press, 1953.

6. BECKER, H. S. "Notes on the Concept of Commitment," *American Journal of Sociology*, 64 (1960), 32.

7. BECKETT, S. *Waiting for Godot*. New York: Grove Press, 1954.

8. BETTELHEIM, B. *The Empty Fortress*. New York: The Free Press, 1967.

9. BIALOS, D. S. "Adverse Marijuana Reactions: A Critical Examination of the Literature with Selected Case Material," *The American Journal of Psychiatry*, 127 (1970), 819.

10. BONIME, W. "Orientational Perception," *The American Journal of Psychiatry*, 125 (1969), 1609.

11. BÖSZÖRMÉNYI-NAGY, I., and J. L. FRAMO, eds. *Intensive Family Therapy*. New York: Hoeber, 1965.

12. BYCHOWSKI, G. "The Archaic Object and Alienation," *International Journal of Psycho-Analysis*, 48 (1967), 384.

13. CAMUS, A. *The Stranger*. New York: Knopf, 1946.

14. CAPPON, D. "Orientational Perception: III. Orientational Percept Distortions in Depersonalization," *The American Journal of Psychiatry*, 125 (1969), 1048.

15. CAPPON, D., and R. BANKS. "Orientational Perception: IV. Time and Length of Perception in Depersonalized and Derealized Patients and Controls under Positive Feedback Conditions," *The American Journal of Psychiatry*, 125 (1969), 1214.

16. CATTELL, J. P. "Depersonalization Phenomena," in S. Arieti, ed., *American Handbook of Psychiatry*, Vol. 3. New York: Basic Books, 1959.

17. CATTELL, J. P., and S. MALITZ. "Revised Survey of Psychopharmacological Agents," *The American Journal of Psychiatry*, 117 (1960), 449.

18. COOK, F. J. *The Warfare State*. New York: Macmillan, 1962.

19. COOLEY, C. H. *Human Nature and the Social Order*. New York: Scribner"s, 1902.

20. DURKHEIM, E. *The Division of Labor in Society*, G. Simpson, transl. New York: Macmillan, 1933.

21. ———. *Suicide*, J. A. Spaulding, and G. Simpson, transl. New York: The Free Press, 1951.

22. ERIKSON, E. H. "Youth, Fidelity and Diversity," *Daedalus*, 5 (1962), 27.

23. ———. *Childhood and Society*, 2nd Ed. New York: W. W. Norton, 1963.

24. FROMM, E. *Escape from Freedom*. New York: Rinehart, 1941.

25. ———. *The Sane Society*. New York: Rinehart, 1955.

26. HARTUNG, F. "Behavior, Culture and Symbolism," in G. E. Porle, and R. L. Carneiro, eds., *Essays in the Science of Culture*. New York: Crowell, 1960.

27. HENDIN, H. Personal Communication.

28. HENRY, J. *Culture Against Man*. New York: Random House, 1963.

29. HOMANS, G. C. *The Human Group*. New York: Harcourt, Brace, 1950.

30. JACOBSON, E. "Depersonalization," *Journal of the American Psychoanalytic Association*, 7 (1959), 581.

31. KAFKA, F. *The Trial*. New York: Knopf, 1937.

32. KATONA, G. *The Powerful Consumer*. New York: McGraw-Hill, 1960.

33. KEELER, M. H. "Motivation for Marihuana Use: A Correlate of Adverse Reaction," *The American Journal of Psychiatry*, 125 (1968), 386.

34. LAING, R. D. *The Divided Self*. Baltimore: Penguin Books, 1965.

35. LIDZ, T., S. FLECK, and A. R. CORNELISON. *Schizophrenia and the Family*. New York: International Universities Press, 1965.

36. LUDWIG, A. M. "Altered States of Consciousness," *Archives of General Psychiatry*, 15 (1966), 225.

37. McGLOTHLIN, W. H., and D. O. ARNOLD. "LSD Revisited," *Archives of General Psychiatry*, 24 (1971), 35.

38. McLUHAN, M. *Understanding Media: The Extensions of Man*. New York: McGraw-Hill, 1964.

39. MAILER, N. "What I Think About Artistic Freedom," *Dissent*, 2 (1955), 98.

40. MARCUSE, H. *One-Dimensional Man*. Boston: Beacon Press, 1964.

41. MAY, R., ed. *Existence*. New York: Basic Books, 1958.

42. MAYER-GROSS, W. "On Depersonalization," *British Journal of Medical Psychology*, 15 (1935), 103.

43. MEAD, G. H. *Mind, Self and Society*. Chicago: University of Chicago Press, 1934.

44. MELGES, F. T., J. R. TINKLENBERG, L. E. HOLLISTER, and H. K. GILLESPIE. "Temporal Disintegration and Depersonalization During Marihuana Intoxication," *Archives of General Psychiatry*, 23 (1970), 204.

45. MERTON, R. K. *Social Theory and Social Structure*. Glencoe: The Free Press, 1949.

46. MILLER, A. *Death of a Salesman.* New York: The Viking Press, 1949.

47. MILLS, C. W. *White Collar.* New York: Oxford University Press, 1953.

48. MIRLIN, S. M. et al. "Casual Versus Heavy Use of Marijuana: A Redefinition of the Marijuana Problem," *The American Journal of Psychiatry,* 127 (1971), 1134.

49. PACKARD, V. *The Hidden Persuaders.* New York: McKay, 1957.

50. PARSONS, T., and R. F. BALES. *Family, Socialization and Interaction Process.* Glencoe: The Free Press, 1955.

51. POTTER, D. M. *People of Plenty: Economic Abundance and the American Character.* Chicago: The University of Chicago Press, 1954.

52. ———. "The Quest for the National Character," in J. Higham, ed., *The Reconstruction of American History.* New York: Harper and Row, 1962.

53. RIESMAN, D. *The Lonely Crowd.* New Haven: Yale University Press, 1950.

54. ROBERTS, W. W. "Normal and Abnormal Depersonalization," *Journal of Mental Sciences,* 106 (1960), 478.

55. ROSEN, J. N. "The Treatment of Schizophrenic Psychosis by Direct Analytic Therapy." *Psychiatric Quarterly,* 2 (1947), 3.

56. ROSEN, V. H. "The Reconstruction of a Traumatic Childhood in a Case of Derealization," *Journal of the American Psychoanalytic Association,* 3 (1955), 211.

57. ROSHCO, M. "Perception, Denial and Depersonalization," *Journal of the American Psychoanalytic Association,* 15 (1967), 243.

58. SARLIN, C. N. "Depersonalization and Derealization," *Journal of the American Psychoanalytic Association,* 10 (1962), 784.

59. SARTRE, J.-P. *Nausea.* New York: New Directions, 1959.

60. SCHMAHL, J. A. *Experiment in Change.* New York: Macmillan, 1966.

61. SCHWING, G. *A Way to the Soul of the Mentally Ill.* New York: International Universities Press, 1951.

62. SEARLES, H. F. *Collected Papers on Schizophrenia and Related Subjects.* New York: International Universities Press, 1965.

63. SECHEHAYE, M. A. *Symbolic Realization. A New Method of Psychotherapy Applied to a Case of Schizophrenia.* New York: International Universities Press, 1951.

64. SHIBUTANI, T. *Society and Personality.* Englewood Cliffs: Prentice-Hall, 1961.

65. SIMMEL, G. *The Sociology of Georg Simmel.* Translated and edited by Kurt Wolff. Glencoe: The Free Press, 1950.

66. ———. "Fashion," *American Journal of Sociology,* 62, (1957), 541–548.

67. STANTON, A. H., and M. S. SCHWARTZ. "The Management of a Type of Institutional Participation in Mental Illness," *Psychiatry,* 12 (1949), 13.

68. ———. "Observations on Dissociation as Social Participation," *Psychiatry,* 12 (1949), 239.

69. STEWART, W. A. "Panel on Depersonalization, 1963," *Journal of the American Psychoanalytic Association,* 12 (1964), 171.

70. STRODTBECK, F. L., and J. L. SHORT, JR. "Aleatory Risks versus Short-Run Hedonism," *Social Problems,* 12 (1964), 127.

71. SULLIVAN, H. S. *Conceptions of Modern Psychiatry.* Washington: The William Alanson White Psychiatric Foundation, 1947.

72. ———. *The Interpersonal Theory of Psychiatry.* New York: W. W. Norton, 1953.

73. TOCQUEVILLE, A. DE. *Democracy in America,* Vol. I. New York: Knopf, 1948.

74. WALTZER, H. "Depersonalization and Self-destruction," *The American Journal of Psychiatry,* 125 (1968), 399.

75. WEBER, M. *The Protestant Ethic and the Spirit of Capitalism,* T. Parsons, transl. New York: Charles Scribner's Sons, 1958.

76. WHYTE, W. H., JR. *The Organization Man.* New York: Simon and Schuster, 1956.

77. WINNICOTT, D. W. *The Maturational Processes and the Facilitating Environment.* New York: International Universities Press, 1965.

78. WITTELS, F. "Psychology and Treatment of Depersonalization," *Psychoanalytic Review,* 27 (1940), 57.

CHAPTER 35

MOTOR SYNDROMES OF FUNCTIONAL OR UNDETERMINED ORIGIN:

Tics, Cramps, Gilles de la Tourette's Disease, and Others

Eduard Ascher

MOTOR DISTURBANCES HAVE ALWAYS been of special interest to the clinician, because they can be readily observed and serve as indicators of the status of an underlying illness.[5,23] In addition, their origin is frequently obscure, as psychogenic motor syndromes often are undistinguishable from those of an organic nature. They may affect almost every part of the body and vary in severity from mild twitchings of a single muscle group to extensive involvements of nearly every striated muscle of the body. Since the affliction of certain muscle groups is of special clinical significance, they will be sin-gled out in this discussion, while keeping it general with respect to all other motor disturbances.

⟨ Tics[50,58,76]

Tics are seemingly purposeless, repetitive, short-lasting, sudden contractions of striated muscles. They are involuntary and may affect but a few bundles. In severe cases, almost every part of the body is involved. The age incidence is highest among children and most commonly affected are the face and neck.

HISTORY AND CLASSIFICATION

The origin of the term was attributed by Brissaud[13] to popular use and considered onomatopoetic by Meige and Feindel.[50] The sound of the word conveying meaning is supported by the fact that several other languages use similar terms (*ziehen, zucken,* and *ticken* in German, tug and tick in English, *tico* in Spanish, *ticchio* in Italian).

The classification of tics depends on location and the extent of the functional determinant. "Habit tics" are those of primarily psychogenic nature and "psychic tics" of solely functional origin. Attitude tics[49] are longer-lasting habit spasms which resemble catatonic symptoms.

Classification according to location is employed by Olson[55] who divides children's tics into five categories: face and neck tics, those of arms and hands, shoulder and gait muscles, alimentary and respiratory, and a miscellaneous group that includes echolalia and coprolalia.

While the controversy of psychic versus organic origin continues unabated, there have been few clinicians who have failed to recognize that the functional component is ever present in tics and should be given serious consideration.[34,35,50,72]

Tics are generally classified to be a hysterical conversion reaction or a compulsive disorder. Hysterical tics are similar to mannerisms and twitchings of normal individuals, according to Cameron,[16] who considered them remnants of an attempt to adjust to anxiety while expressing through their sign language repressed conflicts of current and past significance.

According to Fenichel,[30] tics are hysterical conversion phenomena when a well-circumscribed area of the body is affected and the patient's ego is intact. He calls the more complex tics conversion reactions also, but of a nonhysterical quality. When there is evidence of regression in such patients, he refers to them as compulsive and resembling catatonic states.

According to Bockner,[9] tics differ from acts of a compulsive nature by the fact that they are involuntary, poorly organized, and only partially influenced by conscious effort of control. Purves-Stewart and Worster-Drought[60] point out that tics occur automatically without the subject's attention drawn to them, while compulsive acts are very much in the awareness of the individual who cannot resist performing them.

PSYCHOPATHOLOGY

Because of the uncertain origin of tics, theories to explain them are diverse and numerous. Meige and Feindel[50] saw in them evidence of congenital, organic, and psychological deficits, while stressing the importance of studying each case individually. They felt that they were compulsive, inopportune, defensive, and automatic in nature.

Friedreich[32] believed tics to have been purposive, co-ordinated acts which became involuntary and repetitive. Muncie[54] calls them a motor neurosis resulting from "rut formation." After a period of "legitimate" reaction to discomfort, the movements lose their original meaning and purposiveness by becoming habitual.

Wilder and Silbermann[76] failing to cure tiqueurs by psychotherapy were reluctant to attribute them to psychic causes, while psychoanalysts found in them much to support their libido theory. Ferenczi[31] believing them to be similar to catatonic stereotypes and the result of libidinal displacement named tics "cataclonia." Deutsch,[24] Reich,[63] and Aarons[1] viewed tics as masturbatory equivalents, the latter also expressing the belief that the twitchings were symbolic of a need to ward off the danger of submitting to passive wishes.

TORTICOLLIS

Because torticollis is of relatively frequent occurrence, it is described here separately. It is also known as "wryneck" and is a tic involving the neck muscles, especially the sternocleidomastoid on one or both sides. The tic is complex and consists of quick elevations of the chin while the head is turned to one side as a result of spasmodic contractions of the neck musculature. When the contractions are quick and brief, torticollis is classified as a tic, when protracted and tonic it is considered a cramp.

While tics in general affect children more frequently, psychogenic torticollis is more common among adults. Patterson[57] warns that torticollis in a child must be considered organic, unless proven to the contrary.

The psychodynamics of torticollis is often indicative of expressing the emotion of aversion,[16,54] while Fenichel[30] sees the condition as resulting from anal retentive tendencies, suppressed rage, and castration anxiety.

⟮ Cramps

A cramp is defined as a protracted, tonic muscular contraction of functional origin. It affects a well-circumscribed area of the body, often an extremity. Classified as being of a hysterical nature, it is related to muscular tremors in general.

Cramps are of particular interest in certain occupational groups, because they frequently interfere with a person's ability to carry out his occupational duties, especially when his livelihood is dependent on his work performance. A common form is cramp of the writing hand in individuals who may be able to use the hand for every purpose other than writing. The condition is thought to be the result of ambivalent feeling the patient has towards his occupation; however, it may also be overdetermined and indicative of sexual conflicts that are close to conscious awareness. The sexual nature of the problem is more apparent in *blepharospasm*, which may be an expression of a defense mechanism to prevent voyeuristic impulses from becoming conscious.

Other occupation groups affected are musicians, especially pianists and violinists, seamstresses, typists, and watchmakers.

The relationship of cramps and catatonic symptoms has been the subject of much discussion. Meige[49] described a condition which he called "tic variables" or "attitude tics." This patient shows prolonged spastic contractions of body areas and the condition may progress to catatonia.

Treatment of Tics and Cramps

The nature of the treatment will depend on the degree of impairment and what one hopes to accomplish. Many simple tics are transient and need no special care, other than rest. Other tics are very complex and require intensive psychotherapeutic intervention, often with disappointing results.

Methods of treatment may therefore be divided in those aimed at symptomatic relief and others bringing about changes in attitude and personality structure.

Symptomatic Therapy. Includes the use of rest, massage, heat, autogenous training,[68] progressive muscular relaxation, hydrotherapy, surgery (torticollis), counterirritants, suggestion, hypnotherapy, and relaxant drugs (meprobamate, Valium, Robaxin). Some clinicians have used bed rest with isolation; others found re-education methods of some help. Yates,[78] Rafi,[61] and Clark[20] used behavior modification techniques to reduce the frequency and severity of tics. They reported good results by building up the negative habit of not performing the tic, Rafi using an apparatus based on the conditioned response principle.

The symptomatic treatment of tics has received a big boost through the introduction of the drug, haloperidol, which has proven to be highly effective in the control of tics.[11,44]

The evaluation of therapeutic results is complicated by the fact that tics have a tendency to fluctuate in severity or even disappear spontaneously on occasions. It may be said, however, that the prognosis is directly related to the mental state of the tiqueur[59] and is favorable if there is little mental deterioration. Others factors, such as chronicity and extent of muscular involvement, are also of significance as illustrated by such conditions as the variable chorea of Brissaud and Gilles de la Tourette's disease, which are described below.

Because of the ready availability of motor symptoms for study and observation, their use for evaluation of therapeutic results has been advocated,[5] and as body language they are considered a valid indicator of unconscious processes since they emerge and are expressed in the psychoanalytic procedure.[23]

(Variable Chorea of Brissaud

In 1899, Brissaud[13] described a condition that resembled Sydenham's chorea in its motor movements, but differed from it through its polymorphous manifestations; the choreiform movements lack uniformity, show no regularity in their evolution, and no constancy in their duration. "They come and go, increase and decrease, stop suddenly, recur suddenly, appear to be quick at one time and slow at another."

Meige and Feindel[50] consider the syndrome to be a separate clinical entity, but this view is opposed to that of Gilles de la Tourette, who believed the condition to be a form of the *maladie des tics*. The prognosis of the syndrome is said to be grave, even though there may be prolonged periods of remission.

(Gilles de la Tourette's Disease

History and Clinical Manifestations

First described by Itard[37] in 1825, a clinical syndrome of multiple tics was reported by Gilles de la Tourette who presented case studies of nine patients suffering from a motor disorder which he defined as "nervous affliction characterized by motor inco-ordination accompanied by echolalia and coprolalia."[73] The publications of his case reports aroused considerable interest at the time and various motor disturbances were thought to be evidence of this syndrome. The "latah"[2,74] of Malaya, the "myriachit" of Siberia,[35] and the "Maine jumpers"[74] showed sufficient similarity in their behavior to consider them victims of this motor syndrome.

Anthropological studies by Aberle[2] have since shown that latah differs from it in certain basic characteristics.[74] *Schlaftrunkenheit*, a condition prevalent in Germany, was also attributed to this condition which had become known as Gilles de la Tourette's disease, because of the author's original reports of his clinical observations.[73,74,49]

The syndrome is also mentioned as *maladie des tics,*[17] *koordinierte Erinnerungskraempfe,*[39] *myospasia impulsiva, maladie des tics convulsifs,*[33] *maladie des tics impulsifs, maladie des tics dégénerés,*[38] and *mimischer Krampf.*[12]

According to Gilles de la Tourette, the first symptoms occur in childhood and show no sex preference. Before the age of ten, the child develops tics of the face and extremities which vary in severity and are undistinguishable from other forms of tics or basal ganglia disease. The symptom which is characteristic of the disease is the emergence of a vocal tic. It may sound like a barking noise at first, which is inarticulate. As the condition progresses, words may be formed either of a coprolalic quality or designed to censure the obscene utterances. Such expressions as "keep quiet," "shut up," "don't say it," are not uncommon. On occasions, echolalia may be present, although this is not as frequent as Gilles de la Tourette thought it to be. The same applies to coprolalia, which he considered pathognomonic of the disease, but which other authors[4,71] discount as a requirement to establish the diagnosis of Gilles de la Tourette's disease.

The course of the disease differs from patient to patient. Gilles de la Tourette believed that the condition invariably leads to mental deterioration. More recent reports indicate that there may be general improvement in symptoms during late adolescence and that "spontaneous" remissions are not uncommon.[48,39] With the advent of effective methods of control of the symptoms, there is increasing evidence that mental deterioration is the exception rather than the rule in the outcome of such cases.[29]

Etiology

The cause of the disorder is unknown. Gilles de la Tourette[73] believed it to be a hereditary disease, as did Koester[39] and Oppenheim.[56] Because of the similarity to symptoms of chorea, organic lesions of the brain, especially of the basal ganglion, were held responsible for the syndrome.[45,62,76] Autopsy reports have not been conclusive, but they have been sparse and incomplete.[8,25] EEG tracings indicate that there is abnormality in about 50 percent of the cases, but there is no characteristic pattern for the disease. Concurrent with "organic" theories were psychogenic ones, such as by Guinon[33] who saw little difference between Gilles de la Tourette's disease and hysteria. Other psychogenic theories were advanced by Mahler,[46,47] Ascher,[6] and others.[28,29,75] On the other hand, Wilder and Silbermann[76] expressed the belief that the resistance of patients with Gilles de la Tourette's disease to psychotherapy was proof that it was an organic disease.

RECENT DEVELOPMENTS

After Gilles de la Tourette's publication, there were only occasional case reports in the literature, until Kovacs[40] described the analysis of a case and Wilder and Silbermann[76] discussed the condition in their monograph on tics. They were the first to systematically treat such patients by psychotherapy, followed by Wilson[77] and Mahler and Rangell[47] who used psychoanalysis in the therapy of several children.

In 1948, Ascher[6] reported his cases and reviewed the literature. It was followed by an increasing number of case reports which indicated that the condition was not as rare as was formerly believed. The controversy of organic versus psychogenic continued in most publications; however, there emerged a tendency to consider all possible factors in the management of patients suffering from Gilles de la Tourette's disease.

Ascher[6] investigated psychodynamic factors and concluded that many of the symptoms could be understood in terms of the patient's relationship to authority figures. He considered coprolalia as a dissociative phenomenon, as had Meige and Feindel[50] previously, by which the patient diverts his aggressive impulses toward the authority figure to the world in general.

Mahler and Rangell[47] also considered conflict between repressive force and instinctual process as significant, although they could not accept psychodynamic factors alone to be responsible for the condition. They believed that such patients have a constitutionally inferior subcortical structure with a reduction in their ability to withstand "overwhelming emotional and psychodynamic forces."

Other dynamic factors were introduced by Dunlap[28] whose patient had parents with severe tics, and by Aarons[1] who, like Fenichel,[30] considered the muscular twitchings to be masturbatory equivalents.

In recent years, the interest in Gilles de la Tourette's disease has increased and there are more case reports appearing in the literature. This is partly due to the nature of the disorder, but to a greater extent, to the effectiveness of psychotropic drugs in the control of its symptoms. Investigators have polled their information in panel discussions at national conventions,[71] and an international registry has been established in an attempt to record all cases diagnosed as Gilles de la Tourette's disease.[4]

The effectiveness of one psychotropic drug, haloperidol, has introduced a new factor in explaining the etiology of the syndrome. Because it is a potent blocker of dopamine receptors, it is suggested that hyperactivity of dopamine systems may be a factor in the pathophysiology of Gilles de la Tourette's disease.[7]

Titration of severity of symptoms has been achieved in one case by altering the disposition of the brain catecholamine, norepinephrine.[51]

TREATMENT

The variety of treatment methods employed is an indication of the confusion as regards the etiology of the disorder. Gilles de la Tourette treated his patients with sedatives, tonics, hydrotherapy, and isolation, the latter producing the best results, though temporary. Psychotherapy has been used with discouraging results, but there are reports indicating that psychotherapy was more successful.[29] Hypnotic therapy and electro-convulsive treatment have been ineffective; however, leucotomy,[7] carbon dioxide inhalation,[52] and sleep therapy are reported as having been helpful in controlling symptoms. The question is unanswered whether the improvement was the result of the treatment or represents a spontaneous remission.

The results of drug administrations have not been consistent. Bockner[9] and MacDonald[45] used chlorpromazine, which reduced anxiety, but it has to be given in large amounts to be effective.[42] Amphetamine helped one patient,[53] but this is in sharp conflict with the experience of Meyerhoff and Snyder.[51] Seignot[69] used haloperidol and his success with the drug was subsequently confirmed by Challas and Brauer.[18] Lucas[44] and Chapel[19,43,44] maintained their patients on daily doses of 1.5 mg. and 3.2 mg., respectively. There are a number of other reports describing the effective use of haloperidol.[11,44,51,71] Clark[20] successfully treated three by behavior therapy.

Although the focus of treatment has been on the patient and his symptoms, there is an increasing awareness of the importance of helping family members as well to understand the nature of the disease. This led to a publication of a guide for parents.[4]

The upsurge in interest in Gilles de la Tourette's disease invariably will result in better diagnosis and earlier treatment. This offers great promise that fewer patients will suffer the psychotic deterioration Gilles de la Tourette prognosticated.

(Bibliography

1. AARONS, Z. A. "Notes on a Case of *Maladie des Tics*," *Psychoanalytic Quarterly*, 27 (1958), 194–204.
2. ABERLE, D. F. "Arctic Hysteria and Latah in Mongolia," *Transactions of the New York Academy of Sciences*, II, 14 (1952), 291–297.
3. ABRAHAM, K. "Contribution to a Discussion on Tic," in *Selected Papers on Psychoanalysis*. New York: Basic Books, 1953.
4. ABUZZAHAB, F. S., SR., and K. J. EHLEN. "Tourette's Syndrome, A Guide for Parents." Private publication of University of Minnesota Hospitals, 1970.
5. ASCHER, E. "Motor Attitudes and Psychotherapy," *Psychosomatic Medicine*, II (1949), 228–234.
6. ———. "Psychodynamic Considerations in Gilles de la Tourette's Disease (*Maladie des Tics*)," *The American Journal of Psychiatry*, 105 (1948), 267–276.
7. BAKER, E. F. W. "Gilles de la Tourette's Syndrome Treatment by Bunedial Frontal Leucotomy." *Canadian Medical Association Journal*, 86 (1962), 746–747.
8. BALTHASAR, K. "*Über das anatomische Substrat der generalisierten Tic-Krankheit*," *Archiv für Psychiatrie und Nervenkrankheiten*, 191 (1954), 398.
9. BOCKNER, S. "Gilles de la Tourette's Disease," *Journal of Mental Science*, 105 (1959), 1078–1081.
10. BOJANOVSKI, J., and K. NAHUNEK. "Gilles de la Tourette Syndrome," *Ceskoslovenská Psychiatrie*, 58 (February 1962).
11. BORIS, M. "Gilles de la Tourette's Syndrome: Remission with Haloperidol," *Journal of the AMA*, 205 (1968), 102–103.
12. BRESLER, "*Beitrag zur Lehre von der Maladie des Tics Convulsifs*," *Neurologisches Zentralblatt*, 21 (1896), 965.
13. BRISSAUD, E. "Chorée Variable," *Presse Medicale*, 13 (1899).
14. ———. Quoted in Meige, H., and E. Feindel, Ref. 50.
15. BROWN, E. C. "Tics (Habit Spasms) Secondary to Sinusitis," *Archives of Pediatrics*, 74 (1957), 39–46.
16. CAMERON, N. *The Psychology of Behavior Disorders*. Boston: Houghton, Mifflin, 1947.
17. CHABERT, L. "*De la Maladie des Tics*," *Archives de Neurologie*, 25 (1893), 10.
18. CHALLAS, G., and W. BRAUER. "Tourette's Disease: Relief of Symptoms with R1625," *The American Journal of Psychiatry*, 120 (1963), 283–284.
19. CHAPEL, J. L., N. BROWN, R. L. JENKINS. "Tourette's Disease: Symptomatic Relief with Haloperidol," *The American Journal of Psychiatry*, 121 (1964), 608–610.
20. CLARK, D. F. "Behavior Therapy of Gilles de la Tourette's Disease," *British Journal of Psychiatry*, 112 (1966), 771–778.
21. CLARK, L. P. "Some Observations upon the Aetiology of Mental Torticollis," *Medical Record*, (February 1914).

22. DESHAN, P. W., JR. "Gilles de la Tourette Syndrome; Report of a Case," *Journal of the Oklahoma State Medical Association*, 54 (1961), 636–638.

23. DEUTSCH, F. "Analysis of Postural Behavior," *Psychoanalytic Quarterly*, 16 (1947), 195.

24. DEUTSCH, H. "Zur Psychogenese Eines Tic Falles," *Internazionale Zeitschrift für Psychoanalyse*, 11 (1925), 325–332.

25. DEWULFE, A., and L. VAN BOGAERT. "*Études Anatomocliniques des Syndromes Hypercynétiques Complexes*," *Monatsschrift für Psychiatrie und Neurologie*, 104 (1941), 53.

26. DIETHELM, O. *Treatment in Psychiatry*. New York: Macmillan, 1936.

27. DOLMIERSKI, R., and M. KLOOS. "Gilles de la Tourette Disease," *Annales Médicopsychologiques*, 120 (1962), 225–232.

28. DUNLAP, J. R. "A Case of Gilles de la Tourette's Disease (*Maladie des Tics*): A Study of the Intrafamily Dynamics," *Journal of Nervous and Mental Disease*, 130 (1960), 340–344.

29. EISENBERG, L., E. ASCHER, and L. KANNER. "A Clinical Study of Gilles de la Tourette's Disease (*Maladie des Tics*) in Children," *The American Journal of Psychiatry*, 115 (1959), 715–723.

30. FENICHEL, O. *The Psychoanalytic Theory of Neurosis*. New York: Norton, 1945.

31. FERENCZI, S. "*Psychoanalytische Betrachtungen über den Tic*," *Internazionale Zeitschrift für Psychoanalyse*, (1921), 33–62.

32. FRIEDREICH, N. *Über koordinierte Erinnerungskrämpfe*," *Virchows Archiv für pathologische Anatomie und Physiologie und für Klinische Medizin*, 86 (1881), 430–434.

33. GUINON, G. "*Sur la Maladie des Tics Convulsifs*," *Revue de Médicine*, 6 (1886), 50.

34. ———. "*Tic Convulsif et Hysterie*," *Revue de Médicine*, 7 (1887), 509.

35. HAMMOND, G. M. "Convulsive Tic, Its Nature and Treatment," *Medical Record*, 41 (1892), 236.

36. HEUSCHER, J. "*Beiträge zur Atiologie des Maladie Gilles de la Tourette und zum Regressionsproblem*," *Schweizer Archiv für Neurologie und Psychiatrie*, 66 (1950), 123–158.

37. ITARD, J. M. G. "Memoirés sur quelques functions involuntairs des appareits de la locomotion de la préhension et de la boix," *Archives générale de Medicine*, 8 (1825), 403.

38. KANNER, L. *Child Psychiatry*, 3rd ed. Springfield: Charles C. Thomas, 1960.

39. KOESTER, G. "*Über die Maladie des Tics Impulsifs (Mimische Krampfneurose)*," *Deutsche Zeitschrift für Nervenheilkunde*, 15 (1899), 147.

40. KOVACS, V. "*Analyse eines Falles von Tic Convulsif*," *Internazionale Zeitschrift für Psychoanalyse*, 11 (1925),

41. KROUT, M. "Autistic Gestures, an Experimental Study in Symbolic Movement," *Psychological Monographs*, 46 (1935), 208.

42. LEVY, B. S., and E. ASCHER. "Phenothiazines in the Treatment of Gilles de la Tourette's Disease," *Journal of Nervous and Mental Disease*, 146 (1968), 36–40.

43. LUCAS, A. R. "Gilles de la Tourette's Disease in Children: Treatment with Phenothiazine Drugs," *The American Journal of Psychiatry*, 121 (1964).

44. ———. "Gilles de la Tourette's Disease in Children; Treatment with Haloperiodol," *The American Journal of Psychiatry*, 124 (1967), 243–245.

45. MACDONALD, I. J. "A Case of Gilles de la Tourette Syndrome with Some Aetiological Observations," *British Journal of Psychiatry*, 109 (1963), 206–210.

46. MAHLER, M., and J. A. LUKE. "Outcome of the Tic Syndrome," *Journal of Nervous and Mental Disease*, 103 (1946).

47. MAHLER, M., and L. RANGELL. "A Psychosomatic Study of *Maladie des Tics* (Gilles de la Tourette's Disease)," *Psychiatric Quarterly*, 17 (1943), 519.

48. MAZUR, W. P. "Gilles de la Tourette's Syndrome," *Edinburgh Medical Journal*, 60 (1953), 427.

49. MEIGE, H. "Tics Variables, Tics d'Attitude," *Société de Neurologie de Paris*, July 4, 1901.

50. MEIGE, H., and E. FEINDEL. *Les Tics et leur Traitement*. Paris: Masson et Cie., 1902.

51. MEYERHOFF, J. L., and S. H. SNYDER. "Gilles de la Tourette's Disease and Minimal Brain Dysfunction," (in press).

52. MICHAEL, R. P. "Treatment of a Case of Compulsive Swearing," *British Medical Journal*, 1 (June 29, 1957), 1506–1508.

53. MILMAN, D. H. "Multiple Tics," *The Ameri-*

54. MUNCIE, W. *Psychobiology and Psychiatry.* St. Louis: Mosby, 1939.

55. OLSON, W. C. *The Measurement of Nervous Habits in Normal Children.* Minneapolis: University of Minnesota Press, 1929.

56. OPPENHEIM, Quoted in Koester, G. Ref. 39.

57. PATTERSON, M. "Spasmodic Torticollis," *Lancet*, 249 (1945), 556.

58. PESCETTO, G., and G. MAFFEI. *I Tics, Etiopatogenesi Clinica e Terapia.* Edizione Minerva Medica, 1969.

59. PRINCE, M. "Case of Multiform Tic Including Automatic Speech and Purposive Movements," *Journal of Nervous and Mental Disease*, 33 (1906), 29.

60. PURVES-STEWART, J., and C. WORSTER-DROUGHT. *The Diagnosis of Nervous Disease*, 10th ed. 1952.

61. RAFI, A. A. "Learning Theory and the Treatment of Tics," *Journal of Psychosomatic Research*, 6 (1962), 71–76.

62. RAPOPORT, J. "*Maladie des Tics* in Children," *The American Journal of Psychiatry*, 116 (1959), 177–178.

63. REICH, W. "*Der Psychogene Tic als Onanie Äquivalent*," *Zeitschrift für Sexualwissenschaft*, 11 (1925), 302–313.

64. RODENBERG, L. VON. "*Psychische Faktoren bei einigen Motorischen Störungen*," *Zeitschrift für Psychosomatische Medizin*, 8 (1962), 77–94.

65. ROUMAJON, Y. "*Un Cas de Psychothérapie Instituée pur des Tics*," *Revue Française de Psychanalyse*, 21 (1957), 707–714.

66. SALMI, K. "Gilles de la Tourette's Disease: The Report of a Case and Its Treatment," *Acta Psychiatrica et Neurologica Scandinavica*, 36 (1961), 156–162.

67. SCHNECK, J. M. "Gilles de la Tourette's Disease," *The American Journal of Psychiatry*, 117 (1960), 78.

68. SCHULTZ, J. H. *Das Autogene Training*, 6th ed. Stuttgart: Georg Thieme, 1950.

69. SEIGNOT, J. N. "A Case of Tic of Gilles de la Tourette Cured by R1625," *Annales Médico-Psychologiques*, 119 (1961), 578–579.

70. SINGER, K. "Gilles de la Tourette's Disease," *The American Journal of Psychiatry*, 120 (1963), 80–81.

71. SNYDER, S. H., K. M. TAYLOR, J. T. COYLE, and J. L. MEYERHOFF. "The Role of Dopamine in Behavioral Regulation and the Actions of Psychotropic Drugs," *The American Journal of Psychiatry*, 127 (1970), 117–125.

72. TOBIN, W. G., and J. B. REINHART. "Tic de Gilles de la Tourette," *American Journal for Diseases of Children*, 101 (1961), 778–783.

73. TOURETTE, GILLES DE LA. "*Étude sur une Affection Nerveuse, Caractérisée par de l'Incoordination Motrice, Accompagnée d'Écholalie et de Coprolalie*," *Archives de Neurologie*, 9 (1885), 159.

74. ———. "*Jumping, Latah, Myriachit*," *Archives de Neurologie* (1884), 68.

75. WALSH, P. J. "Compulsive Shouting and Gilles de la Tourette's Disease," *British Journal of Clinical Practice*, 16 (1962), 651–655.

76. WILDER, J., and J. SILBERMANN. "*Beiträge zum Tic Problem*," *Abhandlungen aus der Neurologie, Psychiatrie*, 43 (1927), 1.

77. WILSON, S. A. K. *Neurology.* Baltimore: Williams & Wilkins, 1941.

78. YATES, A. J. "The Application of Learning Theory to the Treatment of Tics," *Journal of Abnormal Social Psychology*, 56 (1958), 175–182.

CHAPTER 36

THE BORDERLINE PATIENT

Richard D. Chessick

⟮ Development of the Concept

THE CONCEPT of the borderline patient, poorly understood and vague, has become lost in a semantic morass; it well illustrates the poor quality of much psychiatric and psychoanalytic literature. Authors combine clinical description and dynamic formulations and using the method of psychoanalytic reconstruction have paid little attention to what others have already included under the term "borderline." As Grinker et al.[16] point out, ". . . the reports are repetitive, discursive and not well documented by empirical references."

Nevertheless, the concept of the borderline patient appears worthwhile and can be saved from the semantic morass. It represents a frequently encountered type of patient in our era, posing special problems for the psychotherapist, the general physician, and for those interested in the etiology and nosology of mental illness.

Although the term "borderline" appears from time to time in the classical psychiatric writings, major credit for delineating the concept and making it clinically respectable goes

to Stern. In three papers,[44,45,46] the first in 1938, he painted the clinical and psychodynamic picture, and discussed special problems in the treatment. He regarded "narcissism" (used by him according to the Freudian definition) as the basic underlying character component of these patients, leading to the development of a person with typical personality features. These are: (1) "psychic bleeding"—the patient goes down in a heap at each occurrence of stress in his life; (2) inordinate hypersensitivity—the patient is constantly insulted and injured by trifling remarks; (3) rigidity; (4) "negative therapeutic reaction"—a response of depression and anger to any interpretation, which is experienced as an injury to the patient's self-esteem; (5) feelings of inferiority and lack of self-assurance; (6) "masochism and wound-licking"—a tendency to self-pity and depression; (7) a strange "pseudo-equanimity" or outward calm, in spite of the inward chaos, may be present (although not always); and (8) a tendency to use projection, especially with people in authority, and corresponding peculiarities in reality-testing. Stern regarded the entire problem as a developmental injury caused by lack of spontaneous affection from the mother. Such patients were described as "traumatized pre-oedipal children," with a profound "affect-hunger."

The second author to make an important contribution to the subject was Deutsch,[14] who—without reference to Stern—described the "as-if" personality. The "as-if" patient is a subclass of the borderline patient group. In general, he is an extreme caricature of Riesman's[39] "other-directed" personality. Although he appears outwardly amiable, he has no identity of his own and is not capable of forming any genuine emotional attachment to people or moral principles. While there is a poverty of object relationships and much narcissism, no obvious defect in reality-testing is present—yet these patients certainly do not belong in the typical clinical "neurotic" category. Deutsch was suspicious of a "schizophrenic predisposition," but admitted that the relationship of "as-if" patients to neurotic and psychotic patients was not clear.

The subject of the borderline patient gained tremendous prominence due to the introduction of a number of new terms by well-known and highly respected authors. The first of these was the concept of "pseudoneurotic schizophrenia," introduced and investigated by Hoch and his co-workers.[19,20,21] Patients suffering from this disorder are characterized by "pan-anxiety"—they are made anxious by everything conceivable—and "pan-neurosis"—they present all varieties of neurotic symptoms, shifting back and forth over our nosological classifications. Furthermore, they may at times show clear-cut psychotic manifestations and even psychotic episodes, but these do not last and the patients as a rule *do not* deteriorate into chronic schizophrenic psychoses.

Grinker et al.[16] point out that Hoch vigorously opposed including pseudoneurotic schizophrenic patients among borderline patients. He considered them a variety of paranoid or catatonic schizophrenia, and opposed the use of the borderline concept altogether. However, clinical experience and common usage have tended to include "pseudoneurotic schizophrenic" patients among borderline patients because their pan-anxiety and pan-neuroses make it impossible to classify them as either neurotic or psychotic and, more importantly, because these conditions usually do not deteriorate into schizophrenia, indicating a certain remarkable stability to the condition. The same narcissism and poverty of object relations previously described for "as-if" and borderline patients are typically present in these patients. Since little further work has been done on this concept, except for Weingarten and Korn,[47] and since the term is used in such different, vague, and general ways, it is perhaps best to drop it altogether.

At this point, it is possible to see how the concept of borderline patient may become confused with "ambulatory schizophrenia"[51] or "latent schizophrenia,"[6] and many other such terms, generally designating schizophrenic patients who are not so sick as to require hospitalization. Thus, ambulatory or latent schizophrenics show the typical symptoms of schizophrenia, except to a less obvious degree; careful clinical examination may be necessary to pick up the classical schizophrenic syndrome, and a diagnosis can then be accurately established.

Knight[25,26,27] gave impetus to the serious psychoanalytic investigation of borderline cases, by discussing them in terms of a variable impairment of ego functions. This provided a partial theoretical explanation for the nosologic confusion, although his term, "borderline schizophrenias," again tended to blur the distinction between borderline patients and ambulatory schizophrenia patients. At any rate, in the borderline patient, as Knight put it, "the ego is laboring badly." The superficial clinical picture of a variety of neurotic symptoms, etc., "may represent a holding operation in a forward position, while the major portion of the ego has regressed far behind this in varying degrees of disorder." The great danger to the clinician is to misunderstand these "forward holding positions" as constituting the illness, and attempt to treat them—when they represent the healthiest part of the patient's ego functioning! Knight emphasizes the major point that only a careful face-to-face clinical examination, sometimes consisting of several interviews, in contrast to quickly putting such patients on the couch at one extreme, or quickly coming up with psychopharmacologic remedies on the other, will enable the physician to assess the "*total* ego functioning" of the patient. He offers details on how to conduct such an examination.

The final major accretion to the concept of borderline patient was added by Boyer,[4] Bender,[3] Schmideberg,[43] and others. Not only may the borderline patient show a variety of neurotic symptoms, but he may show a variety of delinquent, or "acting-out," or "pseudo-psychopathic" symptoms, involving him in all kinds of difficulty with society. This would be logically expected if the condition, as explained by Knight, represented the impairment of various ego functions. Such patients, for example, may involve themselves in all sorts of delinquent activity at various times in their lives, ranging from business chiseling to overt theft and criminal behavior, but it is unusual to find them engaged in major brutal crimes. In our era, they most typically appear in the general physician's office due to the syndrome of "periodic hyperingestion," as described by Chessick.[8] To the despair of their physicians and the panic of their families, these patients may consume large quantities of substances or combinations of substances, including opiates, barbiturates, marijuana, meprobamate, various phenothiazines, and other "tranquilizers," mescaline, alcohol, amphetamines, and food. At other times, there may be complete or almost complete abstention.

Certain physical and psychic symptoms may periodically become intense; these include aches and pains, gnawing and weird abdominal sensations, insomnia, anxiety attacks, epileptiform seizures, tics and twitchings, and depression. They are sometimes followed by an explosion of hyperingestion in which the patient is functionally partly or completely paralyzed and concentrates all his energy on a compulsive "stuffing in" of various substances while other activities are neglected. The substances hyperingested may vary from episode to episode, and the diagnosis of alcoholism or addiction may be mistakenly made at this point. However, although the patient may shift back and forth, he is on the whole able to function reasonably effectively in society and does not deteriorate.

A clear clinical delineation of the borderline patient emerges from this historical review. It includes the following characteristic features:

1. *Any* variety of neurotic, psychotic, psychosomatic, or sociopathic symptoms in any combination or degree of severity may be part of the presenting complaint. Either a bizarre *combination* of such symptoms cuts across the standard nosology, or the relative preponderance of any given symptom group is constantly changing or shifting. Thus, at least two and preferably three diagnostic interviews at intervals of at least a week apart are mandatory in establishing the diagnosis, in addition to a careful history-taking, including details of all symptoms and their vicissitudes. The "psychosomatic" symptoms must be taken seriously, as irreversible tissue damage can occur if proper treatment is not instituted promptly.[12] They should never be dismissed as "merely hysterical."

2. Vagueness of complaint or even a bland, amazingly "smooth," or socially successful personality may be encountered. Careful investigation in such cases will reveal a well-hidden poverty of genuine emotional relationships, behind an attractive and personable social façade. Thus, the patient may present either a very chaotic or stormy series of relationships with a variety of people, or a bland and superficial but relatively stable set of relationships; in both cases, a lack of deep emotional investment in any other person may be carefully, consciously or unconsciously, concealed.

3. The capacity for reality-testing and the ability to function in work and social situations is not seriously impaired, although the degree of functioning may vary from time to time. On the whole, these patients are able to maintain themselves, raise families, and otherwise fit into society (or even the prison environment). They do not present as drifters, chronic hospital or long-term prison cases, totally antisocial personalities, or chronic addicts. On the other hand, they may have tried

everything, and may present a variety of sexual deviations, but they are not functionally paralyzed by these or by their neurotic symptoms or anxieties, at least not for long periods of time.

4. These patients do not deteriorate. The borderline patient suffers from a relatively stable and enduring condition. He may suffer transient psychotic episodes either for no apparent reason or as a result of stress, alcohol, drugs, improper psychotherapy, etc., but he does not remain psychotic for long. He "snaps out of it"; often, he learns what will "snap" him out of it and administers a self-remedy. At times, this remedy simply consists of dropping out of an improper psychotherapy; at other times, it involves all varieties of bizarre rituals or behavior. Sometimes, his marital partner or friends know about this and will even apply his self-remedies for him; they consider this just his "hang-up."

Similarly, when the borderline patient is in one of his pan-neurotic, pan-anxiety, hyperingestive, or psychopathic states, he causes tremendous alarm in those around him, and appears to be in a terrible condition. At the same time, he may frustrate all efforts to "help" at that point, or if "helped" he may show a surprising lack of gratitude. Those borderline patients who suffer from various dramatic transient episodes soon acquire a reputation in the family and are often rejected by physicians as "crocks" or bad patients. They stimulate many unconscious and not-so-unconscious maneuvers by both family and physicians to get rid of them, for example, by sending them to a "sanitarium" for a "rest."

Further outstanding descriptions of the borderline patient are best found in literature, for example in the characters of Sartre[41] or Camus[7] or, as Litowitz and Newman[30] point out, in the "theatre of the absurd."

❲ Recent Areas of Investigation

Four recent areas of investigation of the borderline patient may be called to the attention of the interested reader. These involve more profound recent psychodynamic studies, sociocultural considerations, clinical-descriptive research, and possible biological determinants.

The first current area of investigation involves the use of the psychoanalytic method to develop an increasingly profound understanding of the psychodynamics and genesis of the borderline patient. One of the pioneers in this study was Albrecht Meyer who presented at least two papers on the subject, which to my knowledge have never been published (although mimeographed copies are available), and who organized the study group of psychoanalysts from the Chicago Institute for Psychoanalysis, now headed by Gamm. Some of the findings of this group have been reported by Grinker et al.,[16] and by Chessick.[10,12] Meyer was impressed by the work of Leuba[28] on what was called the "phobia of penetration," later described in a different terminology by Little[31] as "psychotic anxieties" regarding annihilation, identity, and existence itself. Because of this, for example, the patient may either pretend to get well or leave treatment, in order to avoid the resurgence of these fears in the transference.

Meyer also called attention to the work of Odier[36] who presented a little-known but major contribution to understanding the borderline patient in his concept of the "neurosis of abandonment." Odier emphasizes the role of anxiety as described above, which he maintains is directly proportional to the amount of insecurity in early childhood, and produces regression to the prelogical stage of infantile thinking. He describes the magic thinking in detail as involving either (a) objectification of fear—"whatever threatens me is wicked and whatever protects me is good"; (b) objectification of anger—toward animistic malevolent objects, as chosen; and (c) identification with the aggressor. The "objectification" is the magical defense, placing the anxiety and fear and anger *outside* of the psyche onto external objects, as in phobias, or onto fantasy objects, as in nightmares or religion.

In the "neurosis of abandonment," the anxiety is objectified onto a human being, instead of a cosmic image or a transitional object, who is then given the power of creating or abolishing abandonment, insecurity, and helplessness. This individual is seen as all-powerful, sometimes benevolent and sometimes malevolent. In this situation, the oscillation between love and hate, security and insecurity, dependency and paranoia, and the rapid transitions from euphoria to depression, all as a function of the minor provocations or reassurances from the chosen object, lead to the typical picture of the borderline patient.

Modell,[32,33] without reference to Odier, developed the same theme. He stressed the importance of a core of positive sense of identity, of "a sense of beloved self," which develops in infancy as a response to adequate mothering. Without this inner sense—which is probably related to Saul's[42] recent concept of "inner sustainment"—thinking remains magical and object relations remain primitive, just as described by Odier. These defects soon become manifest in psychotherapy in the relationship to the therapist, and represent the fundamental problem in the healing process, described in detail by Chessick.[13]

These concepts are placed into formal psychoanalytic terminology in an important paper by Murray,[34] who stresses the deep narcissistic "sense of entitlement" that pervades the thinking of the borderline patient. The patient lives in a "narcissistic world of omnipotence, with its unlimited power of magical thinking and unlimited entitlement to the lusts and destructions of pregenital excitements." A classic description of this may be found in the progressive deterioration of the heroine as protrayed in Tolstoy's *Anna Karenina*.

The most profound and thorough current attempt to delineate the borderline patient in classical psychoanalytic terminology is presented by Kernberg.[22,23,24,49] He stresses the patient's lack of anxiety tolerance, lack of impulse control, and lack of developed sublimatory channels, and contends that oral aggression plays a crucial role in the psychodynamics. There is a premature development of oedipal conflicts as an attempt to escape from the oral rage, with a subsequent condensation of pregenital and genital conflicts. There is a "pathology of internalized object relationships" and "an intensification and pathological fixation of splitting processes" in the ego functions of these patients, as well as a lack of sublimatory channels.

The mothers of borderline patients have been described by a variety of the clinical authors mentioned above. In general, they are described as intelligent and overfeeding mothers, who were able to hide the emotional impoverishment of their personalities behind pseudo-giving. This is combined with a stern, almost cruel, often unverbalized demand that the child live up to their expectations. This combination of overfeeding and pseudo-giving accompanied by the hidden stern demands produces a chaos in the child's mind that Leuba[28] has called "deception" and Chessick[10,13] a "pre-verbal disaster," leading to severe defects in ego development and an immersion in narcissistic consolation fantasies. These fantasies can pervade the patient's entire behavior, producing a sharp clash with reality, as magnificently portrayed in many of the plays of Eugene O'Neill. The further understanding and delineation of the borderline patient remains an important current area of psychoanalytic investigation.

A second recent area of investigation is a by-product of the current interest in "social psychiatry." The impact of social conditions upon the development of the personality is given major emphasis in this kind of investigation, in contrast to the psychoanalytic focus on the mother-child interaction. An important pioneer in this area is Wheelis[48] who, building on Riesman[39] and others, emphasizes the major change in presenting symptomatology found in psychoanalysts' offices over the recent years. Nowadays, the presenting complaints deal with "vague conditions of maladjustment and discontent"—in short, they sound more like the borderline patient and less like the "classical" neuroses. The lack of identity in these patients is linked to the collapse of institutional absolutes and values, leading to a sense of futility, emptiness, and longing. Chessick[13] also emphasizes the mechanism of externalization as underlying the "existential anguish" commonly presented by these patients.

There are many theoretical and methodological difficulties in this kind of approach, since the "linkage" between cultural-social and psychological systems remains unclear. Grinker et al.[16] devote a chapter in their book on the borderline syndrome to the questions: "Are there some factors in our rapidly changing western society and/or culture which spawn or facilitate the development of the borderline? Do these act directly on the developing personality at various critical periods such as adolescence or young adulthood or indirectly by influencing the maternal child-rearing practices or both?" They are unable to go beyond what might be called an "educated guess" that "in some way social and cultural conditions plus some other variables contrive together to produce the overt syndrome." The opportunity remains for much neglected and much needed interdisciplinary co-operation in understanding the borderline patient.

It is important to keep in mind that the complaints of the borderline patient often resemble a caricature or exaggeration of the complaints and behavior of so-called normal people in our current society; in fact, many "as-if" and other borderline patients are quite successful in the superficial social and business world. This is in marked contrast to the "latent" or "ambulatory" schizophrenic whose complaints are more bizarre and who is usually a generally unsuccessful person, by society's standards of "success."

Grinker et al.[16] and a corroborative study by Gruenewald,[17] from the same institution, have pioneered another area of investigation of the borderline patient, that might be called "clinical-descriptive research." In this study, *hospitalized* patients with the diagnosis of "borderline" were observed by various personnel, and the behavioral observations were rated for specific variables chosen "within an ego-psychology framework" and in terms of "allocated ego-functions." Obviously great care and attention by a team of experienced investigators were given to developing the methodology of this project. The ratings were then analyzed statistically in a sophisticated manner, resulting in a definition of the borderline syndrome and its subcategories.

The over-all characteristics found were: (1) anger was the main effect experienced by such patients; (2) a defect in affectional relationships was present—"these are anaclitic, dependent or complementary, but rarely reciprocal"; (3) indications of consistent self-identity were absent; and (4) depression was based on loneliness rather than guilt. Four subgroups were further delineated.

The investigators consider the borderline syndrome to be based on "the basic defects in maturation and early development expressed in ego-dysfunctions," discussed in psychoanalytic detail by Wilson.[49] A variety of factors are believed to contribute to the development of this defect, but cannot be elucidated at this time. The results of the study show an excellent clinical "fit" with the psychoanalytic office practice concept of the borderline patient described above. This kind of study, which much needs repeating in other institutions and in outpatient settings, helps to distinguish the borderline patient from the "latent" or "ambulatory" schizophrenic patient, and from other conditions.

A final important contemporary area of research concerns the biological determinants of mental illness, especially possible genetic links between schizophrenic and borderline conditions. A problem similar to that found in studying sociocultural factors also exists in these areas of research—to develop a "linkage" between the various factors. Rosenthal,[40] for example, presents several "models" of the "heredity-environmental interaction" that leads to the clinical picture of schizophrenia. He distinguishes between monogenic-biochemical theories of the etiology of schizophrenia, life-experience theories, and diathesis-stress theories, and points out that, "those who emphasize the genetic contribution seldom consider in earnest the role that environment might play, and environmentalists usually pay lip service to the idea that hereditary factors may eventually have to be considered as well."

It is the diathesis-stress theories that bring in the concept of the borderline patient. In this view, a constitutional predisposition to schizophrenia is seen as being inherited, usually on a polygenic basis. An extreme example of this is presented by Heston[18] who utilizes the concept of "schizophrenic spectrum" to include schizophrenia, schizoid conditions, ambulatory, latent *and* borderline schizophrenias. He considers the borderline area around schizophrenia to be clinically fuzzy because it is "biologically unreal," since "schizoidia" and "schizophrenia" are genetically linked conditions. This interesting concept deserves further investigation, but it should be clear from the previous discussion that the borderline patient, as here described, *cannot* be lumped under the "schizophrenic spectrum" and does not belong under "schizoidia." Otherwise, as some authors argue, there would be no point in retaining the concept at all and it would be indistinguishable from "latent" or "ambulatory" schizophrenia, etc.

However, both psychoanalytic clinical research and clinical descriptive research strongly support the presence of a large group of borderline patients who are clearly distinguishable from both ends of the "schizophrenic spectrum" on the one hand, and from the neuroses on the other. Perhaps Stern's original concept of these patients as "traumatized pre-oedipal children" is still valid, if one is willing to accept the psychoanalytic idea that the classical neuroses are based primarily, although certainly not entirely, on disasters during the oedipal period of development. The presence or absence of genetic and biochemical factors in the etiology of these disorders remains unknown and much less investigated than in schizophrenia.

⟨ Treatment of the Borderline Patient

There are almost as many varieties of recommendations for the treatment of the borderline patient as there are authors on the subject. General agreement is found only on a few basic issues. First, ordinary encouragement or supportive therapy as practiced in the general physician's office produces either no effect at all or a dramatic remission soon followed by relapse with the same or new symptoms, accompanied by the angry demand for more

magic. Second, the typical administration of various psychopharmacological agents to these patients often complicates the situation in many ways. They abuse the dosage instructions, and the side-effects produced by improper dosage complicate the symptom picture. They collect medication from various physicians and take these in varying amounts and combinations. Suicide attempts with these medications pose a definite risk.

Consultation of an understanding psychiatrist is mandatory in the management of these patients. It is obvious how intensely frustrating they can be, in spite of the best efforts of the well-intentioned physician. Either the patient is shifting back and forth between a puzzling variety of neurotic and psychosomatic symptoms with possible lapses into delusional material, such as ideas of reference accompanied by the realization that his suspicions "can't really be true," or he is shifting back and forth into various sociopathic behavior forms with the possible additional complication of periodic hyperingestion.

These rapid shifts, with all the excitement, storm, and panic they cause the patient and those around him, usually accompanied by either the missing of appointments, failure to pay the bill, or spending session after session in talking about various symptoms, and the constant introduction of new problems and extraneous matters, can soon make both physician and patient feel that no progress is being made. There is typically an increasing exasperation on the part of the therapist, as well as a developing barrage of complaints about the treatment from the patient, which usually leads to an impasse and a referral either for chronic hospitalization or to a psychiatrist "who works with addicts." A variety of ways are employed to get rid of these patients.

However, if one is willing to put up with a great deal of frustration and disappointment, it is possible to successfully treat many borderline patients. Four basic approaches to the psychotherapy of the borderline patient are found in the literature. It is assumed that the treatment is carried out either directly by an experienced psychiatrist or under careful supervision. There are great opportunities for doing harm, as well as an ever-present serious suicidal risk that must be recognized and cannot be avoided by constant hospitalization. As Little[31] eloquently points out, "Analysis of these patients is a life-and-death matter, psychically, and sometimes somatically as well. The analyst, or some extension of him is all that stands between the patient and death; and at some point he has to stand aside, and simply be there, while the patient takes his life into his own hands, and becomes a living human being—or a corpse."

The first type of psychotherapy recommended is advocated, for example, by Schmideberg.[43] She emphasizes a very authoritative and directive approach, with much psychological pushing and shoving of the patient "to get him moving." She makes it a point to appear involved and "nonprofessional," and emphasizes controls, socialization, and reality-testing. This reminds one of the "total push" type of treatment often used for schizophrenics; it deals mainly with the symptoms and tends to produce an "as-if" personality who modifies himself either to please the therapist or to escape the psychotherapy. Unless interminable contact is maintained with the patient, relapse is to be expected, especially when life stress arises. If this approach can be made to work, it is certainly quicker and cheaper than the long-term intensive therapies.

The second type of approach is formal psychoanalysis. Some argue this to be the treatment of choice, for example, Boyer and Giovacchini,[5] while others see it as a desperate "heroic" measure.[23] Most psychotherapists reject this approach out of clinical experience in which many borderline patients show a complete intolerance to the ordinary psychoanalytic situation, reacting with suicidal attempts, transitory psychoses, or dramatic and chaotic symptoms and acting out that finally interrupt the treatment. Even placing such patients on the couch where they cannot see the psychotherapist may produce an explosive reaction, although in certain cases it may be suprisingly beneficial, as illustrated in Chessick's[11] series of patients. To say the least, a formal psychoanalysis of the borderline patient should not be attempted by anyone except the most experienced and well-trained psychoanalyst who is willing to assume great risks.

The third type of psychotherapy attempts to combine an uncovering psychotherapy with providing a direct "corrective emotional experience" for the patient. This "corrective emotional experience" can range from taking the patient's hand[31] to examining the patient in the nude or letting her bite and suck on the therapist's hand,[2] in a direct attempt to provide better mothering experiences within the particular psychodynamics of the patient. Needless to say, the danger of massive countertransference acting out is quite acute in these situations, and the most hair-raising and destructive behavior by the therapist can be excused as attempting to provide a "corrective emotional experience." Here, again, considerable training and experience is necessary for the psychotherapist to know what he is doing, and repeated consultation with colleagues is required.

From a theoretical point of view, there is the important additional danger that the use of such heroic measures, which must invariably be experienced as primary-process interchange, works directly against the stated aim of converting the patient's ego functioning away from primary process and towards secondary process based on thinking and behavior. The patient, as in the directive and authoritative psychotherapies, can become easily "hung up" on the primary-process gratifications involved, leading to a demand for more, and subsequent stalemate. I have seen this occur repeatedly when attempted by inexperienced or poorly trained psychotherapists.[9]

However, the line between primary-process phenomena and secondary process is not an easy and distinct one, and, "Primary-process phenomena are not necessarily pathological, nor are they always maladaptive," as Arlow and Brenner[1] point out. There are undoubtedly times in every psychotherapy when this type of communication makes all the difference, and fear of such communication can lead to a rigid and withdrawn psychotherapist who surely will fail with borderline patients. Self-understanding, training, and experience are the crucial factors in success or failure with borderline patients who are generally less forgiving of pathology in the therapist than most patients.

Except for the unusually qualified therapist, the treatment offering the greatest potential with the least serious risk for borderline patients goes under the various names of "psychoanalytically oriented psychotherapy" or "psychoanalysis with parameters," the latter a controversial and horrendous term. The most complete and thorough review of "psychoanalysis with parameters" for the borderline case has been presented by Kernberg[23,24] and summarized by Wilson.[49] Chessick[10,13] has explored the psychoanalytically oriented psychotherapy of the borderline patient in a less formal language. I will conclude this chapter by reviewing the psychoanalytically oriented psychotherapy of the borderline patient, which is often a face-to-face psychotherapy, depending on the anxiety level of the patient. In this therapy, the proper understanding and management of the transference is critical, and poses many special problems.[37]

The initial problem of the therapy is getting the patient to form a therapeutic alliance, in spite of all the *Sturm und Drang* which his symptoms can provide for the relationship. In fact, the patient must first be very tightly locked into the therapy, in order to enable him to maintain it when terrific anxieties of abandonment and annihilation arise and must be worked through. A very long period of "being there" from a psychotherapist with a high empathic capacity and great frustration tolerance is necessary before the patient begins to build a sense of confidence and becomes locked into a symbiotic relationship with the therapist. This is facilitated by concentration on reality problems, instead of getting lost in fancy or highly intellectual dream interpretations or psychodynamic formulations, and also by a certain "deep inner attitude"[35] towards one's patients, which is difficult to characterize in detail.

If this locking in takes place, strong trans-ference manifestations appear, affording the opportunity to correct the "pre-verbal disaster" without dangerous heroic measures. This correction takes place in the context of the transference through empathic understanding and interpretation by the therapist, as well as through a deep emotional interaction between therapist and patient, described in detail elsewhere.[10,13] *Success or failure in the treatment depends on this process.* As one might expect, the transference manifestations can be extremely frightening and strong, so that the patient resorts to many unusual measures to deal with them.

Two of the most typical of these measures seen in the psychotherapy of the borderline patient are the "erotized transference"[38] and the involvement of a third person in the transference,[29] both of which must be quickly recognized and dealt with, or the treatment will be ruined. The erotized transference, which was recognized by Freud early in the development of psychoanalysis, manifests itself in borderline cases by the stormy demand for genital contact. When this is rejected, the patient experiences deep and sincere hurt and humiliation. He does not accept interpretations and rather persists in the demands for gratification. Empathy, consistency of approach, patience in understanding the patient's sense of rejection, and not reacting with fear or hostility to his demands, can eventually lead to a resolution of the problem.

Similarly, borderline patients often cannot stand the intensity of their longings for the therapist in the transference, and they may quickly dump all of this on a third person, and engage in massive acting out. If this is not recognized and interpreted and stopped, sometimes forcibly, situations such as marriage or pregnancy may result. Alertness to the problem and consistent concentration on the patient's life situation are necessary. The use of a third person is not always undesirable to help the patient withstand the intense transference longings; it depends on to what extremes the patient has to go. Too energetic interpretations of transference longings can throw the patient into a chaotic panic and disrupt the treatment entirely.

If disruption does not occur, and the transference is properly understood and interpreted, the anxieties are gradually worked through, and in this protective atmosphere the patient is able to uncover his narcissistic core fantasies and sense of "entitlement" (Murray[34]). Meyer's unpublished series of "fifteen to eighteen cases" psychoanalyzed by him demonstrated the presence of this narcissistic core fantasy when the fear of penetration was reduced. This clinical experience was supported by findings from a series of twenty patients studied in psychoanalytically oriented psychotherapy by Chessick.[8,9] The patient lives around a fantasy (or fantasies) which permeates and contaminates all the ego operations. This narcissistic fantasy, for example, being a famous professor or a saint of the church or a great artist, and so on, represents a consolation for the profound early and chronic deprivation of affect from the mother, and also attempts to produce the longed-for affect through satisfying her expectations. The patient often lives as if he has secretly accomplished these things, producing a set of unrealistic responses to life. Sometimes, these core fantasies are apparent even at the beginning of treatment, but direct assault upon them simply results in denial or break-up of the treatment, since they represent substitutes for gratifying human relationships and cannot be given up until the annihilation and abandonment fears are worked through in the transference.

It follows that the basic factor in the successful psychotherapy of borderline patients is how the psychotherapist responds to and handles the "crucial dilemma" (Chessick[9]) produced by the intense transference longings and also the associated deep fears, and forcing the problem of "parameters"[23,24] upon the therapist. The therapist must have an empathic grasp of how the patient perceives and how he feels, and he must be able to both interpret in an empathic fashion and also emotionally respond to the patient, without using the patient to gratify his own needs. At the appropriate time, he must be able to draw back and allow the patient to develop his own identity, providing throughout the psychotherapy Winnicott's[50] well-known "good-enough holding situation."

Working with borderline patients is not easy, but it is extremely rewarding in many ways. It provides a deeper and deeper understanding of the development of ego functioning and warps in ego development that can be applied to all areas of psychopathology. It forces the therapist to constantly pursue and achieve a deeper understanding of himself and demands an ever-increasing maturity from him. Most important of all, when successful, it brings the patient back to life from a situation of psychic death, a state of unparalleled suffering portrayed with great skill in modern theater and literature, beginning perhaps with Dostoyevsky:[15]

But it is just in that cold, abominable half despair, half belief, in that conscious burying oneself alive for grief in the underworld for forty years, in that acutely recognized and yet partly doubtful hopelessness of one's position, in that hell of unsatisfied desires turned inward, in that fever of oscillations, of resolutions determined for ever and repented of again a minute later—that the savour of that strange enjoyment of which I have spoken lies. It is so subtle, so difficult of analysis, that persons who are a little limited, or even simply persons of strong nerves will not understand a single atom of it.

(Bibliography

1. ARLOW, J., and C. BRENNER. *Psychoanalytic Concepts and the Structural Theory.* New York: International Universities Press, 1964.

2. BARRY, M., D. ROBINSON and A. JOHNSON. "Ego Distortions: Some Modifications in the Therapeutic Technique," *American Journal of Psychotherapy*, 13 (1959), 809–825.

3. BENDER, L. "The Concept of Pseudopsychopathic Schizophrenia in Adolescents," *American Journal of Orthopsychiatry*, 29 (1959), 491–512.

4. BOYER, L. "Uses of Delinquent Behavior by a Borderline Schizophrenic," *Archives of Criminal Psychodynamics*, 2 (1957), 541–571.

5. BOYER, L., and P. GIOVACCHINI. *Psycho-analytic Treatment of Characterological and Schizophrenic Disorders*. New York: Science House, 1967.

6. BYCHOWSKI, G. "Psychic Structure and Therapy of Latent Schizophrenia," in A. Rifkin, ed., *Schizophrenia in Psychoanalytic Office Practice*. New York: Grune and Stratton, 1957.

7. CAMUS, A. *The Stranger*. New York: Alfred A. Knopf, 1957.

8. CHESSICK, R. D. "The Psychotherapy of Borderline Patients," *American Journal of Psychotherapy*, 20 (1966), 600–614.

9. ———. "The 'Crucial Dilemma' of the Therapist in the Psychotherapy of Borderline Patients," *American Journal of Psychotherapy*, 22 (1968), 655–666.

10. ———. *How Psychotherapy Heals*. New York: Science House, 1969.

11. ———. "Use of the Couch in the Psychotherapy of Borderline Patients," *Archives of General Psychiatry*, 25 (1971), 306–313.

12. ———. Angiospastic retinopathy: Development during the intensive psychotherapy of a borderline patient, *Archives of General Psychiatry*, 27 (1972), 241–244.

13. ———. *The Technique and Practice of Intensive Psychotherapy*. New York: Jason Aronson Books, 1973.

14. DEUTSCH, H. "Some Forms of Emotional Disturbances and Their Relationship to Schizophrenia," in *Neuroses and Character Types*. New York: International Universities Press, 1965.

15. DOSTOYEVSKY, F. *Notes From Underground*. New York: Dell Publishing Co., 1960.

16. GRINKER, R., B. WERBLE and R. DRYE. *The Borderline Syndrome*. New York: Basic Books, 1968.

17. GRUENEWALD, D. "A Psychologist's View of the Borderline Syndrome," *Archives of General Psychiatry*, 23 (1970), 180–184.

18. HESTON, L. "The Genetics of Schizophrenic and Schizoid Disease," *Science*, 167 (1970), 249–256.

19. HOCH, P., and J. CATTELL. "The Diagnosis of Pseudoneurotic Schizophrenia," *Psychiatric Quarterly*, 33 (1959), 17–43.

20. HOCH, P., J. CATTELL, O. STRAHL and H. PENNES. "The Course and Outcome of Pseudoneurotic Schizophrenia," *The American Journal of Psychiatry*, 119 (1962), 106–115.

21. HOCH, P., and P. POLATIN. "Pseudoneurotic Forms of Schizophrenia," *Psychiatric Quarterly*, 23 (1949), 248–276.

22. KERNBERG, O. "Borderline Personality Organization," *Journal of the American Psychoanalytic Association*, 15 (1967), 641–685.

23. ———. "The Treatment of Patients with Borderline Personality Organization," *International Journal of Psycho-Analysis*, 49 (1968), 600–619.

24. ———. "Treatment of Borderline Patients," in P. Giovacchini, ed., *Tactics and Techniques in Psychoanalytic Therapy*. New York: Science House, 1972.

25. KNIGHT, R. "Borderline States," in R. Lowenstein, ed., *Drives, Affects, Behavior*. New York: International Universities Press, 1953.

26. ———. "Borderline States," in *Psychoanalytic Psychiatry and Psychology*. New York: International Universities Press, 1962.

27. ———. "Management and Psychotherapy of the Borderline Schizophrenic Patient," in *Psychoanalytic Psychiatry and Psychology*. New York: International Universities Press, 1962.

28. LEUBA, J. "*Introduction a l'Étude Clinique du Narcissisme*," *Revue Française de Psychanalyse*, 13 (1949), 456.

29. LIPSHUTZ, D. "Transference in Borderline Cases," *Psychoanalytic Review*, 42 (1955), 195–200.

30. LITOWITZ, N., and K. NEWMAN. "Borderline Personality and the Theatre of the Absurd," *Archives of General Psychiatry*, 16 (1967), 268.

31. LITTLE, M. "Transference in Borderline Cases," *International Journal of Psycho-Analysis*, 47 (1966), 476–485.

32. MODELL, A. "Primitive Object Relations and the Predisposition to Schizophrenia," *International Journal of Psycho-Analysis*, 44 (1963), 282–292.

33. ———. *Object Love and Reality*. New York: International Universities Press, 1968.

34. MURRAY, J. "Narcissism and the Ego Ideal," *Journal of the American Psychoanalytic Association*, 12 (1964), 477–511.

35. NACHT, S. "The Non-Verbal Relationship in Psychoanalytic Treatment," *International Journal of Psycho-Analysis*, 44 (1963), 328–333.

36. ODIER, C. *Anxiety and Magic Thinking*. New York: International Universities Press, 1956.

37. RAMANA, C. "Preliminary Notes on Transference in Borderline Neurosis," *Psychoanalytic Review*, 43 (1956), 129–145.

38. RAPPAPORT, E. "The Management of an Erotized Transference," *Psychoanalytic Quarterly*, 25 (1956), 515–529.

39. RIESMAN, D., R. DENNEY and N. GLAZER. *The Lonely Crowd*. New York: Doubleday, 1955.

40. ROSENTHAL, D. ed. *The Genain Quadruplets*. New York: Basic Books, 1963.

41. SARTRE, J. *Nausea*. New York: New Directions, 1964.

42. SAUL, L. "Inner Sustainment," *Psychoanalytic Quarterly*, 39 (1970), 215–222.

43. SCHMIDEBERG, M. "The Borderline Patient," in S. Arieti, ed., *American Handbook of Psychiatry*, Vol. 1 New York: Basic Books, 1959.

44. STERN, A. "Psychoanalytic Investigation of and Therapy in Borderline Group of Neuroses," *Psychoanalytic Quarterly*, 7 (1938), 467–489.

45. ———. "A Psychoanalytic Therapy in the Borderline Neuroses," *Psychoanalytic Quarterly*, 14 (1945), 190–198.

46. ———. "Transference in the Borderline Neuroses," *Psychoanalytic Quarterly*, 17 (1948), 527–528.

47. WEINGARTEN, L., and S. KORN. "Psychological Test Findings on Pseudoneurotic Schizophrenics," *Archives of General Psychiatry*, 17 (1967), 448–453.

48. WHEELIS, A. *The Quest for Identity*. New York: W. W. Norton & Co., 1958.

49. WILSON, C. "On the Limits of the Effectiveness of Psychoanalysis: Early Ego and Somatic Disturbances," *Journal of the American Psychoanalytic Association*, 19 (1971), 552–564.

50. WINNICOTT, D. *The Maturational Process and the Facilitating Environment*. New York: International Universities Press, 1965.

51. ZILBOORG, G. "Ambulatory Schizophrenias," *Psychiatry*, 4 (1941), 149.

CHAPTER 37

MINOR MALADJUSTMENTS
OF THE AGED

Alvin I. Goldfarb

ONE PERSON IN TEN in the United States is now sixty-five years of age or older. About 1½ million of these 20 million people are between sixty-five and seventy-four years old, 6 million are from seventy-five to eighty-four and 1½ million are eighty-five or more years old. They are obviously a heterogeneous group ranging in age from sixty-five to over ninety years of age, in various states of physical health, functional status and vigor, who vary in education, occupation, ethnic group, and cultural background. They reside in private homes, hospitals, nursing homes, or old age homes, are for the most part poor, but differ widely in economic supports and social status. Many have had psychological or emotional problems over a long period of time and bring into old age mental diseases first noted in youth; others become mentally impaired or psychiatrically ill for the first time in their old age. In some of them, it is a previously existing disorder that emerges as significantly troubling or troublesome because of age related changes in social status, role, or health. In the past twenty-five years there has been increasing interest in the treatment of old persons with psychiatric disorders of all kinds, including those which reflect brain damage.

There are many reasons for the increased attention to the psychiatric disorders of the chronologically old. Among them is the vast number of the disorders, the public health problem created by the depressed old and those with syndromes reflecting brain dysfunction or damage. Medicare financing has increased the demand for services and has helped make more service available. Also, there is growing interest in long-term illness and the deteriorative or degenerative diseases of aging now that infections, metabolic disorders, and many acute conditions are coming under better control. In addition, the sudden rapid advance in pharmacotherapy and the expansion of knowledge about the biochemistry of the psychoses have made possible greatly improved care of disturbing, disturbed and depressed old people, and have added to the efficacy and safety of electroconvulsant treatment. Of special importance is the impact created by the availability of phenothiazines and similar "antipsychotic" drugs since the mid 1950s, and the revolution in the treatment of depressive disorders with the introduction of monoamineoxidase inhibitors and the antidepressant, tricyclic, drugs in 1957 and 1958.

At the same time, there has been growing recognition that drugs and physical modes of treatment, even when they can be specifically helpful, are not entirely sufficient for best results. Moreover, in a host of conditions medication is at best merely adjunctive. To this has been added the confrontational attitude of the departments of mental hygiene, or their equivalents, on a country-wide basis, to discourage the use of state hospitals for persons who may become problems of long-term care, who appear to have serious and acute physical illness, or are not clearly "psychotic." Right or wrong, such action has pressed "back to the community"—to general hospitals, community mental health centers, private physicians, nursing homes, old age homes and various agencies a host of new problems.

Activities programs, special services and dyadic or group therapies are expanding because they appear to improve sociability, social integration, and the mood of old persons with psychological or emotional problems, even when they are also brain-damaged as reflected by accurately measured brain syndrome. This has led to expansion of efforts, over the past twenty-five years, to provide psychotherapeutic relationships in private practice and for old persons in hospitals, old age, or nursing homes, as well as by way of clubs, centers, and educational facilities. New subdivisions of old disciplines are emerging to help manage, care for, and provide special services for the old and aged.

At the present time psychiatrists, psychologists, social workers, nurses, administrators, and even laymen acting as volunteers or by way of self-appointment to quasi-professional status are engaged in such activities. This chapter will discuss, from the psychiatric point of view, some of the problems, views and solutions emerging.

A conceptual scheme useful in the practice of psychiatry with elderly persons is outlined. This scheme permits the organization of information in an eclectic way without sacrificing opportunities for understanding of psychodynamic factors or opportunities for psychodynamically oriented psychotherapy. It encourages treating the disturbed or disturbing behavior of elderly and aged persons, whether with brain damage or without, as if it were motivated and purposive goal-seeking. It also places emphasis upon the therapeutic value of the personal relationship, and upon the importance of the relationship for the initiation, maintenance, and supplementation of other modes of treatment required by a special condition. The schema around which this chapter is developed is outlined in Figure 37–1. As noted in Figure 37–1 many factors may reduce the adaptive capacity of old persons.

Figure 37–1. Components of disorder: psychodynamic sequence.

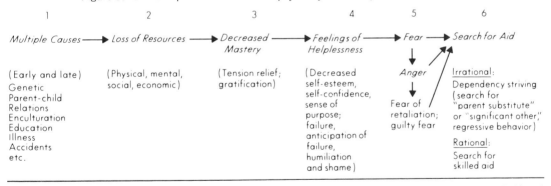

1. Multiple causes or initiating factors that occur either early in life and are reinforced or modified with aging, or occur late in life and are peculiar to old age, several of which may combine forces and some of which may be necessary but insufficient alone, result in
2. an absence or loss of resources for minimally adequate functioning, so that
3. there is decreased mastery of problems, challenges, and adjustments posed by internal changes (biologically determined drives or acquired needs), external changes and threats, with resulting
4. feelings of helplessness or actual powerlessness, and consequent
5. fear with accompanying or subsequent anger, with consequent
6. "rationally" or "irrationally" aimed and elaborated search for aid which becomes patterned in terms acceptable to the individual in terms of his personality organization based upon his past, his present, and his expectations; and contingent on his perception of what is acceptable to and likely to work in "his world," as well as by the social response it receives. In this search there are observable constellations of motivated personal action which range from apathy through pseudoanhedonia, display of helplessness, somatization, hypochondriasis, depression, and paranoid states to the most open and manipulative behavior. In predisposed persons there may be a physiologic shift to a new and relatively inefficient homeostatic level with depressive states, which are then revealed by altered appetite, bowel function, sleep, and other vegetative signs.

From Goldfarb, A.I. (Feb. 1968). Clinical perspectives. *Psychiatric Research Report 23.* Reproduced with permission of American Psychiatric Association.

([Geropsychiatry

A part of the burgeoning of interest in the old and impaired has been the growth of a subspecialty of psychiatry called "geropsychiatry" in the United States and "psychogeriatrics" in Great Britain. The latter term is preferred by the World Health Organization. This small group of specialists has been concerned with defining how psychiatrically or psychodynamically oriented health care delivery as well as specific psychotherapy can be most clearly delineated for the purpose of training, effective application, and advances through research.[193,194]

Geropsychiatry is the branch of psychiatry concerned with the mental disorders of old age, but particularly with those that first emerge as significant in the chronologically old. Defined in this way, the field of the geropsychiatrist may include those persons who have aged in the hospital because of schizophrenia, manic-depressive psychosis, or other disorders resistive to treatment, whose course was complicated by institutional neglect, or for whom there has been necessary provision of either a protective hospital community life or hospital-type care in the community. The psychiatric problems that are related to aging, which first emerge in old age, or which having existed before first emerge as significant, or take on new and special importance in old age, are the geropsychiatrist's chief area of interest. Many of these disorders are not yet easily classified. They occur in the old and in the aged under a variety of conditions, and in various residential settings.

The major psychoses and specific disorders that occur in the aged, although within the field of geropsychiatry, are covered elsewhere in this volume. Consequently, the emphasis here is on the variety of disorders that have not been nosologically specifically dignified, and upon psychodynamic factors common to all.

Psychodynamic or interpersonal factors, as now understood, may play no, or only a small, contributing role to the genesis and development of mood-cyclic, recurrent depressive or schizophrenic reactions. The afflicted person, his family or his physicians, however, may see logical connections between such factors and the disease, which actually do not exist and alterations of which make no prophylactic or therapeutic difference.

Mood-cyclic disorders, recurrent depressions, and schizophrenic episodes, whatever their original causes, may in old age be equivalent to and provoke the same responses as disabling accidents, illness, material or social loss. They contribute to decrease in the person's adaptive capacity and also may exacerbate or aggravate other illnesses or impairments and may themselves be exaggerated or exploited in the reconstituted adaptational pattern.

Old Age

Chronologically old persons, as the term is used here, are persons more than sixty-four years of age. This choice of age is an arbitrary one but it has legal and traditional basis and it does indicate that point of life at which time impairment of mental and physical functions, decline, and changes stigmatic of aging, become increasingly manifest.

The Aged

The truly aged are persons who when chronologically old have also suffered a decline in physical or mental functional status to a degree that interferes with the socially acceptable performance of routine activities. Aging is decline in functional status based upon irreversible structural change. Examples are changes in the lens of the eye which limit function and create a need for prosthesis, deafness related to sensory neural changes, loss of connective tissue elasticity, decline in homeostatic efficiency, loss in muscle fibers and strength, and probably of greatest importance, the loss of cells in the central nervous system. Also, the effects of disease may grossly decrease functional capacity. Decrease in the functional status of the heart, lungs, kidneys, bladder, or bowel in old age may result in poor support of the brain. The loss of functioning neurones in the central nervous system may be sufficiently great to give rise to organic brain syndrome. Other losses, the loss of income, even of savings, and the loss of status, role, and the prestige and power these carry, may be psychologically and emotionally traumatic, and also mean that real protective or comforting services and alliances are removed. With old age, there are losses of persons by death, geographical removal, illness or preoccupation with personal problems; these losses may constitute the disappearance of protective, reassuring, and supportive relationships without which the individual feels abandoned, vulnerable, and weak. To the socioeconomic, psychological, physical, and mentational losses are usually added losses or absences of resources for optimal adaptive functioning that occurred prior to old age. Genetic factors, enculturation, education, occupation, the experience and special social factors which were operative early in life play a part in determining the adaptive status in late life. There are therefore differences in individual ability to substitute for losses with aging, to be flexible in the choice of ends or goals with change in status, and to make optimal use of remaining assets when loss of resources has occurred.

The Well-Adjusted Old

The well-adjusted aged appear to have carried into late life the capacity to gain gratifications, to relieve their tensions—both the biologically determined and those acquired through enculturation and life experience—so as to maintain their self-esteem, self-confidence, purposivity, and a satisfying sense of personal identity and social role despite losses that may occur with aging. This differs from the maladjusted who, either because of earlier influences upon their personality development or differences in life experience at whatever age, do not have the resources to deal constructively and efficiently with life problems.

Well adjusted persons of sixty-five or over appear to have emotional needs that do not

differ greatly from those of younger persons. They have a minimum of complaints. They desire friendships, of varying types of intensity of intimacy, with both sexes. They want to keep busy at work, or at play equivalents, which are within their physical capacities, are commensurate with their intelligence and background of training, and from which they derive a sense of accomplishment. They look for, and object to frustration of, opportunities for the relief of biological tensions, such as hunger and sexual desire. In addition, they may crave, in varying degrees, appreciation, marks of affection, and reassurance that they have made an impression upon this world by means of words, deeds, or by having reproduced themselves. In this way, self-esteem, which in the past rested upon and was reinforced by current performance, can be maintained by the assumption of special status or personally gratifying "life-review." In all this, there may be some difference from adjustment in youth, characterized by mellowness—a lack of haste or pressure, an inner patience, and a philosophic tolerance growing out of a satisfied curiosity. Obviously, emotional problems may be encountered among elderly well-adjusted people. They may meet these successfully alone or may require counsel, guidance, information, or even psychotherapy, as may any younger person under social stress.

Relatively well-adjusted older persons usually are found in their own homes. Old persons who live with relatives usually do so because of financial, physical, or psychiatric need for care. There are many relatively well-adjusted persons in old age homes or other protective settings, but, again, such residence usually denotes need for care and associated psychological problems. The use of a protective setting even when the indication appears to have been physical is usually a clue to the coexistence of psychiatric problems. Persons in nursing homes or other protective settings for the ill are often psychologically and emotionally disturbed—sometimes, in reaction to the illness, often, because there have been such problems long preceding the illness or impairment, which appear to have led to the use of a congregate care facility, because these result in excess disability[91] and to complications in the provision of care.

Protectors Against Low Morale and Maladaptive Behavior

Genetic factors undoubtedly have an influence upon early development. The fortunate child has healthy and well-to-do parents who tend to provide the nurturance which favors nature and leads, through the provision of good schooling, helpful enculturation, and assistance toward remunerative and sustaining occupation, to health-reinforcing experiences. Even in the absence of optimal inheritance,

good nurture favors healthy development. Thus, good mechanisms of physical, mental, emotional, and social adaptation when taught and encouraged early in life tend to become well established, automatized, and to persist throughout the lifetime into late old age.

Relative affluence, high educational level, relatively high or respected social status, and good physical health appear to favor good social integration, minimal complaining by the persons, and a minimum of complaints about them. This is summarized in Table 37–1.

Not only are money, well-established adaptive patterns, and health instrumental in maintaining an individual's good feelings about himself and his world, but these factors ap-

TABLE 37–1.   **The Factors Which Protect Against Low Morale**

FACTOR	PROTECTIVE DEVICE	PROTECTIVE EFFECT	RESULT
Relative Affluence	Economic security: food, shelter, services, mobility, medical care	Freedom from fear and anger	
			Limited need for family and friends
	Physical security: power physical comfort pleasure	Assertiveness	
High Educational Level	Well established mechanisms of: psychological, social and emotional adjustment	Self-confidence Self-esteem Self-direction: interests purpose	Responsiveness to needs of family
	Diversity and range of interests	(Sense of identity)	
Social Status	Social security	Social independence	Capacity for solitary self-enjoyment
Good Health	Power Mobility Physical comfort or pleasure Physical security	Physical independence	Ability for independent production or pleasurable activity

High morale in the aged is favored, not guaranteed, by early opportunity in finances, education, social position, and health. Goldfarb, A. I. "Responsibilities to Our Aged," *Amer. J. of Nursing*, Vol. 64, no. 11 (1964) 78–82.

pear to be closely related to how he presents himself and to the social relationships he has established. All of these factors—and particularly social relationships—may be highly protective against personal neglect and a need for congregate facilities. Protective factors defend him from losing self-sufficiency and becoming more openly dependent upon others.

In sum, good adjustment in old age is characterized by relatively good physical and mental functional status in which the person evidences that good personal habits of physical, psychological, emotional, and social action have been well established or automatized; these in turn favored and were reflected by past good occupation and role acceptance and achievement, which themselves have usually stemmed from the existence of favorable early opportunities and good education. The persons who do best in old age appear to have had good endowment and favorable socioeconomic and personal circumstances that enabled them to develop and continue adaptive ways of life.

The Maladjusted Old Person

In contrast to the well-adjusted chronologically old are those we identify as maladjusted, who have "low morale," as evidenced by many complaints: physical, emotional, economic, domestic, personal, psychological. These may be elaborated and organized in special ways which we identify as psychiatric disorders or syndromes. But also, the maladjusted are persons who express distress and malcontent, and about whom there are complaints by the family and often by social community, as well. Also, as put by Meyer, the physician, in labeling these persons as being ill with this or that disorder, then signals his professional complaint about the patient, which he elaborates in medical terms, to denote what is wrong about the patient that needs, as he sees it, correction.

Poverty, physically or emotionally determined strong needs for support from relatives, friends, or other persons, especially when these decrease self-sufficiency and make for overt material need in addition to implicit and emotional dependency contribute to low morale, and to complaints of loneliness, boredom, mental distress, and pleas for aid. Contrary to general ideas about the importance of physical health, from the point of view of protection against low morale and maladjusted behavior, it is better to be rich and sick than poor and healthy. While this is undoubtedly related to the protective powers of material wealth, it probably also is so because relative affluence and social class are indices of education, prior occupation and habits, and ways of life that contribute to intrapsychic homeostasis and good social relations.

There is a wide range of maladjusted behavior in old persons. These difficulties are not always clearly part of recognized psychiatric disorders or syndromes. Their association with poverty, physical impairment, disability, and illness makes for their higher frequency in protective congregate residential settings of all kinds and poses great administrative, special medical, and comprehensive health care problems of such sites.

Minor Maladjustments

There is now a trend to categorize the predominant number of psychiatric disorders of the old as minor, in the sense that they do not primarily require psychiatric attention because they are related to physical or mental impairment, are social problems, in that they require long-term protective care or appear to fall into the category of psychoneurotic and character disorders modified or accentuated by aging and the problems of the old. Many of the minor maladjustments of the aged may in actuality be major disorders that are being relatively well handled by old persons, that are well tolerated by their social environment, or which are mistakenly diagnosed, but well treated, or which are ignored and, beneficially or otherwise, neglected.

Traditionally, psychoneuroses have been considered the minor, and psychoses the major, mental disturbances. However, an individual may be psychotic from the medical and psychiatric point of view and yet make a good, or at least passable, socioeconomic adjustment, whereas, on the other hand, many persons whose disorder is defined as psychoneurotic may undergo extreme suffering and may present great problems of disability requiring long-term care. Brought along into old age are many mental disorders which did not trouble the family or the community, or which were tolerated or even protected, because of special circumstances or the person's occupational adjustment or special skills. Psychoses, psychoneuroses, and behavior disorders of every variety may be revealed late in life when circumstances change or when attractive appearance, opportunity, skill, or position is lost. Also, an old person may be chronically or acutely ill or malnourished. Any one of these troubles, or a combination of them, adversely affects cerebral functioning. This adds to the problem of differentiating between what is to be considered a minor and what a major disorder. Symptomatic evidence of organic brain syndrome, associated memory loss and confusion seemingly related to cerebral arteriosclerosis or senile sclerosis may incorrectly be assumed to be a major disturbance of mentation premonitory of inevitable progression to disability, emotional dyscontrol, personality change, behavioral disorganization, and the loss of productive capacity and social adaptability. Strong emotion alone, however, may result in exaggeration of relatively minor defects of comprehension, orientation, memory, and judgment—and may lead to a mistaken impression about the severity of the disorder and to the belief that treatment is useless. With minimal brain damage, fear and anger may be so floridly elaborated as to descriptively appear to warrant the label "psychosis." Conversely, persons who appear to have moderate to severe brain damage, and whose behavior is grossly maladjusted, may improve on the establishment of good patient-doctor relationships in a properly supportive environmental setting or in response to relatively minor medical procedures, because the disorder is actually of the functional variety, expressed chiefly by way of exaggeration or exploitation of the impairment. In addition, mood-cyclic disorders or recurrent depressions themselves may be, in old persons, trouble-

some episodes which limit their adaptability, the nature of which they understand and to which they react as to any handicaps or losses of effectiveness. Insightfully or not, they simply respond with depression about the depression. For these reasons, it is better to talk of behavior disorders or disturbed behavior in older persons with or without vegetative nervous system signs and with or without chronic brain syndrome, rather than to attempt to make differentiation between psychoneuroses and psychoses.

Traditional diagnostic procedures, however, are not to be discarded as useless. The measures of depression, especially the presence or absence of vegetative signs—appetite, bowel, sleep disturbance, and diurnal variation of mood—are clues to therapy and of great psychotherapeutic importance. The cognitive defects found in depressive disorders which appear to be chiefly related to preoccupation, decreased attentiveness and poor concentration are not the same as those which reflect brain damage. Evidence pointing to severe brain damage is a grave prognostic sign. From a practical point of view evaluation should include (1) whether potentialities to harm self or others exist; (2) to what extent nuisance value is present; (3) the extent and quality of the patient's suffering; and (4) to what extent they may be modifiable.

In all cases, a psychotherapeutic trial, in addition to good nursing and medical care, is indicated. A detailed knowledge of the symptomatology is less important than data which point to the modifiability of those medical, environmental, or personality factors that influence and maintain the disorder. Of utmost importance is the fact that many disorders are indistinguishable from those seen in younger persons and respond equally well to the same treatment procedure, even when a relatively mild degree of organic brain syndrome is actually present.

There is a great difference in outlook, as well as need for treatment, of persons with severe degrees of brain syndrome, as compared to those with lesser degrees of the syndrome. The needs of persons who have organic brain syndrome with affective disorder also differ on the basis of the type and severity of the mood disturbance. Consequently, all persons who work with old people, whether in their own homes or residential care facilities, should have knowledge of how persons with no, little, or considerable amount of brain syndrome can be differentiated, and of how brain damage complicates or is complicated by mood disorders.

Brain Damage or Brain Dysfunction and Maladjustment

The sufferer, his family, or the social environment and the doctor usually agree that the patient's loss of resources for good adjustment is serious when there is brain damage.

Patients with moderate to severe brain damage may mistakenly be thought to be depressed if they are listless, lacking in initiative, and relatively meek and mild; in actuality, depression may be present in the moderately brain-damaged. Brain damage and its reflection brain syndrome, however, may not be faced by family or friends until it causes gross disturbances; it is not uncommon to be presented with a complaint that the patient has shown decreased memory for one year, when careful history-taking reveals five or more years of decline in functional status.

The declines in functional capacity related to cerebral damage or dysfunction can be measured in a variety of ways to help determine the degree of impairment or disability. Such measure can help in planning care and predicting the course of illness and longevity.

By impairment is meant the loss or limits of function, determined by the structural damage or biochemical disturbance. By disability is meant the decreased capacity of the impaired individual to function as a self-sufficient, sociable, and socially integrated person. Persons with a high degree of physical impairment may be minimally disabled; persons with a slight degree of physical impairment may be severely disabled because of the coexistence of brain damage, or because there are emotional and psychologically motivated exploitation or exaggeration of the impairment; not infrequently impairment of cerebral type is uti-

lized in this way and masquerades as more severe than the lesions dictate. Such states can be termed conditions of "excess disability."

Consequently, it is imperative that there be careful definition of the impairments, disabilities, or syndromes in terms of how they are measured if the treatment approaches are to make sense and be properly evaluated in respect to their value, and if the outlook for improvement or recovery is to be fairly evaluated.

ORGANIC BRAIN SYNDROME

This is the term now preferred for the psychiatric constellations of signs and symptoms that reflect brain dysfunction or brain damage. This term covers what was previously simply called "brain syndrome" and includes all the conditions at one time categorized as "senile dementia"—variously subdivided—and "cerebral arteriosclerosis with psychosis, type specified." It is also referred to by some, chiefly neurologists, as "organic mental syndrome." The World Health Organization has recently advocated calling it the "psychogeriatric syndrome" and agrees that every effort should be made to evaluate its degree of severity, when present.[194]

Organic brain syndrome may be *acute*, that is to say transitory and reversible—or at least partially so—because the cognitive disorder is a reflection of central nervous system dysfunction or, it may be *chronic*, because the brain is permanently and irreversibly damaged; the damage reflected by brain syndrome is a diffuse cortical loss of brain cells, often especially marked in both hippocampal areas. Many investigators are convinced that chronic organic brain syndrome is pathologically indistinguishable from Alzheimer's disease.

ORGANIC BRAIN SYNDROME, ACUTE

Acute organic brain syndrome is an acute confusional state which may reflect cerebral tissue dysfunction. Examples are infections with fever, tachycardia, or other effect which may affect the brain, alcohol or drug intoxication, or withdrawal; avitaminosis—as in the Wernicke-Korsakolf syndrome (thiamine chloride)—and pellagra (nicotinic acid); hepatic dysfunction, renal disease or electrolyte imbalance, especially when there is a low potassium level; poor support of cerebral nutrition, metabolism, circulation, or oxygenation, as in diabetic or hypoglycemic states, and with low blood pressure related to myocardial infarction, shock, or surgery; interference with circulation on account of stenosed carotid vessels, polycythemic vera, cerebral edema, or poor oxygenation with severe anemia, pulmonary disease, or cardiac failure. These causes of brain dysfunction are potentially reversible states and the brain recovers, if intervention is timely. Usually, the underlying disorder can be quickly identified by physical examination or laboratory study, and therapists must be alert to indications of fever, cardiac or pulmonary dysfunction, dehydration or electrolyte disturbance, as well as to a history of head trauma, drug ingestion, surgical operation, and the like. At times, a cryptogenic disease, such as carcinoma of a bronchus, or carcinoma of the colon (especially if cortisone-producing), or pancreatic insulin-producing tumors may result in cerebral dysfunction. Multiple drug use is a very frequent cause of acute organic brain syndrome. Medications for diabetes, hypertension, glaucoma, and Parkinsonism, the antihistaminics, antidepressants, or antipsychotic drugs are common offenders, as are digitalis, sedatives, hypnotics, and analgesics. Overmedication, errors made in self-medication, and often the simultaneous intake of medicines prescribed by a number of different physicians who know nothing of each other but are seen by the patient over the same period of time, make iatrogenic acute organic brain syndrome a common syndrome. Also, alcoholism is not uncommon in the old.

ORGANIC BRAIN SYNDROME, CHRONIC

Organic brain syndrome, chronic, is the irreversible disorder which reflects brain damage. It may follow repeated episodes of acute cerebral dysfunction or may be the result of insidiously progressive cerebral cellular loss—cell loss which undoubtedly occurs with aging in all persons and whose rate probably varies from time to time. It probably also varies from person to person and may increase in old age

either for reasons of genetic origin, or because of disease of early onset but late effect, or with the diseases in later life.

The organic brain syndrome is characterized by disorientation for time, place, person, and situation; memory loss, both remote and recent; inability to recall, learn, and to retain for recall general information of the simplest type, and inability to do calculation of the simplest type. In the American Psychiatric Association Diagnostic Manual of 1968 the syndrome is described as also including poor judgment and shallow, labile affect. These are, however, not invariably present and are quite difficult to measure, and do not appear to be valid reflectors of brain damage.

Organic brain syndrome, chronic, is not a psychosis or disease, it is an impairment which reflects damage to the brain; it is a deficit which can be compounded and complicated by emotion, so that disability may exceed the basic defect. Affect, thought content, and behavior may be seriously disturbed in the presence of or in reaction to this cognitive defect with variable symptomatology. It is of paramount importance to recognize its presence, so that the type of relationship that reassures, supports, and sustains such persons can be established.

The Measurement of Organic Brain Syndrome

There are a number of ways in which organic brain syndrome can be measured. Among the best is the Mental Status Questionnaire and the double simultaneous stimulation of face and hand (the Face-Hand Test). This has been validated and found to be reliable by the simultaneous examination of over 1200 institutionalized patients by psychologists, psychiatrists, and internists who followed the patient's course over a nine-year period.

The Mental Status Questionnaire is shown together with its relation to the areas tested in Table 37-2.

Scoring, recently modified on the basis of continuous clinical experience with non-institutionalized patients, is shown in Table 37-3.

TABLE 37–2.   **Mental Status Questionnaire—"Special Ten"***

QUESTION	PRESUMED TEST AREA
1. Where are we now?	Place
2. Where is this place (located)?	Place
3. What is today's date-day of month?	Time
4. What month is it?	Time
5. What year is it?	Time
6. How old are you?	Memory-recent or remote
7. What is your birthday?	Memory-recent or remote
8. What year were you born?	Memory-remote
9. Who is president of the U.S.?	General information-memory
10. Who was president before him?	General information-memory

* Modified from Mental Status by Kahn, Pollack and Goldfarb. Goldfarb, A. I. "The evaluation of geriatric patients following treatment," in P. H. Hoch and J. Zubin, eds., *Evaluation of Psychiatric Treatment*. New York: Grune & Stratton, 1964.

It should be noted that the Mental Status Questionnaire can do more than evaluate the degree of brain syndrome. It can provide information about behavioral patterns. Patterns of evasion, defensiveness, hostility, and confabulation are discernible when the Mental Status Questionnaire is properly annotated and interpretively reviewed. Misnaming of place or mistakes about time can yield considerable information about the emotional state and adaptational striving of the person.

THE FACE-HAND TEST

The Face-Hand Test is a brief, simple procedure of double, simultaneous stimulation, first described by Fink, Green and Bender as a diagnostic test for brain damage in which errors of response are reliably associated with brain damage in adults. The subject sits facing the examiner, hands resting on knees. He is touched or brushed simultaneously on one cheek and the dorsum of one hand, the order shown in Table 37–4.

A patient who learns to report correctly, consistently—verbally or by sign—where he is touched after the bilaterally symmetrical touching trials, Numbers 5 and 6 in the table, is presumed to be free of brain damage. Persons may not report the touch to a hand (extinction), may localize the hand touch to the cheek, the knee, or elsewhere (displacement), may point to the examiner's hand (projection), or outside himself in space (exomethesia). All of these are errors.

TABLE 37–3.   **Scoring of M.S.Q.**

NO. OF M.S.Q. ERRORS	PRESUMED DEGREE OF O.B.S.
0–2	Absent or Mild
3–5	Moderate
6–8	Moderate to Severe
9+	Severe
Nontestable*	Severe

* In the absence of deafness, language difficulty, or other impairment of rapport. Goldfarb, A. I. "The evaluation of geriatric patients following treatment," in P. H. Hoch and J. Zubin, eds., *Evaluation of Psychiatric Treatment*. New York: Grune & Stratton, 1964.

TABLE 37–4.   **Order of Stimulation Used in Face-Hand Test***

1. Right cheek—left hand
2. Left cheek—right hand
3. Right cheek—left hand
4. Left cheek—left hand
5. Right cheek—left cheek
6. Right hand—left hand
7. Right cheek—left hand
8. Left cheek—right hand
9. Right cheek—right hand
10. Left cheek—left hand

* As modified from Bender, Fink and Green by Kahn and Pollack. Goldfarb, A. I. "The evaluation of geriatric patients following treatment," in P. H. Hoch and J. Zubin, eds., *Evaluation of Psychiatric Treatment*. New York: Grune & Stratton, 1964.

The test is done first with the patient's eyes closed, and if he makes errors it is repeated with eyes open. It is of interest that when incorrect replies are made with eyes closed, there is only infrequently improvement with eyes open. The test is very highly correlated with brain syndrome as measured by the Mental Status Questionnaire, and as determined by psychiatric impression. It is somewhat less reliable in alert, well-educated persons, and persons with depression, agitation, or hypomania, than is the Mental Status Questionnaire. The fact that the patient may respond to this test correctly, although a cursorily done Mental Status Questionnaire suggests severe chronic brain syndrome, should influence the examiner toward hopefulness about affecting functional ability despite impairment. Decrease of any affective disorder present may reveal more resources and adaptability than the history or the present mental status otherwise suggests.

In addition to these simple measures, the patient may be asked to first spell simple words—cat, dog, let—forward and backward. This can usually be done when mild to moderate brain syndrome is present, but is difficult for the more severe. Ability to spell such words as tract, crowd, left, seven, or banana, is impaired with moderately severe and severe brain syndrome and may prove to be stumbling blocks for the mild to moderately impaired. The subtraction of seven from 100, the repetition of more than four digits backwards, the recall and recounting of short, simple anecdotes are usually beyond the capacity of persons with organic brain syndrome. However, difficulty with these tests may be indicative of depression of affect alone and may not signify organic brain syndrome if the M.S.Q., Face-Hand Test, and tests of spelling are well performed.

Measures of Decreased Functional Capacity

Measures of how well the person can conduct himself in *the activities of daily life* can be used as an adjunctive measure of organic brain syndrome. Ability to travel alone, to shop and cook; to do ordinary housework; to

bathe oneself; dress, undress, and wash independently; get about on foot or by wheel chair unassisted; transfer from bed to chair alone; be continent of bowel and bladder, and tend to one's toilet needs is one such list of routine daily activities. By this list, the incontinent and bedfast are considered severely impaired, the nonambulatory are often moderately to severely functionally impaired, those who can dress, undress, and wash may be moderately impaired, but those who can bathe, shop, and cook are usually mildly to moderately impaired, while those who can travel alone probably have no or only minimal mental impairment.

"Functional" versus "Organic" Disorder

As noted, many tests of cognitive functioning that are part of the psychiatric mental status actually measure deficiencies in memory, abstraction, attention, concentration, that accompany or are part of depressive syndromes. Thus, difficulty in doing serial seven abstractions, in attending to, recalling, and repeating a short story, in repeating digits forward and backward, or in associating freely to specific words, are not measures which necessarily reflect brain damage.

Depression, Mistaken for Organic Brain Syndrome

The discussion of organic brain syndrome is somewhat detailed because in the heterogeneous group of old persons who have no obvious "major" maladaptive process are not only those with problems related to social, economic, and health losses, but also many whose difficulties are related to loss of mentational capacity.

It is of great importance to know whether the mentally ill person who appears to be bewildered, puzzled, indecisive, helpless, does or does not have organic brain syndrome, and to what degree. This can usually be determined at once, in the first interview, although psychiatrists unfamiliar with the patterns of organic brain syndrome may need a longer "period of observation" which should be, actually a period of physically, mentally, and emotionally supportive treatment.

In the purely functional disorders, there is no true confusion—there is no disorientation—although memory and cognitive capacity may be below par along with attention, concentration, initiative, and motivation to respond, learn, and perform well. A functional disorder in the presence of measurable organic brain syndrome generally indicates that the degree of organic brain syndrome may test as more severe than its actuality. Affective disorder, paranoid or other schizophrenic reactions with organic brain syndrome are usually as responsive to treatment as when there is no organic brain syndrome. It is important to recognize that cognitive defects may be present with depression but depression does not explain disorientation or, in the ambulatory, physically well patient, incontinence. Attributing diagnosis of an entity which can be termed "pseudodementia" it constitutes a mistake in diagnosis.

Organic Brain Syndrome

Organic brain syndrome may begin with decreased recent memory and inability to learn, and then, rapidly or slowly, go on to include deficits of remote memory which are fully as great. It is in the early, developing phase that confabulation is most obvious. It seems true, however, that confabulation is evidenced more by some types of persons than others. In many, it appears to be a masking from the self, as well as from others, of the deficits, the acknowledgment of which is impossible in the same sense that the loss of a loved one cannot initially be believed. A part of the self has gone, has been taken away; this is grievous and must be mourned, but is first greeted with disbelief, later with anger, still later dealt with constructively piecemeal, and perhaps finally accepted, in that preoccupation and concern with the defect is relinquished and, if adequate assets remain, attention and engagement in the pursuits possible are more wholeheartedly resumed.

As shown in Table 37–5, the various ways of assessing intellectual, that is to say, cogni-

tive, defects, performed by well-trained and experienced clinicians, are generally concordant, and these measures do appear to be directly related to brain damage as assessed by post mortem, course of illness, and longevity, the electro encephalogram, pneumoencephalogram, and arteriogram. In the recent past, based chiefly on Rothschild's data,[150] it has been stated that the degree of organic brain syndrome is not directly related to brain damage, gross or microscopic. However, when the clinically determined intellectual deficits of the cases cited by Rothschild are compared to the pathologic findings, there is concordance. When the degree of disturbance of overt behavioral reaction is compared to pathology, then concordance is absent. In short, brain damage is related to cognitive defect, but not to disturbance of mood, thought content, and overt behavior. This is in keeping with the evaluation and longitudinal follow-up of the large series of cases reported by Roth, Kay,[102,103] Norris and Post, and with the clinical assessments and follow-up studies of Goldfarb, Kahn, Fisch, and Gerber.[80] In all these studies, severe cognitive defects were predictive of poor outlook, shortened life, and evidence of damage to the brain.

In persons with organic brain syndrome, mood or content disorder may be absent. When it is present, it may be inversely related in severity to the measurable degree of organic mental syndrome: "It takes brains," to elaborate psychotic or psychoneurotic behavior. The absence of mood or content disorder is not informative of the degree of brain syndrome. The degree of overt behavior disturbance, however, can be severe with any degree of organic mental syndrome; when organicity is severe, the person may be anything from quiet and co-operative to violently excited in a disorganized, restless, uncontrollable way.

It may at times be difficult to do satisfactory testing. When one measure is of questionable validity, others may be more helpful. It is wise, in general, to make a number of different assessments, so as to clarify the needs of the patient and to make more accurate evalua-

TABLE 37–5.   The Expected Relationship of Special Characteristics of the Aged

CHARACTERISTIC	DEGREE OF DEFECT				
Intellectual Deficit, clinical	None	0–to Mild	Mild to Moderate	Moderate to Severe	Severe
Mental Status Questionnaire No. of errors	0	0–2	3–5	6–8	9+
Face Hand Test Errors					
eyes closed	0	0	0–2	2–4	4
eyes open	0	0	0	1–3	4
Activities of Daily Life (self-sufficiency)	Good	Good	Fair	Poor	Very poor
Mood Disturbance	0–4+	0–4+	0–3+	0–1+	0
Thinking Disorder	0–4+	0–4+	0–2+	0–1+	0
Behavior Disorder Overt	0–4+	0–4+	1+–4+	2+–4+	2+–4+
Incontinence					
Bladder	0	0	0–1+	0–2+	1+–4+
Bowel	0	0	0	0–2+	1+–4+
Electroencephalogram Amount of slow waves	Normal	Normal to Minimal Abnormality	Normal to Minimal Abnormality	Diffuse Abnormality	Normal or Diffuse Abnormality
Ventricular (Angiogram or P.E.G.)	Normal	Normal	Moderate Dilitation	Moderate to Considerable Increase	Great Enlargement
Air Over Cortex (P.E.G.)	None	None	Slight Amount	Slight to Considerable Amount	Slight to Considerable Amount
Average Brain Weight, Grams*	1300	1221	1221	1153	1025
Life Expectancy (for age)	Normal	Normal	Normal	Usually Decreased	Decreased

* Calculated from the post mortem data of D. Rothschild by Goldfarb and Jahn.

tions of the probable outcome. Functional disorders—the affective or content disturbance—should be treated vigorously even when brain syndrome is present. Drugs, psychotherapy, even electroshock therapy may be given, as in younger persons with similar conditions. The physical state of the brain reflected by organic brain syndrome is taken into account when pharmacotherapy is used, since it may require special caution, and if EST is given, special attention is paid to the premedication, anesthesia, curarization, oxygen needs, and to comfort in the recovery periods, not only as a protection of life and physical integrity, but also to avoid disturbances that can lead to acute organic brain syndrome. The advent of acute organic brain syndrome may lead to excess enthusiasm in treatment if it is mistaken for worsening of the functional disorder. In the group which shows moderately severe to severe organic signs, the general medical condition must be very carefully investigated and meticulous attention to symptomatic as well as specific medical care is required while the presence of fear, anger, and its elaborations are taken into account; comprehensive care should be provided with psychiatric "know-how."

OPERATIONAL DEFINITION OF CHRONIC BRAIN SYNDROME

Organic brain syndrome, chronic, can be defined as that point at which the deficit in function of a person with brain damage emerges as disruptive of the personality for the individual, for society, or both. It probably emerges first as a loss of resources, to which the person reacts or which he attempts to integrate into his way of life; at a later point of progression, it becomes manifest as "maladjustment." Our tests appear to be "positive" at this point.

The feelings of helplessness that follow or are associated with the decreased ability to cope with life's problems is a complex component of decreased feelings of worth, loss of self-confidence, loss of the sense that one can achieve pleasures, and the loss of sense of purpose. This may be felt as a sense of failure compounded by humiliation or shame because of poor performance, as well as by guilt for failure to perform as one should. This is followed by fear and anger, further complicated by guilty fear and fear of retaliation. The helplessness and emergency emotion are then generally revealed by complaints of types and patterns determined by the person's value systems and concept of social responsibilities and responses.

The Patterns of Complaints

Chronologically old persons commonly referred to the psychiatrist are complaining, quarrelsome, restless, negativistic, depressed, agitated, or angry; some may be regarded as threatening on a verbal or physical level, suicidal, or assaultive. Somatic complaints and paranoid ideas are common, and suicidal attempts are not infrequent. Less frequently than is popularly believed, sexual behavior unacceptable to the community is the reason for referral. This may vary from exhibitionism to not unreasonable desires to remarry. Not uncommon are complaints that a chronologically old husband is overly assertive sexually; this is often joined by complaints that he accuses his wife of disloyalty and infidelity. Complaints about impotence are also common, as is advice sought about how to handle a rejecting mate who says about sex, "You [or we] or I am too old for that now."

Quiet, subjective suffering on the part of older persons is often missed or neglected, even as it is in younger ones. Psychoneurotic behavior of all kinds is found in aged persons; dramatization, exploitation, and aggravation of disability or weakness are common, and obsessional characteristics are frequently troublesome. Among somatic expressions of emotional distress commonly encountered are headaches and vertigo, constipation, anorexia, insomnia of various types, including early morning waking—these may be the sole manners in which the presence of an actually severe depressive reaction is communicated. A sense of heat in or burning of the skin, intermittent sweats, flushing, and fatigability are frequent complaints. Subjective depression with guilt, self-depreciation, hostile and paranoid thoughts are frequent open complaints. Frank anxiety does occur, but it is far less openly than covertly expressed. The most common reason for referral in shelters for the aged appears to be behavior which has "nuisance" value; noisiness, querulousness, physical complaining, and somatic preoccupation which is unresponsive to the usual medical and nursing care available, and clinging, demanding, or hostile behavior. These seemingly unrelated and heterogeneous complaints in the individual can be understood as complaints of a frightened or angry person whose feelings of helplessness have led to an adaptive maneuver—of a person's search for aid, dependency striving, or attempts to establish personal relationships promissory of protection, care, and security. The evolution of such patterns and their relation to the losses that occur with aging were suggested in Figure 37–1.

The host of complaints about mood, physical functioning, and the behavior of others to oneself, their variability in persons who appear to suffer from the same basic disorder, and their shift, sometimes with great rapidity even in the same persons, with time, circumstances and social environment, become more easily understood if they are listed under a number of headings. They are *apathy, pseudoanhedonia, somatization, display of helplessness, depression,* either relatively pure, or with psychomotor retardation or agitation, *elated* (manic) *states, paranoid states, exploitive-manipulative behavior,* and *coercive behavior.* These patterns may overlap, coexist, occur in sequence or clusters. The patterns alone or in combination, from the adaptational point of view, can be regarded as motivated attempts at problem-solving. Each of the patterns as a whole, and its parts, can be described— "understood"—in psychodynamic terms. That is, the patterns can be regarded as symptoms which symbolize the patient's problems and wishes, justify his search for aid or emotional support, are of a type that he believes can and will earn the kind of care desired, and are also extrapunitive, as though to punish a selected social target for neglect and into action. This is illustrated in Figure 37–2. These common patterns, then, can be discerned to contain all of the intrapsychic elements of the so-called hysterical reaction. They are listed in an order which, at least roughly, is related to the degree in which they appear to be influenced by the emergency emotions, fear and anger. The influence and amount of fear decrease as one moves from apathy to depression, where the influence of degree of anger present is quite large and then tends to increase as the patterns tend to change or include depression, elation, paranoid trends, and conditions that are more clearly manipulative or coercive. These common patterns, obviously, cut across formal nosologic-diagnostic lines. This is because individuals apparently differ first in the genetic predisposition to elaborate emotion pathophysiologically. Some persons appear to have recurrent or cyclic pathophysiologic events which are reflected by mood or behavior changes that tend to be adaptationally elaborated, as here described. In them, the intrapsychic determinants of the pattern appear to give rise to physiologic changes which then reinforce the behavioral disorder. In others, the pathophysiologic changes are akin to the hormonal metabolic changes of the hypertensive or the diabetic and act as causes for the elaboration and emergence of the adaptive syndromes.

These patterns are briefly defined and discussed below.

APATHY

Apathetic patients are listless, enervated, without initiative or spirit; behavior is predictable and stereotyped. They complain of weakness, lethargy, poverty of feeling, loss of interest and initiative. They tend to be withdrawn, slow in speech and movement, to remain seated quietly, or to retreat to bed, usually assuming the same spot and the same posture. Conversation is entered into reluctantly. Problems are denied. Pressure to speak or to take part in activity may receive token compliance followed by protests and possibly angry resistance. Apathetic states in which the individual withdraws are common and such patients are frequently referred to as "regressed."

As used at present, the term "regression" appears to be more a lay blanket than a scientific concept. Even when used to denote one of several concepts—as return to a prior level of psychosexual development and libidinal cathexis, as abandonment of developed or acquired ego functions, or as the use of early developed defenses against anxiety—it lacks

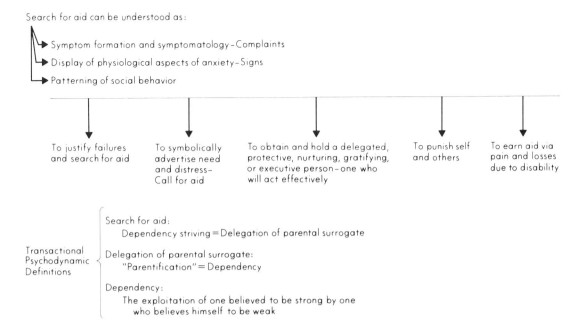

Figure 37–2.   Motivational components of "the search for aid."

precision unless properly qualified. The lay use of the term to describe and explain away withdrawal, sullen or negativistic behavior, and incontinence or slovenliness of complex etiology, as a return to the pleasures of infancy, is unwarranted. This is true even when brain damage complicates the behavior.

The concept of regression can possibly be helpful when it is clearly defined to mean that the aged patient may make use of a developing deficit, such as that related to brain damage, as a means of protest, or to signal distress, despair, or helplessness, and that the defect or disorder may become integrated with the pattern of behavior. The human tendency to integrate symptoms of physical illness and impairment into the personality as a mode of communication and to solve an interpersonal conflict is actually either repair, growth, compensatory action, or an attempt at problem-solving by fight or withdrawal—alone or in combination—its efficiency or adaptive value and its details should not be obscured by a blanket term.

Weinberg[191] has suggested that patients with decreasing ability to contend with the world withdraw as a defensive maneuver to avoid being overwhelmed. More recently, in analogy to computer failure, Dovenmuehle[48] has spoken about "information overload" and patients' attempts to avoid this. Also, the theory of disengagement advanced by Cummings and Henry[45] is a similar concept envisioning that aging persons tend to relinquish their involvement, or "engagement" with their social world, while simultaneously society removes itself from them in a transactional process.

Apathy would seem to be the caricature of such "natural, acceptable" behavior—however, recognizing apathy as an adaptive, signaling maneuver adds a dimension which provides a clue to therapy. In the case of Mrs. B., the apathetic state masked a depression. She mourned the death of her eldest son, was angry at his son—her grandson—for "deserting her" and at her younger son for not meeting her emotional expectations. Her history was one of mood-cyclic disorder. The withdrawn, "apathetic," listless behavior is part of a search for assistance by the suffering patient.

She behaves as though she could bring back a dead son, change her grandson, improve her remaining son, so that he can replace the lost one, by signaling her grief in an uncomplaining, disarming, yet emphatic and forceful way, while suffering the disadvantage and pain of her helplessness and at the same time pursuing her less admired son by being burdensome, and in this way pressing him to do better—for and with her. In this, like all of the patterns of search for aid described, apathy as a symptom complex has the characteristics of the hysterical neurosis, whether or not it is itself part of the so-called psychotic condition.

Pseudo-Anhedonia

The pseudo-anhedonic patient behaves and talks as if to say, "I have no feeling. Nothing matters. Do what you will, and do what you will to me. Nothing can bother me any more; you can't hurt me, you can't please me, nothing matters." That the anhedonic protest is not real is evidenced by the patient's insistence on being "left alone"—not pressed or pushed into activities—by his reluctance to follow instruction and the tendency to skillfully resist, and explain away the value of efforts to help him. As with apathy, the behavior as a symptom is punitive, self-punitive, symbolic, justifies its own existence, and "earns" sympathy.

Display of Helplessness

A third pattern is display of helplessness. The patient points to his weakness, his ineptitude, his "anxiety," or his mental impairment. Physical impairment is exploited, exaggerated, illness is exacerbated by ill-advised behavior and self-neglect. The somatic concomitants of fear and anger are experienced as further frightening, and frustrating, and enraging, and are paraded, pointed to, demonstrated, queried about. For example, Mrs. E., a seventy-six-year-old widow complains of palpitations, of discomfort in the left shoulder and midspine, of weakness, and of intermittent tingling of the fingers. She holds herself tensely, the right shoulder much higher than the left, has labile blood pressure with a diastolic that never exceeds 98 m.hg., but has intermittent tachycardia without irregularity. She fears to live alone and has a companion for as many hours a day as she can afford. She feels alone, neglected, visits the one child who has room for her as often as possible, and stays "as long as I can feel welcome." She is sure she has a serious illness which affects her

spine and her heart, that she should not exert herself, cannot tolerate social activity, cannot lead a normal life. This pattern of invalidism and complaining has persisted for eleven years. It began two years after the loss of her husband, grew slowly worse, and was accentuated on the death of a son. She "tried" but left four physicians. She now visits her psychiatrist monthly and appears to feel gratified by his monitoring of her pulse, blood pressure, and his noncommittal contribution of mild sedative medication.

Subjective distress is denied by Mrs. E. A concomitant or strong emotion has become her obsessive rumination and complaint.

Similarly, Mrs. U. complained about inability to swallow and ascribed all of her personal problems to this somatic difficulty. Other patients may complain of shortness of breath, a weak feeling in the chest, tingling in the fingers and toes, giddiness or sinking feelings, abdominal (frequently hypochondriacal) pain, pain in the back, in the thigh, down the leg, or in the arm. These appear to be preferred communications about concomitants of fear or anger, which emotions the patient ignores or fails to report.

Somatization

With somatization the patient appeals for aid on the basis of bodily disease, discomfort, or impairment for which no adequate nonpsychiatric medical basis can be found. Frequently, complaints of pain, impairment, or disability are related to actual sensory or motor losses, and systemic or organ decline. Among these are osteo- or rheumatoid arthritis, cardiac malfunction and angina pectoris, emphysema, gall bladder disease, hiatus hernia, osteoporosis with vertebral collapse, herniated nucleus polyposus, and meralgia paresthetica. But, with time, it becomes obvious that despite the importance of the somatic changes present, there is, as in display of helplessness, exploitation, aggravation, and sometimes exacerbation of an underlying structural disorder because of the fear or anger of the patient. Included under somatization may be the seemingly fear-free insistence that the whole problem is the pain in the back, arm, or chest. Weakness of extremities, of sight, hearing, or brain function may be paraded as disabling in the absence of any impairment. The difference from display of helplessness is that it is not always the concomitants of fear, anger, or impairment that are displayed but there is seeming displacement of concern to bodily functions and the use of impairment to explain and account for disability to oneself without clear expression of feelings of helplessness.

HYPOCHONDRIASIS

A fifth pattern is hypochondriasis. Here, the motor pain or harmless symptom, or lesion visible or palpable only to the patient, is seized upon as evidence of life-threatening disease or disorder. The wart or harmless sebaceous cyst becomes, in the mind's eye, a cancer. Similarly, rectal pain or emotionally caused constipation is interpreted as proof of the presence of malignancy, urinary frequency is interpreted as related to intractable diabetes or to probably malignant prostatic hypertrophy. Headache, to the sufferer, presages brain tumor. Also common, and sometimes unfortunately shared by physicians, is the patient's conviction the cognitive defects which go along with depression of affect are caused by, and proof of, senility, or cerebral arteriosclerosis, and impending social death.

DEPRESSION

In depressive states, there is usually a subjective and reported sense of low spirits, "depression," and at times of actual sadness. There is inertia, loss of interest, loss of purposivity and motivation to act; there is preoccupation with distress and malaise, and with somatic symptoms, such as heaviness in the chest, dry mouth, bad taste; attention is decreased, thinking may be slow and labored, as may movements, or there may be racing, anxious thoughts and motor agitation. There are also one or more of the other patterns described together with subjectively experienced and reported feelings of despair, hopelessness, loneliness, boredom, feelings of being neglected, abandoned, unwanted; a lowering of mood. In predisposed persons, this pattern

may have been preceded by, although it is usually considered to be followed by and come to include, specific vegetative signs. These are anorexia or bulimia, constipation or diarrhea, a longing for sleep, prompt falling asleep at night followed by insomnia of premature or early morning waking type with depressive rumination, diurnal variation of mood—the worst being in the morning. When the vegetative signs, diurnal variation of mood, and cognitive signs of depressive affect are present, the condition is usually labeled as psychotic. History of prior attacks is almost always elicitable (although many may have masqueraded as physical illness, such as arthritis, or gall bladder trouble, or spastic colitis), and in many such persons there is a clear history of mood-cyclic disorder, which may or may not have been previously recognized and/or treated.

PARANOID IDEATION OR BEHAVIOR

Paranoid ideation or behavior is common with depression of any severity, with or without the genetic predisposition to the so-called psychotic varieties, but may also be seen in relatively "pure culture." It may be the emergence in old age, of a schizophrenic disorder previously subclinical in its manifestations. The patient is openly or covertly angry, is convinced he has been, is, or will be taken advantage of, has been maltreated, or is threatened and vulnerable; he feels he is referred to, talked about, avoided, rejected, and neglected. Frequently, complaints of boredom and loneliness may mask paranoid trends; they are often developed as more or less subtle accusations about spouses, children, relatives, neighbors, or society. At times the paranoid nature of complaints is blatant, yet not truly schizophrenic, but rather the florid elaborations of fear and anger in a patient whose discriminatory capacity has been reduced by brain damage—the loss of cerebral neurons in appreciable degree.

Mr. K., a sixty-nine-year-old man, was disoriented for time and place although he masked it well; he failed to recall appointments, promised and incurred obligations. He was forgetful at home about lights, the stove, appliances, doorlocks, and misplaced money and objects. He questioned repetitiously about minor matters, and rationalized in a confabulatory way about his behavior. This led to verbal explosions on the part of his wife. These appeared to offend, hurt, and finally to anger him, and led to sharp outbursts on his part about her nagging, often culminating in statements that perhaps they should separate for a while. Mr. K. then began to state with apparent conviction, and maintained for several hours at a time, that Mrs. K. was not his wife but an impostor, a member of his wife's family who was attempting to mislead and misinform him. Shortly after such an outburst, during which he asked Mrs. K. to leave, I saw them together in my office. She asked him why he treated her in that way. At first, he denied doing so, then, "You acted like I was a stranger," he said, blushing and smiling in an embarrassed way. "So I acted like you're a stranger. I thought you were one of them" (her family, whom he dislikes). "And now," said she, "you recognize me as your wife of forty years?" "Yes," he replied with a laugh. After a pause he went on to say: "You see, I'm a man. I want to be the man in the family. If you treat me like we aren't . . . like I'm not . . . then I feel depressed." "Did I ever . . ." she asked. "No," he interrupted her and said with remarkable yet truthful inconsistency, "I never let you."

In the presence of mental deficit, which decreases his capacity to perform routine daily tasks, and which lowers his self-esteem, erodes his confidence, leaves him feeling lost, alone, and in need of a helpful wife, this man appears to pay little attention to, or tries to forget his difficulties. When, as he sees it, they are harshly pointed out to him by his wife, he feels doubly distressed. He is a man in need, without the helper he had believed was there, and more, she has changed into the opposite, a critic, a demanding person, an impatient female who is the converse of friend, ally, intimate, reassurer, or supporter. This stranger must be driven away, so that the space she occupies can once more be filled by his wife.

Mr. K. demonstrates what has been described as the "illusion of doubles" described by Capgras and Reboul-Lachaux in 1923.[38] As later outlined by Todd[181] in "Capgras' syndrome" the identity of a person well known to the patient is challenged with the statement that a double has replaced the original.[186] Vie later expanded ideas about the syndrome by calling attention to the "illusion of positive doubles" in which there is an affirmation of imaginary resemblance leading to false recognition, in contrast to the illusion of negative doubles where imaginary differences lead to negation of identity. The perception of "imaginary differences" and "imaginary resemblances" is frequent in the aged and can be understood as based upon their subjective distress, their unhappiness with an existing relationship, their desire to change it, and their attempts to signal their needs to alter the transactions and to find in others what is now lacking in the people about them. In this, we see an elaboration of the ideas expressed by Hughlings-Jackson in 1886,[89] when he spoke of the man with a damaged brain who called his nurse by the name of his wife. He ascribed the failure to recognize the nurse to organically determined decrease in discriminatory capacity (dissolution); he attributed the mistaken identification to elaborations by the intact brain (evolution) based on experientially determined aspects of personality.[89] Past experience, response to the present situation, and hopes or expectations, all contribute to the patterning of behavior.

Exploitive-Manipulative Behavior

Exploitive-manipulative behavior is frequently regarded as "normal," as part of "a way of life." Nevertheless, it is often a seemingly new symptomatic pattern which is akin to, often a component, a precursor, or sequel of a clear-cut depressive disorder.

Coercive Behavior

Coercive behavior is most easily epitomized by the often openly, but sometimes disguisedly stated, "Love me; if you won't love me I'll kill myself." It is manifested in innumerable and at times highly complex ways. A common form is that of the dominating, controlling person whose coercive behavior is masked as parental or marital concern or filial devotion. It may be obvious, as in confrontational antisocial dependency when the person states that he is simply taking by force what should have been freely given, although its emotional core and basis may be forgotten because of the anger it provokes in the social community. At times, coercive behavior becomes clearly homicidal. It is as though the patient said, "On second thought, if you don't love me I won't kill myself, I'll kill you, and then maybe also myself." For example, a man hospitalized for help because of drug abuse pleaded he was not receiving adequate care. While shaving, he was pressed by a nurse to go out on a unit walk, despite his remonstrances that he was not sufficiently well. He turned on her, razor in hand, and said, "Leave me alone or I'll cut my wrists. No. I think I'll cut your throat." More subtle were his refusals to take medicine, to eat, to care for himself hygienically unless he "could gain the proper co-operation of the staff to ease him by medicines."

Coercive, exploitive, paranoid, and complexly elaborated depressive reactions are only seen when brain syndrome is mild to moderate. With moderately severe brain syndrome, apathy, pseudo-anhedonia, and display of helplessness are seen, but even these become less clearly elaborated as severity increases. With severe organic syndromes, fear and anger tend to disorganize behavior or to lead to immobilization. The degree of brain syndrome, however, should not be determined by qualitative evaluation of behavior and never by the quantitative level of disturbed or disturbing behavior, except "paradoxically"—i.e., the more complexly elaborated and seeming severely "psychotic" the disturbance of mood or thought content, the more likely it is that the organic mental severity is of relatively slight degree.

Treatment, Care, and Management

The goals of psychiatric therapy are to decrease the complaints of the patient by increasing comfort, and productivity in work, within the limits of the person's past capacities and current limitations, restore sociability and social integration, and to restore the capacity for self-provision of pleasure to the greatest degree possible.

Review of Figure 37–1 suggests that we can approach treatment, care, and prevention from the viewpoint of etiology, both early and late, by seeking assets to replace, substitute, or compensate for loss; by decreasing challenges to mastery; by dealing with the subjective state called "helplessness"; and by treating the emergency emotions and the behavior to which these lead.

It is not required, however, that a specific etiologic factor or group of factors be determined for rational and definitive treatment. This is fortunate because identification of the necessary factor may be difficult or impossible at this time.

The events of infancy or childhood that decrease or distort resources for personal comfort and social adaptation or genetic factors may be factors of great importance in the evolution and maintenance of many of the maladjusted patterns in the aged. Such factors can be subsumed under what Berezin[13] points to as "the timelessness of the unconscious." They are theoretically modifiable by psychodynamically oriented psychotherapy whether reconstructive (psychoanalytic) or brief. But, few old persons may have the physical strength and time to avail themselves of such benefits, should they be available. Even when such factors are strongly presumed present, expediency may require search for and attention to other factors, the modification of which will make a beneficial difference.

From this point of view, the decrease in self-assertion that can be traced to enculturation "at the mother's knee" may be the necessary but not sufficient factor contributory to accessions of anger seen in an old person who otherwise cannot override the psychological inhibitions which seriously limit his activity for relief of tension from biologic or acquired needs. Therefore, modification of circumstances to eliminate the contributory factors may yield much improvement.

Thus, it may be more expedient to decrease challenges that create difficulties or social obstructions to the realization of goals desired than to re-educate the patient emotionally. This is akin to saying what was once said about effective treatment of certain psychosomatic disorders; that the therapist was effective when he helped the patient to achieve a satisfactory marriage—satisfactory in that the troubled patient found a parentally supportive mate. Much success in psychotherapy, although otherwise rationalized, may be achieved in these "incidental" ways. In fact, the psychiatrist, as noted below, may become the supportive figure with cost of little time and effort.

Also, unless "a complete physician" he will do well to work as part of a team which includes an internist and a neurologist to assist in the search for factors which are most easily dealt with to the benefit of the patient. Examples are awareness of effect of antihypertensive medication upon catecholamines and of the effect of most medical conditions upon cerebral functioning. Moreover, because psychological and emotional changes may be most easily brought about through the use of special services other than psychiatric, they are themselves vehicles for psychotherapy; therefore, the psychiatrist must be ready and able to work with others. For the sake of brevity, the various components are illustrated and the type of treatment indicated is charted. The social and material supports available to the patient have bearing on the provision of treatment.

Good basic services are essential before special programs and psychiatric skills can be brought to bear meaningfully on the patient's problems. Where the patient lives, with whom, and under what conditions, is of considerable importance in dealing with his specific problems. Many old persons live in their own homes. Others live in congregate settings for reasons of health, finances, or because of housing problems.

Own Home

Old people in their own homes include a large number of persons who have problems of pre- and post-retirement for which they may need little more than skilled counseling.

There may be psychological and emotional complications of financial, housing, social, and domestic problems.

Old persons in their own homes who accept referral or who themselves call on a psychiatrist for help can usually be managed and helped with as little, or as much, family involvement as younger individuals.

A large number of old persons, however, are brought by family or friends or have psychiatric consultation or aid thrust upon them by personnel of an agency or residential setting. Under such conditions, the question often arises as to "who is the patient": The referred and the referrers alike appear to be suffering and treatment procedures must often be flexibly and tactfully moulded to suit. At times, a spouse or child of the old person needs treatment and can accept it only in the guise of conversation about treatment of the other, or because of its value to the elderly "patient." Frequently, one encounters *folie à deux*, in which both husband and wife share paranoid trends and depression, and one or both has organic brain syndrome as well. Here, both must usually be treated, each with the necessary medication, and conversation either sequentially in the same "hour" or together. It is usually wise to see first one, then the other, and then—even if briefly—both together, at which time interchange between them may offer valuable clues to therapy needed, as well as an occasion to provide opportunities for controlled ventilation of each, and support and reassurance to both.

Work with family members may be the most important aspect of treatment. For example, the old person may desire to live—however unrealistic this may be—with a selected child as a solution to the health, housing, or financial problem. The available child, although capable and willing, does not suit the parent, who may express this verbally or nonverbally. Another problem is a variance of views as to how the problem of the parent should be resolved. These examples illustrate that parent-child conflicts, sibling rivalry, and interfamilial processes may make the older person the focus of a family fight.

Many social agencies are helpful to old per-

TABLE 37–6.   **Components of Disorder and Psychiatric Treatment Approaches***

COMPONENT	ILLUSTRATIVE EXAMPLE	TREATMENT APPROACH OR METHOD OF PSYCHIATRIC VALUE
Multiple Causes		
(a) Remote (early)	(a) 1. Genetic factors 2. Familial, educational, and cultural influences 3. Occupational effects 4. Diseases	(a) Psychoanalytic, reconstructive or distributive analysis for recognition and correction of genetically-dynamically caused disorders, psychotherapy, counsel, guidance

(b) Recent (in old age)	(b) 1. Physical—disease, accidents, aging
	2. Mental—psychological brain syndrome
	   acute mild
	   chronic moderate
	   severe
	   Emotional concomitants of structural change
	3. Social and economic factors
		(b) Disease prevention
		Accident prevention
		Avoidance of smoking, air and water pollution
		Specific and symptomatic treatment of disease
		
		In youth and middle life, development or reinforcement of good habits of psychological, emotional and social adjustment
		Preparation for change of role, status, or income

Loss of Resources for Action and Protection	(a) 1. Temperament Depressive diathesis 2. Decreased self-assertion "Psychologic inhibition" (Decreased capacity for sexual activity and pleasure) "Psychotic" or "neurotic," traits or specific character, psychophysiologic, or psychiatric disorders 3. "Way of life," well established mechanisms of psychological and emotional reaction	1. Pharmacotherapy or physical therapy for shift in "homeostatic level" 2. & 3. Psychotherapy of an "insight developing," "character changing" type
	(b) Cardiovascular-renal disease: angina, failure, etc. Sensory disturbances Musculoskeletal impairments	(b) Medical treatment: nursing aids Surgical corrections Prostheses, spectacles, hearing aids, dentures, artificial limbs

TABLE 37–6.   (*cont'd.*)

COMPONENT	ILLUSTRATIVE EXAMPLE	TREATMENT APPROACH OR METHOD OF PSYCHIATRIC VALUE
	Prostatism Cystocele Brain syndrome, acute or chronic Reactions to losses Neuro-endocrine (homeostatic) impairment Environmental demands Loss of family, friends Change of status, of role Loss of prestige Decreased income	Psychiatric treatment Environmental changes Clubs, organizations Social service aids Community organization toward occupation and social use of aged Social Security; Medicare, Medicaid, etc.
Decreased Capacity for Mastery	Decreased ability: to relieve tensions of biologic or acquired origin to obtain gratification to experience pleasure based on successful action or thought	See above Medical assistance with regard to bowel and bladder function, etc. Information about sex Social service aid in reaching groups, occupational and recreational facilities Educational programs
Feelings of Helplessness as evidenced by: Fall in self-esteem, and in self-confidence Loss of purpose and sense of identity	"I can't do . . ." (self-confidence) "I am no good" (self-esteem) "I have no role, use . . ." (sense of purpose; loss of identity) "I will fail" (am failing) "How humiliating . . ." "I am ashamed of myself" "What is the meaning of it all?" "What good am I?"	Decrease of feeling of helplessness by way of above and below
(*a*) Fear and Anger (and subsequent guilt; fear of retaliation; depression of mood, with physical shift and vegetative signs in the predisposed) (*b*) Affective Disorder	Signs of emergency emotion immobilization in thought or action Disorganization of thought or action Agitation or retardation Depression or elation	Pharmacologic treatment Electroshock treatment Treatment via relationship: dyadic or group

TABLE 37–6. (*cont'd.*)

COMPONENT	ILLUSTRATIVE EXAMPLE	TREATMENT APPROACH OR METHOD OF PSYCHIATRIC VALUE
Search for Aid A patterning of signs and "symptoms" consistent with the person's experience and acceptable to him as likely to succeed in the actual or fantasied milieu that he perceives	Patterns of sign and symptom display which symbolize: "I hurt" "I'm bored" "I'm lonely" "I'm blue," i.e., I want him (her, my parent, daughter, husband) to care for me as I was cared for by my father (brother, mother, husband, this daughter, etc.) in the past "I'll love you, therefore you must love and help me" "I need a friend (lover, confidante, husband, wife, parent, child, boss, assistant, secretary, companion) to understand, love, fulfill, work with, join with, play along with, enjoy things with (etc.) me."	Response to "dependency strivings" Provision of a paternal figure (significant other), "magician," sheltered milieu, friend, ally, dominatee, confidante, etc.
Dependency Striving Patterned Symptoms and Signs	Apathy Pseudo-anhedonia Display of helplessness Somatization	Controlled personal relationship
Delegation of another to parental role (Significant other)	Hypochondriasis Depressive, paranoid, and exploitive-manipulative states Psychiatric Syndromes and Disorders	Acceptance of delegation of another to parental role (Significant other) Pharmacotherapy Electroshock treatment Milieu, total push, and special hospital services

* Prepared for "The Dependency Construct as an Aid to Psychiatric Care of the Aged" paper presented at the American Psychiatric Association Meeting in Detroit, May, 1967.

sons in their own homes. Under this term can be included the family services of social service organizations, their special division for old persons, church organizations, "Y's," and some special subdivisions of governmental departments of welfare, health, or hygiene.

Some social agencies offer specialized services to impaired and ill persons; these include "meals on wheels," day centers or senior citizens' clubs, counseling, group therapy, homemaker and nursing services. The population served varies and includes many seriously impaired and disabled persons, as well as old persons with a wide variety of psychiatric disorders.

Old persons with moderately severe or severe brain syndrome usually require protection. This is usually best provided in a good old-age home or good nursing home. That such places today are not as good as they should be means that they should be improved, not that this truth can be ignored. Where money is freely available, a one-bed nursing home or hospital can be set up; at best, these usually do not provide the opportunities for social integration and for the various vehicles for psychotherapy that a congregate setting can provide. An old person with brain syndrome kept "at home" may not recognize his own home for what it is and may complain as frequently and bitterly that he wants to leave and go home as he will when in the residential hospital or home. "Home is where the heart is," and his wishes are for thirty years ago, wherever he may now be geographically located; it is the problem of staff in protective settings to establish those relationships which help the patient feel at home. In this sense, it is easier to make a supportive community in a hospital than it is to make a hospital of the community. "Community," in any case, has no meaning for the brain-damaged aged who can in no sense be an active citizen, however much he may have been in the past.

Old Age Homes

Old age homes are, in the United States, voluntary, nonprofit institutions, usually under sectarian auspices, but nonsectarian in admissions for the residential care of old persons. For the most part, they exclude the obviously mentally ill, the severely mentally impaired, and the physically acutely ill. They range in size from very small—ten to twelve beds—and with limited facilities, to very large—500 or more beds—with infirmary facilities of general hospital quality. Waiting periods for admission to such homes are usually too long for the impaired, disabled, and chronically ill, be-

cause of the high demand by such persons for services and the limited number of beds available. Fully ambulatory aged with little need for personal care have shorter waiting periods. Old age homes constitute protective settings in that they offer a structured, safe environment with readily available medical care, and are prosthetic milieus in that they serve to replace, substitute for, and compensate for the losses in physical, mental, and functional status in aged persons. Residents of old age homes theoretically have gone there for social reasons; in actuality, it is need for medical and nursing care, or emotional support and supervision that lead to application and admission. Many are obviously psychiatrically ill. At least 10 percent have a disabling degree of mental impairment (organic brain syndrome). Financing of patients is chiefly from welfare funds. The age of patients on admission is now close to eighty years, and the average age of residents is of course above this.

Nursing Homes

Nursing homes are proprietary institutions for the long-term care of chronically ill or permanently impaired persons. They vary widely in quality of care provided. The best are similar to good, large old-age homes, but do not directly provide medical care, which must be independently arranged. Old people in nursing homes range from the physically ill and impaired to the obviously mentally impaired (persons with organic brain syndrome). Many have depressions or paranoid conditions. One study in the New York City metropolitan area revealed that about 50 percent of the residents, strictly speaking, could be considered certifiable for psychiatric hospital care. About 50 to 80 percent of the patients are paid for by welfare funds, so that nursing homes are basically subcontractors to government agencies for long-term care. The average age of admitted persons is close to eighty years of age. Medicare financing has resulted in a change of many nursing homes to "extended care facilities." These are merely nursing homes which are enjoined by law for reimbursement eligibility to have a certain minimum of rehabilitative services for persons acceptable from general hospital stays on the basis of likelihood to recover and return to their own homes; in general, this excludes persons who have come to hospitals with a psychiatric diagnosis of any kind. There are some public nursing homes. Large public institutions often actually resemble old age homes in their character, quality, staffing, and programs.

SENIOR CITIZENS' HOTELS

In recent years, there have been emerging facilities that purport to be "retirement hotels." They have become "welfare-approved" and accept Old Age Assistance stipends in payment. They have in actuality become old age homes of poor quality because of small staffs and the paucity or lack of trained staff, such as nurses and aides; also, no medical care is available, except by personal arrangement. As it is in old age and nursing homes, the population of such "hotels" is becoming progressively older and more impaired and ill.

STATE HOSPITALS

State psychiatric hospitals do not require definition. There is currently debate about which old persons should be served by these units. Goldfarb[72] in 1959 recommended that State Departments of Mental Hygiene or their equivalents should undertake supervision of the problems of infirm and mentally impaired and emotionally disturbed aged persons, that this should be achieved by way of the expansion of State Hospital systems. Included would be small, geographically well-placed geropsychiatric diagnostic treatment centers with a strong medical treatment component, as well as special psychiatric services. It should be stated, however, that in recent years these social institutions have been closing their doors to the chronologically old who need, or would seem to need, long-term "custodial care." This is essentially a device not to provide for the long-term comprehensive health care needs of mentally impaired and usually also physically ill, as well as poor and bereft of family, aged persons. For purportedly benign and enlightened reasons, but actually because such care is expensive and difficult to organize

and administer, these patients are being thrust back to the community, which is encouraged to develop, with local and federal funds, as well as some help from the state, the agencies and facilities for care.

The best place for psychotherapy of those with relatively severe organic brain syndrome is usually within a good protective setting. The twenty-four-hour care needed by these persons and the capacity to tolerantly and constructively deal with their demanding, hostile, clinging, or angry behavior is too much for family members, and also tends to embitter them and endanger the best of prior relationships.

There should be no debate as to whether old persons should remain in their own homes or go to protective group residences, such as old age homes, nursing homes, or long-term-care hospitals. Such debates are usually based on generalizations which cannot apply to each individual. If they are in relatively good health or, when they are not, have an able and protective family, or enough money to purchase the staff and aids they require, they can remain at home. Remaining at home, however, under all circumstances may not, in balance, be as wise as use of a modern, well-staffed, well-equipped, comfortable old-age home. Prejudice against "institutional life" may deprive an old person of social, recreational, and material benefits he cannot gain in his own residence or community. These may not be good enough at best and at worst may keep him prisoner with a minimum of aids in an unpleasant domicile in a dangerous neighborhood.

Also, physically or mentally ill persons may constitute problems of twenty-four-hour care that can physically and emotionally exhaust the ablest, strongest, best-intentioned, and most available family members. Many persons with brain damage of even greater severity may be meek, mild, free of troublesome stormy episodes, and with a great capacity for congeniality and enjoyment of their homes. Such persons usually can make a good and happy adjustment to a good institution. Others with the same or less brain damage may be bitter and unhappy wherever they may be. In the latter event, the institution is preferable to the private home, if the congregate care facility is staffed by persons with the understanding of how to respond to the emotional, as well as physical needs.

Psychiatric Assistance to Staff

Close and constant caretaking relationships to old persons may provide anxiety and anger, because of the burdens of the task and the fears brought on by close contact with very old age, illness, and death.

Also, there may be fear or anger because of recapitulation in actuality or thought of unpleasant relations with one's own parents, and because of its demonstration of what, one day, may happen to all who live long enough. Overwhelmed and angry personnel may take a seemingly reasoned but actually resentful, nihilistic view toward the care and treatment of the old, or, conversely, may react by over-solicitousness and ingratiating, seductive, flattering, and infantilizing behavior. The old emotionally ill person may be viewed as a worthless, cantankerous "bitch," an "oversexed dirty old man," or as a fetchingly cute and eccentric little doll or a droll, amusing, likeable old rake. Whatever basis for either view, such hostility masked as compassion and sentimentality masked as sentiment often prevent professional appraisal and may be obstructive to proper relationships for treatment.

In hospitals and congregate-care settings, the psychiatrist is usually more useful as a guide, advisor, and therapist for staff than he is on a dyadic basis with individual patients; seminars, conferences, individual meetings with staff members, based on brief contacts with the patients, are often the best means of delivering good care to old persons.[73]

The psychiatrist can also be of aid to general physicians, internists, and surgeons, by directly and indirectly helping them to evaluate the degree of brain syndrome and the intensity of affective disorder in their patients. He helps them by clarifying the differences in the management of predominantly organically impaired persons.

In a residential setting for protective care, the influence of the psychiatrist in guiding personnel toward these ends is of importance; of great value is his work with staff to maintain their morale and optimal emotional health as it may be affected by their work.

Psychotherapy

Historical Background. It has been said that the history of science is science itself. It is tempting to believe that a history of psychotherapeutic approaches to older persons would be revealing of the complete art. Unfortunately, the number of authors and their works is too large to be listed. Like philosophies, they appear to be "the products or expressions of the general condition[19] of society" and their times. For example, Liébault and Beaunis, as quoted by Bernheim in 1886,[19] were interested in the susceptibility of old persons to hypnotism. Table 37–7, modified from Bernheim,[19] compares the suggestibility of an old-age group in this respect with five other age groups in their series of 1012 persons. In persons sixty-three years of age and over (the number of these is not specified), they found that in 11.8 percent somnambulism, in 8.4 percent very deep sleep could be hypnotically achieved, and in only 13.5 percent was there no influence possible.

Bernheim calls attention to the fact that in childhood and up to age fourteen all subjects without exception can be influenced by suggestion of the hypnotic type, and that the proportion of somnambulists is very high; by contrast, in old age the number of somnambulists is observed to decrease, but always remains at a relatively high figure (7 to 11 percent).

Hughlings-Jackson's 1886[89] discussion of the *Factors of Insanities* emphasized that many maladies could be recognized as the combined effect of dissolution and continuing evolution in the nervous system. "The shallower the dissolution the higher the range of evolution remaining, conversely the deeper the dissolution and the lower the range of evolution remaining." The elaboration of symptoms in a mental condition in which the brain is damaged is illustrated by the man who imagines his nurse to be his wife. His "not

TABLE 37-7.   **Suggestibility to Hypnotism, by Age Group (percentages)**

AGE	SOMNAM-BULISM	VERY DEEP SLEEP	DEEP SLEEP	LIGHT SLEEP	SOMNO-LENCE	NO INFLUENCE
Up to 7 years	26.5	4.3	13	52.1	4.3	
7–14 years	55.3	7.6	23	13.8		
28–35 years	22.6	5.9	34.5	17.8	13	5.9
42–49 years	21.6	4.7	29.2	22.6	9.4	12.2
56–63 years	7.3	8.6	37.6	18.8	13	14.4
63 onward	11.8	8.4	38.9	20.3	6.7	13.5

knowing" is a sample of the result of the disease (dissolution): his "wrong knowing" is a sample of what is left intact of his highest cerebral centers. Illusions, delusions, extravagant conduct, and abnormal emotional states in an insane person signify evolution, not dissolution, they signify the elaboration of thought by the remaining intact brain where misinterpretation must occur because of damage to the brain and these must vary "according as the person . . . is a child or an adult or an old man, clever or stupid, intelligent or unintelligent, educated (trade, etc. included) or non-educated." This variance from person to person must be obvious when the damage is not so great as to obscure it ("when the dissolution is but of little depth"). Hughlings-Jackson also forecast our information about confabulation, which is usually prominent early in brain damage and tends to disappear later, by pointing out that with rapid "dissolution" there is greater activity in the remaining "range of evolution." In discussing drug intoxication, he emphasized that not only could there be direct action on the central nervous system, but also indirect action by poisons through their effects on supportive systems. Unfortunately, he illustrated this by the actions of belladonna upon the supportive systems and eyes. This last may serve to show how brilliant observations may be "explained" by incorrect theories derived from convictions of a period of time.

Freud,[55] in 1898, said, "The psychoanalytic method demands a certain nature of clearsightedness and maturity in the patient and is therefore not suited for youthful persons or for adults who are feeble-minded or uneducated."

The newer attitudes were foreshadowed by Byrne,[36] who, in 1916, opened a lecture on the "Psychotherapy of Old Age and Chronic Invalidism" with the words:

In spite of the fact that methods have long since been reduced to principle, it is amazing to find scientific psychotherapy so little utilized by the profession in the treatment of old age and chronic invalidism. This is all the more shocking when one considers the not inconsiderable success obtained without and within the profession by individuals who realize the value of optimism and healthful suggestion, even though they know practically nothing about the scientific application of even these psychotherapeutic measures.

Byrne reminded his audience that where cure is not possible, suffering can be alleviated and destructive processes retarded; the fundamental of treatment, he felt, "*is adjustment of the individual's life and activities to the capacity of his organs*"—to be achieved by optimal activity and "the influence of mind upon body" . . . of emotion upon the circulatory and digestive mechanisms. He spoke of the importance of understanding, patient, supportive staff who would be reassuring, encouraging, attentive, and constructive in helping the aged to live, to make optimal use of their remaining assets and he detailed "how to do it." He did not advocate "tender loving care," but outlined that old persons should be addressed by last name and their dignity maintained, their illnesses meticulously attended, and their social integration encouraged.[36]

In the psychoanalytic literature, there was a lack of clear definition of what is meant by old age. In 1919, Abraham,[1] for example, referred to persons in their forties and fifties as being of "advanced age." Perhaps this is because he was himself at the time only thirty-one years old. He recommended psychoanalytically oriented therapy for older persons, but was careful to point out that poor vocational and sexual past performance, as well as early onset of symptoms, were unfavorable prognostic signs. He emphasized the tendency of many older persons to regard the doctor as a father figure from whom will come suggestions and guidance. In 1925, Jelliffe[90] encouraged psychiatric interest in the psychotherapy of persons in the seventh or eighth decades of life. With only one exception, however, his illustrations of successfully treated persons are in the sixth decade of life. Of interest is the exception, a seventy-two-year-old merchant whose temper improved, and whose hypertension appeared meliorated, through therapeutic sessions. He advocated treatment, saying, "Pessimism closes the door—optimism, even if an illusion, is worth the effort." Kaufman[99] and Atkin,[8] in 1940, appeared to regard the climacteric as the onset of old age, and they too referred to persons in their forties and fifties as old or aged.

The importance of considering the older person in relation to the family and to the community was emphasized by Flügel[52] in 1921; in his *Psychoanalytic Study of the Family*, he made clear that it is for the well-being of society that there be respectful and helpful attitudes toward older persons, and that the success of a culture may be measured by the extent and quality of its provision for its aged. Kardiner,[96] in 1937, outlined the social forces which underlie attitudes toward the aged. The relationship of the subsistence economy to the ability and willingness of the family to protect and preserve the aged, and the occurrence of a child-parent reversal in attitude and action, were cogently discussed by him. He gave an example of successful treatment of one older person, which included manipulation of the social environment. Unfortunately, the ages of the persons used as illustrations were not given.

Psychiatric difficulties of the fifth and sixth decades, to which many of these workers referred, are now better understood as problems of the middle years when many a person sees, or thinks he sees, the true trajectory in life, and views it with disappointment, horror, or fright, without being able significantly to alter his course. This development has nothing to do with involution, either physical or mental, as some have claimed, but it may nevertheless herald the beginning of chronic invalidism or of a mental state, which, even if not itself chronic, may create a social situation which steadily worsens.

After World War II, however, a number of authors, notably Cameron,[37] Rockwell,[144] Wayne,[189] Herkimer[76] and Meerloo.[123] Grotjahn,[84] Stern[169,170] and Goldfarb,[71] reported specifically on the individual psychotherapy of the aged. Others, among them Zeman,[196,197] Ginzberg,[61] Allen,[5] Clow,[40] Linden,[119] Silver,[163] and Hollender,[88] reported on hospital, group, and milieu treatments. A number of reviews of theoretical and practical value have appeared and a number of investigators, notably Busse, Birren, Stotsky,[173–179] Berezin,[13] Goldfarb, Perlin,[133] made sound medical-psychiatric contributions on which therapy can learn.

The fruitfulness of basic study of this age group was affirmed many years ago by the following findings in one institution for the aged. Klopfer[106] deduced that brief psychotherapeutic sessions would be effective; Perlin[133] noted that psychiatric interview was not always helpful in the proper selection of residents; Ballard[10] observed that certain types of older persons do not repeat suicide attempts; Shrut[162] noted that change of residence to an institutional type was related to increased anxiety and fear of death. The continuation of youthful attitudes and tendencies to remain active into old age, despite illness, was demonstrated by Oberleder.[127] Also, Kahn[91] noted that alert, assertive individuals seemed less prone to develop physical symptoms; and Pollock[135] reaffirmed the importance of good early socioeconomic circumstances and of at least minimal education in preserving intellectual ability with the progression of years.

Since then a great deal of work has come from the Geropsychiatric Institute at Duke

University under the direction of Busse[34] and later Eisdorfer. Verwoerdt's[185] study proved that sexual activity persists until late life and confirmed the information gathered by Rubin[152] that those who begin early and continue activity throughout the lifetime, tend to finish later. Palmore[129] and Pfeiffer have shown that persons with "a good start" may fall into an elite group who in later life do well. Pfeiffer confirmed the usefulness of psychotherapy in older persons. The investigative team headed by Simon, Lowenthal, and Epstein have contributed much information on the "paths to the mental hospital" demonstrating, as did Blau,[22] that families do not "dump their aged" into such institutions; illness and need for care result in appeals for such aid after a long history of other attempts at solution. These studies have expanded the work done by Birren[20] and his group at NIMH and that of Goldfarb[72] in New York State.

Rechtschaffen[142] wrote an excellent critical review of the literature on psychotherapy of the aged through 1959. In his discussion he stated,

. . . current thinking seems weighted toward the belief that most older persons, as compared with younger, profit most from supportive approaches in which the therapist plays a more active role. Therapeutic approaches might be arranged along a continuum of the degree of patient participation, as follows: (1) insight approaches, (2) supportive approaches, (3) direct gratification and environmental modification, (4) illusion-of-mastery therapy.

In general the trend has been to use approaches toward the last-named end of the continuum with the following characteristics of the aged being offered as reasons: the increased dependency which arises from realistically difficult circumstances; the immodifiability of external circumstances to which a neurosis may be an optimal adjustive mechanism; irreversible impairment of intellectual and learning ability; resistance (or lack of resistance) to critical self-examination; the economics of therapeutic investment when life expectancy is shortened. There is considerable disagreement as to what weight the various factors actually carry.

The "illusion-of-mastery" therapy of Goldfarb[142] in actuality was a description of what appeared to be taking place in effective dyadic or group psychotherapy with aged persons. It was not advocacy of foisting an "illusory relationship" on the patient. The therapist accepts the patient's delegation to parental status, does nothing to destroy this illusion, and permits the patient to feel secure, protected, triumphant, and in control of the powers he believes this chosen figure possesses. If the therapist fails to permit this, he "loses" the patient who goes on to seek out one he can regard as a parental surrogate in whom he can confide, for whom he can confess, or from whom he may believe he has produced punitive action, or whatever response he must see as present if he is to be convinced he has found the desired, potentially protective person. He may search for and find this in his spouse, a confidante, a friend, a mistress, his barber, a physician, or a charlatan. Further, Goldfarb was convinced that with persons of any age most, if not all therapy, other than that which can become completed "reconstructive" (to use Rado's term) or psychoanalytic therapy, is actually hypnoid in type. That is to say, in all psychotherapy the suggestibility of the patient is wittingly or unwittingly increased by the therapist even as by Liébault, Beaunis and Bernheim,[19] who then makes use of the powers delegated to him to the benefit of the patient. In psychoanalytic or reconstructive therapy, this comes to be understood, "worked through," by the analysand, and the therapist as a figure who has been parentified is relinquished in reality, although his influence and precepts may be psychically incorporated. Viewed in this light, many so-called insight approaches are actually merely reassuring and supportive, and provide direct gratification or constitute environmental modification through the existence of the psychotherapist as a special figure in the patient's social environment who fulfills the patient's need to find and hold him.

What kind of a parental surrogate the patient needs to feel reassured, what kind of behavior he will regard as supportive is signaled by the associational flow of the patient. It is my opinion that the common denominator of the wide variety of successful therapeutic methods is that they provide the patient with an illusion of mastery. If the therapist has come to understand what reassures and what supports the particular patient, the patient comes to feel "loved" and feel assured of protective aid, should he ask for it. This may lead some therapists to try to play a role, but the therapist should be chameleon-like. His "coloring" is determined by what the patient wishes to see, and he need play no role but merely avoid destroying the patient's illusions about him. In our society, with middle-class patients, behaving "like a doctor" may suffice.

Sprague[167] stated, "The therapist may serve the patient in a number of ways," and divided the roles of the therapist into active and passive. Among the passive roles are those of listener and target for the patient's ventilation of emotions. Among the active roles are those of indicator, comforter, explainer, desensitizer, analyzer, lecturer, negotiator, manager, decider, and philosopher. But, in Goldfarb's opinion, the therapist is first the listener and target, and then may permit the patient to believe that he is a reflecting mirror, or comforter, punisher, forgiver, by following the patient's symbolic productions and responding to this as required to maintain the relationship. With time and patience, he can also provide active direction of "helpful" nature through the trust and power placed in him as the parental surrogate, not thereby playing a role but by being the wiser, more constructively oriented person who is sought for.

In group therapy, the same general principles also apply. Stimulating improved social relationships in brain-damaged persons requires a special type of staff leadership. Patients establish relationships first with the leader, just as in dyadic therapy, and later, if at all, with peers through the common bond with the leader.

For an aged person, a relationship such as is described here is the important factor in the prevention or mitigation of fear and anger. They help him to cope with the disorganizing, or personally and interpersonally disturbing effects of emergency emotion. It is true that many aged institutional residents are more frightened and angry than truly demented; their behavior is disorganized by emergency emotion. The best restraint or corrective for confused, agitated patients appears to be the presence of interested, alert attendants who recognize that much, if not all, of the seemingly meaningless behavior of even brain-damaged aged persons can be managed if such behavior is regarded as a motivated and socially directed problem-solving attempt. Careful testing for intellectual assets may reveal their presence. Structured, flexible, nondemanding and nonthreatening group programs may reveal the patients' resources in even more gratifying ways—by encouraging and eliciting constructive behavior.

FEELINGS OF HELPLESSNESS AND DEPENDENCE

The recognition of helplessness and dependency in persons as making therapy possible has clarified some of the problems of psychiatric treatment of aged persons and has contributed to their solution. Although some aged persons are in a position to review their patterns of behavior and gain insight into their dynamic determinants so as to make sweeping changes in themselves, most must be helped to regain or to utilize more efficiently their old effective patterns of action and to do so with a sense of purpose, restored interest, and pleasure. The psychotherapeutic interrelationship in which the older person regards the therapist as the parent or child-parent, and the utilization of this relationship for the patient's benefit, have been demonstrated. The need for flexibility in the approach to treatment has been repeatedly emphasized. Appointments may be infrequent, sessions brief. Environmental manipulation and the role of ancillary personnel in treatment may be even more important than the sessions with the therapist. The need to work with the family or the persons who have assumed responsibility for the care of the relatively dependent person and the usefulness of the social worker in this respect have been emphasized.

Therefore, there is now increasing need for the instruction of personnel of all types in the care of aged persons with mental disorder.

Some current teaching of theory and practice, however, may lead to misguided therapeutic efforts with the chronically ill and aged. Emphasis, in teaching and practice, upon the patient's achievement of self-sufficiency and independence may result in the therapist's failure to recognize the patient's helplessness and dependency as a motivational force and nucleus for socially acceptable, effective patterns of behavior.

Therapists at all levels can be helped to grasp that psychiatric care of the aged can be directed toward (1) the correction of factors which initiate or maintain the mental suffering and social disturbance; (2) decreasing the environmental obstructions to gratification or relief from tension; (3) assisting the individual toward gratifying experience and aid in relief from tension; (4) decreasing feelings of helplessness, anxiety, and anger, or altering mood; (5) converting socially disturbing reparative patterns to more acceptable behavior, or (6) responding to the irrational as well as rational search for assistance and emotional support, so as to decrease personal suffering and environmental disturbance, and to favor increase in functional efficiency. Not all of these are equally feasible or desirable with aged persons. While each of these may increase capacity for "mastery," the first three may actually do so, but the second three may be achieved on an illusory basis.

This is so because with increased age, added socioeconomic losses, and physical or mental decline of the individual, personal opportunities and activities may be limited and sociomedical opportunity to exert corrective action is decreased. There remains the continuing opportunity to respond appropriately to the irrational aspect of the patient's search for aid: his dependency. The concept of dependency as a transaction cultivated by the person because it is emotionally gratifying, eliminates or decreases fear, anger, and feelings of helplessness, contributes to self-confidence and self-esteem, and lends meaning or purpose to life, assists the therapist in the beneficial use of this relationship. Professional awareness and judicious acceptance of the patient's dependency leads to diminution of its overt manifesta-

tions, to increased self-sufficient behavior, and quasi-independent action.

For its proper use, the dependency relationship must be clearly defined. It must be understood that life experiences, including that called psychotherapy, may yield a shift from one pattern of dependency to another, or of one pattern of nondependent function to another, but that the shift from dependent personality functioning to nondependency may not be feasible. Dependent psychodynamic patterns can be distinguished from nondependent patterns by their focus upon the instrumental use of others to elicit and maintain self-esteem, self-confidence, and a sense of purpose of personal identity. Subcategories of dependent and nondependent social relationships—simple, masked, pseudo-, and asocial or antisocial, can be defined as shown in Table 37–8. A socially desirable and personally helpful strengthening of a pattern or a shift from one pattern to one more socially acceptable can often be achieved.

Recognition that helplessness and emotional dependency of patients is of value for therapy helps to define goals of therapy on a practical, realistic basis, rather than in mystical terms, or within an ill-defined framework which is contemptuous of the patient's weakness, regards him as regressed, or depreciates his search for magic or for a powerful parental figure.

PSYCHOTHERAPEUTIC APPROACH

As suggested by the schematic representation, an old person who has lost resources for adequate, gratifying mastery of material, intrapsychic, or interpersonal problems may, because of feelings of helplessness, fear, and anger, search for aid, that is, strive to find and hold a person in relationship to whom he may regain feelings of ability "to do," about which he feels proud, which restores his sense of purpose, and gives him pleasure. This postulate points to the psychotherapist to help the patient to feel he has found the desired person and won the longed-for relationship. This can be achieved if the therapist can behave so as not to destroy the person's belief he has found and won what he seeks; this is done without role-playing if the therapist simply does noth-

TABLE 37–8.   **Personality and Social Characteristics of Dependent and Nondependent Personalities**

NONDEPENDENT PERSONALITY	DEPENDENT PERSONALITY
PERSONALITY CHARACTERISTICS	
Sense of Purpose is geared to internalized desire for self-realization and biologic drive for survival and reproduction; thus self-assertion serves to improve self and society.	*Sense of Purpose* is focused on seeking, winning, and controlling a "strong" protector with useful attributes.
Self-Esteem is enhanced by recognizing self as an effective individual with ability to gratify own needs, and to engage in mutually rewarding social relationships with others.	*Self-Esteem* is contingent on gaining and maintaining the approval of others, or from belief that intrinsic worth derives from class, clan, or family association.
Self-Confidence is achieved by mastery of his environment, and augmented by outside recognition of his ability and achievements.	*Self-Confidence* is based on success in attracting and holding others, on ability to gain a friend, ally, and helper through own efforts.
Pleasure comes from relief of tensions and satisfaction of needs in a personally and socially approved manner, and from contributing to tension relief and gratification of others on a cooperative problem-solving or sensual level.	*Pleasure* comes from accomplishments and services designed primarily to please others, in order to dominate and manipulate them.
SUBTYPES AND SOCIAL CHARACTERISTICS	
1. *Independent:* Rational, cooperative functioning in social relationships; actions and emotions attuned to individual goals and appropriate to the situation.	1. *Simple:* Transparent, easily recognized and freely admitted, usually without guilt or shame and sometimes with pride.
2. *Masked Independent:* Same as above, but less obtrusive.	2. *Masked Dependent:* Exploitation of others is disguised or rationalized as virtuous and socially useful, self-imposed subservience to delegated parent figure as "martyrdom."
3. *Pseudo-Dependent:* Rational social functioning modified by outward conformity to dependent behavior to avoid interpersonal complications.	3. *Pseudo-Independent:* Brave facade of masculinity or femininity and maternity; when disappointed in delegated parent figure, defiant self-assertion usually with controlled anger.
4. *Asocial:* Openly exploitive behavior aimed at individual gratification with little regard for its effect on others.	4. *Antisocial:* Demands the help of others as his right, resorts to force or takes what is not given freely.

Taken from Goldfarb, A. I., "The Psychodynamics of Dependency and the Search for Aid," *Occasional Papers in Gerontology*, No. 6., Institute of Gerontology, The University of Michigan-Wayne State University, August, 1969. Pp. 1–15.

ing to contradict the patient's verbal or non-verbal indication that the therapist does fulfill that role. This is tantamount to saying that the child-like submissive state of mind of the patient, the sufferer, the helpless one, is one of readiness to accept suggestion. The noncontradictory acceptance of the patient's readiness to be directed is an implicit suggestion to the patient that he continue in this role; this heightens the patient's suggestibility. Implicitly, the relationship enjoins the patient to be on his good behavior, to work to win and hold the therapist's good will. This is the state of craving for magic from the magician in which the patient seeks to learn and use the rites which will bring the magic-maker under his control. Improved behavior results, and then the improved behavior tends to increase self-confidence, self-esteem, and to connote that the therapist has been helpful. This heightens motivation to use the therapist and the pursuit of his help becomes a more and more important goal, giving the patient a sense of purpose. Feeling successful in this, and feeling successful in following the implicit but unstated suggestions of the therapist to do well so as to win him, so as to have him, is essentially a hypnotic relationship which leads to successful activity outside the therapeutic relationship, within the limits of the patient's resources. An added dimension is that the patient, in going through his behavioral struggle to win the therapist, comes to feel understood. This, as Stekel put it, is to feel loved, and as we may now put it, it is to feel secure, to have the power to control another. If the therapist goes on to utilize the states of parent-magician-the-one-to-be-obeyed, he may constructively instruct the patient to examine his own behavior so as to improve it. Such discriminatory self-examination may be beyond the capacity of persons with even mild brain damage, but is more likely beyond the capacity of most persons because of their fear to become acquainted with their dependency-striving outside, not to speak of inside, the therapist's office.

Put in practical terms, a number a factors can be singled out as having a therapeutic influence. These are:

1. The delegation to the therapist of great powers.

2. The patient's belief in the therapist's increasing interest in him.

3. The rise of satisfaction that goes with the belief in the therapist's interest and understanding, which are believed to be, or responded to as, love.

4. The belief that the therapist's interest is based on understanding and guarantees continued care.

5. The rise of satisfaction from having an ally, friend, protector, or parental figure who is more or less constantly present, since the feelings are carried along and incorporated. It is as though a magician had been found and was being controlled.

6. Gratification from having won over or triumphed over the therapist; this is life proof of one's own strength, wit, or cunning, and may be equated with the idea that one knows or has learned the complex rites that gain control over the magician's powers. This gratification is often gained when the therapist gives some specific practical aid, such as prescriptions for medication, recommendation of special diet, or helps make minor changes in the environment, such as a shift in room or roommate, in an institution, or in an item of family care.

7. Gratification from feeling favored by the therapist over another—the patient before, the patient after, or the colleague who is not a patient—a victory in sibling rivalry, gratification in lording it over others, silently or aloud, because one has been "chosen."

8. Gratification from true success in performances that were motivated by a desire to please the therapist but that have real value. For example, success in occupational therapy —the making of a rug or an ashtray about which the therapist can be told, or that can be given as a gift to the doctor—or success in a sheltered workshop, as evidenced by output and remuneration.

9. The similar gratifications obtained with others about which the therapist may be told, or that may be kept as a secret to tell the therapist some day, or that are referred to the incorporated therapist-parent in the conversa-

tions with him that take place only in the thoughts of the patient between visits.

10. Triumphant feelings on the part of the patient from having withheld information of hidden trouble; pride in self-sufficiency as evidenced by silently and uncomplainingly enduring pain, in relation to the approving incorporated parent, because this is what could please the therapist—if he knew about it.

11. Accentuation of guilt fear (conscience) with some decrease in aggressiveness, because the angry feelings are becoming known to another. Pride and rise in self-esteem on the basis of self-control because of this, and an increase in self-confidence of this self-control.

12. Decrease in the guilty fear because of the permissive or reassuring attitude of the therapist who appears to regard the discomfort of guilty fear as expiatory self-punishment which earns forgiving.

13. The change of disorganizing fear to organizing anger as there is decrease in the fear of punishment and of the belief that anger is best.

14. The change of disorganizing anger to organizing fear, and the alerting of self to dangers; self-propulsion toward best behavior on the basis of exposure to the consensus, to the leader's comments, and to one's own second thoughts.

PHARMACOTHERAPY

Pharmacotherapy is dealt with in detail elsewhere in this book. In older persons with no brain damage the same medications are useful as in younger persons for similar conditions, but the doses are usually smaller and medications such as anti-depressants started more cautiously. Antihistaminics and analgesics, sedatives and hypnotics, are also useful to decrease fear and anger with good effect. The choice of medication can sometimes be made on the basis of whether fear predominates and is accompanied by anger, or whether anger now predominates and contributes to fear. At times, trial and error can clarify whether an antianxiety (fear-decreasing) medication is necessary or a tranquilizer (sedative, anger-decreasing, antipsychotic) meliorative is the

most useful. Also, for persons whose autonomic nervous system concomitants of emergency emotion appear to have triggered a sustained shift in biochemistry or homeostasis, anticholinergic antidepressants or phenothiazines may be helpful, depending upon whether the reaction is depressive or schizophrenic in type.

(Bibliography

1. ABRAHAM, K. (1919), "The applicability of psychoanalytic treatment to patients of advanced age," in *Selected Papers*, pp. 312–317, Basic Books, New York, 1953.

2. ALLEN, E. B. "Psychological orientation in geriatrics," *Geriatrics* 4:67, 1949.

3. ———. "Psychiatric aspects of cerebral arteriosclerosis," *New England J. Med.*, 245:677, 1951.

4. ALLEN, E. B., and CLOW, H. E. "Paranoid reactions in the aging," *Geriatrics* 5:66, 1950.

5. ———. "The psychiatrist's role in the care of the aging," *Geriatrics* 7:117, 1952.

6. ———. "Psycho-physical compensatory adjustment in the aged," *J. Am. Geriatrics Soc.*, 1:785, 1953.

7. ARONSON, J. "Psychiatric management of disturbed behavior in a home for the aged," *Geriatrics* 11:39, 1956.

8. ATKIN, S. "Discussion of old age and aging: The psychoanalytic point of view," *Am. J. Orthopsychiat.*, 10:79, 1940.

9. BALLARD, A. B. "Suicide in old age," unpublished paper, 1956.

10. ———. "Psychiatric emergencies in a home for the aged," paper presented at Annual Meeting, Assoc. of Psychoanalyt. Med., May 7, 1957.

11. BARNACLE, C. H. "Psychiatry for senescence," *Southwestern Med.*, 30:137, 1949.

12. BENDER, M. B. *Disorders in perception*, Charles C. Thomas, Springfield, Illinois, 1952.

13. BEREZIN, M. A. "Some intrapsychic aspects of aging," in N. E. Ainsberg, ed. *Normal Psychology of the Aging Process*, pp. 93–117, New York, International Universities Press, 1963.

14. ———. "Partial grief in family members

and others who care for the elderly patient," *J. Geriat. Psychiat.* 4:53–64, 1970.

15. ———. "Sex and old age: a review of the literature, *J. Geriat. Psychiat.* 2:131–149, 1969.

16. BEREZIN, M. A. and D. J. FERN. "Persistence of early emotional problems in a seventy-year-old woman," *J. Geriat. Psychiat.* 1:45–60, 1967.

17. BEREZIN, M. A., and B. A. STOTSKY, H. Grunebaum (ed.), *The geriatric patient, in the Practice of Community Mental Health.* Boston: Little, Brown and Co., 1970, pp. 219–244.

18. BERGMANN, K., D. W. K. KAY, E. M. FOSTER, A. A. MCKECHNIE, and M. ROTH. "A further study of randomly selected community residents to assess the affects of chronic brain syndrome and cerebrovascular disease." Paper read at World Psychiat. Assoc. Conf. in Mexico City at 5th World Congress of Psychiatry, 1971.

19. BERNHEIM, H. *Suggestive therapeutics, a treatise on the nature and uses of hypnotism*, translated by Christian S. Haerther, Edinburgh and London, 1890.

20. BIRREN, J. E., R. N. BUTLER, S. W. GREENHOUSE, L. SOKOLOFF, and M. R. YARROW. *Human aging—a biological and behavioral study.* U.S. Dept. of Health, Education and Welfare. Public Health Service Publication 986, 1963.

21. BIRREN, J. E., ed., *Handbook of Aging and the Individual.* Chicago: University of Chicago Press, 1959.

22. BLAU, D. "The role of community physicians in the psychiatric hospitalization of aged patients." Paper presented at the 14th. annual meeting of the Gerontological Society, Pittsburgh, Pa., Nov. 1961.

23. ———. "Psychiatric hospitalization of the aged." *Geriatrics*, 1966, 21, 204–210.

24. BRENNAN, M. and R. P. KNIGHT. "Hypnotherapy for mental illness in the aged: Case report of hysterical psychosis in a seventy-one year old woman," *Bull. Menninger Clin.*, 7:188, 1943.

25. BROOKS, L., "A case of eroticized transference in a 73-year-old woman," *J. Geriat. Psychiat.* 2:150–162, 1967.

26. BROTMAN, H. B. "Every tenth American: Adding life to years," *Bulletin of the Institute of Gerontology* (University of Iowa) 15 (suppl. 10):3–7, 1968.

27. BUSSE, E., "Research on aging: Some methods and findings." in *Geriatric Psychiatry: Grief, Loss and Emotional Disorders in the Aging Process.* New York: International Universities Press.

28. BUSSE, E., R. H. BARNES, A. J. SILVERMAN, G. M. SHY, M. THALER, and L. L. FROST. "Studies of the process of aging: Factors that influence the psyche of elderly persons," *Am. J. Psychiat.*, 110:897, 1954.

29. BUSSE, E., R. H. BARNES, A. J. SILVERMAN, M. THALER, and L. L. FROST. (1955), "Studies of the process of aging X: The strength and weaknesses of psychic functioning in the aged." *Amer. J. Psychiat.*, 111: 896–903, 1955.

30. BUSSE, E., R. H. BARNES, and L. D. COHEN. "Factors Producing Ego Disintegration in the Aged," *North Carolina M.J.*, 16:528, 1955.

31. BUSSE, E., R. H. DOVENMUEHLE, and R. G. BROWN. (1960), "Psychoneurotic reactions of the aged." *Geriatrics*, 15:97–105.

32. BUSSE, E. and C. N. NICHOLS. "Emotional Disturbances of Older People," *Medical Times*, 86 (1958) 263–268.

33. BUSSE, E., and E. PFEIFFER. (1969), "Functional psychiatric disorders in old age," in Busse and Pfeiffer (eds.), *Behavior and Adaptation in Late Life*, Little, Brown & Co., Boston.

34. BUSSE, E., and E. PFEIFFER, (1973). "Mental illness in later life," in Busse and Pfeiffer (eds.), *Amer. Psychiat. Assoc. Publ.*

35. BUTLER, R. N. "Aspects of survival and adaptation in human aging," *Amer. J. Psychiat.* 123:1233–1243, 1969.

36. BYRNE. J. "Psychotherapy of old age and chronic invalidism." *Hospital Bulletin of the New York City Department of Charities*, 1:103–107, 1951.

37. CAMERON, N. "Neuroses of later maturity," in O. J. Kaplan, (ed.), *Mental disorders in later life*, Stanford Univ. Press, Stanford, Calif. 1945.

38. CAPGRAS, J. and J. REBOUL-LACHAUX. *Illusion des sosies dans une délire systématisé chroniqué, Bull. Soc. Clin. de Méd. Ment.,* January, 1923.

39. CLAMAN, A. D. "Introduction to panel discussion: sexual difficulties after 50." *Canad. Med. Ass. J.* 94:207, 1966.

40. CLOW, H. E., "A study of 100 patients suf-

fering from psychosis with cerebral arterio-sclerosis," *Am. J. Psychiat.*, 97:16, 1940.

41. CLOW, H. E., and E. B. ALLEN. "Manifestations of psychoneuroses occurring in later life," *Geriatrics*, 6:31, 1951.

42. COLEMAN, S. "The phantom double. Its psychological significance," *Brit. Jour. M. Psychol.* 14:254, 1934.

43. COMMISSION ON CHRONIC ILLNESS. *Chronic illness in the United States*, Vol. II, Harvard Univ. Press, Cambridge, Mass., 1956.

44. COSIN, L. Z., F. POST, and M. ROTH. "Discussion on geriatric problems in psychiatry," *Proc. Roy. Soc. Med.* 49:237, 1956.

45. CUMMINGS, E. and W. E. HENRY. "Growing old: the process of disengagement," Basic Books, New York, 1961.

46. DAVIDSON, G. *Psychiat. Quart.* "The Syndrome of Capgras," 15:513, 1941.

47. DIAMOND, O. K. "New developments in the care of the aged mentally ill," *New York J. Med.* 51:2375, 1951.

48. DOVENMUEHLE, R. H. personal communication, 1969.

49. EHRENTHEIL, O. F. "Differential diagnosis of organic dementias and affective disorders in aged patients," *Geriatrics*, 12:426, 1957.

50. FENICHEL, O. *The Psychoanalytic Theory of Neurosis*, Norton, New York, 1945.

51. FERENCZI, S., "Stages in the development of the sense of reality," in J. S. Van Teslaar (ed.), *An Outline of Psychoanalysis*, 108–127, Random House, New York, 1925.

52. FLÜGEL, J. C. *Psychoanalytic Study of the Family*. Hogarth, London, 1950.

53. FOWLIE, H. C., C. COHEN, and M. P. ANAND. (1963). "Depression in elderly patients with subnutrition." *Geront. Clin.*, 5:215–225.

54. FREEDMAN, A. M., and H. I. KAPLAN. (eds.), *Comprehensive Textbook of Psychiatry*. Williams and Wilkens, Baltimore, 1967.

55. FREUD, S. (1915). "Further recommendations in the technique of psychoanalysis; observations on transference love," in *Collected Papers*, Vol. 2, pp. 377–391, Basic Books, New York, 1953.

56. ———, (1904). "On psychotherapy," in *Collected Papers*, Vol. 1, pp. 249–271, Basic Books, New York, 1959.

57. ———, (1898). "Sexuality in the aetiology of the neuroses," in *Collected Papers*, Vol. 1, pp. 220–248, Basic Books, New York, 1959.

58. ———, (1919). "Turnings in the ways of psychoanalytic therapy," in *Collected Papers*, Vol. 2, pp. 392–402, Basic Books, New York, 1959.

59. FROMM-REICHMANN, F. (ed.). *The Philosophy of Insanity*, p. 85, Greenberg, New York, 1947.

60. GAITY, C. H. ed. *Aging and the Brain*. Plenum Press, New York, 1972.

61. GINZBERG, R. "Geriatric ward psychiatry: techniques in the psychological management of elderly psychotics," *Am. J. Psychiat.*, 110:296, 1953.

62. GINZBERG, R., and C. W. BRINECAR. "Psychiatric problems in elderly residents of county homes," *Am. J. Psychiat.*, 110:454, 1953.

63. GITELSON, M. "The emotional problems of elderly people," *Geriatrics*, 3:135, 1948.

64. GOLDFARB, A. I. "Psychotherapy of aged persons: I. The orientation of staff in a home for the aged," *Men. Hyg.*, 37:76, 1953.

65. ———. "Recommendations for psychiatric care in a home for the aged," *J. Gerontol.* 8:343, 1953.

66. ———. "A psychiatric approach to institutional work with the aged," in H. Turner, (ed.), *Community Service Society Seminar*, Nat. Welfare Assembly, New York, 1955.

67. ———. "Psychiatric problems of old age," *New York State J. Med.*, 55:494, 1955.

68. ———. "Psychotherapy of aged persons: IV. One aspect of the therapeutic situation with aged patients," *Psychoanalyt. Rev.*, 42:180, 1955.

69. ———. "Psychotherapy of the aged: The use and value of an adaptational frame of reference," *Psychoanalyt. Rev.*, 43:68, 1956.

70. ———. "The rationale for psychotherapy with older ersons," *Am. J. M. Sc.*, 232:181, 1956.

71. ———. "The rationale for psychotherapy with older persons." *American Jrnl. of Medical Sciences*, 232, No. 2, 1956.

72. ———. "Report to the commissioner of N.Y. State, Summarization of activities for the year 1958 from the office of the consultant on services for the aged," unpublished report, 1959, mimeo, N.Y. State Department of Mental Health, Albany, N.Y.

73. ———. "Current trends in the management

of psychiatrically ill aged," in *Psycho-pathology of Aging*, Paul H. Hoch and Joseph Zubin. (eds.), 248–265, Grune and Stratton, New York, 1961.

74. ———. "A psychosocial and sociophysiological approach to aging, in N. I. Zinberg, and I. Kaufman. (eds.) *Normal Psychology of the Aging Process*, pp. 72–92, International Universities Press, New York, 1963.

75. ———. "Geriatric psychiatry," in H. I. Kaplan, and A. M. Freedman, (eds.), *Comprehensive Textbook of Psychiatry*, Williams & Wilkins, Baltimore, Md., 1967.

76. ———. "Predicting mortality in the institutionalized aged," *Arch. Gen. Psychiat.*, *21*, Aug. 1969.

77. ———. "Group therapy with the old and aged," in H. I. Kaplan, and B. J. Sodock, (eds.), *Comprehensive Group Psychotherapy*, Williams & Wilkins, Baltimore, Md., 1971.

78. GOLDFARB, A. I. and J. SHEPS. "Psychotherapy of aged persons: III. Brief therapy of interrelated psychological and somatic disorders," *Psychosom. Med.* *16*:209, 1954.

79. GOLDFARB, A. I. and H. TURNER. "Psychotherapy of aged persons: II. Utilization and effectiveness of 'brief' therapy," *Am. J. Psychiat.*, *109*:916, 1953.

80. GOLDFARB, A. I., M. FISCH, and I. E. GERBER. "Predictors of mortality in the institutionalized aged." *Diseases of the Nervous System*, *27*:21–29, 1966.

81. GRANICK, S. "Studies of psychopathology in later maturity," *J. Gerontol.*, *5*:361, 1950.

82. GREENLEIGH, L. "Some psychological aspects of aging," *Soc. Casework*, *36*:99, 1955.

83. GROTJAHN, M. "Psychoanalytic investigation of a seventy-one year old man with senile dementia," *Psychoanalyt. Quart.* *9*:40, 1940.

84. ———. "Analytic psychotherapy with the elderly," *Psychoanal. Rev.*, *42*:419–427. 1955.

85. GROUP FOR THE ADVANCEMENT OF PSYCHIATRY, *Psychiatry and the Aged: An Introductory Approach*, Vol. 5, Report 59. Group for the Advancement of Psychiatry, New York, 1965.

86. HALLIDAY, J. L. *Psychological Medicine*, Norton, New York, 1948.

87. HERKIMER, J. H. and J. A. M. MEERLOO. "Treatment of mental disturbances in elderly women," *Soc. Casework*, *32*:419, 1951.

88. HOLLENDER, M. H. "The role of the psychiatrist in homes for the aged," *Geriatrics*, *6*:243, 1951.

89. JACKSON, J. H. "Factors of insanities," in James Taylor (ed.), *Selected Writings of John Hughlings Jackson*, Vol. 2 Medical Press and Circular, 1894.

90. JELLIFFE, S. E. "The old age factor in psychoanalytic therapy," *Med. J., and Record*, *121*:7, 1925.

91. KAHN, R. L., F. D. ZEMAN, and A. I. GOLDFARB. "Attitudes toward illness in the aged," *Geriatrics*, *13*:246, 1958.

92. KANT, A. P. "An experiment in the counseling of older people," *Geriatrics* *11*:44, 1956.

93. KAPLAN, H. I., and B. V. SADOSK, eds. *Comprehensive Group Psychotherapy*, Williams and Wilkins, Baltimore, 1971.

94. KAPLAN, O. J., (ed.), *Mental Disorders in Later Life*, Stanford Univ. Press, Stanford, Calif., 1945.

95. KARDINER, A. *The Individual and Society*, Columbia, New York, 1939.

96. ———. "Psychological factors in old age," in *Mental Hygiene in Old Age*, pp. 14–26. Family Service Assoc. of America, New York, 1937.

97. KARDINER, A. and L. OVESY. *The Mark of Oppression*, Norton, New York, 1951.

98. KARDINER, A., and H. SPIEGEL. *War Stress and Neurotic Illness*, 2nd ed., Hoebar, New York, 1947.

99. KAUFMAN, M. "Old age and aging: The psychoanalytic point of view," *Am. J. Orthopsychiat.*, *10*:73, 1940.

100. KAY, D. W. K. (1959). "Observations on the natural history and genetics of old age psychoses: A Stockholm material, 1931–1937 (abridged)," *Proc. Roy. Soc. Med.*, *52*:791.

101. KAY, D. W. K., P. BEAMISH, and M. ROTH, (1964). "Old age mental disorders in Newcastle-upon-Tyne, Part 1: A study of prevalence," *Brit. J. Psychiat.*, *110*:146–158.

102. ———, (1964), "Old age mental disorders in Newcastle-upon-Tyne, Part 2," *Brit. J. Psychiat.*, *110*:668–682.

103. KAY, D. W. K., V. NORRIS, and R. POST, (1956). "Prognosis in psychiatric disorders of the elderly," *J. Ment. Sci.*, *102*:129.

104. KAY, D. W. K., M. ROTH, and B. HOPKINS,

(1955), "Affective disorders in the senium: (1) Their association with organic cerebral degeneration." *J. Ment. Sci.*, 101:302–316.

105. KENT, D. P., R. KESTENBAUM, and S. SHER-WOOD, (eds.). *Research Planning and Action for the Elderly*, Behavioral Publications, New York, 1972.

106. KLOPFER, W. G. "The role of a clinical psychologist in a home for the aged," *Geriatrics*, 6:404, 1951.

107. KRAMER, M., C. TAUBE, and S. STARR. (Feb. 1968). "Patterns of use of psychiatric facilities by the aged: current status, trends and implications." *Psychiatric Research Report 23*, American Psychiatric Assoc.

108. LAWTON, G. "Psychotherapy with older persons," *Psychoanalysis* 1:27, 1952.

109. LECKY, W. E. H. *History of European Morals*, Braziller, New York, 1955.

110. LEVIN, S. "Depression in the aged," in M. A. Berezin, and S. H. Cath, (eds.), *Geriatric Psychiatry: Grief, Loss, and Emotional Disorders in the Aging Process*, pp. 203–225, International Universities Press, New York, 1965.

111. LEVIN, S. and R. J. KAHANA. *Psychodynamic Studies on Aging, Creativity, Reminiscing, and Dying*, International Universities Press, New York, 1967.

112. LIN, T. (1953). "Mental disorder in Chinese and other cultures," *Psychiatry.* 16:313–36.

113. LINDEMANN, E. "Symptomatology and management of acute grief," *Amer. J. Psychiat.* 101:141–148, 1944.

114. LINDEN, M. E. "Emotional problems in aging," *Jewish Soc. Service Quart.* 31:1, 1954.

115. ———. "The significance of dual leadership on gerontologic group psychotherapy: Studies in gerontologic human relations, III," *Internat. J. Group Psychotherapy*, 4:262, 1954.

116. ———. "Tensions created by the increasing span of life," paper read before the Atlantic County Assoc. for Mental Health, May 9, 1955: privately printed, Philadelphia, 1955.

117. ———. "Transference in gerontologic group psychotherapy: Studies in gerontologic human relations IV," *Internat. J. Group Psychotherapy*, 5:61, 1955.

118. ———. "The older person in the family: Studies in gerontologic human relations, VII," *Soc. Casework* 37:75, 1956.

119. LINDEN, M. E. and D. COURTNEY. "The human life cycle and its interpretations: A psychological hypothesis: Studies in gerontologic human relations I," *Am. J. Psychiat.*, 109:906, 1953.

120. LOWENTHAL, M. F. *Lives in Distress*, Basic Books, New York, 1964.

121. LOWENTHAL, M. F., P. BERKMAN, and associates (1967). *Aging and Mental Disorder in San Francisco*, Jossey Bass Inc., San Francisco.

122. MADDOX, G. L. "Adaptation to retirement," *Gerontologist*, 10:14–18, 1970.

123. MEERLOO, J. A. M. "Psychotherapy with elderly people," *Geriatrics*, 10:583, 1955.

124. NEW YORK STATE DEPT. OF MENTAL HYGIENE, MENTAL HEALTH RESEARCH UNIT. *A Mental Health Survey of Older People.* State Hospitals Press, Utica, N.Y. 1960, 1961.

125. NORRIS, V. (1969). "Mental Illness in London," *Maudsley Monograph, 6.* Oxford University Press, London.

126. NORRIS, V. and F. POST (1954). "Treatment of psychiatric patients: Use of a diagnostic classification." *Brit. Med. J.*, 1, 675.

127. OBERLEDER, M. "Attitudes related to adjustment in a home for the aged," Ph.D. Thesis, Teachers College, Columbia University, 1957; study conducted at the Home for Aged and Infirm Hebrews, New York, N.Y.

128. OVERHOLSER, W. "Mental disease," Chap. 17 in E. J. Stieglitz, (ed), *Geriatric Medicine*, 2nd ed., Saunders, Philadelphia, 1949.

129. PALMORE, E., ed. *Normal Aging: Reports from Duke Longitudinal Study, 1955–1969.* Duke University Press, Durham, N.C., 1970.

130. PALMORE, E. and F. C. JEFFERS, eds. *Prediction of Life Span.* Heath, Lexington, Mass., 1971.

131. PAMPIGLIONE, G., and F. POST. (1958). "The value of electroencephalographic examination in psychiatric disorders of old age," *Geriatrics*, 13:725.

132. PECK, A. "Psychotherapy of the aged," *J. Amer. Geriat. Soc.* 14:748–753, 1966.

133. PERLIN, S. Personal communications.

134. POLLACK, M. "Psychiatric screening in a home for the aged," I.A. Followup Study, *Geriatrics* 13:747, 1958.

135. POLLACK, M., R. L. KAHN, and A. I. GOLD-

FARB. "Cultural and environmental factors affecting complex perception in institutionalized aged," *J. Gerontol. 12*:4, 1957.

136. POST, F. (1959). "Early treatment of persistent senile confusion," *Geront. Clin. 1*: 114.

137. ———. (1962). "The Significance of Affective Symptoms in Old Age," *Maudsley Monograph 10*, Oxford University Press, London.

138. RADO, S. "Mind, unconscious mind, and brain," *Psychosom. Med., 11*:165, 1949.

139. ———. "Emergency behavior," Chap. 9 in Hoch, P. H. and J. Zubin, (eds.), *Anxiety*, Grune & Stratton, New York, 1950.

140. ———. "Recent advances of psychoanalytic therapy," Chap. 15 in "Psychiatric Treatment," *A. Res. Nerve & Ment. Dis., Proc. 21*:42, 1953.

141. ———. "The relationship of patient to therapist," *Am. J. Orthopsychiat. 12*:542, 1942.

142. RECHTSCHAFFEN, A. "Psychotherapy with geriatric patients: a review of the literature." *Jrnl. of Geront., 14*, No. 1, Jan. 1959.

143. ROCHLIN, G. "The loss complex," *J. Amer. Psychoanal. Ass., 7*:299–316, 1959.

144. ROCKWELL, F. V. "Psychotherapy in the older individual, in O. J. Kaplan, (ed), *Mental Disorders in Later Life*, Stanford Univ. Press, Stanford, Calif. 1954.

145. ROTH, M. "Some psychiatric aspects of senescence: A review of the literature," *Psychiatric Quart., 28*:93, 1954.

146. ———. (1955). "The natural history of mental disorders in old age," *J. Ment. Sci., 101*:281–301.

147. ———. (1959). "Mental health problems of aging and the aged," *Bull. Wld. Hlth. Org., 21*:527–561.

148. ROTH, M. and D. W. K. KAY, (1956). "Affective disorders arising in the senium, II: Physical disability as an aetiological factor." *J. Ment. Sci. 102*:141.

149. ROTH, M. and J. O. MORRISSEY, (1952). "Problems in the diagnosis and classification of mental disorder in old age: With a study of case material." *J. Ment. Sci., 98*:66.

150. ROTHSCHILD, D. "Pathological changes in senile psychoses and their psychobiologic significance," *Am. J. Psychiat., 93*:757, 1937.

151. ROTHSCHILD, D. "Senile psychoses and psychoses with cerebral arteriosclerosis," in

O. J. Kaplan, (ed.), *Mental Disorders in Later Life*, Stanford Univ. Press, Stanford, Calif., 1945.

152. RUBIN, I. *Sexual Life After Sixty*, Basic Books, New York, 1965.

153. RUESCH, J. *Chronic Disease and Psychological Invalidism: A Psychosomatic Study*, Univ. of California Press, Berkeley, 1951.

154. SAND, R. *The Advance to Social Medicine*, Staples, London, 1952.

155. SANDS, I. J. "The neuropsychiatric disorders of the aged," *New York J. Medicine, 51*:2370, 1951.

156. SANDS, S. L. and D. ROTHSCHILD. "Sociopsychiatric foundations for theory of reactions to aging," *J. Nerv. and Mental Dis., 116*:233, 1952.

157. SAVITSKY, E. "Psychological factors in nutrition of the aged," *Soc. Casework, 34*:435, 1953.

158. SCHUSTER, D. B. "A psychological study of a 106 year old man," *Am. J. Psychiat., 109*:112, 1952.

159. SELIGER, R. V. "Alcoholism in the older age groups," *Geriatrics, 3*:166, 1948.

160. SHANAS, E. "Health and adjustment in retirement," *Gerontologist, 10*:19–21, 1970.

161. SHELDON, J. H. (1948). *The Social Medicine of Old Age: Report of an Inquiry in Wolverhampton*, Oxford University Press, London.

162. SHRUT, S. "Old age and death attitudes," Ph.D. Thesis, New York University, 1955, study conducted at the Home for Aged and Infirm Hebrews, New York.

163. SILVER, A. "Group psychotherapy with senile psychotic patients," *Geriatrics, 7*:1, 1952.

164. SIMON, A. "Psychological problems of aging," *California Med., 75*:73, 1951.

165. ———. "Screening of the aged mentally ill," *J. Geriat. Psychiat., 4*:5–17, 1970.

166. SIMON, A., L. EPSTEIN and L. REYNOLDS. "Alcoholism in the geriatric mentally ill," *Geriatrics, 23*:125–131, 1968.

167. SPRAGUE, M. B. "The psychiatrist's role with his patient." *Amer. J. Psychiat., 95*:135, 1938.

168. STENBACH, A. "Object Loss and Depression," *Arch. Gen. Psychiat., 12*:144–151, Feb. 1965.

169. STERN, K. "Observations in an old age counseling center," *J. Gerontol., 3*:48, 1948.

170. ———. "Problems encountered in an old

age counseling center. Conference on problems of aging," Josiah Macy Foundation, Transactions, New York, 1950.

171. ———. "Reactive depressions in later life," Chap. 10 in P. H. Hoch, and J. Zubin, (eds.), *Depression*, Grune & Stratton, New York, 1954.

172. STERN, K., G. H. WILLIAMS, and M. PRADOS, (1951). "Grief reactions in later life," *Amer. J. Psychiat.*, 108:289–294.

173. STOTSKY, B. A. "Nursing homes: A review," *Amer. J. Psychiat.*, 123:249–258, 1966.

174. ———. *The Elderly Patient*, New York, Grune & Stratton, 1968.

175. ———. "Discussion of emotional problems of patients in nursing homes," *J. Geriat. Psychiat.*, 1:167–173, 1968.

176. ———. *The Nursing Home and the Aged Psychiatric Patient*, New York, Appleton-Century-Crofts, 1970.

177. ———. "Discussion of the screening of the mentally ill," *J. Geriat. Psychiat.*, 4:18–22, 1970.

178. STOTSKY, B. A. and J. P. DOMINICK. "The psysician's role in the nursing and retirement home," *Gerontologist*, 10:38–44, 1970.

179. STOTSKY, B. A. and S. LEVEY. "Issues in planning for geriatric services," *J. Amer. Geriat. Soc.*, 17:459–468, 1969.

180. TILKIN, L. "Clinical evaluation of psychiatric disorders in the aged," *Geriatrics*, 7:56, 1952.

181. TODD, J. "The syndrome of Capgras." *Psychiatric Quarterly*, pp. 250–265, 1968.

182. TUCKMAN, J. and I. LORGE. "Older people's appraisal of adjustment over the life span," *J. Pers.*, 22:417, 1954.

183. TUCKMAN, J., J. LORGE, and F. D. ZEMAN. "Retesting older people with the Cornell Medical Index with the Supplementary Health Questionnaire," *J. Gerontol.*, 9:306, 1954.

184. TURNER, H. "Promoting understanding of aged patients," *Soc. Casework*, 34:428, 1953.

185. VERWOERDT, A. "The physician's role in retirement counseling," *Gerontologist*, 10:22–26, 1970.

186. VIÉ, J. "Les méconnaissances systématiques." *Ann. Méd. Psych.*, 31:440–455, 1944.

187. VISCHER, A. L. *Old Age—Its Compensations and Rewards*, Macmillan, New York, 1947.

188. WATTERS, T. A. "The neurotic struggle in senescence," *Geriatrics*, 3:301, 1948.

189. WAYNE, G. J. "Psychotherapy in senescence," *Ann. West. Med. & Surg.*, 6:88, 1952.

190. ———. "Work as therapy, with special reference to the elderly," *Ment. Hyg.*: 39–79, 1955.

191. WEINBERG, J. "Research in aging." Veterans Administration, 1959.

192. WOLK, R. L. and A. I. GOLDFARB. "The response to group psychotherapy of aged recent admissions compared with long-term mental hospital patients," *Amer. J. Psychiat.*, 123:1251–1257, 1967.

193. WORLD HEALTH ORGANIZATION, Technical Report Series No. 171. "Mental Health Problems of Aging and the Aged," *Sixth Report of the Expert Committee on Mental Health*, Geneva, 1959.

194. ———, Technical Report Series No. 507. "Psychogeriatrics," Report of a WHO Scientific Group, Geneva, 1972.

195. ZEMAN, F. D. "Infectious diseases in old age," *Clinics*, 4:5, 1946.

196. ———. "Constructive programs for the mental health of the elderly," *Ment. Hyg.*, 35:221, 1951.

197. ———. "The institutional care of the aged: The scope and function of the modern home for the aged" (mimeo), Home for Aged and Infirm Hebrews, New York, 1952.

198. ———. "Common clinical errors in the care of the elderly," *Practitioner*, 174:556, 1955.

199. ———. "Recent contributions to the medical problems of old age," *New England J. Med.*, 257:317, 369, 411: 1957.

200. ZIMBERG, S. "The psychiatrist and medical home care; geriatric psychiatry in the Harlem community." *Amer. J. Psychiat.*, 127:1062–1066, 1971.

NAME INDEX

Note: Bold face figures indicate chapter pages.

SUBJECT INDEX

Hysteriform borderline personalities, 186

Hysterogenic zones, 169

Iatmul, morbidity among, 724

Iatrogenic lesbianism, 338

Iatrogenic suggestion, in hysterical disorders, 169–170

Ibogaine, 410, 411

ICD-8 (see International Classification of Diseases (ICD-8) [World Health Organization])

Id: anxiety in, 103; childhood hysteria and, 182; hysteria and, 164; schizophrenia and, 528, 629

Ideal masochism, 320

Ideas, Freud's work with hidden meanings in, 18

Identical twin studies (see Monozygotic twin studies)

Identification: adolescent, 434; bisexual, 356; childhood hysteria and, 182; in episodic psychotic reactions, 244; exhibitionism and, 361; in female homosexuality, 308; in homosexuality, 295, 296, 298, 301, 303; in hysteria, 178–179, 187; with masochistic parents, 326; in monozygotic twins, 591; neurosis of abandonment and, 811; paranoid conditions and, 232, 691; in phobias, 116–117; primary, 355; projective, in psychoses, 630; schizophrenia and, 560; splitting of self-representation in gender, 356; suggestibility and, 179

Illness: class and type of, 149–150; distortions (symptoms) in, 5–6; freedom to change and, 4–5; genetic predisposition to, 220; obsessive dread of, 330; phobias about, 114; as social role, 24; stress from, 50

Imageless thought, 5

Imipramine, depression treatment with, 80, 494, 495

Immigrants, manic-depressive psychoses among, 480

Immobilization, as response to danger in animals, 167

Immunoglobulin levels in schizophrenia, 610

Implicit culture, 19

Implosive therapy, phobia treatment through, 129–131

Impotence: among aged, 833; masochism and, 323; sadistic acts and, 316

Impulse neuroses, 238

Impulsive dyscontrol, 241–242; intentions of, 244

Inadequate personality, 228–229

Incest taboo, establishment of, 183

Incestuous wishes: hysteria and

identification with, 187; hysteria in men and, 186; manic-depressive psychoses development in childhood and, 466; phobic symbolism reflecting, 120

Incipient schizophrenia, 542

Independence, adolescent conflicts over, 18

India: manic-depressive psychoses in, 478; marginality and role conflicts among untouchable caste in, 28

Indian Hemp Commission, 421, 422

Indians (see American Indians)

Individual psychotherapy: for alcoholism, 382–383; for depersonalization, 793; neuroleptic pharmacotherapy compared with, for schizophrenia, 663; for paranoid conditions, 689–691; for schizophrenia, 627–651

Individuation: hysteria treatment and, 190; in homosexuality, 296, 297; primary identification and, 355; in schizoid personality, 227

Indoclon, neurophysiological treatment of schizophrenia with, 667

Indoctrinated paranoia, 331

Indoleamines: depression studies of, 80, 496–498; for involutional depression, 701; schizophrenia studies on, 604–607, 618

Indole (tryptamine) derivatives, 410, 412–414

Industrial accidents: psychic reactions to, 40; stress from, 49

Industrialism, alienation and, 431

Infancy: awareness of sex differences in, 339–340; differences between American and Japanese infants during, 18–19; fear reactions in, 112; gender identity emergence in, 336; hysteria related to sexuality in, 174; neurotic process in, 4; paranoid conditions and, 679, 687; sadism in, 688; schizoid personalities in, 227; transexualism origins in, 342; unconscious fantasies of sadism in, 68

Infectious disease, simulation of psychiatric disorders by, 725–726

Inhibition, masochism and, 329, 330

Inhibitions, Symptoms, and Anxiety (Freud), 18

Inner-directed personality, 467, 770; manic-depressive psychoses and, 479–480

Inorganic ions, schizophrenia studies of, 617–618

Insight psychotherapy: LSD and, 425; for obsessive behavior, 221, 222

Insomnia: among aged, 837; amphetamines and, 415; barbiturates

for treatment of, 107; in depression, 61; hyperingestion and, 810; during manic attack, 460; neurasthenia and, 142

"Instincts and Their Vicissitudes" (Freud), 321–322

Instinctual dyscontrol, 240–241; intentions of, 244

Instinctual processes, early childhood conflicts and, 14

Institutionalized behavior patterns, culture and, 23–24

Insulin: Capgras' syndrome treatment with, 713; malingering and use of, 276; schizophrenia studies of, 613, 614, 618

Insulin coma therapy for schizophrenia, 652–653, 663

Insulin hypoglycemia, depression studies of, 501, 502

Integration, development of self and, 772

Intellectualization, obsessive behavior development and, 210

Intercourse, sadism in, 316–317

Interference pattern of tension discharge, 200

Intermittent psychoses, 461

International Classification of Diseases (ICD-8) (World Health Organization): anxiety under, 93; borderline syndromes in, 542; episodic behavioral disorders in, 238; schizophrenia in, 536, 545

Interpretation: borderline patients and, 816; in paranoid conditions, 690; in schizophrenia treatment, 630

Interpretation of Dreams, The (Freud), 18, 120, 571

Intersexualism: sex reassignment and, 337–339; surgical repair in, 336–337; see also Hermaphroditism; Transexuality

Intrauterine life: fantasies of, 116; schizophrenia beginnings in, 551

Introductory Lectures (Freud), 118

Introjected psychological causality, 580, 581–582

Introjection: ego ideals and, 452; in melancholia, 703; projection and, 578, 579; suicide and, 746

Introversion, in hysteria, 187

Inventory of Somatic Complaints, 65

Involuntary movements, in hysteria, 166–169

Involutional depression, 694–709; genetics of, 702–703; menopause and, 700–701; psychological aspects of, 703–705; psychopharmacology for, 701–702; symptomatology of, 705; suicide and, 755

Involutional melancholia, 64; classical picture of, 694–695; defini-

cholia, 703; sexual bondage to, 321; suicide and introjected, 746

Lower classes: hysteria among, 183; hysteria treatment in, 190; neuroses among, 182; social evaluation of deviant behavior among, 25–26; suicide attempts among, 750; symptomatic behavior among, 20

LSD (lysergic acid diathylamide): adverse effects of, 418–420, 423–424; alcoholism treatment with, 382, 424, 425; alertness with, 409; antinomian personality of hippie and, 435; cultural factors in use of, 423; flashback experience and, 422; group emphasis in use of, 432; habitual use of, 428; latent psychoses and, 726; marijuana and, 432; mescaline and, 413–414; mutogenic and teratogenic effects of, 420; pharmacology of, 412; prevalence and patterns of use of, 426–428; psychedelic experience of, 406–407; psychological reactions of, 418–420; schizophrenia diagnosis and, 546, 608; social or recreational use of, 428; tetrahydrocannabinols and, 417; therapeutic use of, 424–425; wave-like quality of experience with, 408

Lubin Scale, 67

Lues, schizophrenia symptoms similar to, 597

Lycanthropy, collective psychoses and, 719–720

Lying, malingering and, 281, 284

Lymphocytes, schizophrenia studies of, 610

Lysergic acid diethylamide (*see* LSD (lysergic acid diethylamide))

S$_{19}$ macroglobulin, schizophrenia studies on, 610

Macy Foundation Conferences on Cybernetics, 7

Magic, childhood hysteria and, 181

Magic thought, obsessive behavior and, 202–203

Magnesium: alcoholism and, 381; depression studies of, 492, 504, 506

Maintenance therapy, for schizophrenia, 654, 658, 659

Majeptil, schizophrenia treatment with, 655

Major tranquilizers, schizophrenia treatment with, 654

Maladie de Lucy, 280

Malamud-Sands Psychiatric Rating Scales, 67

Malaria, psychiatric disorders simulated by, 725

Malaria treatment of dementia paralytica, 652

Malaya, latah syndrome in, 717

Mal de Pelea, 729

Malingering, 270–287; definitions in, 271; etiology and psychodynamics of, 273–275; Ganser Syndrome and, 279–280, 711; historical aspects of, 271–273; management of, 283–284; Manchausen's Syndrome and, 280–281; prevalence of, 273; psychological tests for, 281–283; role-playing and, 275–276; symptomatology of, 276–277

Manchausen's Syndrome, 717–719; malingering and, 271, 274, 276, 280–281, 284

Manganese, dementia praecox treatment with, 652

Mania: acute, 461; in African patients, 724; akinetic, 461; delirious, 461; delusional, 461; depression and, 506–507; depressive, 461; euphoric experience in, 407; historical notes on, 451–452; 5-hydroxyindoleacetic acid (5-HIAA) levels in, 80; lithium therapy for, 482; mutism and, 278; overinclusive thinking in, 531; possession symptoms in, 180; postpartum, 471; unproductive, 461; varieties of, 460–461

Manic-depressive psychoses, 449–490; among aged, 822; alcoholism and, 382; Capgras' syndrome in, 713; catatonic schizophrenia and, 582; childbirth and, 569; childhood and, 464–467; circular type of, 64; classification of, 64; course of, 461–462; cyclic AMP in, 500; definition of, 451; diagnostic criteria for, 463; ecological distribution of, 481; existentialist school approach to, 454–455; genetic predisposition to, 220; historical notes on, 451–455, 525, 676, 697; among Hutterites, 76; identical twin studies of, 78; involutional melancholia and, 699, 706; love object and, 68; manic attack in, 459–461; paranoid delusions in, 687; prepsychotic personality and, 467–474; psychoanalytic approaches to, 452–454; psychodynamic mechanisms of, 463–467; psychotherapy for, 482–488; psychotic attack in, 472–474; schizophrenia differentiated from, 526; schizophrenia following, 543; schizophrenia genetically related to, 596; suicide and, 755, 756; symptomatology of, 455–467; therapy for, 481–488; X chromosome transmission of, 493

Manic excitement, general paresis and, 726

Manic stupor, 461

MAO inhibitors, depression and, 79, 80

Maoris, lesbianism among, 733

Marginal individuals, depersonalization and, 779; role conflicts among, 28–29

Marijuana: adverse effects of, 420; alcohol compared with, 409; amotivational syndrome and, 419–420, 435; classification of, 411; depersonalization and, 767n; determinants of use of, 429–430; euphoric experience of, 407–410; flashback experience with, 422; group emphasis in use of, 432; habitual use of, 428; heroin addiction and use of, 397; hyperingestion of, 810; learning process in use of, 432; legal control of, 394; LSD and, 419, 432; masochistic tendencies and dependence on, 327; obsessive behavior treatment with, 222; pharmacology of, 415–417; prevalence and patterns of use of, 426–428; social or recreational use of, 428

Marijuana Tax Act (1936), 416

Marital schism, 786–787

Marital status: depression and, 76; paranoid conditions and, 679; suicide rates and, 755

Marriage: as achieved status, 27; dominant other in, 468; drinking among women and, 371; excessive drinking patterns in, 374; female homosexuals and, 305–306; heterosexuality supported by, 291; homosexuality and, 300; of hysterical women to obsessive men, 218; marital schism in, 786–787; as precipitating event in psychotic episode, 569; schizoid personality and, 227

Marxism, 430

Masculinity, sadism and agressiveness in, 317–318

Masochism, 318–322; alcoholism and, 374; anxiety and, 329–330; in borderline patients, 808; definition of, 318–319; delusional, 688; dependency and, 331–332; depression and, 331; depression and dreams revealing, 73; goals in, 325–326; homosexuality and, 296, 302, 305; humor and, 328–329; in hysteria, 190; ideal, 320; love and, 326–327; malingering and, 275; manic-depressive psychoses development in childhood and, 466; moral, 324; nonsexual, 324–325; obsessive behavior and, 330–331; paranoid mechanisms and, 331; power in, 317–318, 319–320; suicide and, 329; treatment of, 332

Massachusetts, witchcraft in, 157

Mass democracy, alienation and, 431

Mass hysteria, 155

Neuroses: acute or chronic stress as determinant in, 39–60; antisocial behavior classified as, 257; antisocial behavior differentiated from, 261–262; class and prevalence of, 182; compensation, (*see* Compensation neurosis); cybernetic chain and, 10–11; depersonalization in, 767; episodic reactions in, 247; essential qualities of, 6; experimental, 12; female homosexuality and, 306; Freud's work with, 142–143; hypnosis for induction of dissociations in, 8; hypochondriasis and, 151; limited regression in, 584; malingered, 277, 279, 284; neurasthenia and, 151; obligatory repetition in, 8–9; overinclusive thinking in, 531; oversimplifications in description of, 6; parent-child relationship and origination of, 198; phobic symptom formation and predisposition to, 122; pseudoneurotic schizophrenia and, 809; psychotic disorganization and, 13–15; regression to phallic stage of development in, 175; repetition in, 4, 5; schizophrenia genetically related to, 595; sexual etiology of, 147; symbolization and, 7–8; treatment of, 232; variational homosexuality in, 301; war, 40; *see also specific neuroses*

Neuroses of abandonment, 811

Neutralization of drives, 354

New Haven study of patients, 149–150

New Left sociology, counterculture and, 430

New York City, drug addiction treatment programs in, 395

Nexus, as conceptual scheme, 149

Niacin, schizophrenia studies of, 605, 617

Nialimide, depression studies and, 494

Nicotinamide, schizophrenia treatment with, 664, 665

Nicotinamide adenine nucleotide (NAD), schizophrenia treatment with, 664, 665

Nicotinic acid: pellagra and, 827; schizophrenia treatment with, 653, 664, 665

Night phobias, 114

Nitrous oxide, delirious effect of, 410, 411, 417

Noncombat military neuroses, 49

Noncomformity, drug usage and, 423

Noradrenaline, depression and, 79

Norepinephrine: anxiety and release of, 94; depression studies of, 79, 492, 494, 495, 496, 498, 499, 503; emotional responses related

to, 99–100; pheochromocytoma and, 106; reserpine and, 656; schizophrenia studies on, 607, 608, 614; suicide and concentrations of, 495

Norlestrin, sex reassignment as male and, 346

Normetanephrine, depression studies and, 79, 495

Notensil, schizophrenia treatment with, 655

Nozinan, schizophrenia treatment with, 655

Nuclear families, attachments and rivalries within, 18

Numerology, 430

Nurses, schizophrenia treatment and, 629, 646

Nursing homes, 844

Nutmeg, psychotomimetic properties of, 411

Nutritional deficiencies, psychiatric disorders simulated by, 726

Object relations: antisocial behavior and, 261; depression and loss in, 69; development of self and, 772; ego libido and, 143; identification in, 179; involutional melancholia and, 699; mother-child relationship and differentiation in, 355; narcissistic, in psychoses, 630; reconstitution in trauma and, 55; in schizophrenia, 544, 562

Obligatory repetition, neurotic process and, 8–9

Obotestis, 335

Obsessional neurotic, obsessional personality differentiated from, 225–226

"Obsessions and Phobias: Their Psychical Mechanisms and Their Aetiology" (Freud), 111

Obsessive behavior, 195–223; childhood, 219–220; chronic brain syndrome and, 219; as class-linked behavior, 20; clinical picture of, 196–197; course of, 221; defenses in, 225; depression differentiated from, 218; differential diagnosis of, 215–220; early work with, 111; fear-anger conflict in, 212; Freud's work with, 195–196, 198, 207; genetics of, 220–221; hypochondriasis as precursor of, 143; incidence of, 221; love object and, 68; as manifestation of maladjustive processes, 148; masochism and, 330–331; neurasthenia as precursor of, 143; obsessional neurotic differentiated from, 225–226; pathology of, 197–207; phenomenological (existential) model for, 209–215; phobic symptoms in, 126; riddance phenomena in, 329; schizo-

phrenia and, 218–219; symptom development in, 238; treatment of, 221–222

Obsessive-compulsive behavior: as adaptive behavior, 22; catatonic schizophrenia and, 581; as category of character-personality syndromes, 226; in depression, 485; psychosurgery for, 669; in spasmodic torticollis cases, 169

Obsessive-compulsive neuroses: anxiety in, 94; anxious character and, 97; cultural factors in, 733; diagnosis of, 478; schizophrenia genetically related to, 595

Obsessive-compulsive psychoses, depression and, 699

Oceanic feelings, in schizophrenia, 544

Occult, youthful preoccupation with, 430

Occupation, as achieved status, 27

Occupational cramps, 169

Odyssey House, 401

Oedipal phase of development: gender identity during, 336; negative, 355

Oedipal type of homosexuality, 298–299, 300

Oedipism, 276

Oedipus complex: animal phobias and, 122; childhood hysteria and, 181; homosexuality and, 295, 298, 303, 311; hysteria related to, 174, 178, 187; manic-depressive psychoses and resolution of, 453; obsessive behavior related to, 210; oral level of development and, 175; phobic fears in, 116; sadistic phallic wishes of, 165; sex differences in, 183

Ojibwas: mental disorders among, 724; whitico psychosis among, 180, 731

Old age homes, 844

Older people (*see* Aged)

Old Testament, 294

Olfaction, sexuality and, 319n

Olfactory hallucinations, in schizophrenia onset, 535

Omnipotence, obsessive behavior and sense of, 212, 215

Oneirophrenia, 245

"On Narcissism" (Freud), 143

Ontogeny, primary process thinking and, 571, 572

Operant conditioning, drug addiction and, 399

Ophthalmological conditions, in malingering, 276

Opium and opiates: euphoric experience of, 407; hyperingestion of, 810; mental deterioration from use of, 397; naloxone treatment for addiction to, 382

Oppositional behavior, 199n

230; childhood experiences and, 234; as descriptive category, 226

Passive-parasitic type of antisocial behavior, 260–261

Passivity: conflicts in oral and anal phases and, 355; drug usage and, 423; male transexual's conception of femininity and, 345; masochism and, 329; in traumatic experiences, 47

Pathomimes, 272

Pathomimie de Dieulafoy, 280

Patient role: cultural conditioning of, 28; symptomatic behavior in hospitals and, 29–31

Patuxent Institution, Jessup, Maryland, 265, 266

Pavlovian conditioning, of fear, 104–105, 112

Peccatiphobia, 114

Pedarasty, among ancient Greeks, 294

Pedophilia, as modified sexual pattern, 292

Pellagra: among aged, 827; psychiatric disorders simulated by, 726

Penetration, phobia of, 811

Penfluridol, schizophrenia treatment with, 659

Penis: female homosexuality and fantasy of, 308; homosexual sexuality and, 296; koro syndrome and, 730; phobias about, 345

Penis envy, in Electra situation, 183

Pentobarbitol, psychotomimetic properties of, 419

Peptic ulcer, stress and, 57

Perinatal stress, paranoid conditions and, 678, 679, 687

Perphenazine, schizophrenia treatment with, 655, 657, 658

Persecution delusions, amphetamine use and, 424, 546

Personality character syndromes, 227–232

Personality disintegration, 744

Personality types, definition of, 226–227

Personalization, development of self and, 772

Peru, sense of powerlessness among Andean Indian serfs in, 32

Peyote, psychotomimetic properties of, 411, 413, 420, 429

Phallic phase of development: castration anxiety during, 355; hysteria in women and, 183; hysterical symptoms from fixation at, 175

Phantasmic thinking, 557

Pharmacotherapy: for aged, 854; for anxiety, 107; electro-convulsive therapy and, 667, 668; schizophrenia treatment with, 653–664, 670

Pharmacothymia, 374

Pharyngeal anesthesia, in hysterical convulsive attacks, 187

Phenmetrazine, psychotomimetic properties of, 411, 414, 415

Phenomenological school: obsessive behavior theories of, 209–215; schizophrenia theories in, 529

Phenothiazines: for aged, 854; anxiety treatment with, 107; depersonalization treatment with, 796; depression treatment with, 506, 821; for episodic behavioral disorders, 252; hyperingestion of, 810; LSD panic reaction and, 412, 419; for obsessive behavior with schizophrenia, 219; schizophrenia treatment with, 655, 656–657, 660, 661, 662

Phenylcyclidine, psychotomimetic properties of, 417, 418

Phenylethylamine derivatives, psychotomimetic properties of, 411, 413

Phenylketonuria, schizophrenia-like psychosis with, 546

Pheochromocytoma, anxiety differentiated from, 106

Phobias: behavior therapy for, 105, 126–129; cannibalism in whitico syndrome and, 731; counterphobias and, 123; deconditioning for, 107; derivation of term, 110; early work with, 110–111; existential therapy for, 132–133; fear differentiated from, 112–114; hypnotherapy for, 133–135; identification in, 116–117; implosive therapy for, 129–131; incidence of, 221; masochism and, 331; modeling in treatment of, 131–132; obsessive behavior differentiated from, 216; pathogenesis of, 114–115; penetration, 811; of penis, 345; physiological symptoms in, 110; psychoanalytic approach to, 123–126; regression in, 116–117, 584; symbolism in, 117–120; therapy for, 123–135; variables in, 9; *see also specific phobias*

Phobic neuroses: anxiety as central feature of, 94; anxiety differentiated from, 106; anxious character and, 97

Phobic reactions, 110–140

Phoenix House, 401

Phonemes, in schizophrenic hallucinations, 535, 539

Phosphaturia, neurasthenia and, 142

Photophobia, 114

Photosensitivity, neuroleptic treatment for schizophrenia and, 660, 662

Phrenology, antisocial behavior and, 256–257

Phylogeny, in primary process thinking as, 571, 572

Physical therapies, for schizophrenia, 627–628, 652–675

Pibloktok hysteria, 180, 728

Pigmentary retinopathy, neuroleptic treatment for schizophrenia and, 660, 662

Piltatropine, psychotomimetic properties of, 411

Piperacetazine, schizophrenia treatment with, 655

Piperazine derivatives, schizophrenia treatment with, 655, 656–657, 660, 661

Piperidine derivatives, schizophrenia treatment with, 655, 657, 660

Piper methysticum, psychotomimetic properties of, 411

Piperyddil-benzilates, psychotomimetic properties of, 411, 417

Piptadenia peregrina, cohaba from, 410

Pithiatism, in hysterical disorders, 169, 179

Pituitary: depression studies of, 501, 502; schizophrenia studies of, 616

Placebo effect, in phobia treatment, 135

Plants, psychotomimetic properties in, 410–411

Plasma proteins, schizophrenia and, 601–604, 618

Plasma studies, of depression, 79, 80–81

Plasmatestosterone, depression studies of, 502

Play: androgen-determined behavior manifested in, 336; sex differences in, 349

Pleasure principle, masochism and, 321

Political meetings, group hysteria in, 180

Polymorphous perverse sexuality, antisocial behavior and, 261

Polysurgery addiction, 277, 283

Possession, religious excitement and, 180

Postpartum depression, 471, 502, 506

Postpartum manic states, 471

Portpartum psychoses, 569

Postprandial state in dreams, 163

Potassium: depression studies of, 492, 503, 504; electrolyte imbalance in aged and, 828; schizophrenia studies of, 615

Power: alcoholism and, 374; dependence and erotization of, 324; masochism and, 317–318, 319–320, 324, 325; sadism and, 317–318

Preconscious, symbolic distortions and conflict in, 10

Preconscious stream, 4

Predicate thinking, in schizophrenia, 532

Reverberating processes in cns, influence of drugs on, 15
Reversal, symbolic distortions as, 9–10
Riddance phenomena, 329
Rio de Janeiro, deviant behavior and hospitalization in, 26, 32, 33
Risk-taking: anxiety in ego-syntonic behavior and compulsive, 24; masochistic tendencies and, 328
Ritalin psychotomimetic properties of, 411, 414
Ritual-making, in obsessive behavior, 196, 200, 201, 202
Robaxin, cramps treated with, 802
Rockefeller University Hospital, New York City, 399
Roles: malingering and, 275–276; marginality and conflicts in, 28–29; patient, 28; sexuality and, 772–773; symptomatic behavior and, 26–29; women's, 28
Romans: homosexuality among, 294; malingering among, 272; manic-depressive psychoses in, 451; opium use in, 394
Rorschach tests: antisocial behavior under, 258; among hospital patients, 32; malingering tested under, 282; phobia diagnosis through, 112n; psychodelic experiences and, 406
Running amok syndrome, 729–730

Sachs mechanism, 296, 298, 299
Sadism, 316–318; definition of, 316; homosexuality and, 309; infant, 68, 688; intensification of masculine sexual character and, 321; phobic symbolism reflecting, 120
Sadistic anal phase of development, 323
Sadistic tendencies: manic-depressive psychoses development in childhood and, 466; melancholia and, 703; of oedipal situation, 165; in spider phobias, 114; torticollis and, 174
Sadomasochism: melancholia and, 699; in obsessive behavior, 198; primary, 355
St. Vitus' dance, collective psychoses in, 719
Salem, Massachusetts, witchcraft in, 157
Salivation, depression and reduction in, 506
Schema, in depression, 72–73
Schizoaffective psychoses, 539
Schizoid personality, 227–228; alcoholism and object relations in, 373; as category of character-personality syndrome, 226; desocialization in, 577; free-floating anxiety in, 533; as prepsychotic personality, 561–562, 564

Schizoid psychopathy, 595
Schizophrenia: abreaction, affectualization, and emotional flooding in treatment for, 170; active concretization in, 572–573; age and, 75; among aged, 822; alcoholism and, 382; alpha-methyl-paratyrosine (AMPT) studies on, 498; ambivalence in, 204, 455; ambulatory (see Ambulatory schizophrenia); amines and, 604–609; amphetamine psychoses and, 424; antibodies and, 609–611; anxiety in, 94, 106, 107; biochemistry of, 601–626; borderline syndromes and, 542; carbohydrate metabolism and, 611–614; casuality and action in, 580–582; catatonic (see Catatonic schizophrenia); cerebrospinal fluid studies of, 597; childhood beginnings of, 555–564; chronic (see Chronic schizophrenia); chronic undifferentiated, 539–540; clinical concept of, 546–547; cognition in, 531, 571–572; cognitive approach to, 529; contamination obsessions in, 211; delusions in, 217, 457; desymbolization and desocialization in, 577–580; diagnosis of, 478, 542–545; differential diagnosis in, 545–546; dissociative process in, 8; double bind in, 774–776; ecological distribution of, 481; electro-convulsive therapy for, 627, 628, 653, 667–668, 669; episodic psychotic reactions and, 244; episodic symptoms in, 245; existential approach to, 529; familial genetic studies of, 589–591; family and, 552–555; female homosexuality and, 307; first use of term, 141, 526; formal view of, 571–584; Freud's theories of, 628–630; Ganser's syndrome and, 280, 711–712; genetic predisposition to, 220; genetics of, 588–600; genetic unity of, 595–596; hebephrenic (see Hebephrenic schizophrenia); hemolytic factors in, 611, 618; historical introduction to physical treatment for, 652–653; historical review of, 525–533; historical survey of psychotherapy for, 628–634; homosexuality and, 292, 296, 302; hormones and, 614–616; among Hutterites, 76; hyperglycemic coma treatment for, 652–653, 666–667; hypochondriasis as precursor of, 143, 144, 148; hysteria and multiple fixations in, 175; hysteria differentiated from, 188–189; hysteria transitional to, 159; inadequate personality differentiated from, 228, 229; incipient, 542; individual psychotherapy

for, 627–651; inorganic ions and, 617–618; involutional psychoses and, 702; larval, 542; late, 541–542; latent (see Latent schizophrenia); literature on, 477; logical processes in, 532–533; LSD reactions and, 419; LSD treatment of, 424; lycanthropy and, 719; maintenance therapy for, 654, 658, 659; manic-depressive psychoses and, 462n; marijuana and, 421; mental set in, 531–532; metabolic treatment for, 664–666; 3-methoxy-4-hydroxyphenylglycol (MHPG) concentrations and, 496; neurasthenia as precursor of, 143, 147; neurophysiological treatment of, 653, 667–668; obsessive behavior differentiated from, 211; obsessive symptoms in, 218–219; onset of, 533–535; overinclusion in, 530–531; paleologic thought in, 574–577; paranoid (see Paranoid schizophrenia); paranoid conditions and, 677; paranoid delusions in, 687; phenothiazines for anxiety in, 107; phobic symptoms in, 126; physical therapies for, 627–628, 652–675; plasma proteins in, 601–604; possession symptoms in, 180; preadolescent forms of, 595; process, 543, 568; prognosis in, 367–368, 545; progressive teleologic regression in, 583–584; pseudo-communities in, 683; pseudoneurotic (see Pseudoneurotic schizophrenia); pseudopsychopathic, 595; psychoanalytic approach to, 527–529; psychodynamic analysis for, 643–646; psychodynamics of, 551–571; psychostructural view of, 571–584; reactive, 543, 568; recurrences of, 535–536; residual, 541; schizoid personality and, 227, 228; Schneider's diagnostic criteria for, 543–544; simple (see Simple schizophrenia); stimulus filtration in, 531–532; suicide and, 755, 756; suicide attempts and, 749, 751; suicide rates for, 67; symbolic transformation in, 450; symptomatology of, 524–550; syphilophobia and, 114n; termination in therapy for, 647–648; three-day, 245; transexualism and, 347; types of, 536–540; vitamins and, 616–617
Schizophrenic spectrum, 814
Schizophreniform psychoses: introduction of term, 543; LSD use and, 419
Schizophrenogenic mothers: family disturbances and, 554–555; genetic studies of, 591
Schlaftrunkenheit, 803
School: antisocial behavior patterns

in, 754–755; psychiatric disorders and, 756; suicide compared with, 744–745; treatment and, 759–760

Sumerian civilization, opium use in, 393

Superego: antisocial behavior and, 261, 263, 264, 266; anxiety in, 103; depersonalization and, 164; homosexuality and, 300, 311; incest taboo establishment in, 183; involutional melancholia and, 695; learned cultural values as core of, 19; mania and, 452–453; nonsexual masochism and, 324; obsessive behavior development and, 210, 215; paranoid conditions and, 682, 688, 691; sadistic, in obsessive behavior, 198; schizophrenia and, 544, 631; suicide and, 747; suicide attempts and, 750

Supportive therapy: for anxiety, 107; for obsessive behavior, 221

Surgery: ambiguous gender identity and sex reassignment through, 337–339; masochistic behavior and desire for, 329; polysurgery addiction to, 277, 283; psychiatric, 653, 663, 668–670; sex assignment, 336-337, 339; stress during, 50, 52; transexual, 347–348

Survival guilt, 40, 50

Susto syndrome, 731

Sweating, in phobias, 110

Sweden, suicide rates in, 748, 751

Sydenham's chorea: hysterical mimesis differentiated from, 168; variable chorea of Brissaud differentiated from, 803

Symbiotic phase of development, 354

Symbolic displacement, 133

Symbolic processes: illness and disturbances in, 6; vulnerability to neurotic distortions in, 4

Symbolic realization in psychoses, 632

Symbolism: Freudian view of, 575; in language, 177; in phobias, 117–120

Symbolization: distortions in, 9–10, 12; in hysteria, 187; neurotic processes and, 7–8; in thinking, 577–578

Sympatomimetic amines, psychotomimetic disorders and, 411, 414

Symptomatic behavior: adaptive behavior as, 21–22; cross-cultural approach to, 31; defense mechanisms as, 17–23; as distortions in illnesses, 6; Freudian view of, 19; hospital milieu and, 29–33; Midtown Manhattan Study of prevalence of, 76; minority status and, 32–33; role and, 26–29; social and cultural appraisal of, 23–26;

socioeconomic level and, 32–33; status and, 26–29

Symptomatic schizophrenia, 245

Synanon, 401

Syphillis, psychiatric disorders simulated by, 726

Syphilophobia, 114n

Systematic desensitization, phobia treatment with, 126–127, 129, 130, 131

Systems concepts, alcoholism and, 375

Taboos: sex, 733; voodoo death and, 732

Tachycardia: among aged, 827; amphetamines and, 415; anxiety and, 94, 106; education and literacy levels and, 33; in phobias, 110

Tactile hallucinations, in schizophrenia onset, 535

Taractan, schizophrenia treatment with, 655

Tarantism, collective psychoses in, 719

Taraxein, schizophrenia studies on, 609

Tardive dyskinesia, neuroleptic treatment of schizophrenia and, 661

TAT (see Thematic Apperception Test (TAT))

Teleologic thought, progressive regression in, in schizophrenia, 532, 583–584

Temperature regulation by infant, 353

Temporal lobe epilepsy: folic acid and, 617; gender behavior disturbances and, 349; hypochondriasis and, 246; schizophrenia symptoms similar to, 546, 597

Tendon reflexes, hysteria and changes in, 188

Tenuate, psychotomimetic properties of, 411, 414

Teratogenicity in LSD use, 420

Termination, in schizophrenia treatment, 647–648

Terror, as central affective position, 10

Testicular-feminizing syndrome, 338

Testosterone: female hermaphrodites and therapy with, 339; among homosexual males, 293

Testosterone enanthate, sex reassignment as female and, 346

Tests: for malingering, 281–283; for phobia diagnosis, 124; see also specific tests

Tetrahydrocannabinol (THC): classification of, 411; effects of, 409–410; euphoric experience and, 407; LSD and, 412; memory impairment with, 408, 409; phar-

macology of, 415–417; sympathetic emotions and, 222

Tetrahydroharmine, psychotomimetic properties of, 410

Thalamotomies, schizophrenia treatment through, 668

Thalamus, as locus of emotions, 99

Thallium poisoning, schizophrenia-like psychosis with, 546

Thanatomania, 732

Theater of the Absurd, 770, 811

Thematic Apperception Test (TAT): among hospital patients, 32; malingering in, 282

Theosophy, 430

Therapeutic alliance: with borderline patients, 816; homosexuality and, 309–310; with paranoid personalities, 232

Therapist, in phobia treatment, 129

Thiamine, alcoholism treatment with, 381

Thiamine chloride, Wernicke-Kosakoff syndrome and, 827

Thiopropazate, schizophrenia treatment with, 655

Thioproperazine, schizophrenia treatment with, 655

Thioridazine: ECG abnormalities and, 661; schizophrenia treatment with, 655

Thiothixene, schizophrenia treatment with, 655

Thioxanthenes, schizophrenia treatment with, 655, 657, 660

Thorazine: depression treatment with, 488; schizophrenia treatment with, 655

Thought processes: in classical depression, 456–457; during depression, 476; psychedelic experience and, 406

Three-day psychosis, schizophrenia differentiated from, 545

Three-day schizophrenia, 245

Three Essays (Freud), 295

Threshold effect, schizophrenia and, 598

Thumb-sucking, as obsessive behavior, 216

Thyroid hormones: depression studies on, 499, 502; malingering and use of, 276; schizophrenia studies of, 614–615

Tics, 800–802; hyperingestion and, 810; hysteria and, 168; in obsessive behavior, 202; paresis and, 166

Time perception, LSD and marijuana use and, 406–407, 408

Tindal, schizophrenia treatment with, 655

TMA (3,4,5-trimethoxyamphetamine), psychotomimetic properties of, 411, 414

Tobacco dependence, masochistic behavior and, 327, 328

Weaning: infantile convulsions and, 182; manic-depressive psychoses development and, 465

Wechsler-Bellevue Intelligence Scale: antisocial behavior related to scores on, 262; malingering tested with, 281

Weeping: conversion reactions and, 178; in hysterical disorders, 170–171

Weight, somatic preoccupation with, 149

Wernicke-Korsakoff's psychosis, alcoholism and, 377

Wernicke-Korsakoff syndrome, among aged, 827

Wernicke's syndrome, prevention and treatment of, 381

Whipping, sadism and, 317, 319

White-collar crimes, 256

Whites: depression among, 75–76; education and literacy levels and symptomatic behavior among, 33; marginality and role conflicts among, 28–29; social evaluation of deviant behavior among, 25–26; suicide rates among, 755

Whitico psychoses, 180, 731

William Wilson (Poe), 715

Will to survive, during stress situations, 40

Wilson's disease, schizophrenia-like psychosis with, 546

Witchcraft, hysteria seen as, 157

Withdrawal treatment of drug addiction, 399

Wittenborn Scales, 67

"Wolf Man" case, animal phobias in, 121n

Wolves, lycanthropy and, 719–720

Womb theory of hysteria, 156, 157

Women: alcoholism and, 371, 374; ambiguous gender identity and sex reassignment as, 337–338;

Cotard's syndrome in, 716; cultural factors in somatic preoccupations of, 149; culturally conditioned role of, 28; depersonalization among, 767; depression and crying in, 62, 64; depression in, 493, 502; differences between men and (*see* Sex differences); dominant other in therapy and, 484; endogenous depression among, 75; episodic schizophrenic symptoms and menstrual cycle in 245; female hermaphrodites assigned as, 339; histrionic character features among, 186; homosexuality among (*see* Lesbianism); hormonal sex reassignment as, 346-347; hysteria in, 156, 175, 183, 218, 261; involutional depression at menopause in, 700–701, 704–705; involutional melancholia in, 695; latah syndrome among, 727–729; male homosexual's relationship with, 311; Manchausen's syndrome in, 718; manic-depressive psychoses in, 462; masochism in, 320, 322; as masochistic power figure, for men, 323–324; melancholia in, 699; pain thresholds among, 24; passive-defensive sexual role of, 316–317, 320–321; pederasty in ancient Greece and status of, 294; reactive depression among, 75; sadism in, 317; social evaluation of deviant behavior as symptomatic among, 26; suicide attempts among, 750, 754; suicide rates for, 75, 751, 755

Word association tests, for schizophrenia, 527, 531

Words: characteristics of, 578; evolution from paleosymbol of, 578; magic of, 202

Work: self and, 768–769; stress of adjustment to, 50

World Health Organization (WHO): addiction definition of, 393; *International Classification of Diseases* (*see International Classification of Diseases* (World Health Organization)); psychogeriatrics and, 822, 827; suicide study by, 744, 754, 757, 759

World War I, 40; anxiety studies during, 93, 94

World War II, 8, 40; anxiety in, 93–94; three-day schizophrenia during, 245

Writer's cramps, 169, 802

Wryneck syndrome, 801

Würzburg School, imageless thought of, 5

Xanthurenic acid, depression studies with, 497

X chromosome: depression transmission through, 493; Klinefelter's syndrome and, 342

XXY chromosome pattern, antisocial behavior and, 262

XYY chromosome pattern: antisocial behavior and, 262; schizophrenic disorders and, 597

Yaws, psychiatric disorders simulated by, 726

Yin and yan, shook yong syndrome and, 730

Yoruba people, depression among, 76

Youth: marijuana and LSD use among, 423; schizophrenic development during, 564–566

Zen Buddhism, 430

Zwangsneurose (obsessional neurosis), 195n